W9-DFE-233

Endovascular Intervention: Today and Tomorrow

Series Editor

Frank J. Criado, MD

Volume 3

Endovascular Intervention: Today and Tomorrow

Series Editor
Frank J. Criado, MD
Director, Center for Vascular Intervention
Chief, Division of Vascular Surgery
Union Memorial Hospital/MedStar Health
Baltimore, MD

Volume 3

Endovascular Intervention: *New Tools and Techniques for the 21st Century*

Edited by

Frank J. Criado, MD
Director, Center for Vascular Intervention
Chief, Division of Vascular Surgery
Union Memorial Hospital/MedStar Health
Baltimore, MD

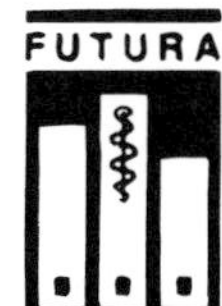

Futura Publishing Company, Inc.
Armonk, New York

Library of Congress Cataloging-in-Publications Data

Endovascular intervention: new tools and techniques for the 21st century / edited by Frank J. Criado.
p. ; cm.—(Endovascular intervention ; v. 3)
Includes bibliographical references and index.
ISBN 0-87993-459-6 (alk. paper)
1. Blood-vessels—Surgery. 2. Blood-vessels—Endoscopic surgery. 3. Surgical instruments and apparatus. I. Criado, Frank J. II. Series.
[DNLM: 1. Vascular Surgical Procedures—trends. 2. Surgical Procedures, Minimally Invasive—trends. 3. Vascular Surgical Procedures—instrumentation. 4. Vascular Surgical Procedures—methods. WG 170 E5612 2002]
RD598.5 .E525 2002
617.4′13—dc21

2001054466

Published by
Futura Publishing Company
135 Bedford Road
Armonk, NY 10504
www.futuraco.com

LC#: 2001054466
ISBN#: 0-87993-495-6

Printed in the United States of America on acid-free paper.

Introduction

This is the third volume of Futura's monograph series *Endovascular Intervention: Today and Tomorrow*. The chosen theme "new tools and techniques" should prove timely and of considerable interest to practicing vascular specialists. Developments in endovascular technologies continue to have an overpowering influence in the vascular world. My own specialty of vascular surgery is undergoing a process of transformation that is both fast paced and profound. New therapeutic options and innovative strategies for management of aortic aneurysms and carotid artery disease constitute the two most glaring examples of changes that can be appropriately termed "revolutionary." Infrainguinal revascularization may be next as catheter-based femoropopliteal recanalization reemerges at the dawn of a new wave of explosive growth in intervention fueled by the availability of drug-eluting stents which promise to become 'game changers'—even if 'early results' prove to be half true only!

As with the previous volumes in this series, I owe a debt of gratitude to Futura Publishing for their continued support, and to all contributors, whose effort and unselfish willingness to share insight and experience constitute the real foundation of this publishing venture.

Contributors

Marcos F. Barnatan, MD Endovascular Associate, Center for Vascular Intervention, Union Memorial Hospital/MedStar Health, Baltimore, MD

Hugh G. Beebe, MD Clinical Professor of Surgery, University of Michigan Medical School, Ann Arbor, MI; Director, Jobst Vascular Center, Toledo, OH

Nancy S. Clark, MD Co-Director, Vascular Laboratory, Union Memorial Hospital/MedStar Health, Baltimore, MD

Frank J. Criado, MD Director, Center for Vascular Intervention, Chief, Division of Vascular Surgery, Union Memorial Hospital/MedStar Health, Baltimore, MD

Edward B. Diethrich, MD Medical Director, Arizona Heart Institute and Arizona Heart Hospital, Phoenix, AZ

Yves-Marie Dion, MD, MSc, FACS, FRCSC Associate Professor of Surgery, Centre Hospitalier Universitaire de Québec, Pavillon St-François d'Assise, Université Laval, Québec, Québec, Canada

Tom W. Duerig, PhD President of Nitinol Devices and Components, Cordis Corporation, Fremont, CA

Gustav R. Eles, DO Pittsburgh Vascular Institute, Shadyside Hospital, Pittsburgh, PA

Thomas J. Fogarty, MD Professor of Surgery, Stanford University School of Medicine, Division of Vascular Surgery, Stanford University Hospital, Stanford, CA

Carlos R. Gracia, MD, FACS Medical Director, Minimally Invasive Surgery, ValleyCare Health System, Pleasanton, CA

Robin H. Heijmen, MD, PhD Surgical Resident, Department of Vascular Surgery, St. Antonius Hospital, Nieuwegein, The Netherlands

Isabelle Henry, MD Interventional Cardiologist, U.C.C.I., Polyclinique, Essey-Les-Nancy, France

Michel Henry, MD Interventional Cardiologist, U.C.C.I., Polyclinique, Essey-Les-Nancy, France

Bradley B. Hill, MD Assistant Professor of Surgery, Stanford University School of Medicine, Division of Vascular Surgery, Stanford University Hospital, Stanford, CA; Attending Vascular Surgeon, Kaiser Permanente Medical Center, Santa Clara, CA

Michael R. Jaff, DO, FACP, FACC Director, Vascular Medicine, Co-Director, Vascular Diagnostic Laboratory, The Heart and Vascular Institute, Morristown, NJ

Chester R. Jarmolowski, MD Pittsburgh Vascular Institute, Shadyside Hospital, Pittsburgh, PA

Boonprasit Kritpracha, MD Department of Surgery, Prince of Songkla University, Hat-Yai, Songkla, Thailand; Visiting Research Scientist, University of Michigan, Ann Arbor, MI; Jobst Vascular Center, Toledo, OH

Frans L. Moll, MD, PhD Vascular Surgeon, Department of Vascular Surgery, St. Antonius Hospital, Nieuwegein, The Netherlands

Amir Motarjeme, MD Director, Midwest Vascular Institute of Illinois, Downer's Grove (Chicago), IL

Francisco J. Osse, MD Associate Professor of Vascular and Endovascular Surgery, Department of Endovascular Surgery, Santa Casa de Misericórdia de São Paulo, São Paulo, Brazil

Youssef Rizk, DO Endovascular Associate, Center for Vascular Intervention, Union Memorial Hospital/MedStar Health, Baltimore, MD

Walter Tan, MD Pittsburgh Vascular Institute, Shadyside Hospital, Pittsburgh, PA

Joep A.W. Teijink, MD, PhD Vascular Surgeon, Department of Vascular Surgery, Atrium Medical Centre, Heerlen, The Netherlands

Patricia E. Thorpe, MD Professor of Radiology, Chief, Vascular and Interventional Radiology, Director, University Venous Center, University of Iowa, Iowa City, IA

Deborah E. Tolomeo, PhD Principal Engineer, Cordis Corporation, Fremont, CA

Kiril Tzvetanov, MD Cardiologist, U.C.C.I., Polyclinique, Essey-Les-Nancy, France

Jos C. van den Berg, MD, PhD Radiologist, Department of Radiology, St. Antonius Hospital, Nieuwegein, The Netherlands

Frank J. Veith, MD The William J. von Liebig Chair in Vascular Surgery, Professor and Vice Chairman, Department of Surgery, Montefiore Medical Center, The University Hospital for the Albert Einstein College of Medicine, Bronx, NY

Reese A. Wain, MD Chief of Vascular Surgery, Albert Einstein Hospital; Medical Director, Vascular Laboratories, Montefiore and Albert Einstein Hospitals; Assistant Professor of Surgery, Albert Einstein College of Medicine, Bronx, NY

Cecilia F. Wang, MS Medical Student, Center for Vascular Intervention, Union Memorial Hospital/MedStar Health, Baltimore, MD

Mark H. Wholey, MD Chairman, Pittsburgh Vascular Institute, UPMC-Shadyside; Clinical Professor of Radiology, University of Pittsburgh School of Medicine, Pittsburgh, PA

Michael H. Wholey, MD, MBA assistant Professor, Chief, Department of Cardiovascular and Interventional Radiology, University of Texas Health Science Center at San Antonio, San Antonio, TX

Contents

1

Vascular Surgery and Endoluminal Intervention:

An Overview of Vascular Therapies at the Turn of the Century

Edward B. Diethrich, MD

Introduction

Treatment of vascular disease has been revolutionized by endovascular surgical techniques. The growth of this new field has been characterized by innovations that include balloon angioplasty, atherectomy, stenting, and endoluminal grafting (ELG). All of these techniques permit us to restore patency and flow in occluded vessels either percutaneously or with a minimal incision. This allows for treatment of a wide spectrum of patients with minimally invasive procedures that may reduce hospital stay, expense, and recovery time.

The introduction of stent technology has been a major breakthrough in the treatment of coronary and peripheral lesions. There is now a substantial body of research detailing the successful use of stents in the iliac, renal, and subclavian regions. Experience with these devices in the coronary arteries and vessels of the extremities has led to their use in the carotid region as well. Although stents are not yet approved for use in the carotid or in most other arterial locations, a number of investigators have published the results of early clinical studies. Results are encouraging and indicate that improvements in device design and delivery techniques may reduce complications.

One of the most exciting new endovascular technologies is ELG, which incorporates covered stent designs that are now being used to treat aneurysms. ELG technology is proliferating at an unprecedented rate, and clinical trials are in progress at institutions throughout the world; two devices have received approval from the US Food and Drug Administration (FDA) for marketing in

From Criado FJ (ed): *Endovascular Intervention: New Tools and Techniques for the 21st Century.* Armonk, NY: Futura Publishing Co., Inc.; ©2002.

the US. A great deal of progress has been made in ELG design, and advancements in deployment technique have also been realized. ELG technology has already changed the indications for treatment in many centers, and we can anticipate numerous opportunities for additional investigation with this exciting treatment modality.

In this chapter, we examine the influence of some of the new therapies that have shaped the technical revolution in endovascular surgery and provide an overview of stenting and ELG in the treatment of aneurysms and iliac and carotid artery disease.

Endovascular Treatment of Abdominal Aortic Aneurysmal Disease

Overview

Exclusion of abdominal aortic aneurysms (AAAs) using nonsurgical, endoluminal technology has attracted worldwide attention. Initially, the procedure was designed for use in patients with cardiac pathologies, pulmonary insufficiency, a hostile abdomen, or other conditions that heighten the risks associated with classic surgical intervention.[1] The use of endoluminal techniques for exclusion of AAAs has now been proposed in patients without comorbid conditions and even in those with small, asymptomatic aneurysms.[2] The more recent proposal, however, must be tempered in view of the paucity of long-term data and the complications that have been seen with ELG technology. Still, in older patients who have large aneurysms and severe comorbidities, endovascular treatment offers an appealing alternative to surgical intervention. Indeed, the incidence of AAA rupture does not appear to be declining, and a study of ruptured AAAs in the state of Maryland (n=527) indicates that open surgical repair continues to be risky, particularly in the elderly.[3] The risk of rupture in patients with AAAs (n=218) detected through ultrasound screening revealed that the rate of actual rupture plus the elective surgery rate for AAAs 3.0 to 4.4 cm was 2.1% per year and for AAAs 4.5 to 5.9 cm it was 10.2%. The authors concluded that the operative mortality rate for a procedure should be weighed carefully against the probability of rupture.[4]

One of the major drawbacks to endovascular repair has been the problem of incomplete exclusion of the aneurysm, which causes endoleaks and complicates a significant number of cases. The endoleak rate is influenced by anatomical variations, the type of graft used, and the method of insertion.[5] Endoleaks have been categorized as follows: type 1, which is related to the graft device itself; type 2, which is retrograde flow from collateral branches (called a "retroleak"); type 3, comprising fabric tears, graft disconnection, or disintegration; and type 4, which is flow through graft wall because of porosity.[6]

A variety of ELG devices are in use, and clinical results from a number of centers are now available. The following review of devices and results allows comparison of preliminary data and an overview of some of the complications that have been encountered. This information will form the basis for comparison of results with third- and fourth-generation devices that will become available in the next few years. Indeed, in reviewing these related data, one must keep in mind that the ELG development process is ongoing and that many early devices have or will transition into more sophisticated models in the near future. For example, early Mintec and Stentor prototypes led to the development of a new generation of devices called Vanguard (Boston Scientific, Natick, MA). The Vanguard III device was recently introduced in Europe. The Talent (Medtronic AVE, Santa Rosa, CA) and Endovascular Technologies (EVT) devices were purchased by Guidant (Menlo Park, CA), and the Guidant Ancure ELG device was one of the two initial entrants into the US marketplace. Johnson & Johnson (Warren, NJ), W.L. Gore & Associates (Flagstaff, AZ), Cook Inc. (Bloomington, IN), Endologix (Irvine, CA), and several other companies are rapidly developing new prototypes and advancing their designs into the field.

Clinical Results

The 3-year experience with a modular stent-graft device was reported by Stelter and colleagues.[7] A total of 201 patients were treated; 178 with the Stentor or Vanguard device and 23 with the Talent endograft. The technical success rate was 89%; a total of 7 patients died in the perioperative period, and 5 renal artery occlusions were encountered. There were 18 primary endoleaks and 19 late endoleaks. The authors concluded that liberal patient selection contributed to a "seemingly high" complication rate.

In another study conducted over a 3-year period, 28 of 30 patients underwent endovascular repair, and these results were compared with outcomes of conventional open repair.[8] Endovascular repair was associated with less blood loss (408 mL versus 1287 mL), shorter intensive care unit (0.1 days versus 1.8 days) and hospital (3.9 days versus 10.3 days) stays, and more rapid recovery (11 days versus 47 days). The rate of postoperative complications was the same in both groups, but complications in patients treated with endovascular techniques tended to be less severe.

Endoluminal repair of AAAs with the EVT and Stentor ELGs in 29 patients yielded successful results in 24 procedures (83%).[9] Two deaths from microembolization were reported, and there were 5 conversions. Endoleaks occurred in 4 patients, and continued aneurysm expansion was present in 3 patients. In another study, EVT investigators also evaluated the effect of preexisting thrombus on changes in aneurysm size following endovascular grafting.[10] Measurements of AAA diameters pre- and postprocedure and at 1 year were made via computed tomography (CT). There was no statistically significant relationship between the preexisting thrombus fraction and the rate of change in aneurysm size. Thus, the authors concluded that failure of the aneurysm to shrink after the procedure should not be attributed to preexisting thrombus and should be investigated. Incomplete exclusion of the aneurysm is the more likely cause. Observations such as these are important, but it is critical to realize that substantially longer follow-up of the morphologic changes subsequent to AAA ELG exclusion is needed before any final conclusions can be made.

Conversion to open repair constitutes failure of the ELG technique as exhibited in a 5-year review of endoluminal repair of AAAs in 156 patients.[11] Primary conversion during the original operation was required in 14 patients, and secondary conversion was necessary in 9 patients. The most common reasons for primary conversion are rupture of the aorta, migration of the ELG that obstructs the iliac arteries, and irreversible twisting of a bifurcated ELG. Reasons for secondary conversion include persistent endoleak, persistent aneurysm expansion, and infected ELG.

The continued enlargement of AAAs has been demonstrated after conventional surgical repair (Fig. 1) and endovascular intervention. A morphometric analysis[12] of aortic neck size was completed in 59 patients who had received straight tube ELGs, and demonstrated significant enlargement that persisted for at least 24 months after the procedure. Surprisingly, enlargement was most

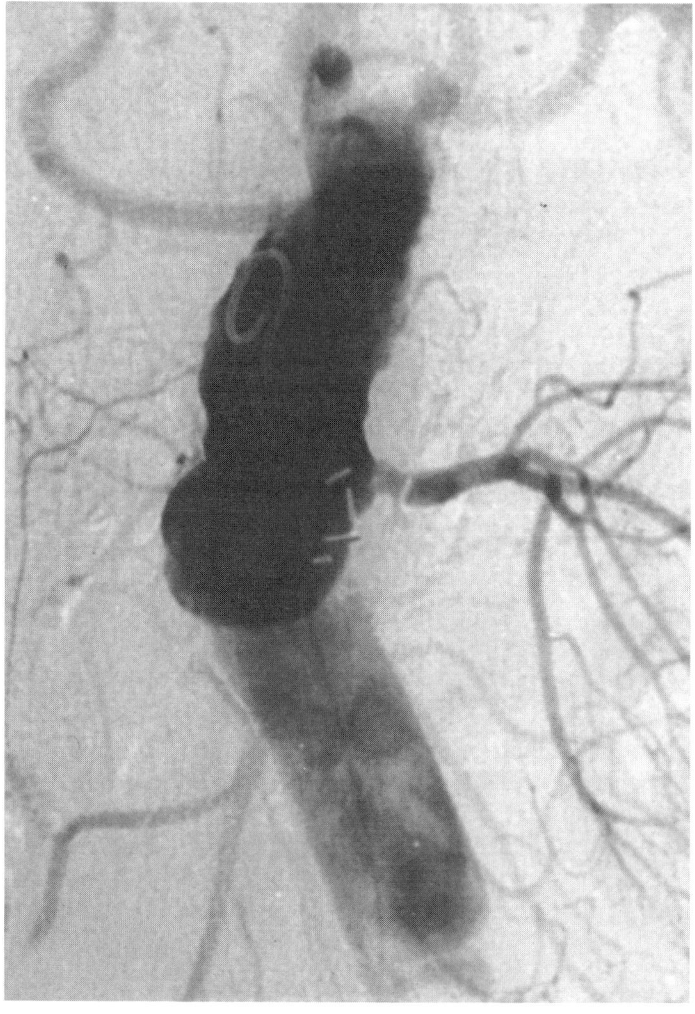

Figure 1. Aortogram performed several years after classic resection and Dacron graft repair of an infrarenal abdominal aortic aneurysm. The study shows significant aneurysmal dilatation between the cephalad end of the graft and the renal arteries.

pronounced in the distal neck. Migration of the device was seen in 3 patients in whom the minor diameter of the distal neck was greater than 6 mm larger than the preimplant diameter of the ELG. Observations of this kind indicate that the best method for ELG fixation is still in question. In one cadaver study,[13] longitudinal traction was applied to devices to compare fixation of hooks and barbs with radial force alone. Hooks and barbs added anchoring strength, while the radial force of stents had no impact. One of the latest ELG designs (Zenith, by Cook Inc.) incorporates 2.5 cm of bare stent with hooks that are intended to be placed above the renal arteries (Fig. 2).

The incidence of renal complications in patients who have undergone endovascular repair of AAAs was studied in 149 patients with normal renal function.[14] Approximately 6% of patients developed renal dysfunction. In patients who had preoperative renal impairment, the perioperative mortality associated with endovascular AAA was high (27%).

At this point, it should be clear that ELG designs are in their infancy and that an enormous amount of further development will be required over the next several years to allow broad clinical application of this important endovascular therapy.

Clinical Results from the Arizona Heart Institute

Our own experience at the Arizona Heart Institute and Heart Hospital parallels that of other investigators in a variety of ways. Beginning in January of 1994, the Arizona Heart Institute surgical team instituted a protocol

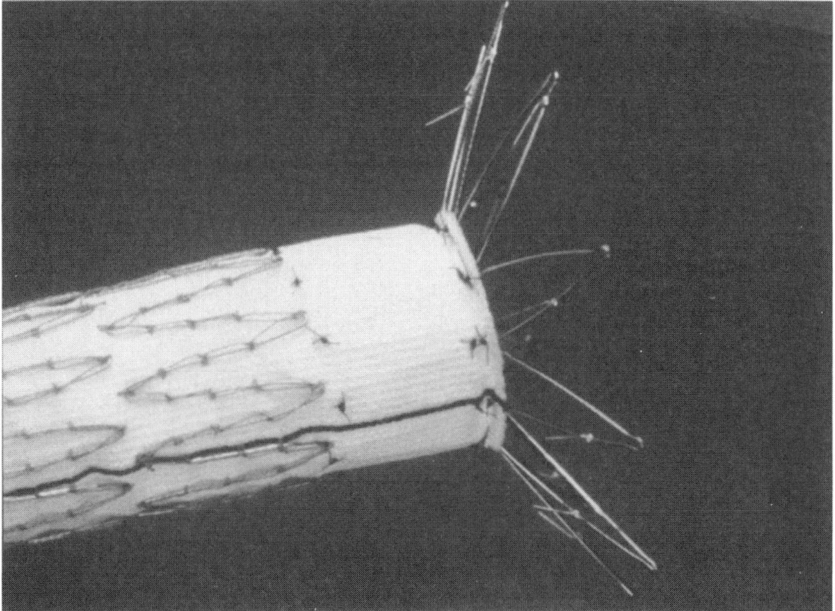

Figure 2. Photograph of the new Cook Zenith endoluminal graft with barbed bare stent placed above the renal arteries.

to study ELG exclusion of AAAs. The initial devices studied were constructed of commercially available polytetrafluoroethylene (PTFE) graft material and Palmaz stents (Cordis Endovascular, a Johnson & Johnson Company, Miami Lakes, FL) at the cephalad and caudal ends for graft anchoring (Fig. 3). The majority of the body of the device was unsupported. This design concept was originated by Parodi, and most of the early work worldwide embraced this basic design principle. In treating 54 patients over a 2-year period, it became clear to us that the use of grafts without support throughout the entire body created problems with delivery as well as migration of the device. The new "total support" concept in ELG design (Fig. 3) has been adopted in almost all of the current investigations and certainly accounts for some of the improvements we have seen in technical success. Controversy over partial versus total support in ELGs used for AAA exclusion continues, however, and there are other investigators who prefer to use partially supported grafts.

After our initial study period, an FDA Investigational Device Exemption was obtained. Under this single-center protocol and in additional corporate-sponsored protocols, patient enrollment began in January of 1997. During 1997

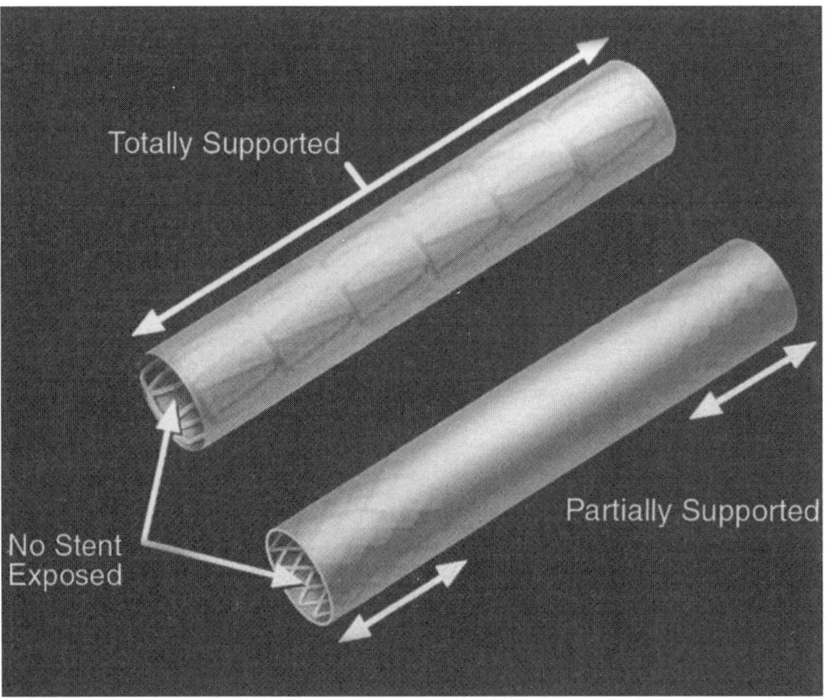

Figure 3. Bottom: Early design from Arizona Heart Institute that was similar to Juan Parodi's endoluminal graft (ELG) design; polytetrafluoroethylene was substituted for Dacron as the covering material in our device. Top: A second-generation ELG design incorporating full stent support over the entire length of the graft. ELGs in development now all use the "total support design."

and 1998, a total of 223 patients were treated. The periprocedural and short-term results have been exceptionally satisfactory as evidenced by conversion in only 4 patients (1.8%). One conversion was due to a device failure, another to excessive angulation of the artery, the third as a result of extensive plaque formation at the caudal end of the aorta that caused inappropriately high deployment of the ELG, and the fourth because of difficulty accessing the lesion. There were 2 deaths (0.9%) within the 30-day postprocedural period. Late mortality included 10 patients (4.5%). One patient died from a procedure-related incident, and 9 deaths resulted from causes not associated with the procedure. The most common periprocedural complication was access related; the small size and torturous and calcific nature of the iliac arteries made it difficult to deliver the device in some cases. Distal embolization was observed in only 1 patient. Ten endoleaks were identified; 2 sealed spontaneously, 3 were sealed with endovascular intervention, and 5 have persisted. These results are clearly better than some of the earlier studies reported, and are indicative of the potential for further improvement in the future.

Discussion

Although we have seen reductions in complications in our series, recent study seems to indicate that the incidence of adverse events after AAA repair is not necessarily related to iatrogenic complications that are a result of the learning curve for using new devices. In a study by May and colleagues,[15] patients who underwent endovascular treatment in the initial 3-year period (n=75) were compared with those had procedures in the subsequent 2.5-year period (n=115). There was no significant difference in the incidence of adverse events between groups. The authors concluded that despite improvements in technology and experience, the adverse event rate (45%) was relatively high in patients undergoing endovascular repair of AAAs.

It is clear that patients require close follow-up after endovascular treatment of AAAs, even if no endoleaks are detected (Fig. 4). Rupture of an AAA 16 months after placement of an endograft was reported by Torsello and colleagues.[16] Although there had been no evidence of an endoleak, CT demonstrated enlargement of the aneurysm sac 7 months after the procedure.

As we have emphasized, it is important to recognize that the results of current trials are generally restricted to outcomes with first- and second-generation devices. These results must therefore be reviewed with the understanding that the typical development process includes observation of these early devices with an eye toward improving design and delivery strategies. This is clearly evidenced in ELG programs for exclusion of AAAs. Already we have seen dramatic improvements in the single-stage, unibody ELG that we are developing with the Endologix company (Fig. 5). Operative time, complications, and endoleaks, as well as ease of use, are all very favorable with the third-generation device. Similar improvements are likely to be apparent with other devices as well.

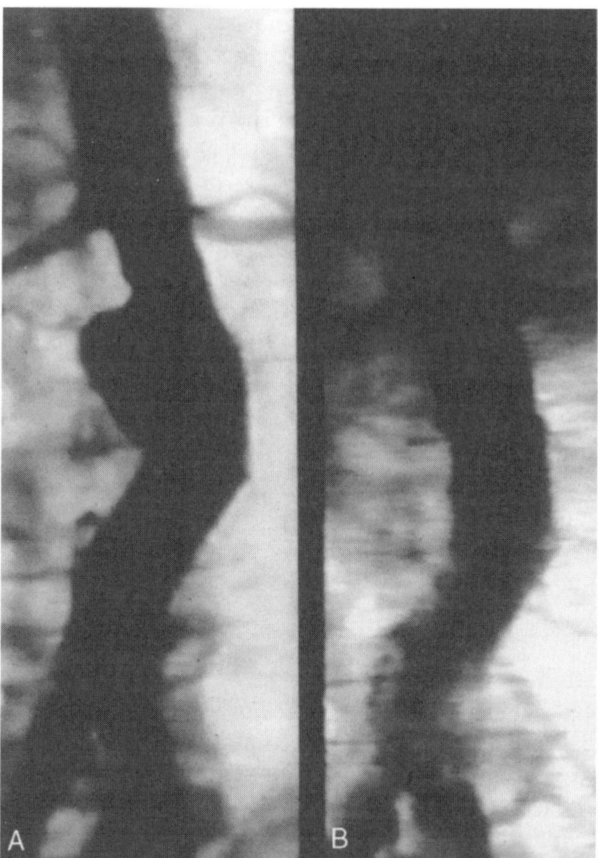

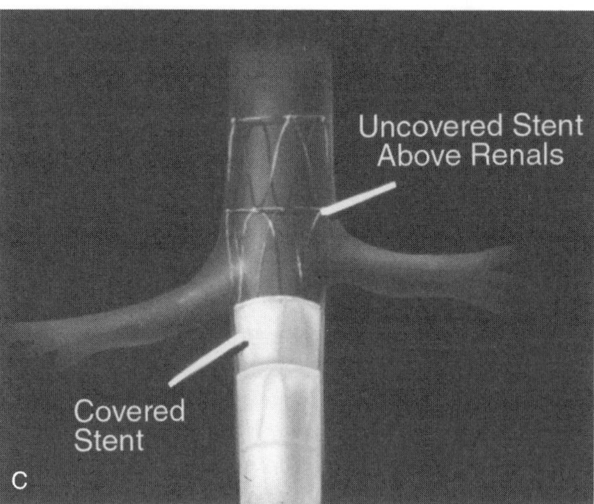

Figure 4. A. Angiogram illustrating development of an aneurysm cephalad to an endoluminal graft 14 months after its deployment. **B.** Illustration of technique used to isolate the proximal aneurysm—repair of aneurysm that shows complete exclusion of proximal dilatation with stent access across the renal arteries. **C.** Illustration of technique used to exclude aneurysm with an uncovered stent placed across the renal arteries.

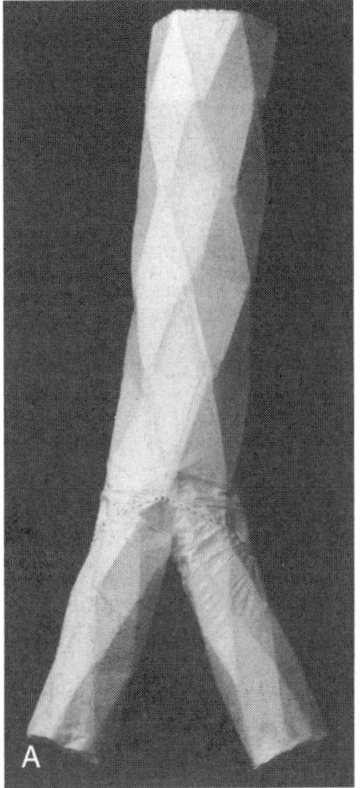

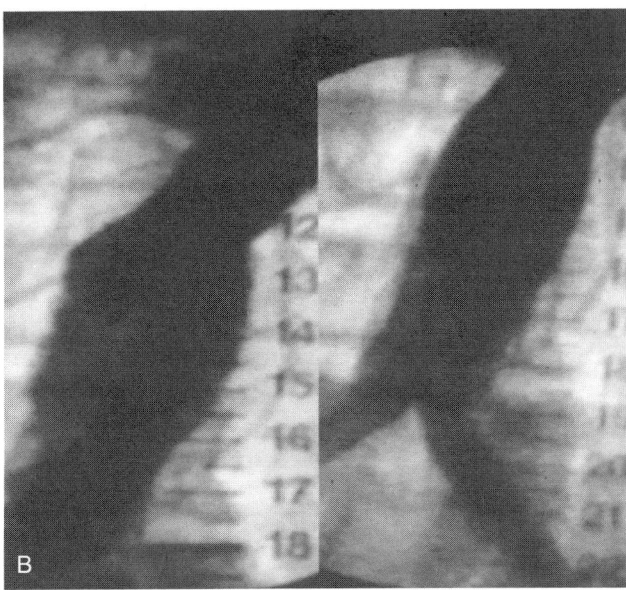

Figure 5. A. A new, single-stage unibody endoluminal graft developed at the Arizona Heart Institute for exclusion of abdominal aortic aneurysms (AAAs). **B.** Pre- and post-procedural angiogram showing exclusion of the AAA. This device has already enhanced delivery and reduced complications in 50 patients.

Endovascular Treatment of Lower Extremity Ischemia

Overview

Aortoiliac occlusive disease is a frequent cause of lower extremity ischemia. Stents are often used in the extremities to correct inadequacies or complications of balloon angioplasty, including dissection, acute or chronic occlusion, significant residual gradients, and restenosis.[17] As one approaches the arterial pathologies from the iliac to the popliteal, however, the results of interventions become less favorable. It has become clear that treatment of lesions below the inguinal ligament is considerably less successful than that in lesions in the more proximal arterial locations.

ELGs are a new approach to treatment of occlusive disease in the extremities. The successful evolution of simple tubular aortic endografts to more complex modular designs lies in providing a series of devices that are flexible enough to allow in situ customization based on operative and fluoroscopic findings.[18]

Clinical Results

The long-term efficacy of iliac artery stent placement with the Palmaz stent was reported by Murphy and colleagues in 1995.[19] In this series, a total of 83 patients underwent 108 iliac artery stent placements, and 80 of the patients were followed clinically for a mean of 25.8 months (range 1 to 70 months). Thirty patients were followed with angiography for a mean of 10.4 months (range 1 to 48 months). Clinical success was 98.9% immediately after the procedure and 86.2% at 48 months. A primary patency rate of 87.5% was demonstrated arteriographically at the latest follow-up period; there were 5 occlusions (12.5%) and 2 restenoses (5.0%). The overall complication rate was 9.7%, and 30-day mortality was 1.2%.

The results of an FDA phase II multicenter trial of the Wallstent (Schneider/Boston Scientific, Natick, MA) in the iliac and femoral arteries were also reported in 1995.[20] A total of 225 patients (mean age 64.2 years, range 32 to 88 years) entered the trial, and iliac and femoral stents were placed in 140 and 90 patients, respectively. Angiographic patency at 6 months in the iliac was 93%, and primary clinical patency was 81% and 71% at 1 and 2 years, respectively. Secondary clinical patency was 91% at 1 year and 86% at 2 years. Results in the femoral system were less favorable, with a 6-month angiographic patency of 80% and a primary clinical patency of 61% and 49% at 1 and 2 years, respectively (Fig. 6). Secondary patency was 84% at 1 year and 72% at 2 years. Major and minor complications occurred more frequently in stenting of the femoral artery. Overall, major complications (hematoma, pseudoaneurysm, arteriovenous fistula, distal embolus, acute thrombosis, and cerebrovascular and other hemorrhagic complications) were seen in 9.3% of patients. Minor complications were seen in 11.3% of all patients.

In another series, Wallstents were also used to treat 103 patients with iliac artery occlusions.[21] A total of 99 of these patients demonstrated clinical improvement. Embolization was seen in 5 patients, and complications that required further intervention were seen in 6 patients. Primary patency was 87% at 1 year, 83% at 2 years, and 78% after 4 years. Secondary patency was 94%, 90%, and 88% at 1, 2, and 4 years, respectively.

The results of follow-up of stenting in iliac artery stenoses over 6 years were reported in 1996 by Nöldge and colleagues.[22] A total of 141 patients received stents, and successful results were seen in 140 patients. The mean trans-stenotic gradient fell from 29.5 to 6.7 mm Hg. The cumulative 6-year angiographic patency was 64.6%, and the clinical success rate was 72.7%. There were 23 late failures, and 17 of these resulted from progressive restenosis of the treated lesion. In this series, a comparison of results with stenting and angioplasty was made. Stenting proved statistically significantly better in terms of early- and long-term success and patency and resulted in significantly fewer complications than angioplasty. In general, stenting of the popliteal and superficial femoral arteries has not provided satisfactory long-term results, and the use devices that provide new alternatives for treating these vessels is under study.

Covered stents have been used in the iliac artery to repair rupture resulting from balloon dilatation. While this type of injury would normally require correction via an open surgical procedure, use of the covered stent is a less aggressive means of treating this complication.[23]

Endovascular grafts fashioned from Palmaz stents and PTFE have been used successfully,[24–26] with primary and secondary patency of 89% and 100%, respectively, at 18 months.[24] Grafts are particularly useful in treating patients with iliac artery aneurysms. In a study by Dorros and colleagues,[25] 80% of the

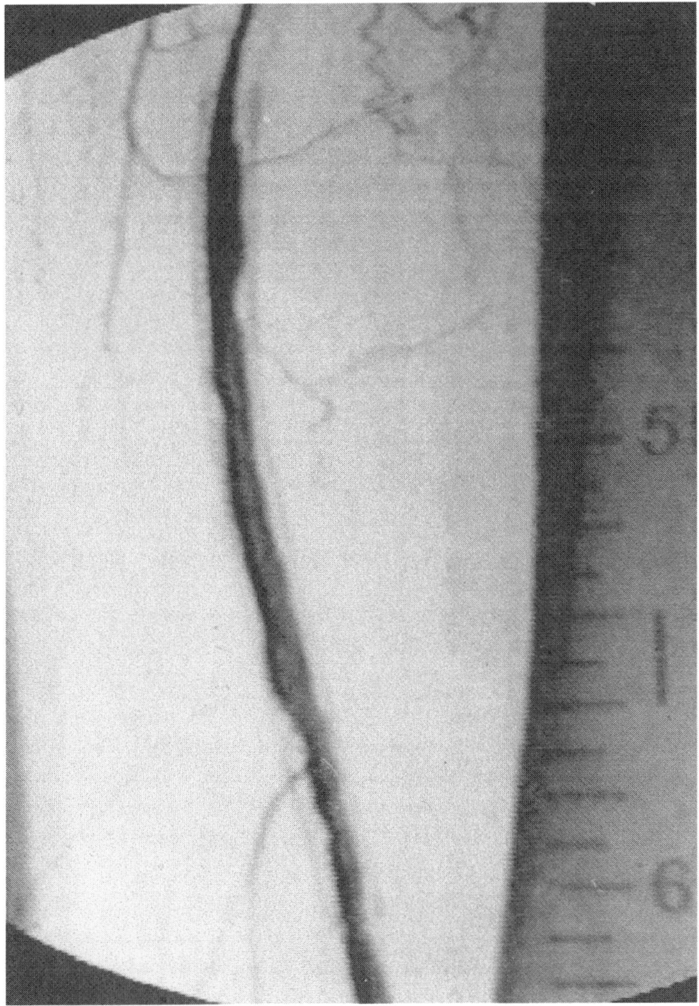

Figure 6. Arteriogram of superficial femoral artery 6 months after a Wallstent was deployed. The diffuse intimal hyperplasia observed here is typical when stents are placed in the lower extremity; long-term patency is rare in these cases.

grafts were patent and free of endoleaks at a mean follow-up of 14 months.

In another study, 24 patients received 29 endovascular stent-grafts for treatment of claudication or limb-threatening iliofemoral occlusive disease.[27] The majority of the grafts originated from the aortoiliac junction or the common iliac arteries. Outflow procedures (profundaplasty or femorodistal grafting) were performed in all cases. Operative mortality was 9%, and 1 occlusion was noted postoperatively. Cumulative primary and secondary patency rates at 1 year were 85% and 95%, respectively, and the limb salvage rate was 95%.

The Wallgraft (Schneider/Boston Scientific) is the first commercially available product of this category and has been approved in the US (Fig. 7). This device is very user-friendly and is deployed in a manner similar to that of the Wallstent.

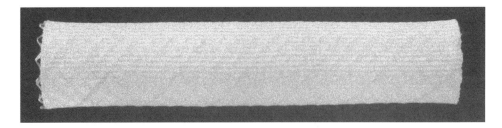

Figure 7. Photograph of the Wallgraft, which is currently being studied in clinical trials. This device is made by Schneider/Boston Scientific, which received FDA approval for use in the trachea-bronchial tree.

Endovascular Treatment of Carotid Artery Disease

Overview

In patients with carotid stenoses and transient ischemic attacks, the cumulative 5-year risk of stroke is 30% to 35%.[28,29] Treatment of the condition has traditionally employed carotid endarterectomy, a surgical technique that is considered the gold standard of therapy.[30] Recently, however, endovascular intervention in lesions originating in the great vessels of the aortic arch, the left subclavian, innominate, and right subclavian arteries has been relatively prevalent.[31–37] More recently, endoluminal treatment of lesions in the common carotid and at the cervical bifurcation into the internal carotid artery has been reported by a number of investigators.[38–44]

Technological advances in endoluminal equipment have changed treatment strategies for vascular disease in these anatomical regions. While the successful results of intervention in the subclavian and innominate arteries are well documented, our experience in the carotid arterial region is still in the early stages, and investigators are proceeding slowly because of the potential for neurologic complications. We now find ourselves in the position of comparing the results of endovascular intervention with those of what has become a classic, gold standard procedure, carotid endarterectomy. The field of endovascular surgery is evolving rapidly, and the goal of endovascular treatment is to provide a favorable outcome with fewer or equal complications as compared to the classic surgical procedure. Because of the potential for successful treatment of this particular disease entity with endovascular techniques, we believe carotid stenting will be in frequent use in the coming years. Accordingly, we review the recent clinical results of carotid stenting and outline our own experience at the Arizona Heart Institute.

Clinical Results

Results of carotid stenting by Wholey and colleagues[45] reveal that carotid stents were successfully placed in 108 of 114 lesions in 108 patients. There were 6 technical failures that were due to access problems (n=5) and 1 seizure during balloon inflation. Complications included 2 major and 2 minor strokes, 5 transient ischemic attacks, and 2 seizure episodes. The overall stroke or death rate was 5.3%, and in the 6-month follow-up period, there was 1 restenosis that was successfully treated.

In a more recent update presented at International Congress on Endovascular Interventions XII (Scottsdale, AZ; February 1999), Dr. Wholey reviewed his most recent accumulated experience in 315 carotid procedures (Table 1). The rates of major and minor stroke were 1.7% and 1.4%, respectively, and the death rate was 0.7%. Dr. Wholey estimated that at clinical experimental sites, the annualized rate of stent deployment is increasing 30% each year. At the 1999 American College of Cardiology (ACC) meeting in New Orleans, LA, Dr. Wholey stated that an interventionist typically requires 20 carotid procedures in the learning curve before an acceptable stroke/death rate of 3% is achieved.

In a study by Teitlebaum and colleagues,[46] a 96% technical success rate was achieved in 25 carotid lesions in 22 patients. One death from MI occurred 3 weeks after stenting, and the 30-day combined death, stroke, and ipsilateral blindness rate was 27% (6 of 22 patients); however, only 2 strokes were directly related to the procedure. One month after the procedure, 91% of the surviving patients were ambulatory and independent. In 6-month follow-up, there was a 14% rate of occlusion or restenosis.

A 1998 global survey of carotid stenting in 24 medical centers throughout the world indicates that 2048 procedures had been performed with a technical success rate of 98.6%.[47] Complications included 63 minor strokes (3%), 27 major strokes (1.3%), 28 deaths within 30 days (1.4%), and restenosis of 4.8% at 6 months. The authors concluded that the periprocedural risks for major and minor strokes and death were acceptable given the early stage of development in this discipline. More recent results of this collaborative effort are detailed in Table 2; these results were presented at the International Congress on Endovascular Interventions XII and at the ACC.

Comparative results of carotid stenting by Roubin and colleagues (Table 3) were also presented at the International Congress on Endovascular Interventions XII and indicate a trend toward reduction in complications over time as experience with patient selection and technical procedures is gained.

Table 1

Carotid Stenting: Results from the Pittsburgh Vascular Institute*

	(n=315)
Major stroke	1.7%
Minor stroke	1.4%
Death	0.7%
Total stroke and death	3.8%

*Includes "learning curve" data (n=20).

(Wholey and colleagues, as presented at the International Congress on Endovascular Interventions XII.)

Table 2

Carotid Stenting: Results of 28-Center International Registry*	
(n=3500)	
Periprocedural stroke and death	3.5%–8%
Symptomatic	69%
Asymptomatic	31%

*85% of patients had comorbidities that would have excluded them from the NASCET trial.

(Wholey and colleagues 1999, as presented at the International Congress on Endovascular Interventions XII.)

Clinical Results from the Arizona Heart Institute

General Observations

At the Arizona Heart Institute, our carotid stenting program includes only those patients in whom we believe the benefits of the endoluminal intervention potentially outweigh the risks. We have defined four specific subgroups of patients in whom it seems the endovascular approach is either comparable with or superior to the classic endarterectomy procedure:

- Patients with high internal carotid artery lesions
- Patients who have undergone radiation to the cervical carotid area and/or a radical node dissection
- Patients who have previously undergone one or more carotid endarterectomy procedures
- Patients with combined or sequential lesions

Patients who present with lesions in the distal internal carotid artery (at the base of the skull) are often candidates for stenting, as these lesions are dif-

Table 3

Progression of Experience with Carotid Stenting

	1994–1995	*1995–1996*	*1996–1997*	*1997–1998*
Total # of patients	89	100	132	88
Total # of vessels	97	119	137	97
Deaths from neurologic complications	0	0	3	0
Major strokes	1	2	1	0
Minor strokes	7	8	6	2

(Roubin and colleagues 1999, as presented at the International Congress on Endovascular Interventions XII.)

ficult to access surgically without otolaryngeal and neurologic sequelae. Lesions in the high internal carotid are frequently short and often appear as an "hourglass" configuration located well beyond the bifurcation, where atherosclerotic debris is common. The pathology of these lesions is usually well localized, smooth walled, and free of loose debris. In some cases, the midportion of the lesion may be extremely narrow, requiring small balloon dilation at low pressure before stent application. Short stents can be deployed across the lesions, keeping them completely distinct from the bifurcation area. This form of treatment is certainly preferable to a complex surgical procedure that may entail subluxation of the mandible and its requisite wiring for fixation.[48,49]

Radiation treatment of the cervical carotid area and/or a radical node dissection frequently causes extensive scarring and radiation damage, making surgical intervention technically difficult. Endovascular treatment may be an attractive alternative to classic surgical intervention in these cases. Indeed, in some patients it is nearly impossible to locate the carotid artery surgically, and the potential for arterial trauma and neurologic damage is considerable. Stents may be used in these situations to correct diffuse lesions along the entire course of the artery. The device traps plaque and debris against the artery wall and may eliminate the potential for embolic events frequently associated with these types of lesions.

Although endarterectomy has demonstrated considerable success in the treatment of carotid artery stenosis, there are patients who require reoperation. The reported incidence of restenosis with endarterectomy varies from 1.2% to 36%,[50,51] but it is generally agreed that only approximately 10% of the recurrent cases are clinically significant.[52,53] Unless the recurrence is creating a stenosis ≥80% or a contralateral internal carotid artery is occluded, reintervention may not be indicated in the absence of specific symptoms. In those patients who do require reintervention, stenting may be an appealing option because accessing the lesion surgically is often difficult due to scarring, adherence of nerve tissue, and cephalad extension of disease.

Our experience reveals that lesion characteristics vary considerably from patient to patient. Nevertheless, a number of general observations about recurrent lesions are apparent. Lesions that recur in the first 12 to 18 months following endarterectomy are usually the result of myointimal hyperplasia or a technical problem associated with the operation. Myointimal hyperplasia typically causes smooth, firmly adherent lesions with localized thickening. When technical errors occur during a procedure, the resultant pathology generally appears as a flap of plaque or a suture line that narrows the artery. These irregularities can be corrected using stents, and the results are usually excellent and the complication rate low. Lesions that recur several years after the original operation, however, are far more likely to present with plaque that is similar to the original lesion, and endovascular manipulation within these lesions may provoke embolization.

Lesions are sometimes seen in two locations, one or both of which may be amenable to endovascular therapy. We have encountered high-grade stenosis of the left common carotid artery at the aortic arch in combination with an occlusive process of the left carotid bifurcation. Treatment of the proximal lesion is required before or in concert with the more cephalad intervention. In general, the proximal lesions are easily corrected with stents and are not particularly prone to embolization. Treatment of bifurcation lesions depends on their morphologic characteristics; classic endarterectomy should be employed in friable lesions with loose debris (Fig. 8).

Results of Endovascular Treatment

Our single-center experience with endovascular treatment of cerebrovascular lesions encompasses a 5-year period from 1993 to 1998 (Fig. 9). The results of our initial experience with carotid stenting in 110 patients were published in February of 1996.[43] In this series, both asymptomatic and symptomatic patients with ≥70% arteriographically defined carotid stenoses or ulcerative lesions were treated. The procedures were performed either via direct-stick percutaneous access to the cervical common carotid artery or through a retrograde femoral artery approach.

Minor complications included 4 cases of spasm (successfully treated with papaverine), 1 flow-limiting dissection (stented); and 6 access-site problems. There were 7 strokes (2 major, 5 reversible) (6.4%) and 5 minor transient events (4.5%) that resolved within 24 hours. Three patients were converted to endarterectomy (2.7%) prior to discharge. One stroke patient expired (0.9%), and another patient died of an unrelated cardiac event in the hospital. In the 30-day postprocedural period, 2 internal carotid artery stents occluded (patients asymptomatic).

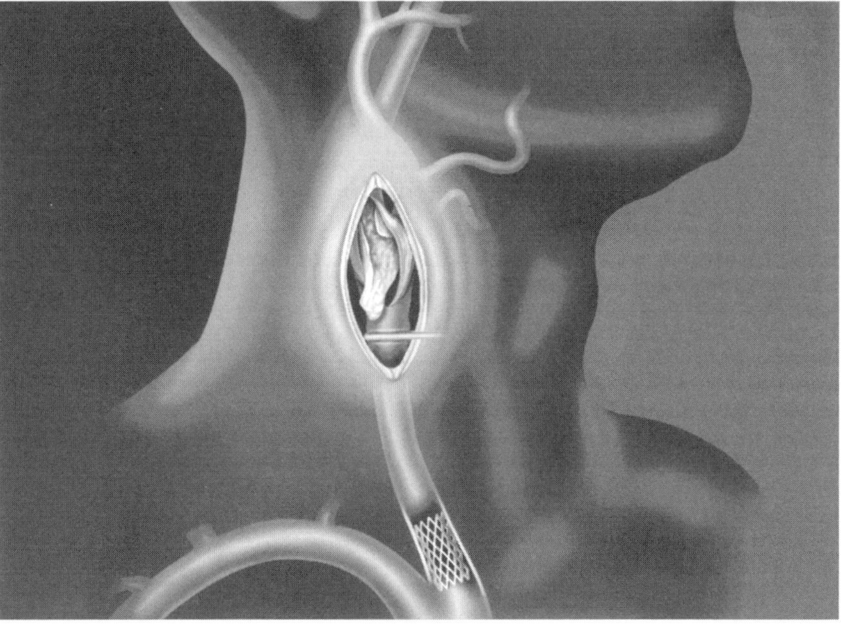

Figure 8. Illustration showing a combined procedure to correct a proximal carotid artery lesion with an endoluminal stent and repair a bifurcation lesion with endarterectomy. The lesions were treated accessed via a short cervical incision.

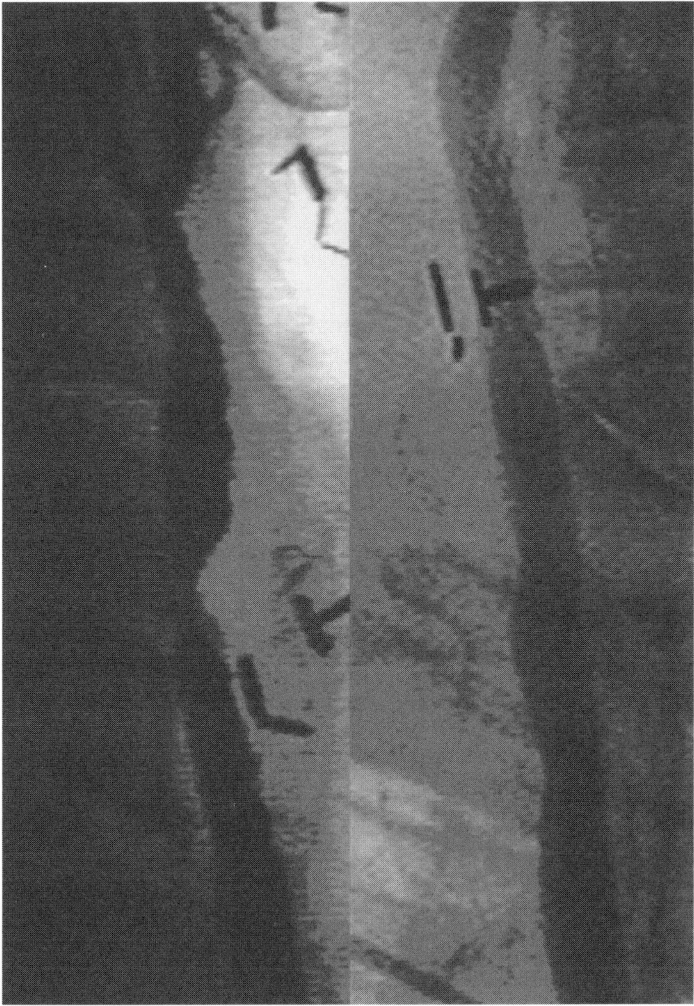

Figure 9. Left: Angiogram of our first carotid stent case, which was placed in 1993. Right: Follow-up 5 years later shows intact patency without any intimal hyperplasia in the Palmaz 294 stent.

Clinical success at 30 days (no technical failure, death, endarterectomy, stroke, or occlusion) was 89.1% (98 of 110). Life-table analysis showed an 89% cumulative primary patency rate at 18 months. Several important changes in both patient selection and technique have dramatically reduced the incidence of complications in the more recent series.

In the more recent series, a total of 179 patients were treated with carotid angioplasty and stenting between September 1995 and April 1998. Approximately 70% of the patients were asymptomatic and 30% were symptomatic or were being stented prior to a major operative procedure. A total of 18 patients presented with recurrent carotid stenosis following a previous carotid endarterectomy. In this series, there was a nearly equal distribution of Palmaz stents and Wallstents.

Analysis of results in the series of 179 patients indicates a procedural success rate of 96% and a dramatic reduction in complications as compared to the initial series. Neurologic complications occurred in 4 patients (3.6%) in the current series. One patient suffered a spasm that resolved; the CT scan was negative. In 3 other patients, embolization was suspected, and all 3 patients had positive CT scans.

The overall rate of death and neurologic complications declined from 10.9% in the initial series to 6.2% in the current series. Of the 3 deaths in the current series, 1 was clearly preventable. The patient had an open exposure of the carotid artery for internal carotid artery stenting. Shortly after she was returned to the intensive care unit, her blood pressure increased suddenly to nearly 300 mm Hg systolic. Swelling in her neck caused tracheal compression, and she arrested despite a tracheotomy. The second death occurred in a patient who received an Integra stent (investigational device; Boston Scientific/Meadox) and died from distal embolization. A third patient died several hours after the procedure from a distal dissection of the internal carotid artery that occurred well above the location of the stent and resulted in complete thrombosis of the artery.

Discussion

The results of the current series indicate acceptable rates of technical success and complications with endovascular intervention=mparticularly given that a subset of these patients had combined lesions. Had classic surgical intervention been used, it is doubtful that comparable results could have been obtained. Nevertheless, one of the greatest concerns about carotid angioplasty and stenting remains the potential for cerebral embolization and neurologic complications.

Our frequent use of the Wallstent in the current series was not due to concern about the potential for deformation with the Palmaz stent, which we have observed in only 3 cases, but rather because it is easier to deploy in situations in which there is excessive tortuosity of the arch vessels (Fig. 10). We have also deployed the Symphony stent (Boston Scientific) successfully in 3 patients and have placed 2 Integra stents.

We have found that stent deployment via open exposure of the carotid artery is indicated in some patients due to difficult arch vessel configuration. In our initial series, difficulties with stent compression and hematoma at the sheath site were associated with direct, percutaneous puncture of the carotid artery, and we have abandoned the technique in favor of open exposure. When access is problematic, the majority of patients are now stented using a retrograde femoral approach with a direct puncture technique that incorporates a short, cervical incision.

As we have indicated, there are major differences in complication rates and postprocedural results, depending on the exact location of the intervention. The potential for periprocedural embolization is greatest in lesions at the level of the carotid bifurcation. Loose atherosclerotic debris is frequently present here, and passing a wire and balloon and deploying a stent under these circumstances may dislodge it.

Clearly, our goals for endovascular intervention should include the pre-

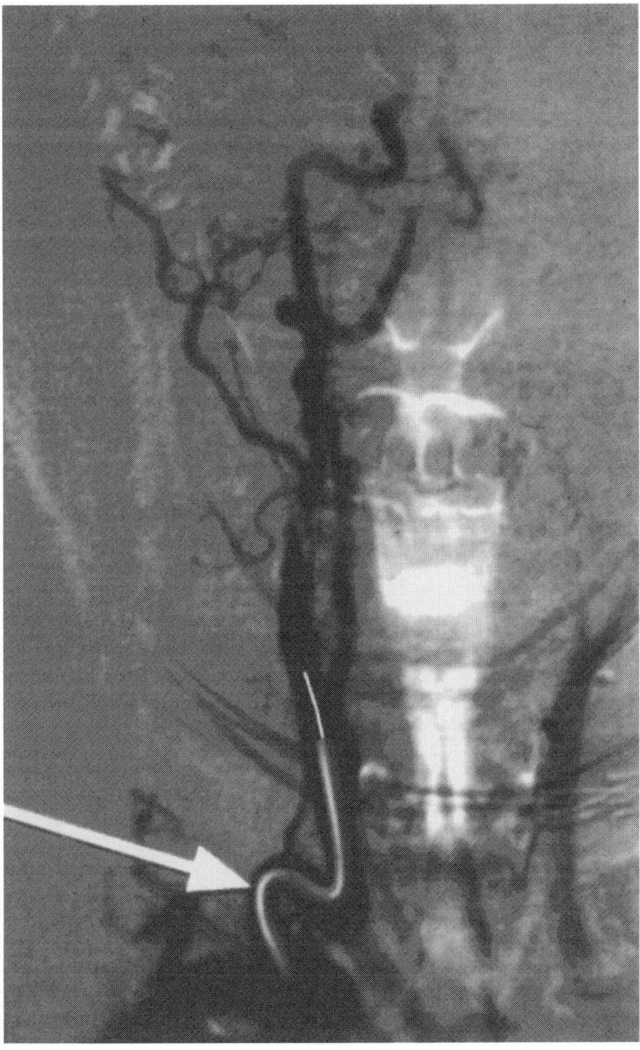

Figure 10. Angiogram with catheter superimposed; this image illustrates a technical problem associated with delivery of a rigid stent across the tortuous arch vessels.

vention of complications. The use of duplex scanning to identify lesions with potential for embolization is under study[54,55] and at our institution, we routinely perform a duplex scan before angioplasty and stenting procedures. The duplex scan often reveals pathology that predisposes the patient to embolization. Further refinement of imaging techniques and equipment will continue to aid patient selection for endovascular therapy.

Restenosis has proven to be a major limitation of angioplasty and stenting in other vessels but, as yet, there are no comprehensive studies of incidence in patients who have undergone carotid procedures. Thus far, our own experience indicates that the restenosis rate in carotid lesions treated with angioplasty and stenting has been quite low.

Summary

The field of endovascular surgery is constantly changing as new techniques and devices are adopted. Stenting has been an extremely important advance, and ELG technology is proliferating at an unprecedented rate. A great deal of progress has been made in device design, and advancements in deployment technique have also been realized. The use of stents and ELGs has already changed the indications for treatment in many centers, and we can anticipate that further innovation will broaden the scope of endovascular treatment of vascular disease. The continual problem of "instant restenosis," particularly in the superficial femoral artery (SFA), may be influenced positively by the use of radiation, which is currently under study for this indication. Gene therapy may have a future role not only in angiogenesis, but also perhaps in combating restenosis.

The use of ELGs in AAAs has proven quite successful in many cases. While there are still improvements to be made, device modifications and changes in deployment techniques have reduced the rate of endoleaks, which have been one of the most prevalent complications. The results of stenting in the iliac artery have been favorable, and the procedure is now a well-accepted alternative to open surgical intervention. Although our experience with carotid endovascular procedures is relatively recent, it has already become evident that some anatomical locations within the region are more amenable to endovascular treatment than others. Neurologic event rates, for example, may be unacceptably high in endovascular treatment of complicated bifurcation disease, while stenting in aortic arch lesions, high internal carotid artery lesions, and restenotic lesions in patients with damage from radical neck dissection and/or radiation have been more encouraging.

The future of endovascular intervention is very bright, and the introduction of new devices and surgical techniques is certain to ensure additional success in endovascular intervention into the next century.

References

1. Parodi JC, Palmaz JC, Barone HD. Transfemoral intraluminal graft implantation for abdominal aortic aneurysms. *Ann Vasc Surg* 1991;5:491–499.
2. May J, White G, Yu W, et al. Concurrent comparison of endoluminal repair versus no treatment for small abdominal aortic aneurysms. *Eur J Vasc Endovasc Surg* 1997;13:472–476.
3. Dardik A, Burleyson GP, Bowman H, et al. Surgical repair of ruptured abdominal aortic aneurysms in the state of Maryland: Factors influencing outcome among 527 recent cases. *J Vasc Surg* 1998;28:413–420.
4. Scott RA, Tisi PV, Ashton HA, Allen DR. Abdominal aortic aneurysm rupture rates: A 7-year follow-up of the entire abdominal aortic aneurysm population detected by screening. *J Vasc Surg* 1998;28:124–128.
5. Wain RA, Marin ML, Ohki T, et al. Endoleaks after endovascular graft treatment of aortic aneurysms: Classification, risk factors, and outcome. *J Vasc Surg* 1998;27:69–68.
6. White GH, May J, Waigh RC, et al. Type III and type IV endoleak: Toward a complete definition of blood flow in the sac after endoluminal AAA repair. *J Endovasc Surg* 1998;5:305–309.

7. Stelter W, Umscheid T, Ziegler P. Three-year experience with modular stent-graft devices for endovascular AAA treatment. *J Endovasc Surg* 1997;4:362–369.
8. Brewster DC, Geller SC, Kaufman JA, et al. Initial experience with endovascular repair: Comparison of early results with outcome of conventional open repair. *J Vasc Surg* 1998;27:992–1003.
9. Nasim A, Thompson MM, Sayers RD, et al. Is endoluminal abdominal aortic aneurysm repair using an aortoaortic (tube) device a durable procedure? *Ann Vasc Surg* 1998;12:522–528.
10. EVT Investigators. Preexisting thrombus and aortic aneurysm size change after endovascular repair. *J Surg Res* 1999;81:11–14.
11. May J, White GH, Yu W, et al. Endovascular grafting for abdominal aortic aneurysms: Changing incidence and indication for conversion to open operation. *Cardiovasc Surg* 1998;6:194–197.
12. Matsumura JS, Chaikof EL. Continued expansion of aortic necks after endovascular repair of abdominal aortic aneurysms. EVT investigators. Endovascular Technologies, Inc. *J Vasc Surg* 1998;28:422–430.
13. Malina M, Lindblad B, Ivancev K, et al. Endovascular AAA exclusion: Will stents with hooks and barbs prevent stent-graft migration? *J Endovasc Surg* 1998;5:310–317.
14. Walker STR, Yusuf SW, Wenham PW, Hopkinson BR. Renal complications following endovascular repair of abdominal aortic aneurysms. *J Endovasc Surg* 1998;5:318–322.
15. May J, White GH, Waugh R, et al. Adverse events after endoluminal repair of abdominal aortic aneurysms: A comparison during two successive periods of time. *J Vasc Surg* 1999;29:32–39.
16. Torsello GB, Klenk E, Kasprzak B, Umscheid T. Rupture of abdominal aortic aneurysm previously treated by endovascular stentgraft. *J Vasc Surg* 1998;28:184–187.
17. Cikrit DF, Dalsing MC. Lower-extremity arterial endovascular stenting. *Surg Clin North Am* 1998;78:617–629.
18. Marin ML, Hollier LH, Avrahami R, Parsons R. Varying strategies for endovascular repair of abdominal and iliac artery aneurysms. *Surg Clin North Am* 1998;78:631–645.
19. Murphy KD, Encarnacion CE, Le VA, Palmaz JC. Iliac artery stent placement with the Palmaz stent: Follow-up study. *J Vasc Interv Radiol* 1995;6:321–329.
20. Martin EC, Katzen BT, Benenati JF, et al. Multicenter trial of the Wallstent in the iliac and femoral arteries. *J Vasc Interv Radiol* 1995;6:843–849.
21. Vorwerk D, Guenther RW, Schürmann K, et al. Primary stent placement for chronic iliac artery occlusions: Follow-up results in 103 patients. *Radiology* 1995;194:745–749.
22. Nöldge G, Richter GM, Rören T, et al. A randomized trial of iliac stenting versus PTA in iliac artery stenoses and occlusions: Updated 6-year results. *J Endovasc Surg* 1996;3:99–100. Abstract.
23. Formichi M, Raybaud G, Benichou H, Ciosi G. Rupture of the external iliac artery during balloon angioplasty: Endovascular treatment using a covered stent. *J Endovasc Surg* 1998;5:37–41.
24. Sanchez LA, Wain RA, Veith FJ, et al. Endovascular grafting for aortoiliac occlusive disease. *Semin Vasc Surg* 1997;10:297–309.
25. Dorros G, Cohn JM, Jaff MR. Percutaneous endovascular stent-graft repair of iliac artery aneurysms. *J Endovasc Surg* 1997;4:370–375.
26. Quinn SF, Sheley RC, Semonsen KG, et al. Endovascular stents covered with preexpanded polytetrafluoroethylene for treatment of iliac artery aneurysms and fistulas. *J Vasc Interv Radiol* 1997;8:1057–1063.
27. Nevelsteen A, Lacroix H, Stockx L, Wilms G. Stent grafts for iliofemoral occlusive disease. *Cardiovasc Surg* 1997;5:393–397.
28. Whisnant JP, Wiebers DO. Clinical epidemiology of transient cerebral ischemic attacks on the anterior and posterior circulation. In Sundt TM Jr (ed): *Occlusive Cerebrovascular Disease: Diagnosis and Surgical Management.* Philadelphia: W.B. Saunders Co.; 1987:60–65.

29. Dennis M, Bamford J, Sandercock P, et al. Prognosis of transient ischemic attacks in the Oxfordshire Community Stroke Project. *Stroke* 1990;21:848–853.
30. Zarins CK. Carotid endarterectomy: The gold standard. *J Endovasc Surg* 1996;3;10–15.
31. Diethrich EB. Initial experience with stenting in the innominate, subclavian, and carotid arteries. *J Endovasc Surg* 1995;2:196–221.
32. Kumar K, Dorros G, Bates MC, et al. Primary stent deployment in occlusive subclavian artery disease. *Cathet Cardiovasc Diagn* 1995;34:281–285.
33. Martinez, R, Rodriguez-Lopez J, Torruella L, et al. Stenting for occlusion of subclavian arteries: technical aspects and follow-up results. *Texas Heart J* 1997;24:23–27.
34. Mathias K. Ein neues Kathetersystem zur perkutanen transluminalen Angioplastie von Karotisstenosen. *Fortschr Med* 1977;95:1007–1011.
35. Motarjeme A. Percutaneous transluminal angioplasty of supra-aortic vessels. *J Endovasc Surg* 1996;3:171–181.
36. Queral LA, Criado FJ. The treatment of focal aortic arch branch lesions with Palmaz stents. *J Vasc Surg* 1996;23:368–375.
37. Sullivan TM, Bacharach M, Childs MB. PTA and primary stenting of the subclavian and innominate arteries. *Circulation* 1995;92:I383. Abstract.
38. Kachel R, Basche S, Heerklotz I, et al. Percutaneous transluminal angioplasty of supra-aortic arteries, especially the internal carotid artery. *Neuroradiology* 1991;33:191–194.
39. Kachel R. Results of balloon angioplasty in the carotid arteries. *J Endovasc Surg* 1996;3:22–30.
40. Theron J. Angioplastie carotidienne protegee et stents carotidiens. *J Mal Vasc* 1996;21(suppl A):113–122.
41. Gaines P. The European carotid angioplasty trial. *J Endovasc Surg* 1996;3:107. Abstract.
42. Gaines PA. Carotid angioplasty and CAVATAS update. *J Endovasc Surg* 1997;4(suppl I):I12. Abstract.
43. Diethrich EB, Ndiaye M, Reid DB. Stenting in the carotid artery: Initial experience in 110 patients. *J Endovasc Surg* 1996;3:42–62.
44. Iyer SS, Roubin G, Yadav S, et al. Elective carotid stenting. *J Endovasc Surg* 1996;3:105–106. Abstract.
45. Wholey MH, Wholey M, Jarmolowski CR, et al. Endovascular stents for carotid artery occlusive disease. *J Endovasc Surg* 1997;4:326–338.
46. Teitlebaum GP, Lefkowitz MA, Giannotta SL. Carotid angioplasty and stenting in high-risk patients. *Surg Neurol* 1998;50:300–311.
47. Wholey MH, Wholey M, Bergeron P, et al. Current global status of carotid artery stent placement. *Cathet Cardiovasc Diagn* 1998;44:1–6.
48. Fisher DF, Clagett GP, Parker JL, et al. Mandibular subluxation for high carotid exposure. *J Vasc Surg* 1984;1:727–733.
49. Rossi PJ, Myers SI, Clagett GP. Reoperative approaches for carotid restenosis. *Semin Vasc Surg* 1994;7:195–200.
50. Gagne PJ, Riles TS, Jacobowitz GR, et al. Long-term follow-up of patients undergoing reoperation for recurrent carotid artery disease. *J Vasc Surg* 1993;18:991–1001.
51. Carbello RE, Towne JB, Seabrook GR, et al. An outcome analysis of carotid endarterectomy: The incidence and natural history of recurrent stenosis. *J Vasc Surg* 1996;23:749–754.
52. Mansour MA, Kang SS, Baker WH, et al. Carotid endarterectomy for recurrent stenosis. *J Vasc Surg* 1997;25:877–883.
53. Raithel D. Recurrent carotid disease: Optimum technique for redo surgery. *J Endovasc Surg* 1996;3:69–75.
54. El-Barghouty N, Geroulakos G, Nicolaides A, et al. Computer-assisted carotid plaque characterization. *Eur J Vasc Endovasc Surg* 1995;9:389–393.
55. El-Barghouty N, Nicolaides A, Tegos T, et al. The relative effect of carotid plaque heterogeneity and echogenicity on ipsilateral cerebral infarction and symptoms of cerebrovascular disease. *Int Angiol* 1996;15:300–306.

2

Noninterventional Management of Peripheral Vascular Disease:

Advances and Limitations

Michael R. Jaff, DO

Introduction

Endovascular therapy has revolutionized the management of peripheral arterial occlusive disease. Although proposed more than 35 years ago by Dotter and Judkins[1] and initially applied only to the coronary arteries, it was not until the 1980s that interest in endovascular therapy for peripheral arterial occlusive disease gained enthusiasm by the practicing interventionist. This interest has rapidly increased, and has become a primary therapeutic option for patients with peripheral vascular disease.[2]

Although the technology and devices available for endovascular therapy of arterial occlusive disease have become more sophisticated and reliable, the data comparing angioplasty and stenting to surgical revascularization or noninterventional therapy are lacking in many clinical scenarios. In addition, endovascular therapy is not without risk. Early experience with angioplasty for peripheral vascular disease in 352 patients (453 angioplasties) resulted in 59 complications in 53 patients.[3] Although the majority of these were access site hematomas, acute arterial occlusion, other complications such as arterial dissection, distal embolization, and vessel wall rupture were also observed. The advent of endovascular stents led to improved patency, but not with significant reduction in complications. Of 147 iliac artery stents deployed in 98 limbs, there were 29 (19.4%) complications.[4]

Most physicians still recognize noninterventional therapy as the first option for patients without emergent need for revascularization. Unfortunately, noninterventional therapy has generally included only smoking cessation, control of hypertension, hypercholesterolemia, diabetes mellitus, and unsuper-

From Criado FJ (ed): *Endovascular Intervention: New Tools and Techniques for the 21st Century.* Armonk, NY: Futura Publishing Co., Inc.; ©2002.

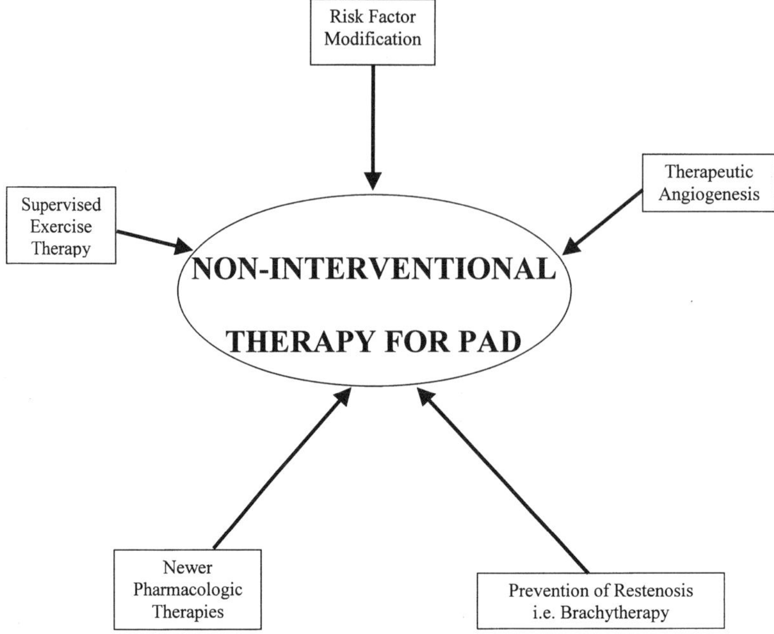

Figure 1. Noninterventional therapy for peripheral arterial occlusive disease (PAD).

vised exercise therapy, options that are only occasionally used by patients, and methods which offer variable benefit. Historically, physicians have viewed these options as temporizing measures for patients who will ultimately come to revascularization or limb loss.

Noninterventional therapy for peripheral arterial occlusive disease is much more than unsupervised walking. Options for noninterventional therapy have now come to include supervised exercise therapy, new pharmacologic agents for intermittent claudication, novel angiogenic growth factors, and vascular brachytherapy to promote patency after intervention (Fig. 1). Certainly, aggressive risk factor modification, including tobacco cessation, normalization of hypercholesterolemia, control of hypertension, and aggressive glycemic control in diabetes mellitus, is an important primary maneuver in the care of patients with vascular disease, and should represent the cornerstone of treatment, even if revascularization is required.[5] Position papers reviewing the role of percutaneous revascularization for peripheral arterial occlusive disease support the initial role of risk factor modification and exercise.[6]

Exercise Therapy

Exercise therapy has been well established as a primary treatment for peripheral arterial occlusive disease. Many vascular physicians, however, have a skeptical view of the true efficacy of this therapy. Historically, when patients with moderate lower extremity arterial occlusive disease are told to embark on an exercise program, a formal prescription is rarely provided. Patients are told to "walk" for 20 to 30 minutes 5 to 7 times weekly; however, these patients are not told the pace of walking, and there is no supervision provided. There are many social reasons for this, although the most prevalent is the lack of reimbursement by government or private insurance plans.

A review of the published series prior to 1993 demonstrated impressive improvement in pain-free walking distances, despite the fact that two of these series reflected unsupervised exercise.[7] One early series of supervised exercise therapy for 4 to 6 months in 148 patients demonstrated a mean increase in walking ability of 234%, with 88% of patients demonstrating significant walking improvement.[8] Comparisons of supervised versus home exercise therapy among more current series have consistently revealed marked benefit in both the time to onset of intermittent claudication and maximum walking time among patients receiving supervised exercise therapy.[9,10] Supervised exercise therapy also offers improvement in functional status as measured by walking impairment questionnaires and physical activity recall surveys.[11] Addition of pentoxifylline[12] or strength training to exercise therapy[13] has not offered significant additive benefits in pain-free walking distance.

In vascular laboratories, exercise treadmill testing is routine during evaluation for intermittent claudication, and the classic protocol is a treadmill speed of 2 miles per hour at an incline of 12% for a maximum walking distance of 5 minutes. Alternate treadmill protocols have been studied in an effort to improve the accuracy and reproducibility of treadmill exercise as *treatment* for intermittent claudication.[14] More recent protocols suggest increasing treadmill speed and adapting graded exercise testing as opposed to constant load testing, using either the Gardner or Hiatt protocol.[15] These modifications may result in less patient variability and diminish the placebo response.

A recent meta-analysis of published studies of exercise rehabilitation programs for the treatment of intermittent claudication revealed an increase in initial claudicating distance (ICD) of 179% and absolute claudicating distance (ACD) of 122%.[16] This analysis also suggested that an optimal exercise program should consist of three 30-minute sessions per week for at least 6 months, supervised walking as the primary exercise modality, and near-maximal claudication pain as the pain endpoint (Table 1).

Direct comparisons between exercise and endovascular therapy are sparse in the medical literature. In one series of 368 consecutive patients over 4 years,

Table 1

Components of a Successful Exercise Rehabilitation Program For Chronic Peripheral Arterial Occlusive Disease

- Direct patient supervision
- Six-month program duration
- (Three) 30-minute sessions per week
- Walking as the exercise modality
- Near-maximal claudication pain as the pain endpoint

patients were retrospectively asked to complete the SF-36 Health Survey and the Walking Impairment Questionnaire. Fifty-four percent of patients responded. Only 80 patients received invasive therapy after their initial evaluation (39 percutaneous transluminal angioplasty [PTA], 28 bypass, 13 both). Statistical analysis revealed that patients who underwent surgical bypass reported improvement in physical functioning and leg symptoms as compared to patients who underwent exercise or endovascular therapy.[17] Multiple flaws exist in this trial, including the retrospective nature of the study, lack of supervised exercise, lack of use of endovascular stents, and no stratification to location or severity of arterial disease. A more statistically sound comparison of these three modalities is required.

Pharmacologic Therapy for Intermittent Claudication

Drug therapy for lower extremity arterial occlusive disease, and specifically intermittent claudication, has been viewed as ineffective. Between 1965 and 1985, 75 trials studied 33 pharmacologic agents to assess efficacy as primary therapy for intermittent claudication. Unfortunately, 75% of these trials were flawed by lack of a placebo-controlled arm, no double-blinding, inaccurate endpoints, or small sample sizes.[18]

Chelation therapy has generated many unsubstantiated claims of dramatic improvements in ACDs; however, one double-blind, randomized, controlled trial of 32 patients with intermittent claudication demonstrated no clinically significant increase in subjective and measured walking distances or ankle-brachial index (ABI).[19] A thorough review of the published literature confirms the lack of scientific data supporting the use of a chelating agent as primary therapy for patients with intermittent claudication.[20]

A number of promising new agents are undergoing intense investigation as pharmacologic therapy for patients with lower extremity arterial occlusive disease (Table 2).

Vasodilator therapy has been disappointing as treatment for patients with peripheral arterial occlusive disease. The overall benefit of vasodilator therapy

Table 2

New, Promising Pharmacologic Agents for the Treatment of Chronic Stable Intermittent Claudication

- Prostaglandin E_1 (Iloprost)
- Propionyl-L-carnitine
- L-arginine
- Cilostazol*

*Recently received approval from the US Food and Drug Administration.

has been weak. One recent short-term trial, however, suggests that patients with intermittent claudication who receive sublingual glyceryl trinitrate prior to exercise have a greater maximal walking distance and a decrease in the fall in the ABI after exercise.[21] Verapamil has been shown to increase oxygen extraction in an ischemic limb. One short-term dose-ranging trial of slow-release verapamil in patients with moderate distance intermittent claudication showed a statistically significant increase in maximal walking distance of 49% in those patients receiving verapamil as compared with placebo.[22] These and other vasodilator agents will require large-scale trials before their use in patients with peripheral arterial occlusive disease will be widely accepted.

In patients with peripheral arterial occlusive disease, antiplatelet therapy has been used predominantly as a method of preventing coronary and cerebrovascular events and death.[23] Ticlopidine and clopidogrel are thienopyridine derivatives that inhibit platelet aggregation. Ticlopidine has been shown to decrease the incidence of myocardial infarction, stroke, and transient ischemic attacks in patients with intermittent claudication.[24] In addition, as therapy for intermittent claudication, ticlopidine has demonstrated increases in the initial and ACDs when compared with placebo.[25] Finally, in comparison with placebo, ticlopidine has been shown to improve the long-term patency of lower extremity saphenous vein bypass grafts. Patients assigned to placebo had a 2-year cumulative patency rate of 63%, compared to 82% in the patients treated with ticlopidine.[26]

The Clopidogrel versus Aspirin in Patients at Risk for Ischemic Events (CAPRIE) trial evaluated 19,000 patients with history of ischemic stroke, myocardial infarction, or symptomatic peripheral arterial occlusive disease, randomized to either clopidogrel or aspirin. Patients assigned to clopidogrel had a statistically significant reduction in the primary endpoint of stroke, myocardial infarction, or vascular death compared to aspirin. The patients enrolled with symptomatic peripheral arterial occlusive disease gained the greatest benefit using clopidogrel as compared to aspirin.[27] Clopidogrel appears to be an important adjunct in the care of patients with peripheral arterial occlusive disease to prevent cardiovascular events and vascular death.

There has been considerable interest in the role of prostaglandin E_1 (PGE_1) as treatment for intermittent claudication. Studies comparing intravenous PGE_1 to exercise therapy or pentoxifylline have revealed significant benefits of PGE_1 over comparable therapies. One outpatient study of 213 patients with intermittent claudication randomized the patients to daily intravenous infusions of PGE_1 or placebo for 2 months, and revealed an increase in treadmill walking distance of 101% with PGE_1 compared to 60% in placebo-treated patients.[28] Studies with oral forms of PGE_1 are ongoing.

L-carnitine has biochemical effects that may offer significant advantages for patients with intermittent claudication. Administration of L-carnitine in ischemic muscle causes an increase in total carnitine concentration in the muscle, as well as a decrease in plasma lactate levels. It appears that patients with severe intermittent claudication have the highest concentration of short-chain acylcarnitines in muscle and plasma. Higher total carnitine levels can deplete acetyl-coenzyme A, which activates the acyl scavenger system and aids in removal of these acylcarnitines.[29]

Propionyl-L-carnitine is effective in increasing walking capacity. In one double-blind dosing trial of 245 patients with intermittent claudication, the use of propionyl-L-carnitine caused a marked increase in walking capacity, and in the patients' view of quality of life, when compared with placebo.[30] A large-scale North American trial is under way to further study the benefits of this therapy.

L-arginine has effects on nitric oxide formation, which restores endothelium-induced vasodilation. Nitric oxide is synthesized from L-arginine, and is critical to blood pressure regulation and vascular tone. A recent study of 39 patients with intermittent claudication, comparing intravenous infusions of L-arginine, PGE_1, or placebo, revealed not only a marked increase in pain-free walking distance by both active agents over placebo, but also a normalization of endogenous nitric oxide formation with L-arginine therapy. This was not seen with PGE_1 or placebo infusions.[31] The clinical utility of L-arginine therapy remains unclear.

Pentoxifylline is the only medication that has been approved by the US Food and Drug Administration for treatment of stable intermittent claudication. Porter and Bauer[32] evaluated 128 patients in a randomized, double-blind, placebo-controlled fashion, and demonstrated a statistically significant increase in initial and ACDs in patients assigned to pentoxifylline over placebo. Given the large number of clinical trials of varying scientific merit, a meta-analysis was performed to determine the true benefit of pentoxifylline in patients with intermittent claudication.[33] A total of 12 studies met the criteria set forth by the authors. The analysis suggests that pentoxifylline is effective in improving walking capacity of patients with moderate intermittent claudication; however, when all trials, and all 'high-quality' trials, were reviewed, the results were not statistically significant.

The most exciting advance in pharmacologic therapy for patients with intermittent claudication has been the advent of cilostazol. Cilostazol is a chemically unique compound with several mechanisms of action, the most important being inhibition of platelet aggregation and vasodilation. Clinical data have emerged demonstrating marked improvement in walking distances over both placebo and pentoxifylline.

In a multicenter, randomized, double-blind, placebo-controlled trial of 81 patients with chronic stable intermittent claudication, 54 were assigned to cilostazol, and 27 received matching placebo. All patients were evaluated with a constant speed and a constant grade treadmill test, and all were followed for 12 weeks. There was a 35% increase in ICD, and a 41% increase in ACD among patients who received cilostazol.[34]

A dose-ranging trial of cilostazol compared doses of 50 mg twice daily versus 100 mg twice daily versus placebo in 394 patients with chronic stable intermittent claudication. After 24 weeks, both doses of cilostazol demonstrated superiority in ACD and ICD when compared with placebo, with the 100-mg twice-daily dose achieving optimal results.[35]

In another randomized, prospective, double-blind trial of 239 patients with intermittent claudication, 119 received cilostazol 100 mg orally twice daily, and 120 received matching placebo. All patients were studied with constant speed and variable grade treadmill examinations, and all were followed on their assigned medications for 16 weeks. In addition, standardized quality of life indicators were assessed. Patients receiving cilostazol demonstrated significant improvements in ACD. Those assigned to cilostazol had a 96.4-m increase in ACD, compared to only 31.4 m in the placebo group.[36]

Finally, a 24-week, multicenter, randomized, double-blind trial compared the effects of cilostazol 100 mg twice a day, pentoxifylline 400 mg three times a day, and placebo in 698 patients with chronic stable claudication. Constant speed, variable grade treadmill testing was performed at 4-week intervals. Compared to placebo, cilostazol demonstrated a statistically significant increase in ICD (98.3% versus 55.1%) and ACD (53.9% versus 33.5%), whereas pentoxifylline did not (ICD 68.4% versus 55.1%; ACD 30.4% versus 33.5%). In addition, cilostazol was clearly and statistically significantly more effective in improving ICD and ACD than pentoxifylline.[37] As a result of these data, cilostazol has recently gained US Food and Drug Administration approval for use in patients with chronic stable intermittent claudication.

Therapeutic Angiogenesis for Peripheral Arterial Occlusive Disease

Angiogenic growth factors have been isolated, identified, and generated by recombinant gene technology in an effort to increase collateral arterial development in animal models of critical limb ischemia. This began with the development of fibroblast growth factor and basic fibroblast growth factor, which were administered intramuscularly to rabbits with acute hindlimb ischemia. After 14 days, there was marked augmentation of collateral vessel development compared to control limbs.[38]

A similar animal model was used to investigate the role of vascular endothelial growth factor (VEGF) in improving collateral arterial development. Using naked plasmid DNA encoding for VEGF applied to the hydrogel polymer coating of a balloon angioplasty catheter, the balloon was delivered percutaneously to the femoral artery. Not only did augmentation of collateral vessels occur, but improvement in calf blood pressure ratios was found in those limbs treated with VEGF.[39]

Direct intramuscular injection of naked plasmid DNA encoding for VEGF has been performed in the ischemic rabbit hindlimb model, and has demonstrated dramatic augmentation in vascularity and improved perfusion to the ischemic limb.[40]

As a result, human studies have been performed. Again using naked plasmid DNA encoding for VEGF, 10 limbs in 9 patients with chronic critical limb ischemia and nonhealing ulcers and/or ischemic rest pain underwent direct intramuscular injection. Although improved ABIs and augmentation in collateral vessel growth on contrast and magnetic resonance arteriography were found, the most impressive results were clinical. Ischemic ulcers either healed or improved markedly in 4 of 7 limbs, with limb salvage in 3 patients who were previously advised to undergo below-knee amputation.[41]

Experimental models of bypass grafts have been performed in New Zealand white rabbits. Reversed jugular vein to common carotid artery vein grafts were submerged in solution containing VEGF or saline, implanted, and then removed and histologically examined after 28 days. The vein grafts submerged in VEGF had a marked reduction in intimal thickness compared to saline-treated grafts, suggesting that VEGF and other angiogenic growth factors may aid in graft patency.[42] A predictor of clinical efficacy of intramuscular VEGF therapy appears to be a patent dorsalis pedis artery, especially in patients with ischemic ulcerations.[43]

Adjunctive percutaneous balloon angioplasty (PTA) and intra-arterial delivery of naked plasmid DNA encoding for VEGF has been performed in a small series of patients who underwent PTA of the superficial femoral artery. Of 19 patients in this cohort, VEGF was applied directly to the angioplasty site. After a mean follow-up of 9 months, 75% of angioplasty sites demonstrated no restenosis or minimal intimal hyperplasia.[44]

A small series of patients with thromboangiitis obliterans (Buerger's Disease) and ischemic ulcerations and/or ischemic rest pain received two intramuscular injections of phVEGF165 within 4 weeks. All 5 patients with digital gangrene demonstrated complete ulcer healing. One patient with rest pain had complete resolution. The 2 remaining patients with extensive gangrene of the forefoot required below-knee amputation, despite having evidence by contrast and magnetic resonance arteriography of new collateral vessel growth.[45]

Many planned controlled trials will provide further information on the clinical role and efficacy of angiogenesis, not only in patients with advanced peripheral arterial occlusive disease, but in patients with lifestyle-limiting disease as well.

Vascular Brachytherapy

Although not truly "noninterventional," vascular brachytherapy is emerging as a potentially important method of decreasing or preventing restenosis after revascularization in the peripheral arteries. Radiation prevents neointimal proliferation and vessel constriction after injury.[46] There is interest in delivering endovascular radiation by either catheter-based systems or radioactive stents. Issues of choice of radioactive isotope, dosimetry, and dwell times are beyond the scope of this chapter. In one series of 28 patients who suffered restenosis or occlusion of an infrainguinal artery within 6 months of an endovascular revascularization procedure, intravascular brachytherapy with a 10-Ci ^{192}Ir source was positioned within a stent used to recanalize the area of stenosis or occlusion. Of 25 patients who underwent follow-up, 21 had no evidence of restenosis within the treated segment.[47]

A feasibility trial of 40 patients who underwent ^{192}Ir therapy for peripheral arterial occlusive disease after PTA of an infrainguinal vessel has been completed. The arteriographic restenosis rates after 6 months was only 11.6% (Waksman R, personal communication, 1999).

The ultimate role of vascular brachytherapy to prevent restenosis after endovascular therapy is unclear, and further research is required.

Summary

Despite the enthusiasm for novel endovascular methods to revascularize patients with lower extremity arterial occlusive disease, the data documenting long-term improvement are somewhat limited. In addition, these procedures are accompanied by a small, but definite, risk of complications.

The role of risk factor modification (tobacco cessation, control of hypertension/hyperlipidemia/diabetes mellitus) must remain the cornerstone of therapy. In addition, supervised exercise rehabilitation, new pharmacologic agents (i.e., cilostazol), angiogenesis, and potential methods to prevent restenosis (i.e., brachytherapy) may play an increasingly important role in the management of this complex condition.

References

1. Dotter CT, Judkins MP. Transluminal treatment of arteriosclerotic obstruction: Description of a new technique and a preliminary report of its applications. *Circulation* 1964;30:654–670.
2. Isner JM, Rosenfield K. Redefining the treatment of peripheral artery disease. Role of percutaneous revascularization. *Circulation* 1993;88:1534–1557.
3. Gardiner GA, Meyerovitz MF, Stokes KR, et al. Complications of transluminal angioplasty. *Radiology* 1986;159:201–208.
4. Ballard JL, Sparks SR, Taylor FC, et al. Complications of iliac artery stent deployment. *J Vasc Surg* 1996;24:545–555.
5. Weitz JI, Byrne J, Clagett GP, et al. Diagnosis and treatment of chronic arterial insufficiency of the lower extremities: A critical review. *Circulation* 1996;94:3026–3049.
6. Pentecost MJ, Criqui MH, Dorros G, et al. Guidelines for peripheral percutaneous transluminal angioplasty of the abdominal aorta and lower extremity vessels. A statement for health professionals from a special writing group of the councils on cardiovascular radiology, clinical cardiology, and epidemiology and prevention, the American Heart Association. *Circulation* 1994;89:511–530.
7. Ernst E, Fialka V. A review of the clinical effectiveness of exercise therapy for intermittent claudication. *Arch Intern Med* 1993;153:2357–2360.
8. Ekroth R, Dahllof AG, Gundevall B, et al. Physical training of patients with intermittent claudication: Indications, methods, and results. *Surgery* 1978;84:640–643.
9. Williams LR, Ekers MA, Collins PS, Lee JF. Vascular rehabilitation: Benefits of a structured exercise/risk modification program. *J Vasc Surg* 1991;14:320–326.
10. Patterson RB, Pinto B, Marcus B, et al. Value of a supervised exercise program for the therapy of arterial claudication. *J Vasc Surg* 1997;25:312–319.
11. Regensteiner JG, Steiner JF, Hiatt WR. Exercise training improves functional status in patients with peripheral arterial disease. *J Vasc Surg* 1996;23:104–115.
12. Scheffler P, de la Hamette D, Gross J, et al. Intensive vascular training in stage IIb of peripheral arterial occlusive disease. The additive effects of intravenous prostaglandin E_1 or intravenous pentoxifylline during training. *Circulation* 1994;90:818–822.
13. Hiatt WR, Wolfel EE, Meier RH, Regensteiner JG. Superiority of treadmill walking exercise versus strength training for patients with peripheral arterial disease. Implications for the mechanism of the training response. *Circulation* 1994;90:1866–1874.
14. Hiatt WR, Nawaz D, Regensteiner JG, Hossack KF. The evaluation of exercise performance in patients with peripheral vascular disease. *J Cardiopulmonary Rehabil* 1988;12:525–532.

15. Hiatt WR, Hirsch AT, Regensteiner JG, et al. Clinical trials for claudication. Assessment of exercise performance, functional status, and clinical end points. *Circulation* 1995;92:614–621.
16. Gardner AW, Poehlman ET. Exercise rehabilitation programs for the treatment of claudication pain. *JAMA* 1995;274:975–980.
17. Reifler DR, Feinglass J, Slavensky R, et al. Functional outcomes for patients with intermittent claudication: Bypass surgery versus angioplasty versus noninvasive management. *J Vasc Med Biol* 1994;5:203–211.
18. Cameron HA, Waller PC, Ramsay LE. Drug treatment of intermittent claudication: A critical analysis of the methods and findings of published clinical trials, 1965–1985. *Br J Clin Pharmcol* 1988;26:569–576.
19. van Rij AM, Solomon C, Packer SGK, Hopkins WG. Chelation therapy for intermittent claudication. A double-blind, randomized, controlled trial. *Circulation* 1994;90:1194–1199.
20. Ernst E. Chelation therapy for peripheral arterial occlusive disease. A systemic review. *Circulation* 1997;96:1031–1033.
21. Walker SR, Tennant S, MacSweeney ST. A randomized, double-blind, placebo-controlled, crossover study to assess the immediate effect of sublingual glyceryl trinitrate on the ankle-brachial index, claudication, and maximum walking distance of patients with intermittent claudication. *J Vasc Surg* 1998;28:895–900.
22. Bagger JP, Helligsoe P, Randsback F, et al. Effect of verapamil in intermittent claudication. A randomized, double-blind, placebo-controlled, cross-over study after individual dose-response assessment. *Circulation* 1997;95:411–414.
23. Antiplatelet trialists' collaboration. Collaborative overview of randomised trials of antiplatelet therapy-I: Prevention of death, myocardial infarction, and stroke by prolonged antiplatelet therapy in various categories of patients. *Br Med J* 1994;308:81–106.
24. Janzon L, Bergqvist D, Boberg J, et al. Prevention of myocardial infarction and stroke in patients with intermittent claudication: Effects of ticlopidine. Results from STIMS, the Swedish Ticlopidine Multicentre Study. *J Intern Med* 1990;227:301–308.
25. Balsano F, Coccheri S, Libretti A, et al. Ticlopidine in the treatment of intermittent claudication: A 21-month double-blind trial. *J Lab Clin Med* 1989;114:84–91.
26. Becquemin JP. [Effect of ticlopidine on the long-term patency of saphenous-vein bypass grafts in the legs.] Etude de la Ticlopidine apres Pontage Femoro-Poplite and the Association Universitaire de Recherche en Chirurgie. *N Engl J Med* 1997;337:1726–1731.
27. A randomised, blinded, trial of clopidogrel versus aspirin in patients at risk of ischaemic events (CAPRIE). CAPRIE steering committee. *Lancet* 1996;348: 1329–1339.
28. Diehm C, Balzer K, Bisler H, et al. Efficacy of a new prostaglandin E1 regimen in outpatients with severe intermittent claudication: results of a multicenter placebo-controlled double-blind trial. *J Vasc Surg* 1997;25:537–544.
29. Brevetti G, di Lisa F, Perna S, et al. Carnitine-related alterations in patients with intermittent claudication. Indication for a focused carnitine therapy. *Circulation* 1996;93:1685–1689.
30. Brevetti G, Perna S, Sabba C, et al. Effect of propionyl-L-carnitine on quality of life in intermittent claudication. *Am J Cardiol* 1997;79:777–780.
31. Boger RH, Bode-Boger SM, Thiele W, et al. Restoring vascular nitric oxide formation by L-Arginine improves the symptoms of intermittent claudication in patients with peripheral arterial occlusive disease. *J Am Coll Cardiol* 1998;32:1336–1344.
32. Porter JM, Bauer GM. Pharmacologic treatment of intermittent claudication. *Surgery* 1982;92:966–971.
33. Hood SC, Moher D, Barber GG. Management of intermittent claudication with pentoxifylline: Meta-analysis of randomized controlled trials. *Can Med Assoc J* 1996;155:1053–1059.
34. Dawson DL, Cutler BS, Meissner MH, Strandness DE. Cilostazol has beneficial effects in treatment of intermittent claudication. *Circulation* 1998;98:678–686.

35. Strandness DE, Dalman R, Panian S, et al. Two doses of cilostazol versus placebo in the treatment of claudication: Results of a randomized, multicenter trial. Presented in abstract form at: 71st Scientific Session, American Heart Association, November 1998; Dallas, Texas.
36. Money SR, Herd JA, Isaacsohn JL, et al. Effect of cilostazol on walking distances in patients with intermittent claudication caused by peripheral vascular disease. *J Vasc Surg* 1998;27:267–275.
37. Dawson DL, Beebe HG, Davidson MH, et al. Cilostazol or pentoxifylline for claudication? Presented in abstract form at: 71st Scientific Session, American Heart Association, November 1998; Dallas, Texas.
38. Baffour R, Berman J, Garb JL, et al. Enhanced angiogenesis and growth of collaterals by in vivo administration of recombinant basic fibroblast growth factor in a rabbit model of acute lower limb ischemia: Dose-response effect of basic fibroblast growth factor. *J Vasc Surg* 1992;16:181–191.
39. Isner JM, Walsh K, Symes J, et al. Arterial gene therapy for therapeutic angiogenesis in patients with peripheral artery disease. *Circulation* 1995;91:2687–2692.
40. Tsurami Y, Takeshita S, Chen D, et al. Direct intramuscular gene transfer of naked DNA encoding vascular endothelial growth factor augments collateral development and tissue perfusion. *Circulation* 1996;94:3281–3290.
41. Baumgartner I, Pieczek A, Manor O, et al. Constitutive expression of $phVEGF_{165}$ after intramuscular gene transfer promotes collateral vessel development in patients with critical limb ischemia. *Circulation* 1998;97:1114–1123.
42. Luo Z, Asahara T, Tsurumi Y, et al. Reduction of vein graft intimal hyperplasia and preservation of endothelium-dependent relaxation by topical vascular endothelial growth factor. *J Vasc Surg* 1998;27:167–173.
43. Isner JM, Blair R, Vale P, et al. Patency of dorsalis pedis artery as a predictor of clinical outcome after intramuscular gene transfer of phVEGF165 in patients with non-healing ischemic ulcers. Presented in abstract form at: 71st Scientific Session, American Heart Association, November 1998; Dallas, Texas.
44. Vale PR, Wuensch DI, Rauh GF, et al. Arterial gene therapy for inhibiting restenosis in patients with claudication undergoing superficial femoral artery angioplasty. Presented in abstract form at: 71st Scientific Session, American Heart Association, November 1998; Dallas, Texas.
45. Rauh G, Baumgartner I, Pieczek A, et al. Treatment of Buerger's Disease by intramuscular gene transfer of phVEGF165. Presented in abstract form at: 71st Scientific Session, American Heart Association, November 1998; Dallas, Texas.
46. Waksman R. Endovascular brachytherapy: Overcoming 'practical' obstacles. *Am J Cardiol* 1998;81:21E-26E.
47. Schopohl B, Liermann D, Pohlit LJ, et al. ^{192}IR endovascular brachytherapy for avoidance of intimal hyperplasia after percutaneous transluminal angioplasty and stent implantation in peripheral vessels: 6 years of experience. *Int J Radiat Oncol Biol Phys* 1996;36:835–840.

3

How and When Will Carotid Angioplasty and Stenting Replace Surgical Endarterectomy?

Michael H. Wholey, MD, MBA, Mark H. Wholey, MD, Gustav R. Eles, DO, Chester R. Jarmolowski, MD, and Walter Tan, MD

Introduction and Historical Background

Stroke is the most common and disabling neurologic disorder in the elderly population.[1] In the US, more than one half million people have strokes annually, accounting for more than 2 million stroke survivors with varying degrees of disability.[1,2] After heart disease and cancer, cerebrovascular disease is the third leading cause of death, with 1.5 deaths per 1000 people.[2] Carotid artery occlusive diseases are responsible for approximately 20% to 30% of strokes.[3,4]

The traditional standard of care in treating cervical carotid artery stenosis has been carotid endarterectomy. The procedure was initially performed in the 1950s by such pioneers as Eascott, DeBakey, and Cooley.[4] With the landmark North American Symptomatic Carotid Endarterectomy Trial (NASCET) and Asymptomatic Carotid Atherosclerosis Study (ACAS), carotid endarterectomy has been proven beneficial in reducing the stroke risks for symptomatic and asymptomatic patients with significant carotid artery stenosis.[5–8]

As an alternative to the traditional surgical treatment of carotid artery occlusive disease, there has been much interest in the use of carotid artery stent placement[9,10] (Figs. 1 through 4). This has grown naturally from the early work in angioplasty of carotid arteries that was performed by the groups of Theron,[11] Mathias,[12] and Kachel[13] in the 1980s. With the advent of stent

From Criado FJ (ed): *Endovascular Intervention: New Tools and Techniques for the 21st Century.* Armonk, NY: Futura Publishing Co., Inc.; ©2002.

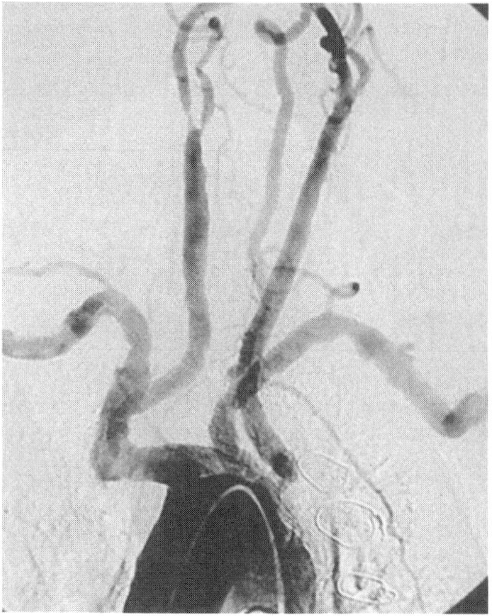

Figure 1. Right anterior oblique projection of thoracic angiogram in an 85-year-old female with history of transient ischemic attacks revealing an atherosclerotic aorta with marked tortuosity of the great vessels and high-grade (80%) stenosis of the right internal carotid artery.

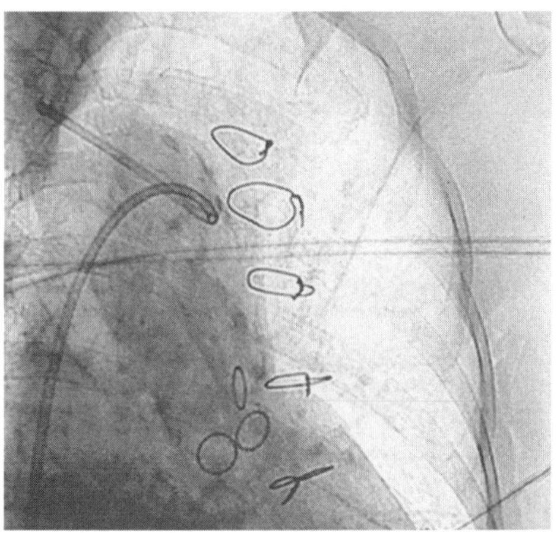

Figure 2. Right anterior oblique projection revealing take-off of innominate artery with the 7F Brite Tip sheath (Cordis Endovascular, a Johnson & Johnson Company, Miami Lakes, FL) placed at origin of common carotid artery. We could not safely advance the sheath past this point.

technology, interventional management of carotid artery disease began to develop as a practical new technique, as shown in early work by the groups of Wholey,[14] Yadav,[15] and Diethrich.[16] Stents provided key improvements compared to angioplasty alone; stents helped reduce restenosis, prevented disastrous dissections, and helped to contain lesion surfaces that are susceptible for thromboemboli.

Discussion

How and when will carotid stent placement replace surgical endarterectomy? In order to answer this question, certain aspects of carotid stenting and its alternative, carotid endarterectomy, must be addressed. These include the following:

- How does carotid stenting compare to the gold standard of carotid endarterectomy in terms of technical success, complications, and long-term results?
- What are current indications and contraindications for carotid stent placement?
- How quickly has carotid stenting grown, and what are its factors for growth?

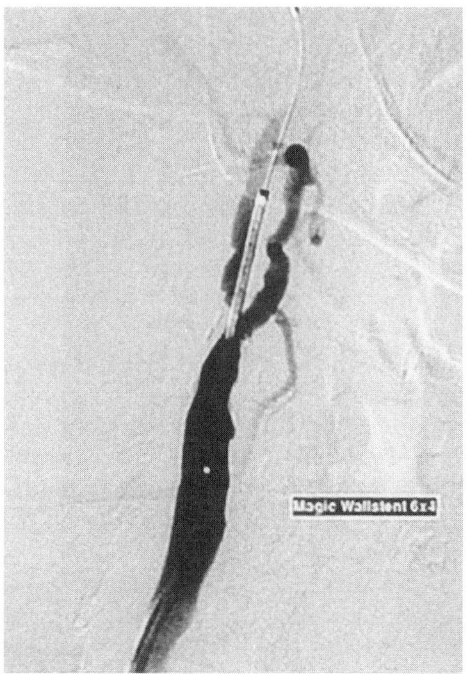

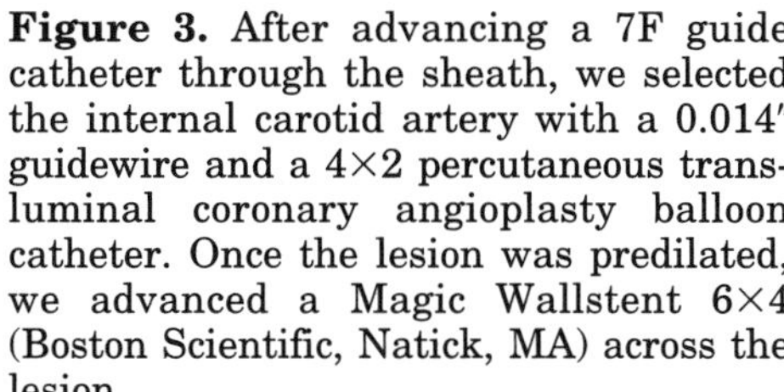

Figure 3. After advancing a 7F guide catheter through the sheath, we selected the internal carotid artery with a 0.014″ guidewire and a 4×2 percutaneous transluminal coronary angioplasty balloon catheter. Once the lesion was predilated, we advanced a Magic Wallstent 6×4 (Boston Scientific, Natick, MA) across the lesion.

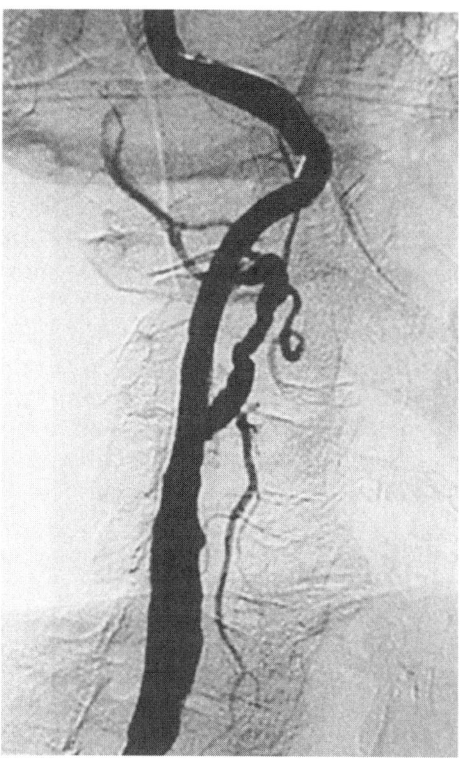

Figure 4. Final angiogram obtained after deployment and 5×2 angioplasty revealing good position of stent with minimal residual stenosis.

Comparison of Carotid Stent Placement to Endarterectomy

Whenever a new procedure is developed, there are always questions regarding its safety, efficiency, and long-term results. How does carotid stent placement compare with endarterectomy prior to any major randomized trials? Similar to endarterectomy, the technical success of carotid stenting exceeds 98% in most studies.[9,10,14–17] The limiting factor for technical success has been the inability to gain safe access into the common carotid artery with guide catheters and sheaths.

The risks of perioperative stroke from carotid endarterectomy vary from 1.5% to 9% depending on the published series.[18,19] The perioperative stroke/death rate is 7.5% in the European Carotid Surgery Trial (ECST), and 5.8% in NASCET.[5–8,18,19] Also, the NASCET perioperative stroke/death rate for contralateral occlusions is 14.3%.[20] The risks for cranial nerve palsies occur in 7.6% to 27%, and are frequently not recorded as morbidity in surgical publications.[17,18,21]

In the Pittsburgh Vascular Institute (PVI) series, which involved 345 patients, we found a 4.4% rate of minor and major strokes and all deaths in a 30-day postprocedure period; this is comparable to other endovascular stent centers.[22] Henry et al[23] reported a 1.7% major and 2.8% minor neurologic complication rate in their series of 174 cases. Roubin et al[24] reported a 6.3% incidence of death and neurologic complications (1 death, 2 major strokes) in their series of 238 carotid procedures. An updated questionnaire to 36 centers worldwide revealed that in 5210 carotid stent procedures performed in 4757 patients, there were 129 (2.83%) minor and 72 (1.58%) major strokes and 41 (0.88%) procedure-related deaths for an overall rate of 5.29%.[10] If non-procedure-related deaths are included, then the overall rate is 6.29%.[10]

Though it is difficult to compare endarterectomy with endovascular stent placement, especially with generally higher risk patients in the latter group, some early comparisons can be made. The rate of neurologic complications and deaths with endovascular stent placement of 4.5% to 6.3% has been acceptable for a newly developed procedure.[10,23,24] It generally falls within the American Heart Association's 6% to 7% perioperative stroke and death rate established for symptomatic patients undergoing endarterectomy.[25]

The Carotid And Vertebral Artery Transluminal Angioplasty Study (CAVATAS) was established to investigate the risks and benefits of cerebrovascular percutaneous transluminal angioplasty (PTA).[26] Twenty-four centers in Europe, Australia, Canada, and the US collaborated to randomize 504 patients (mean age 67 years; 69% men) with carotid stenosis to surgery (n=253) or angioplasty (n=251) between 1992 and 1997. Approximately 90% of the patients had recently been symptomatic. PTA was carried out using balloon catheters, with the adjunctive use of stents in 26%. There was no difference in the primary outcome measure of disabling stroke or death within 30 days (surgery 6%, PTA 6%). Cranial nerve injury and myocardial ischemia were only reported at the time of treatment in the surgical group. Long-term survival curves showed no difference in ipsilateral stroke during follow-up. Carotid surgery and angioplasty are equivalent in safety and efficacy, but angioplasty has advantages with respect to nerve injury and cardiac complications.

The Carotid Endarterectomy versus Stent Trial (CREST) is a study currently under way that is funded by the National Institutes of Health and industry. This study, under the directorship of Doctors Hobson and Ferguson,[27,28] involves self-expandable stents. Once a credential phase is complete, an anticipated 2800 patients will be randomized between stent placement and endarterectomy procedures. This randomized trial will be important in determining the future of carotid stenting.

Based on the early technology and limited development, carotid stenting has proved relatively safe with symptomatic patients. There are limited data on carotid stent placement for asymptomatic patients. Among the 148 asymptomatic patients in the PVI series, there was a 4.1% occurrence of strokes and deaths.[22] In a particular subset of 1361 world carotid survey patients, there was a 3.38% occurrence of strokes and deaths.[10] These numbers are slightly higher than the accepted 2.3% in ACAS.[6,7]

There is limited information regarding the long-term results of carotid stenting. We reported a restenosis rate of 4.8% and a freedom of neurologic death and any stroke of 98% for 1 year, which is similar to that reported by other centers.[22] The world survey of the 36 centers reported a 1-year patency of 3.36%.[10] In their series of 18 patients treated for carotid endarterectomy restenosis, Lanzino et al[29] reported a 5.5% rate at 3 years. Vitek et al[30] reported a restenosis rate of 5% and a freedom from neurologic death or stroke of 92% at 3 years in their series of 345 patients who underwent carotid stent placement. Hence, compared with surgical endarterectomy, stent placement has equivalent technical success and complication rates for symptomatic patients. Little information is known on the long-term patency, though this appears likewise comparable to surgical data.

In asymptomatic patients, carotid stent placement is associated with slightly higher risks than surgery. This will be one of the major areas for improvement that could be provided by effective and safe embolic filters and catheters.

Current Indications and Contraindications for Carotid Stent Placement

There are a substantial number of clinical scenarios in which carotid endovascular stenting could benefit patients in terms of being potentially less risky under, less traumatic, and likely to cause less discomfort.[31,32] These include the following:

1. In nonsurgical lesions that were inaccessible for technical reasons in patients with high or low internal carotid artery cervical segment stenoses as well as those patients with short, obese necks.
2. In patients with metastatic disease or other comorbidity processes that would make them high surgical risks.
3. In patients with significant restenosis following prior successful carotid endarterectomy. Incidentally, these patients comprised 27% of the PVI series.
4. In patients undergoing aorto-coronary bypass surgery or thoracic and/or aneurysmal surgery with coexistent significant internal carotid artery stenosis (>70%).
5. In cervical carotid arterial lesions secondary to fibromuscular dysplasia or from post radiation associated with radical neck dissections.
6. In patients with contralateral occlusions or incomplete circle of Willis.
7. Carotid endarterectomy studies have not addressed patients with simultaneous cardiac and cerebrovascular disease and the safety of combined serial carotid endarterectomy and coronary artery bypass surgery.[28–30] In Shawl's series, 63% of the patients underwent, staged or at the same setting, coronary intervention because of Class III or IV angina.[31]

The following criteria were used to exclude 12 patients (bringing the number of participants in the PVI carotid stent study to 345):

1. Stenosis less than 70%. Two patients had color Doppler ultrasound examinations from other institutions, which reported "severe stenosis";

but diagnostic angiograms revealed less than 70% narrowing and these patients were excluded. Additionally, 2 patients with reportedly severe stenosis on outside angiograms were excluded when angiograms at our institution revealed minimal narrowing.
2. Prior life-threatening contrast reaction.
3. Patients who were at high risk for nephrotoxicity from contrast secondary to underlying renal disease and were not yet on dialysis (2 patients).
4. Patients with uncorrected bleeding disorders.
5. Presence of intracranial tumor or arteriovenous malformation.
6. Lesions not technically feasible via a percutaneous approach (2 patients).
7. Patients or their legal representatives who were unable to give informed consent.
8. Patients with long multiple neck lesions or complex lesions with ulcerative and/or active thrombotic changes at the carotid bifurcation (4 patients) as diagnosed with previous angiograms.

Prior to consideration for entry into the carotid stent study, informed consent was obtained from all patients and family members. Careful counseling was provided regarding risks and complications of the stent procedure as well as therapeutic options including carotid endarterectomy. Institutional Review Board and Institution Device Committee approval had been appropriately obtained prior to the start, and was maintained throughout the study.

The Growth of Carotid Stent Placement

Already, carotid stent placement is growing. A review of previous numbers of carotid stent procedures in the global carotid stent survey revealed in June 1997 that 2047 stent procedures had been done by the original 24 centers.[10] The number of stent procedures increased to 2591 in January 1998 for a 27% per annum growth rate, and to 3379 by January 1999 for an 18% per annum growth rate.[10] The current number of 4135 procedures by the original 24 centers represents a 47% per annum growth rate.[10]

What is the potential growth of carotid stent placement? In the US alone there are more than 210,000 strokes per year possibly attributable to carotid artery disease. The number of carotid endarterectomies per year exceeds 130,000 in the US, which includes primarily symptomatic patients and barely addresses the asymptomatic patient population.[32]

Endovascular stent placement will grow in application as technological improvements are made in devices and equipment and as more training and education of physicians and patients occurs. Improvements in technology will be a major trend. Developments have been made in carotid-based self-expandable stents. The current designs have problems in size, requiring 9F and 10F guide catheters, as well as in stiff distal ends, causing difficulty in advancement past tortuous carotid arteries; however, as new designs become more streamlined, lower profile, and more trackable, these technological improvements will result in fewer complications. Other major improvements will be made in guide catheter technology—in the PVI series, 6 of the 8 technical failures came from inadequate guide catheter positioning.

The need for cerebral protection from thromboemboli has been a major development that will impact the growth of carotid angioplasty and stent placement. The majority of major carotid centers are just beginning to employ cerebral protection. The technique described by Theron et al[11,33,34] involved the use of an occlusion balloon that is attached to a guidewire; the balloon is inflated once past the lesion and occludes flow until the intervention is completed and a catheter is used to aspirate material proximal to the balloon. Henry et al[35] have completed a small series, and reported marked improvement in complication rates with the use of the balloon occlusion technique. A different approach has been the use of embolic filters, which are placed at the end of the guidewire. Once past the lesion, the filter is deployed and then retrieved when the procedure is completed. Early results with the use of embolic filters have been very encouraging as well.

With the advent of embolic protection, there has been a decrease in complications from carotid stenting. At Pittsburgh Vascular Institute, Wholey et al[36] reviewed immediate complications with and without embolic protection and found fewer strokes and neurologic-related deaths: 2.4% with protection versus 4.2% without protection. This occurred despite a relatively high rate of technical failures. Others have reported similar improvements in neurologic events with cerebral protection. Reimers et al[37] reported a stroke and death rate of 1.2% in 86 patients with cerebral protection, Al-Mubarak et al[38] revealed a 2% stroke and death rate for 162 patients in a multicenter study, and Henry et al[35] reported a stroke and death rate of 2.7% for 167 patients. With the impressive results achieved with cerebral protection, it is becoming the standard of care to employ protection in carotid stent procedures.

Technical issues on the use of IIb/IIIa inhibitors in conjunction with stenting are still debated. Likewise, an issue on the need for poststent dilatation has also been raised. As with all new procedures, standard techniques and methods are still evolving.

As shown in the literature, there is a significant learning curve for carotid stent placement.[9,10,30] In the world survey, we found that experience with 50 procedures was necessary to achieve optimal proficiency.[9,10] In order for complication rates to be acceptable, it is important that key centers play a dominant role in the early stages.

Physician and patient education will also provide important contributions to growth. The acceptance of carotid stenting as a viable alternative to surgical treatment will grow as patients and referring physicians become aware of the procedure and its benefits.

Another set of factors that will help determine the growth of carotid stenting includes economics. Currently in the US, carotid stent placement is not reimbursable; some centers had billed it as subclavian angioplasty and stenting, but this is no longer permitted. Appeals are now under way with various governmental sections. Reimbursement problems exist similarly in Europe depending upon the country.

Conclusion

How and when will carotid stent placement replace surgical endarterectomy? Endovascular stent placement for carotid artery occlusive disease is evolving from its initial controversial position to that of an alternative treatment for extracranial carotid artery disease. Carotid stent placement is already serving as an alternative in symptomatic patients, especially those with high surgical comorbidities and other conditions. How will carotid stenting replace endarterectomy? Economic, technological, and patient/physician education factors will help propel this new procedure. Its high technical success as well as the relatively few complications involved makes carotid stenting impressive at such an early stage. As stent design, guide catheters, and cerebral protection devices improve, the technical success, patency, and complication rates will improve. Still, the important test for carotid stent placement will be its long-term (1-, 3-, and 5-year) patency as well as the results of randomized studies against the "gold standard," carotid endarterectomy.

Will carotid stenting replace endarterectomy? It is the authors' opinion that it will not. Just as percutaneous transluminal coronary angioplasty and stenting did not replace bypass surgery, neither will carotid stenting replace endarterectomy. The low rate of complications in experienced hands, short hospital stay, and referral patterns associated with carotid endarterectomy will keep it in strong growth. Carotid stenting will augment endarterectomy as both procedures increase in numbers. Will it overshadow endarterectomy? Possibly, but again this will depend on technology to reduce the complication rates, especially for asymptomatic patient populations. When will the number of carotid stenting procedures equal that of endarterectomy? In an optimistic scenario with a growth rate of 50% per year, it will take approximately 8 years for the carotid stenting to approach 130,000 procedures per year. At a more realistic 25% rate, it will require 15 years.

References

1. Patient outcomes research teams study groups. In *Stroke Clinical Updates*. Englewood, CO: National Stroke Association; 1994;5:9–12.
2. The American Heart Association. *Heart and Stroke Facts Statistical Supplement.* Dallas: 1994:12.
3. Dorros G. Carotid arterial obliterative disease: Should endovascular revascularization (stent supported angioplasty) today supplant carotid endarterectomy? *J Intervent Cardiol* 1996;9:193–196.
4. DeBakey MH. Carotid endarterectomy revisited. *J Endovasc Surg* 1996;3:4.
5. Beneficial effect of carotid endarterectomy in symptomatic patients with high-grade carotid stenosis: North American Symptomatic Carotid Endarterectomy Trial collaborators. *N Engl J Med* 1991;325:445–453.
6. Asymptomatic Carotid Atherosclerosis Study Group. Endarterectomy for asymptomatic carotid artery stenosis. *JAMA* 1995;273:1421–1428.
7. Clinical advisory: Carotid endarterectomy for patients with asymptomatic internal carotid artery stenosis. *J Neurol Sci* 1995;129:76–77.
8. Clinical advisory: Carotid endarterectomy for patients with asymptomatic internal carotid artery stenosis. *Stroke* 1994;25:2523–2524.

9. Wholey MH, Wholey M, Bergeron P, et al. Current global status of carotid artery stent placement. *Cathet Cardiovasc Diagn* 1998;44:1–6.
10. Wholey MH, Wholey M, Mathias K, et al. Global experience in cervical carotid artery stent placement. *Cathet Cardiovasc Interv* 2000;50:160–167.
11. Theron J, Courtheroux P, Alachkar F, et al. New triple coaxial catheter system for carotid angioplasty with cerebral protection. *AJNR Am J Neuroradiol* 1990;11:869–874.
12. Mathias KD, Jaeger MJ, Sahl H. Internal carotid stents-PTA: 7 year experience. *Cardiovasc Intervent Radiol* 1997;20(suppl):I46. Abstract.
13. Kachel R, Basche ST, Heerklotz I, et al. Percutaneous transluminal angioplasty (PTA) of supra-aortic arteries especially the internal carotid artery. *Neuroradiology* 1991;33:191–194.
14. Wholey MH, Wholey M, Eles G, et al. Endovascular stents for carotid occlusive disease. *J Endovasc Surg* 1997;4:326–338.
15. Yadav JS, Roubin GS, Iyer S, et al. Elective stenting of the extracranial carotid arteries. *Circulation* 1997;95:376–381.
16. Diethrich EB, Ndiaye M, Reid DB. Stenting in the carotid artery: Initial experience in 100 patients. *J Endovasc Surg* 1996;3:42–46.
17. Yadav JS, Roubin GS, King P, et al. Angioplasty and stenting for restenosis after carotid endarterectomy. *Stroke* 1997;27:2075–2079.
18. Lusby RJ, Wylie EJ. Complications of carotid endarterectomy. *Surg Clin North Am* 1983;63:1293–1302.
19. Zarins CK. Carotid endarterectomy: The gold standard. *J Endovasc Surg* 1996;3:10–15.
20. Gasecki AP, Eliasziw M, Ferguson GG, et al. Long-term prognosis and effect of endarterectomy in patients with symptomatic severe carotid stenosis and contralateral carotid stenosis or occlusion: Results from NASCET. North American Symptomatic Carotid Endarterectomy Trial (NASCET) Group. *J Neurosurg* 1995;83:778–782.
21. Diethrich EB. Cerebrovascular disease therapy: The past, the present, and the future. *J Endovasc Surg* 1996;3:7–9.
22. Wholey MH, Wholey M, Tan WA, et al. Review and management of neurologic complications related to carotid artery stent placement. *J Endovasc Ther* 2001;8:343–351.
23. Henry M, Amor M, Masson I, et al. Angioplasty and stenting of the extracranial arteries. *J Endovasc Surg* 1998;5:293–304.
24. Roubin GS, Vitek J, Iyer S, et al. Carotid stenting: Current status. Future prospects. *J Vasc Interv Radiol* 1997;8(suppl):25–28.
25. Moore WS, Barnett HJM, Beebe HG, et al. Guidelines for carotid endarterectomy: A multidisciplinary consensus statement from the ad hoc committee, American Heart Association. *Stroke* 1995;26:188–200.
26. Brown MM, Venables F, Clifton A, et al. Carotid endarterectomy vs carotid angioplasty. *Lancet* 1997;349:880–881.
27. Hobson RW. Status of carotid angioplasty and stent trials. *J Vasc Surg* 1998;27:791.
28. Hobson RW, Brott T, Ferguson R, et al. CREST: Carotid Revascularization Endarterectomy versus Stent Trial. *Cardiovasc Surg* 1997;5:457–458.
29. Lanzino G, Mericle RA, Lopes DK, et al. Percutaneous transluminal angioplasty and stent placement for recurrent carotid artery stenosis. *J Neurosurg* 1999;90:688–694.
30. Vitek J, Iyer S, Roubin G. Carotid stenting in 350 vessels: Problems faced and solved. *J Invasive Cardiol* 1998;10:311–314.
31. Diethrich EB. Indications for carotid stenting: A preview of the potential derived from early clinical experience. *J Endovasc Surg* 1996;3:132–139.
32. Hopkins LN, Lanzino G, Mericle RA, Guterman LR. Carotid intervention: A neurosurgeon's perspective. *J Invasive Cardiol* 1998;10:279–291.
33. Theron J, Dorros G. A rationale for endovascular therapy with balloon occlusion during extracranial atherosclerotic carotid artery stenosis. *J Intervent Cardiol* 1996;9:209–213.

34. Theron JG, Payelle GG, Coskun O, et al. Carotid artery stenosis: Treatment with protected balloon angioplasty and stent placement. *Radiology* 1996;201:627–636.
35. Henry M, Henry I, Klonaris C, et al. Benefits of cerebral protection during carotid stenting with the PercuSurge GuardWire System: Midterm results. *J Endovasc Ther* 2002;9:1–13.
36. Wholey MH, Wholey M, Tan WA, et al. Long term follow up comparing balloon-mounted and self-expandable stents. *J Endovasc Ther* 2002. In press.
37. Reimers B, Corvaja N, Moshiri S, et al. Cerebral protection with filter devices during carotid artery stenting. *Circulation* 2001;104:12–15.
38. Al-Mubarak N, Colombo A, Gaines PA, et al. Multicenter evaluation of carotid stenting with a filter protection system. *J Am Coll Cardiol* 2002;39:841–846.

4

Evolving Strategies and New Techniques to Determine Morphology and Precise Measurements for Endograft Planning

Hugh G. Beebe, MD and Boonprasit Kritpracha, MD

Introduction

As endovascular therapy moved beyond the focal application of balloon angioplasty and stents to treat lesions of relatively short length and into the expanding field of endovascular grafting for complex lesions that extend over large segments of the vascular tree, new imaging problems and limitations became apparent. This chapter discusses evolving techniques for measurement of the aortoiliac arterial segment morphology to achieve both precision and accuracy in planning and follow-up for endovascular surgery.

Carefully controlled trials of aortic endografts were undertaken in the US during the mid 1990s, and problems with imaging methods became a central focus of their methodology.[1] Even experienced interventional radiologists learned that new levels of difficulty existed in determining the dimensions of vessels that were to receive endografts. The introduction during that time of graduated marker catheters to help compensate for magnification errors and to attempt length estimation is an example of this. The difficulty of assuring that each patient's anatomy met arterial size, angulation, and length inclusion and exclusion criteria led some trials to mandate a second independent review of preoperative planning images before acceptance of each patient into the treatment cohort. Debate sprang up over whether treatment planning could be accomplished accurately enough by conventional imaging methods in patients

From Criado FJ (ed): *Endovascular Intervention: New Tools and Techniques for the 21st Century.* Armonk, NY: Futura Publishing Co., Inc.; ©2002.

with complex anatomy. Some authorities preferred to repeat measurements by alternative methods such as intravascular ultrasound in an attempt to be certain of the data.[2]

Now, as endografting has just seen its tenth anniversary,[3] general consensus has formed on the most important artifacts that can mislead enough to impact on patient outcome, and on the methods for obtaining essential morphology data. Most endovascular therapists rely on the combination of computed tomography (CT) radiographs and contrast arteriography (CA) for procedure planning to identify patients appropriate for endografting of aortoiliac aneurysms and selection of devices to be used. In practice, the artifacts and shortcomings of each of these standard imaging methods are different from each other.[4] Thus, their combination provides a useful database for planning.

An alternative that appears to be increasingly valued for accuracy and cost saving is the use of CT angiography (CTA) together with use of three-dimensional (3D) image processing. This approach allows a single image acquisition step to provide a variety of postprocessing images that can be used dynamically in a personal computer workstation to view and measure the relevant arterial segments. Both approaches, combined use of CT and CA or CTA with specialized 3D reconstruction, are validated by widespread successful clinical use by a variety of specialists[5–7] and are described here with emphasis on avoiding artifact-related problems.

Contrast Arteriography

Since the 1930s arteriography has been the mainstay of predicting the luminal status of arteries. The most valuable application of CA is in occlusive disease, but even there, important misrepresentation may occur because of projection angles together with dense contrast obscuring luminal filling defects. In aneurysm treatment planning, the well-known thrombus artifact is much on the mind of any observer and represents a primary reason for obtaining CT scan images in addition to CA (Fig. 1). The thrombus artifact may result in a false representation of aortic size because thrombus prevents complete circulation of contrast in the aneurysmal segment. The aorta may appear to have adequate proximal or distal attachment sites, when in reality one or both may make the morphology unacceptable for endovascular repair. Even a thin crescent of thrombus in the proximal aortic neck presents an undefined risk of late failure. Evaluation of the iliac arteries is also negatively affected because the presence of aneurysms cannot be confidently ruled out due to thrombus artifact.

Although diameter measurements can be obtained with the use of graduated marker catheters, when placed within the segment to be measured, there are special requirements for getting the most out of this compensation for arteriography artifacts. First, careful attention must be made to the precision with which measurement devices are applied to the catheter markers and to whether the catheter calibration marks appear perpendicular to the plane of the radiograph. Regardless of whether computer workstation cursors or calipers applied to cut film images on a view box are used, attention must be paid to standardized positioning on the catheter markers. Variation here can yield errors as large as 3 mm that are further multiplied by intraobserver er-

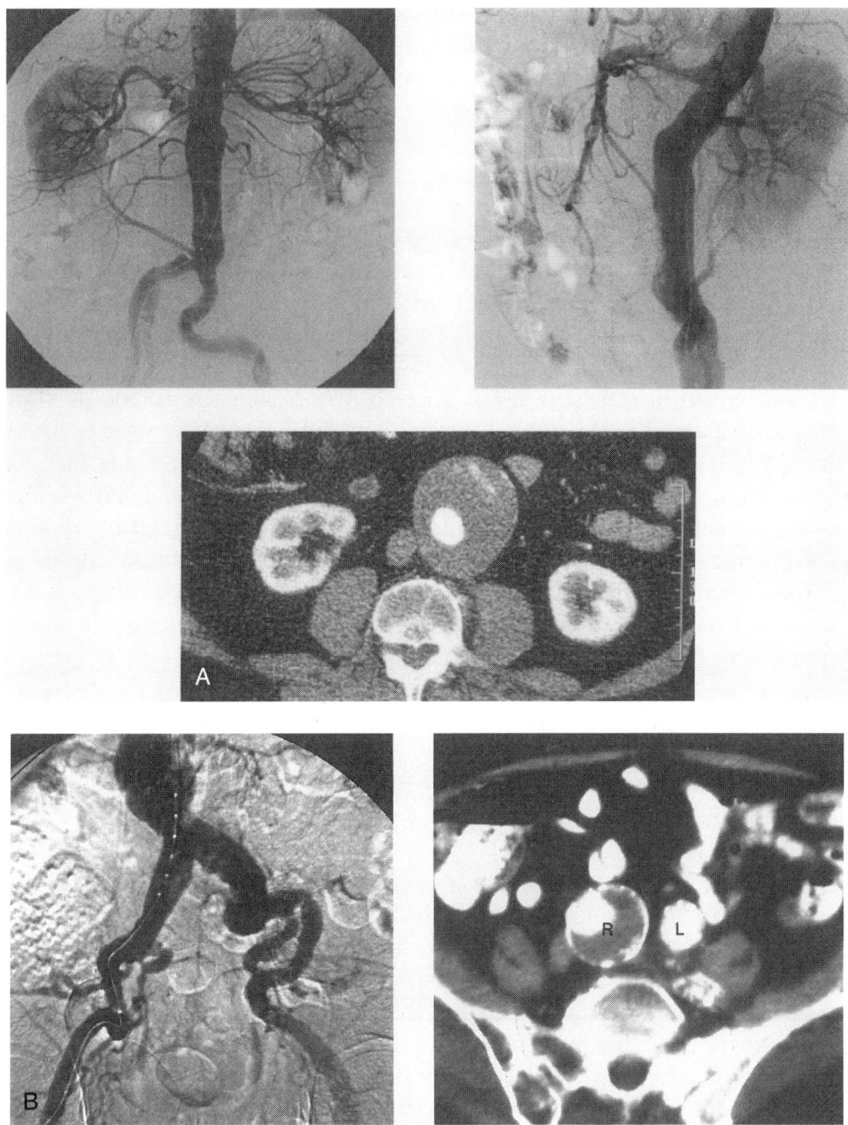

Figure 1. A. The arteriogram, seen above in biplanar views, does not show direct evidence of aortic aneurysm. Angulation of the proximal infrarenal aorta, seen on the lateral view above right, suggests aneurysm but does not reveal it. Proof of aneurysm as well as explanation for the false appearance of the arteriogram is seen in the computed tomography (CT) slice below. **B.** Another striking example of misleading information from arteriography with implications for endografting. The right common iliac aneurysm, shown in the CT slice on the right (R), is not seen on the arteriogram.

ror. In addition, careful checking of the distance between marks is needed to avoid undermeasuring when the scale is lying at an angle to the x-ray beam.

There are two other problems associated with CA that have major significance and must be taken into account when planning endografts: projection angle errors and length artifacts. Determination of proximal aortic neck angulation is critically important for endograft planning because extreme tortuosity in this segment is an independent risk factor for primary endoleak. The most important inherent limitation of CA is that it provides a two-dimensional representation of anatomy that exists in three dimensions. Therefore, in considering vessel tortuosity, the angle of projection can yield widely variable results. The standard method of assessing this in the aorta is to obtain both anteroposterior and lateral projections. This is of help, aided by the fact that proximal neck angulation is mostly perpendicular to the lateral plane, but not always satisfactory. Problems include combination of anterior and lateral displacement of the proximal infrarenal aorta by the aneurysm distal to it and, in the lateral projection, superimposed vessels making the exact location of the renal artery orifices difficult or impossible to ascertain (Fig. 2).

Vessel length inaccuracy in CA derives from two sources: the path of angiographic catheters within blood vessels and foreshortening of the proximal aortic neck and iliac arteries. Catheters traverse large, curved vessels in a relatively straight line that cuts across the actual centerline of blood flow. For the same reason, aortic endografts also do not always lie in the centerline of blood flow, but they tend to move toward it when they are deployed as the forces of blood flow are applied to them in a pulsatile manner. So an estimation of how the endograft will probably lie in vivo is part of the art of endograft planning. To some extent, this is dependent on the prosthesis that is used. There is wide variation in the contour and conformity to vessel shape among endografts that are fully stented and those that are not. Even the fully stented modular endografts vary considerably in their rigidity or resistance to lateral displacement. Making allowances for this and compensating for the straight-line path of the arteriographic catheter is not easy or exact, especially in the case of a large aneurysm (Fig. 3).

Because the aortic neck segment is of critical importance in endograft planning and may be a cause of procedure failure directly attributable to inaccurate preoperative planning, its accurate length measurement is a subject of serious concern. But, when the aorta is assessed by CA, the x-ray tube is usually perpendicular to the body axis in an anteroposterior projection, not to the axis of an aorta that has been displaced by the growth of the aneurysm below it. Thus, foreshortening may occur, giving a false impression of aortic neck length that is actually longer than it appears.

Fortunately, length measurement of the entire aortoiliac segment is not always critical. Usually there is an endpoint range within the iliac arteries that forgives imprecision in preoperative measurement, but this is not always so. The need to cross one common iliac artery because it is aneurysmal places emphasis on precise knowledge of the length of the contralateral common iliac artery to avoid bilateral internal iliac artery occlusion. Here again, device differences may enter into consideration. Modular endograft types that allow considerable placement range (so-called trombone effect) make length measurement a relatively easier problem to solve. In addition, as data accumulate from long-term endograft follow up, it is apparent that some late failures from secondary endoleak have occurred when an iliac limb pulled out of its host vessel and up into the dilated aorta or when the common iliac artery has become further dilated. This has most often occurred in patients having the combination

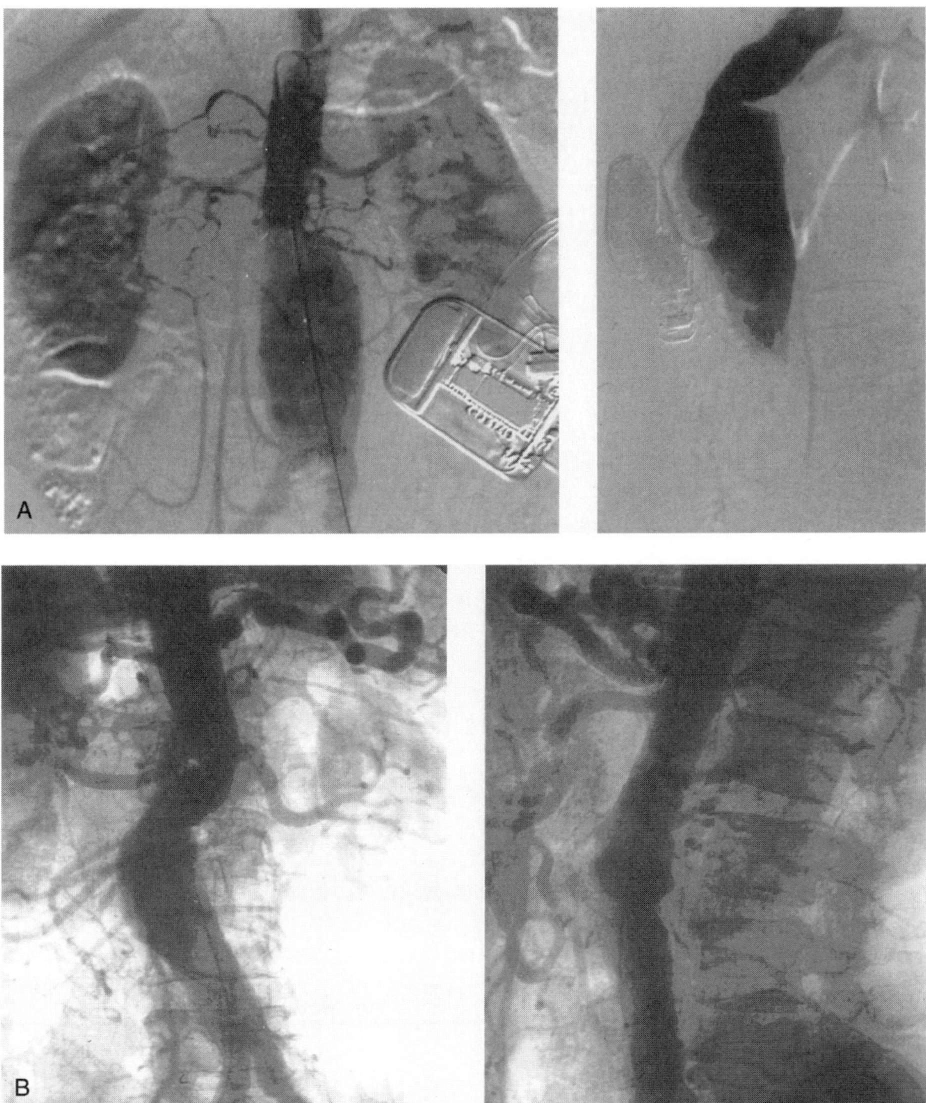

Figure 2. A. Biplanar aortogram showing the degree to which the measurement of aortic tortuosity is affected by projection angle of the arteriographic view. While the frontal projection (left) looks straight, there is actually highly significant angulation of 52° seen on the lateral view (right). From these views, there is no way to assess whether this is the maximum angulation or not. **B.** Aortic angulation is quite variable, and not always shown accurately by any one view or pair of views. For example, this patient's greater degree of angulation is shown in the frontal projection (left) and looks straight on the lateral view (right) in contrast to the patient shown in panel A.

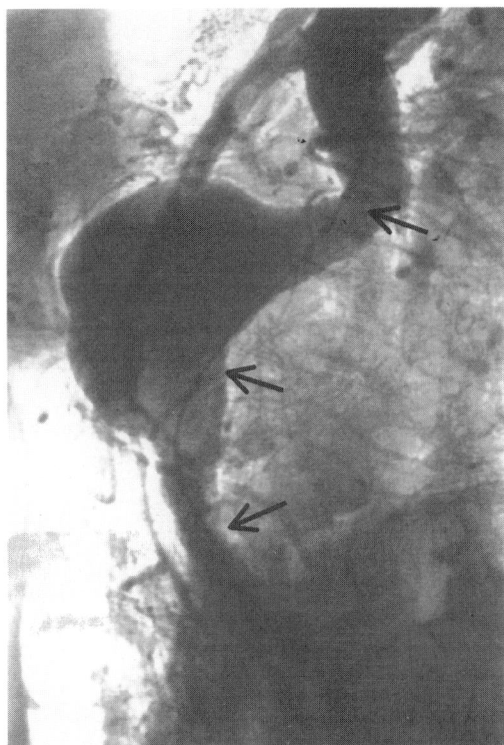

Figure 3. The path taken by the angiographic catheter (arrows) can be seen to cut across the short axis of this curved aorta. Measurement of length is inaccurate by this method for several reasons, of which this is the major one.

of late endograft angulation and a minimal length of common iliac artery insertion of the endoprosthesis. Recognition of such late problems can be expected to increase emphasis on inserting endografts as far distally into the common iliac artery as possible. This will also increase the need for accurate length measurement in the iliac vessels and of the entire length of the segment to be excluded with the endograft.

The practice of obtaining the "planning" arteriogram at the time of performing the procedure is sometimes employed. While this has the appeal of making the preoperative evaluation process simpler and, depending on the patient care reimbursement scheme in use, making cost shifting possible, the idea may not be a good one for several reasons. First, it means that the patient is already on the operating table when the rest of the data are first obtained. This has three flaws: CA may reveal adverse anatomy not previously appreciated and review of the new CA information adds to time of the procedure in a very expensive setting. Second, the contrast load during the procedure is needlessly increased. Third, the CA measurement process will not be conducted under ideal circumstances, indeed often seen to be inferior because of the use of fluoroscopy monitors instead of either workstation or cut film images. When using the combination of CT and CA for endograft planning, the ideal approach is to look at both images together and obtain measurements while moving from one to the other as needed so as to obtain maximum benefit from their dissimilar artifacts.

Computed Tomography

CT scans are the best overall method of assessing aneurysm disease in the aorta and iliac arteries, but they have limitations, too. They are most often viewed in axial slice projections, each of these individually representing in two dimensions an aggregate of the anatomy contained in the slice thickness. There is an abundance of potential problems contained in the details of the CT process. Important anatomical features may be blurred and "averaged out" in slices as thick as only 5 to 7 mm, let alone the commonly used 8- to 10-mm slices in general diagnostic CT scans. Length measurement, always a problem in CT of any slice thickness, is not possible with relatively thick sections (Fig. 4).

Another shortcoming of axial CT scans is of major importance in endograft planning. The axial projection does not accurately depict the cross-sectional shape of any structure that curves across the plane of the slice. The usual artifact produced is that a blood vessel with a circular cross section is shown as being elliptical or ovoid in shape because its tortuous course is tangent to the x-ray beam (Fig. 5). Thus, when a curved vessel is seen in an axial projection, an artifact is present that must be compensated for when measurements are obtained. This is often of critical importance in two locations that directly affect

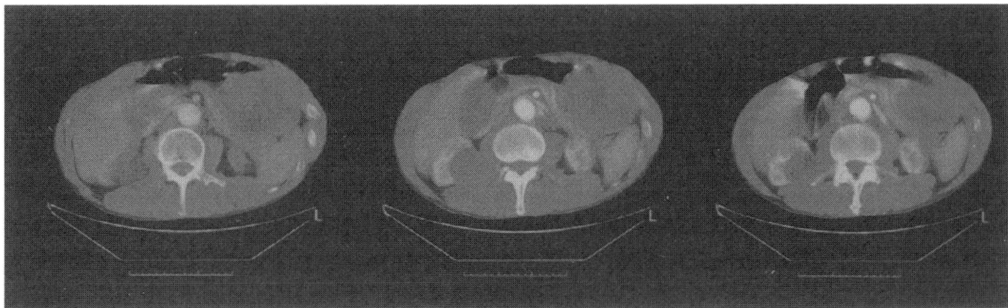

Slice Thickness 10 mm

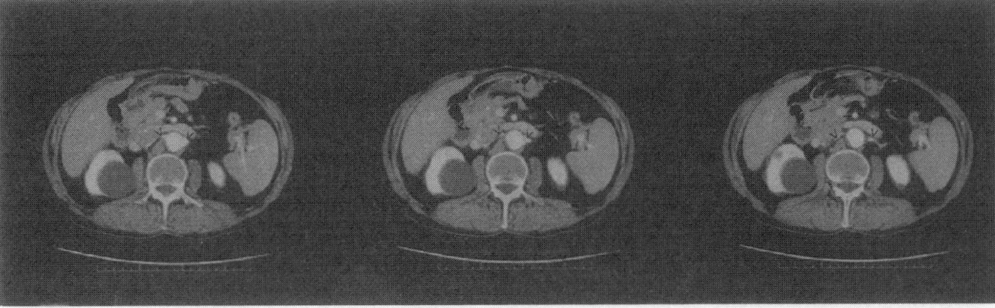

Slice Thickness 2 mm

Figure 4. The axial computed tomography (CT) sections seen in the top row are 10 mm in thickness and traverse the full length of the aorta containing the renal arteries; but nowhere can the renal arteries be seen because they are lost in the volume averaging of these thick slices. On the bottom row of CT slices with a thickness of 2 mm, through the same area in the same patient, the renal artery origins are clearly identified bilaterally (arrowheads).

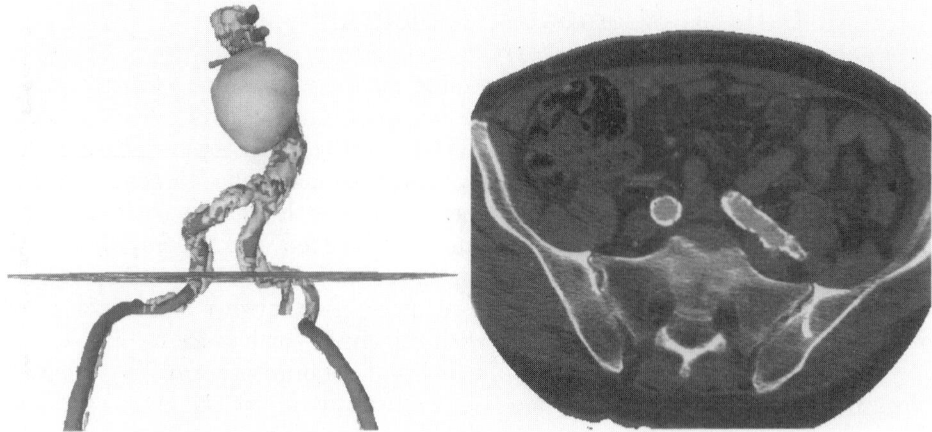

Figure 5. On the right can be seen the large difference between appearances of the right common iliac artery (circular) and the left common iliac artery (elongated ellipse). In reality, these vessels have identical, almost circular shapes. This also shows the great difficulty of measuring length by computed tomography scan even within this single 2-mm-thick slice.

clinical success in aortic endografting, the proximal aortic neck diameter and the size of the iliac artery at the distal extent of the endograft.

The usual method of compensating for this problem is to measure the least diameter at the site of interest and use this as the basis for sizing. The underlying assumption must be that the vessel has a circular cross section. Otherwise, if the vessel is not actually circular in shape, a significant error may occur. The use of reformatted CT sections that are perpendicular to the vessel axis (discussed below in the section on 3D models) has revealed strikingly the relatively common occurrence of proximal infrarenal aortic necks that are not circular in shape.[8]

Length measurement by axial CT is very difficult and problematic. In patients with aortoiliac anatomy that is aligned in a relatively straight path with the body sagittal axis, length of the aorta can be estimated by simply multiplying the number of contiguous sections between two points by their slice thickness. This process cannot be used for the iliac arteries, however, because they normally curve through the true pelvis in an anteroposterior plane. Moreover, aortic aneurysms are not always straight in line with the body axis. Thus, the deviation from that axis by the vessel centerline cannot be measured directly by axial CT scans. This problem is a good example of how the artifacts of the two imaging methods, CT and CA, are not the same and compensate for each other when used in combination.

Spiral CTA with 3D Reconstruction

With acquisition of an image data set by spiral CT scan that includes skillful use of contrast medium, computerized postprocessing can add greatly to the understanding of aortoiliac morphology. The value of this approach derives from use of multiple computer-reconstructed views and highly precise measurement tools to obtain accurate dimensions of vascular anatomy. When used carefully, the combination of good quality spiral CT data and vascular imaging software provides complete information required for endograft planning obtained from a single examination. In this approach, the need for arteriography is eliminated, thus avoiding the attendant morbidity, expense, and possible complications. Further, the use of modern 3D software allows the interpreter to overcome artifacts that are present in both arteriography and axial CT images.

This method of describing aortoiliac morphology measurement requires an understanding of the importance of spiral CT scanning techniques and a critical approach to use of computerized postprocessing of images. The ideal spiral CT scan will be free of motion artifact and have an appropriate amount of contrast present within the vessels of interest. Too little contrast makes it difficult to distinguish the flow lumen from thrombus or atheroma, so for CTA dense contrast in the vessels of interest is desirable. Very dense contrast is a problem for viewing CT scans on cut films because, to the unaided eye, it may appear undistinguishable from adjacent calcium in the vessel wall. But use of the viewing tools in the software described here allows the viewer to adjust the intensity range to take advantage of density differences between contrast-containing blood and vascular calcification during later observation.

There are several sources of computerized images for viewing vascular anatomy through CTA. The proprietary workstations that are an accessory part of CT scanner equipment can generate automated shaded surface display or volume renderings and curved planar reformation when the appropriate software is available. This software is highly efficient in terms of rapid function because it uses automated techniques for selecting regions of interest. It also uses semiautomated techniques for making measurements when the observer places cursors on selected points in the image while operating the software at the workstation. In general, these images are limited in the measurement tools they provide and in the accuracy of an automated process for rendering the anatomy. Also, most automated systems do not directly overcome the artifacts mentioned above in the discussion of CT, because they do not reformat CT slices perpendicular to the vessel axis. Also, the measurement of length is most accurate when made along the vessel center within the virtual space of the 3D model, not as a line on the surface as is usual with automated software.

A different approach involves use of proprietary software together with operator-guided creation of the 3D model (Preview™, Medical Media Systems, West Lebanon, NH). This is a more time-consuming process that needs skilled technologist participation in creation of the model by computerized processing and yields a patient-specific compact disc containing anatomical images. The interpreting physician can use these images in many ways with a variety of tools provided by the program. With minimal experience, complete anatomical measurements can be made throughout all points of the aortoiliac segment. In addition, computer simulation by use of virtual endograft models can be placed within the patient-specific anatomy to determine whether device selection is appropriate.

Using any personal computer that has a compact disc reader, the physician can quickly gain intuitive familiarity with the aortoiliac segment to be treated by continuously rotating the 3D model to be viewed from any perspective either externally or from within the lumen of the model. The Preview technology is not designed for use as a "fly through" kind of software and, in the usual case, there is very little to be learned from attempting this. However, for specific indications such as borderline tapered shape of the proximal aortic neck, calcified atheroma in or adjacent to the neck, narrow aortic bifurcation, or endograft migration, the intraluminal view may provide added insight. The patient shown in Figure 6 developed an endograft migration problem and secondary endoleak 1 year after implantation of a straight graft. The aneurysm shrunk and traction forces, kinking the endograft severely, caused upward migration of the distal end. Explantation was planned, but after study of the severely kinked (72°) endograft with endoluminal views and virtual endograft modeling, an endovascular procedure was planned. A second and bifurcated endograft was successfully placed, resolving the endoleak.

Following qualitative inspection, detailed measurements can be made using the tools provided in the proprietary software. This allows creation of reformatted slices lying perpendicular to the vessel axis to be dropped into the model for documented location when obtaining accurate diameter data. A series of diameter measurements can then be taken showing the diameter at points throughout the intended proximal attachment zone of the endograft, the largest diameter of the aneurysm, and diameters of the distal aorta or il-

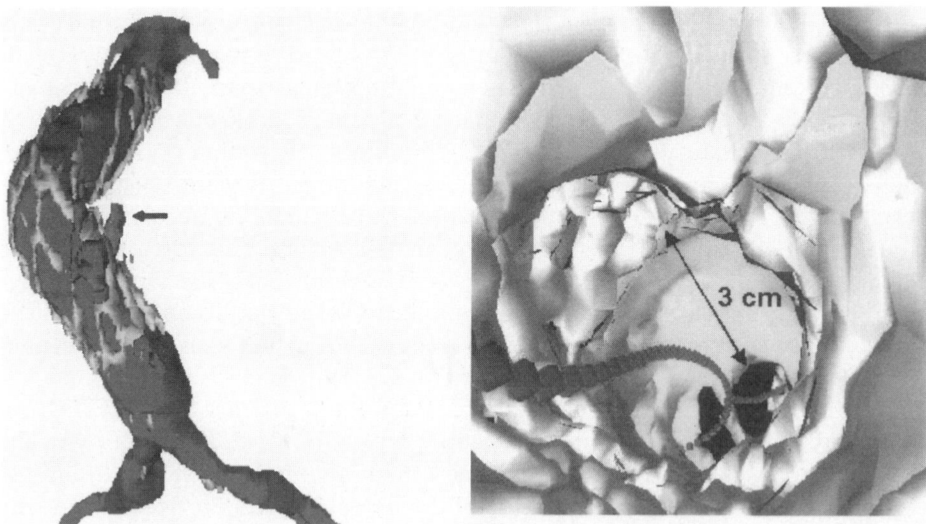

Figure 6. The follow-up image of this patient at 1 year post implant revealed the extent of endograft migration and development of secondary endoleak (left, arrow). The straight endograft migrated up from the aortic bifurcation for a distance of 3 cm, well seen in the intraluminal view on the right. In this view the centerline of the lumen is shown as a three-dimensional dashed line looking distally through the aortic bifurcation and into the right iliac artery. This type of information changed the clinical treatment plan, see text.

iac arteries to assess where available endoprostheses will be adequate for distal sealing.

Length measurement is obtained along the center of the blood flow lumen and is automatically calculated by the computer program when the endpoints have been specified, generally the lowermost renal artery, aortic bifurcation, and common iliac artery bifurcation. It is important to understand the significant difference of a measurement made by computer on the surface of a 3D rendering and a measurement that is actually taken from "within" using the voxels that comprise the space representing the lumen (Fig. 7). The former is very much similar to holding a ruler along a curved garden hose, while the latter is analogous to a string that lies in the center of the garden hose along its length. The iliac arteries are then measured similarly to determine their length to the bifurcation, their maximum and minimum diameters, and, if relevant, the angles to quantify tortuosity. This software option avoids the two most common causes of length measurement errors, inaccurate identification of the sites for length measurement and the tendency for intravascular catheters to follow straight-line paths through curved structures (Fig. 8).

The availability of sagittal and coronal slices that can be dropped into the model is often revealing in a qualitative manner when assessing angulation, but precise angle measurement is also done by automatic calculation when the

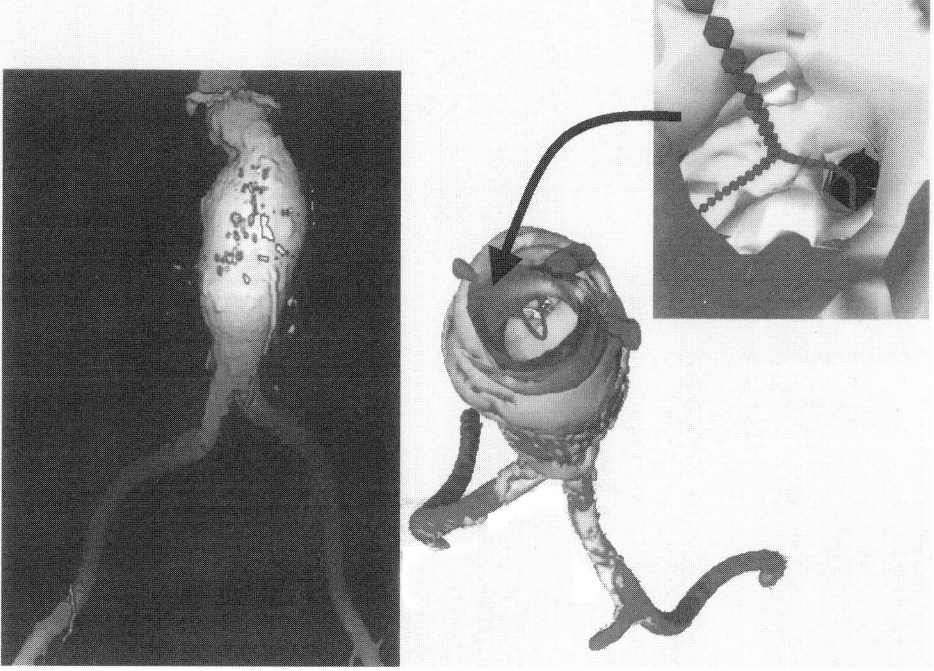

Figure 7. Left: One projection of a three-dimensional (3D) rendering from automated processing in a computed tomography scanner workstation. Right: A 3D model made using the Preview system described. An intraluminal view shows the dashed line that accurately depicts the center of flow along the vessel axis. Lighter areas in the model represent thrombus while dark areas show the blood flow lumen.

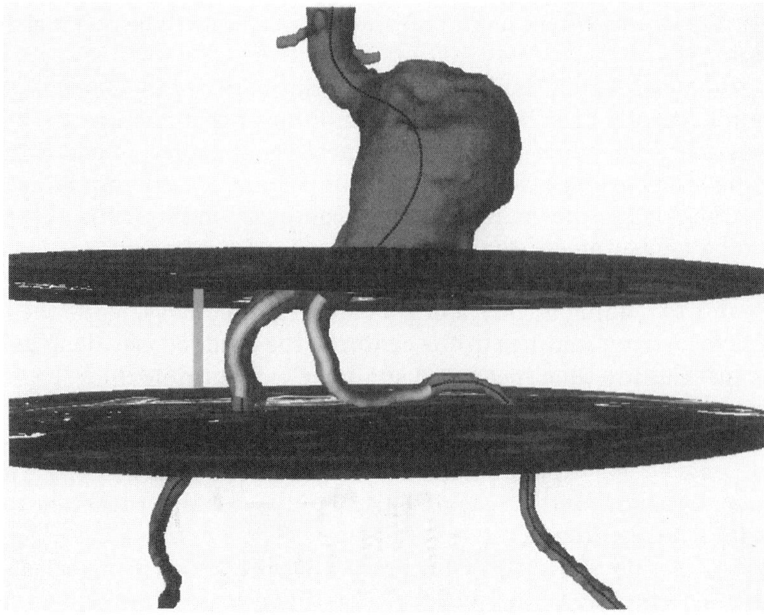

Figure 8. Notice the difference in length between the right and left iliac arteries. Simple calculation by multiplying numbers of slices by their thickness does not result in accurate estimation of length when vessels are curved in the computed tomography plane.

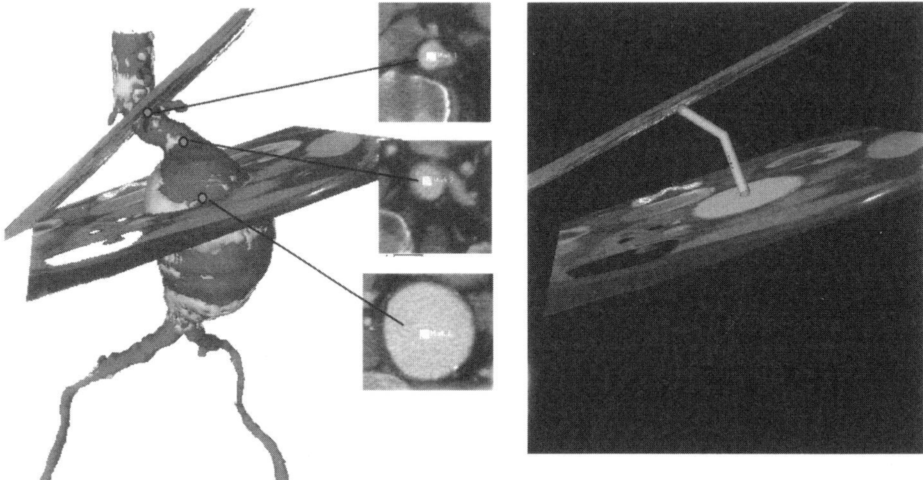

Figure 9. Measurement of angles is virtually impossible from axial computed tomography (CT) slices and subject to error of projection angle when attempted by arteriogram. Here, after the observer has placed marks within the model lumen using CT slices (shaded circles on left), the software automatically calculates an accurate result.

user specifies the endpoints through which the program is to measure. This feature, combined with precise diameter information, allows informed decisions to be made about the proximal aortic neck in particular, since both of the measurement parameters are independent influences on the risk of direct endoleak (Fig. 9).

Use of CTA and 3D Modeling in Clinical Practice

We have used CTA and 3D modeling with confidence as a stand-alone, complete imaging method for preoperative planning of aortic endografts for several years.[9] In a study from August 1997 to April 1998, 25 consecutive patients with abdominal aortic aneurysm were treated by endovascular aortic grafting in which all were evaluated with spiral CT scan (2-mm slice thickness) with computerized 3D model construction using the Preview software program. The primary research question was whether direct measurement within the 3D model provides accurate and complete morphology assessment overcoming the artifacts and errors of conventional imaging.

No additional imaging for planning was performed. From the 3D model of the aortoiliac segment, diameter, length, thrombus, calcification, and vessel tortuosity were measured and evaluated. These data were used for patient selection, selection of the type, diameter, and length of endograft components, and attachment sites for deployment. Results showed that endografting procedural success was 100%. There were no conversions to open repair and all endografts were deployed as planned. Mean endovascular aortic grafting procedure time was 91 minutes (range 24 to 273 minutes). Endoleak from side branches occurred in two cases and both sealed spontaneously within 1 month. Six patients required adjunctive procedures for delivery system access or iliac aneurysm exclusion, and all were predicted by the 3D model. No graft-related complications or death resulted within 30 days. We concluded that the computerized 3D model provided accurate data for preoperative evaluation of the aortoiliac segment for endovascular aortic grafting. Satisfactory patient outcomes can be achieved without use of invasive imaging procedures prior to surgery.

Another valuable clinical use for CTA with 3D modeling is endograft planning for the patient whose anatomy is marginally suited to the use of an available endograft. The usual anatomical factors that make aortic aneurysm treatment by endovascular exclusion a marginal choice include diameters in the attachment zone that are at the borderline of upper limit, angulation between the proximal neck and the aneurysm that is extreme enough to predict technical difficulty in delivery or misaligned deployment of the prosthesis, and length overall that is either too long or too short. After these measurements have been made, the physician will have a set of accurate digital descriptors that provide useful information, but the use of "virtual endografts" solidifies the judgment for or against an endovascular solution to the clinical problem.

Placing a simulated endograft into the model allows the operator to make a visual assessment from all angles to see how the intended prosthesis will reside within the excluded segment (Figs. 10 and 11). This virtual graft simula-

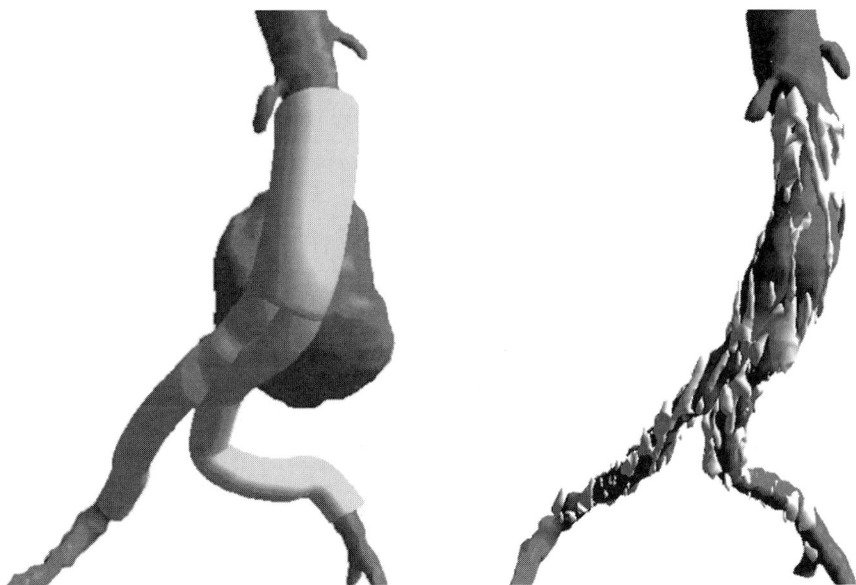

Figure 10. Left: Virtual endograft modeling using the Preview software to plan an endograft in a patient with an unusually short aortoiliac segment. Concern over covering both internal iliac arteries even using the shortest available endograft was present until this modeling step provided convincing evidence of satisfactory sizing without a margin of error. Right: Follow-up scan showing the actual endograft in position just beneath the right renal artery and just above the left internal iliac artery as predicted by the model.

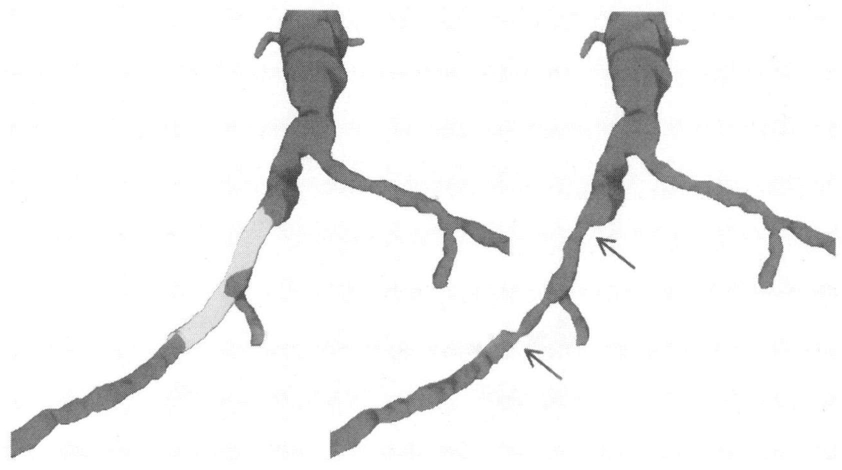

Figure 11. The degree of difficulty in passing an endograft delivery system through stenotic iliac arteries is often an issue. Left: Virtual rendering of the delivery sheath is shown as light area. Since the sheath is seen outside the flow lumen, its passage is predicted to be difficult or impossible. Right: The actual flow lumen can be seen including several stenotic areas in the same segment (arrows).

tion technique can also be used to predict the degree of difficulty of inserting a sheath of any dimension into iliac arteries that are stenotic. This type of simulation is valuable for predicting the need for adjunctive pre-endograft angioplasty and/or stenting. It also often aids in choosing the side through which to insert the larger diameter sheath in the delivery system of a modular graft that requires bilateral access using devices with significantly different diameter sheaths.

Summary

Planning aortic endografts requires precise definition of anatomical factors that exert a profound influence on results of treatment in both early and late follow-up. Failure to know the required measurements thoroughly is to trust to luck or to assume that over-dimensioned, self-expanding prostheses will make up for detailed planning. The well-informed, careful observer can achieve adequate knowledge of aortoiliac anatomy by using CT and CA together with devices such as marker catheters to compensate for inherent errors. Alternatively, CTA and computerized 3D modeling has a broader range of inherently accurate features that provide greater information from a single, low-morbidity examination. In recent years, attention at our center has been directed exclusively to the latter process, with satisfactory clinical results.

References

1. Beebe HG, Jackson T, Pigott JP. Aortic aneurysm morphology for planning endovascular aortic grafts: Limitations of conventional imaging methods. *J Endovasc Surg* 1995;2:139–148.
2. Cavaye DM, Diethrich EB, Santiago OJ, et al. Intravascular ultrasound imaging: An essential component of angioplasty assessment and vascular stent deployment. *Int Angiol* 1993;12:214–220.
3. Parodi JC, Palmaz JC, Barone HD. Transfemoral intraluminal graft implantation for abdominal aortic aneurysms. *Ann Vasc Surg* 1991;5:491–499.
4. Broeders IA, Blankensteijn JD, Olree M, et al. Preoperative sizing of grafts for transfemoral endovascular aneurysm management: A prospective comparative study of spiral CT angiography, arteriography, and conventional CT imaging. *J Endovasc Surg* 1997;4:252–261.
5. May J, White GH, Yu W, et al. Concurrent comparison of endoluminal versus open repair in the treatment of abdominal aortic aneurysms: Analysis of 303 patients by life table method. *J Vasc Surg* 1998;27:213–220.
6. Rubin GD, Paik DS, Johnston PC, Napel S. Measurement of the aorta and its branches with helical CT. *Radiology* 1998;206:823–829.
7. Rubin GD, Walker PJ, Dake MD, et al. Three-dimensional spiral computed tomographic angiography: An alternative imaging modality for the abdominal aorta and its branches. *J Vasc Surg* 1993;18:656–665.
8. Kritpracha B, Wolfe J, Beebe HG. CT artifacts of the proximal aortic neck: An important problem in endograft planning. *J Endovasc Ther* 2002;9:103–110.
9. Beebe HG, Kritpracha B, Serres S, et al. Endograft planning without preoperative arteriography: A clinical feasibility study. *J Endovasc Ther* 2000;7:8–15.

5

Endovascular Grafting in the Treatment of Extensive Aortoiliac Occlusive Disease:

Will it Replace Conventional Surgery?

Reese A. Wain, MD and Frank J. Veith, MD

Introduction

Atherosclerotic aortoiliac lesions are currently treated with endarterectomy, angioplasty, and stenting and anatomical as well as extra-anatomical bypass procedures. The appropriate treatment of a given lesion depends not only on the patient's symptomatology and coexisting medical problems, but on the local extent of the lesion and the presence of bilateral and outflow disease as well. Over the past several years, endovascular grafts have been investigated as alternatives to conventional techniques for managing occlusive aortoiliac lesions. The goal of endovascular graft treatment of these lesions is identical to that of more conventional procedures: the effective long-term relief of a patient's symptoms. When a new technique such as endovascular grafting demonstrates clinical feasibility, its merits and limitations must be carefully judged relative to those of existing procedures of known durability and efficacy. This chapter presents an overview of the current status of endovascular grafting for aortoiliac occlusive disease and compares the advantages and disadvantages of this new technique with those of conventional surgical procedures. Through this process, we hope that the reader will be able to decide whether endovascular grafting can replace conventional surgery for the treatment of aortoiliac occlusive disease.

From Criado FJ (ed): *Endovascular Intervention: New Tools and Techniques for the 21st Century.* Armonk, NY: Futura Publishing Co., Inc.; ©2002.

Endovascular grafting is a technique whereby lesions distant from the site of arterial access can be treated with an endoluminally deployed bypass graft. Endovascular grafts are typically constructed from metallic stents that expand and fix a prosthetic graft to the luminal surface of a blood vessel. Once deployed, the graft effectively replaces the diseased intimal surface of a vessel with a smooth prosthetic lining.

Of late, two different types of endovascular grafts have been used clinically to treat patients with aortoiliac occlusive disease. One type of graft is inserted percutaneously and consists of a short self-expanding stent, which is attached throughout its length to a prosthetic covering. After the offending lesion is identified radiographically, standard angioplasty balloon catheters are used to dilate the occlusion or stenosis and one of these "covered stents" is inserted across the lesion. After the associated deployment device is retrieved, prograde blood flow is restored within the lumen of the graft and recoil of the native arterial wall is countered by the stent.

Our focus at the Montefiore Medical Center in New York has been on an operative rather than a percutaneous approach to the endovascular treatment of aortoiliac lesions. In an operating suite, open access to the relevant vasculature, usually the common femoral artery, is achieved via a standard arteriotomy. Under fluoroscopic guidance, guidewire- and catheter-based techniques are used to insert a device consisting of a conventional prosthetic graft attached proximally to a Palmaz balloon-expandable stent (Cordis Endovascular, a Johnson & Johnson Company, Miami Lakes, FL). The stent portion of the endovascular graft is affixed to the native arterial wall proximal to the lesion being treated, and the end of the graft is retrieved from within the arteriotomy. Next, the distal anastomosis is individually tailored to treat the patient's pattern of outflow disease. In contrast to covered stents, this type of device is not supported along its entire length. These devices, however, can bypass long segments of diseased vessels and can be used to treat patients with a wide range of disease patterns.

Covered Stents

Representative early series using covered stents have been reported by groups working with the Cragg Endopro System 1 (Boston Scientific, Natick, MA)[1–3] and the Hemobahn endograft (W.L. Gore & Associates, Flagstaff, AZ).[4] In Nancy, France, Henry et al[3] treated 19 patients with symptomatic iliac artery stenoses ranging in length from 3 to 20 cm. Although the patients in this group had the usual risk factors for vascular disease, they were primarily claudicants and had covered stents placed to treat recurrent or ulcerated lesions and residual stenoses or dissections following balloon angioplasty.

With the patients under local anesthesia, Nitinol self-expanding stents covered with woven polyester were inserted in an antegrade fashion following percutaneous access to the femoral artery ipsilateral to the lesion. The lesion was crossed with a guidewire and an angioplasty balloon was used for dilatation purposes. Next, an appropriately sized covered stent was chosen and inserted through a 50-cm-long, 9F Cragg introducer sheath. A coaxial positioning catheter held the endograft in place as the sheath was removed, and the graft was allowed to expand. Finally, balloon dilatation of the covered stent was performed to improve fixation of the device to the vessel wall.

Technical success was achieved in all of the treated patients as assessed by a reduction in the percent stenosis of the treated lesion, a decreased pressure gradient across the lesion, and noninvasive vascular laboratory studies. With up to 8 months of follow-up, patency was maintained in all cases. One patient required a stent in the contralateral iliac artery when a covered stent partially protruded into the aorta and obstructed flow in the unaffected extremity. Based on these good initial and short-term results, the authors concluded that covered stents do appear promising for the treatment of long iliac lesions. They cautioned, however, that analysis of long-term results would be required before this new technique could be compared to conventional operative bypass procedures.

In France, Pernes et al[2] have also had considerable early clinical success using the Cragg Endopro System. This group treated 10 patients with iliac artery lesions more than 6 cm in length with 15 separate covered stents. Similar to the aforementioned study, these patients were treated primarily for claudication. In this group, immediate technical success was achieved in 9 patients. One patient experienced a rupture of the external iliac artery during balloon angioplasty. Although this iatrogenic lesion was fixed with a covered stent, the vessel thrombosed the following day and the patient required an extra-anatomical bypass. Two patients experienced recurrence of their symptoms in the postprocedure period; one required repeat balloon dilatation of a proximal graft lesion and the fate of the second was not reported. Additionally, one patient was found to have an asymptomatic stenosis within his graft that was also effectively treated by balloon dilatation during the follow-up period.

In 1998, Allen and associates[4] reported on their early clinical experience using the Hemobahn endograft (an expanded polytetrafluoroethylene [PTFE] tube externally supported by Nitinol wire) to treat 7 patients with chronic lower extremity ischemia caused by iliac artery occlusive disease. The patients in this series were treated for a mix of claudication and limb-threatening ischemia and had lesions averaging only 4.6 cm in length. They, too, achieved a 100% technical success rate and significant postoperative improvements in the ankle-brachial index in all patients. Three patients, however, experienced iliac artery dissections, and one patient suffered an embolus to the contralateral extremity at the time of surgery and required additional endovascular treatment.[4]

Endovascular Grafts

The Montefiore Experience

Between January of 1993 and December of 1997 we used endovascular grafts to treat 52 patients with aortoiliac occlusive disease.[5–14] Most of the patients (81%) were treated for limb-threatening ischemia (gangrene or ulceration) and the remainder suffered from rest pain. Almost one third of the patients we treated had synchronous disease involving the contralateral lower extremity that also required treatment, and half of the patients required infrainguinal bypasses at the time of their inflow procedure.

Our endovascular grafts consist of 30-mm Palmaz balloon-expandable stents and 6-mm PTFE grafts (W.L. Gore & Associates). The stents are attached to the proximal end of the graft with CV-6 PTFE sutures (W.L. Gore & Associates) so that one half of the stent's predeployment length remains uncovered. The stent-graft devices are then mounted on 8-mm by 3- or 4-cm angioplasty balloons (Blue Max or PMT, (Medi-tech/Boston Scientific, Watertown, MA). Next, the graft-balloon complex is inserted into a delivery sheath containing a second balloon catheter. When inflated, this "tip balloon" gives a smooth taper to the device and allows the sheath to be pressurized with saline to facilitate its insertion (Fig. 1).

In contradistinction to percutaneous insertion of a covered stent, our technique of endovascular grafting is more similar to an operative bypass than an interventional procedure. Our endovascular grafts are inserted in the operating room, with the patient under general, regional, or local anesthesia. Following conventional exposure and control of the relevant common femoral artery, a standard introducer sheath is inserted directly into the vessel. Stenotic iliac

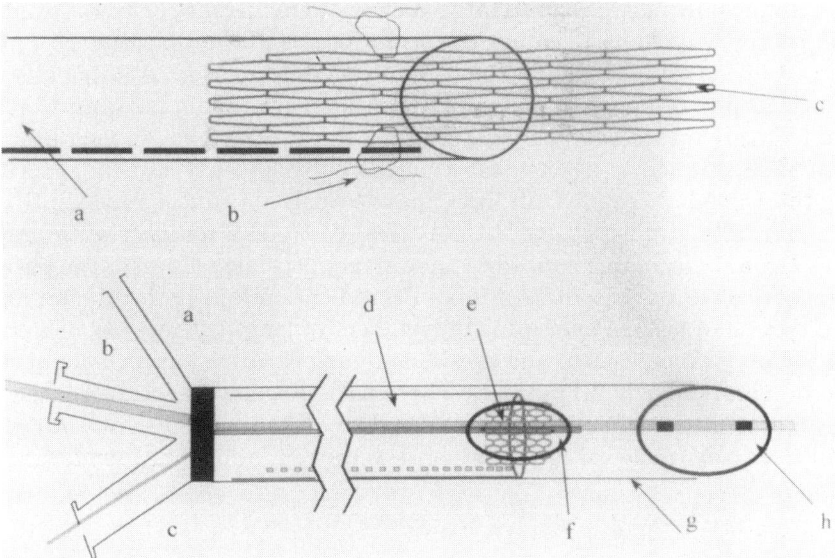

Figure 1. Construction of an endovascular graft. Top: Thin-walled polytetrafluoroethylene (PTFE) graft (a) is sutured with interrupted PTFE sutures (b) to a 30-mm Palmaz balloon-expandable stent (c). Bottom: Endovascular graft consisting of a PTFE graft (d) and Palmaz stent (e) is mounted on an 8-mm by 30-mm angioplasty balloon (f) and placed within a 20F delivery sheath (g). The delivery sheath contains a second "tip balloon" (h), which gives it a smooth tapered profile. The distal end of the delivery sheath has a hemostatic port for saline infusion (a) and for egress of the "tip" (b) and endovascular graft (c) balloon catheters.

artery lesions are then crossed with a guidewire under fluoroscopic guidance. Occluded arteries require recanalization, which is preferentially undertaken via a percutaneously inserted guidewire introduced through a patent contralateral femoral artery. When this guidewire can be advanced up and into the contralateral common iliac artery, a recanalization plane is often obtained with the lumen of the vessel requiring treatment. When the contralateral vasculature is also occluded, a retrograde approach is used.

Once a guidewire is successfully placed across the diseased segment, the full length of the iliac artery being treated as well as the proximal common femoral artery is dilated with an 8-mm angioplasty balloon. This technique allows the delivery sheath housing the endovascular graft to be inserted without undue friction, which could damage an already calcified and inelastic vessel. After the delivery sheath is inserted, the tip balloon is deflated and the proximal aspect of the endovascular graft is positioned in the appropriate location. After the sheath is partially withdrawn, the balloon underlying the proximal stent is inflated to seal the graft against the wall of the vessel. After the graft is secured proximally, the introducer sheath is withdrawn and the distal unsupported portion of the prosthetic graft is manually retrieved from within the femoral artery. Next, a balloon catheter is inflated sequentially throughout the length of the prosthetic graft to fully expand the graft and prevent kinking (Fig. 2).

Once the device is successfully inserted, the distal anastomosis can be fashioned. In the absence of infrainguinal disease, an endoluminal anastomosis is created within the femoral artery. Early in our experience, the arteriotomy was closed primarily; however, we currently perform a patch repair of the arteriotomy to prevent anastomotic stenoses. In the presence of significant multilevel or bilateral disease, the arteriotomy can be covered with the proximal hood of a distal or crossover bypass graft. Alternatively, the graft can be anastomosed in a conventional extraluminal fashion to a more distal vessel or existing bypass graft.

We routinely perform completion arteriograms in the operating room to exclude the presence of midgraft stenoses, which can result from incomplete expansion of the endovascular graft or extrinsic compression of the graft from the diseased native arterial wall. Once discovered, these lesions are corrected with repeat balloon dilatations of the offending segment with or without placement of additional intragraft stents.

Using this technique, we were able to achieve 3-year primary and secondary endovascular graft patency rates of 66% and 72%, respectively. The limb salvage rate over this same interval was 89% and patient survival was approximately 50%, highlighting the advanced comorbid disease in the cohort of patients we treated. We believe that our early results obtained in patients with severe coexisting medical conditions and multilevel occlusive disease justified further evaluation of endovascular grafts as an alternative to conventional operative procedures for the treatment of aortoiliac occlusive disease (Figs. 3 and 4).

Other Series

Using an approach similar to our own, Nevelsteen[15] recently reported preliminary results in 24 patients who underwent endovascular grafting for aor-

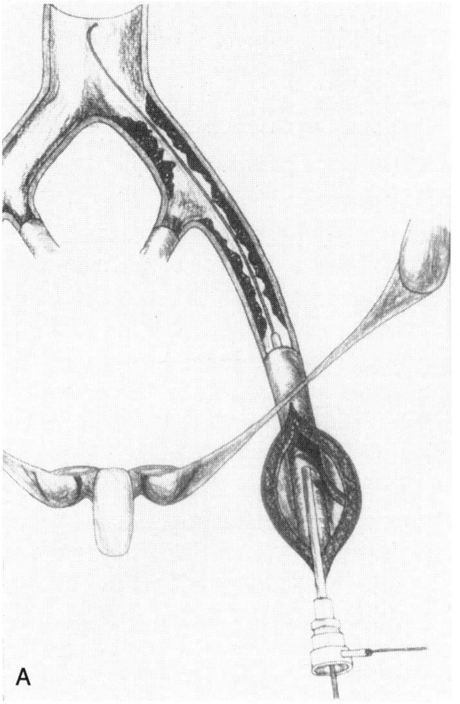

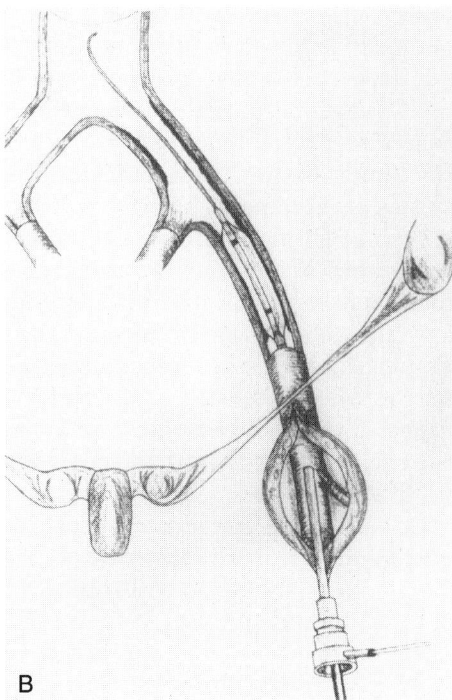

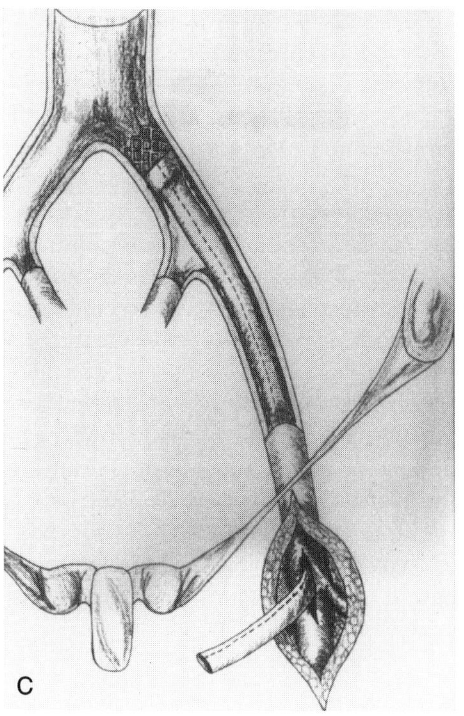

Figure 2. Endovascular grafting techniques. **A.** After femoral artery cut-down, a guidewire has been used to traverse a diffusely diseased iliac segment. **B.** Once the diseased artery has been recanalized (in this case via a retrograde approach), a balloon angioplasty catheter is used to dilate the entire length of the iliac artery to the level of the femoral arteriotomy. **C.** An endovascular graft has been inserted within the diffusely dilated vessel. The origin of the graft is within the proximal common iliac artery and the distal aspect of the graft is retrieved from within the arteriotomy.

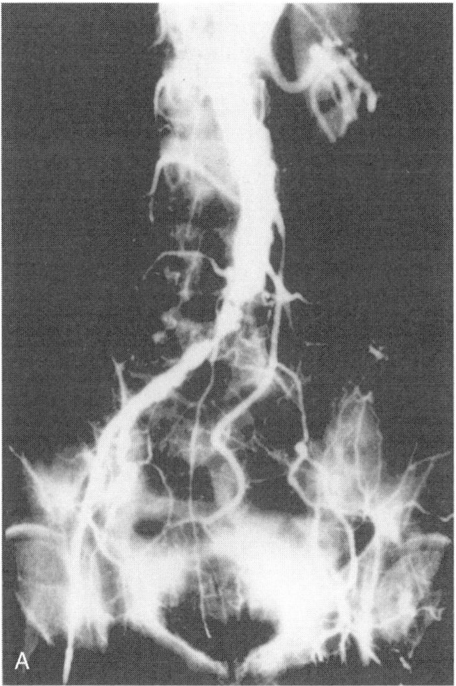

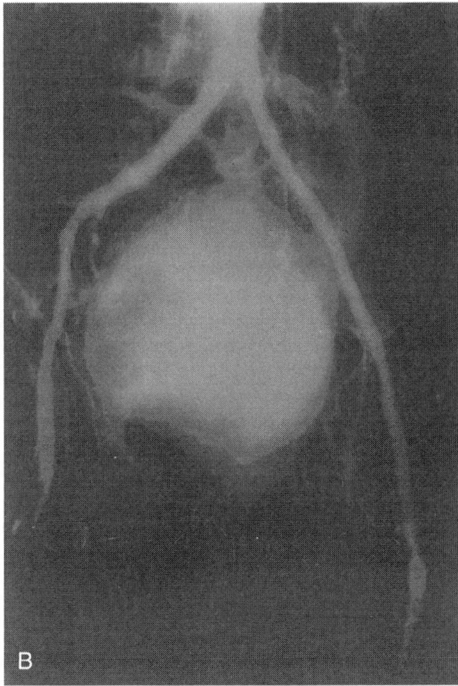

Figure 3. An endovascular graft inserted for limb-threatening ischemia. **A.** An angiogram obtained in an 86-year-old patient reveals severe disease within the right common iliac artery and an occluded left iliac artery. **B.** The left iliac system was successfully recanalized and dilated with an angioplasty balloon. Next, an endovascular graft was inserted from the aortic bifurcation to the femoral artery. The patient also required a concurrent femoropopliteal bypass and underwent angioplasty and stenting of her right iliac artery stenosis.

toiliac occlusive disease. They inserted 29 endovascular grafts to treat limb-threatening ischemia in 17 patients and claudication in 7. Their technical success rate was 93%, and the 2 patients in whom treatment failed had iliac artery occlusions that could not be successfully recanalized. In this series, follow-up ranged from 2 to 22 months with a mean of 13 months. Two patients experienced loss of endovascular graft patency in the follow-up period, and the primary and secondary cumulative 1-year patency rates of 85% and 95%, respectively, were similar to our own results. The authors recognized that further experience with this developing technique was necessary before its widespread use could be advocated, but they espoused its advantages in patients who were at high risk for conventional procedures.

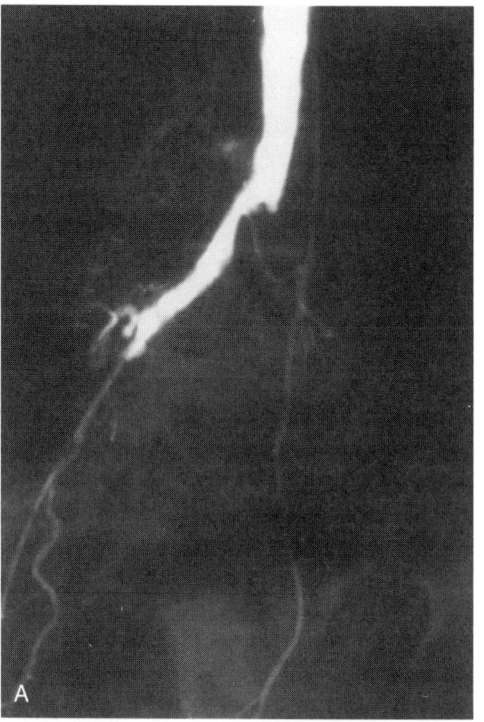

Figure 4. Endovascular graft insertion as a prelude to femorofemoral bypass grafting. **A.** Preoperative angiogram of a 77-year-old patient with foot gangrene revealing bilateral long-segmental iliac artery occlusions. **B.** An endovascular graft was inserted from the aortic bifurcation to the right femoral artery. **C.** The hood of a femorofemoral bypass graft was used to close the femoral arteriotomy and reperfuse the contralateral extremity.

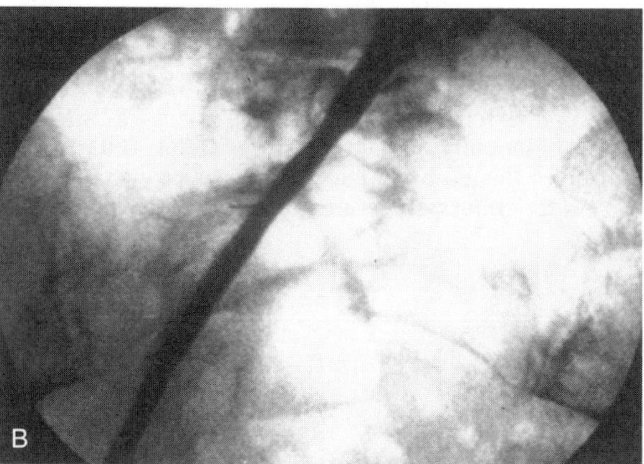

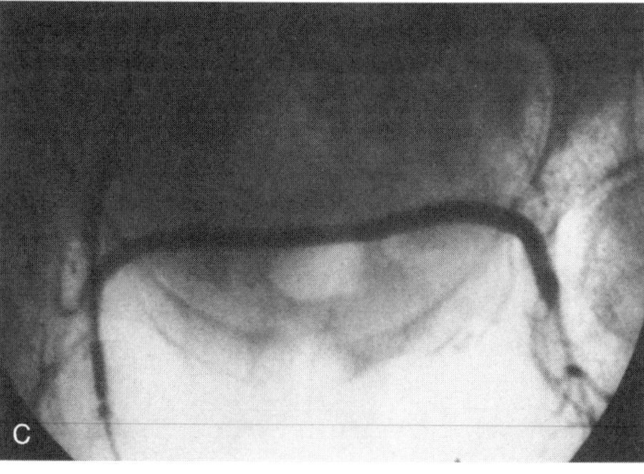

Comparison of Endovascular Grafting and Conventional Vascular Bypasses for the Treatment of Aortoiliac Occlusive Lesions

Endovascular Grafting and Aortobifemoral Bypass Grafting

Aortobifemoral bypass grafting has achieved the most widespread and enduring success in the treatment of aortoiliac lesions and is therefore the procedure against which newly emerging techniques must be compared. The ascendancy of aortobifemoral grafting as the gold standard for treating these lesions is in large part explained by the ability of this procedure to effectively treat disease in the aorta and common iliac arteries as well as disease involving the external iliac, common, and deep femoral vasculature. The ability of one standardized procedure to treat a gamut of inflow lesions and provide unsurpassed flow contributes to its durability and lasting popularity. Large series conducted over extended intervals have demonstrated 5-year cumulative patency rates between 75% and 90%.[16–19]

Endovascular grafting, similar to aortofemoral grafting, can provide patients with excellent inflow when the proximal limb of the graft is secured at the aortic bifurcation. Anchoring the graft in this location negates the effect of disease progression proximal to the origin of the graft. Just as an aortofemoral graft is typically anastomosed to the femoral vasculature to avoid disease progression within the external iliac arteries, so too is the endovascular graft. In both cases, disease within the common or deep femoral artery can also be addressed during the primary bypass procedure. Endovascular grafting, like aortofemoral grafting, allows a standardized approach to the treatment of a range of aortoiliac lesions. Although the distal anastomosis is typically tailored for the pattern of disease of each individual patient, the remainder of the procedure and the construction of the endovascular device itself are identical in all cases. The presence of bilateral disease can also be adequately addressed with an endovascular graft by performing a femorofemoral bypass after a unilateral aortofemoral endovascular graft is inserted.[9] Although our initial patency data for patients with limb-threatening ischemia are slightly inferior to those seen on early follow-up in patients undergoing conventional aortobifemoral grafting, the analysis of long-term results must be undertaken before a comparison of the durability of the two procedures would be meaningful.

The conventional aortobifemoral bypass has been the procedure of choice for treating patients with combined renal and aortoiliac occlusive disease and for patients experiencing emboli from ulcerated aortic lesions.[20] Although we have not inserted endovascular grafts to treat aortic lesions producing atheroemboli, these grafts can be adapted to treat such lesions. With similar techniques to those used to treat infrarenal abdominal aortic aneurysms in an endovascular fashion, these lesions can be effectively excluded from the circulation. To accomplish this, the proximal end of an endovascular graft is affixed to the infrarenal aorta. Next, the distal aspect of the graft is anastomosed in an endoluminal fashion to the femoral artery and a femorofemoral bypass is performed. Finally, an endovascular occlusion device is inserted within the contralateral iliac artery to prevent retrograde filling of the aorta. In this fashion, the ulcerated lesion is "covered" by the endovascular graft, and its embolic potential is negated. Concomitant renal artery stenoses cannot currently be treated with endovascular grafts; however, many such lesions can be treated at the time of endovascular grafting with balloon angioplasty and stents.

Depending on how an aortofemoral bypass is performed, blood flow through accessory renal arteries, the inferior mesenteric artery, and both hypogastrics might be sacrificed with an increased risk of end organ damage. In contrast, our endovascular grafts originate within the proximal common iliac artery and end within the femoral artery and sacrifice only the ipsilateral hypogastric artery. In our experience, covering the orifice of this vessel with the side of a prosthetic graft has not been a problem.

Aortobifemoral bypass grafting with aortic endarterectomy has a well-defined role in the treatment of patients with infrarenal aortic occlusion. Currently, endovascular grafting is contraindicated in this setting because of the risk of occluding or embolizing the renal vasculature. However, if the aorta is occluded at a distance from the renal arteries, endovascular grafting remains an important option if the occlusion can be recanalized.

Aortobifemoral grafting is an invasive procedure requiring general anesthesia and aortic clamping, both of which may impose a significant cardiac stress on patients who are frequently also afflicted with ischemic heart disease. In fact, 30% and 60% of patients requiring surgery for aortoiliac occlusive disease will die within 5 and 10 years of surgery, respectively. Not surprisingly, the leading cause of death in these patients is a cardiac event.[21] In addition, cardiac complications are the among the most common perioperative complications occurring in patients undergoing aortofemoral bypasses. Although still hotly contested, several reports suggest that reductions in morbidity and mortality in surgical patients can be achieved using regional as opposed to general anesthesia.[22–24] It is therefore necessary to carefully consider a patient's preexisting medical comorbidities before choosing to undertake an aortofemoral bypass, which requires general anesthesia, versus an alternative procedure that does not.

Likewise, patients with considerable pulmonary dysfunction may not be candidates for aortofemoral bypass grafting because of the need for general anesthesia and the fear that the patient may remain dependent on a ventilator. In addition, patients with a "hostile abdomen" may be denied an aortofemoral graft if they have undergone multiple prior abdominal procedures, have an ostomy, or have been irradiated in the past. Finally, surgeons may choose not to pursue conventional aortofemoral bypasses in patients with limited life expectancies based on advanced age, cancer, or other severe comorbid illnesses.

One of the greatest potential advantages of endovascular grafting is that it can be performed without an abdominal incision and without general anesthesia. Our devices were inserted through a modest groin incision in all cases, and regional anesthesia was used 80% of the time. In this fashion, we feel that we were able to limit both the cardiac and the pulmonary stress associated with general anesthesia and aortic cross-clamping. Similarly, patients who are denied aortofemoral bypasses because of a limited life expectancy or a hostile abdomen can also be treated with an endovascular graft. In our series, almost one third of the patients treated had at least one previous abdominal procedure that would have complicated a transperitoneal aortic approach to standard aortofemoral grafting.

Up to 20% of all patients undergoing aortobifemoral bypasses experience graft limb occlusions within 10 years of surgery. In addition, 5% of patients can be expected to have an anastomotic aneurysm and just less than 2% an aortic graft infection over this same interval.[25] In fact, in a series of 1647 patients reviewed by Szilagyi and colleagues,[18] 26% required reoperation to treat a complication of an aortobifemoral graft. Therefore, although these grafts have documented durability, the high rate of reoperation required to treat a complication of the initial procedure must be viewed as a limitation of aortobifemoral grafting.

Patients treated with endovascular grafts will also experience graft limb thrombosis due to distal disease progression. However, the short-term follow-up of endovascular grafts precludes a meaningful comparison on the propensity of these grafts to thrombose relative to aortofemoral grafts. An additional unknown factor related to endovascular grafts is the effect of dilating the entire iliac artery prior to endovascular graft insertion. It is possible that this technique may accelerate disease progression within the native iliac artery leading to constriction and thrombosis of the endovascular graft in the future.

Anastomotic pseudoaneurysms have not been seen to complicate endovascular procedures because, in most instances, the distal anastomosis is purely endoluminal and the proximal anastomosis is stented and not sutured. In addition, patients with endovascular grafts are not immune from bloodborne pathogens, which could cause a graft infection. These grafts, however, are inserted entirely within the vasculature and infections caused by intra-abdominal processes should not occur because the peritoneum is not violated at the time of surgery.

Another potential complication of aortobifemoral bypasses is that of postoperative male sexual dysfunction. Disruption of the pelvic autonomic nerves during dissection of the aorta may occur in between 15% to 25% of patients.[19] Although an endovascular procedure does not damage these nerves, potency may be adversely affected by sacrifice of hypogastric blood flow. Therefore, a more detailed study is necessary to elucidate which procedure may least affect sexual function.

Endovascular Grafts and Extra-anatomical Bypass Grafting

Extra-anatomical bypasses were first performed to treat patients with infected prosthetic aortic grafts and those with severe coexisting medical problems. The single most important benefit of these procedures when used to treat aortoiliac occlusive disease is that they do not carry the risks associated with general anesthesia and aortic cross-clamping. A femorofemoral bypass graft can be quickly performed under local or regional anesthesia in a patient with limb-threatening ischemia and medical comorbidities severe enough to contraindicate general anesthesia. Similarly, axillobifemoral bypasses, although not easy to perform under local anesthesia, are also less stressful to patients with severe cardiac, pulmonary, and renal disease than are major aortic procedures.

Often quoted comparisons of morbidity and mortality rates between extra-anatomical bypasses and aortofemoral bypasses are probably unjust because the latter are used primarily to treat high-risk patients. Nonetheless, several major series have reported operative mortality rates between 0% and 8% in these complicated patients.[26–32] Our experience with endovascular grafting using regional or local anesthesia in these seriously ill patients is concordant with these reports. In our series, only 3 patients died within the perioperative period. Two succumbed to myocardial infarctions and one died as a result of diffuse microembolization.

The usefulness of axillofemoral and femorofemoral bypass grafting is also highlighted in patients who have multiply reoperated abdomens or colostomies and in those who have undergone radiotherapy for an intra-abdominal malignancy. In addition, they may be the only operative option for patients with infected aortic grafts or those with intraperitoneal inflammatory processes. We have not used endovascular grafting extensively in the treatment of aortic graft infections, and we cannot currently recommend it as a viable alternative for more conventional modalities. The potential role of endovascular grafting in the presence of a hostile abdominal wall or peritonitis, however, should not be dismissed.

Extra-anatomical bypasses are often used to treat patients with symptomatic aortoiliac occlusive disease with failed aortobifemoral bypasses in whom a redo aortic procedure is considered too dangerous secondary to scarring or a patient's medical comorbidities. In this setting, endovascular grafting could become the procedure of choice if the endovascular graft can be deployed within the limb of a recanalized aortofemoral bypass. Balloon dilatation of a chronically thrombosed graft may result in a widely patent lumen, whereas a conventional thrombectomy may prove fruitless. In these cases, unlike extra-anatomical bypasses, it is possible to restore aortic inflow without performing a more invasive redo aortic procedure or implicating an unaffected extremity.

One of the most frequently discussed limitations of extra-anatomical bypasses is decreased long-term patency rates when compared to aortobifemoral bypasses. Reports published in the 1970s and 1980s reveal 5-year primary patency rates varying between 40% and 85% for axillobifemoral bypasses, with the predominance of the results at the lower end of this range.[29,31–35] A more recent study reported on 3-year primary patency rates for low-risk patients receiving aortofemoral or femorofemoral bypasses and found rates of 87% and 61%, respectively.[36] Our initial patency rates do compare favorably with those reported in large series of patients undergoing extra-anatomical bypasses; however, longer term follow-up is necessary in a larger cohort of patients before lasting conclusions can be derived.

A potential cause for the decreased patency rates associated with extra-anatomical bypass may relate to hemodynamic factors within the bypass and associated donor vasculature.[36–38] The impaired hemodynamics when compared to bypasses that provide aortic inflow through large-caliber conduits may relate to the long length of an axillobifemoral graft or the small size and presence of disease within axillary and femoral donor arteries. Endovascular grafts, like aortobifemoral grafts, are shorter than axillofemoral grafts and revascularize an ischemic extremity with straight-line aortic inflow. Therefore, they should not experience the same hemodynamic limitations that may compromise grafts originating from smaller peripheral vessels. In addition, grafts originating at the femoral or axillary level may be adversely affected by proximal disease progression, which would not occur to such an extent in a graft of aortic origin.

Axillofemoral and femorofemoral grafts are also potentially disadvantageous because they implicate an unaffected extremity in a revascularization procedure. The formerly uninvolved limb is therefore placed at risk for complications such as distal embolization, infection, and steal syndrome, which, although uncommon, can result in limb loss. Contrarily, endovascular grafts originate in vessels that are typically already diseased and therefore do not risk injury to an unaffected extremity.

Conclusion

Presently, we cannot conclude that endovascular grafts are equivalent to existing conventional techniques for the treatment of patients with aortoiliac occlusive disease. In the absence of significant coexisting medical problems or other anatomical limitations, standard balloon angioplasty and stenting or aortofemoral or extra-anatomical bypasses should still first be considered for these patients. However, based on our early results using this new technique, we believe that endovascular grafts represent a valuable option for treating high-risk patients in limb loss situations when contraindications to standard revascularization procedures exist. In the future, improvements in endovascular grafting techniques may expand the indications for this developing minimally invasive procedure.

References

1. Cragg AH, Dake MD. Percutaneous femoro-popliteal graft placement. *Radiology* 1993;187:643–648.
2. Pernes JM, August MA, Hovasse D, et al. Long iliac stenosis: Initial clinical experience with the Cragg endoluminal graft. *Radiology* 1995;196:67–71.
3. Henry M, Amor M, Ethevenot G, et al. Initial experience with the Cragg Endopro System 1 for intraluminal treatment of peripheral vascular disease. *J Endovasc Surg* 1994;1:31–43.
4. Allen BT, Hovsepian DM, Reilly JM, et al. Endovascular stent grafts for aneurysmal and occlusive vascular disease. *Am J Surg* 1998;176:574–580.
5. Marin ML, Veith FJ, Sanchez LA, et al. Endovascular repair of aortoiliac occlusive disease. *World J Surg* 1996;20:679–686.
6. Veith FJ, Marin ML. The present status of endoluminal stented grafts for the treatment of aneurysms, traumatic injuries and arterial occlusions. *Cardiovasc Surg* 1996;4:3–7.
7. Wain RA, Marin ML, Veith FJ, Levine BA. The Montefiore Medical Center experience with endovascular stented grafts. In Szabo Z, Lewis JE, Fantini G (eds): *Sur-*

gical Technology International IV. San Francisco: Universal Medical Press; 1995:366–372.
8. Marin ML, Veith FJ, Cynamon J, et al. Transfemoral endovascular stented graft treatment of aorto-iliac and femoropopliteal occlusive disease for limb salvage. *Am J Surg* 1994;168:156–162.
9. Ohki T, Marin ML, Veith FJ, et al. Endovascular aortounifemoral grafts and femorofemoral bypass for bilateral limb-threatening ischemia. *J Vasc Surg* 1996;24:984–987.
10. Marin ML, Veith FJ. Preliminary experience with endovascular stented grafts for limb-threatening aortoiliac occlusive disease. In Yao JST, Pearce WH (eds): *The Ischemic Extremity: Advances in Treatment*. Norwalk: Appleton and Lange; 1995:363–376.
11. Marin ML, Veith FJ, Sanchez LA, et al. Endovascular aortoiliac grafts in combination with standard infrainguinal arterial bypasses in the management of limb-threatening ischemia: Preliminary report. *J Vasc Surg* 1995;22:316–325.
12. Marin ML, Veith FJ. Clinical application of endovascular grafts in aortoiliac occlusive disease and vascular trauma. *Cardiovasc Surg* 1995;3:115–120.
13. Marin ML, Veith FJ. The role of stented grafts in the management of failed arterial reconstructions. *Semin Vasc Surg* 1994;7:188–194.
14. Marin ML, Veith FJ, Cynamon J, et al. Initial experience with transluminally placed endovascular grafts for the treatment of complex vascular lesions. *Ann Surg* 1995;222:449–469.
15. Nevelsteen A, Lacroix H, Stockx L, Wilms G. Stent grafts for iliofemoral occlusive disease. *Cardiovasc Surg* 1997;5:393–397.
16. Brewster DC, Darling RC. Optimal methods of aortoiliac reconstruction. *Surgery* 1978;84:739–748.
17. Crawford ES, Bomberger RA, Glaeser DH, et al. Aortoiliac occlusive disease: Factors influencing survival and function following reconstructive operation over a twenty-five-year period. *Surgery* 1981;90:1055–1067.
18. Szilagyi DE, Elliott JP, Smith RF, et al. A thirty-year survey of the reconstructive surgical treatment of aortoiliac occlusive disease. *J Vasc Surg* 1986;3:421–436.
19. Brewster DC. Clinical and anatomical considerations for surgery in aortoiliac disease and results of surgical treatment. *Circulation* 1991;83(suppl I):I42-I52.
20. Kempczinski RF. Lower extremity arterial emboli from ulcerating atherosclerotic plaques. *JAMA* 1979;241:807–810.
21. Malone JM, Moore WS, Goldstone J. Life expectancy following aortofemoral arterial grafting. *Surgery* 1977;81:551–555.
22. Baron J, Bertrand M, Barre E, et al. Combined epidural and general anesthesia versus general anesthesia for abdominal aortic surgery. *Anesthesiology* 1991;75:611–618.
23. Christopherson R, Beattie C, Frank SM, et al. Perioperative morbidity in patients randomized to epidural or general anesthesia for lower extremity vascular surgery. *Anesthesiology* 1993;79:422–434.
24. Yeager MP, Glass DD, Neff RK, Brinck-Johnsen T. Epidural anesthesia and analgesia in high-risk surgical patients. *Anesthesiology* 1987;66:729–736.
25. Brewster DC, Meier GH, Darling RC, et al. Reoperation for aortofemoral graft limb occlusion: Optimal methods and long-term results. *J Vasc Surg* 1987;5:303–374.
26. Brief DK, Brener B, Alpert J, Parsonnet V. Crossover femorofemoral grafts followed up five years or more: An analysis. *Arch Surg* 1975;110:1294–1299.
27. Flanigan P, Pratt DG, Goodreau JJ, et al. Hemodynamic and angiographic guidelines in selection of patients for femorofemoral bypass. *Arch Surg* 1978;113:1257–1262.
28. Livesay JJ, Atkinson JB, Baker JD, et al. Late results of extraanatomic bypass. *Arch Surg* 1979;114:1260–1267.
29. Rutherford RB, Patt A, Pearce WH. Extra-anatomic bypass: A closer view. *J Vasc Surg* 1987;5:437–446.
30. LoGerfo FW, Johnson WC, Corson JD, et al. A comparison of the late patency rates

of axillobilateral femoral and axillounilateral femoral grafts. *Surgery* 1977;81:33–40.
31. Ray LI, O'Connor JB, Davis CC, et al. Axillofemoral bypass: A critical reappraisal of its role in the management of aortoiliac occlusive disease. *Am J Surg* 1979;138:117–128.
32. Eugene J, Goldstone J, Moore WS. Fifteen-year experience with subcutaneous bypass grafts for lower extremity ischemia. *Ann Surg* 1976;286:177–183.
33. Chang JB. Current state of extraanatomic bypasses. *Am J Surg* 1986;152:202–205.
34. Ascer E, Veith FJ, Gupta SK, et al. Comparison of axillounifemoral and axillobifemoral bypass operations. *Surgery* 1985;97:169–175.
35. Harris EJ, Taylor LM, McConnell DB, et al. Clinical results of axillobifemoral bypass using externally supported polytetrafluoroethylene. *J Vasc Surg* 1990;12:416–420.
36. Schneider JR, Besso SR, Walsh DB, et al. Femorofemoral versus aortobifemoral bypass: Outcome and hemodynamic results. *J Vasc Surg* 1994;19:43–57.
37. Self SB, Richardson JD, Klamer TW, et al. Utility of femorofemoral bypass: Comparison of results with indications for operation. *Am Surg* 1991;57:602–606.
38. Schneider JR, McDaniel MD, Walsh DB, et al. Axillofemoral bypass: Outcome and hemodynamic results in high-risk patients. *J Vasc Surg* 1992;15:952–963.

6

Role of Covered Stents in Peripheral Arterial Diseases

Michel Henry, MD, Isabelle Henry, MD, and Kiril Tzvetanov, MD

Introduction

The scope of percutaneous vascular intervention has continued to expand over the past two decades, thanks to the advancement of technical developments. Angioplasty is now the first treatment proposed for peripheral vascular diseases and the treatment of choice for simple arterial lesions. Yet, angioplasty alone is limited and has several complications (dissections, acute thromboses, etc.). The problem of restenosis remains, and for long lesions the initial success and the long-term results are not as good as they are for short lesions, particularly in femoropopliteal arteries, in which surgery is often preferred.[1–3]

The concept of vascular stenting originated with Charles Dotter in 1969,[4] but it did not become a clinical reality until the late 1980s. Expandable metallic stents have proved their usefulness in the management of complications related to angioplasty and possibly restenosis[5–7]; for the latter, however, this benefit is debated. The process of restenosis starts when a stent is placed, with a vascular "injury" that is induced by percutaneous transluminal angioplasty (PTA) and/or stent placement; such injuries include deposits of plasma proteins, platelets, and leukocytes on the stent's struts.[8–10] Stents have not proven beneficial, however, at the femoropopliteal level.[11–18]

Endoluminal stent-grafts and covered stents are now being investigated for treatment of both aneurysmal and occlusive peripheral arterial diseases.[19–32] For occlusive diseases, it is postulated that an endoluminal bypass with a stent-graft may limit the ingrowth of intimal hyperplasia along the length of the treated segment thereby improving patency as compared to conventional angioplasty and stenting. For an aneurysmal disease, the stent-graft may be used to bridge the aneurysmal segment and therefore occlude the aneurysm from the native circulation.

From Criado FJ (ed): *Endovascular Intervention: New Tools and Techniques for the 21st Century.* Armonk, NY: Futura Publishing Co., Inc.; ©2002.

Several covered stents are either currently available or in clinical experiment:

1. The Cragg Endopro System 1 (Boston Scientific, Natick, MA)
2. The Passager (Boston Scientific)
3. The Corvita Endoluminal Graft (Boston Scientific)
4. The Hemobahn (W.L. Gore & Associates, Flagstaff, AZ)
5. The Wallgraft (Boston Scientific)
6. The Jostent (Jomed International AB, Helsingberg, Sweden)

We describe below these different covered stents, the results obtained, and their clinical applications.

The Different Covered Stents: Results

Cragg Endopro System 1/Passager

Stent-Graft Construction

The Cragg Endopro System 1/Passager consists of a flexible, self-expandable nitinol stent covered with ultrathin woven polyester fabric (Fig. 1). It has the property of shape memory.[19,20] The design and construction of the stent have been previously described.[15,21,33–35] The fabric is of low porosity and is attached to the stent framework by polyester ligatures. The stent-graft is presented in a compressed form in a loading cartridge. Stent-grafts range from 5

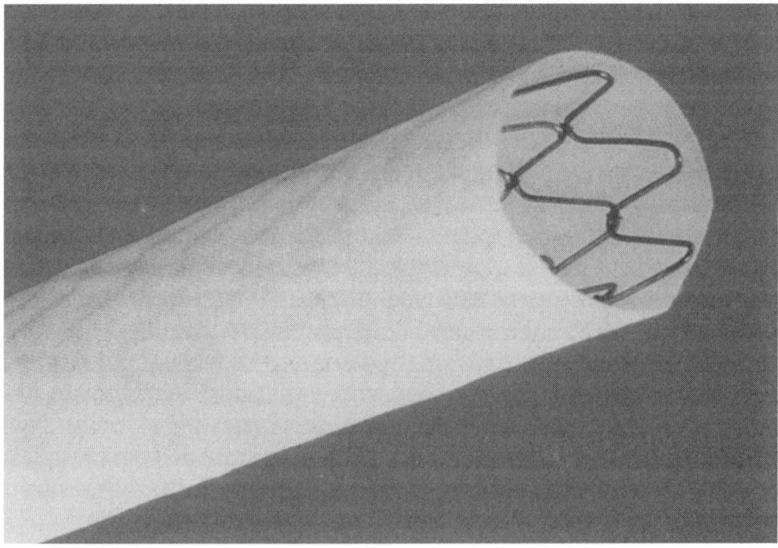

Figure 1. Cragg Endopro System 1/Passager Nitinol stent covered with polyester woven fabric.

to 12 mm in diameter and from 3 to 10 cm in length. They are delivered through 50-cm-long introducer sheaths ranging in diameter from 7F to 10F, depending on the size of the stent-graft to be implanted.

Stent-Graft Introduction Technique (see Fig. 1)

Device delivery is usually accomplished using an ipsilateral retrograde or antegrade femoral artery approach. A retrograde popliteal approach has been used in cases in which femoral artery access was not possible. The rigidity of the delivery device limits the possibilities of implantation using the contralateral access. For occlusive disease, balloon angioplasty is always performed first in order to enlarge the arterial lumen. Occasionally, debulking techniques such as rotational atherectomy are used. The stent-graft is delivered through the 50-cm-long introducer sheath, which is placed across the lesion to be treated. The stent-graft diameter is usually selected to be equal to or 1 mm greater than the nominal arterial diameter.

The stent-graft is positioned fluoroscopically across the treated segment. Platinum markers at each end of the stent assist in positioning the device. Once the stent-graft is in position, the sheath is withdrawn, and an internal positioning catheter is used to fix the stent-graft in place. The stent-graft expands using the thermal memory characteristics of its nitinol frame. The graft is usually then dilated with an angioplasty balloon at high pressure (14 to 16 atm). This fixes the graft against the arterial wall and helps unwrinkle the fabric. When several grafts are needed to cover a long lesion, it is important to overlap the prostheses by at least 5 mm so that the fabric portion of the graft covers the entire arterial lumen. In the middle part of the femoral artery, an overlapping of 1 cm may be better to avoid disjunction of the stents.

Our Experience

Patient Population: One hundred and fifty-six patients (134 males, 22 females), mean age 63.4±10.5 years (range 38 to 88 years) were selected for treatment with the stent-graft. Risk factors included smoking (78), hypertension (57), dyslipidemia (41), and diabetes (21). Sixty-three patients had multiple vascular symptoms including cerebral, cardiac, or renal disease, 37 had prior surgical vascular intervention, and 48 had prior angioplasty. According to Rutherford's classification, 136 patients were in grade I (8 in category 2, 128 in category 3), 12 patients in grade II, and 8 in grade III (category 5). The mean ankle-brachial index (ABI) was 0.56±0.11. Three tibial vessels were patent in 72, two in 74, and one in 10 patients.

Results: Table 1 shows the locations and the types of lesions. We treated 64 iliac arteries (33 for stenoses, 18 for occlusions [Fig. 2], and 13 for aneurysms), 82 femoral arteries (28 for stenoses, 46 for occlusions [Fig. 3], and 8 for aneurysms [Fig. 4]), and 10 popliteal arteries (4 for occlusions, 1 for stenosis, and 5 for aneurysms). Ninety-three lesions were heavily calcified (21 were treated with rotational atherectomy), 17 ulcerated.

Table 1

Lesion Characteristics (1)

Location	*N.*	*Sten.*	*Occl.*	*Aneur.*	*Calc.*	*Ulcerated*
Iliac	64	33	18	13	27	10
Femoral	82	28	46	8	63	6
Popliteal	10	1	4	5	3	1
Total	156	62	68	26	93	17

Tables 2 and 3 detail the lesion characteristics including the mean lesion length, the mean percent stenosis before angioplasty and graft placement, and the mean arterial diameter. Occlusions were recanalized using either a hydrophilic guidewire (33) or Holmium laser (35). Eleven patients had a combination of Holmium laser treatment and rotational atherectomy.

The arterial approaches were as follows: retrograde femoral 64, antegrade femoral 68, and popliteal access 24. In 21 cases, the popliteal access was initially used to approach an otherwise inaccessible superficial femoral lesion. In 3 cases, the popliteal access was used after failure of the antegrade access.

A total of 266 stent-grafts were placed. Lengths ranged from 3 to 10 cm and diameters ranged from 5 to 10 mm. In 33 patients, 2 stent-grafts were placed in the same artery; 7 at the iliac and 25 at the femoral level and 1 at the popliteal level. In 17 patients, 3 stent-grafts were placed in the same superficial femoral artery to treat long occlusions or aneurysms. In 1 patient, 4 stent-grafts were placed to treat a 35-cm-long femoral aneurysm.

Indications for stent-graft placement were postangioplasty residual stenoses (n=70), dissections (n=22), restenoses (n=21), ulcerated lesions (n=17), and aneurysms (n=26).

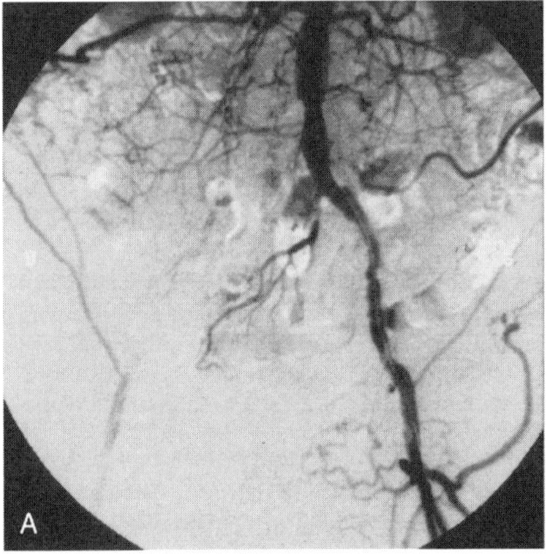

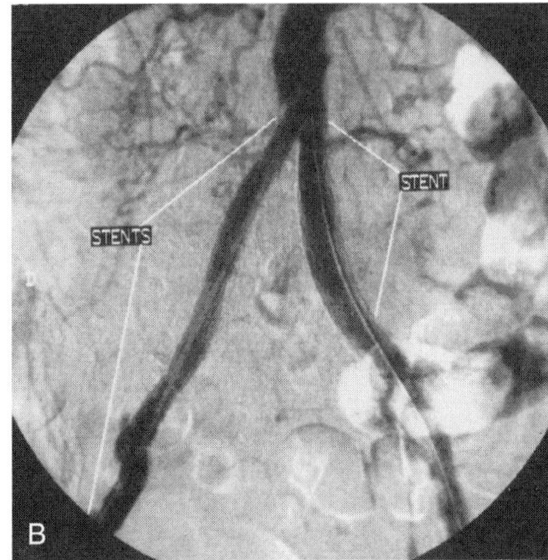

Figure 2. A. Right iliac artery thrombosis. Left iliac artery polystenosis. **B.** Placement of Cragg Endopro System 1/Passager stents.

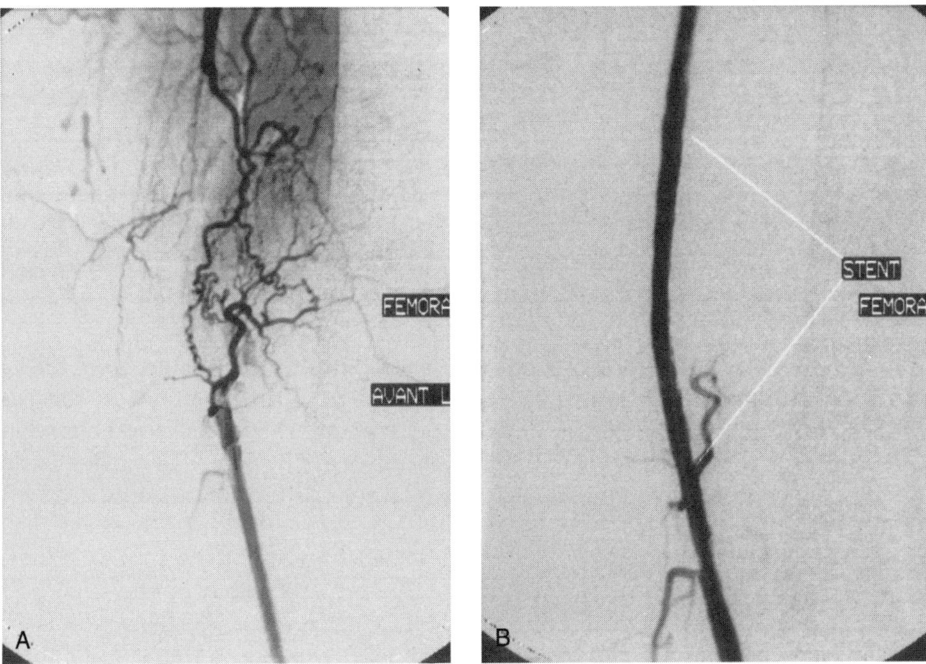

Figure 3. A. Femoral artery thrombosis. **B.** Result after recanalization and placement of Cragg Endopro System 1/Passager stents.

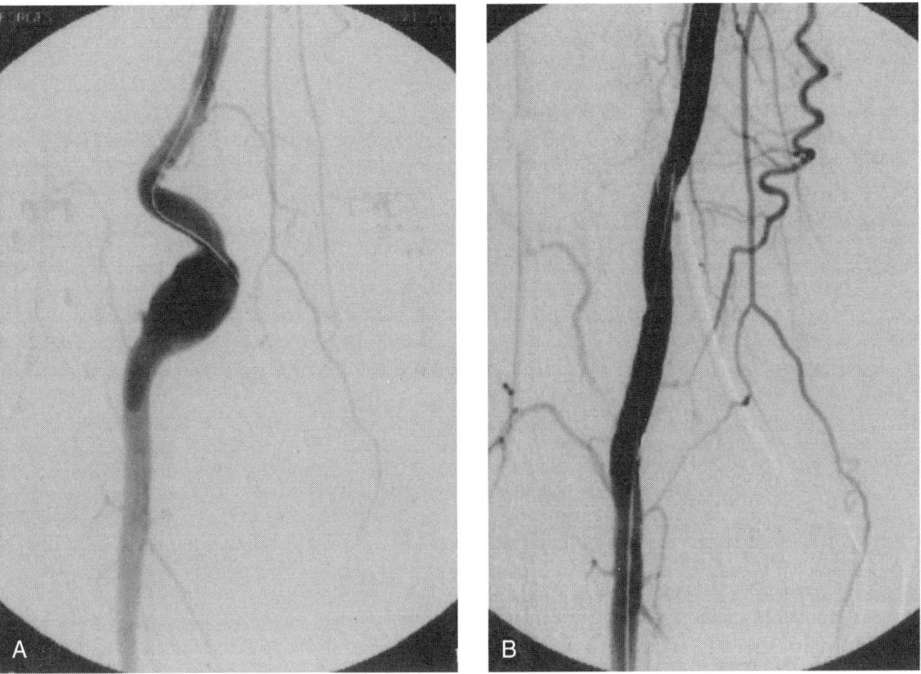

Figure 4. A. Femoropopliteal aneurysm. **B.** Result after placement of a Cragg Endopro System 1/Passager stent.

Table 2

Lesion Characteristics (2) Mean Lesion Length				
Location	*Sten.*	*Occl.*	*Aneur.*	*Range*
Iliac	52.2±26.4	86.7±36.1	38.5±13.9	20–150
Fem.	112.5±69.8	161.1±85.3	125±93.3	20–300
Pop.	80	67.5±15	114±80.5	30–200

Technical success was achieved in all cases but one at the iliac level (98%) and the femoropopliteal level (99%) (83 cases of 84). In this one case, the patient had a large femoral aneurysm, and partial success was achieved but with a persistent arterial leak at the distal part of the aneurysm. This patient was in poor general condition and died of an acute myocardial infarction 4 days after the procedure.

Postangioplasty percent stenoses decreased from 43±3.9% to 0.6±3% after stent-graft implantation, with no significant difference in the iliac and femoropopliteal location (Table 4). No significant residual stenosis was seen even in calcified lesions. The mean length of stent segments was significantly greater at the femoropopliteal level in comparison with the iliac level for occlusions and stenoses (Table 5). The mean stent-graft length for all lesions was 114.7±65.7 mm. Immediate clinical success was obtained in all uncomplicated cases with an increase in the ABI from 0.56±0.11 to 0.95±0.14. All patients were given ticlopidine (250 mg/d) and aspirin (100 mg/d) for 1 month, and aspirin alone thereafter.

Complications: In the first 30 days there were 18 major complications. At the puncture site, 5 complications occurred:

- Two hematomas, 1 requiring surgery.
- Two pseudoaneurysms both requiring surgery.

Table 3

Lesion Characteristics (3)		
Mean % stenosis before PTA		
• SFA:	93±4.1%	(70–100%)
• Iliac:	89±3.7%	(70–100%)
• Popliteal:	92±4.6%	(75–100%)
Mean arterial diameter		
• SFA:	5.95±0.6 mm	(5–7)
• Iliac:		
• Stenosis:	7.8±1.1 mm	(6–10)
• Occlusion:	7.9±1.1 mm	(7–10)
• Popliteal:	5.5±0.6 mm	(5–6)

PTA = percutaneous transluminal angiography; SFA = superficial femoral artery.

Table 4

Results (1)

	Avg. % Stenosis Before PTA	*Avg. % Stenosis After PTA*	*Avg. Stenosis After Stent*
Global pop.	92±3.7	43±3.9	0.6±0.3
Iliac	89±3.7	48±4.3	0
Fem.	93±4.3	45±3.8	0.8±0.8
Pop.	92±4.6	37±2.7	0.5±0.3

PTA = percutaneous transluminal angiography.

- One local thrombosis treated by thrombolysis.

At the iliac level, 4 complications occurred (6.2%):

- One stent-graft thrombosed within 24 hours; this was associated with distal embolization, treated by surgical thrombectomy.
- One patient who had 2 stent-grafts placed for treatment of a right iliac occlusion presented 15 days postprocedure with left leg claudication. Angiography demonstrated partial obstruction of the left common iliac artery by one of the stent-grafts, which protruded slightly into the aorta. A new stent-graft was placed in the left common iliac artery with a good result.
- Two arteries thrombosed and were treated with success by new PTA.

At the femoropopliteal level:

- One patient developed distal embolization after recanalization of an 8-cm-long femoral occlusion, treated by thrombolysis and thrombo-aspiration. This patient died of an acute myocardial infarction on the third postoperative day.
- Seven stent-graft thromboses occurred within 24 hours of the procedure. Three were treated by thrombolysis and thrombo-aspiration and 4 required surgical bypass. Five of the lesions were longer than 15 cm.
- One stent-graft thrombosis occurred on day 8, requiring surgical bypass.

Table 5

Results (2)

	Avg. Lesion Length Before Stent (mm)	*Avg. Stented Lesion Length (mm)*	*Mean % of Covering*
Global pop.	104.1	114.7	110.2
Iliac	59.2	63.8	107.8
Fem.	140.9	155.2	110.1
Pop.	92	112	121.7

Finally, a complication that appears to be directly linked with this type of endoprosthesis is the rapid development of fever along with pain in the region of the implant that can last from 2 to 3 weeks; however, no infection has been found in these cases. Consequently, the etiology of this phenomenon is still uncertain. This was observed 29 times (18.6%) : 25 times at the femoropopliteal level (occlusion n=15, stenosis n=7, aneurysm n=3) and 4 times at the iliac level (occlusion 1, stenosis 3). There could be a relation between this phenomenon and lesion length, as it appears to be more frequent as the lesion length increases; however, the condition appears to be self-limiting.

Follow-Up: All patients were followed up by duplex scan on day 180 and every 6 months thereafter. At 6 months, a follow-up angiography was performed. The maximum follow-up was 60 months, the mean follow-up 36.9±17.9 months.

Restenosis:

- At the iliac level 1 restenosis occurred outside the stent and was treated with success by new PTA.
- At the femoropopliteal level 8 patients (8.6%) developed a restenosis, regardless of the stents placed at this extremity (Fig. 5). Restenosis inside the stent was not observed. Of these 8 restenoses, 7 were treated by new angioplasty and 3 had an additional stent-graft placement. One patient was treated surgically with a bypass.

Pseudoaneurysms: In 3 patients small pseudoaneurysms were detected at the end of the stent-graft. In 2 cases they were treated by the placement of an

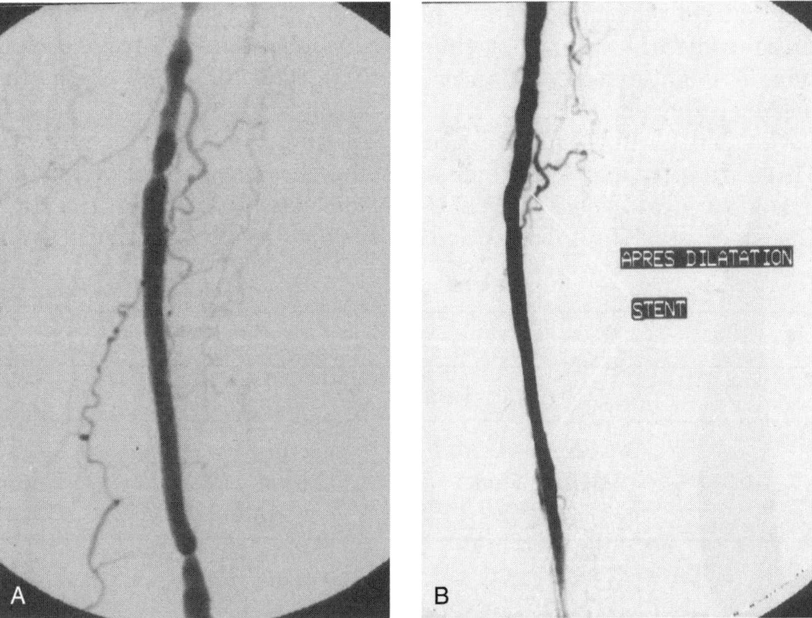

Figure 5. A. Femoral restenosis outside the stent. **B.** Result after repeat angioplasty.

additional short stent-graft. The third patient, however, was only monitored medically due to the small size of the aneurysm.

Late Thrombosis:

- At the iliac level, no late thrombosis was observed.
- At the femoropopliteal level, 18 patients (19.6%) had graft thrombosis. One was recanalized percutaneously, 3 were treated by surgical thrombectomy, 10 required bypass graft placement, and 4 refused surgery and were treated medically. Of these lesions, 12 were longer than 15 cm.

Long-Term Follow-Up: The long-term patencies at 60 months are shown in Tables 6 through 13 (primary patency and secondary patency).

The Corvita Endoluminal Graft[36–38]

Stent-Graft Construction

The Corvita Endoluminal Graft is a self-expanding endoluminal vascular prosthesis with an introducer system that makes it a low-profile device and permits percutaneous delivery and deployment.

The integrated endoluminal graft consists of two components (Fig. 6): 1) a self-expanding cylindrical wire structure, and 2) a highly porous and elastic coating of spun 13-μm thin Corethane (polycarbonate urethane; The Polymer Technology Group Inc., Berkeley, CA) fibers in which blood can coagulate and

Text continues on page 94.

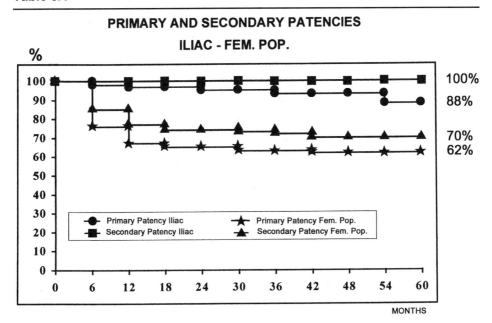

Table 6A

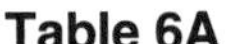

Table 6B

Primary and Secondary Patencies **Iliac-Femoropopliteal**	
60 Months	
Iliac	
Primary patency: 88%	Secondary patency: 100%
Femoropopliteal	
Primary patency: 62%	Secondary patency: 70%

Table 7A

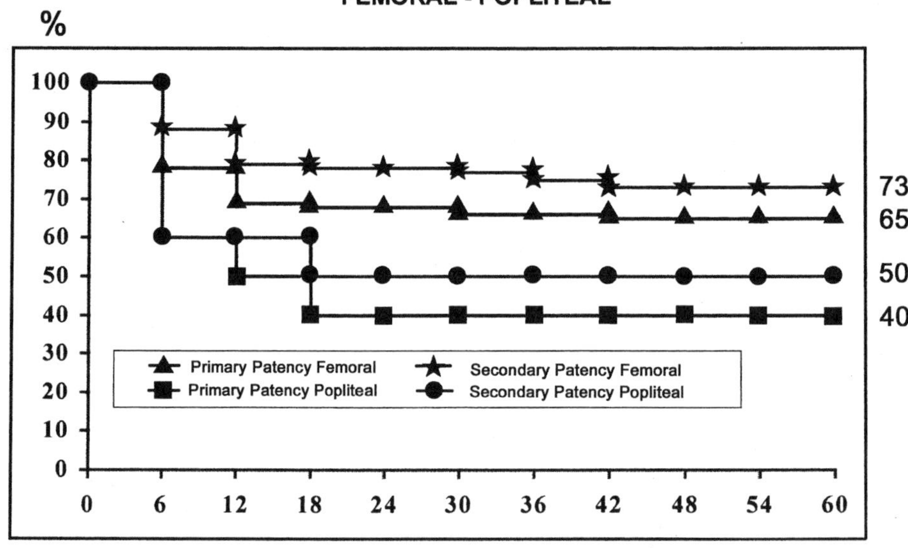

Table 7B

Primary and Secondary Patencies **Femoral—Popliteal**	
60 Months	
Femoral	
Primary patency: 65%	Secondary patency: 73%
Popliteal	
Primary patency: 40%	Secondary patency: 50%

Table 8A

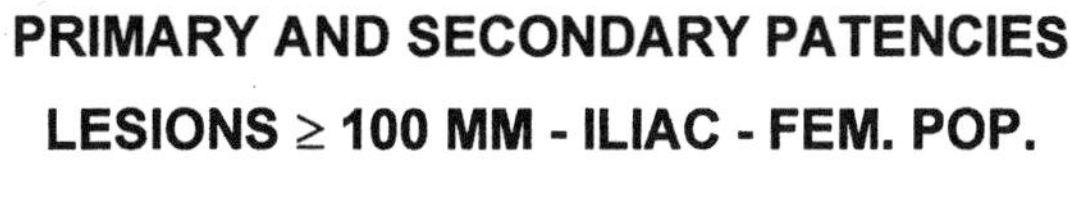

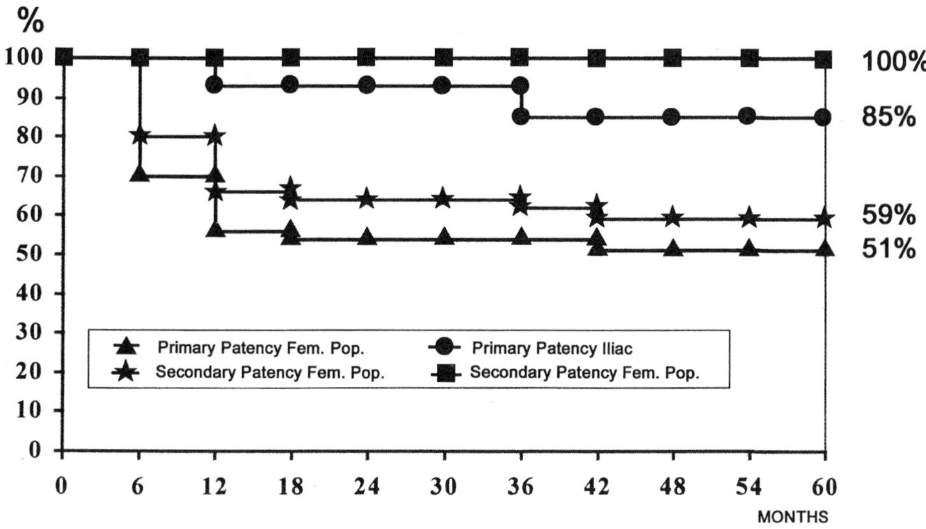

Table 8B

Primary and Secondary Patencies Lesions ≥100 mm, Iliac—Femoropopliteal	
60 Months	
Iliac	
Primary patency: 85%	Secondary patency: 100%
Femoropopliteal	
Primary patency: 51%	Secondary patency: 59%

Table 9A

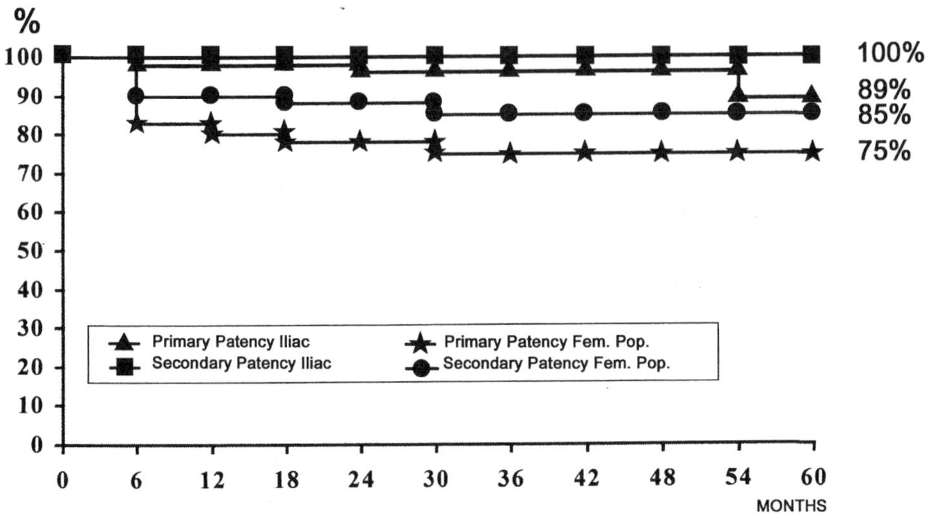

Table 9B

Primary and Secondary Patencies Lesions <100 mm, Iliac—Femoropopliteal	
60 Months	
Iliac	
Primary patency: 89%	Secondary patency: 100%
Femoropopliteal	
Primary patency: 75%	Secondary patency: 85%

Table 10A

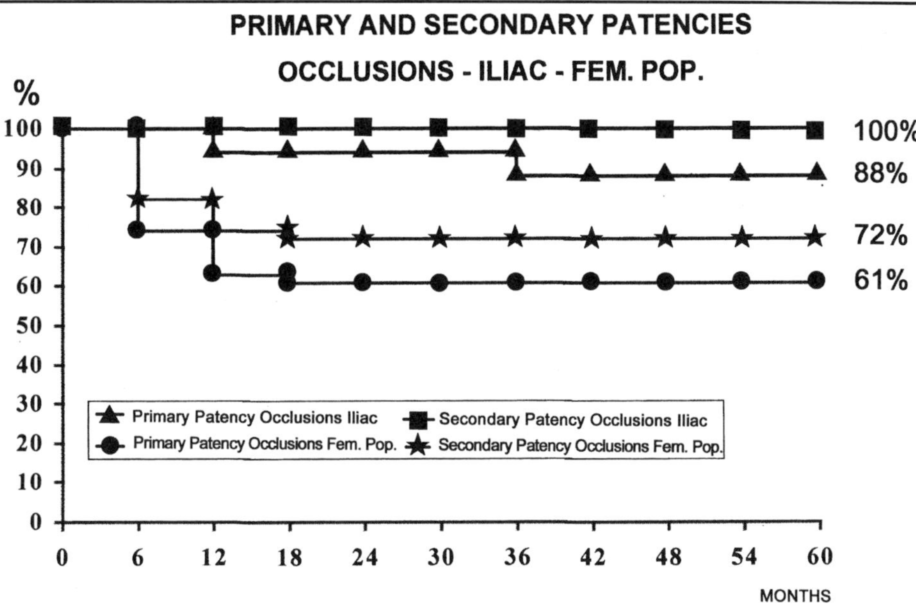

Table 10B

Primary and Secondary Patencies Occlusions, Iliac—Femoropopliteal	
60 Months	
Iliac	
Primary patency: 88%	Secondary patency: 100%
Femoropopliteal	
Primary patency: 61%	Secondary patency: 72%

Table 11A

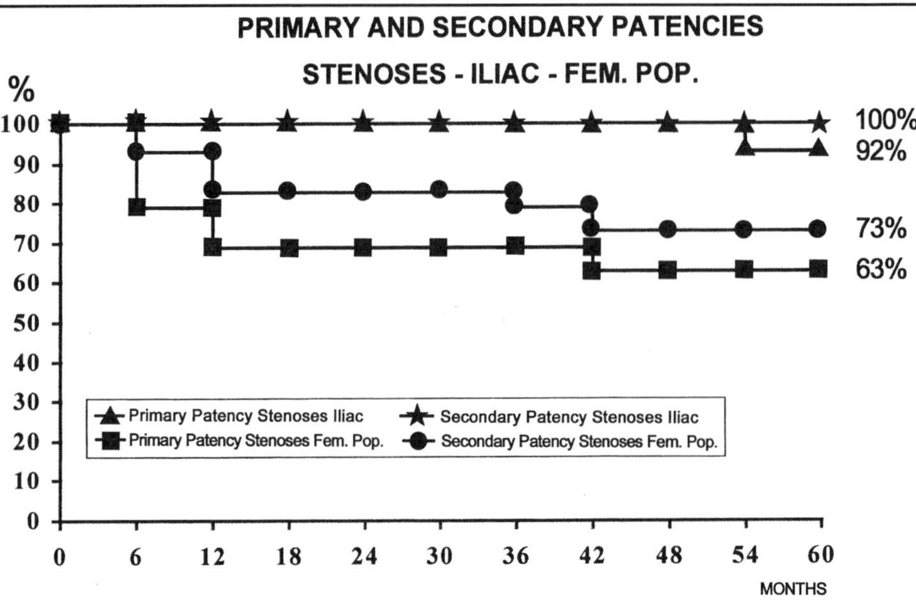

Table 11B

Primary and Secondary Patencies Stenoses, Iliac—Femoropopliteal	
60 Months	
Iliac	
Primary patency: 92%	Secondary patency: 100%
Femoropopliteal	
Primary patency: 63%	Secondary patency: 73%

Table 12A

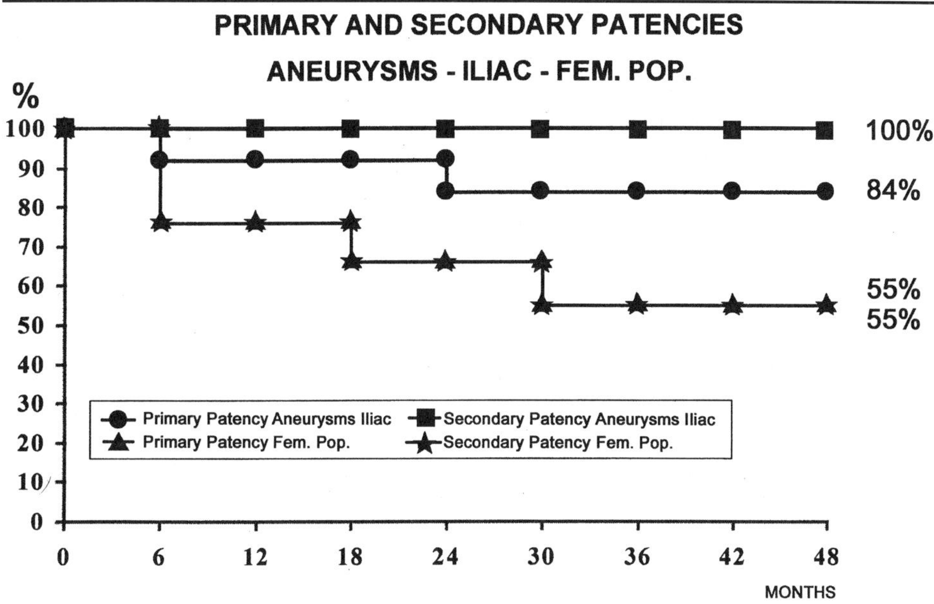

Table 12B

Primary and Secondary Patencies Aneurysms, Iliac—Femoropopliteal	
48 Months	
Iliac	
Primary patency: 84%	Secondary patency: 100%
Femoropopliteal	
Primary patency: 55%	Secondary patency: 55%

Table 13

Long-Term Patencies at 60 Months

	Primary Patency %	*Secondary Patency %*
Iliac		
Global	88	100
Lesions ≥10 cm	85	100
Lesions <10 cm	89	100
Occlusions	88	100
Stenoses	92	100
Aneurysms	84	100
Femoro-popliteal		
Global	62	70
Lesions ≥10 cm	51	59
Lesions <10 cm	75	85
Occlusions	61	72
Stenoses	63	73
Aneurysms	55	55
Femoral	65	73
Popliteal	40	50

seal the Corvita Endoluminal Graft to form a new blood-tight vessel wall. The Corethane coating is glued on the inside of the metallic structure.

Stent-Graft Implantation

The endoluminal graft can be cut to length by the user with surgical scissors and mounted in the tip of an introducer sheath. For that purpose, the Corvita Endoluminal Graft is manually compressed to one fifth or one sixth of its original, expanded diameter and simply inserted by the user into the introducer sheath. Then it is loaded into and deployed from a delivery system consisting of an internal sheath and a coaxial catheter which is introduced inside

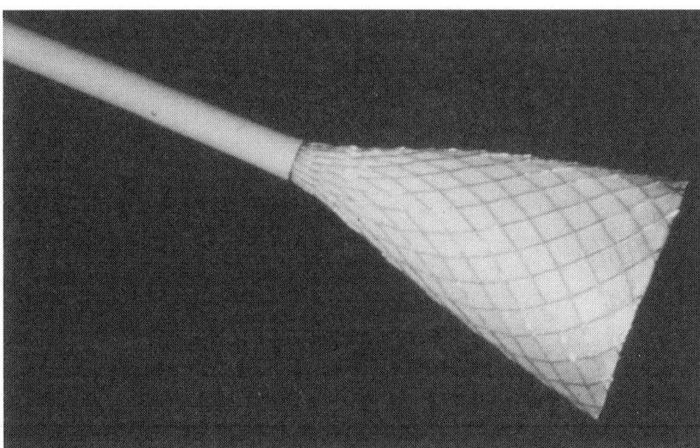

Figure 6. Corvita Endoluminal Graft.

the sheath and therefore helps to release the endoluminal graft precisely at the predetermined placement site. The introducer sheath with the compressed Corvita Endoluminal Graft in the tip can be introduced transfemorally as well as over a guidewire into the arterial system and advanced under continual fluoroscopic visualization to the site of the lesion. The Corvita Endoluminal Graft can be released from the introducer sheath at the intended site by coaxial introduction of a "holding" catheter and by slowly withdrawing the introducer sheath. The exact placement of the Corvita Endoluminal Graft can still be corrected during the initial release process. The flexibility of this device allows its implantation using various approaches such as the ipsilateral femoral, the contralateral or the popliteal approach, and in tortuous arteries.

Our Experience

Population: Sixty-four patients (51 males, 13 females), mean age 65.1±9.8 years (range 39 to 86) were treated with Corvita Endoluminal Graft. All patients presented with lower limb arterial diseases. According to Fontaine's classification, 10 were in stage IIa (patients with aneurysms), 52 were in stage IIb, and 2 were in stage III. At the distal arterial level, 6 patients had only 1 patent leg vessel, 36 had 2 patent vessels, and 22 had 3 patent vessels.

Lesion Characteristics: Table 14 summarizes the localization of the lesions following their etiology. We treated 27 stenoses (iliac n=18, femoropopliteal n=9), 20 occlusions (iliac n=8, femoropopliteal n=12), and 17 aneurysms (iliac n=12, femoropopliteal n=5). The mean length of the lesions was 80.5±55.2 mm (range 20 to 300). At the iliac level, the mean length was 60.5±28.3 (range 20 to 150) and at the femoropopliteal level it was 109.7±70.7 (range 20 to 300). Table 15 shows the average percentage of stenoses and the mean arterial diameter before PTA.

Reasons for Stenting:
- long residual stenoses: 31
- dissections: 7 (Fig. 7)

Table 14

Corvita Endoluminal Graft
Lesion Characteristics (1)

Location	*N.*	*Stenoses*	*Occlusions*	*Aneurysms*
Iliac	38	18	8	12
Femoral	22	8	12	2
Popliteal	3	–	–	3
Bypass	1	1	–	–
Total	64	27	20	17

Table 15

Corvita Endoluminal Graft
Lesion Characteristics (2)

Mean % stenosis before PTA		
• Overall population:	77.9±8.4%	(50–100)
• Iliac:	75.5±8.6%	(50–100)
• Femoropopliteal:	83.3±5.0%	(80–100)
Mean arterial diameter		
• Overall population:	8.1±1.5 mm	(5–14)
• Iliac:	8.5±1.6 mm	(7–14)
• Femoropopliteal:	7.4±1.2 mm	(5–10)

PTA = percutaneous transluminal angioplasty.

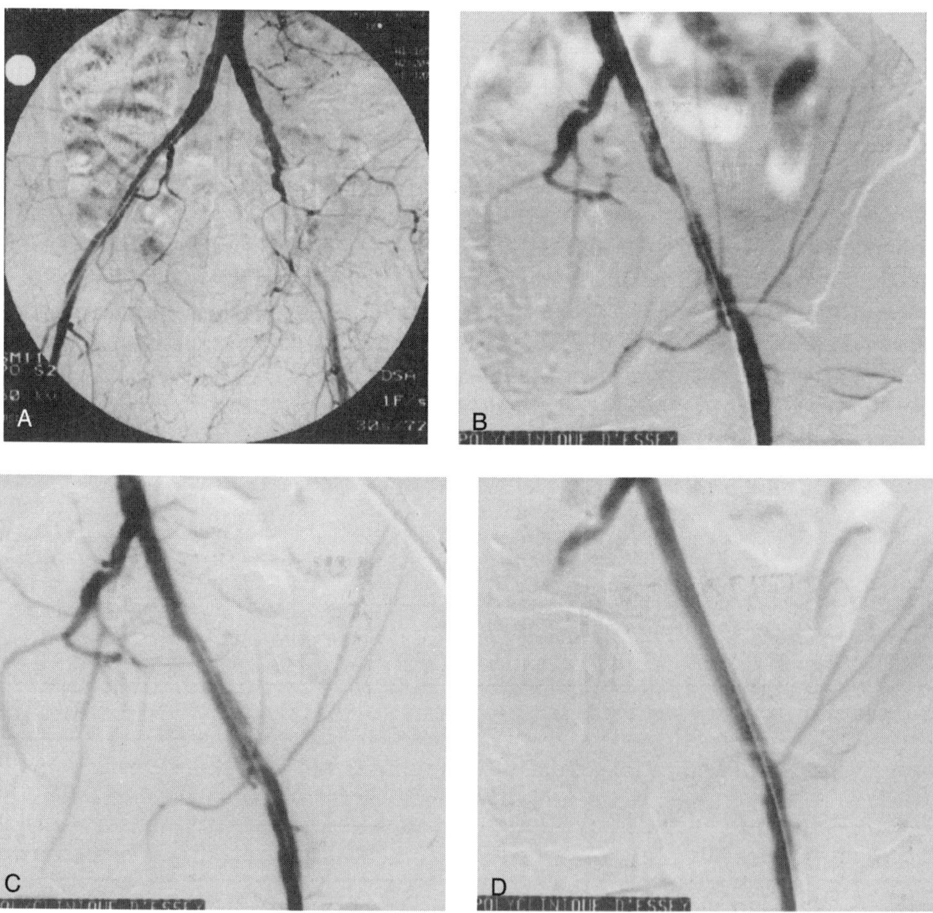

Figure 7. A. Left external iliac artery occlusion. **B.** Result after thrombolysis. **C.** Result after balloon angioplasty. **D.** Final result.

- restenoses: 6 (Fig. 8)
- ulcerated lesions: 3
- aneurysms: 17 (Figs. 9 and 10)

Technique: The lesion was always treated by the percutaneous approach with an 8F to 12F introducer through the following approaches:

- ipsilateral: 52 patients
- contralateral: 12 patients

Treatment of the Lesion: Twenty occlusions were treated either with a hydrophilic guidewire (n=11), or an excimer laser fiber (n=9). Balloon angioplasty was always performed with a balloon diameter equal to that of the artery. Twenty-seven stenoses were treated with balloon angioplasty. Seventeen aneurysms were treated. In 6 cases, an associated stenosis was treated with balloon angioplasty after placement of the Corvita Endoluminal Graft.

The Implanted Stents: Seventy-five stents were implanted (length 40 to 230 mm, diameter 5 to 14 mm). Two stents were implanted in the same artery in 5 femoral and 2 iliac arteries, and 3 stents in 2 iliac arteries.

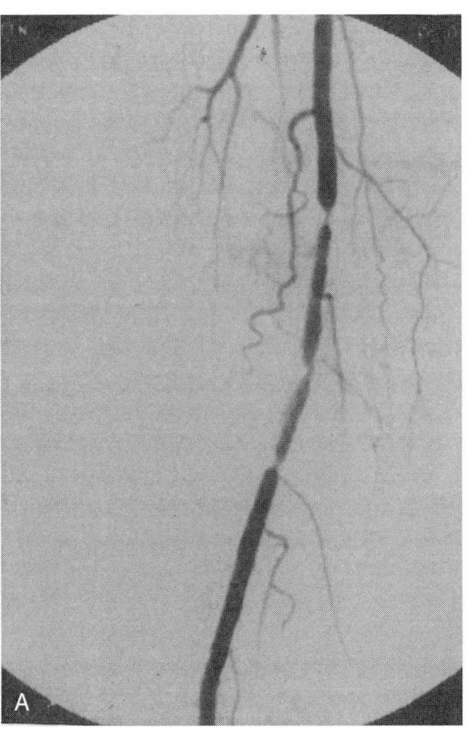

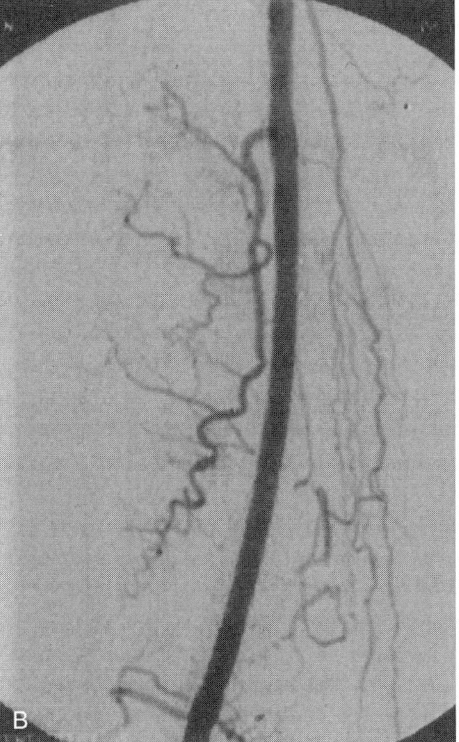

Figure 8. A. Right femoral artery restenosis in two Palmaz stents (Cordis Endovascular, a Johnson & Johnson Company, Miami Lakes, FL). **B.** Result after balloon angioplasty and implantation of a Corvita stent (10 cm long).

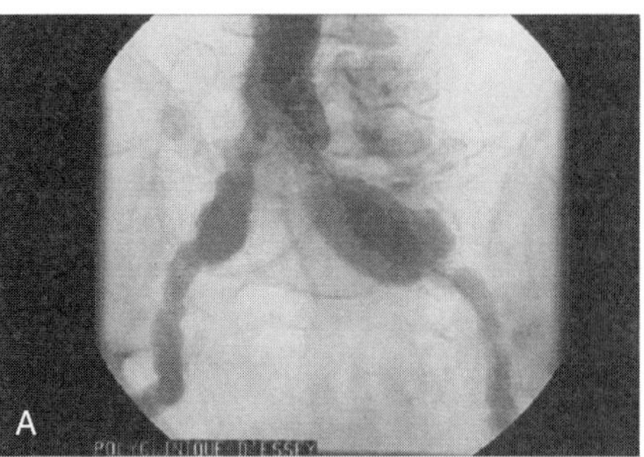

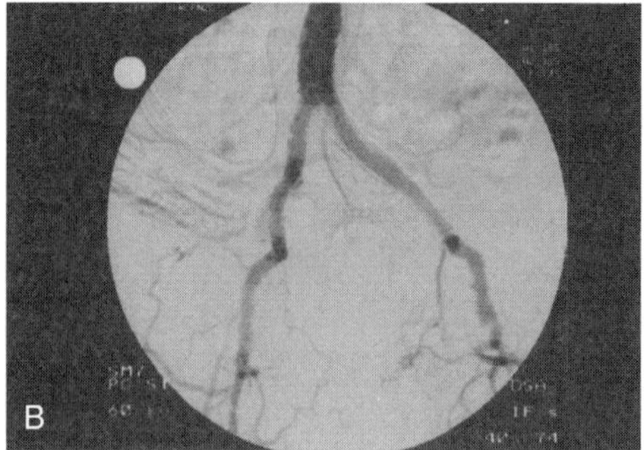

Figure 9. A. Bilateral iliac aneurysm. **B.** Result after placement of a Corvita stent.

The diameter of the stent was chosen so that it was 10% to 20% larger than the diameter of the artery. Its length was at least equal to the length of the lesion, because it is important to cover the entire length of the lesion. Also, the stent should be implanted on a safe segment.

The stent was always dilated at the end of the procedure so as to obtain a good expansion and a good anchorage to the arterial wall. An endovascular ul-

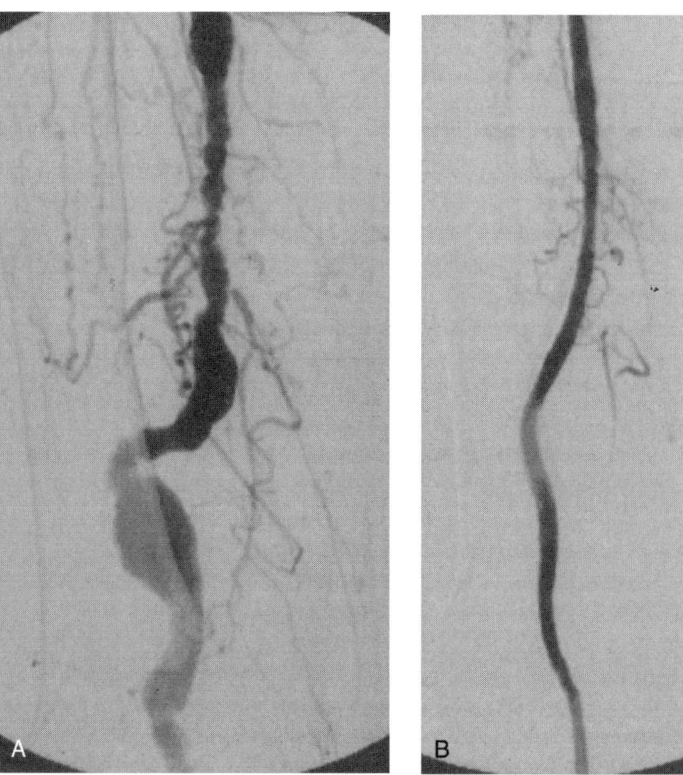

Figure 10. A. Long femoropopliteal aneurysm. **B.** Result after implantation of a Corvita stent (2.5 cm).

trasound study was performed during and at the end of the procedure in several cases to check the expansion of the stent and to look for residual lesions.

Patient Follow-Up: All patients were followed up by echo Doppler the day after the procedure, on day 30, and on day 180, and every 6 months thereafter. At 6 months, a follow-up angiography was performed.

Adjunct Treatment: All of our procedures were performed using 5000 to 10,000 units of intravenous heparin as bolus. The patients were given ticlopidine (250 mg/d), and aspirin (100 mg/d) for 1 month. Thereafter, they were given aspirin alone (250 mg/d).

Results

Immediate Results: Immediate technical success was obtained in all patients (100%). The ABI increased from 0.60±0.05 to 0.98±0.03.

Table 16 shows the mean stenosis percentage at the iliac and femoropopliteal level before and after PTA and after stenting. Significant stenosis still persisted after PTA, but there was no significant stenosis after stent placement.

Early Complications: We reported:

- Seven early thromboses:
  - ❖ Two at the iliac level: 1 after treatment of a large aneurysm, which was treated using a Fogarty catheter (Edwards Lifesciences Corp., Irvine, CA) and patency was rapidly restored, the other after treatment of a long stenosis, which was successfully treated by new PTA.
  - ❖ Four at the femoral level after treatment of lesions longer than 15 cm. Three were treated by bypass and 1 by new PTA.
- One at the popliteal level after treatment of an aneurysm; it was successfully treated by thromboaspiration and repeat angioplasty.
- One distal embolism in the deep femoral artery after treatment of an iliac aneurysm; it was successfully treated using a Fogarty catheter.

Table 16

Corvita Endoluminal Graft
Immediate Results

	Mean % Stenosis Before PTA	*Mean % Stenosis After PTA*	*Mean % Stenosis After Stenting*
Overall population	77.9±8.4	39±3.7	3.1±1.9
Iliac	75.5±8.6	41±4.2	3±2.6
Fem. Pop.	83.3±5.0	35±4.9	2±1.9

PTA = percutaneous transluminal angiography.

- Two hematomas at the puncture site that resolved spontaneously.
- One patient with two 12-cm-long prostheses in the superficial femoral artery developed a fever along with pain in the leg for 3 weeks. These prostheses thrombosed at 2 months.

Follow-Up: The maximum follow-up period of our patients was 32 months. The mean follow-up period was 20.3±10 months.

Restenosis: We reported 4 restenoses:

- Two at the iliac level: One was treated by bypass and the other was treated successfully by new PTA.
- One at the femoral level that was treated by bypass.
- One at the popliteal level that was treated by a new PTA and successful placement of an Instent (Medtronic Inc., Minneapolis, MN) stent.

In 3 patients, restenoses were located at extremities of the endoprosthesis, and 1 inside the prosthesis (iliac).

Late Thromboses: We reported 5 late thromboses:

- One at the iliac level treated by bypass.
- Three at the femoral level; 2 were treated by new PTA with success and 1 surgically (bypass).
- One at the popliteal level after treatment of an aneurysm. This patient refused surgery and was treated medically.

Long-Term Follow-Up: Primary patency and secondary patency at 3-year follow-up are listed in Table 17.

Table 17

Primary Patency and Secondary Patency at 3-Year Follow-Up

	Primary Patency %	*Secondary Patency %*
Global	74	86
Iliac		
Global	87	95
Lesion ≥10 cm	100	100
Lesion <10 cm	85	94
Stenosis	83	94
Occlusion	88	88
Aneurysm	92	100
Femoropopliteal		
Global	55	72
Lesion ≥10 cm	55	64
Lesion <10 cm	54	82
Stenosis	78	78
Occlusion	31	64
Aneurysm	57	78

Hemobahn: Results of a Multicenter Feasibility Study[39]

The Prograft Hemobahn is a self-expanding endovascular stent-graft composed of 30-μ internodal ultrathin wall polytetrafluoroethylene graft on the inner surface and a self-expanding Nitinol stent on the outer surface. These devices have excellent flexibility in both the deployed and nondeployed states, excellent kink resistance, and good radial stiffness. Devices available in the initial study ranged from 4.5 to 12 mm in diameter with lengths from 5 to 15 cm.

An initial feasibility study addressing iliac and femoral artery occlusive disease was performed at 3 investigational sites in the US and in 12 European centers. In total, 93 patients had 100 lesions treated (iliac 58, femoral 42). The current mean implant duration was 5.4 months. The primary technical success in this group was 99%. The primary and secondary iliac patency at 1 month (n=49), 3 months (n=43), and 6 months (n=24), was 96% at all intervals. The primary patency for treated femoral arteries at 1 month (n=37), 3 months (n=24), and 6 months (n=7) was 100%, 91%, and 80%, respectively. The corresponding secondary patency in the femoral region was 100%, 94%, and 82% at 1 month, 3 months, and 6 months of follow-up.

Procedure-related complications have included distal embolization in 5%, groin hematoma in 2%, and iliac artery rupture in 1%. The latter case was successfully managed with deployment of a second stent-graft without clinical sequelae.

The Wallgraft

This prosthesis (Figs. 11 and 12) consists of a Wallstent coated with polyester yarn (PET). The available diameters range from 6 to 12 mm, and the lengths from 5 to 7 cm. Its flexibility allows use in tortuous arteries and even through a contralateral approach. Its shortening, however, may render precise placement difficult. We have used this prosthesis in the iliac and femoral arteries.

Indications of this device for treatment of occlusive disease are at best unclear, and await availability of outcome data from well-controlled clinical studies.

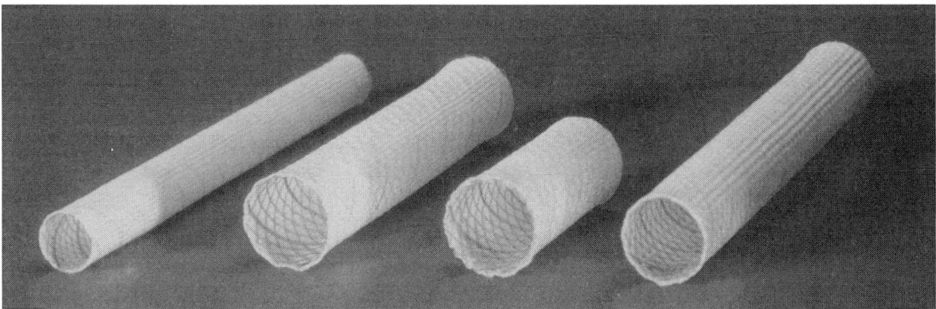

Figure 11. The Wallgraft stent.

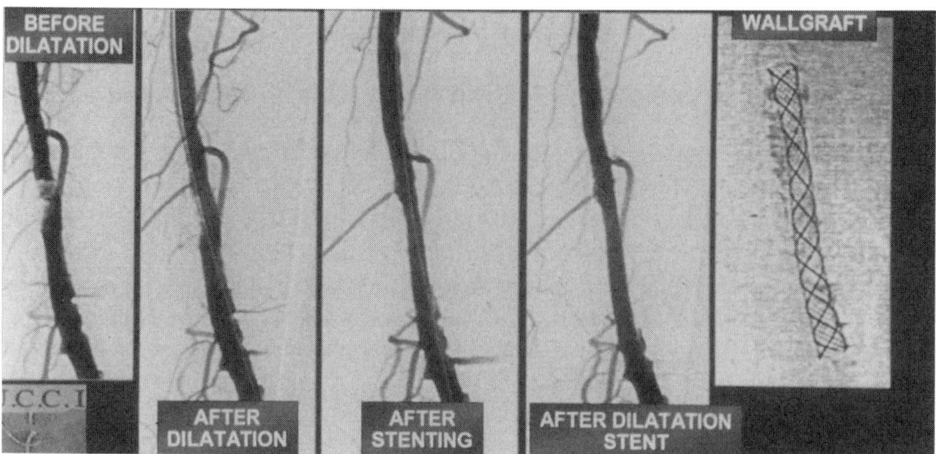

Figure 12. Calcified stenosis of the left superficial femoral artery. Result after dilatation and placement of a Wallgraft stent.

The Jostent Stent

The Josent stent (Figs. 13 and 14) is a balloon-expandable prosthesis that recently became available. It is available in lengths ranging from 28 to 58 mm and its expansion diameter ranges from 5 to 10 mm. It consists of a double thin stainless steel prosthesis. There is a polytetrafluoroethylene coating between the two prostheses.

We have successfully implanted it with success in the iliac and femoral arteries in 20 patients with the same indications as for other covered stents. A popliteal implantation in a flexion area such as the popliteal artery should be avoided because of potential compression. Follow-up is too short for a better appreciation. Longer term follow-up and larger series are expected.

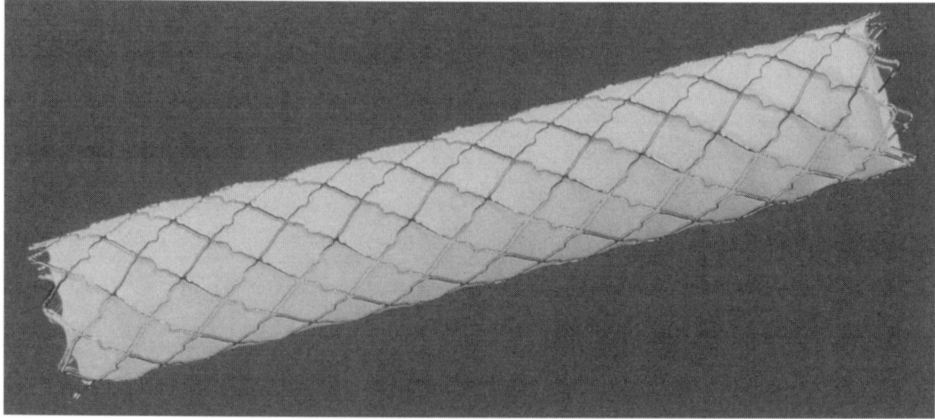

Figure 13. The Jostent peripheral stent-graft.

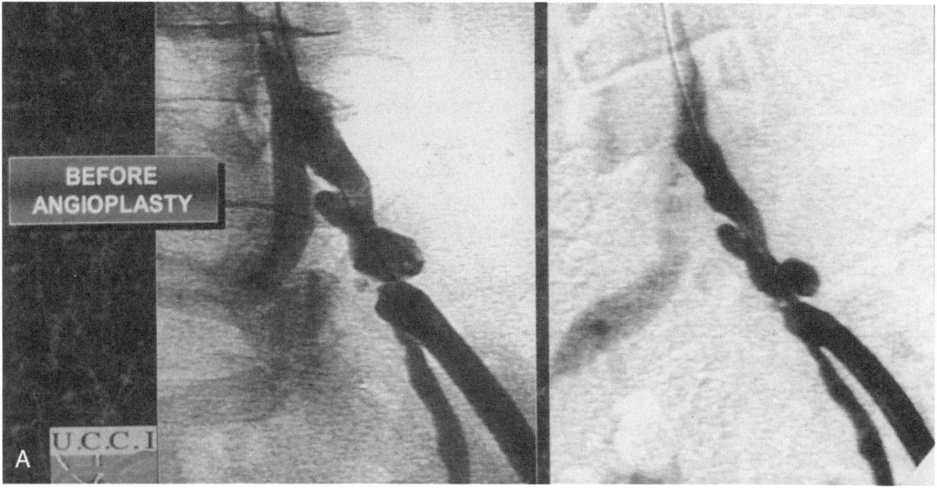

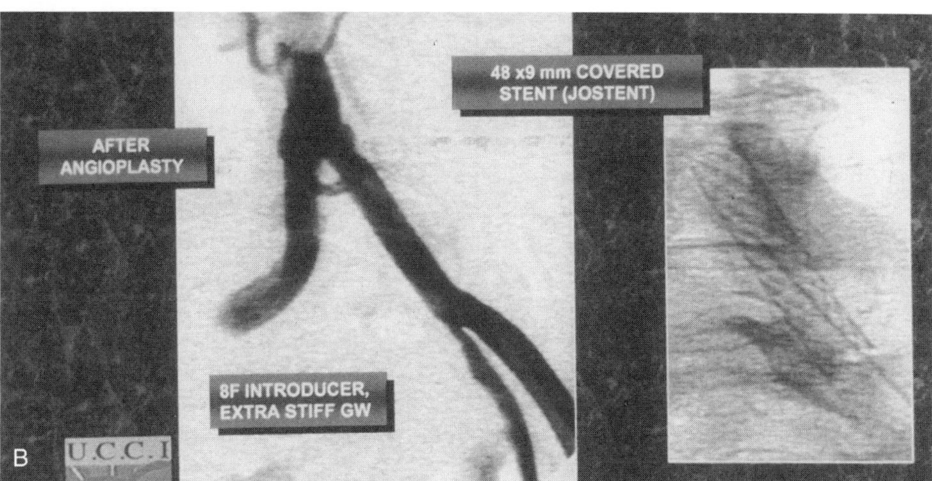

Figure 14. A. Stenosis and ulceration in the left iliac artery. **B.** Result after angioplasty and placement of a Jostent stent.

Discussion

PTA is still the most common method for percutaneous revascularization of peripheral arterial occlusive disease. Long-term results are now available for this treatment modality. In general, patients with short lesions in larger vessels (>6 mm diameter) do well, with restenosis rates of less than 30% at 1 year. It is also known, however, that patients with long lesions (>10 cm), particularly in the superficial femoral artery, or patients with poor initial angioplasty results, such as dissection, do much worse, with patency rates as low as 20% at 5 years.[40–43] Restenosis rates are also lower in concentric lesions instead of eccentric nonostial stenoses and higher in ostial lesions and occlusions (given equal lesion length and for claudication rather than for limb salvage).

Alternative revascularization methods such as laser and atherectomy have not, in general, improved the midterm patency of long occlusive lesions.[44–48] Owing to these results, endoprostheses have been placed at different levels to deal with acute problems of angioplasty to try to improve the long term-results. In the iliac artery, intraluminal noncovered stents have been shown to improve the midterm patency compared to traditional PTA.[5,13,14,49–51]

Implantation of prostheses of the Palmaz or Wallstent type in these arteries has become an efficient method of treatment. Long-term results are good although they are less favorable for long lesions.[51]

Use of conventional stents at the femoropopliteal level is more controversial and is limited because of long lengths of the lesion, smaller arterial diameters, and exposed nature of the femoral artery, which may lead to the compression of rigid stents.

Favorable results were reported for short lesions and particularly for lesions in the upper and middle part of the superficial femoral artery.[18,49,52] In general, the results depended on the length of the lesions and the number of stents placed, with patencies dropping as both of these factors increased.

Long segment covered stents or stent-grafts have a role in the endoluminal treatment of peripheral vascular occlusive diseases and peripheral aneurysms. Since the concept of vascular stenting was first presented, a number of techniques have been proposed and developed to treat lesions at the iliac, femoral, and popliteal levels and aneurysms.[4,19,20,22–32,53–58]

In the iliac artery, the use of endoprostheses may be not considered as a determining factor except for long and/or ulcerated aneurysms and/or after recanalization. In our series, the iliac lesions were longer (5 to 9 cm) than those of series that are usually reported with noncovered stents. Despite the length of the segments, primary and secondary patencies were excellent, regardless of the prosthesis used.

In femoropopliteal arteries, covered prostheses were used for long lesions greater than 10 cm (3 to 4 times longer than noncovered endoprostheses). The results obtained with these long covered endoprostheses in femoropopliteal arteries are still linked with high thrombotic complication rates. These complications were usually treated by an interventional technique (thrombolysis or angioplasty). The secondary patency therefore remains satisfactory with regard to the treated lesions. However, the results seem more favorable for lesions smaller than 10 cm, and also more favorable for femoral lesions than for popliteal lesions. The use of covered endoprostheses in femoropopliteal arteries is therefore crucial, first, in the interest represented by the use of the stent itself, and second, for the surface it covers. The stent portion of the device provides mechanical enlargement of the arterial lumen. The stent-graft is flexible and expandable so that compression and moderate bending in the femoropopliteal segment do not compromise the integrity of the graft. Since the stent is fully supported, kinking and external compression, which can occur with a rigid stent, do not happen with these prostheses. The graft covering acts as a barrier to smooth muscle ingrowth. In this fashion, a true endoluminal bypass can be created.

Nevertheless, restenosis is still possible despite this type of stent. With the Cragg Endopro System 1 or Passager, we have only seen restenoses at the extremities of the prosthesis, which could be easily dilated, whereas with the

Corvita Endoluminal Graft, in-stent restenoses were possible due to its greater porosity.

Our technique for graft placement has evolved with our experience. The following are important points that we have learned during our initial stent-graft experience. Prior to stent-graft implantation, the target lesion should be predilated with a balloon approximately 1 mm larger than the nominal arterial diameter. In some cases, such as calcified lesions, rotational atherectomy may be useful to debulk the arteries. It is important to cover the entire lesion with the stent-graft and, if possible, to implant a sufficiently long stent-graft so that both ends are implanted in a relatively normal segment of the artery. Angioplasty should not be performed outside of the target lesion, to avoid restenosis. Accurate placement of the endoprosthesis can be obtained with the Cragg Endopro System1/Passager and the Hemobahn, due to the minimal shortening, but can sometimes be difficult with the Corvita Endoluminal Graft, because its distal end may be precisely placed but its proximal end may not because of its significant shortening during its expansion. After stent implantation, it is important to dilate the stent-graft to its nominal diameter. This helps to fully expand the stent and to remove any wrinkles in the fabric that may have occurred during compression and delivery of the graft. When long lesions must be treated with several prostheses, grafts should overlap approximately 5 to 10 mm to prevent them from separating from each other. Separation may lead to a false aneurysm that could thrombose, as had happened in one of our cases with the Corvita Endoluminal Graft.

In our experience, better results were obtained with the placement of the stent-graft in the iliac artery versus the femoropopliteal arteries. A number of short-term and midterm thrombotic episodes have occurred that may be related to the thrombogenic nature of the graft, poor flow during ipsilateral compression after sheath removal, inadequate anticoagulation, or other factors. Generally, these episodes were readily treated with a secondary interventional technique such as thrombolysis, mechanical thrombectomy, and PTA. The global secondary patency for these endoprostheses may be considered as encouraging due to the length of the lesions, regardless of the graft used. Nonetheless, significant improvements must be made in the short- and midterm patency of longer endoluminal grafts. Issues that must be addressed include the short-term thrombogenicity of the implanted graft and the development of restenosis at the ends of the graft. A powerful antiaggregant protocol associating ticlopidine and aspirin given several days before the procedure seems to have limited early thromboses. In the future, pharmacologic or radiation inhibitors of intimal hyperplasia may allow a broader application of these devices for long segment revascularization of the peripheral arterial circulation.

The treatment of aneurysms with covered stents in the iliac and femoropopliteal arteries seems rather easy. The results of our series are very favorable at the iliac level but less favorable at the femoropopliteal level, regardless of the graft used. The simplicity of their use should make these covered grafts the treatment of choice for aneurysmal lesions. We wish to insist that even after a stent occlusion at the femoropopliteal level, there have been no serious ischemic complications or limb loss in our experience.

The phenomenon of pain and fever encountered after implantation of Cragg Endopro System/Passager is a complication that we still do not fully understand. The phenomenon does not seem to be related to local infection, but it is clearly an inflammatory response to graft implantation.[59] It is likely that the stent-graft itself or one of its fabric or metal components may be an inducer of cytokinins from neutrophils.[59]

The indications for covered stents are still debated; however, the following indications are not debatable:

- aneurysms
- arteriovenous fistulae
- arterial traumas
- arterial rupture

Covered stents should be available in all catheterization laboratories in order to quickly treat arterial ruptures that may occur during an angioplasty procedure and thus avoid surgical repair.

Certain indications are more questionable:

- long occlusions or stenoses
- long dissections

We have obtained excellent results with certain prostheses at the iliac level and we think that their indications are licit at this level. And yet, implantation of a covered stent at the femoropopliteal level is more debatable, taking into account the rather high rates of occlusion.

One should, however, keep in mind the very high restenosis rates obtained with some noncovered stents for the treatment of femoropopliteal lesions of more than 5 cm (Wallgraft, for instance). Results obtained with covered stents seem encouraging and the use of new prostheses, with lower embolic risks, should allow the treatment of long lesions with success rates and results that are at least as good as those obtained with surgery. Results obtained with the Hemobahn seem promising. New antiplatelet agents will probably improve long-term patencies.

Conclusion

Covered endoprostheses allow the operator to perform true internal bypass using the percutaneous access. The indications for their use should broaden and they could become an alternative to surgery. Improvements should come about, particularly with respect to thrombogenicity and the method of implantation. Randomized studies versus surgery and other types of stents are expected in order to confirm the interest of these new prostheses and their place as compared to noncovered prostheses.

References

1. Johnston KW. Femoral and popliteal arteries: Reanalysis of results of balloon angioplasty. *Radiology* 1992;183:767–771.

2. Capek P, McLean GK, Berkowitz HD. Femoropopliteal angioplasty. Factors influencing long-term success. *Circulation* 1991;83(suppl I):I70-I80.
3. Moore WS. Therapeutic options for femoropopliteal occlusive disease. *Circulation* 1991;83(suppl I):I91-I93.
4. Dotter CT. Transluminally placed coil-spring endarterial tube grafts: Long-term patency in canine popliteal artery. *Invest Radiol* 1969;329–332.
5. Richter GM, Roeren TH, Loeldge G, et al. Superior clinical results of iliac stent placement versus percutaneous transluminal angioplasty: Four-years success rates of a randomized study. *Radiology* 1991;181(suppl):161. Abstract.
6. Henry M, Amor M, Ethevenot G, et al. Palmaz-Schatz stent in the treatment of peripheral vascular diseases: Two year follow up. A single center experience. *Circulation* 1992;86:4. Abstract.
7. Henry M, Amor M, Ethevenot G, et al. Le stent de Palmaz dans le traitement des artériopathies périphériques. *Techno Coeur* 1993;117–130.
8. Schatz RA. A view of vascular stents. *Circulation* 1989;79:445–457.
9. Palmaz JC. Intravascular stents: Tissue-stent interactions and design considerations. *AJR Am J Roentgenol* 1993;160:613–618.
10. Parsson H, Cwikiel W, Johansson K, et al. Deposition of platelets and neutrophils in porcine iliac arteries after angioplasty and Wallstent placement compared with angioplasty alone. *Cardiovasc Intervent Radiol* 1994;17:190–196.
11. Hallisey MJ, Parker BC, von Breda A. Current status and extended applications of intravascular stents. *Curr Opin Radiol* 1992;4:7–12.
12. Palmaz JC, Garcia OJ, Schatz RA, et al. Placement of balloon-expandable intraluminal stents in iliac arteries: First 171 procedures. *Radiology* 1990;174:969–975.
13. Raillat C, Rousseau H, Joffre F, et al. Treatment of iliac artery stenoses with the Wallstent endoprosthesis. *AJR Am J Roentgenol* 1990;154:613–616.
14. Zollikofer CL, Antonuci F, Pfyffer M, et al. Arterial stent placement with the use of the Wallstent: Midterm results of clinical experience. *Radiology* 1991;179:449–456.
15. Hausegger KA, Lammer J, Hagen B, et al. Iliac artery stenting. Clinical experience with the Palmaz stent, Wallstent and Strecker stent. *Acta Radiol* 1992;292–296.
16. White GH, Liew SCC, Waugh RC, et al. Early outcome and intermediate follow-up of vascular stents in the femoral and popliteal arteries without long-term anticoagulation. *J Vasc Surg* 1995;21:270–281.
17. Bray AE, Liu WG, Lewis WA, et al. Use of the Strecker stent in the femoropopliteal arteries. *J Endovasc Surg* 1995;2:150–160.
18. Bergeron P, Pinot JJ, Poyen V, et al. Long-term results with the Palmaz stent in the superficial femoral artery. *J Endovasc Surg* 1995;2:161–167.
19. Cragg AH, Lund G, Rysavy JA, et al. Nonsurgical placement of arterial endoprostheses: A new technique using nitinol wire. *Radiology* 1983;147:261–283.
20. Cragg AH, Lund G, Rysavy JA, et al. Percutaneous arterial grafting. *Radiology* 1984;150:45–49.
21. Cragg AH, De Jong SC, Barnhart WH, et al. Nitinol intravascular stent: Results of pre-clinical evaluation. *Radiology* 1993;189:775–778.
22. Cragg AH, Dake MD. Percutaneous femoropopliteal graft placement. *J Vasc Intervent Radiol* 1993;4:445–463.
23. Parodi JC. Endovascular repair of abdominal aortic aneurysms and other arterial lesions. *J Vasc Surg* 1995;21:549–557.
24. Diethrich EB, Papazoglou CO, Lundquist P, et al. Early experience with aneurysm exclusion devices and endoluminal bypass prostheses. *J Intervent Cardiol* 1994;7:108–109. Abstract.
25. Diethrich EB, Papazoglou CO, Rodriguez-Lopez J, et al. Endoluminal grafts for percutaneous aneurysm exclusion and intraluminal bypass. *Circulation* 1994;90:I206.
26. Papazoglou C, Lopez-Galarza L, Rodriguez-Lopez J, et al. Endoluminal grafting: The Arizona Heart Institute experience. *J Endovasc Surg* 1995;2:89–90. Abstract.
27. Diethrich EB, Papazoglou CO. Endoluminal grafting for aneurysmal and occlusive disease in the superficial femoral artery: Early experience. *J Endovasc Surg* 1995;2:225–239.
28. Papazoglou C, Diethrich EB, Lopez-Galarza L, et al. Percutaneous endoluminal

grafting for iliofemoral aneurysmal and occlusive disease. *J Vasc Intervent Radiol* 1995;6:40. Abstract.

29. Marin ML, Veith FJ, Cynamon J, et al. Transfemoral endovascular stented graft treatment of aortoiliac and femoropopliteal occlusive disease for limb salvage. *Am J Surg* 1994;168:156–162.
30. Bergeron P. Stenting and endoluminal grafting of femoral and popliteal arteries. *J Endovasc Surg* 1995;2:197–198. Abstract.
31. Bray A. Superficial femoral endarterectomy with intra-arterial PTFE grafting. *J Endovasc Surg* 1995;2:297–301.
32. Sanchez LA, Marin ML, Veith FJ, et al. Placement of endovascular stented grafts via remote access sites: A new approach to the treatment of failed aortoiliofemoral reconstructions. *Am Vasc Surg* 1995;9:1–8.
33. Henry M, Amor M, Ethevenot G, et al. Initial experience with the Cragg Endopro System 1 for intraluminal treatment of peripheral vascular disease. *J Endovasc Surg* 1994;1:31–43.
34. Henry M, Amor M, Cragg A, et al. Occlusive and aneurysmal peripheral arterial disease: Assessment of a stent-graft system. *Radiology* 1996;201:717–724.
35. Henry M, Amor M, Henry I, et al. Application d'une nouvelle endoprothèse couverte au traitement des artériopathies périphériques occlusives et anévrismales. *Arch Mal Coeur* 1997;90:953–960.
36. Donayre CE, Scoccianti M. Applications in peripheral vascular surgery: Traumatic arteriovenous fistulas and pseudoaneurysms. In Chuter TAM, Donayre CE, White R (eds): *Endoluminal Vascular Prostheses*. Boston: Little, Brown and Company; 1995:217–255.
37. Dereume JP, Ferreira J, El Douaihy M, et al. Clinical experience with an integrated self-expandable stented graft (Corvita) for the treatment of various arterial lesions. In Veith FJ (ed): *Current Critical Problems in Vascular Surgery, Vol. 6*. St. Louis: Quality Medical Publishing Inc; 1995.
38. Dereume JP. Clinical experience with a self-expanding endoluminal vascular prosthesis. Presented at: Symposium of Vascular Surgery; September 1–2, 1995; Berlin, Germany.
39. Dake MD, Semba CP, Kee ST, et al. Hemobahn: Results of a multicenter feasibility study. Presented at: International Symposium on Vascular Diagnosis and Intervention. January 11–15, 1998; Miami, FL.
40. Krepel K, Vanadel T, Van Erp F, et al. Percutaneous angioplasty of the femoropopliteal artery: Initial and long-term results. *Radiology* 1985;156:325–328.
41. Jeans WD, Armstrong S, Colese A, et al. Fate of patients undergoing transluminal angioplasty for lower-limb ischemia. *Radiology* 1990;177:559–564.
42. Murray RR, Hewes RC, White RL, et al. Long segment femoropopliteal diseases: Is angioplasty a boon or a bust? *Radiology* 1987;162:473–476.
43. Capek P, McLean GK, Berkowitz HD. Femoropopliteal angioplasty: Factors influencing long-term results. *Circulation* 1991;83(suppl O):170–180.
44. Cragg AH, Gardiner GA, Smith TP. Vascular applications of laser. *Radiology* 1989;172:925–935.
45. Henry M, Amor M, Ethevenot G. L'angioplastie périphérique par laser saphir de contact. Expérience à propos de 113 lésions ilio-fémorales. *Techno Coeur* 1992:35–44.
46. Huppert PE, Duda SH, Helbert U, et al. Comparison of pulsed laser assisted angioplasty in femoropopliteal occlusions. *Radiology* 1992;184:363–367.
47. Katzen BT, Becker GJ, Benenati JF, et al. Long-term follow-up of directional atherectomy in the femoral and popliteal arteries. *J Vasc Intervent Radiol* 1992;3:38–39.
48. Henry M, Amor M, Ethevenot G. Percutaneous peripheral rotational ablation using the Rotablator: Immediate and mid-term results. Single center experience concerning 146 lesions treated. *Int Angiol* 1993:231–244.
49. Martin EC, Katzen BT, Benenati JF, et al. Multicenter trial of the Wallstent in the iliac and femoral arteries. *J Vasc Interv Radiol* 1995;6:843–849.
50. Sapoval MR, Chatellier G, Long AL, et al. Self-expandable stents for the treatment

of iliac artery obstructive lesions: Long term success and prognostic factors. *AJR Am J Roentgenol* 1996;166:1173–1179.
51. Murphy TP, Webb MS, Hass RA, et al. Percutaneous revascularization of complex iliac artery stenoses and occlusions with use of Wallstents: Three-year experience. *J Vasc Interv Radiol* 1996;7:21–27.
52. Henry M, Amor M, Ethevenot G, et al. Palmaz stent placement in iliac and femoropopliteal arteries: Primary and secondary patency in 310 patients with 2–4 years follow-up. *Radiology* 1995;197:167–174.
53. Dotter CT, Buschmann RW, McKinney MK, et al. Transluminal expandable nitinol coil stent grafting: Preliminary report. *Radiology* 1983;147:259–260.
54. Balko A, Piasecki GI, Shah DM, et al. Transfemoral placement of intraluminal polyurethane prosthesis for abdominal aortic aneurysm. *J Surg Res* 1986;40:305–309.
55. Volodos NL, Shekhanin VE, Karpovich IP, et al. Self-fixing synthetic prosthesis for endoprosthetics of the vessels. *Vestn Khir Im II Grek* 1986;137:123–125.
56. Parodi JC, Palmaz JC, Barone HD. Transfemoral intraluminal graft implantation for abdominal aortic aneurysms. *Ann Vasc Surg* 1991;5:491–499.
57. Parodi JC, Criado FJ, Barone HD, et al. Endoluminal aortic aneurysm repair using a balloon-expandable stent-graft device: A progress report. *Ann Vasc Surg* 1994;8:523–529.
58. Laborde JC, Parodi JC, Clem MF, et al. Intraluminal bypass of abdominal aortic aneurysm: Feasibility study. *Radiology* 1992;184:185–190.
59. Hayoz D, DoDai DO, Mahler F, et al. Acute inflammatory reaction associated with endoluminal bypass grafts. *J Endovasc Surg* 1997;4:354–360.

7

Endoluminal Treatment of Extensive Disease in the Superficial Femoral Artery:

The Remote Endarterectomy

Joep A.W. Teijink, MD, PhD, Robin H. Heijmen, MD, PhD, Jos C. van den Berg, MD, PhD, and Frans L. Moll, MD, PhD

Introduction

Compared to other similar sized arteries, the superficial femoral artery (SFA) appears to have a high affinity for atherosclerotic disease. Differences in hydrostatic pressures, marked variations in flow rate depending on physical activity, and mechanical trauma caused by the adductor magnus tendon are possible explanations for this phenomenon.

The existing alternatives for venous femoropopliteal bypass surgery for treatment of occlusions or multiple stenosed segments in the SFA are disappointing, in both primary technical success rate and patency after successful recanalization or bypass surgery. Green et al[1] recently showed that both polyester and expanded polytetrafluoroethylene (ePTFE) above-knee femoropopliteal bypass grafts have primary and secondary patency rates at 5 years of 45% and 68%, respectively. Given this, venous bypass surgery may be considered the first option of treatment; however, many surgeons believe that for the above-knee bypass it is better to spare autologous venous material for future cardiovascular or peripheral surgery. Finally, there is a group of patients who have no available venous material of sufficient quality to perform a peripheral bypass.

The introduction of a new technique becomes of interest when it has at least comparable results to existing techniques, as well as added patient bene-

From Criado FJ (ed): *Endovascular Intervention: New Tools and Techniques for the 21st Century.* Armonk, NY: Futura Publishing Co., Inc.; ©2002.

fit. The final decision for the intervention of preference will be based on the durability of the procedure, life expectancy, and general condition of the patient. In the last decade several alternative techniques were introduced, some of which have already been abandoned.

Conservative Treatment

The majority of patients with stable intermittent claudication can be treated in a conservative way. Cessation of smoking, regular exercise, and weight loss are the cornerstones of treatment, supplemented by antiplatelet and lipid-lowering therapy as well as strict regulation of diabetes (if applicable).

Most patients with intermittent claudication who are treated in this way do not need further treatment. When bypass surgery was the only option to treat patients with intermittent claudication due to SFA disease, many surgeons claimed that they accepted this approach. Quite a few patients, however, were operated on what was called disabling claudication, clearly illustrating the need for less invasive treatment modalities in multiple stenosed or occlusive SFAs.

Percutaneous Treatment

Initial success rate and long-term patency with femoropopliteal angioplasty are disappointing in comparison to iliac angioplasty.[2] Short occlusions or stenoses can be treated by percutaneous transluminal angioplasty (PTA); however, long-term patency results for longer (>10 cm) occlusive lesions are disappointing. Despite close surveillance and early reintervention, the use of stents in combination with angioplasty has not altered these results. Optimal lesions for femoropopliteal PTA are short stenoses (<2 cm) with a good run-off. Hunink et al[3] found an increase in quality-adjusted lifetime with reduced expenditures if a PTA was performed on a 65-year-old man with intermittent claudication due to a femoropopliteal stenoses or occlusion.

To enhance the results of femoropopliteal PTA, numerous laser devices have emerged in the last 20 years. Despite promising early results, patency rates appeared disappointing.[4,5] The use of stents in femoropopliteal disease lacks randomized studies to support this expensive treatment adjunct.

In the pursuit of improvements in percutaneous techniques of SFA recanalization, it was observed that a successful outcome could be achieved if the false lumen created by accidental subintimal passage was pursued and a reentry into the true lumen beyond the occlusion obtained. The technique of deliberate subintimal angioplasty, the so-called "Bolia technique" or "PIER technique," has some strong proponents[6,7]; however, although several centers have been attempting this technique for several years, the paucity of published results can be interpreted as a reflection of the difficulty of the technique. Whether centers other than the two major proponents can reproduce similar good results remains to be seen.

Minimally Invasive Surgery

Transluminal surgical endarterectomy dates back more than 50 years to 1946, when the Portuguese surgeon Joao Cid dos Santos performed the first thromboendarterectomy.[8] The first procedure was performed through two arteriotomies in a 66-year-old male patient with atherosclerotic occlusive disease of the SFA. One year later, when dos Santos published this new technique for treating arterial occlusive disease, a new treatment concept was born. The American surgeon Jack Wylie introduced this technique in the US.[9]

The initial enthusiasm was followed by the awareness of the limitations and complications associated with this technique. Despite promising early results, open and semiclosed endarterectomies were largely abandoned in the 1970s. Several reports suggested inferior results of an endarterectomy in comparison with femoropopliteal venous bypass grafting.[10,11] These retrospective, nonrandomized studies, often with historical control groups, compared patency rates of vein bypass and endarterectomy. Most series comprised small numbers of patients, and most did not differentiate between open and semiclosed endarterectomy. Several other important variables that could have influenced patency rates (e.g., run-off score) were not evaluated. In addition, one must realize that autologous venous material for bypass surgery is not always available.

The advantages of endarterectomy over arterial bypass surgery include:

1. Less invasive surgery without harvesting and use of autologous venous material, which could be saved for later cardiovascular or peripheral surgery.
2. Long-term patency rates approach patency rates of venous bypass surgery.
3. Conversion to bypass surgery in case of technical failure remains possible.

There are two main reasons for abandoning the technique of endarterectomy. One is the relatively high surgical skills necessary for this technique in comparison to the extra-anatomical femoropopliteal bypass from prosthetic or biological material; the other is the occurrence of unexpected restenoses and occlusions in the endarterectomized artery. The latter remains a point of dispute, because even recent publications show not much difference in patency between endarterectomy and prosthetic bypass graft.[12,13] So far no data are available from randomized trials to resolve this discussion.

Our reason for reappraisal of the endarterectomy is the availability and application of new intraoperative technology to improve results from the past. With the help of digital subtraction angiography, angioscopy, and intravascular ultrasound, the semiclosed endarterectomized artery can be inspected more accurately and intraoperative endoluminal corrections can be made. Postoperatively, the onset of initial intimal hyperplasia and restenosis can be detected in time noninvasively by duplex scanning. Early restenosis can be treated by angioplasty, which can thus create better primary assisted patency rates.

Remote Endarterectomy with the MollRing Cutter

With the use of the MollRing Cutter (Vascular Architects, Inc., San Jose, CA), which is a modification of the single ring stripper, the surgeon is able to cut the endoluminal atheroma core remotely (Fig. 1). The surgical exposure of the superficial and common femoral artery can be limited to a small single arteriotomy at the origin in the groin. Because the atheroma core can be transected using the MollRing Cutter, distal open exposure of the popliteal artery at the endpoint of the endarterectomized segment becomes unnecessary. Weinstein and Krupski[14] describe the technique of closed endarterectomy. We prefer to call this technique a remote endarterectomy (REA) because it is not a closed technique—a small incision in the groin remains necessary. We also prefer not to make an arteriotomy in the common femoral artery but rather in the proximal part of the SFA. This enables flow through the profunda femoris artery during the actual procedure. This is advantageous for two reasons. First, it obviously shortens the duration of ischemia to the leg. Second, backflow through the endarterectomized SFA prevents distal embolization during the REA.

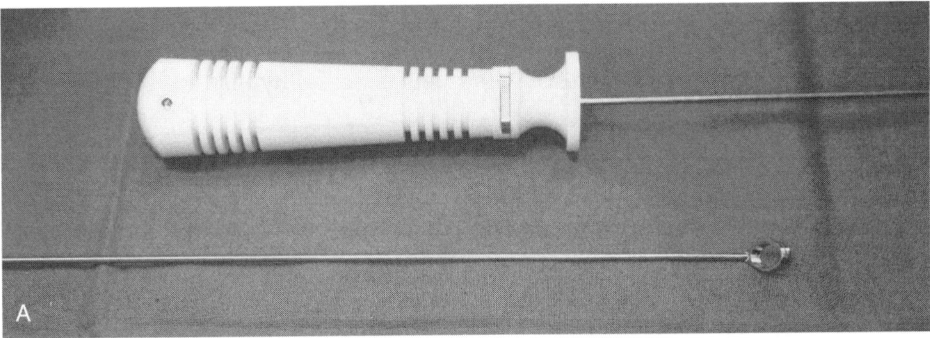

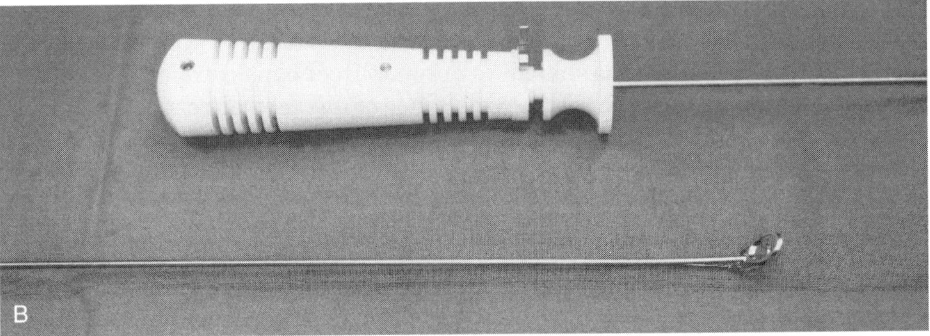

Figure 1. The MollRing Cutter in closed (**A**) and semiopened (**B**) position. The proximal end of the MollRing Cutter consists of a handle and knob that are locked together by a small metal tab (A). To unlock the handle and knob, the metal tab must be set in a vertical position (B). While holding the knob portion firmly, the handle portion must be pulled toward the surgeon. The cutting occurs as the rings pass each other. When the handle portion is returned to its original position flush with the knob, the rings return to the original overlapped position.

The MollRing Cutter is a modified ring dissector with two shafts that telescope into each other. Two symmetrical single ellipse-shaped rings at a 135° angle are attached at the most distal part of each shaft. The ellipse-shaped rings come in different sizes, ranging from 5 to 10 mm inner diameter. Both parallel rings have sharpened inner edges that cut like a pair of scissors when both rings shear along each other. The remote cutting mechanism is activated with a handle at the end of the shafts. The technique of REA is illustrated in Figures 2 through 10.

The minimally invasive approach of REA with the avoidance of a second distal incision and dissection of the popliteal artery creates less operative trauma and a reduction of postoperative discomfort, leading to earlier recovery and discharge of the patient. In our clinic, more than 200 REA procedures have been performed. The cumulative 2-year primary, primary assisted, and secondary patency rates were 73%, 86%, and 86%, respectively.[13]

Routine postoperative surveillance of the endarterectomized SFA is mandatory. All patients treated by REA in the femoropopliteal artery are entered in a duplex scanning surveillance program. This program consists of duplex scanning within 6 weeks postoperatively and after 3, 6, 9, and 12 months. In our series, only 25% of all recurrent stenosis after REA were associated with deterioration of clinical symptoms or a decrease of ankle-brachial indices. In 82% of all restenoses, time of onset was within the first year. The locations of these restenoses were equally distributed within the SFA and were not restricted to the stent or distal SFA region. Preliminary studies on the results of revision indicate that early restenosis may be treated successfully with balloon

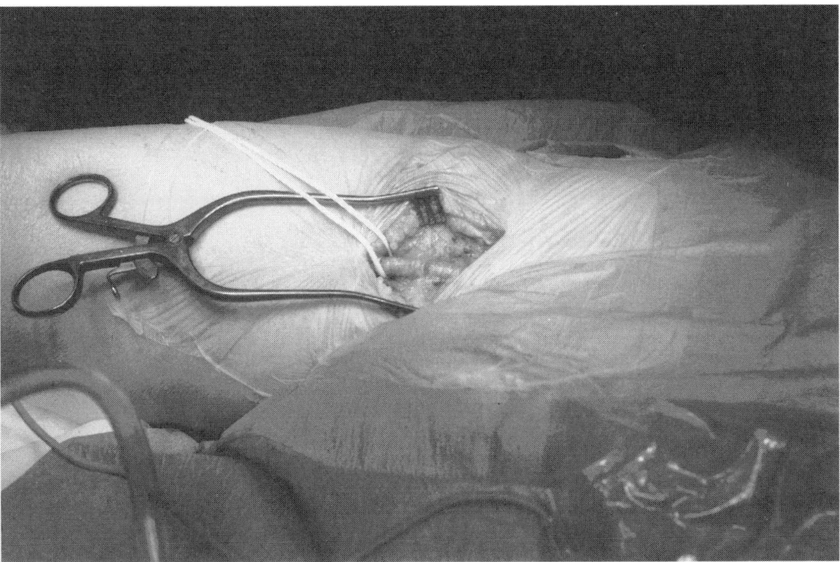

Figure 2. Exposure of the proximal superficial femoral artery (SFA) should be performed according to standard surgical technique. The dissection should allow for control of the distal common femoral artery (CFA), the profunda femoris artery (PFA), and the proximal segment of the SFA. A doubled vessel loop is placed around the distal portion of the SFA to control anticipated backbleeding after successful endarterectomy.

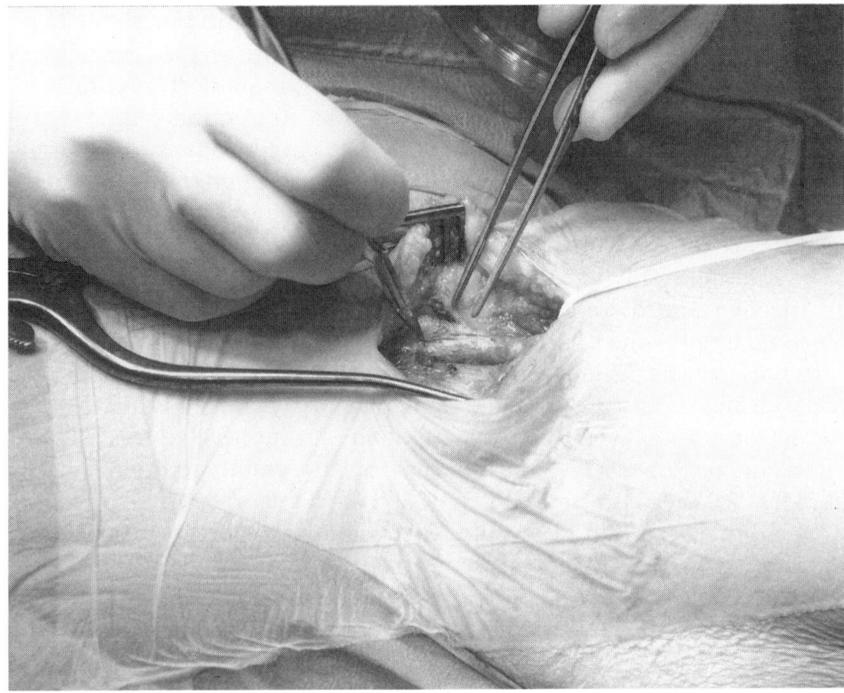

Figure 3. With the use of a #11 scalpel blade, a 3- to 4-cm incision of the adventitia of the proximal SFA is made in order to enter the subadventitial plane.

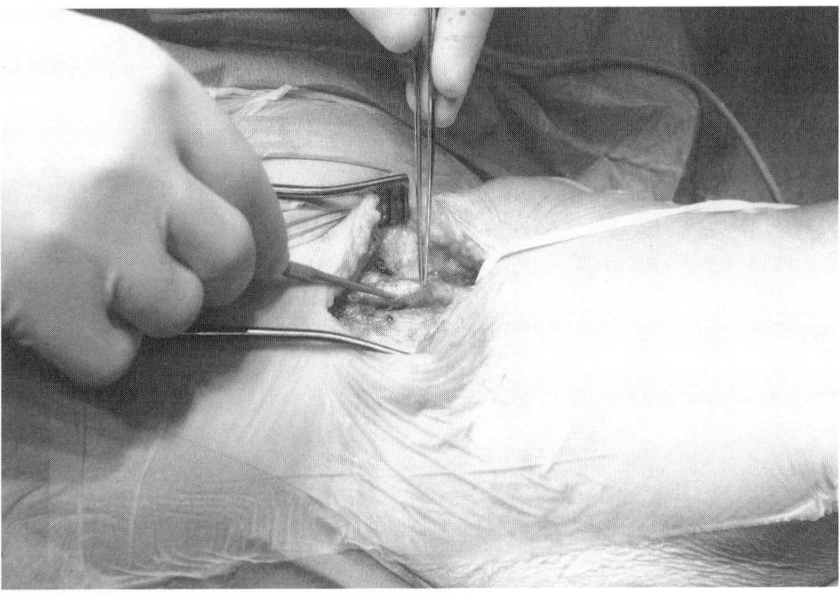

Figure 4. With the use of a Halle or Freer elevator, the establishment of a subadventitial dissection plane is facilitated. The vessel wall is dissected away from the core in the arteriotomy and 1 to 2 cm distally.

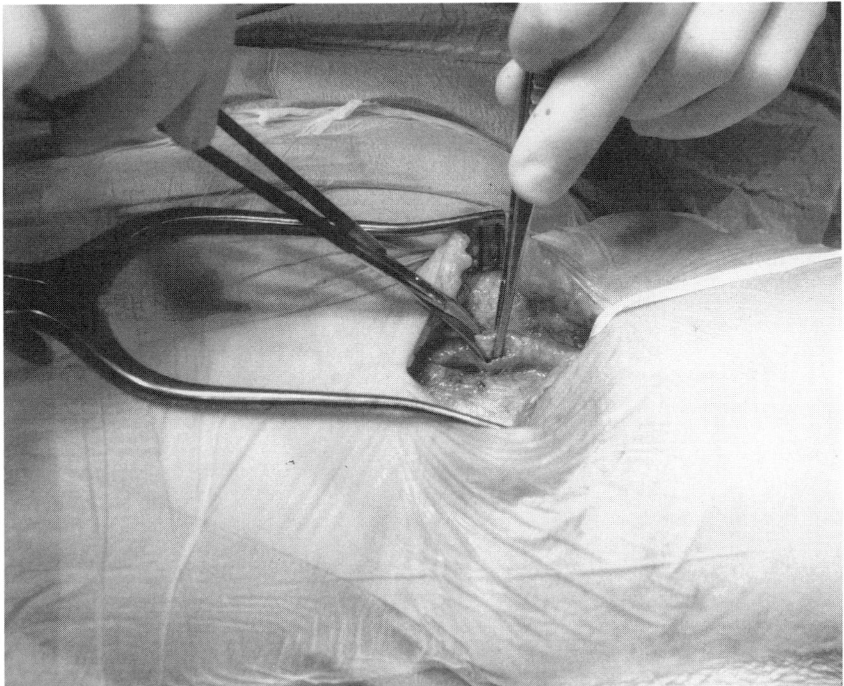

Figure 5. The core is transected proximally in the arteriotomy. The resulting core should be long enough to be grasped by the assistant during both the ringstripper dissection and removal of the core after transection.

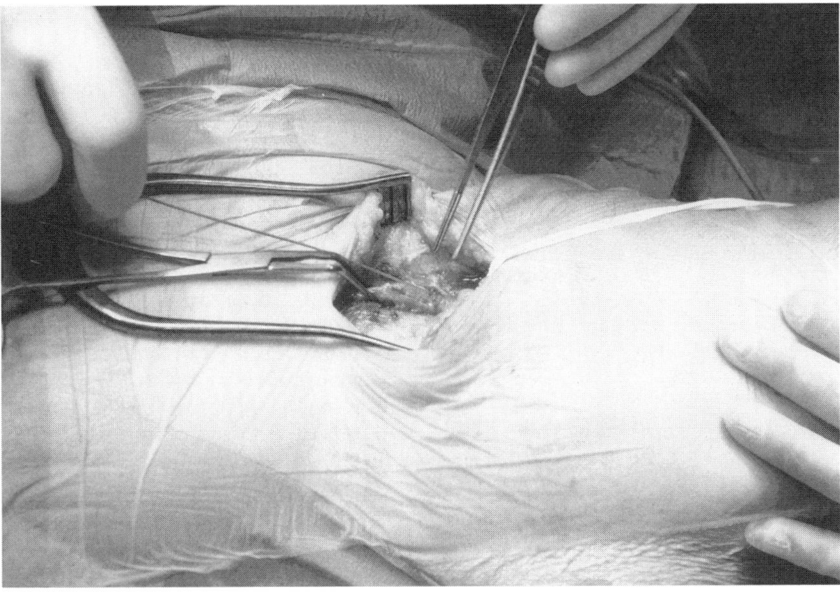

Figure 6. The ringstripper is advanced distal to the vessel loop that is then gently retracted to prevent backbleeding. Dissection of the core distally is continued with a slow and controlled to-and-fro motion of the dissector handle. Alternating use of a different size ringstripper can be useful if localized calcification of the core is encountered resulting in different core diameters.

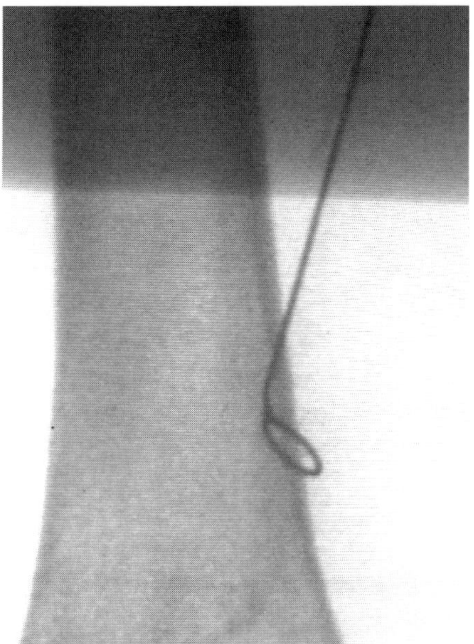

Figure 7. Under fluoroscopy the dissection of the core is continued to the area 1 cm above a previously chosen endpoint of the core.

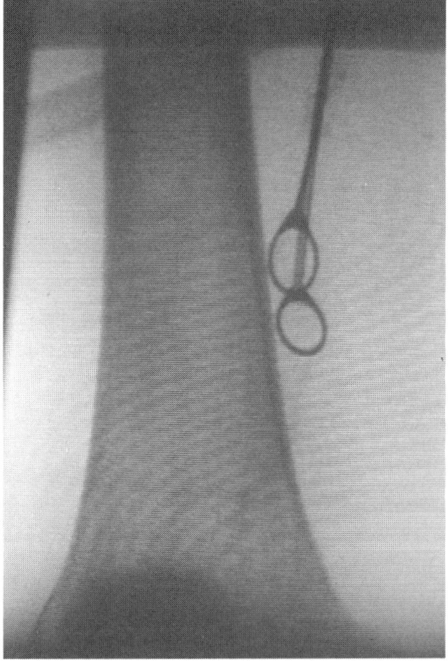

Figure 8. The selected MollRing Cutter is placed over the core and advanced distally to the endpoint of the previous dissection. Once the initial endpoint is confirmed, the MollRing Cutter is advanced 1 to 2 cm beyond that point. The MollRing Cutter should be oriented so that the distal angulation is pointing ventrally; since most of the residual plaque is usually located on the posterior wall of the vessel, this orientation will allow transection of the least diseased area distally. The plaque is transected. With the MollRing Cutter returned to a position where the rings are one third deployed (Fig. 1B), the distal end of the core will be grasped. Using DeBakey pick-ups or a mosquito clamp on the proximal part of the intima core and simultaneous pulling, the core is removed.

Figure 10. With the use of a 0.035″ angled glide wire and a multipurpose angiographic catheter, the popliteal artery lumen is catheterized. At the level of the transected endpoint, the distal intima is secured with a short stent, either balloon expandable or self expandable. Endoluminal stenting prevents further intimal dissection and provides a smooth transition zone to the normal intima in the reconstituted popliteal artery.

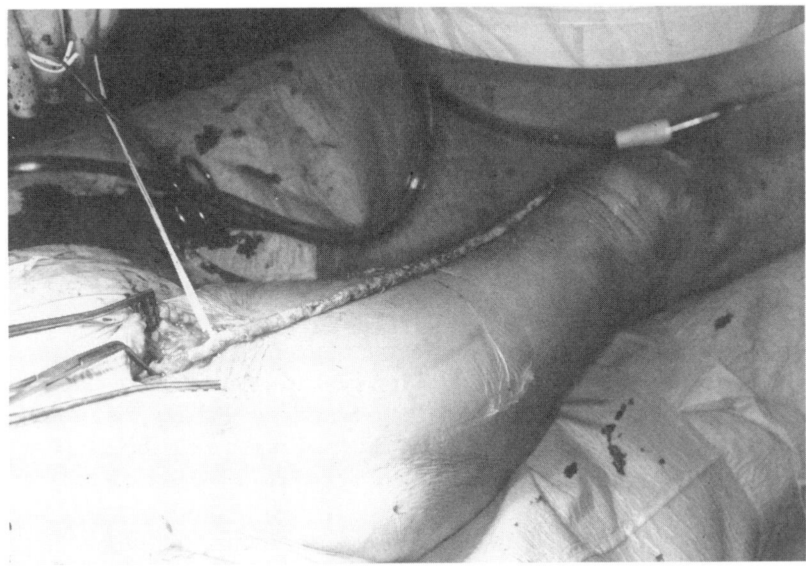

Figure 9. The removed intima core placed on the patient's leg. Note the tightened vessel loop to control backbleeding.

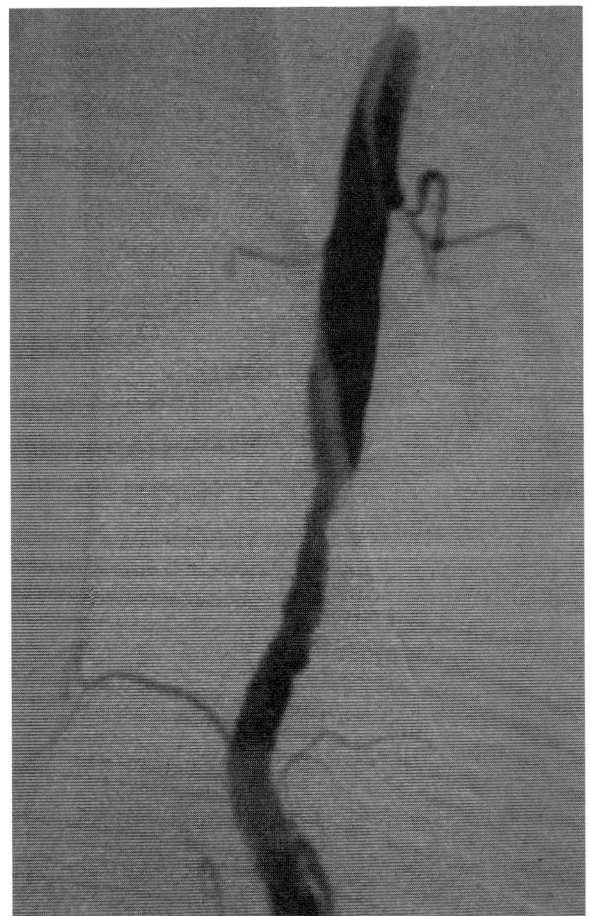

angioplasty. Recurrent stenoses developing after 1 year seem to have a different natural history and require intervention only for clinical symptoms. Controversy exists with regard to the use of antiplatelet drugs or warfarin. The authors give all patients an antiplatelet drug (ASA 100 mg daily).

REA Followed by Endolining

The unfortunate finding of a high incidence (46%) of early restenoses after REA, dispersed over the entire endarterectomized SFA, made us look for alternatives or adjuncts to improve results. Four directions of research to prevent restenosis can be distinguished: gene and drug therapy, cell seeding, radiation or brachytherapy, and endoluminal grafting or a combination of those. Gene and drug therapy as well as cell seeding research is making progress, but is still not in clinical use.

In 1997, in the US and The Netherlands, randomized studies for gamma irradiation after PTA of the SFA have been started. On theoretical grounds, irradiation might be even more effective if, prior to the irradiation, debulking of the atheromatous plaque is performed instead of angioplasty. After debulking by means of atherectomy or REA, it is more likely to get an equal dose distribution to the adventitia of the artery, because centering of the source seems more accurate. This concept has not yet been investigated.

In 1997 we started the application of endolining, which has the theoretical advantages of being anatomical, delivering a concentric anastomosis, and thus giving a minimal loss of compliance. The concept of endovascular grafting in stenotic or occlusive arterial disease, isolating the flow surface of the arterial segment, is not new. Most experience of endovascular grafting, however, has been gained with recanalization and predilatation only prior to endograft insertion, and hence without removing the atherosclerotic intimal core.[11–13] It is conceivable that the natural tendency for elastic recoil of the arterial wall after dilatation may result in endograft compression, jeopardizing patency in the longer term. In addition, extensive smooth muscle cell proliferation within compressed atherosclerotic plaques external to the endovascular graft may encroach on the lumen and increase the risk of reocclusion. In concordance with the approach of Bergeron et al[15] and Morris et al,[16] we advocate debulking of the atherosclerotic artery by means of (remote) endarterectomy prior to graft insertion, to theoretically eliminate the risk of external graft compression.

Since 1998, we have been performing REA followed by endolining of the SFA with a distensible and radially enforced ePTFE endovascular graft (Enduring, WL Gore & Associates, Flagstaff, AZ) (Fig. 11).[17] Despite a high initial technical success rate as documented by completion angiography, we have encountered a relatively high number of reocclusions, resulting in primary and secondary patency rates of 46% and 66%, respectively.[18] The relatively high number of early reocclusions in our study must be further addressed. In contrast to REA alone, no recurrent stenoses were detected in the central part of the graft, suggesting adequate resistance to the compressive force of the artery.

In conclusion, insertion of the new balloon-expandable, radially enforced, ePTFE endovascular graft (Enduring) following REA of the SFA effectively results in a less invasive treatment for femoropopliteal occlusive disease. Addi-

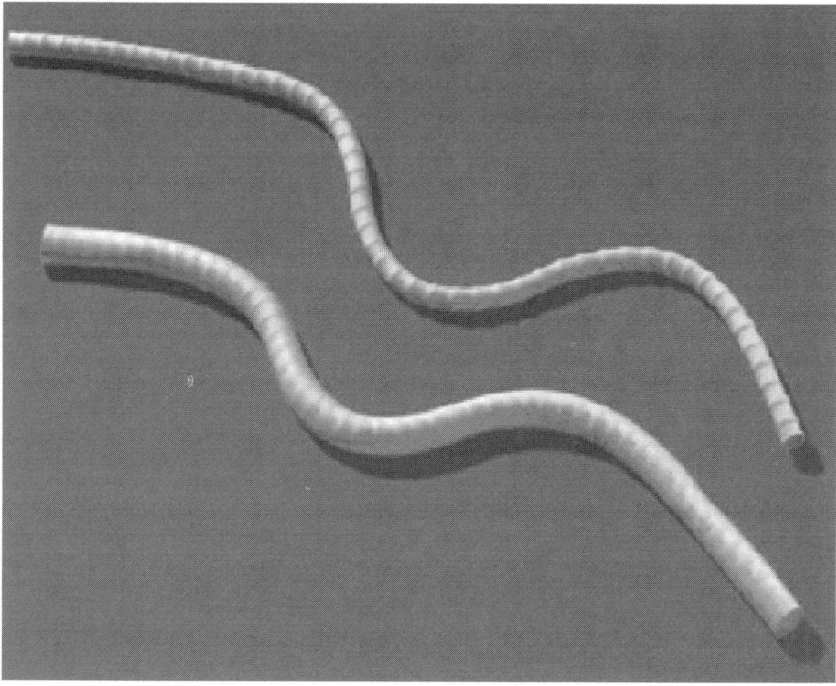

Figure 11. The Enduring expanded polytetrafluoroethylene endovascular graft.

tional technical refinements of the procedure, however, are required to avoid procedure- and graft-related early failures.

Future Perspectives

The MollRing Cutter device enables the surgeon to perform an REA of virtually any occluded peripheral artery. The REA procedure can also be performed in iliac and popliteal arteries. Both procedures have already been successfully performed in our institution, using a retrograde approach for the iliac artery. The results of this procedure may approach those of grafts for femoral supragenicular popliteal bypasses and can be chosen as a first option for treatment of SFA occlusive disease when a minimally invasive procedure is desirable for the individual patient. If, in the future, the occurrence of restenosis after endarterectomies can be reduced, the role of bypass grafting turns into a bailout procedure for failed minimally invasive techniques.

References

1. Green RM, Abbott WM, Matsumoto T, et al. Prosthetic above-knee femoropopliteal bypass grafting: Five-year results of a randomized trial. *J Vasc Surg* 2000;31:417–425.
2. Johnston KW. Femoral and popliteal arteries: Reanalysis of results of balloon angioplasty. *Radiology* 1992;183:767–771.

3. Hunink MGM, Wong JB, Donaldson MC, et al. Revascularization for femoropopliteal disease. A decision and cost-effectiveness analysis. *JAMA* 1995;274:165–171.
4. Sandborn TA, Cumberland DC, Greenfield AJ, et al. Percutaneous laser thermal angioplasty: Initial results and 1-year follow-up in 129 femoropopliteal lesions. *Radiology* 1988;168:121–125.
5. Ashley S, Brooks SG, Gehani AA, et al. Percutaneous laser recanalization of femoropopliteal occlusions using continuous wave Nd YAG laser and sapphire contact probe delivery system. *Eur J Vasc Surg* 1994;8:494–501.
6. Bolia A, Miles KA, Brennan J, Bell PRF. Percutaneous transluminal angioplasty of occlusions of the femoral and popliteal arteries by subintimal dissection. *Cardiovasc Intervent Radiol* 1990;13:357–363.
7. Reekers JA, Kromhout JG, Jacobs JHM. Percutaneous intentional extraluminal recanalization of the femoropopliteal artery. *Eur J Vasc Surg* 1994;8:723–728.
8. dos Santos JC. Sur la desobstruction des thromboses arterielles anciennes. *Mem Acad Chir* 1947;73:409–411.
9. Wylie EJ, Kerr E, Davies O. Experimental and clinical experience with the use of fascia lata applied as a graft about major arteries after endarterectomy and aneurysmography. *Surg Gynaecol Obstet* 1951;93:257–272.
10. DeWeese JA, Barner HB, Mahoney EB, Rob CG. Autogenous venous bypass grafts and thromboendarterectomies for atherosclerotic lesions of the femoropopliteal arteries. *Ann Surg* 1966;163:205–214.
11. Darling RC, Linton RR. Durability of femoropopliteal reconstructions. *Am J Surg* 1972;123:472–479.
12. Ho GH. *Endovascular Remote Endarterectomy: Initial Experience with a New Technique in the Treatment of Superficial Femoral Artery Occlusive Disease.* [Thesis]. Utrecht, The Netherlands: University of Utrecht; 1999. ISBN 90-393-2010-1.
13. Ho GH, Moll FL. Remote endarterectomy in SFA occlusive disease. *Eur J Radiol* 1998;28:205–210.
14. Weinstein ES, Krupski WC. Thromboendarterectomy for lower extremity arterial occlusive disease. In Rutherford RB (ed): *Vascular Surgery*. Philadelphia: W.B. Saunders Co.; 2000:972–981.
15. Bergeron P, Chiarandini S, Nava G, Roth O. Femoral artery endoluminal bypass grafting: Indications and early results. *J Endovasc Surg* 1997;4:404–405.
16. Morris GE, Ahn SS, Quick CRG, et al. Endovascular femoropopliteal bypass: A cadaveric study. *Eur J Vasc Endovasc Surg* 1995;10:9–15.
17. Ho GW, Moll FL, Tutein Nolthenius RP, et al. Endovascular femoropopliteal bypass combined with remote endarterectomy in superficial femoral artery occlusive disease: Initial experience. *Eur J Vasc Endovasc Surg* 2000;19:27–34.
18. Heijmen RH, Teijink JAW, van den Berg JC, et al. A distensible, radially enforced ePTFE endograft following remote endarterectomy of the superficial femoral artery: A single institution's one year experience. *J Endovasc Ther* 2001, in press.

8

Devices and Techniques for Mechanical Clot Removal

Bradley B. Hill, MD and Thomas J. Fogarty, MD

Introduction

Embolization of clot and in situ arterial thrombosis are the most common causes of acute arterial insufficiency. Before the advent of catheter-mediated therapies, emboli were removed surgically by opening the blood vessel and directly removing the clot, as first described by Labey in 1911.[1] Technically successful procedures had high associated morbidity and mortality because they required extensive tissue dissection, because most patients had serious comorbidities, and because the surgeon was usually consulted only after significant ischemic tissue injury had occurred.

The surgical treatment of acute arterial occlusion was greatly simplified in 1961 with the introduction of the balloon catheter thromboembolectomy technique.[2] Early experience typically involved removal of embolic material and soft propagated thrombus from otherwise healthy arteries. Today, many patients still have emboli of cardiac origin; however, an increasing number have in situ thrombosis of atherosclerotic arteries, thrombosed bypass grafts, or arteriovenous grafts.[3] In situ thrombosis frequently involves adherent laminated clot that cannot be removed with the standard thromboembolectomy balloon catheter.

The trend toward minimally invasive treatments and the challenge of removing organized clot material have led to recent advances in clot management. Instrumentation for transluminal clot removal now includes a variety of thrombectomy balloon catheters, pullback thrombectomy devices, clot aspiration catheters, and devices that ablate clot by means of hydrodynamic, ultrasonic, and electromagnetic energy.

From Criado FJ (ed): *Endovascular Intervention: New Tools and Techniques for the 21st Century.* Armonk, NY: Futura Publishing Co., Inc.; ©2002.

Acute Arterial Occlusions: General Considerations

The treating physician must understand the basic pathophysiology of acute arterial occlusion. Preoperative diagnostic work-up, operative technique, and perioperative management are the determinants of successful therapy. These basic considerations merit review.

Pathophysiology

The heart is the most common source of arterial emboli. Other sources include aneurysms of the aorta, iliac, or extremity arteries, and atherosclerotic lesions. Ninety percent of patients who present with surgically treatable emboli have lower extremity ischemia. The most common location of embolic arterial occlusion is the common femoral bifurcation. The common iliac bifurcation is the next most frequent site followed by the terminal aorta and popliteal artery (Fig. 1). Multiple emboli are common, and more than one limb is involved in 10% of patients. "Silent emboli" may occur in tissue beds with well-developed collateral blood supply.

The tissue effects of acute arterial occlusion are fairly consistent and involve anaerobic metabolism and lactic acidosis (Fig. 2). Necrosis of nerve and muscle occurs within 6 to 12 hours in cases of profound ischemia. The duration and magnitude of ischemia and the sensitivity of the tissue determine the degree of injury. Nerve tissue is most sensitive to hypoxia and the earliest symptoms of ischemia typically are pain, numbness, and paresthesias.

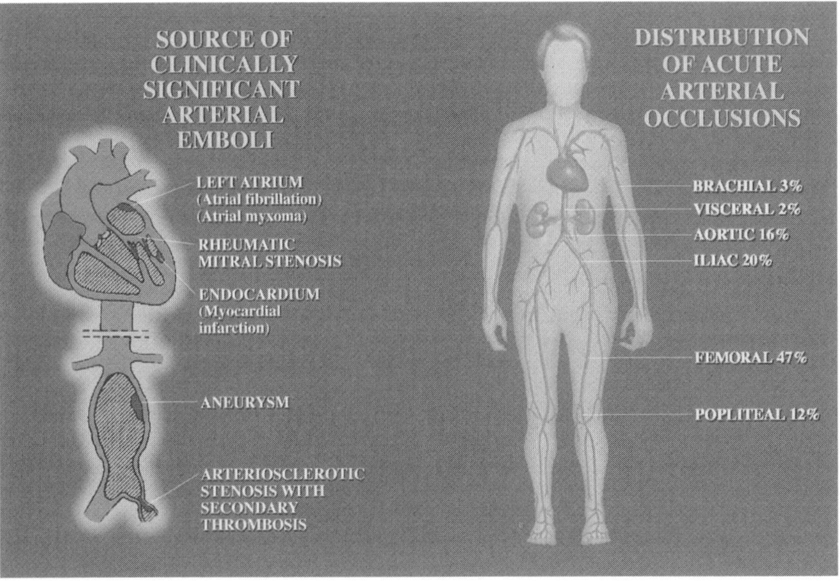

Figure 1. Source and distribution of clinically significant arterial emboli.

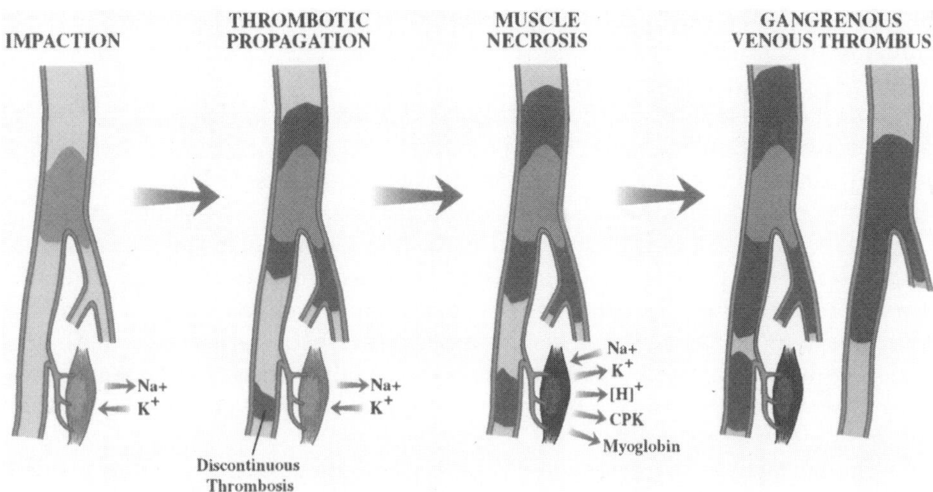

Figure 2. Pathophysiology of acute embolic arterial occlusion. Embolus leads to propagation of thrombus and formation of discontinuous thrombus distally. Ischemia causes cellular dysfunction and eventual tissue necrosis.

Diagnosis

The diagnosis of acute arterial occlusion can almost always be made based on the history and physical examination. An acute embolus often occurs without warning and the characteristic presentation is the syndrome of the 5 "P's": pain, pallor, paresthesia, paralysis, and pulselessness. A history of atrial fibrillation, recent myocardial infarction, or aortic aneurysm is typical. In situ thrombosis is typically associated with symptoms of chronic arterial occlusive disease such as claudication, pain at rest, nonhealing wounds, or previous arterial bypass procedures.

Documentation of physical examination should include the presence and amplitude of arterial pulsations. Examination of pulsations is critical because the site of embolic occlusion is typically the major arterial bifurcation above the most proximal absent arterial pulsation. The color, temperature, and the presence or absence of sensation, proprioception, and motor function of the effected limb should be documented. The location and quality of Doppler signals and ankle-brachial indices should be documented in cases of lower extremity arterial occlusion.

If patients have suspected visceral or renal artery occlusion, or evidence of significant arterial occlusive disease, they should be evaluated angiographically, either preoperatively or intraoperatively, so that the arterial anatomy can be defined and the operative procedure planned. Prompt assessment of cardiac status is essential because many of these patients have coexisting heart disease.

Perioperative Management

All patients with acute arterial occlusions should be promptly anticoagulated to prevent further embolization and propagation of thrombus at the site of embolization. A heparin bolus of 100 U/kg followed by a continuous heparin infusion to maintain the partial thromboplastin time 21/2 times control will generally produce adequate anticoagulation.

The goals of treatment should be patient survival, limb salvage, and avoidance of toxic systemic effects. Prompt thromboembolectomy and restoration of arterial perfusion is critical in the setting of profound ischemia. Delaying the operative procedure in order to complete preoperative assessment must be weighed against the risk of irreversible tissue ischemia and the systemic consequences of reperfusing ischemic tissue. The most important determinant of a successful outcome is the condition of the ischemic limb preoperatively and the ability to remove the clot and restore arterial perfusion. Absence of both sensation and motor activity often indicates a nonviable extremity. In such cases, thromboembolectomy may improve success of a lower level amputation than would otherwise be possible.

The surgical preparation should be from nipples to toes to allow arterial exploration from the abdominal aorta to the pedal arteries if needed. Pharmacologic myocardial protective measures such as β-blocker and nitrate administration may be prudent in patients with cardiac disease. Fortunately, mechanical clot removal can usually be accomplished with infrainguinal incisions under spinal anesthesia with limited physiologic stress on the patient.

Reperfusion of ischemic tissue can result in hyperkalemia and acidosis severe enough to cause myocardial dysfunction. Oxygen free radicals and cytokines released from ischemic tissue upon reperfusion can provoke a state of systemic inflammation and multiorgan dysfunction or failure. The benefit of reperfusing ischemic tissue may not justify the risk of systemic toxicity, especially if the patient has no sensory function or motor activity in the extremity preoperatively. If operation is performed, fasciotomies may be required if compartment pressures are 25 mm Hg or higher before or after reperfusion.

Postoperative anticoagulation may be indicated in instances of incomplete thrombectomy, especially if a proximal source of emboli is identified. Anticoagulation with heparin within 6 to 12 hours after thromboembolectomy is usually feasible, and conversion to oral warfarin is recommended if a cardiac source of emboli is present, an arterial abnormality such as aneurysm or an ulcerated plaque is identified and remains untreated, or a hypercoagulable state is diagnosed.

If the source of emboli is unknown, thorough cardiac evaluation is indicated, including electrocardiography, echocardiography, and 24-hour cardiac telemetry to identify possible anatomical or electrophysiologic conditions that may predispose to thrombus formation. If a pulsatile mass is palpable in the abdomen, abdominal ultrasonography may confirm the presence of an aneurysm. Angiography, from the aortic valve to the site of arterial embolization, may be indicated if no obvious cardiac source or aneurysm is identified. Conventional angiography, computed tomographic angiography, and magnetic resonance angiography are all effective in identifying arterial sources of emboli. The decision to use a particular modality depends on the available resources and the expertise of those reconstructing the image data if computed tomographic angiography or magnetic resonance angiography is used.

Patients with hypercoagulable states may present with acute arterial occlusion from emboli and in situ thrombosis of otherwise normal arteries. The same work-up for proximal sources of emboli applies in these cases. If no explanatory cardiac or proximal arterial abnormality is identified, or if otherwise normal appearing proximal artery has adherent thrombus, a thorough work-up for hypercoagulability is indicated.

Conventional Thromboembolectomy

Thromboembolectomy performed remotely through open surgical incisions and small arteriotomies has been the mainstay of surgical treatment for acute arterial occlusions since the 1960s. Devices and techniques for "conventional thromboembolectomy" have evolved over the years but the general principles and technical considerations remain the same. The original balloon catheter design is still the most widely used device for thromboembolectomy.

Balloon Catheter Thromboembolectomy

The original balloon catheter for thromboembolectomy consisted of a single-lumen catheter with a distensible balloon mounted at its distal end. The balloon was inserted into a blood vessel, advanced beyond the thrombus, expanded with saline or air, and pulled back to extract the clot. The basic catheter design has remained largely unchanged from the original Fogarty design (Edwards Lifesciences Corp., Irvine, CA) (Fig. 3). Sizes range from 2F to 7F and the smaller catheters have a spring tip to decrease the chance of intimal damage or perforation. Each catheter is calibrated for optimal balloon distention and the recommended volume should not be exceeded. Saline is typically used for 4F and larger catheters and air is used for the 2F and 3F catheters. Use of air in smaller devices allows for more rapid inflation and deflation, gives a better sense of feel during withdrawal, and is less likely to damage small, fragile vessels.

Atherosclerotic plaque can hinder the passage of the balloon catheter beyond the thrombus. Maneuvers to improve the chances of successful passage include preforming the catheter tip and rotating at the site of an obstruction, introducing more than one catheter simultaneously, progressively flexing nearby joints to alter the advancement angle of the catheter tip, and inflation of the balloon at the site of obstruction to bring the catheter tip away from the vessel wall followed by gentle advancement during balloon deflation.

After the catheter has been advanced as far as safely possible, the balloon is inflated while the catheter is slowly withdrawn. The operator must 'feel' the resistance during pullback and adjust the balloon volume to maintain a constant degree of resistance and prevent vessel damage as the catheter and clot are removed. This process is facilitated by the balloon catheter, which is constructed such that the initial inflation of the balloon involves only the 1-cm area in the center of the balloon jacket. Increased resistance caused by mild atherosclerotic plaque forces displacement of fluid to the uninflated portion of the balloon. This process of conformability allows the balloon to 'glide' across areas of mild atherosclerotic narrowing without damaging the vessel wall.

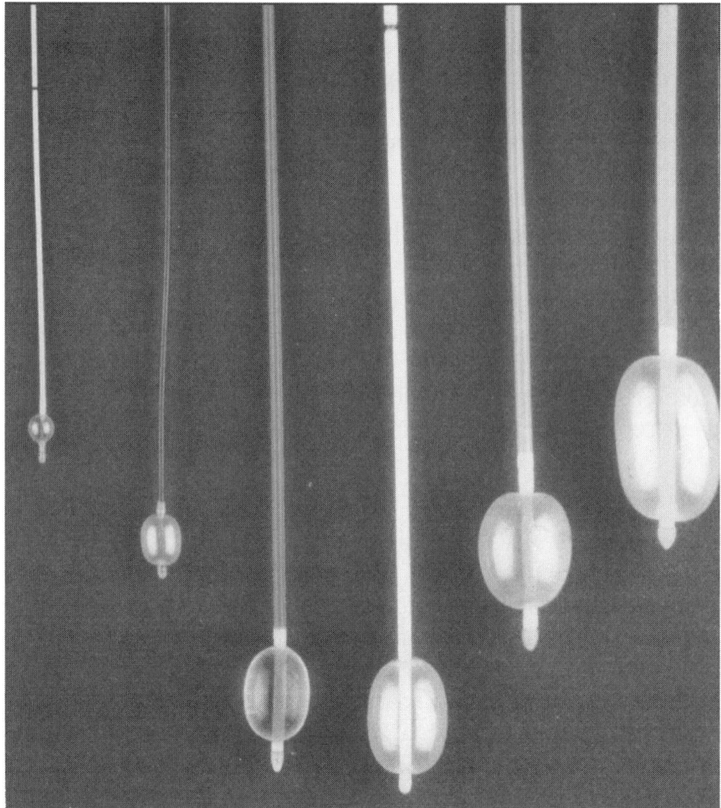

Figure 3. Fogarty balloon embolectomy catheters are available in sizes ranging from 2F to 7F.

Extraction of aortic and iliac artery emboli involves making bilateral groin incisions. The common, superficial, and profunda femoris arteries are mobilized and controlled. The common femoral artery is clamped proximally and a common femoral arteriotomy, usually transverse, is made just proximal to the bifurcation to allow easy entry into the superficial and deep femoral arteries. If significant common femoral atherosclerosis is present, longitudinal arteriotomy, endarterectomy, and patch angioplasty may be required. If no significant atherosclerosis is present, a transverse or oblique arteriotomy is preferable to allow primary closure without narrowing. Distal exploration is initially performed. A 3F or 4F catheter is advanced into the superficial femoral artery as far distally as possible. After successful exploration, 25 to 50 mL heparin-saline (5000 U heparin/250 mL 0.9 % saline solution) is flushed into the vessel that is then occluded with an atraumatic clamp. The profunda femoris artery is explored in likewise fashion, but not more than 25 cm of the embolectomy catheter is advanced into the artery. Proximal exploration is performed with a 6F embolectomy catheter that is advanced into the aorta. The balloon is inflated and withdrawn until forceful antegrade flow is obtained. To avoid excessive blood loss, the catheter can be passed through the jaws of a Fogarty clamp.

After adequate extraction from one side, a similar procedure is performed on the opposite side. If only one iliac artery is occluded, unilateral thromboembolectomy is performed; however, it is best to prepare both limbs for surgery at the outset because of the possibility of dislodging proximal iliac thrombus that can embolize down the opposite side.

The presence of backbleeding during thromboembolectomy is no assurance that the distal artery is patent, since discontinuous thrombus may be present and backbleeding may be profuse through collateral branches. Operative arteriography, intravascular ultrasound, angioscopy, and Doppler flow evaluation may be appropriate for further assessment if there is a question regarding distal arterial patency.

Extraction of femoral and popliteal emboli is best performed through a distal common femoral artery approach as previously described. Tibial vessels can also be explored through the common femoral artery with a 2F or 3F balloon catheter. Thrombus can be extracted from more than one tibial artery by passing two or three catheters into the superficial femoral artery. After passage of the first catheter, the knee is flexed and a second catheter is more likely to enter a vessel orifice not obstructed by the first catheter.

If thrombus remains in a tibial vessel, and attempts at thrombectomy from above are unsuccessful, an incision is made along the medial aspect of the leg below the knee. The distal popliteal and proximal tibial arteries are mobilized. A transverse arteriotomy is made in the distal popliteal artery and 2F and 3F balloon catheters are directed into the tibial arteries. On rare occasions, direct exploration of the dorsalis pedis and posterior tibial arteries may be required to facilitate thrombectomy using 2F balloon catheters.

Adequacy of thrombectomy is assessed by inspecting the retrieved thrombus. A cutoff usually indicates incomplete thrombectomy, whereas a gradual smooth taper is consistent with adequate clot removal. If further assessment is needed, angiography or angioscopy should be performed.

Adherent Clot Catheter

The limitations of the balloon thromboembolectomy catheter became more evident as the pathophysiology of acute arterial occlusion shifted from a predominance of embolic over thrombotic etiologies. This change in disease patterns reflects the decreased prevalence of rheumatic heart disease and the growing number of patients with diffuse atherosclerosis and prosthetic vascular grafts. Chronic organized clot often coexists with fresh thrombus in the setting of thrombotic arterial occlusion. Unlike fresh thrombus that is usually removed with the first pass of a balloon catheter, organized clot often cannot be dislodged with a compressible balloon. The Adherent Clot Catheter (Edwards Lifesciences Corp.) is particularly useful for thrombectomy of native arteries with thrombosis on top of localized stenotic lesions.[4] It consists of a flexible catheter body with an adjustable-pitch, latex-covered corkscrew at the distal tip and a control handle used to adjust the pitch of the corkscrew from completely straight to fully spiraled. The latex cover does not inflate but rather coils to variable diameters to engage and dislodge the clot by frictional force. The Adherent Clot Catheter and its mechanism of action are illustrated in Figure 4.

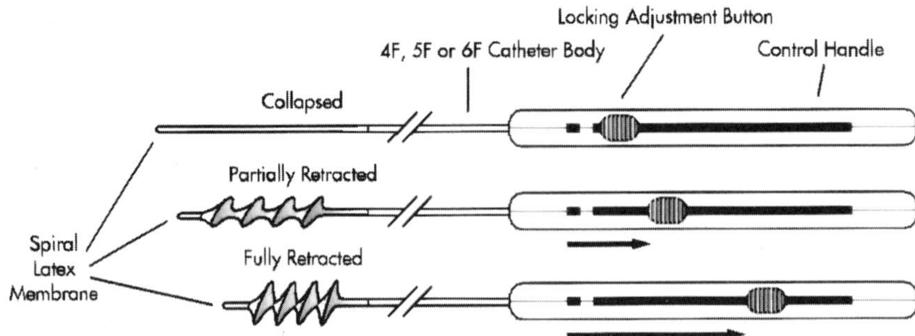

Figure 4. Adherent clot catheter shown in three stages of retraction. Top: In fully extended position for introduction into the thrombus. Middle: Partially retracted to begin trapping adherent clot in its corkscrew mechanism. Bottom: Fully retracted ensnaring clot for withdrawal from the vessel.

Graft Thrombectomy Catheter

The most common late complication associated with aortofemoral grafting, prosthetic lower extremity bypass grafting, and arteriovenous shunting is thrombosis with or without tissue ischemia. The same problem that limits removal of organized thrombus with a compressible balloon is also true for most thrombosed prosthetic grafts. The Graft Thrombectomy Catheter (Edwards Lifesciences Corp.), designed specifically for prosthetic grafts, consists of two helical wires spiraled around the catheter shaft near the distal tip. The wires are bare and can be expanded out from the catheter shaft by controlling a knob on the catheter handle (Fig. 5).

The Graft Thrombectomy Catheter is especially useful for restoring patency in cases of aortofemoral graft occlusion as illustrated in Figure 6. The procedure is performed by mobilizing and controlling the femoral artery on the involved side. An occlusion balloon catheter is placed through the helical wires of the Graft Thrombectomy Catheter, inserted through an arteriotomy in the femoral artery, advanced retrograde into the distal aorta, and inflated to prevent blood flow into the graft limb. Fresh and organized clot is removed from the graft lumen with multiple pullback maneuvers. Angioscopy is useful for assessing the result of thrombectomy. Compromise of arterial outflow is most frequently the etiology of aortofemoral graft occlusion, and correction of the anatomical defect after thrombectomy is crucial for long-term graft patency.

Thru-Lumen Balloon Catheter

A recent modification to the embolectomy balloon catheter was the addition of a coaxial lumen so that the catheter could be advanced over a guidewire. Organized thrombus can be difficult to traverse with a standard balloon catheter if the clot is firm or is superimposed over a stenotic arterial segment.

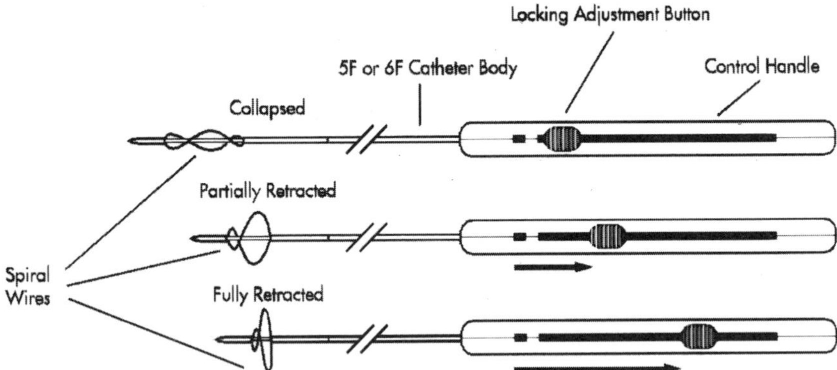

Figure 5. Graft thrombectomy catheter shown in its collapsed profile for introduction into the graft, partially retracted position, and fully retracted position where the wire is expanded against the graft wall to remove adherent material.

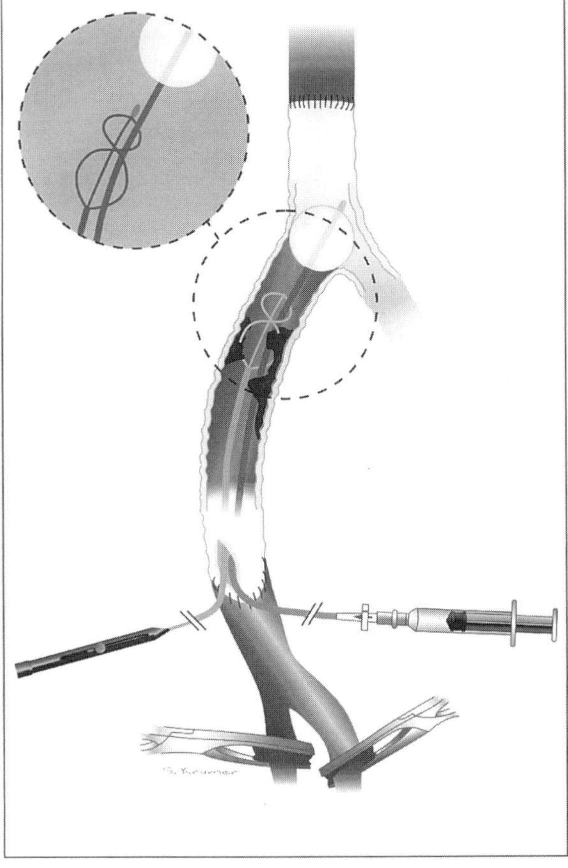

Figure 6. Method of aorto-femoral graft thrombectomy using the graft thrombectomy catheter. An occlusion balloon is threaded through the helical wires of the graft thrombectomy catheter prior to introduction of the occlusion balloon into the vessel. Occlusion balloon is shown in correct position at bifurcation, allowing the thrombectomy catheter to be centered and repeatedly worked up and down the graft to perform thrombectomy.

If the area of thrombosis can be traversed with a guidewire, the thru-lumen balloon catheter can be advanced over the wire to facilitate mechanical thrombectomy.

Large thru-lumen balloon catheters for aortic occlusion can be stabilized over a stiff guidewire when inserted retrograde for proximal arterial control during repair of ruptured aneurysms, or when cross-clamping the aorta is potentially hazardous because of extensive calcification. Thru-lumen aortic occlusion catheters can also be introduced through the left axillary or brachial artery.[5] This is greatly facilitated by introducing a stiff guidewire through the artery into the descending thoracic aorta using fluoroscopic guidance. The aortic occlusion balloon can then be advanced over the guidewire to the desired level to achieve proximal aortic control. Inflation of the aortic occlusion balloon with air or CO_2 will decrease the mass of material inside the balloon, minimize movement of the balloon during the cardiac cycle, and lessen the likelihood of balloon rupture.

Thrombolytic therapy can effectively restore patency to thrombosed arteries and grafts. A problem encountered during thrombolysis is that of keeping the lytic agent in the vicinity of the clot for activation of thrombus-bound plasminogen. Pulse spray catheters were developed to infuse the agent directly into the thrombus. Another method is to use the thru-lumen balloon catheter. The catheter is advanced through the patent lumen of the artery until its tip is near the thrombus. The artery is occluded by inflating the balloon and the lytic agent is infused into the clot without washout through patent collaterals. The thru-lumen catheter can also be used for temporary occlusion over a guidewire and for blood sampling.

Thromboembolectomy with Angioscopic Guidance

Angioscopy has been used as a visual assistance tool during endovascular procedures including angioplasty, stenting, thromboembolectomy, and endoluminal graft assessment. Angioscopy provides full color, three-dimensional views of the arterial lumen that may show residual thrombus after thrombectomy. Angioscopic guidance of thromboembolectomy is performed by first controlling blood flow in the artery of interest. The angioscope is advanced until the area of residual thrombus or debris is in full view. The balloon catheter is then introduced alongside the angioscope and positioned just beyond the thrombus. The balloon catheter is inflated and removed along with the angioscope. This technique can help the surgeon target areas of adherent thrombus or intraluminal debris. Applying the least amount of pressure that is necessary to dislodge and remove the clot can minimize intimal damage.

Percutaneous Thrombectomy

A number of techniques and devices have been developed for percutaneous removal of intraluminal clot. Although a few devices are commercially available in the US and are used mainly for thrombectomy of dialysis access grafts, most are only available outside the US and are considered investigational. Clinical trials are under way to determine safety and efficacy of these devices. An extensive review by Sharafuddin and Hicks[6–8] describes many of these new technologies in detail. A useful classification scheme is as follows:

1. *Percutaneous aspiration thrombectomy* involves the application of suction through a large lumen catheter to remove thromboembolic material.
2. *Pullback thrombectomy and trapping* is a method by which thrombus is retrieved with a balloon or basket and collected into a trapping device for safe removal.
3. *Rotational and hydraulic recirculation thrombectomy* involves the microfragmentation of thrombus by the action of a high shear stress hydrodynamic vortex.
4. *Nonrecirculating mechanical thrombectomy* uses low-speed rotation or cutting blades, or both, without hydrodynamic recirculation to break up clot.
5. Thrombectomy may be achieved by the action of *ultrasound and laser energy* that can produce thrombolysis via two distinct separate approaches.

Percutaneous Aspiration Thrombectomy

Percutaneous aspiration thrombectomy, as first described by Sniderman and associates[9] more than a decade ago, is a technique that involves placing an antegrade vascular sheath into a thrombosed vessel. A guidewire is introduced and advanced through the thrombus. A 5F to 8F guide catheter is passed over the wire until the catheter abuts the leading edge of the thrombus. Aspiration with a syringe or vacuum container is performed to draw the clot into the catheter. Firm clot that will not pass into the guide catheter is withdrawn into the sheath and eliminated.

Three examples of percutaneous aspiration thrombectomy devices that are commercially available in Europe include the Stark Catheter (Angiomed/Bard, Covington, Georgia), SPAT (Balt-Extrusion, Montmorency, France), and Rotating Aspiration Thrombectomy Device (RAT) (Angiomed/Bard, Karlsrube, Germany). Brief descriptions of the products and their intended applications are noted in Table 1.

Pullback Thrombectomy and Trapping

Notable among the aspiration thrombectomy devices is the transvenous embolectomy device introduced by Greenfield in 1969 for the removal of acute pulmonary emboli.[10,11] The modern version of the Greenfield Transvenous Pulmonary Embolectomy Catheter (Medi-tech/Boston Scientific, Watertown, MA) consists of a double-lumen steerable catheter with a vacuum-cup at the distal tip (Fig. 7). The 12F catheter is inserted via a jugular or femoral vein through a venotomy or large sheath and positioned within the pulmonary artery next to the thrombus using fluoroscopic guidance and pulmonary angiography.

Table 1

Selected Percutaneous Thrombectomy Devices

Device	*Company*	*Product Description*	*Applications*
I. Percutaneous Aspiration Thrombectomy (PAT)			
Rotating Aspiration Thrombectomy Device (RAT)	Angiomed/Bard (Covington, GA) www.crbard.com	Dual-lumen catheter (8F); distal rotating spiral 2000 rpm	Chronic adherent thrombus; embolic plaque; intimal flap
SPAT set	Balt-Extrusion (Montmorency, France) www.balt.fr/contact.html	Dual-lumen catheter (8–10F); large lumen for aspiration, small for contrasting, guidewire	Acute thrombosis/thromboembolism peripheral arteries/grafts/veins; visceral arteries; iatrogenic and post-PTA
Stark Catheter	Angiomed/Bard (Covington, GA) www.crbard.com	Thin-walled, nontapered catheter (5–8F)	Acute thrombosis/thromboembolism peripheral arteries/grafts/veins, visceral arteries; iatrogenic and post-PTA
II. Pull-back Thrombectomy/ Clot Trapping			
Ahn thrombectomy catheter	American BioMed (The Woodlands, TX) www.americanbiomed.com	Dual-balloon thrombectomy catheter	Dialysis grafts
Fogarty balloon catheter	Baxter (Deerfield, IL) www.baxter.com	Single-balloon design with single lumen or dual lumen for over-the-wire	Peripheral arteries/grafts/veins
Greenfield Transvenous Pulmonary Embolectomy Catheter	Medi-tech/Boston Scientific (Watertown, MA)	Dual-lumen catheter (12F) with distal vacuum cup	Massive acute pulmonary embolism
Tulip Thrombectomy Sheath	Applied Vascular Devices (Laguna Hills, CA)	Wire mesh tulip (various diameters); 5–10F stem	Peripheral arteries/grafts/veins

(continues)

Table 1 continued.

Selected Percutaneous Thrombectomy Devices

Device	*Company*	*Product Description*	*Applications*
III. Rotational and Hydraulic Recirculation Thrombectomy			
Angiojet Rheolytic Thrombectomy System	Possis Medical (Minneapolis, MN) www.possis.com	Hydraulic recirculation produces thrombolysis and clot removal through effluent lumen (Venturi effect); 5F, 60-cm cath has 7 saline jets; large drive unit; compatible with 0.018″ guidewire	Dialysis grafts, peripheral arteries/ veins/grafts central/iliocaval thrombosis; pulmonary arteries TIPS; coronary arteries; visceral arteries
Clot Buster: Amplatz Thrombectomy Device	MicroVena (White Bear Lake, MN) www.microvena.com	High-speed rotation (100,000 rpm); recessed impeller at catheter tip; 6–8F catheter; 50–120 cm length no aspiration	Dialysis grafts, peripheral arteries/ veins/grafts central/iliocaval thrombosis; pulmonary arteries TIPS
Hydrolyser	Cordis Endovascular, a Johnson & Johnson Company (Miami Lakes, FL)	Hydraulic recirculation produces thrombolysis and clot removal through effluent lumen (Venturi effect) 7F dual-lumen cath, 65 and 100 cm lengths; uses standard power injector; guidewire up to 0.025″	Dialysis grafts, peripheral arteries/ grafts coronary arteries
Kensey (Trac-Wright) Catheter	Dow Corning Wright/Theratek International (Miami, FL) www.dowcorning.com	High-speed rotation (100,000 rpm) of distal end creates hydrodynamic vortex; 5–9F catheter with blunt rotating cam; no aspiration	Dialysis grafts, peripheral arteries/ grafts

(continues)

Table 1 continued.

Selected Percutaneous Thrombectomy Devices			
Device	*Company*	*Product Description*	*Applications*
Oasis	Boston Scientific (Natick, MA) www.bsci.com	Hydraulic recirculation produces thrombolysis and clot removal through effluent lumen (Venturi effect) uses standard power injector, 6F catheter, 65–100 cm length, 0.018″ guidewire, 6F sheath compatibility	Dialysis grafts, peripheral arteries/ grafts
IV. Nonrecirculating Mechanical Thrombectomy			
Without Aspiration			
Castaneda Over the Wire Brush	Micro Therapeutics, Inc. (Irvine, CA) www.microtherapeutics.com	Rotating brush tracks over 0.035″ wire, macerates clot; catheter length 65 cm or 115 cm; catheter diameter 6F; sidehole for infusion	Dialysis grafts
Cragg Brush	Micro Therapeutics, Inc. (Irvine, CA) www.microtherapeutics.com	6-mm nylon brush with 6F brush catheter rotates at 2000 rpm; endhole for simultaneous infusion of thrombolytic agent	Dialysis grafts
Arrow-Treratola PDT Device	Arrow International (Reading, PA) www.arrowintl.com	Rotating basket (3000 rpm) at distal end of 5F, 65-cm catheter	Primarily atherectomy cutter but may be useful thrombosed dialysis grafts
Simpson Atherectomy Device	Mallinckrodt (Saint Louis, MO) www.mallinckrodt.com	6–11F catheter with directional cutting chamber at distal end	Primarily atherectomy cutter but may be useful thrombosed dialysis grafts

(continues)

Table 1 continued.

Selected Percutaneous Thrombectomy Devices

Device	*Company*	*Product Description*	*Applications*
With aspiration			
Transluminal Extraction Catheter (TEC)	Interventional Technologies (San Diego, CA) www.ivt.com	5–14F torque catheter with distal cutting blades; electronic drive at 700 rpm; ball tip guidewire	Primarily atherectomy cutter but may be useful thrombosed dialysis grafts
Gelbfish Endo-Vac Device	NeoVascular Technologies (Brooklyn, NY)	6F sheath with coaxial manually reciprocating "clot spoon" on a drive shaft; percutaneous aspiration of thrombus	Thrombosed dialysis grafts
V. Ultrasound and Laser Thrombectomy Devices			
Clot-Specific Laser Thrombolysis Device	Latis (Horsham, PA)	Catheter delivers clot-specific laser energy that vaporizes thrombus without damaging vessel or surrounding tissues	Cerebral emboli
Ultrasound Thrombolysis Device (Acolysis System)	Angiosonics (Morrisville, NC) www.angiosonics.com	Croronary ultrasound thrombectomy device	Post myocardial infarction thrombosis

PTA = percutaneous transluminal angioplasty; TIPS = transjugular intrahepatic portosystemic stent.

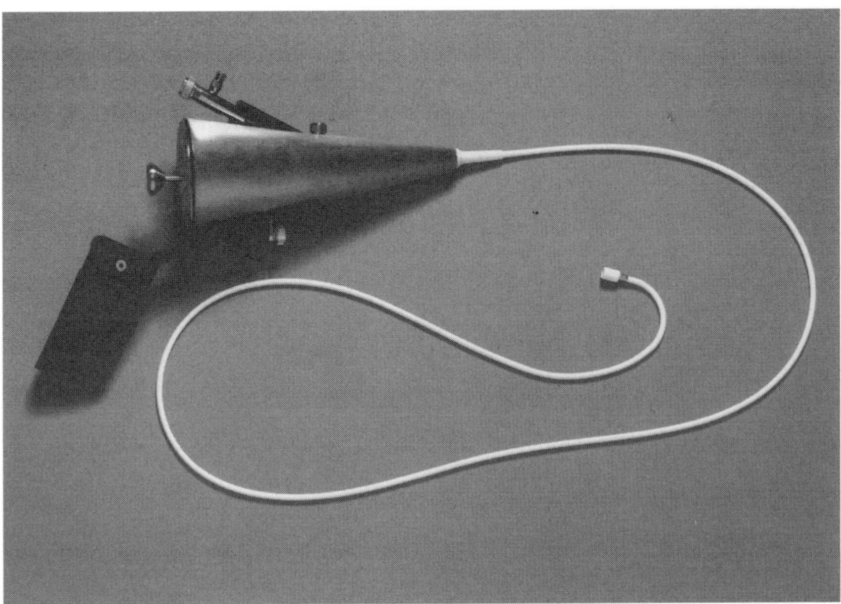

Figure 7. Greenfield Transvenous Pulmonary Embolectomy Catheter consists of a double-lumen steerable catheter with a vacuum-cup at distal tip for extraction of massive acute pulmonary emboli.

Syringe suction is applied to aspirate the embolus into the cup where it is held in place as the catheter is withdrawn. In a series of 32 patients with life-threatening pulmonary embolism, embolectomy was achieved with the device in 29 cases for a technical success rate of 91% and an overall survival rate of 78%.[10] The technique was unsuccessful when the embolus was more than 72 hours old.

Other percutaneous pullback thrombectomy techniques include self-expanding sheaths such as the Tulip Sheath (Schneider Europe, Zurich, Switzerland) and the Ahn thrombectomy catheter (American BioMed; The Woodlands, TX). The Tulip Sheath consists of a coaxial Fogarty balloon catheter that traps thrombus inside a self-expanding Wallstent (Boston Scientific, Natick, MA). The thrombus is compressed and removed as the stent is withdrawn into a 5F to 10F sheath. The Ahn catheter consists of a thrombectomy catheter with dual silicone balloons. The distal balloon traps clot and prevents blood loss after the proximal balloon is removed from the artery.

Rotational and Hydraulic Recirculation Thrombectomy

Recirculation thrombectomy devices create a hydrodynamic vortex at the tip of the catheter that fragments thrombus and pulverizes the resulting particles. The hydrodynamic vortex is generated by either rotational or hydraulic recirculation at the catheter tip.

Devices that create rotational recirculation all consist of a catheter with an impeller or basket at the distal tip that rotates at a high speed (100,000 to

150,000 rpm). The resulting fluid vortex creates a pressure gradient (Venturi effect) that obliterates and evacuates thrombus from the vessel lumen. The Clot Buster (Microvena Corp., White Bear Lake, MN) and the Trac-Wright Catheter (Dow, Corning, Wright/Theratek International, Miami, FL) are examples of rotational recirculation devices (Figs. 8 and 9).

Hydraulic recirculation devices make use of high-pressure fluid jets (source pressures up to 10,000 psi) that create a Venturi effect and pressure differential that results in pulvarization and aspiration of thrombus. These sys-

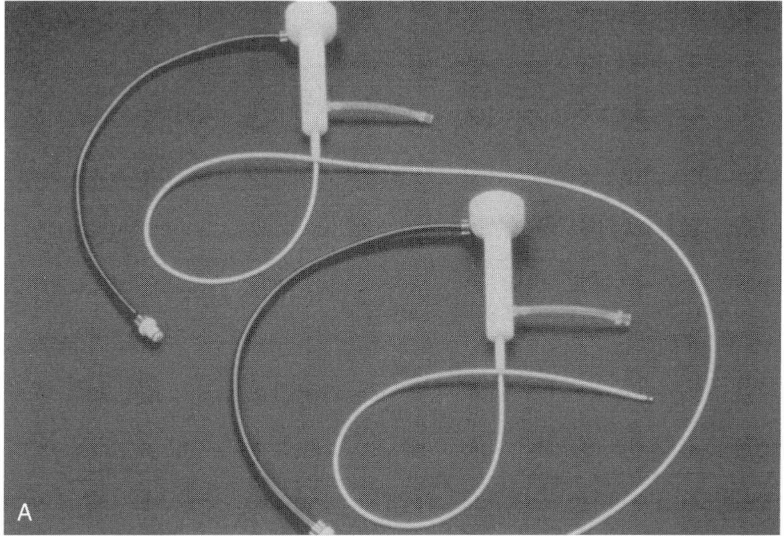

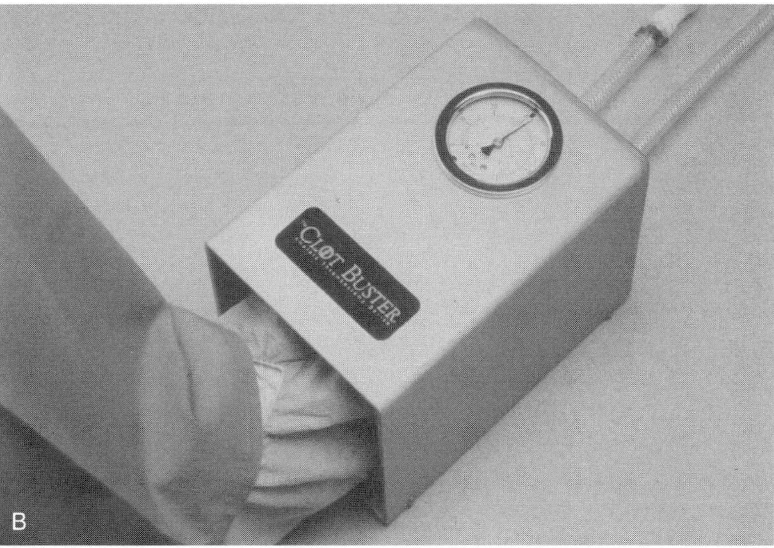

Figure 8. The Clot Buster: Amplatz Thrombectomy Device. **A.** 6F and 8F catheters shown have recessed impeller at the tip that rotates at 100,000 rpm to pulverize thrombus without concomitant aspiration. **B.** Pneumatic drive unit.

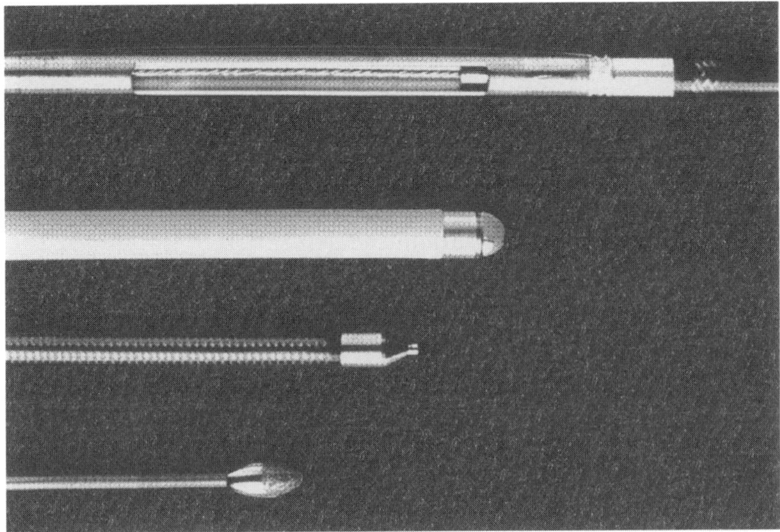

Figure 9. Magnified view of working ends of four atherectomy/thrombectomy devices Top to bottom: Simpson AtheroCath—nonrecirculating mechanical thrombectomy; Kensey (Trac-Wright) Catheter—rotational recirculation thrombectomy; Transluminal Extraction Catheter (TEC) system—nonrecirculating mechanical thrombectomy with aspiration; and Auth Rotablator—atherectomy.

tems require fluid compression control units. The Angiojet Rheolytic Thrombectomy System (Possis Medical, Minneapolis, MN) and the Oasis (Boston Scientific Vascular, Natick, MA) are examples of hydraulic recirculation devices (Fig. 10). Additional rotational and hydraulic recirculation devices are listed in Table 1.

Nonrecirculating Mechanical Thrombectomy

Percutaneous devices that macerate clot by mechanical means without the use of a hydrodynamic vortex are referred to as nonrecirculating mechanical thrombectomy devices. Some produce mechanical maceration without aspiration of particles, and others macerate with particle aspiration. The Arrow-Trerotola Percutaneous Thrombectomy Device (Arrow International, Reading, PA) consists of a 5F, 65-cm-long catheter with a 9-mm fragmentation basket that rotates at 3000 rpm. The device has no aspiration capability. It is approved in the US for thrombosed dialysis grafts. The Simpson Atherectomy Device, or AtheroCath (Mallinckrodt, Saint Louis, MO) is a 6F to 11F catheter with a distal directional cutting chamber that has a cutting side window, a positioning balloon, and an electronically driven inner blade (Fig. 9). The device has been approved by the US Food and Drug Administration (FDA) for recanalization of atherosclerotic peripheral arteries and grafts. Other nonrecirculating mechanical thrombectomy devices without aspiration capability are listed in Table 1.

The Gelbfish Endovac (Neovascular Technologies, Brooklyn, NY) is a per-

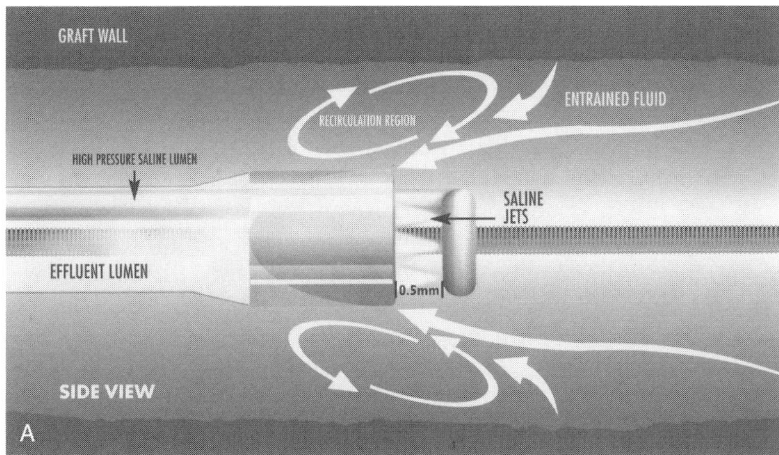

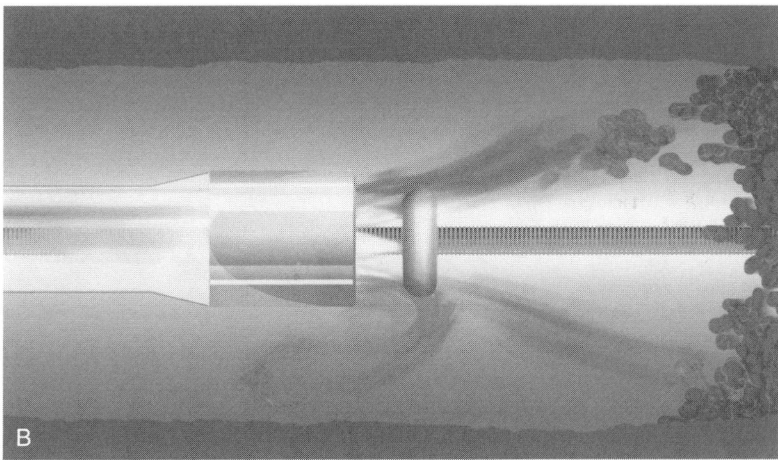

Figure 10. The Angiojet Rheolytic Thrombectomy System. **A.** Diagram depicting device with high-pressure fluid jet action that produces thrombolysis and clot removal through effluent lumen. **B.** Depiction of hydraulic recirculation and clot removal.

cutaneous clot removal system that uses a spoon at the distal end to break up clot, which is then aspirated through a 6F percutaneous sheath. The distal spoon has a retrograde irrigation port to assist in clot fragmentation and removal. The device is FDA approved for use in thrombosed dialysis grafts. The Transluminal Extraction Catheter (TEC) (Interventional Technologies, San Diego, CA) consists of a catheter with distal cutting blades that rotate at 700 rpm. The resulting thrombus particles are aspirated from the vessel lumen.

A number of devices have been investigated that use other forms of energy to destroy or remove thrombus. Ultrasound and laser energy are also used for purposes of eliminating intraluminal thrombus. Two such devices, the Ultrasound Thrombolysis Device, Acolysis System (Angiosonics, Morrisville, NC) and the Clot-Specific Laser Thrombolysis Device (Latis, Horsham, PA), are described in Table 1.

Comment

As the nature of arterial pathology continues to evolve with more patients having complex arterial reconstructions, in situ thrombosis, thrombosed bypass grafts, and occluded dialysis access grafts, there is a need for better devices and techniques for mechanical thrombectomy. Thrombolytic therapy is important, and the development of improved lytic agents with lesser side effects will represent a major advance in therapy. Newer methods of mechanical thrombectomy may prove to be superior to existing modalities. Proper evaluation of these technologies will require careful study and comparison to standard treatments to determine their safety, efficacy, and clinical utility for treating acute arterial occlusions.

References

1. Fogarty TJ, Zarins CK. Fogarty® catheter thromboembolectomy. In Nyhus LM, Baker RJ, Fischer JE (eds): *Mastery of Surgery*. 3rd ed. Boston: Little, Brown and Company. 1996:1887–1898.
2. Fogarty TJ, Cranley JJ, Krause RJ, et al. A method for extraction of arterial emboli and thrombi. *Surg Gynecol Obstet* 1963;116:241–244.
3. Hight DW, Tilney NL, Couch NP. Changing clinical trends in patients with peripheral arterial emboli. *Surgery* 1976;79:172–176.
4. Fogarty TJ, Monfort MY, Hermann GH, et al. Surgical technology—new techniques and instrumentation for the management of adherent clot in native and synthetic vessels. *Curr Surg* 1991;4:123–126.
5. Hyde GL, Sullivan DM. Fogarty catheter tamponade of ruptured abdominal aortic aneurysms. *Surg Gynecol Obstet* 1982;154:197–199.
6. Sharafuddin MJ, Hicks ME. Current status of percutaneous mechanical thrombectomy. Part I. General principles. *J Vasc Interv Radiol* 1997;8:911–921.
7. Sharafuddin MJ, Hicks ME. Current status of percutaneous mechanical thrombectomy. Part II. Devices and mechanisms of action. *J Vasc Interv Radiol* 1998;9(1 pt. 1):15–31.
8. Sharafuddin MJ, Hicks ME. Current status of percutaneous mechanical thrombectomy. Part III. Present and future applications. *J Vasc Interv Radiol* 1998;9:209–224.
9. Sniderman KW, Bodner L, Saddekni S, et al. Percutaneous embolectomy by transcatheter aspiration. *Radiology* 1984;150:357=N361.
10. Langham MR Jr, Greenfield LJ. Transvenous catheter embolectomy for life-threatening pulmonary embolism. *Infect Surg* 1986;5:694.
11. Greenfield LJ, Proctor MC, Williams DM, Wakefield TW. Long term experience with transvenous catheter pulmonary embolectomy. *J Vasc Surg* 1993;18:450–458.

9

Current and Future Innovations in Thrombolytic Therapy

Amir Motarjeme, MD

Thrombolysis

Thrombolytic therapy is being recognized as a well-documented, valid treatment for suitable cases of peripheral arterial occlusions, venous thrombosis, and thrombosed arterial grafts. As endovascular techniques become increasingly applicable in the management of arterial occlusive disease and as interventionists learn more about the natural history of occlusions, thrombolytic history plays an increasingly important role in both pre- and postprocedure treatment.

Historical Background

Tillett and Garner[1] reported their discovery of exogenous thrombolytic activity of streptococcal extract in 1933. Later, the lytic agent streptokinase (SK) was isolated from beta-hemolytic streptococci. Similarly, in 1946 urokinase (UK) was isolated from human urine and shown to have thrombolytic activity.[2] The first report on clinical experience with SK appeared in the literature in 1955,[3] and the first clinical evaluation of UK appeared shortly thereafter. Thrombolysin, a combination of SK and plasminogen, was also used briefly but not as widely in clinical evaluation as SK and UK.

Thrombolytic therapy was first utilized systemically for thromboembolic peripheral occlusions.[4–8] Although complete or partial thrombolysis was achieved in 20% to 50% of the patients, the high incidence of hemorrhagic complications led investigators to explore the effectiveness of selective local treatment of arterial occlusions resulting from thrombotic disease.[9–12] Local intra-arterial infusion of SK was reported as early as 1963 by McNicol et al[13] and

From Criado FJ (ed): *Endovascular Intervention: New Tools and Techniques for the 21st Century.* Armonk, NY: Futura Publishing Co., Inc.; ©2002.

Verstraete et al.[14] In 1974, Dotter et al[15] described the angiographic technique for intra-arterial infusion of thrombolytic agent (SK) in the treatment of arterial thromboembolic disease. Although their success was not nearly as impressive as that of more recent reports,[16] it represented the start of a new therapeutic modality.

Although UK was occasionally used as an alternative to SK,[17–19] it was not used routinely until 1985, when McNamara and Fischer[20] reported their experiences in a series of 85 patients. Subsequently, numerous reports of intra-arterial infusion of UK in arterial and bypass graft occlusions appeared in literature.[20–25] In most reports, UK was considered safer and more effective than SK and was the preferred thrombolytic agent until early 1999, when the Food and Drug Administration (FDA) halted the manufacturing and distribution of UK by Abbott Laboratories because of concerns about the risk of viral transmission. The form of UK (Abbokinase, Abbott Laboratories, Abbott Park, IL) used in the US is obtained from human kidney cells by tissue culture techniques. On January 25, 1999, a drug warning letter was distributed by the FDA alerting physicians to a number of problems related to the manufacturing of Abbokinase.[26] Abbott Laboratories stopped the shipment of Abbokinase in March of 1999.

Out of necessity, UK was replaced by recumbent human tissue-type plasminogen activator (r-TPA, Genentech, South San Francisco, CA) and shortly thereafter by reteplase (r-PA, Retavase, Centocor, Malvern, PA). These two newer thrombolytic agents proved to be as effective as UK in treatment of acute and subacute arterial and venous thrombosis, but they are associated with a slightly higher bleeding complication rate. More recently, tenecteplase (Tankase, Genentech), a new thrombolytic agent, has been introduced. Although experience with this new agent is very limited, it appears to be promising.[27]

The Fibrinolytic System

The fibrinolytic system, which is responsible for clot lysis, is activated when plasminogen is converted to plasmin by mediators such as tissue-type plasminogen activator. Exogenous activators such as UK, SK, actaplase, and reteplase can also initiate fibrinolysis. Plasmin degrades fibrin and fibrinogen into fragments, some of which have antithrombotic activity. The fibrinolytic therapy is most effective on fresh thrombus, but has also been shown to be effective in more organized thromboses.[28]

Plasminogen and plasmin exist in free circulating and thrombus-bound forms. To protect against the development of a generalized fibrinolytic state, the plasma contains antiplasmins: a-2 antiplasmin, which instantly neutralizes free plasmin; a-2 microglobulin, a slower, more stable inhibition of plasmin; a-1-antitrypsin, antithrombin III, and C-1 inactivator. Plasmin bond within thrombus is protected from neutralization by the antiplasmins and therefore is free to degrade fibrin. Thus, the interaction between plasmin and antiplasmin provides a system of selective fibrinolysis.[29]

Thrombolytic Agents

Streptokinase

SK is a purified preparation of a bacterial protein elaborated by group C, B-hemolytic streptococci. It is supplied as a water-soluble, white, lyophilized powder. SK is a foreign protein, capable of inducing resistance and allergic response. It has two distinct peaks of activity, one at 16 minutes and the other at 83 minutes. SK combines with plasminogen to form SK-plasminogen. This complex then unites with another plasminogen molecule to form plasmin. Since each molecule of SK uses two molecules of plasminogen to generate a molecule of plasmin, it is less efficient and also causes greater plasminogen depletion than UK. Because SK-plasminogen is perhaps a more potent activator than UK, fibrinogen degradation is also greater than during UK administration.[29] SK is antigenic, and prior streptococcal infection induces a variety of antibodies, including a specific SK antibody that directly inactivates the agent by forming an irreversible complex in a 1:1 ratio. Therefore, all antibody sites must be saturated by an initial loading dose of SK before subsequent doses can be active systemically. Measured antibody titers differ widely from individual to individual. Calculation of the loading dose required to neutralize all antibody sites should be performed in the initial clinical trial of the drug. Currently, a standardized loading dose of 250,000 units is used, since this dose will neutralize antibodies in 90% of the American population.[30] The antigenicity of SK, thought to cause the occasional pyretic response to the drug (in up to 5% to 10% of patients), has also caused serum sickness.[31,32] Anaphylaxis has been reported,[33] but serious reactions are rare.[34]

Urokinase

UK is an enzyme produced by the kidney and found in the urine. There are two forms of UK, differing in molecular weight but having a similar clinical effect. Abbokinase (injectable UK, Abbott Laboratories, Abbott Park, IL), a thrombolytic agent obtained from human kidney cells by tissue culture techniques, is primarily the low molecular weight form. UK differs significantly from SK in several aspects. First, there are no antibodies to cause inactivation, so no loading dose is necessary. In addition, UK is a direct plasminogen activator and does not form an intermediate activator complex. All plasminogen activated by UK is converted to plasmin. Excessive plasminogen consumption or plasmin activation does not occur.[35] UK is nonantigenic and does not induce an allergic response. Its half-life is relatively short, averaging 14 minutes.

Tissue Plasminogen Activator (TPA)

Alteplase (r-TPA)

Presently, alteplase (Activase, r-TPA Genentech) is used for local thrombolysis in peripheral arterial or bypass graft occlusions.[36] This TPA, produced by recombinant DNA technology, is an enzyme that has the property of fibrin-enhanced conversion of plasminogen to plasmin. It produces limited conversion of plasminogen in the absence of fibrin. When introduced into the systemic circulation at pharmacologic concentration, it binds to fibrin in a thrombus and converts the entrapped plasminogen to plasmin. This initiates local fibrinolysis but also produces some systemic proteolysis. Although a broad range of dosage has been used, the most common dose in arterial occlusions and graft thrombosis is 0.5 to 2 U/h. The length of infusion is commonly 12 to 36 hours, but it may extend to 48 hours, especially in venous cases. A longer infusion is not recommended, especially in elderly patients.

Reteplase

r-PA (Retavase, Centocor) is a nonglycosylated deletion mutein, which contains 355 of the 527 amino acids found in wild-type TPA.

Retavase catalyzes the cleavage of endogenous plasminogen to generate plasmin. The activation of plasminogen is stimulated in the presence of fibrin and is mediated via the kringle-2 domain. Plasmin in turn degrades the fibrin matrix of the thrombus, thereby exerting its thrombolytic action.[36–38] The usual dose of Retavase is 0.5 to 1.0 U/h.

Tenecteplase

Tenecteplase is a triple-combination mutant of alteplase that was developed to circumvent some of the limitations of current fibrinolytic therapies. Tenecteplase has a longer plasma half-life (20 versus 4 minutes), better fibrin specificity, and a high resistance to inhibition by plasminogen-activator inhibitor-1 than alteplase.[27] There is very limited experience with tenecteplase in the treatment of peripheral vascular disease. The usual dosage is one half that of alteplase.

Clinical Application of Thrombolytic Therapy

Thrombolysis has been shown to be an effective treatment for arterial occlusions caused by clots, in the case of thrombosis or emboli. Although all thrombolytic agents are effective in acute thrombosis, both in venous and arterial, there is sufficient experience showing the effectiveness of UK in chronic arterial and synthetic graft thrombosis.[28]

Technical Consideration

Arterial Puncture

For thrombolysis, the arterial puncture must be a clean one-wall puncture. A micropuncture technique is mandatory.

Sheaths

An arterial sheath of 5F or 6F is always used. Insertion of the catheter without a sheath increases the incidence of hematoma at the puncture site. When a contralateral approach is used, a 6F crossover (45 cm) sheath is preferred. This sheath is also needed for angioplasty and stenting following thrombolysis (Fig. 1).

Catheters

A 4F end-hole catheter can be used for a single port. A 4F or 5F catheter with a larger inner diameter such as glide catheter along with an injectable 0.035″ or 0.038″ wire can be used for coaxial infusion (Fig. 2). Multi-sidehole catheters and wires are also available.

Thrombolysis, Iliac Arteries

Approach: Contralateral femoral approach (Fig. 3).

Catheters: Preshaped contralateral catheter (e.g., Motarjeme Tip, Merit Medical Systems, Inc., South Jordan, UT).

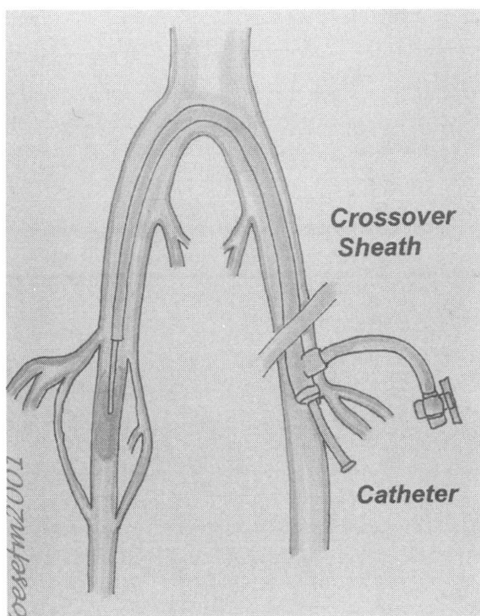

Figure 1. Contralateral approach for thrombolysis of the superficial femoral artery. A 45-cm-long crossover sheath is placed in the common femoral artery, through which a 4F end-hole catheter is inserted and embedded into the thrombus.

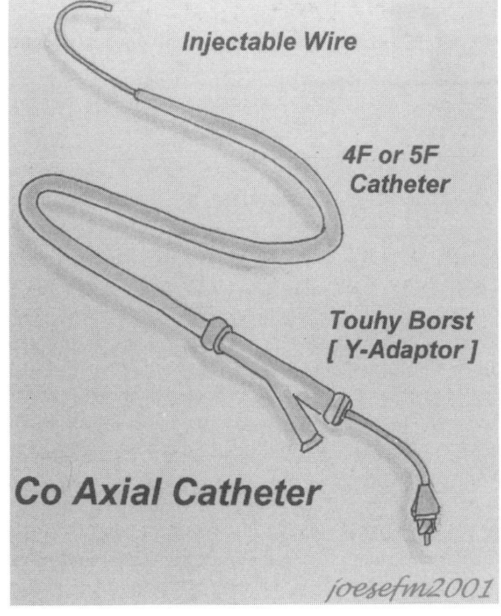

Figure 2. Coaxial catheter system.

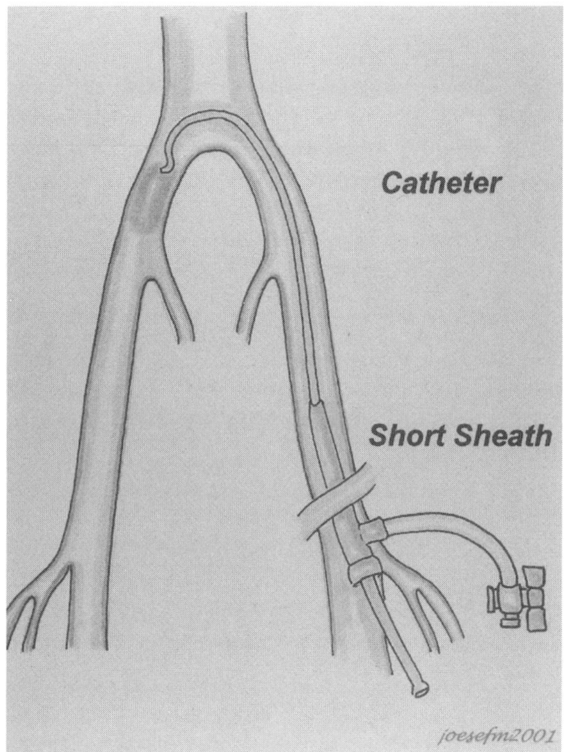

Figure 3. Technique for thrombolysis of the common iliac artery occlusion. A contralateral approach, 10-cm-long, 5F sheath, and a Motarjeme Tip catheter are being used.

Infusion wires: Sos wire (Medtronic Vascular, Danvers, MA). Note: for chronic occlusions, the infusion catheter or wire must be embedded into the occlusion.

Infusion time: 24 hours.
See Figures 4 and 5.

Femoral, Popliteal, and Distal Arteries

Approach: Contralateral or ipsilateral: a contralateral approach is preferred.

Sheath: Crossover (45 cm) sheath.

Catheters: 4F infusion catheter and 0.035″ infusion wire (Fig. 1).

Infusion time: 24 to 36 hours.
See Figures 6 and 7.

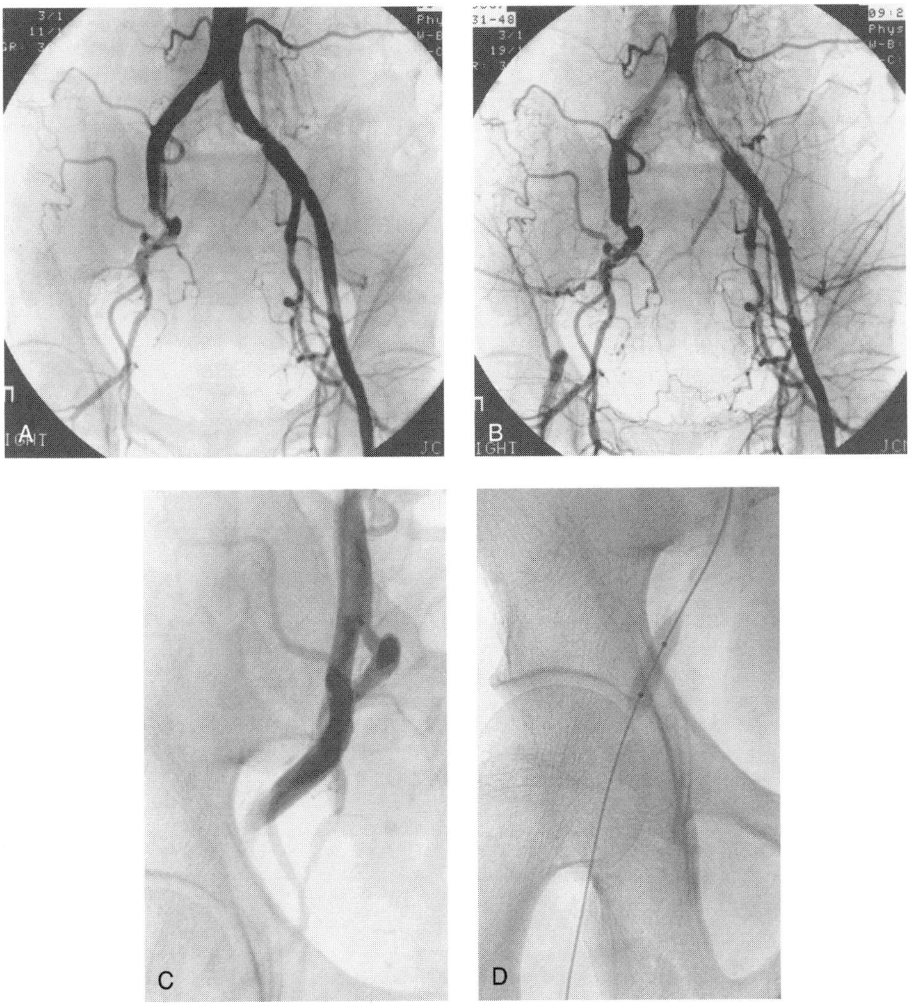

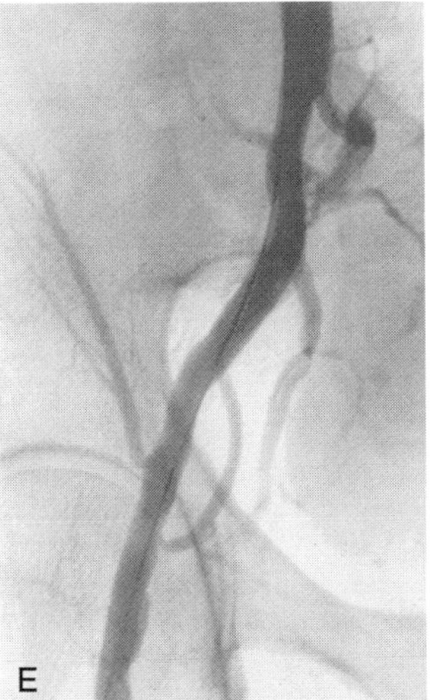

Figure 4. A 54-year-old male having claudication of the right leg for the past 18 months: **A.** and **B.** Abdominal aortogram revealing occlusion of the right external iliac with reconstitution of the common femoral arteries. **C.** Post-24-hour thrombolysis arteriogram showing thrombolysis and patency of the external iliac artery, but there is still occlusion of the junction of the external iliac and the common femoral arteries. **D.** Recanalization and dilatation of a short segment occlusion with a 7×20-mm balloon catheter. **E.** Post-thrombolysis and angioplasty arteriogram showing patent iliac and common femoral arteries.

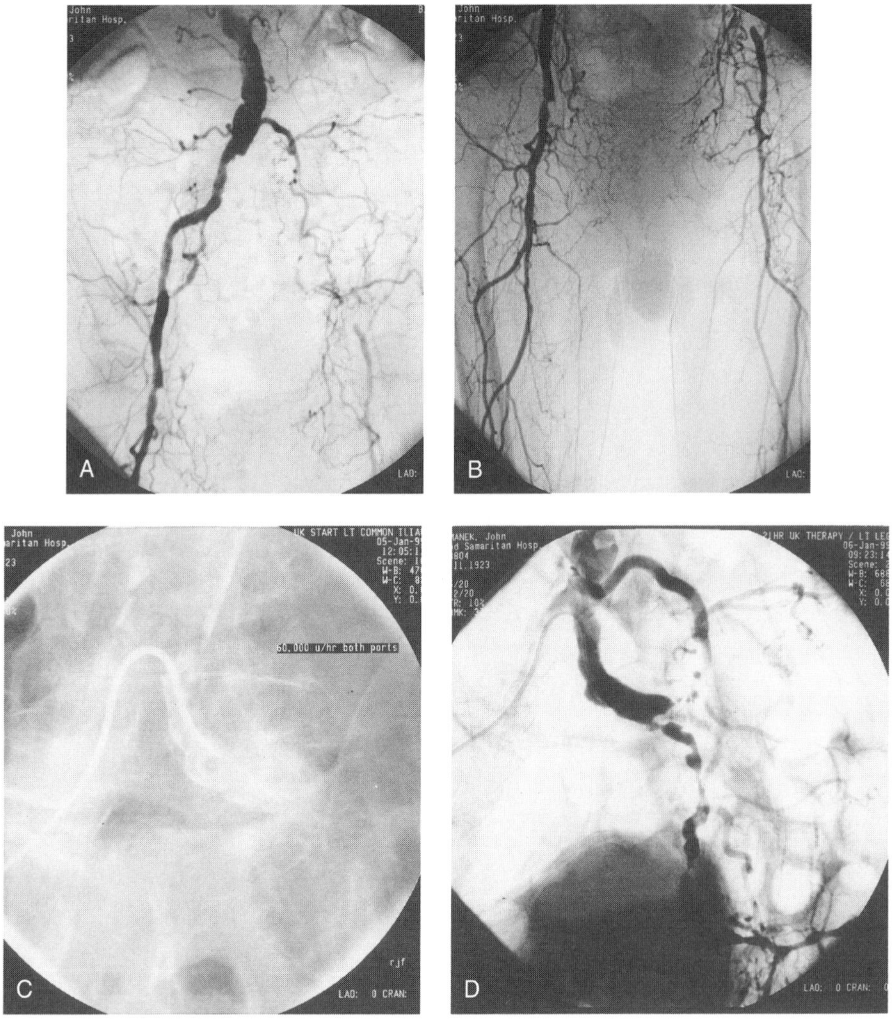

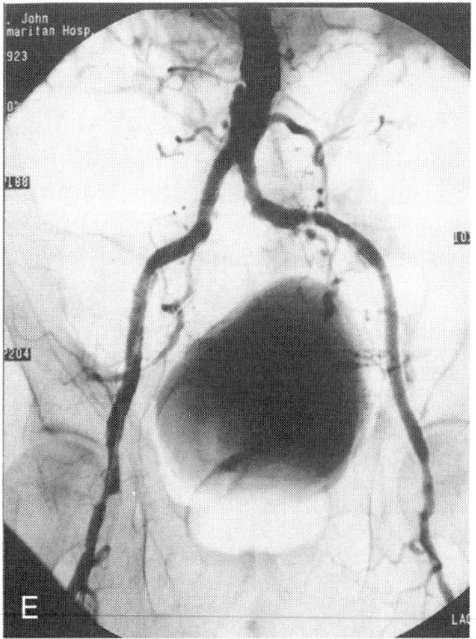

Figure 5. An 85-year-old male with severe ischemia of the left leg: **A.** and **B.** Bilateral iliac and femoral arteriograms showing total occlusion of the left common and external iliac arteries. The common and deep femoral arteries are patent, but the superficial femoral arteries are occluded. **C.** Thrombolytic therapy, a Motarjeme Tip catheter and a Sos wire placed in the common iliac artery and intra-arterial infusion of urokinase, 60,000 U/h per ports was infused. **D.** Twenty-four-hour postinfusion arteriogram showing complete clot lysis and patency of the common iliac artery, but there still is occlusion of the external iliac artery. **E.** Recanalization and stenting of the external iliac artery.

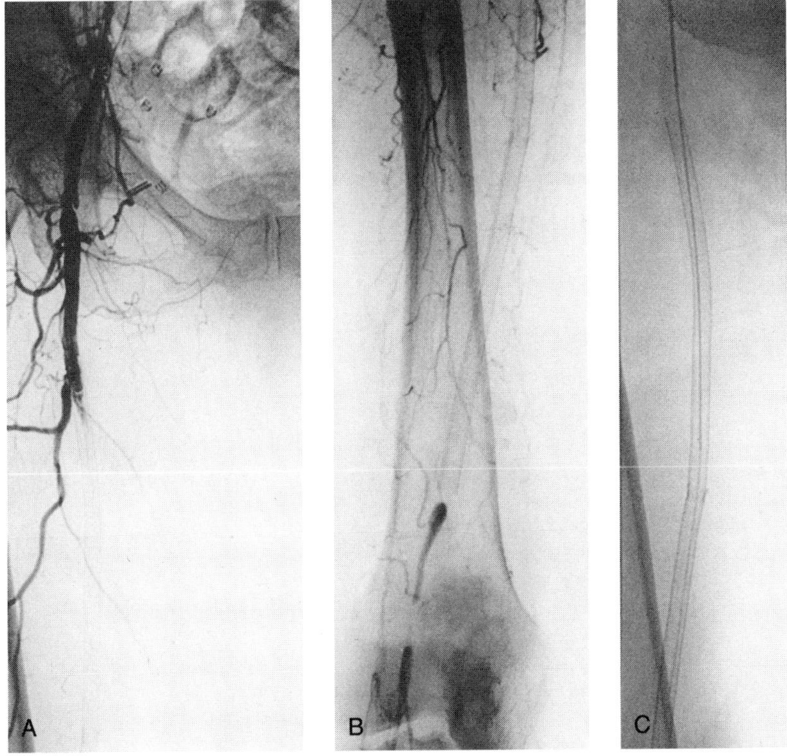

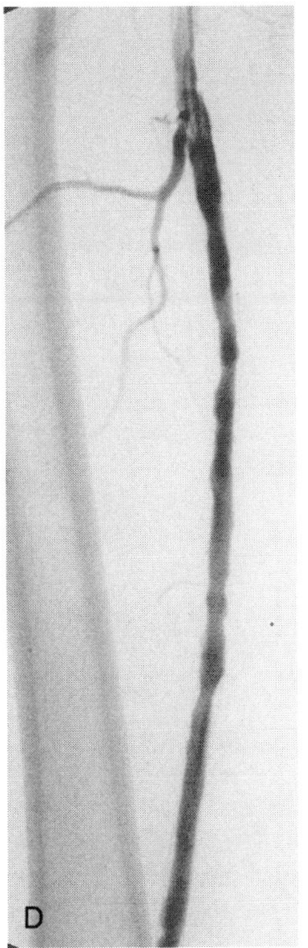

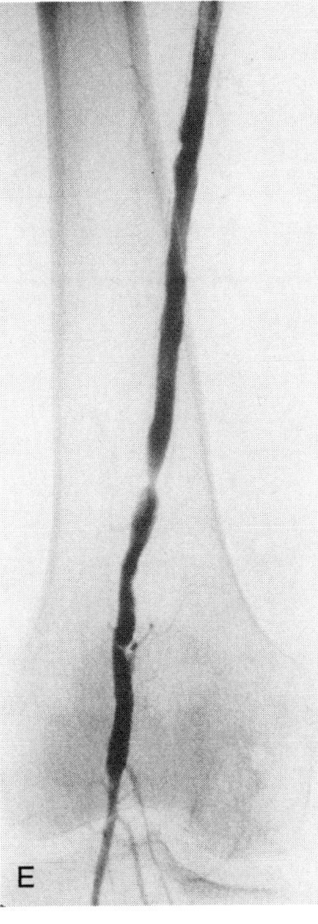

Figure 6. A 76-year-old female with a history of intermittent claudication, s/p angioplasty and stenting of the superficial femoral artery has developed a sudden onset of severe claudication and coldness and numbness of the right leg. **A.** and **B.** Femoral arteriogram showing total occlusion of the superficial femoral artery just proximal to the stent. There is a popliteal run-off above the knee, but there is also very severe stenosis of the popliteal run-off. **C.** Thrombolysis via a contralateral approach. There is a coaxial system in place with catheter just proximal to the stent and the Sos wire in the distal stent. Infusion of Retavase 0.25 U/h proximally and 0.13 U/h distally was started. **D.** and **E.** Post-24-hour infusion arteriogram showing total clot lysis.

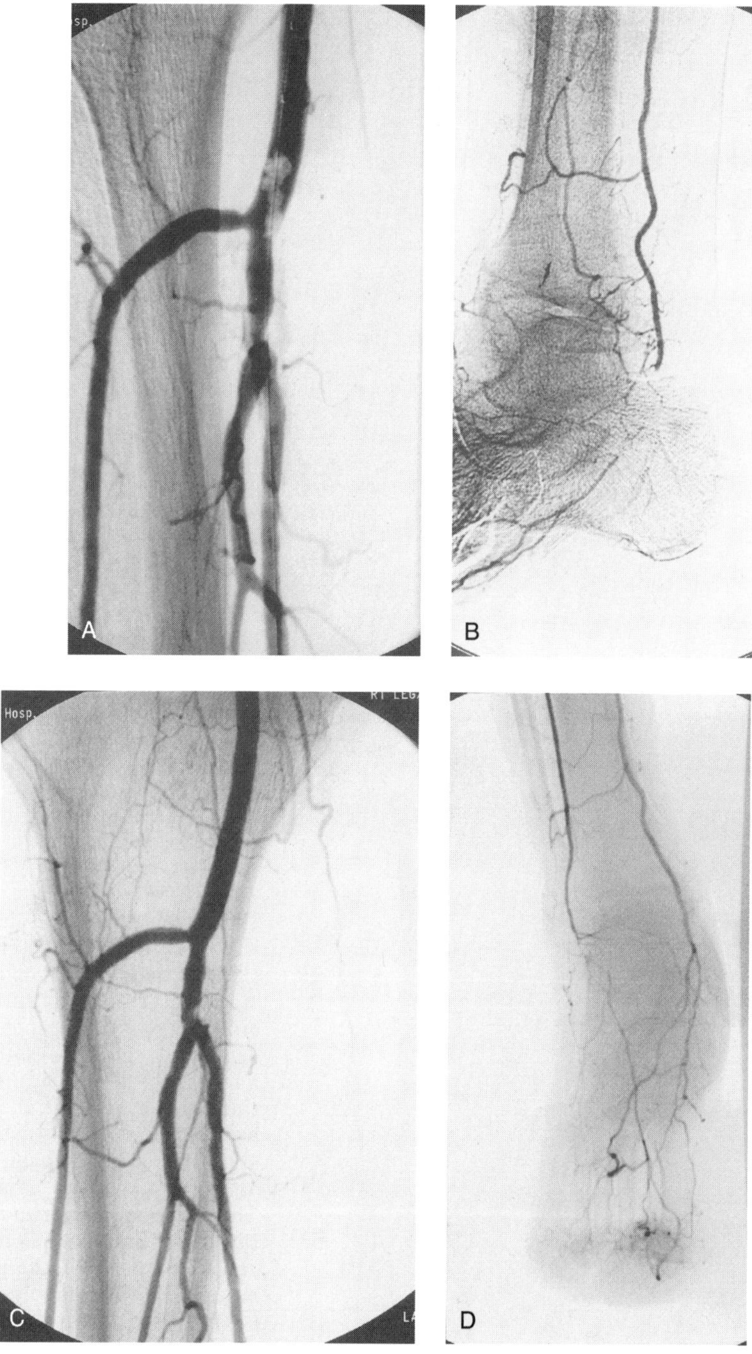

Figure 7. A 62-year-old male with a history of atrial fibrillation developed a sudden onset of pain and some numbness of the foot. **A.** and **B.** Femoral arteriogram performed via a contralateral approach showing a thrombus in the popliteal trifurcation and small embolus occluding the common plantar artery. Thrombolysis with tissue plasminogen activator using a coaxial catheter with a proximal port in the distal popliteal and the distal port in the proximal posterior tibial arteries. **C.** and **D.** Total resolution of the emboli of the popliteal and posterior tibial arteries.

Femoropopliteal Graft (Figs. 8 and 9)

Approach: Contralateral femoral.

Sheath: Crossover (45 cm) sheath.

Catheter and wire: 4F infusion catheter and 0.035″ infusion wire (Fig. 8).

Infusion time: 12 to 24 hours.

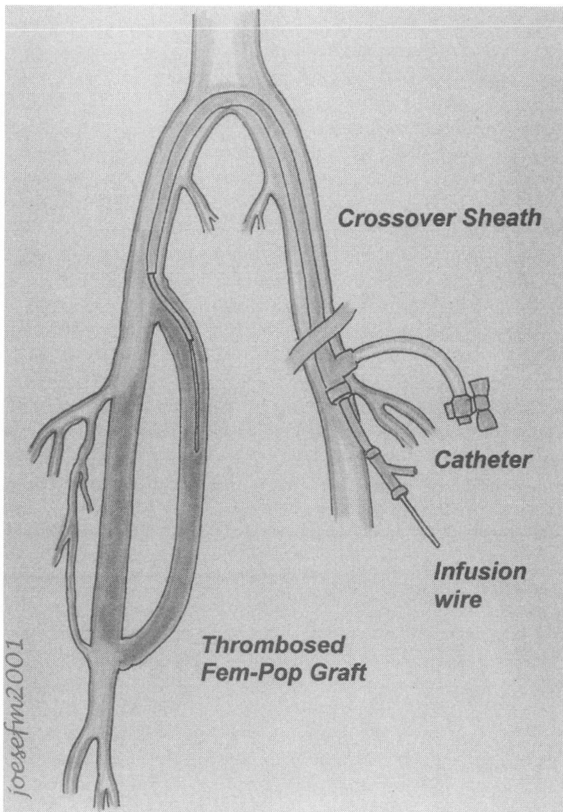

Figure 8. Technique for thrombolysis of a thrombosed femoropopliteal graft. A contralateral approach is used and a crossover sheath is placed in the common femoral artery just above the proximal anastomosis. A coaxial infusion catheter and wires are inserted into the graft. The catheter is embedded into the proximal end of the graft while the wire is placed in the middle or lower one third of the graft. Two thirds of the thrombolytic agent is infused proximally while one third is infused distally.

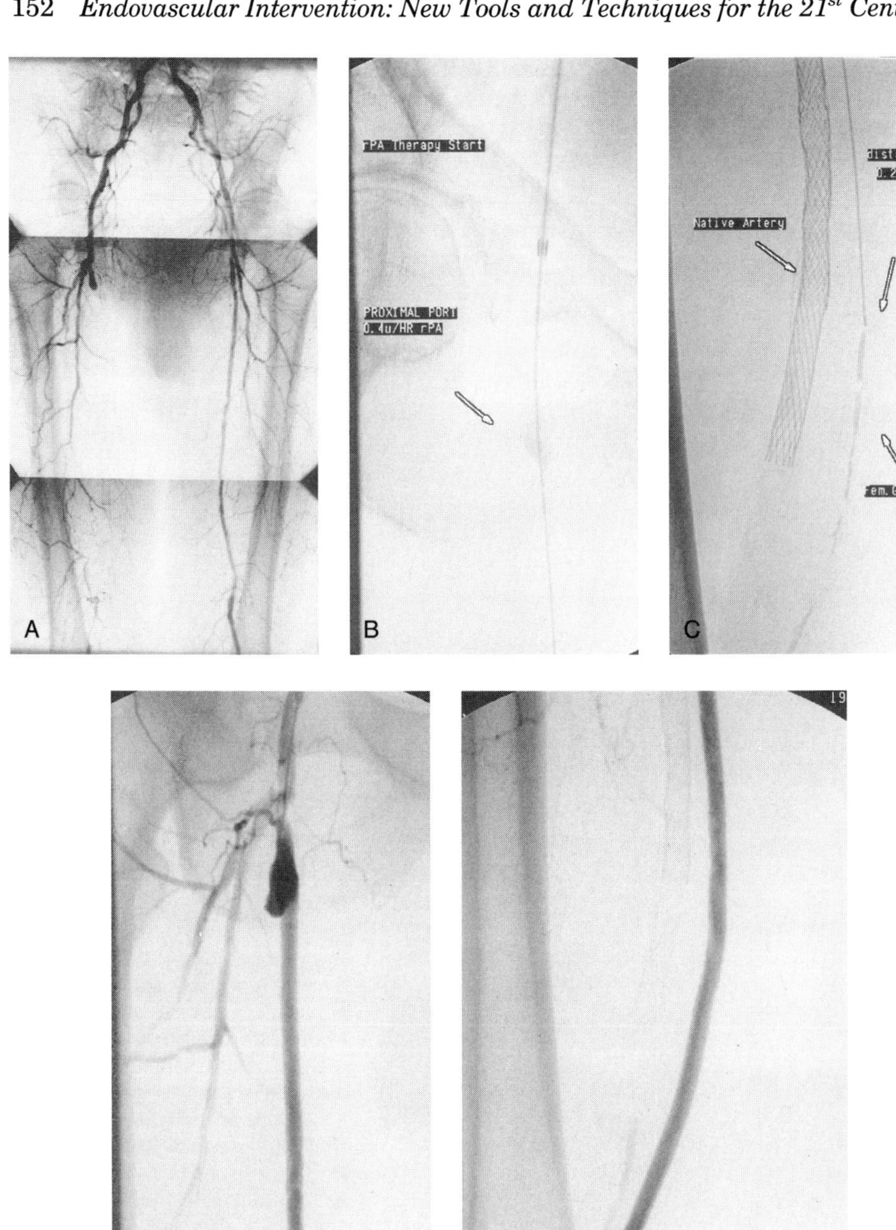
A
B
rPA Therapy Start
PROXIMAL PORT
0.4u/HR rPA
C
Native Artery
distal port
0.2u/HR
Fem.Graft
D
E
19

References

1. Tillett WS, Garner RL. The fibrinolytic activity of hemolytic streptococci. *J Exp Med* 1933;58:485–502.
2. MacFarlane RG, Pilling J. Observations on fibrinolysis: Plasminogen, plasmin and antiplasmin content of human blood. *Lancet* 1946;2:562–565.
3. Tillett WC, Johnson AJ, McCarthy WF. The intravenous infusion of streptococcal fibrinolytic principle (streptokinase) into patients. *J Clin Invest* 1955;34:169–175.
4. Poliwoda H, Alexander K, Buhl V, et al. Treatment of chronic arterial occlusions with streptokinase. *N Engl J Med* 1969;280:689–692.
5. Martin M, Schoop W, Weitler E. Streptokinase in chronic arterial occlusive disease. *JAMA* 1970;211:1169–1173.
6. Amery A, Deloof W, Vermylen J, et al. Outcome of recent thromboembolic occlusions of limb arteries treated with streptokinase. *Br Med J* 1970;4:639–644.
7. Hume M, Gurewich V, Thomas DP, et al. Streptokinase for chronic arterial occlusive disease. *Arch Surg* 1970;101:653–657.
8. Persson AV, Thompson JE, Patman RD. Streptokinase as an adjunct arterial surgery. *Arch Surg* 1973;107:779–784.
9. Weinstein J. Treatment of myocardial infarction with intracoronary streptokinase: Efficacy and safety data from 209 United States cases in Hocchst-Roussel registry. *Am Heart J* 1982;104:894.
10. Ganz W, Ninomiya K, Hashida J, et al. Intracoronary thrombolysis in acute myocardial infarction: Experimental background and clinical experience. *Am Heart J* 1981;102:1145.
11. Reduto LA, Smalling RW, Freund GC, et al. Intracoronary infusion of streptokinase in patients with acute myocardial infarction: Effects of reperfusion on left ventricular performance. *Am J Cardiol* 1981;48:403.
12. Rentrop P, Blanke H, Karsch KP, et al. Selective intracoronary thrombolysis in acute myocardial infarction and unstable angina pectoris. *Circulation* 1981;63:307.
13. McNicol GP, Reid W, Bain WH, et al. Treatment of peripheral arterial occlusion by streptokinase perfusion. *Br Med J* 1963;2:1508–1512.
14. Verstraete M, Amery A, Vermylen J. Feasibility of adequate thrombolytic therapy with streptokinase in peripheral arterial occlusions: I. Clinical and arteriographic results. *Br Med J* 1963;2:1499–1504.
15. Dotter CT, Rosch J, Seamen AJ. Selective clot lysis with low dose streptokinase. *Radiology* 1974;111:31–37.
16. Katzen BT, van Breda A. Low dose streptokinase in the treatment of arterial occlusions. *AJR Am J Roentgenol* 1981;136:1171–1178.
17. Totty WG, Gilula LA, McClennan BL, et al. Low dose intravascular fibrinolytic therapy. *Radiology* 1982;143:59–69.
18. Hurley JJ, Burrell MJ, Auer AL, et al. Surgical implications of fibrinolytic therapy. *Am J Surg* 1984;148:830–835.
19. Flessinger JN, Vayssairat NM, Julliet Y, et al. Local urokinase in arterial thromboembolism. *Angiology* 1980;31:715–720.

Figure 9. A 63-year-old male with a long history of intermittent claudication s/p angioplasty and stenting, which failed after 13 months. The patient was treated with a femoral popliteal graft. The patient developed a sudden onset of pain, coldness, and numbness of the right leg. **A.** Bilateral femoral arteriograms showing thrombosis of the right femoropopliteal graft. **B.** and **C.** Thrombolysis, a 6F crossover sheath is placed in the right common femoral artery through which a coaxial infusion catheter is inserted into the femoropopliteal graft. The catheter is placed at the proximal end of the graft and infusion of Retavase 0.4 U/h is started. The distal port is placed in the distal one third of the graft and infusion of Retavase at 0.2 U/h is started. **D.** and **E.** Total clot lysis and patency of the femoropopliteal graft.

20. McNamara TO, Fischer JR. Thrombolysis of peripheral arterial and graft occlusions: Improved results using high dose urokinase. *AJR Am J Roentgenol* 1985;144:769–775.
21. Belkin M, Belkin B, Bucknam CA, et al. Intra-arterial fibrinolytic therapy: Efficacy of streptokinase. *Arch Surg* 1986;121:769–773.
22. Gardiner GA, Koltun W, Kandarpa K, et al. Thrombolysis of occluded femoropopliteal grafts. *AJR Am J Roentgenol* 1986;147:621–626.
23. Traughber PD, Cook PS, Micklos TJ, et al. Intra-arterial fibrinolytic therapy for popliteal and tibial artery obstruction: Comparison of streptokinase and urokinase. *AJR Am J Roentgenol* 1987;149:453.
24. van Breda A, Katzen BT, Deutsch AS. Urokinase versus streptokinase in local thrombolysis. *Radiology* 1987;165:109.
25. Motarjeme A. Thrombolytic therapy in arterial occlusion and graft thrombosis. *Semin Vasc Surg* 1989;2:155–178.
26. Hartnell GG, Gates JG. The case of urokinase and the FDA: The events leading to the suspension of Abbokinase supplies in the United States. *J Vasc Interv Radiol* 2000;11:841–847.
27. ASSENT-2 Investigators: Single-bolus tenecteplase compared with front-loaded alteplase in acute myocardial infarction: The ASSENT-2 double blind randomized trial. *Lancet* 1999;354:716–722.
28. Motarjeme A. Thrombolysis and angioplasty of chronic iliac artery occlusions. *J Vasc Interv Radiol* 1995;6:665–725.
29. Sasahara A. Fundamentals of fibrinolytic therapy. *Cardiovasc Intervent Radiol* 1988;11:S3-S5.
30. Sharma GVRK, Cella G, Parisi AF, et al. Thrombolytic therapy. *N Engl J Med* 1982;306:1268–1276.
31. Totty WG, Romano T, Benian GM, et al. Serum sickness following streptokinase therapy. *AJR Am J Roentgenol* 1982;138:143–144.
32. Weatherbee TC, Esterbrooks DJ, Katz DA, et al. Serum sickness following selective intracoronary streptokinase. *Curr Ther Res* 1984;25:433–438.
33. Baumgartner TG, Davis RG. Streptokinase induced anaphylactic reaction. *Clin Pharmacol* 1982;1:470–471.
34. van Breada A, Katzen BT. Thrombolytic therapy of peripheral vascular disease. *Semin Intervent Radiol* 1985;2:354–368.
35. Collen D. On the regulation and control of fibrinolysis. *Thromb Haemost* 1980;43:77–89. 36. Risius B, Graor RA, Geisinger MA, et al. Recombinant human tissue-type plasminogen activator for thrombolysis in peripheral arteries and bypass grafts. *Radiology* 1986;160:183–188.
37. Kohnert U, Rudolph R, Verheijen JH. Biochemical properties of the kringle 2 and protease domains are maintained in the refolded t-PA deletion variant BM 06.022. *Protein Eng* 1992;5:93–100.
38. Martin U, Bader R, Böhm E, et al. Boehringer Mannheim 06.022: A novel recombinant plasminogen activator. *Cardiovasc Drug Rev* 1993;11:299–311.

10

Chronic Venous Insufficiency:

The Role for Endovascular Therapy

Patricia E. Thorpe, MD and Francisco J. Osse, MD

Introduction

The term chronic venous insufficiency (CVI) denotes a condition caused by venous hypertension. The signs and symptoms range from minimal postural edema or tiny telangiectasia to unremitting edema, pain, and nonhealing ulcers. Those familiar with CVI recognize that symptoms range from almost nothing to severe.[1] Reporting standards, including CEAP (clinical, etiology, anatomy, pathophysiology) classification, assist in evaluating treatments and procedures. Success or failure of any therapeutic approach translates to quality of life (QOL) for the patient and their family. Mild signs and symptoms of venous insufficiency do not bother many individuals, but there is a large patient population, in almost every nation, that experiences a wide range of disabilities related to venous disease.

The clinical spectrum may be related to primary or secondary valvular dysfunction, thrombotic obstruction, or a combination of occlusion and reflux. The superficial and deep veins may be involved separately or in combination, along with competent or incompetent perforators. CVI affects approximately 3% of the Medicare-aged population.[2] The cost to society for treatment and maintenance of patients with nonhealing venous ulcers due to venous hypertension is estimated to be more than $200 million per year.[3] Effective intervention earlier in the disease could help limit costs and improve the health of thousands of patients with symptomatic venous hypertension. The complexity of venous pathology may, in part, explain why there has been relatively little focus on treatment and research of venous compared to arterial disease. An-

From Criado FJ (ed): *Endovascular Intervention: New Tools and Techniques for the 21st Century.* Armonk, NY: Futura Publishing Co., Inc.; ©2002.

Our efforts were supported by a major grant from the Health Future Foundation of Creighton University, and for that we are grateful.

other factor has been the technical difficulty encountered in attempting to treat reflux or obstruction. Long-term success in solving obstructive problems is frequently plagued with rethrombosis or restenosis due to intimal hyperplasia. Recurrence is a perpetual problem with treatment of reflux and varicosities. Different topical approaches and endoscopic perforator ligation are being investigated for treatment of nonhealing ulcers. The prospect of effective, minimally invasive therapies for any aspect of venous disease is appealing. Since the trend toward minimally invasive therapy has been well accepted, during the past decade techniques that found success in treating arterial disease are being applied in new treatments for venous disease.

Endovenous Therapy: What's New?

Endovenous Reconstruction for Chronic Occlusion

Catheter-directed thrombolysis, developed during the last decade, is safe and effective in treating acute thrombosis.[4] The advantages of early thrombus removal are preservation of valvular integrity and rapid restoration of flow.[5,6] Compared to heparin therapy, without adjunctive thrombolysis, patients treated with urokinase for acute deep vein thrombosis (DVT), reported less post-thrombotic pain in long-term follow-up. The combination of thrombolysis and stent technology has led to significant advancements in endovenous therapy. Primary stenting of clinically significant common iliac vein compression is now performed.[7,8] As an adjunct to thrombectomy and thrombolysis, stenting of the abnormal segment underlying an acutely thrombosed iliac vein has been shown to be more effective than angioplasty and has better lasting results.[9,10] Symptomatic chronic thrombosis of the inferior vena cava continues to pose a challenge to vascular interventionists because of the technical difficulties associated with treating this condition. In addition, there are patients who suffer from chronic isolated tibiopopliteal occlusion, which can be very disabling to some. Chronic occlusion of the subclavian and superior vena cava are, perhaps, less commonly symptomatic than lower extremity thromboses; however, in the context of dialysis access, this is yet another important area for therapeutic intervention with lysis and stents.

Endovenous Saphenous Vein Obliteration to Replace Stripping

Minimally invasive treatment for varicosities and saphenous reflux now includes a new device (Closure®, VNUS Medical Technologies, Inc., Sunnyvale, CA) that uses radiofrequency ablation to eliminate the greater saphenous vein.[11,12] The device comprises a computer-controlled, bipolar generator and a choice of 1.7-mm (5F) and 2.7-mm (8F) catheters that have a sheathable, multiprong electrode tip (Fig. 1). Tumescent anesthesia is used with stab- or ultrasound-guided percutaneous technique. After a 6F sheath is positioned at knee level, the Closure catheter can be passed retrograde in the saphenous vein. Veins between 2 and 12 mm may be treated to produce a controlled radiofrequency injury, which induces contraction of venous wall collagen.

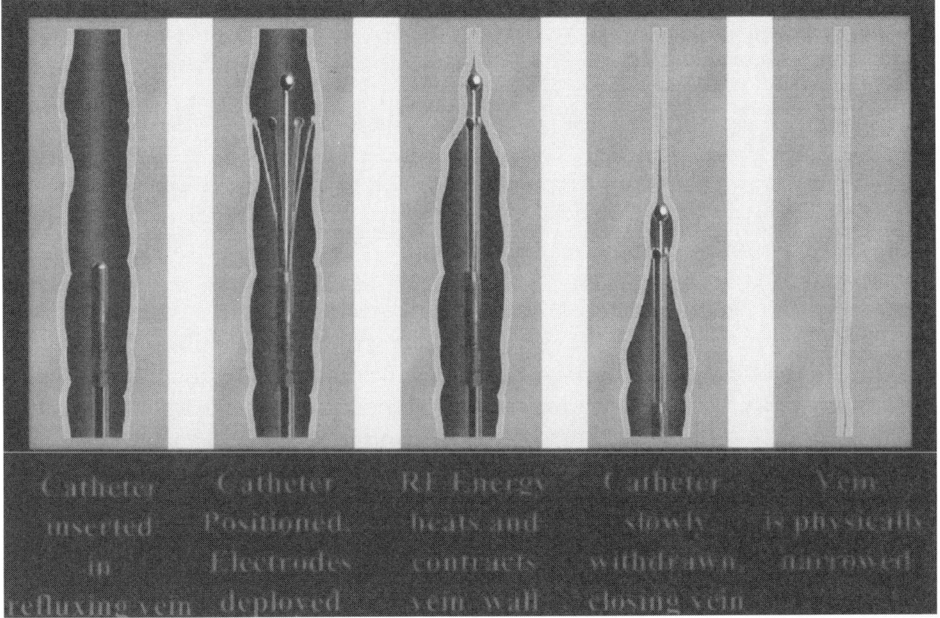

Figure 1. Closure procedure. A minimally invasive alternative to ligation and stripping.

The procedure eliminates saphenofemoral reflux through vein obliteration rather than thrombosis or ligation and stripping. Prior endovenous attempts to eliminate reflux have relied on electrocoagulation of blood to thrombose the vessel. Potential recanalization makes this approach less effective.[11] High ligation was used with catheter application. This procedure is designed to replace vein stripping as a means of treating hypertension and varicosities related to saphenous incompetence (Fig. 1). Chandler et al.[12] reported on treatment of 301 limbs in 273 patients in a multinational registry involving 25 sites. Acute occlusion was achieved in 290 limbs (96%). The procedure failed to yield obliteration in 11 limbs. Paresthesias were reported in 15% of treatments confined to areas above the knee, but this figure increased to 30% in limbs treated below that level. Thermal skin injuries were noted in 8 cases. These complications prompted change from local to tumescent anesthesia. After a mean follow-up of 4.9 months, 21 treated veins demonstrated some degree of recanalization and 11 (3.8%) had demonstrable reflux. Patient satisfaction with the procedure is high, and 91 patients, followed between 6 and 12 months, showed significant improvement in the CEAP class and decrease in symptoms. For appropriately selected patients, this appears to be a promising procedure that is gaining in popularity because it eliminates the need for groin surgery of scars from stab-avulsion sites. The results are more immediately cosmetic, with less bruising and decreased risk of infection. It can be done as an outpatient procedure in less than 2 hours. Patients experience less overall discomfort and faster recuperation than with traditional ligation and stripping procedures. Ultrasound guidance is recommended to facilitate atraumatic, single-wall puncture at the entry site and, to determine the location of the saphenofemoral junction.

Investigation of Valve-Stent Combinations for Valve Replacement

Research is being conducted at several sites to develop a percutaneous procedure whereby a valve prosthesis and stent are combined for the treatment of deep valvular insufficiency.[13–15] Gomez-Jorge et al[13] are working with a glutaraldehyde-treated bovine jugular vein valve combined with a Nitinol stent. Initial, short-term animal data indicated early inflammatory response but continued valve function and patency. Two other groups are combining efforts to develop a prosthetic valve from small intestine submucosa, a material that has been shown effective in vascular repair.[16] The combination of valve-leaflets and modified Z-stent design has been implanted in swine and sheep, in studies designed to achieve a model suitable for clinical trials in the treatment of symptomatic deep venous valvular dysfunction[14,15] (Fig. 2).

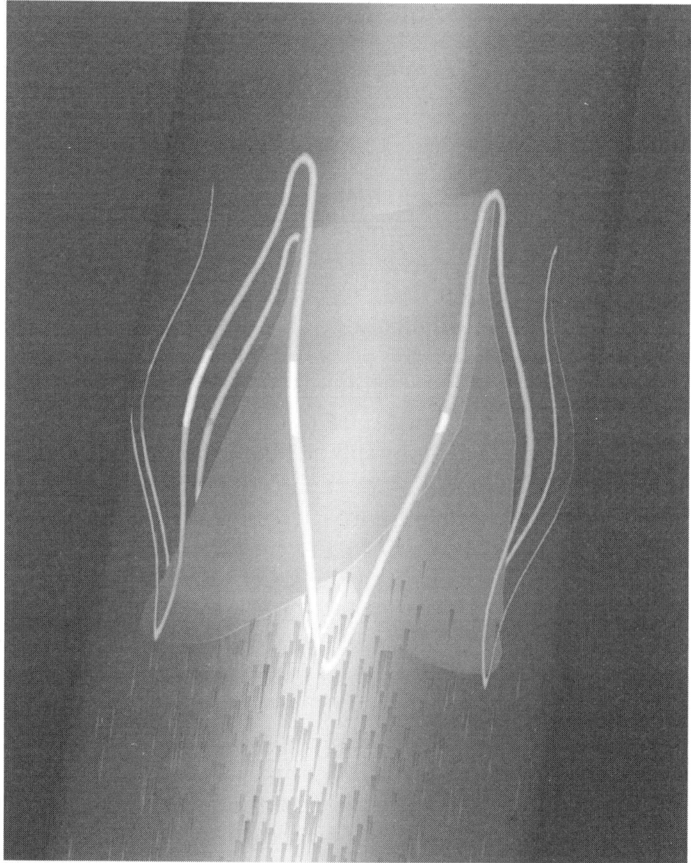

Figure 2. Graphic rendering of a metallic stent adapted to a bulbous configuration similar to the native vein at the valve site.

Sclerotherapy with Microfoam

A new idea for venous intervention is being developed by Dr. J. Cabrera and colleagues in Granada, Spain. They recently reported on ultrasound-guided injection of a microfoam sclerosant made of sodium tetratetradecyl sulfate or polydocanol.[17] The material is slowly injected under direct ultrasound visualization to treat inoperable hemangiomas. The high echogenicity of the foam allows controlled displacement of blood from abnormal vessels. There is less dilution and deactivation of the sclerosant with greater chance of endothelial contact. Overfilling and contact with normal structures can be avoided. Cabrera et al reported on treatment of 33 patients presenting with inoperable venous malformations. All therapies were staged with the number of treatments ranging between 4 and 22, depending on the size and location of the lesion. The formula for the microfoam substance is protected by a patent and is not yet commercially available; however, the technique and results appear to be a significant contribution to endovenous therapy.

Endovenous Therapy for Chronic Venous Occlusion

Patients presenting with severe CVI due to thrombotic obstruction of multiple segments may also have reflux caused by injury to the valves. The standard therapeutic approach, conservative management with graduated compression hosiery, is more or less palliative, depending on the extent of pathology. When phlebography and duplex demonstrate minimal deep flow due to a poorly recanalized deep system, collateral flow via the saphenous system or possibly the profunda, and transpelvic collaterals indicating iliac occlusion, there are few therapeutic options.

The location of thrombotic occlusion in axial veins can cause common patterns of limb edema and pain. When the iliac system is occluded and collaterals are inadequate, the entire leg is symptomatic and the patient often experiences groin discomfort with sitting or ulcer formation (Figs. 3 and 4). When there is isolated obstruction of the popliteal and/or upper calf veins despite normal venous anatomy above this level, the patient complains of edema and discomfort below the knee, while the thigh and pelvic regions remain unremarkable.

Generally, signs and symptoms correspond to the extent and duration of thrombosis, but there may be genetic variability involved in individual ability to autolyse extremity thrombus. Although recanalization occurs in response to thrombosis,[18] the process of reopening veins and recruiting collateral pathways can be inadequate, thus leaving a person with venous hypertension.[19] How prevalent is post-thrombotic disability? We recognize it most in the elderly, but symptomatic venous conditions, more often related to reflux than DVT, are not uncommon in younger patients. The epidemiology of chronic venous conditions among adults between ages 20 and 65 is simply not established; however, we do understand that individuals with short segment, subocclusive DVT do well

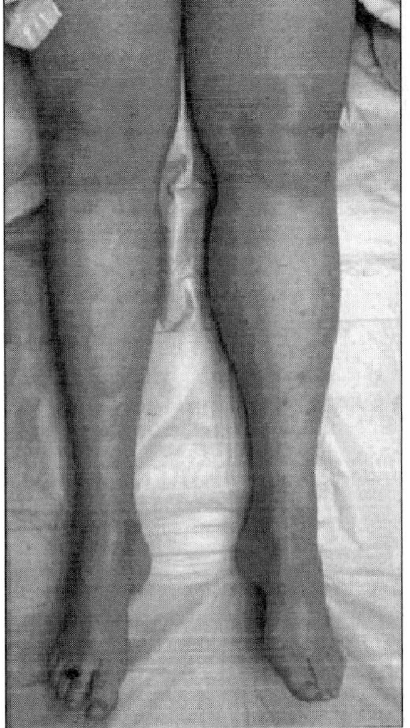

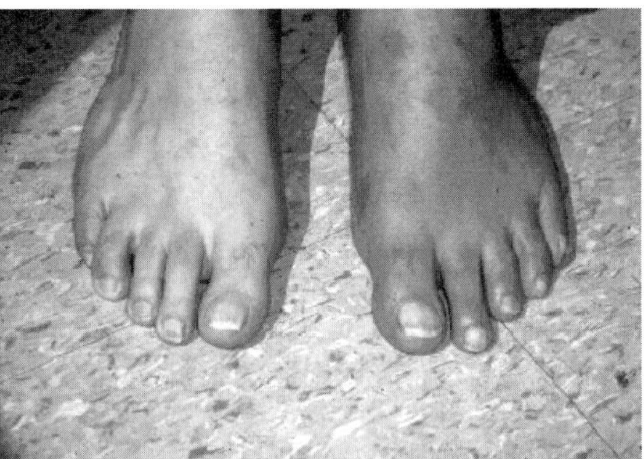

Figure 3. Chronic iliofemoral occlusion. Left leg edema 30 years after initial deep vein thrombosis following motor vehicle accident. The patient experiences no pain at rest, but claudication and dependent discoloration are present.

clinically. Quite possibly, many episodes of minimal DVT are undiagnosed because symptoms and signs are vague and resolve quickly. Multisegmental, occlusive thrombus, on the other hand, is more frequently associated with residual obstruction and associated valve damage or obliteration. These patients comprise the population of symptomatic individuals who have been diagnosed

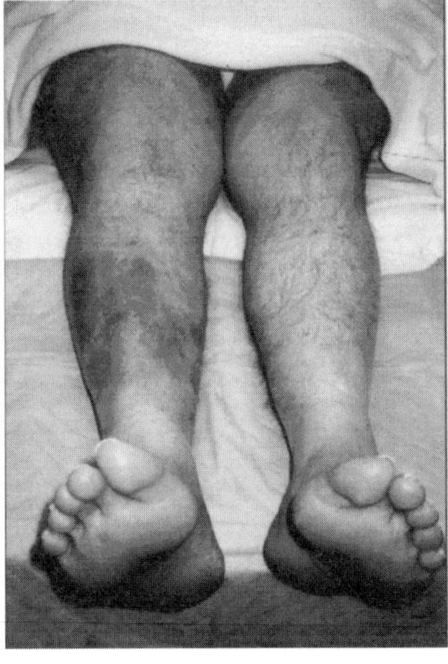

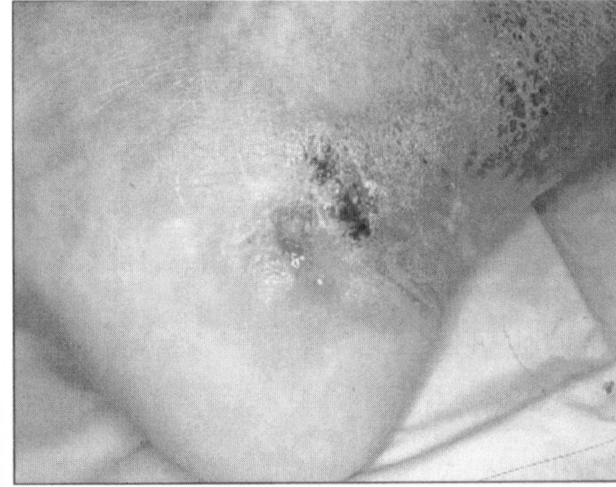

Figure 4. Chronic venous obstruction CEAP Class VI. Hyperpigmentation and recurrent stasis ulcer in a 45-year-old male, 10 years after initial deep vein thrombosis episode.

with DVT and treated with standard therapy. Patients often present with acute thrombosis superimposed on old thrombus (Fig. 5). Many have taken warfarin for 6 months only to have a recurrent episode after termination of the anticoagulation. Some have an underlying hypercoagulability, which remains unknown as long as they take warfarin. Others are almost incapacitated with the pain associated with nerve involvement at the site of nonhealing ulcers. Venogenic pain can be recalcitrant to narcotic medication. This is another dimension to patient care, in addition to time-consuming wound care. Moreover, these individuals are at risk for infection and amputation.

Post-thrombotic disability decreases QOL but is generally not limb threatening. Anyone who works with vascular patients addresses QOL issues daily. Discussion of QOL relative to venous disease has recently appeared in the literature.[8,20,21] Comerota et al[21] state that patients who have undergone thrombolysis for iliofemoral DVT have better functioning and wellbeing than similar patients treated with anticoagulation alone. In clinic, it is important to determine how disabled a patient is by asking 1) how many hours of the day are spent with the leg elevated for relief of discomfort of swelling? 2) How many daily decisions are influenced by this condition? Work? After work? Shopping? 3) What activity does the patient no longer do, or would do, if the leg was more normal? It is also important to observe the patient walking. Some patients complain about pain but walk normally. Others, reluctant to complain or to appear weak of spirit, limp when they walk. It is important for the patient to think about the QOL issues, because after intervention, compliance with compression stocking and warfarin relates to a person's desire to preserve the gains and prevent return to a more disabled state.

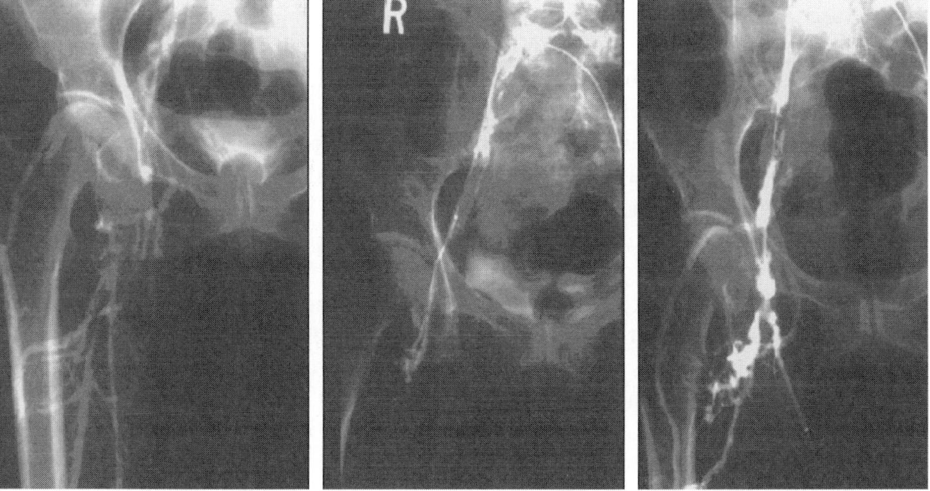

Figure 5. Chronic iliofemoral deep vein thrombosis with acute presentation. Left: Baseline ascending venogram. Center: First injection via catheter placed over bifurcation. Right: Follow-up after 24 hours of catheter-directed lysis with urokinase.

Clinical Patterns of Post-thrombotic Syndrome

We have recognized several different clinical patterns of chronic post-thrombotic venous insufficiency. In the first group (*HF=heparin failure*), patients present with unremitting pain and edema after the initial episode of DVT. Invariably, these patients have sought and received timely diagnosis and anticoagulation but have failed to respond to traditional heparin and warfarin regimens. These patients have significant venous hypertension related to the extent of their thrombosis. They lack sufficient recanalization to prevent edema. They are frequently very disabled and cannot work, drive, or perform normal daily activities. Patients with nonhealing ulcers may be in the heparin failure or recurrent DVT groups. They commonly have chronic compression or occlusion of the left common iliac vein. Individuals in the second group (*AC= acute-on-chronic*) present with an acute episode of thrombosis, without any documented and/or suspected history of DVT. Phlebography, however, reveals anatomical changes consistent with prior thrombosis of indeterminate age. Patients in a third group (*R=recurrent DVT*) have a common history of one or more prior episodes of thromboembolism. Many have been hospitalized more than once for pulmonary embolus and/or DVT. They are routinely readmitted for intravenous heparin therapy and further anticoagulation. Recurrent DVT frequently occurs shortly (1 to 3 months) after discontinuation of oral anticoagulation. A relatively high number of these patients have a family history of thrombosis, suggesting an inherited hypercoagulability disorder. Ulceration is more common in this group.

Selecting Patients for Endovenous Therapy

There is emerging recognition of a symptomatic condition that has previously been ignored and, in many instances, has led to left leg thrombosis. The May-Thurner, or iliac compression, syndrome,[22] caused by compression or occlusion of the left common iliac vein by the right iliac artery, can be clinically occult or cause unilateral leg and ankle edema or discomfort. The diagnosis is unfortunately most often made in association with acute iliofemoral thrombosis (Fig. 6); however, the success of endovascular stents has led to greater awareness of this condition in young women, prior to thrombosis. The diagnosis can be made by a history of unilateral leg or ankle edema or discomfort. The duplex exam, performed to rule out DVT, is often negative. The subtle findings in velocity changes and widening of the common iliac vein are often missed because the pelvis is not included in the exam, or in the presence of obesity or bowel gas, which makes imaging of that area difficult. Phlebography, with contrast injection from the popliteal or femoral level, is the best way to image the abnormality. Iliac occlusion is implied by transpelvic or trans-sacral collaterals (Fig. 7). It is important to exclude other causes of iliac thrombosis such as malignancy or trauma. Cross-sectional imaging can suggest the condition but does

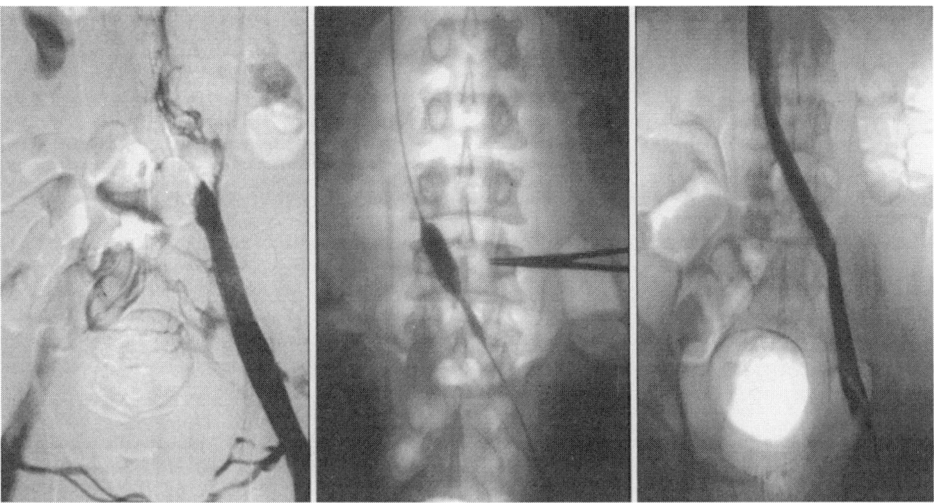

Figure 6. Primary stenting of May-Thurner compression. Left: Chronic iliac occlusion. Center: 12×4-cm balloon. Right: 12×60-mm Wallstent.

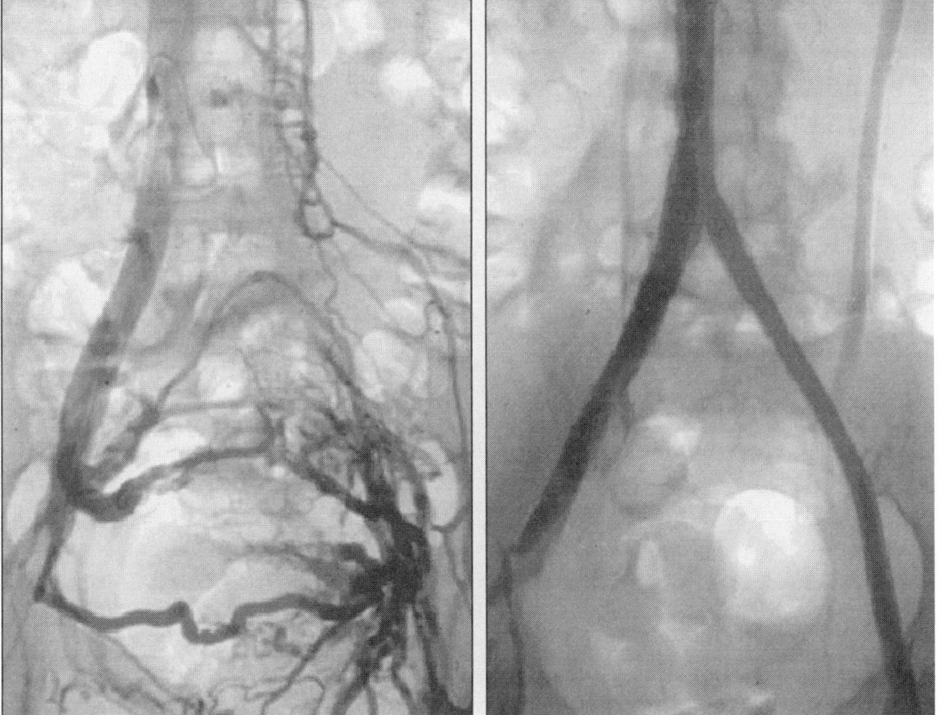

Figure 7. May-Thurner syndrome. Left: 46-year-old female with a 12-month history of debilitating pain and edema after left deep vein thrombosis. Right: Following urokinase and three Wallstents, 10×94, 10×68, and 10×42. Patient at 3 years.

not provide information about the hemodynamic significance of the compression. Everyone has this anatomical relationship of the vein and artery, but in postmortem studies, only 25% to 30% of patients had focal vessel abnormalities.[22]

Regardless of the age of the thrombus or the number of times a patient has been hospitalized with DVT, in our experience subjective and objective improvement can be achieved and sustained with endovascular therapy, provided the patient remains anticoagulated. Therefore, an important criterion for patient selection is ability to be compliant with anticoagulation. As we gain more long-term data on patients with iliac stents, we may be able to identify a profile for patients who do not require lifetime anticoagulation. Our data indicate that this group includes patients with 1 to 3 stents in the suprainguinal location, with excellent inflow from relatively normal distal veins.

The standard contraindications to lytic therapy apply for patients with chronic DVT, especially because the infusions are longer than those for acute DVT. We have performed uncomplicated, prolonged infusions of urokinase in patients within 14 days of major surgery, including gastric bypass (14 days), abdominal hysterectomy (10 days), and total knee arthroplasty (5 days). One patient was treated 14 days after normal vaginal childbirth, and several women have been treated during menses without complication. Because of differences in fibrin affinity, perioperative use of alteplase has not been attempted.

Endovenous reconstruction of chronic thrombosis is contraindicated in patients with renal failure because iodinated contrast is required for this procedure. Whereas acute DVT can be treated with a combination of ultrasound guidance and monitoring, manipulation of catheters and wires in chronic occlusions requires fluoroscopic visualization with iodinated contrast. An alternative contrast agent is carbon dioxide, which can be used to image venous as well as arterial disease.[23] A flow-directed infusion can be performed, with ultrasound assistance used to identify the location of the saphenous pressure sites, for tourniquet placement, and for follow-up monitoring.

Endovenous Tools

Thrombolysis, balloon dilatation, and stent placement comprise the main thrust of endovenous therapy for revascularization. Thrombectomy devices, useful in dialysis fistulae, have not aided the treatment of lower extremity venous thrombosis due to the limited size of the debulking channel.[8] This issue is being addressed by industry, and newer 0.035″ devices will work more effectively in larger vessels. All mechanical devices work best in the presence of acute, not organized thrombus.

Our approach to endovascular therapy for thrombotic occlusion, especially chronic occlusion, is based on the following philosophy. If one considers a limb as an "organ system," in the sense that venous segments exist in continuity with smaller veins below and larger veins above, one can see that, ideally, they should not be treated in isolation. The entire limb concept generally applies to arterial therapy, but few apply this notion to veno-occlusive disease. For example, flow in a stented iliac segment depends on flow from the femoral, popliteal, and infrapopliteal segments. If there is subacute and chronic DVT in the calf and thigh, treating only the superficial femoral vein without addressing the occlusive thrombus in distal veins will result is suboptimal restoration of deep venous flow. If tibial flow is occluded, blood preferentially goes to the superficial veins. This pathway will persist even when the superficial femoral vein is reopened, because blood is being shunted to the saphenous system in the lower calf. The reopened superficial femoral vein will not be the path of least resistance, due to persistent occlusion more distally. The limb will have diminished flow in the deep system, despite perforators, since the saphenous vein remains the path of least resistance. Ignoring strategic distal thrombus can cause early technical failure.[8] A newly reopened femoral system is at greater risk for rethrombosis if there is little deep venous flow channeled into this segment. It is similar to placement of an arterial bypass graft above poor run-off. Patency will be less than in a limb with good run-off. In addition, residual distal thrombus can limit clinical improvement, due to persistent hypertension in the calf. In both venous and arterial reconstruction, interaction among all segments must be taken into account to achieve optimal results. We have found a combination of catheter- and flow-directed therapy is most beneficial for treating multisegmental thrombosis. Improving flow in the whole limb may be essential for good long-term clinical results in patients with thrombus located at every level.

Catheter-Directed Therapy: Tricks and Tips

Venous access for catheter placement to treat iliofemoral and proximal superficial femoral thrombosis is achieved through a contralateral femoral vein or through the ipsilateral femoral or popliteal veins. The right internal jugular approach may be used, but it can be difficult to manipulate catheter tips from such a distance. This approach works better for acute thrombus. The most popular approach to endovascular treatment of the femoral and iliac veins is now via the popliteal vein. The entry point is 3″ to 4″ above the popliteal crease. This can be safely accessed with color duplex or even with a smaller portable unit without color. Micropuncture technique is strongly recommended. We use the Micropuncture set from Cook Inc. (Bloomington, IN), which uses a 21-gauge, 9-cm beveled needle that takes an 0.018″ Nitinol-tipped stainless steel guidewire. A key technique has been the use of a short, clear-plastic connection tube with a 3- to 6-mL syringe. It is easy to puncture both walls without knowing. Therefore, one should gently aspirate with a small syringe that is not directly placed on the needle; hand tremor can inadvertently advance the needle through the back wall or cause it to exit the lumen. Once blood aspirates easily, the wire can be carefully advanced. If the wire does not advance smoothly, it can be coiling outside the lumen. If the wire kinks, it may not withdraw through the 21-gauge needle. If this is the case, the needle and wire must be withdrawn as a unit, or one risks leaving the wire tip in the patient. Once the wire is in place, the coaxial dilators are positioned and, after removing the 3F inner dilator, a 0.035″ wire can be advanced up the femoral vein.

Following placement of a vascular sheath, a multisidehole catheter is directed over a guidewire and positioned in the thrombosed vein. If initial guidewire traversal of the thrombosed segment is difficult, a 5F catheter is positioned into the thrombus as far as possible for initial infusion of lytic therapy. When a subsequent attempt to pass the guidewire is successful, the catheter can be advanced and strategically positioned throughout the thrombosed segment. Chronic obstruction in this region requires tedious manipulation of the catheter and wire to find the best passageway to the upper thigh and pelvis. Finesse is necessary to avoid perforation.

In the event that the wire or catheter perforates the vein, usually a result of pushing too hard, this area should not be dilated. Acutely dilating and/or stenting venous perforations can cause extravasation. However, thrombolysis can be continued above this point, and after 24 to 36 hours a small perforation or false passage is usually not evident or problematic. A variety of multisidehole 5F catheters can be used, including predetermined length (i.e., 10, 20, 30, or 50 cm), or adjustable length, coaxial systems that are also available. The length of the infusion catheter is selected according to the ability to position the catheter across the thrombosed area. A long continuous segment of thrombus is treated with a single catheter when possible. Extensive thrombus often requires repositioning of the catheter at the time of follow-up, so an adjustable length catheter will preclude multiple catheter exchanges. The catheter may be safely advanced over wires in both retrograde and antegrade directions. While it is easier to advance through venous valves from an antegrade approach, the popliteal vein is not always the best approach, as it, too, may be obliterated or occluded. A Roadrunner wire (Cook Inc.) and an angled Glidewire (Meditech/Boston Scientific, Watertown, MA) are the instruments of choice for traversing venous valves, regardless of direction. A 4F or 5F straight or 45° angle catheter can then be advanced over a wire. An alternative coaxial system, consisting of a 5F Mewissen multisidehole catheter (Cook Inc.) in combination with a 0.035″ Katzen (Cook Inc.) wire can be useful. With this system, one can separate the infusions and position the catheter/wire system in different locations for most effective intrathrombus delivery. The AngioDynamics catheter (AngioDynamics Corp., Queensbury, NY) has multiple infusion lengths and works with an end-occluding wire. It works well with the automatic Pulse*Spray pump (AngioDynamics Corp.), which we have found very effective in both acute and chronic occlusions. The coaxial Mewissen-Katzen system requires two infusion pumps with a divided dose of urokinase. The heparin infusion is piggybacked into the catheter. When combined with a flow-directed infusion from a pedal access site, the total dose is divided between the two sites. The amount per infusion is determined by the initial venous flow rate (seen fluoroscopically) and the amount and distribution of thrombus. Laboratory monitoring (using mini samples of <2.5 cc) is done every 4 to 6 hours for evaluation of fibrinogen, prothrombin time (PT) and partial thromboplastin time (PTT), hemoglobin, and platelet count. The fibrinogen level is maintained at greater than 25% of baseline, which is usually more than 100 mg/dL. The PTT range is maintained between 50 and 80 seconds.

Flow-Directed Infusions: When and Why?

This technique is reserved for treating thrombus located in the tibial, soleus, gastrocnemius, and popliteal veins. If the baseline venogram reveals preferential flow in the superficial veins of the calf, one can acquire an idea of the location of the thrombus by injecting contrast with tourniquets in place. The duplex may underestimate the amount of thrombus in the upper calf. If there is no continuity of flow in the deep veins of the calf and the thigh, a lytic infusion from the level can be effective in reopening veins that are untreatable with catheter technique. Acute failure has been attributed to residual thrombus in the popliteal vein, below the sheath entry site. Unfortunately, some interventionists have recognized the importance of treating the distal vein, especially the entire popliteal, after rethrombosis of successfully lysed iliofemoral segments. For this reason, we recommend a baseline and completion venogram, from the foot, before sheath removal.

A 22-gauge inter-cath placed in a dorsal pedal vein for the purpose of performing the baseline venogram is used for the flow-directed infusion. A single puncture in a pedal vein below the ankle is desirable. Although multiple punctures cannot be avoided in certain patients, we attempt to work from a distal-to-proximal direction to avoid infusing urokinase below multiple punctures. A small clear plastic dressing is placed over the 22-gauge catheter to maintain visualization of the site throughout the procedure. It is important to loop the intravenous tubing to prevent inadvertent loss of the site. Infection and/or bleeding are not problems but, as always, care is taken to observe for any extravasation of contrast during each injection. A short, clear plastic connecting tube is used with a three-way stopcock to facilitate interval injection of contrast for follow-up evaluation of progress of lytic therapy. A saline infusion is maintained through the pedal site if urokinase is not being infused. A Velcro-type tourniquet (Tiger Surgical, Portland, OR) is placed at the malleolar level, in combination with a small disc positioned to provide focal compression of the saphenous vein against the medial malleolus (Fig. 8). Under fluoroscopic visualization, a small amount of contrast is injected to ascertain focal compression of the saphenous vein and redirection of flow through a communicating vein into the deep system. The disc position, as well as the upper and lower margins of the tourniquet, is marked on the skin. This allows a nurse to release the tourniquet once every hour and replace it in the correct position. A folded 4×4 gauze is placed under the disc to protect the skin from pressure. The pedal pulse is marked and monitored with blood pressure and pulse; the tourniquet provides adequate redirection of venous flow without any compromise of arterial flow. It is released 10 minutes every hour and reapplied at a specific marked level, which assures proper disc position and tightness.

Normally, blood flows preferentially from the superficial to the deep system. In the presence of DVT, however, one may see contrast reflux through the perforating veins into the superficial system in mid calf or above. When this is fluoroscopically recognized, a second tourniquet is placed at the knee to compress the greater saphenous vein against the femoral condyle to promote redirection of flow into the tibiopopliteal veins.

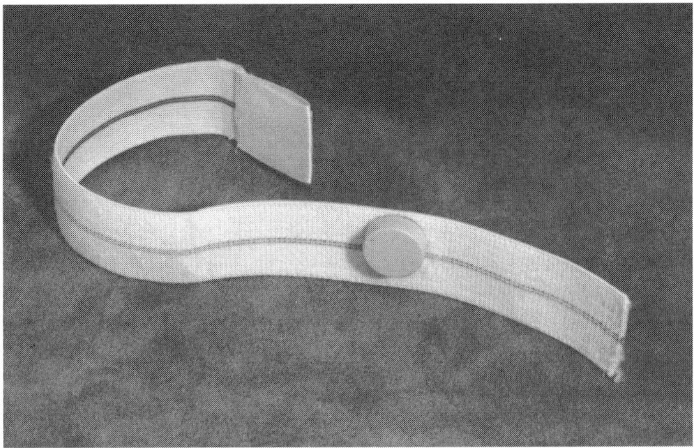

Figure 8. Tourniquet used to compress the saphenous vein against medial malleolus (Tiger Surgical).

After the course of thrombolytic therapy, additional intervention is performed to treat underlying venous stenosis. Persistently narrowed venous channels can be dilated, but the result is often hemodynamically unsatisfactory. This can be documented with pullback pressures through the areas of stenosis. We have noted greater widening of the chronically occluded lumen after overnight use of the pulse spray technique versus drip infusion. In the event of significant lumen irregularity and residual narrowing of the iliofemoral segments, one or more self-expanding metallic stents can be placed to augment outflow. Pullback pressures are always obtained before and after iliac stent placement. Greater than 3 to 4 mm Hg resting pressure differential between the inferior vena cava and the iliac vein is considered significant. Self-expanding metallic stents are placed from the ipsilateral or contralateral approach after maximum thrombolytic therapy. Duplex imaging is used to confirm stent patency and assess flow velocities 1 day post op, at 1, 3, 6, and 12 months, and yearly thereafter. Intravascular ultrasound[7] and angioscopy[24] have been used in several series. Intravascular ultrasound has the advantage of checking on stent position and opening. It is also a useful tool for evaluating hyperplasia.

Patients are systemically heparinized (PTT >50 and <80 seconds) throughout the period of thrombolysis and following angioplasty or stent procedures. Oral anticoagulation is tapered before therapy (2 days off Coumadin before admission) and restarted 1 day prior to stent placement. This allows removal of the sheath before the international normalized ratio (INR) is therapeutic. Upon completion of thrombolysis, heparinization is continued until oral anticoagulation is consistent: PT greater than 20 seconds, and INR 2.5 to 3.0. Oral anticoagulation is monitored cooperatively with the referring physician for several months, as inadequate anticoagulation is the most frequent cause of early failure. Younger patients with chronic conditions may have a hypercoagulable state, making warfarin titration challenging. We can only emphasize the great importance of diligent monitoring of the PT/INR. Whereas a minimum of 6 to 12 months of warfarin is standard in acute DVT, patients with chronic disease and/or stents are prescribed indefinite oral anticoagulation. Compression stockings or leggings are prescribed and fitted for all patients before discharge. Patients are followed with clinic visits, duplex exams, and photoplethysmography and air plethysmography upon completion, at 3-month intervals for 1 year, and yearly thereafter.

A Review of the Literature

Among the larger series in the literature[25] are two reported by the Stanford group in 1994 and in July 2000.[8] In the earlier study, they discussed treatment of 27 limbs in 21 patients (20 acute, 7 chronic) with catheter-directed thrombolysis. The average dose of urokinase was 4.9 million IU (range 1.4 to 16 million IU) infused over an average of 30 hours (range 15 to 74 hours). Sixteen limbs had underlying stenoses that were treated with angioplasty (2) or angioplasty and stent (14). Two chronically occluded iliac veins could not be traversed with a guidewire. Primary patency at 3 months was documented in 11 of 12 (92%). The lack of long-term follow-up in the first study was resolved in the recent study, which details results in 39 patients treated for acute and chronic left iliofemoral thrombosis associated with May-Thurner compression. Median follow-up was 2.6 years. This study includes life-table analysis and a QOL survey of patients treated between 1993 and 1999. Seventy-five percent of the patients were women and the mean age was 46 years. Among the 20 patients treated for post-thrombotic CVI (median duration of symptoms 270 days), 8 patients underwent primary stenting without adjunctive thrombolysis. Initial technical success was achieved in 34 of 39 (87%). In all, 72 stents were used (60 Wallstents [Boston Scientific, Natick, MA] and 12 Palmaz [Cordis Endovascular, a Johnson & Johnson Company, Miami Lakes, FL], with an average of 2 stents per patient; range 1 to 11). Among the 5 technical failures were 2 in which the wire could not be passed, 1 in which poor inflow precluded stenting, and 1 involving a combination of both circumstances. Stented patients with acute symptoms had a 1-year patency rate of 91.6%, while 1-year patency in stented patients with chronic presentations was 93.9%. Combined primary patency at 1 year was 79%. There were no major bleeding complications, death, or pulmonary embolus associated with therapy. Relatively few stents have been placed below the inguinal ligament at most institutions but, as the Stanford report illustrates, continuity of flow from distal to proximal segments is key to long-term clinical improvement. In patients with extensive involvement of the superficial femoral vein, judicious placement of stents may be necessary.

The Minnesota group has also reported their endovascular venous experience.[10,26] Nazarian and colleagues[10] reported on the role of metallic stents after failure of balloon angioplasty or surgery. Over a 4-year period they observed follow-up in 55 patients who received stents in the subclavian veins (9), innominate veins (3), superior vena cava (4), inferior vena cava (3), iliac veins (29), femoral veins (5), and portal veins (6). The series included patients treated for malignant stenoses and benign, chronic iliac occlusions. These investigators noted no significant difference in 1-year patency between patients with a history of DVT and those without, or relative to the type of stent used (i.e., Gianturco [Cook Inc.], Palmaz, or Wallstent). Stenotic lesions had a 1-year primary assisted patency of 74% compared to 57% for veins with prestent occlusions (*P*=.15). Among the iliac veins, 13 were initially occluded. Primary assisted patency for iliac veins was 66% compared to 37% when femoral thrombosis accompanied iliac DVT (*P*=.06). Two-year patency rates were significantly lower in patients with known malignancy. Technical problems were associated with single-module Z-stents that persistently slipped above or below the stenosis. One external iliac Z-stent fracture was identified at 5 months with no adverse outcome.

In 1997, Bjarnason et al[26] reported on treatment of 77 patients, some of whom were included in the paper by Nazarian et al. The majority of the patients (78%) presented with acute DVT symptoms of less than 14 days' duration (69/86,78%), while the others had either subacute thrombus (14 to 28 days) or thrombus older than 28 days. The mean length of symptoms prior to thrombolysis was 15 days (range 0 to 256 days). The average dose of urokinase was 10.5 million IU (range 0.4 to 24 million IU) and the average infusion time was 75 hours (range 8 to 247 hours). They reported greater technical success in treating iliac veins (79%) versus femoral veins (63%). We have seen this pattern, as well. It reflects the fact that subclinical thrombosis is present prior to clinical presentation with acute iliofemoral DVT. Even though the initial technical success was similar between patients undergoing stent placement versus those who were not, it was less for patients with thrombus older than 4 weeks than for those with more acute conditions. Thrombosed superficial femoral veins are often poorly recanalized and respond poorly to thrombolysis, alone. Eighty-six stents were placed in 38 (44%) of the 87 limbs treated for iliofemoral thrombosis. Seventy-five Wallstents were placed in 36 limbs, and 11 Gianturco stents were placed in 2 limbs. Interestingly, they found a lower 6-month primary patency rate between stented (60%) and nonstented (75%) iliac veins and 54% versus 75% at 1 year (*P*=.011). At 1 year, the secondary patency rate was 76% for stented and 82% for nonstented vessels (*P*=.46). The authors hypothesized that patients requiring stents presented with more severe chronic venous disease, accounting for the poorer long-term results. Stented patients were not uniformly maintained on warfarin longer that 6 months.

An important report in the literature regards the National Venous Registry (1994 to 1997),[4] a multicenter registry that collected data on 473 iliofemoral DVT patients treated with endovascular techniques. The study included 287 patients with adequate follow-up. The majority (70%) had acute presentation of iliofemoral thrombosis. The average dose of urokinase was 7.8 million IU, and nearly 50% required placement of an iliac stent. Technical success, including placement of 104 stents, was 97%. Results were reported in terms of lysis grade. Complete lysis was achieved in 60% of patients presenting with acute thrombus (<10 days). Among this group, 90% remained patent at 12 months compared to 70% of those with less than complete lysis. Patients were maintained on warfarin for 4 to 6 months. The study revealed greater long-term patency in patients with iliac stenosis treated with angioplasty plus stent versus stent alone. The study was based on analysis of pre and post phlebograms and duplex ultrasound with minimal follow-up of 12 months.

Neglen and Raju[7] reported their experience treating iliac lesions in 94 consecutive patients with suspected iliac vein obstruction. Fifty-four (57%) were women, and the median age was 48 years. These investigators had a high degree of initial technical success (98%) but reported early rethrombosis in 5 patients. Thrombolysis was not used in any of the initial stent procedures. Two major bleeding complications occurred early in the study. There were no deaths. A total of 118 Wallstents were deployed in 77 veins of 102 limbs that were evaluated. A single stent was placed in 62% and 29% received two stents. The most common stent size was 16 mm in diameter (n=34), followed by 14 mm (n=15) and 18 mm (n=14). Forty-four (55%) of the stenoses were located within the common iliac vein whereas 25 (31%) involved the common and/or the external iliac segments. No stent was placed below the inguinal ligament. Median follow-up in 70 (91%) of the 77 stented limbs was 12 months (range 1 to 21). Only 2 patients had occlusive thrombosis; the majority was treated for stenosis, not obstruction. Neglen and Raju's use of intravascular ultrasound documented the amount of recoil occurring in vein segments with angioplasty. They also performed pressure gradients in all patients and found a resting gradient of greater than 2 mm Hg in 12 of 80 (15%). With papaverine injection, 28 of 80 (35%) demonstrated a pressure gradient greater than 2 mm Hg across the stenosis. Primary, assisted, and secondary patency rates at 1 year were 82%, 91%, and 92%, respectively. Neglen and Raju emphasize the need to extend the stent into the inferior vena cava. Early in our experience, rethrombosis occurred because of this problem of incomplete stenting across the compression site. Neglen and Raju also note that reflux remains an issue in some, but not all, patients. Symptomatic venous hypertension due to post-thrombotic valvular injury or coexisting primary insufficiency may not respond to compression and may require additional intervention. Meissner et al[27] have recently reported that, in addition to DVT-associated damage of valves in the deep veins, similar damage can and does occur in superficial veins when they are thrombosed. But parallel occurrence in the uninvolved limb lends support to Raju's previous suggestion that poorly functioning valves may be, in fact, the cause of thrombosis rather than the result thereof.[28]

Between 1988 and 1998, 84 patients were treated at Creighton with thrombolysis for post-thrombotic CVI.[9] Acute thrombosis characterized 28 patient presentations (30 limbs) while 56 patients (63 limbs) had a chronic history ranging between 2 months and 20 years. These patients had extensive disease, with 98% showing superficial femoral vein involvement and 84% an affected popliteal segment. The mean age was 47.5 years (range 12 to 83 years). The female/male ratio was evenly divided (42F/42M). Physical exam revealed 98% with edema, 39% with skin changes. Nine percent (9) had healed (2) or nonhealing (7) ulcers. Stents were placed in 40 patients (53%). The Wallstent was used 98% of the time. Although we have seen good long-term patency using 10-mm and 12-mm stents, others have begun to use the larger 14- to 16-mm models to reduce the chance of significant intimal hyperplasia. Complications causing death occurred in 2 patients. One 78-year-old male had a successful procedure for extremity and caval occlusion, but had an intracranial hemorrhage 2 days after cessation of urokinase. A 52-year-old woman died of retroperitoneal bleeding leading to disseminated intravascular coagulation. Patients have been followed annually with hemodynamic studies and duplex, to assess stent patency. Early rethrombosis was related to subtherapeutic warfarin levels. Close observation for recurrent edema or discomfort has led to repeat balloon dilatation of the iliac stents in 4 patients between 6 and 18 months after insertion. In each patient, signs and symptoms resolved after reintervention. This was done via a popliteal approach, and was performed on an outpatient basis with use of the low molecular weight heparin (enoxaparin) administered subcutaneously (1 mg/kg twice daily). Stents were placed in infrainguinal segments in 22 patients. Excellent patency was documented in 19 of 22 (86%) at 1 year. Two patients showed no flow on duplex and 1 patient had diminished flow consistent with hyperplasia or thrombosis; however, all patients in this group remain clinically improved compared to before endovascular therapy. Our experience treating multisegmental chronic thrombosis suggests the importance of observing the hemodynamic changes that occur after lytic infusion and stent placement. Venous flow increases as resistance decreases. This can occur despite persistence of an abnormal appearing venogram. Physiologic improvement is best documented with video phlebography, increase in resting flow velocities (cm/s) recorded with ultrasound, or decrease in ambulatory venous pressures.

Alternative Thrombolytic Agents

Urokinase was the preferred lytic agent for peripheral vascular procedure throughout the 1990s. The US Food and Drug Administration (FDA)-prompted withdrawal of urokinase (Abbokinase; Abbott Laboratories, Abbott Park, IL) from the market in early 1999 caused tremendous concern among interventional radiologists and vascular surgeons. The preference for urokinase over streptokinase had been well established. Although cardiologists prefer alteplase, the comfort level with protocols and results achieved in peripheral urokinase administration left the entire community at a loss without a supply of the lytic agent that had been trusted. It became incumbent upon everyone to become familiar with alternative fibrinolytic agents such as alteplase (Activase, Genentec, South San Francisco, CA) and reteplase (Retavase, Centacor, Malvern, PA). Many interventionalists feel that the incidence of fatal and nonfatal bleeding complications associated with thrombolysis increased when we began to use alteplase. The apparent increased incidence of complications was attributed to the learning curve for peripheral applications. Physicians soon realized that coronary dosing recommendations were not ideal for peripheral infusions. Heparin rates were adjusted downward, and smaller doses were used than recommended in the cardiac literature. Empirically, it was established that alteplase, given at a slightly higher dose per hour (e.g., 1 to 2 mg/h) for a short period (4 to 8 hours) worked more effectively, with fewer bleeding problems, than a lower dose infusion for a more prolonged period (Motarjame A. Personal communication, June 2000). There is currently information about dosing protocols featured on Internet web sites, including those of the Society for Interventional Radiology, the Endovascular Forum of the Miami Vascular Institute, the University of California, Los Angeles, and Stanford University.

Reports regarding organized efforts to bring safe and effective dosing strategies to the interventional community were published recently.[29–32] Early data indicate ability to achieve comparable results in treating both arterial and venous occlusions with alternative agents. The accumulated safety and efficacy data represent a relatively small number, compared to the extensive 20-year experience with urokinase. However, the interventional community is to be commended for rapidly and conscientiously addressing an unprecedented dilemma, which had the double jeopardy of denying patients a known drug while substituting agents with almost nonexistent tract records in the peripheral arena. Of interest is a recent report which concludes that appropriately designed clinical trials are essential for future FDA approval of drugs *and* devices designated for use in peripheral vascular disease.

Teaching Case: Acute Multisegmental DVT Superimposed on Chronic Iliofemoral Thrombosis

Recanalization may be ‘too little, too late’ to prevent serious post-thrombotic edema, especially in cases of phlegmasia. This case demonstrates the efficacy of high-dose local lytic therapy when major proximal and distal veins are obstructed. It also demonstrates long-term patency (108 months) of venous stents that cross the inguinal ligament.

In May 1993, a 74-year-old female, recently returned from a transpacific airplane trip, presented with a 1-week history of discoloration and increasing edema in her right lower extremity. She had been treated at a clinic for presumed cellulitis with doxycycline for 7 days. Pain increased with ambulating as the swelling progressed. Because her symptoms continued with no apparent improvement, she was referred to a vascular surgeon. Three months prior to admission, she had been treated for “pneumonia” after she developed shortness of breath. Her chest x-ray revealed an infiltrate and small effusion, but the possibility of pulmonary edema was not considered.

The physical examination revealed a significantly swollen right lower extremity. Her right calf measured 36 cm in circumference compared to 32 cm on the left; the right thigh measured 55 cm, left 53 cm. A palpable cord was noted in the right medial thigh. Normal pulses were palpated distally. When the patient stood, there was distinct discoloration of the foot consistent with venous stasis. No hyperpigmentation was evident. After the duplex, she was diagnosed with phlegmasia cerulea dolens and referred for thrombolysis.

The baseline noninvasive study revealed noncompressible thrombus extending to the confluence of the external and internal iliac veins with nonocclusive mural thrombus in the common femoral segment. The inferior vena cava was normal. The infrainguinal deep system had thrombus in the proximal and distal superficial femoral vein as well as the popliteal and posterior tibial system. Acute thrombus was also seen throughout the greater saphenous vein. We have noted that with phlegmasia, obstruction of the venous outflow can be so extensive that the dorsalis pedis waveform is dampened but the palpable pulse is strong. This paradox of a water-hammer pulse, with an altered, monophasic waveform, is consistent with massive venous obstruction.

The baseline ascending venogram (see left panel of Fig. 5) was performed with a 22-gauge inter-cath placed in a dorsal vein of the right foot. Evidence of acute and chronic DVT was documented and the study confirmed the extensive thrombosis. Initially, only the anterior tibial and superficial veins were visualized below the knee. Superficial femoral and popliteal collaterals to the profunda femoris channeled flow in the thigh, and the greater saphenous vein was not visualized. In the upper thigh, a well-developed collateral system of femoral circumflex to hypogastric veins was vaguely seen, indicating obstructing chronic thrombosis of the common femoral segment. Prolonged stasis was consistent with a low flow state and the possibility of thrombus in the collateral outflow, i.e., hypogastric vein. The saphenofemoral junction could not be distinguished due to chronic changes and acute thrombosis.

A combination of catheter-directed and flow-directed techniques was used in this case. From a contralateral iliac approach, a Mewissen catheter was positioned in the right internal iliac vein. Intraclot thrombolytic therapy with the catheter plus flow-directed urokinase from below was initiated at 300,000 IU/h (150,000 IU/h via each system). Systemic heparinization was maintained by using a three-way stopcock to deliver both heparin and the lytic agent to the deep venous system. The patient received a total of 11,380,600 IU over 72 hours. Follow-up venograms were obtained every 18 to 24 hours to evaluate progress. At 24 hours, thrombus was outlined in the external iliac vein. The catheter was advanced into the common femoral region. At 72 hours, the profunda and superficial femoral vein had improved flow. Furthermore, there was reestablished patency of the greater saphenous vein. A very irregular pattern prevailed in the femoral and iliac veins consistent with chronic DVT. Despite improved flow in the calf and popliteal vein, chronic changes persisted in the upper thigh with the majority of flow being directed through the lateral and medial circumflex veins into branches of the internal iliac system. Although we continued catheter-directed therapy, no further improvement occurred in the femoral area. Balloon dilatation also failed to improve flow through this abnormal anatomy. Therefore, in conjunction with percutaneous transluminal angioplasty, we elected to stent the residual narrowing knowing that the outflow tract would not remain patent if left in this state, even with anticoagulation. Self-expanding Wallstents were positioned between the right distal common iliac and the proximal superficial femoral vein, in serial fashion, with about 1 to 1.5 cm of overlap. Following deployment of the 10-mm×68-mm stents, additional balloon dilatation was performed to fully expand the metallic matrix to appose the irregular vessel wall (Fig. 5). Although not routine, a caval filter was subsequently placed in this elderly patient in the event she would stop warfarin and be at risk for DVT and/or pulmonary edema. Systemic heparin was continued until the PT was therapeutic on a predictable dose of warfarin. She was discharged after 12 days and has continued on 2 mg warfarin per day maintaining the INR at 2.0. Annual duplex follow-up demonstrates continued patency of the stents for more than 7 years. On physical examination, she remains CEAP Class III, with mild edema controlled with compression stockings. No progressive skin changes are noted despite mild popliteal reflux and chronic nonocclusive thrombus in the popliteal and superficial femoral vein. Now, at 81, she recently spent 2 months in her homeland in Asia.

The patient has been closely followed for more than 7 years. She has experienced no recurrent DVT in the right lower extremity. She denies pain in the right leg and continues an active lifestyle. She occasionally has mild edema in the right calf and ankle. She wears a Class I compression stocking most of the time. Annual follow-up color duplex exams have revealed continued stent patency (Fig. 9). A small amount of intimal hyperplasia became evident at 14 months. It has not increased and the flow is not affected. Both immediate post-stent placement and subsequent follow-up have shown reestablished patency of the popliteal, superficial femoral, femoral, iliac, and greater saphenous veins with residual nonocclusive popliteal and superficial femoral vein mural thrombus. Photoplethysmography exam on August 3, 1995 revealed deep venous valvular insufficiency (16 seconds with cuff). Subsequent air plethysmography show the right venous filling index (with superficial femoral vein occlusion) to be 2.7 mL, versus 1.2 mL on the left. She revisited Asia in 1994 and 2000 and had no evidence of recurrent DVT or pulmonary edema after prolonged air travel.

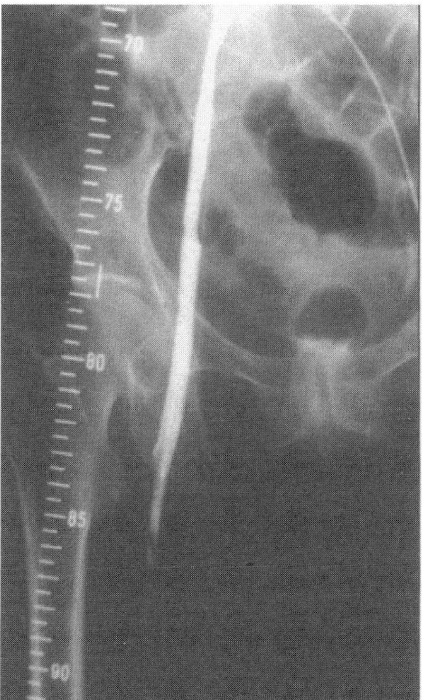

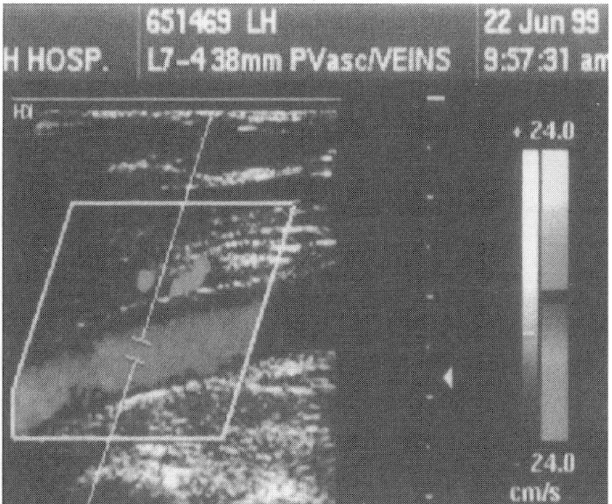

Figure 9. Stent therapy for chronic iliofemoral deep vein thrombosis. Left: Tandem Wallstents placed in superficial femoral vein, common femoral vein, external iliac, and common iliac segments in May 1993. Right: Duplex follow-up after 6 years shows minimal FIH and continued primary patency.

Comments

This case illustrates a very common condition—that of acute thrombosis associated with chronic changes. Although she clinically presented with acute DVT, if we had not elected to stent this patient's abnormal, stenotic iliofemoral veins, she very likely would have developed significant venous insufficiency during the ensuing 7 years. She also represents one of 22 patients with stents placed below the inguinal ligament since 1993. Serial duplex imaging has shown little change in the appearance of the stents over time. May-Thurner compression of the right common iliac vein may have been the etiology of her initial thrombosis. This occurs with a much lower incidence (<2%), but it should be suspected if other causes of iliofemoral DVT are excluded.[16] This case also demonstrates cooperative use of catheter- and flow-directed thrombolysis to achieve optimal results.

Phlegmasia cerulea dolens is a severe form of lower extremity DVT characterized by extraordinary extremity swelling, pain, and cyanosis. This generally reflects the degree of venous congestion caused by massive thrombosis, which can include both the external and internal iliac veins. Such extensive obstruction can progress to gangrene if not relieved.[33,34] Standard therapy includes bed rest, fluid resuscitation, extremity elevation, and systemic heparinization; however, since flow is so compromised, even systemic heparin may not prevent propagation. Recanalization may be 'too little, too late' to prevent gangrene. In the face of such extensive occlusive thrombosis, thrombolytic therapy, selectively administered, has been beneficial.[35] The extent of the thrombus load, however, can be overwhelming to many physicians. Effective lytic therapy may require multiple catheters and flow-directed urokinase. Very often, chronic thrombus and abnormal venous anatomy underlie the "critical mass" of acute thrombus, which causes the presenting symptoms. Stents may be required to augment and maintain outflow after maximum thrombolysis.

Recent studies have shown propagation of thrombus can occur even when patients are known to be appropriately anticoagulated with INR levels above 2. In one series, approximately 30% of patients experienced clot propagation on the standard heparin-warfarin regimen.[36] Persistent thrombus, in addition to obstructing flow, can damage venous valve cusps and lead to CVI.[5,6]

As early as 1980, a National Institutes of Health Consensus Conference advised that with the advent of thrombolytic agents, anticoagulation alone was no longer the optimal therapy for DVT and pulmonary embolism.[37] The first report of phlegmasia cerulea dolens treated successfully with streptokinase was published by Paquet and Popov in 1970.[38] They described 10 cases, of which 9 had excellent results. There was no incidence of pulmonary embolism, gangrene, or death. In 1993, Robinson and Teeitelbaum [39] reported the use of pulse spray technique in treating extensive limb thrombosis.

Phlegmasia can result from the acute onset of a coagulopathy related to trauma, surgery, or malignancy. Many cases occur as a result of chronic subclinical venous obstruction, which remains unsuspected until the limb decompensates. This is due to a "critical mass" of new thrombus, which forms on the surface of old thrombus. Multiple factors may contribute to the clinical presentation, such as prolonged immobilization, dehydration, malignancy, or compression (e.g., pregnancy). The morbidity associated with extensive thrombosis is significant and includes the prospect of life-long disability due to the post-thrombotic syndrome.[40]

How to Evaluate Endovenous Reconstruction

Lytic results in acute thrombosis are classified as follows:

- *complete lysis* when the occluded vein is reopened along its entire length; less than 10% residual thrombus is considered insignificant;
- *partial lysis* if significant change occurs in the venogram, with increased outflow but incomplete (>50% but <90%) removal of residual mural thrombus;
- *minimal lysis* if no change occurs in the venogram or rate of contrast clearance.

In addition to determination of the degree of lysis, most appropriately used in acute thrombosis, *phlebographic improvement* applies to chronic cases. This is measured by the following:

1. decrease in resistance when injecting contrast into the deep system from the pedal site;
2. decrease in stasis of contrast and more rapid clearance of contrast through the calf and thigh;
3. greater visualization of deep veins, particularly in the calf;
4. continuity of flow between segments, i.e., tibial to popliteal to superficial femoral vein.

These improvements are not totally captured on still films. Rather, the "real time" flow pattern, through the entire leg, provides information about increase in flow capacity due to augmentation or retrieval of deep veins that were not open before lytic therapy. As flow in main channels improves, collaterals decrease and it is possible to advance wires and catheters through the thrombosed femoral and iliac veins. Forward progress, i.e., catheter advancement, may be slow in cases of very chronic occlusion. It is important to continue the lytic infusion to open "invisible" channels. Eventually, a wire can be advanced through a retrieved true lumen. Once the probing wire and catheter reach the inferior vena cava, an Amplatz stiff exchange wire (Cook Inc., Bloomington, IN) can be positioned to secure the access. Balloon dilatation and stent placement are then performed to reestablish antegrade flow in the axial veins.

Duplex imaging can provide indication of flow improvement but does not provide any indication of relative stasis or clearance of blood. Duplex does, however, measure flow velocity in the femoral and iliac stents. This can be an important indicator of success. Velocities less than 10 to 15 cm/s indicate too little inflow from the distal veins. Stents with greater than 15 cm/s have a greater likelihood of long-term patency.[26] As with arterial stents, abnormally high velocities indicate stenosis from intimal hyperplasia. Restenosis is uncommon, and not possible to predict. In our experience, it occurs in less than

20% of patients. Recognition and retreatment with balloon dilatation or double stenting have been effective in correcting restenoses.

Although primary stenting is an ideal approach to stenosis, in occlusive disease thrombolysis assists with guidewire access in to permit balloon dilatation and stenting. How does thrombolysis help in treating chronic occlusion? No one can really explain what we empirically observe in some, albeit not all, patients. Sevitt[18] described the process of thrombus recanalization and the creation of small pockets of lysis. From the description, it is clear that thrombus is a dynamic substance, undergoing constant remodeling by interaction of resident cellular components. It is not usually appreciated that chronic thrombus has small channels. These fenestrations are not identified with standard ultrasound and are least of all perceived with phlebography. In addition, there are numerous intermuscular and intramuscular venous channels interfacing with occluded segments of larger veins. In the calf, in particular, patency of these draining veins is important for efficient muscle-pump activity. Although it may not be apparent on serial venograms of chronic DVT, pathology studies show that thrombus is in a dynamic state capable of constant remodeling, even though the overall hemodynamic situation changes slowly. Pousseille's law of fluid dynamics teaches that the amount of flow across any point in a cylindrical tube is proportionate to the fourth power of the diameter. Therefore, a totally occluded vein has a flow unit of zero and a 1-mm venous lumen allows flow. But, a small increment in diameter, to 2 mm, will increase the flow by 16, and at 3 mm the flow is increased to 81. If the numerous unnamed veins and the major veins are augmented by 2 to 3 mm, the change might not be obvious on a phlebogram. The rate of flow will increase, however, because dissolving subacute thrombus (superimposed on older layers adherent to the vessel wall) can enlarge many small channels. Even in therapeutically anticoagulated patients, thrombus propagation has been shown to occur, especially in areas of extremely slow flow. Patients who stop taking warfarin at 3 to 6 months may propagate thrombus on the substrate of residual mural irregularity. Since the clinical course is so indolent, it is hard to believe that dissolvable thrombus exits in CVI. The results of lytic therapy in CVI patients suggest this is indeed the case.

Reluctance to use lytic agents, particularly in young patients, derives from the perceived risk of bleeding complications, as well as the belief that bed rest and anticoagulation provide the same long-term results, e.g., a functional extremity with inconsequential post-thrombotic swelling or discomfort. Few patients are thought to progress to severe, disabling conditions. However, the epidemiology of DVT is poorly documented, and we really do not know the number of persons incapacitated with CVI in the 20- to 60-year age range.

It has been frequently stated in the literature that venous thrombus older than 14 days is not amenable to thrombolysis.[4,8,41] This perception is based on experience with systemic infusion of streptokinase, which has been much less effective than catheter-directed therapy. We are in the midst of an evolution of techniques and ideas about therapeutic intervention for both acute and chronic venous disorders. The very composition of the thrombus is dynamic and reconfigures, over time, with the body's efforts to recanalize and divert venous flow around and through a vascular obstruction. Although relatively little attention has been paid to venous pathology (compared to arterial disease), Sevitt[18] described the pattern of peripheral pockets of autolysis, which characterize older clots. This is a progressive biochemical process, relying on lytic agents secreted by endothelial cells that line the venous lumen. Why then, is it a surprise to many that purposeful, local infusion of additional lytic agent would not augment and facilitate a natural response? The balance between thrombosis and thrombolysis is complex; but the body shows us that recanalization of chronic occlusions does occur. Some say removal of old thrombus is not possible. Systemic infusions, by nature, were very ineffective in delivering a lytic agent to thrombosed veins in the lower limb, since flow is diverted into superficial veins. However, the evolution of catheter techniques and a careful observation of the residual flow patterns in the obstructed extremity provide new avenues for effective adjunctive lytic therapy to supplement the intrinsic lytic process already in motion. Thrombolytic therapy can do much to restore a favorable balance of flow. This, in turn, can relieve venous hypertension and the associated pain and edema. Improving venous outflow can also help heal chronic ulcers, which are refractory to all other therapies. Revascularization with urokinase and stents resulted in progressive healing of venous ulcer in 8 patients in the Creighton series.[9]

The endogenous lytic system is overwhelmed by massive thrombus or rapidly propagating thrombus. Therefore, augmenting lysis in acute thrombosis would be ideal therapy. Upregulation of endothelial secretion of t-PA and urokinase remains a concept for the future. Therefore, we are faced with treating DVT when it is diagnosed; however, since it is often quite difficult to make the clinical diagnosis of DVT, the process may be advanced before the patient becomes symptomatic. A small amount of partially obstructing thrombus may be dissolved by the body's intrinsic lytic capacity. Residual nonobstructing thrombus remains a nidus for subsequent thrombus formation. This can occur with mechanical stasis and/or change in coagulability with trauma or surgery or disease. Generally, a combination of factors results in thrombosis. As stated above, new thrombus forms on top of old, forming a multilayered thrombus composed of various ages and degrees of organization. When thrombus becomes a "critical mass," flow is obstructed and signs and symptoms of DVT occur if collateral compensation is inadequate. Since this entire sequence can be indolent, patients and physicians can be deceived into thinking that there is an "acute event." It is much more likely, however, that "acute" obstruction of the venous channel occurs by a slowly accumulating mass of thrombus, which can be days, weeks, or months old.

The value of lytic therapy, therefore, is the removal of the acute and subacute thrombus, to restore the flow balance. The goal is not to remove all of the oldest thrombus, but to reestablish an adequate system of venous pathways to accommodate throughput of venous blood at a rate that reduces edema and pain. The number of symptomatic limbs, affected with venous pathology, is largely underestimated. The magnitude of venous disease as a clinical entity is, in fact, somewhat ignored. I believe this relates to the sense of futility we have learned from our patients and from medical school teachings regarding our limited ability to treat thromboembolic disorders. Quite simply, there is often a sense of hopeless resignation surrounding chronic venous disorders that

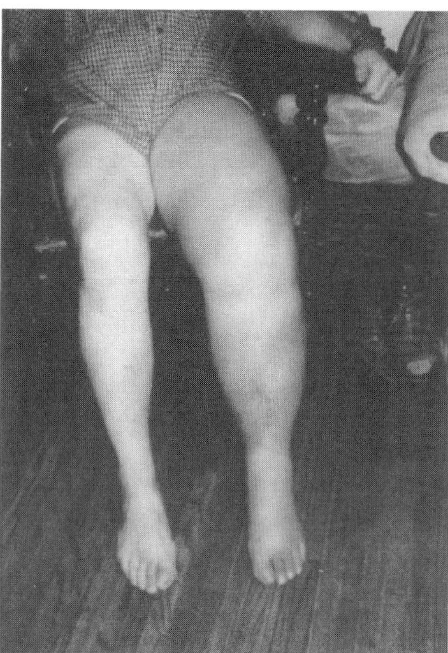
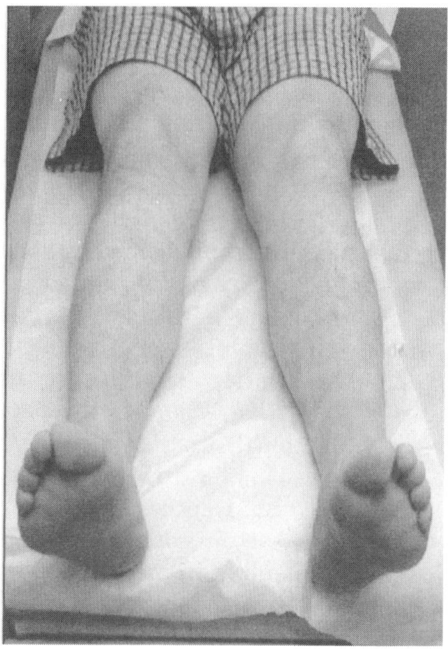

Figure 10. Before (left) and after (right) endovenous reconstruction for chronic iliofemoral occlusion in 1997. This 42-year-old man presented after four hospitalizations for left deep vein thrombosis within 5 years. He now has greater than 3-year follow-up with continued patency. Reflux requires Circ-Aid® (San Diego, CA) compression legging. He remains CEAP Class V.

has been predicated on the difficulties in treatment and the small number of effective therapies. Endovenous therapy may be an option for patients with post-thrombotic syndrome, i.e., chronic swelling, heaviness, numbness, and/or pain. As we have seen, disability may decrease significantly after endovascular intervention (Fig. 10). Furthermore, if improvement can be sustained or, when necessary, maintained with additional therapy, the value of thrombolysis and stents will endure. More importantly, there is increasing appreciation that early intervention in acute thrombosis may reduce the number of persons who develop chronic conditions years after the initial event.

Conclusion

Technological advances have allowed physicians to develop new treatments for venous disorders, such as malformations, nonhealing ulcers, varicosities, reflux, and chronic obstruction, that have challenged physicians and vascular specialists for centuries. What is technically feasible, however, may not always be in the patient's best interest. Endovascular therapy requires great care with patient selection and informed judgment. Above all, new therapies must be governed by responsible scientific research and careful patient follow-up.

Acknowledgments: The work represented in this chapter could not have been accomplished without the dedicated work of a very competent and caring staff including Martin Reece, RT, Shela Stratton, RT, Sandra Woods, RVT, Susan Schubert, BSN, RN, and Jane A. Brown, administrative assistant. Special thanks to Dr. Xiaoxing Zhan for all his thoughtful help and to the Biomedical Graphics Department at Creighton. Last, we wish to express appreciation to all of our patients, whose courage and caring sustain us all.

References

1. Nicolaides AN, Eklof B, Bergan JJ, et al. Classification and grading of chronic venous disease in the lower limbs: A consensus statement. *Phlebology* 1995;10:42–45.
2. Ricotta JJ, Dalsing MC, Ouriel K, et al. Research and clinical issues in chronic venous disease. *Cardiovasc Surg* 1997;5:343–349.
3. Hume M. Venous ulcers, the vascular surgeon and the Medicare budget. *J Vasc Surg* 1992;16:671–673.
4. Mewissen MW, Seabrooke GR, Meissner MH, et al. Catheter-directed thrombolysis for lower extremity deep vein thrombosis: Report of a national multi-center registry. *Radiology* 1999;211:39–49.
5. van Bemmelen PS, Bedford G, Beach K, et al. Status of the valves in the superficial and deep system in chronic venous disease. *Surgery* 1991;109:130–139.
6. Meissner MH, Manzo RA, Bergelin RO, et al. Deep venous insufficiency: The relationship between lysis and consequent reflux. *J Vasc Surg* 1993;18:596–608.
7. Neglen P, Raju S. Balloon dilatation and stenting of chronic iliac vein obstruction: Technical aspects and early clinical outcome. *J Endovasc Surg* 2000;7:79–91.
8. O'Sullivan GJ, Semba CP, Bittner CA, et al. Endovascular management of iliac vein compression (May-Thurner) syndrome. *J Vasc Interv Radiol* 2000;11:823–836.
9. Thorpe PE. Endovascular therapy for chronic venous obstruction. In Ballard JL, Bergan JJ (eds): *Chronic Venous Insufficiency*. New York: Springer; 1999:179–193.
10. Nazarian GK, Austin WT, Wegryn AS. Venous recanalization by metallic stents after failure of balloon angioplasty or surgery: Four-year experience. *Cardiovasc Intervent Radiol* 1996;19:227–233.
11. Goldman MP. Closure of the greater saphenous vein with endoluminal radiofrequency heating of the vein wall in combination with ambulatory phlebectomy: Preliminary 6-month follow-up. *Dermatol Surg* 2000;26:1–5.
12. Chandler JG, Pichot O, Sessa C, et al. Treatment of primary venous insufficiency by endovenous saphenous vein obliteration. *Vasc Surg* 2000;34:201–214.
13. Gomez-Jorge J, Venbrus AC, Magee C. Percutaneous deployment of a valved bovine jugular vein in the swine venous system: A potential treatment for venous insufficiency. *J Vasc Interv Radiol* 2000;11:931–936.
14. Thorpe PE, Osse FJ, Correa LO, et al. Combining a stent and prosthetic valve for percutaneous treatment of femoropopliteal reflux. Presented at: The American Venous Forum; February 4–6, 2000; Scottsdale, AZ.
15. Pavcnik D, Uchida BT, Timmerman HA. Percutaneously introduced prosthetic venous valve: An experimental study. *J Vasc Interv Radiol* 2000;11(suppl):307.
16. Kim SS, Kaihara S, Benvenuto MS, et al. Small intestinal submucosa as a small-caliber venous graft: A novel model for hepatocyte transplantation on synthetic biodegradable polymer scaffolds with direct access to the portal venous system. *J Pediatr Surg* 1999;34:124–128.
17. Cabrera J, Cabrera J Jr, Garcia-Olmedo MA. Treatment of inoperable venous malformations with sclerosants in microfoam form. Paper presented at: The European Venous Forum; June 29–July 1, 2000; Lyon, France.
18. Sevitt J. The mechanisms of canalization in deep vein thrombosis. *J Pathol* 1973;110:153–165.
19. Beyth RJ, Cohen AM, Landerfeld S. Long-term outcomes of deep-vein thrombosis. *Arch Intern Med* 1995;155:1031–1037.
20. Launois R. Construction and validation of a specific health-related quality-of-life questionnaire in chronic venous insufficiency. *Quality Life Res* 1996;5:539–554.

21. Comerota AJ, Throm RC, Mathias SD, et al. Catheter-directed thrombolysis for iliofemoral deep venous thrombosis improves health-related quality of life. *J Vasc Surg* 2000;32:130–137.
22. May R, Thurner J. The cause of the predominantly sinstral occurrence of thrombosis of the pelvic veins. *Angiology* 1957;8:419–427.
23. Sing RF, Cicci CK, LeQuire MH, et al. Bedside carbon dioxide cavograms for inferior vena cava filters: Preliminary results. *J Vasc Surg* 2000;32:144–147.
24. Wohlgemuth WA, Weber H, Loeprecht H, et al. PTA and stenting of benign stenosis in the pelvis: Long-term results. *Cardiovasc Intervent Radiol* 2000;23:9–16.
25. Thorpe PE, Osse FJ, Dang HP. Endovascular reconstruction for chronic iliac vein and inferior vena cava obstruction. In: Gloviczki P, Yao JST (eds): *Handbook of Venous Disorders. 2nd ed. Guidelines of the American Venous Forum.* London: Arnold; 2001:349–360.
26. Bjarnason H, Kruse JR, Asinger DA, et al. Iliofemoral deep vein thrombosis: Safety and efficacy during 5 years of catheter-directed thrombolytic therapy. *J Vasc Interv Radiol* 1997;8:405–418.
27. Meissner MH, Caps MT, Zierler BK, et al. Deep venous reflux and superficial venous reflux. *J Vasc Surg* 2000;32:48–56.
28. Raju S. Venous insufficiency of the lower limb and stasis ulceration: Changing concepts and management. *Ann Surg* 1983;6:688–697.
29. Davidian MM, Powell A, Benenati JF, et al. Initial results of reteplase in the treatment of acute lower extremity arterial occlusions. *J Vasc Interv Radiol* 2000;11:289–294.
30. Semba CP, Murphy TP, Bakal CW, et al. Thrombolytic therapy with use of alteplase (rt-PA) in peripheral arterial occlusive disease: Review of the clinical literature. *J Vasc Interv Radiol* 2000;11:149–161.
31. Semba CP, Bakal CW, Calis KA. Alteplase as an alternative to urokinase. *J Vasc Interv Radiol* 2000;11:279–287.
32. Ouriel K, Katzen B, Mewissen M, et al. Reteplase in the treatment of peripheral arterial and venous occlusions: A pilot study. *J Vasc Interv Radiol* 2000;11:849–854.
33. Brockman SK, Vasco JS. The pathologic physiology of phlegmasia cerulea dolens. *Surgery* 1966;59:997–1007.
34. Weaver FA, Menchum PW, Adkins RB, et al. Phlegmasia cerulea dolens. Therapeutic considerations. *South Med J* 1988;81:306–312.
35. Hood DB, Weaver FA, Modral JG, et al. Advances in the treatment of phlegmasia cerulea dolens. *Am J Surg* 1993;166:206–210.
36. Krupski WC, Bas A, Dilley RB, et al. Propagation of deep venous thrombosis identified by duplex ultrasonography. *J Vasc Surg* 1990;12:467–475.
37. Sherry S, Bell WR, Duckert FH, et al. Thrombolytic therapy in thrombosis: A National Institute of Health consensus development conference. *Ann Intern Med* 1980;93:141–144.
38. Paquet KJ, Popov S. Guidelines and results of consequent fibrinolytic therapy in phlegmasia cerulea dolens. *Dtsch Med Wochenschr* 1970;95:903–904.
39. Robinson DL, Teeitelbaum GF. Phlegmasia cerulea dolens: Treatment by pulse-spray and infusion thrombolysis. *AJR Am J Roentgenol* 1993;160:2188–1290.
40. Strandness DE, Langlios Y, Cramer M, et al. Long-term sequelae of acute venous thrombosis. *JAMA* 1983;250:1289–1292.
41. Hansen MCH, Wollersheim H, van Asten WN, et al. The post-thrombotic syndrome: A review. *Phlebology* 1996;11:86–94.

11

Techniques of Stent-Graft Repair in the Thoracic Aorta

Frank J. Criado, MD, Youssef Rizk, DO, Marcos F. Barnatan, MD, Cecilia F. Wang, MS, and Nancy S. Clark, MD

Introduction

Stent-graft technology has forever changed the management of aortic aneurysms, and has brought about a true revolution in vascular surgery. Since its inception in 1990,[1] treatment of aneurysms in the abdominal aorta has been the main focus of endograft research and development, and progress with the thoracic aorta has lagged behind that of its infradiaphragmatic counterpart. Such asymmetry is about to change as a result of rapidly accumulating endovascular experience in the repair of thoracic aortic pathology.[2–4] Thoracic aortic aneurysms (TAAs) and aortic dissections represent the two most common significant lesions; they seem to occur with an incidence that is clearly higher than previously believed. Both conditions are potentially treatable using a catheter-based endograft strategy, made more attractive by the fact that "conventional" surgical treatment (of both TAAs and aortic dissections) is often accompanied by high mortality and frequent serious morbidity.[5–7] As a result, there is a reluctance on the part of surgeons to treat many, if not most, patients. Less invasive endoluminal intervention is a truly appealing new alternative, likely to have an even greater impact than it has had on the abdominal aorta, where standard surgery offers a low-mortality treatment option for many patients.

Successful arterial segmental exclusion with an endograft—in the thoracic aorta or any other vessel—requires availability of greater than 15 mm proximal and distal "landing (attachment) zones" of nonaneurysmal (cylindri-

From Criado FJ (ed): *Endovascular Intervention: New Tools and Techniques for the 21st Century.* Armonk, NY: Futura Publishing Co., Inc.; ©2002.

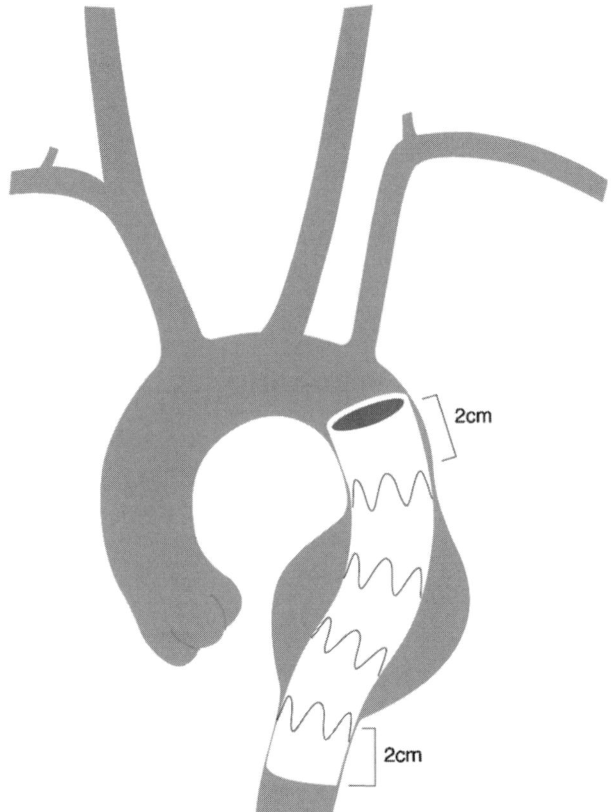

Figure 1. "Ideal" 2.0-cm attachment zones proximally and distally for optimal stent-graft exclusion.

cal) aorta (Fig. 1). Unfortunately, a significant number of lesions likely to benefit from stent-grafting involve the proximal-most portion of the descending thoracic aorta (DTA) or distal aortic arch (Fig. 2). Additionally, the arch itself may be the site of pathology or the target for device deployment and attachment. On both accounts, stent-graft placement is challenged by the presence of the left subclavian artery (LSA) and other arch branches precluding availability of a greater than 15 mm long proximal landing zone. In such case, one may need to use adjunctive surgical bypass or transposition techniques designed to "lengthen the branchless DTA" and enable stent-graft placement in the parasubclavian and paracarotid thoracic aorta, and even within the aortic arch proper. The range of possibilities is relatively wide, and includes simple coverage of the aortic origin of the vessel, transostial crossing with a bare (uncovered) stent, and various options for branch disconnection and revascularization by direct transposition to a neighboring artery or bypass from another vessel.

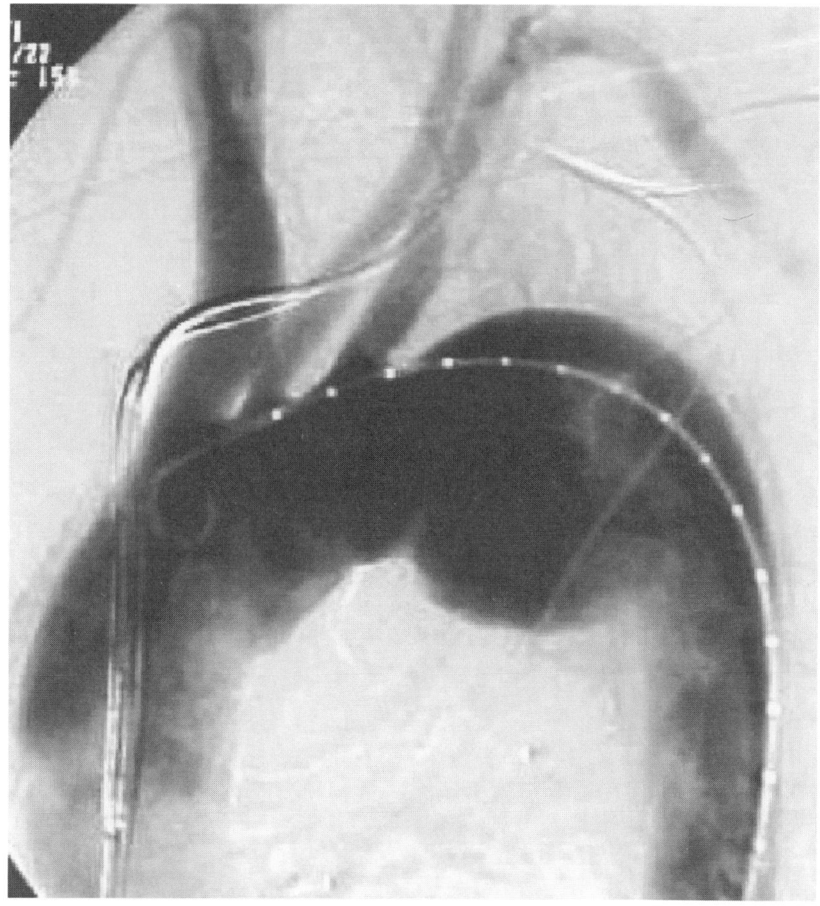

Figure 2. Large juxtasubclavian aneurysm involving the proximal-most portion of the descending thoracic aorta.

The "Parasubclavian" Thoracic Aorta: Management Options for the LSA

The LSA interferes with stent-graft placement when the aneurysm or dissection begins within 15 mm of its origin (Fig. 2), and even more so when the lesion actually involves the LSA (Fig. 3). The latter occurs only infrequently, but the former is more common. Simple vessel coverage by stent-graft, without revascularization, is possible and has been reported to be well tolerated (Fig. 4).[8] The ability to cover-occlude this artery with little or no risk of causing overt arm or vertebrobasilar ischemia is likely related to the rather profuse network of collateral pathways in the area. Should ischemia develop, secondary revascularization can be easily performed by cervical bypass or transposition. Devices that contain an uncovered proximal stent (i.e., Talent Free-Flo,

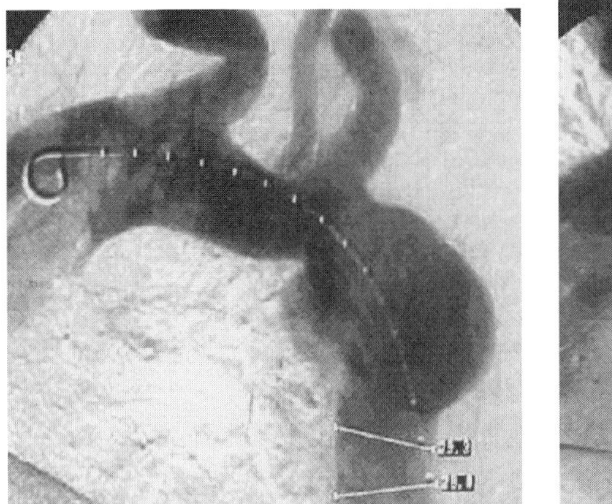

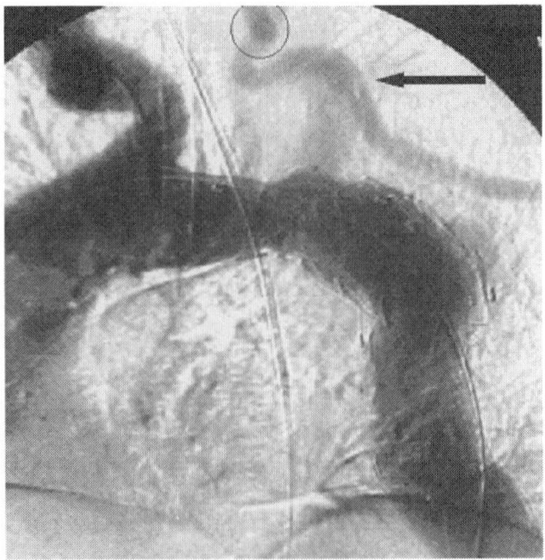

Figure 3. Large aneurysm occurring many years after surgical repair of coarctation of the thoracic aorta (left). Involvement of left subclavian artery and close proximity to left common carotid artery origin required adjunctive procedures (right) to obtain an appropriate segment for proximal stent-graft fixation; crossover right-to-left carotid-carotid bypass (circle) and left carotid-subclavian bypass (arrow), combined with proximal ligation of the left common carotid artery and left subclavian artery achieved such objective.

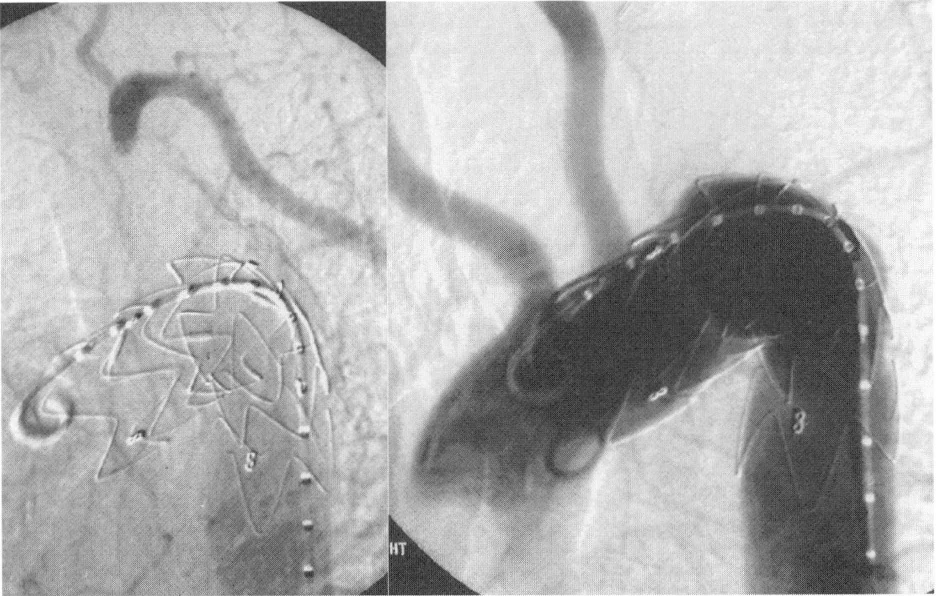

Figure 4. Stent-graft placement across origin of left subclavian artery, causing obstruction of vessel. Note retrograde filling via reversal of flow in left vertebral artery (left).

Medtronic AVE, Santa Rosa, CA) provide the additional possibility of stent-graft placement across the LSA origin with continuing normal flow into the vessel.

Actual involvement of the LSA by an aneurysm brings a new set of issues and challenges; reflux endoleak, not ischemia, is the concern in this setting. In such case, the LSA must be excluded (disconnected) ahead of time in preparation for stent-graft deployment: the techniques of supraclavicular approach to the LSA for ligation (proximal to the vertebral artery origin) and concomitant carotid-subclavian bypass (Fig. 5) are familiar to all vascular surgeons. An LSA-to-carotid transposition (SCT) can achieve both goals in one step, does not use a prosthesis, and should be regarded as the superior option (Fig. 6).

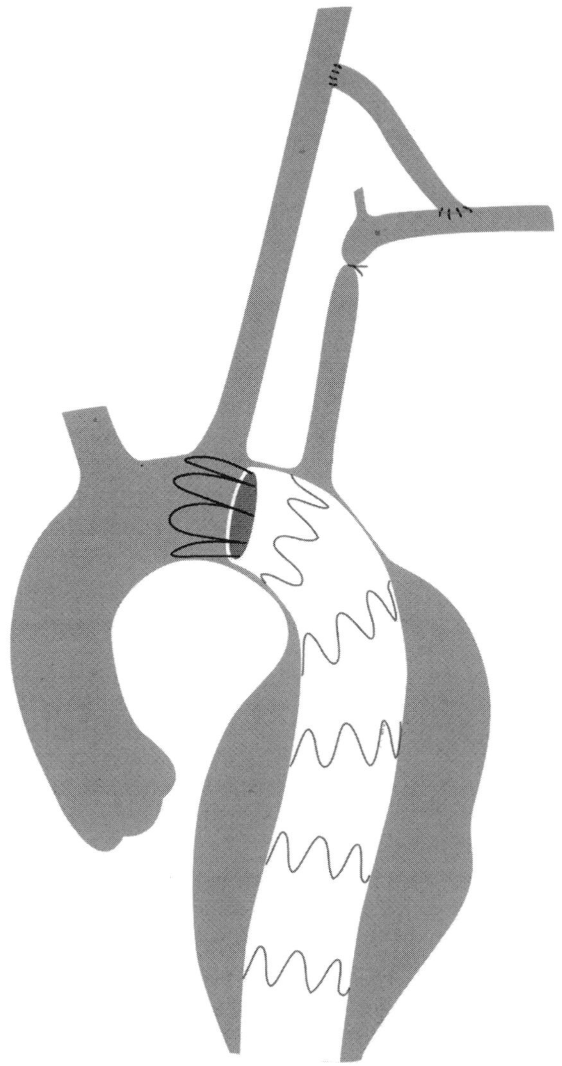

Figure 5. Left carotid-subclavian bypass and proximal ligation of left subclavian artery.

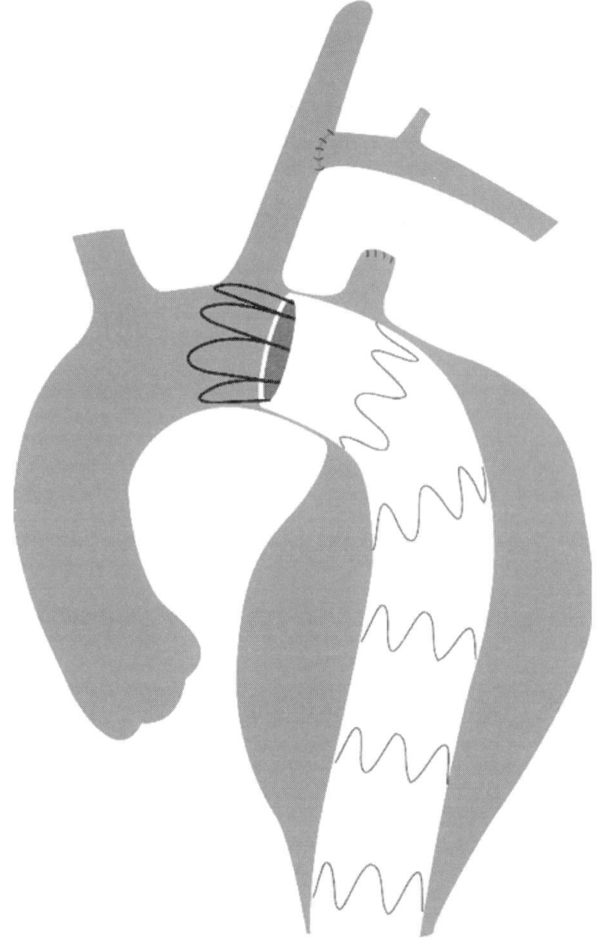

Figure 6. Left subclavian artery-to-carotid transposition.

The Left Common Carotid Artery

The left common carotid artery (LCCA) poses an issue when there is a juxtasubclavian or suprasubclavian aneurysm and close anatomical proximity (<20 mm) between the common carotid and the LSA. Unlike the previously described scenario for the subclavian artery, "simple" graft coverage of the LCCA is not appropriate. Concomitant disconnection and revascularization of the LCCA at the time of LSA operation is the recommended course of action, to "lengthen" the available segment of aorta (to the origin of the innominate artery) for stent-graft fixation. Technical options include:

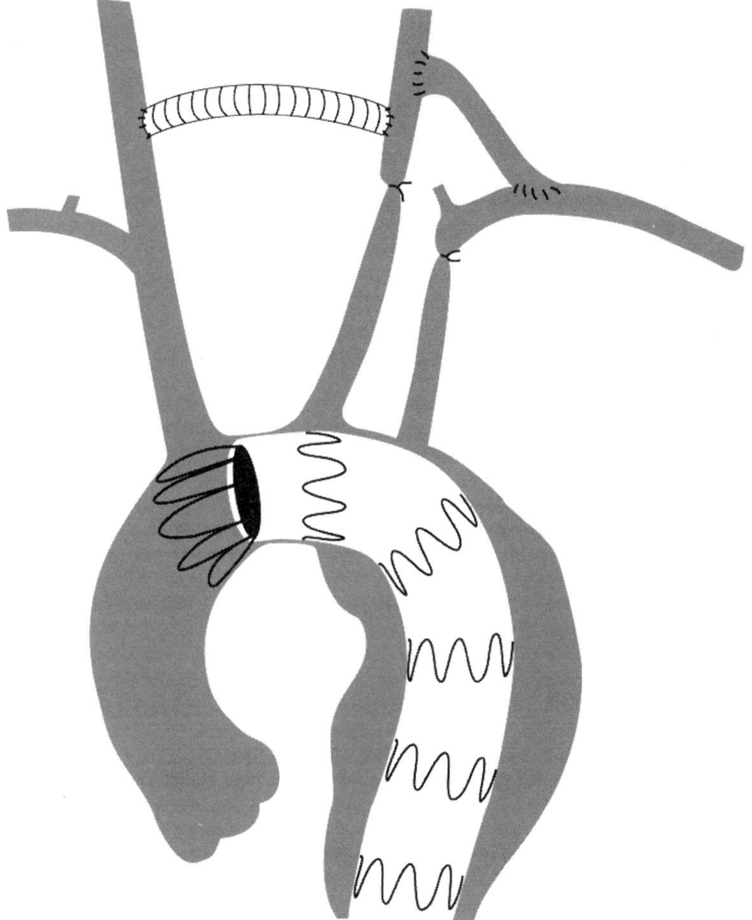

Figure 7. Right-to-left carotid-carotid bypass, left carotid-subclavian bypass, proximal ligation of left common carotid artery and left subclavian artery.

- Crossover (retropharyngeal) carotid-carotid artery bypass, with proximal ligation of the LCCA, simultaneous with LSA ligation and carotid-subclavian bypass or SCT (see above) (Fig. 7).
- On rare occasions it may be necessary to consider femoral-artery-based reconstruction, such as femoral-axillary bypass, plus SCT and carotid-carotid artery bypass with proximal ligation of the LCCA (Fig. 8).

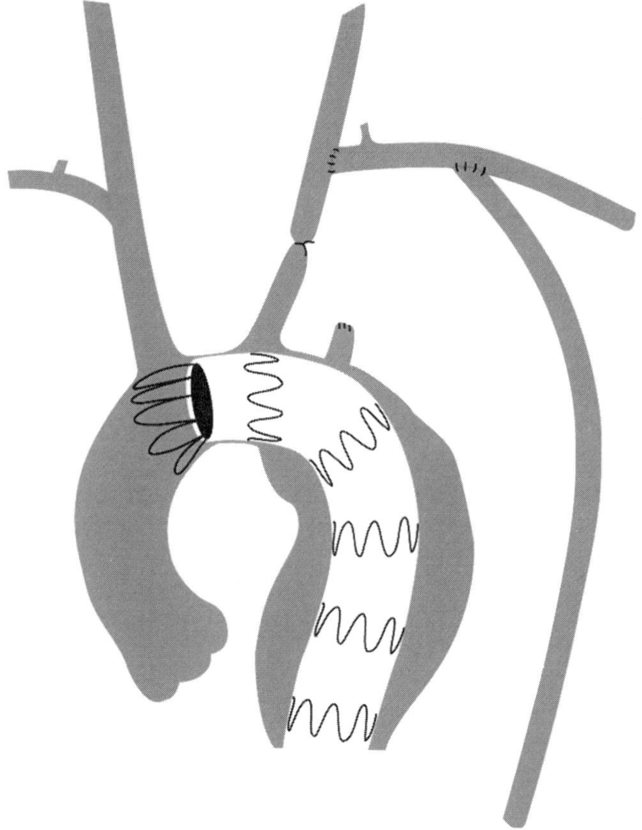

Figure 8. Left femoroaxillary bypass, left subclavian artery-to-carotid transposition, proximal ligation of left common carotid artery.

Management of the Innominate Artery

The innominate artery can also be "relocated" to enable placement of a stent-graft device to cover the entire transverse aortic arch, and even extend it proximally as far as the ascending aorta. We have not yet had personal experience with such an approach, but it is certainly feasible. From a technical and hemodynamic perspective, an ascending aorta-based bypass would constitute the most satisfactory arrangement at the time of innominate artery disconnection, but it would require a transthoracic operation that may not be well tolerated by the patient. Extrathoracic revascularization of all arch branches can be achieved with femoral-axillary bypass and secondary "jump grafts" from the SA to the CCA on the same side, and crossover to the CCA and SA on the other side (Fig. 9).[9,10] Such procedures would be extraordinarily complex and of only exceptional clinical application.

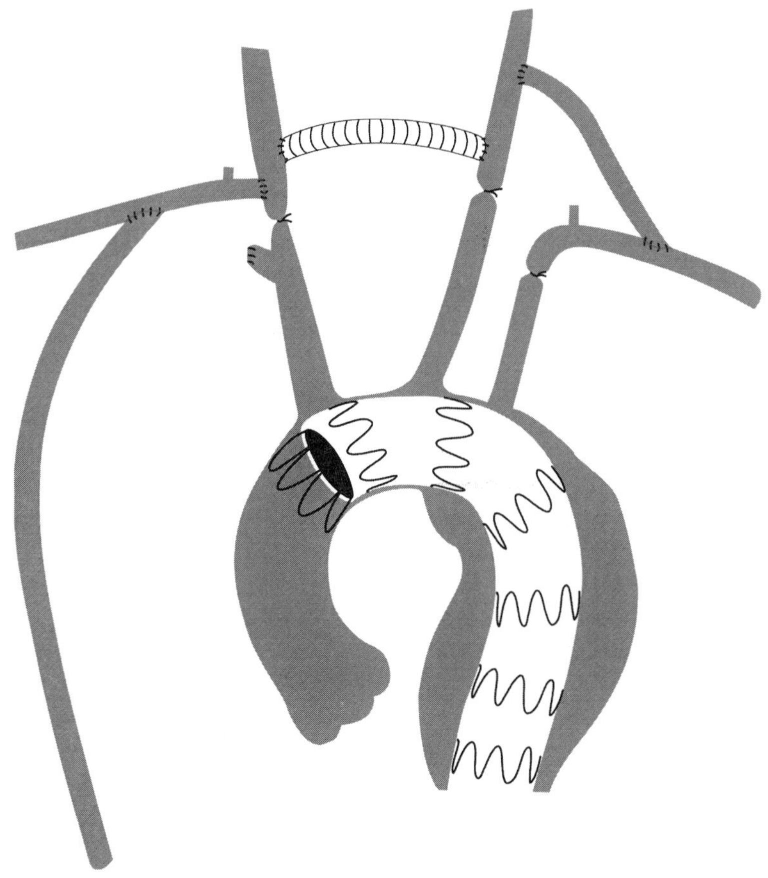

Figure 9. Right femoroaxillary bypass, intercarotid bypass, left carotid-subclavian bypass, ligation of right and left common carotid arteries and left subclavian artery.

Summary of Personal Experience

Forty-two patients received thoracic stent-graft implants in our service during the 44-month period ending December 31, 2001. Twenty-nine patients had aneurysms (TAA) and 13 had type B aortic dissections. In 3 of the TAA patients, a dissecting origin of the aneurysm was suspected but not confirmed. Proximal attachment of the device was in zone 1 in 3, zone 2 in 6, zone 3 in 19, and zone 4 in 14 (Fig. 10). Distal attachment was in the supradiaphragmatic DTA in 38, and in the upper abdominal aorta in 4. The celiac artery origin was covered (occluded) with the graft in 1 and simply crossed with the bare stent (not occluded) in 2. A total of 45 thoracic endograft implants were performed as 3 patients underwent secondary stent-grafting for treatment of endoleaks. Endograft coverage or trans-subclavian placement of the bare stent was performed in 5 instances, and 7 patients underwent preliminary cervical bypass

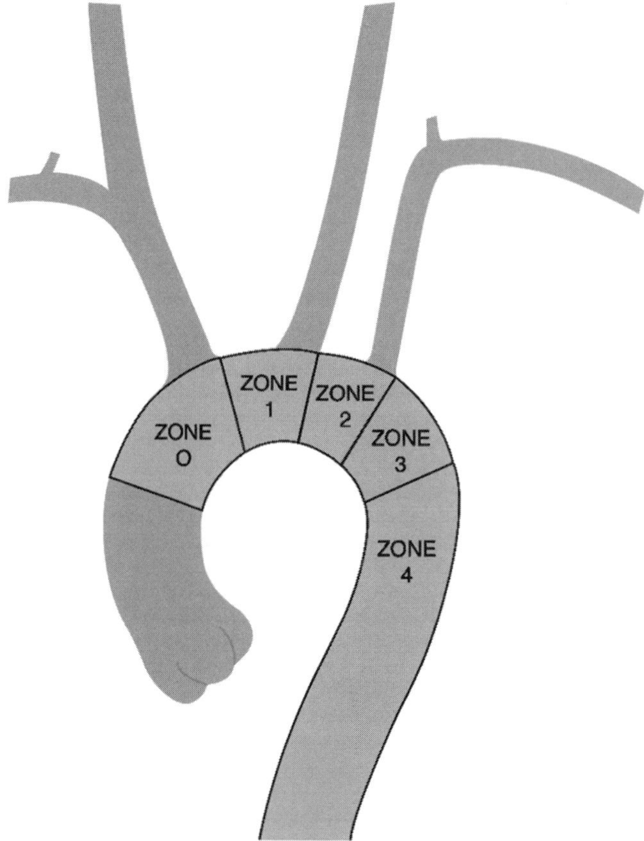

Figure 10. Aortic arch "map" to illustrate proximal fixation site of stent-graft implant.

or transposition operations to enable stent-grafting of aortic arch or proximal DTA lesions. "Zone 1 patients" (n=3) had preliminary crossover right-to-left carotid-carotid artery bypass, proximal ligation of LCCA, as well as left carotid-subclavian bypass (n=2) or SCT (n=1) and ligation of LSA proximal to the vertebral artery origin to allow proximal endograft attachment at or immediately distal to the origin of the innominate artery. Of "Zone 2 patients" (n=6), 4 had preliminary proximal LSA ligations, and carotid-subclavian bypass (n=2) or SCT (n=2). In cases in which endograft attachment was in zone 3, intentional graft coverage with occlusion of the LSA was performed in 2 instances, and transostial placement of the bare stent in 3. One patient (2.4%) died intraoperatively from access-related iliac artery rupture with massive hemorrhage; that was the single 30-day mortality. No patient developed paraplegia or stroke, and none required surgical conversion. Postoperative morbid adverse events occurred in 8 patients (19%), none related to LSA occlusion. One patient died at 60 days from rupture of an infected thoracoabdominal aneurysm with juxtaceliac attachment endoleak.

Discussion and Overview

It is clear that our knowledge base is still quite limited, making it difficult to formulate firm guidelines and even opinions on critical areas such as clinical indications, success rates, and long-term durability of stent-graft endovascular repair in the thoracic aorta. Such doubts are even more significant as they relate to decision making in the treatment of aortic dissections. However, we must keep in mind that many of these are often "neglected" because of surgeons' reluctance to undertake transthoracic aortic reconstruction for fear of serious morbidity and unacceptable risks of perioperative mortality. Minimally invasive stent-graft intervention offers an exciting and truly innovative treatment strategy for a significant number of patients with TAAs, dissections, and other related conditions which, interestingly and somewhat unfortunately, seem to involve the proximal DTA and parasubclavian aorta with predilection. The adjunctive techniques described in this chapter allow expansion of stent-graft indications to include lesions in close proximity to or actually involving one or more branches of the aortic arch. This is especially important for individuals who are at high risk for major thoracic aortic surgery—that is, the majority of patients!

References

1. Parodi JC, Palmaz JC, Barone HD. Transfemoral intraluminal graft implantation for abdominal aortic aneurysms. *Ann Vasc Surg* 1991;5:491–499.
2. Dake MD, Miller DC, Semba CP, et al. Transluminal placement of endovascular stent-grafts for the treatment of descending thoracic aortic aneurysms. *N Engl J Med* 1994;331:1729–1734.
3. Mitchell RS, Miller DC, Dake MD. Stent-graft repair of thoracic aortic aneurysms. *Semin Vasc Surg* 1997;4:257–271.
4. Temudom T, D'Ayala M, Marin ML, et al. Endovascular grafts in the treatment of thoracic aortic aneurysms and pseudoaneurysms. *Ann Vasc Surg* 2000;14:230–238.
5. Greenberg R, Resch T, Nyman U, et al. Endovascular repair of descending thoracic aortic aneurysms: An early experience with intermediate-term follow-up. *J Vasc Surg* 2000;31:147–156.
6. Greenberg R, Risher W. Clinical decision making and operative approaches to thoracic aortic aneurysms. *Surg Clin North Am* 1998;78:805–826.
7. Rizzo JA, Coady MA, Elefteriades JA. Interpreting data on thoracic aortic aneurysms. Statistical issues. *Cardiol Clin* 1999;17:797–805.
8. Hausegger KA, Oberwalder P, Tiesenhausen K, et al. Intentional left subclavian artery occlusion by thoracic aortic stent-grafts without surgical transposition. *J Endovasc Ther* 2001;8:472–476.
9. Moore WS, Malone JM, Goldstone J. Extrathoracic repair of branch occlusions of the aortic arch. *Am J Surg* 1976;132:249–257.
10. Criado FJ. Extrathoracic management of aortic arch syndrome. *Br J Surg* 1982;69(suppl):S45-S51.

12

Superelastic Stent Designs

Tom W. Duerig, PhD, Deborah E. Tolomeo, PhD, and Mark H. Wholey, MD

Introduction

Superelasticity refers to an attribute of Nitinol and certain other metals to return to their original shape after severe deformations. As such, it is an extension of the conventional elasticity that all metals exhibit to varying degrees: stainless steel can return to its original length if stretched up to 0.3% of its original length, certain high-strength titanium alloys up to 2%, and superelastic Nitinol more than 10%. While a superelastic material appears macroscopically to be simply 'very elastic,' the mechanism of deformation is in fact quite different than conventional elasticity or simply the stretching of atomic bonds. When a stress is applied to Nitinol superelastic, Nitinol changes its crystal structure from austenite to martensite.* This stress-assisted phase transition allows the material to change shape as directed by the applied stress. When the stresses are removed, the material reverts to the original austenite and recovers its original shape.

Nitinol is a nearly equiatomic composition of nickel and titanium and is one of very few alloys that is both superelastic and biocompatible. Moreover, the narrow temperature range within which Nitinol's superelasticity is exhibited includes body temperature. Thus, Nitinol has become the 'material of choice' for designers of self-expanding stents. Self-expanding stents are manufactured with a diameter larger than that of the target vessel; they are crimped and restrained in a delivery system, then elastically released into the target vessel. Performance of self-expanding stents is therefore limited by the ability of the material to store elastic energy while constrained in the delivery system; this makes Nitinol the ideal choice. While the exact mechanisms of superelasticity in Nitinol are well understood,[1] the application of Nitinol to stents is relatively new.[2]

From Criado FJ (ed): *Endovascular Intervention: New Tools and Techniques for the 21st Century.* Armonk, NY: Futura Publishing Co., Inc.; ©2002.

*The austenite, or "parent," crystal structure is cubic in nature; the martensitic "daughter" structure is a complex monoclinic structure.

The most dramatic and demonstrable attribute of Nitinol stents is their crush recoverability. Most, if not all, Nitinol stents can be crushed fully flat and still elastically recover their original shape without clinically relevant loss of lumen diameter. This attribute is important in superficial indications subject to external crushing such as the carotid artery. Crush recoverability is surely the easiest way one can distinguish Nitinol from stainless steel, but differences between balloon-expandable and self-expanding stents are far more numerous and important.

Terminology and Definition of Forces

As a preamble, it is necessary to define some terminology regarding vascular forces, and cylindrical shapes in general. Blood vessels experience loads from a variety of sources, such as the pulse pressure of the cardiac cycle, spasms, angioplasty balloons, the placement of a stent, etc. Pressures applied to any cylindrical structure, such as a blood vessel, result in hoop, or circumferential, loading of the vessel (Fig. 1a). Both the applied pressure and the resulting hoop stress have units of 'force per unit area,' but differ in direction. Pressure refers to the force normal to the vessel wall divided by the surface area of the lumen (circumference times length), while hoop stress is the circumferential load in the vessel wall divided by the cross-sectional area of the vessel wall (length times wall thickness). By analogy, water pressure within a pipe results in a tensile hoop stress within the metal pipe itself. The pressure

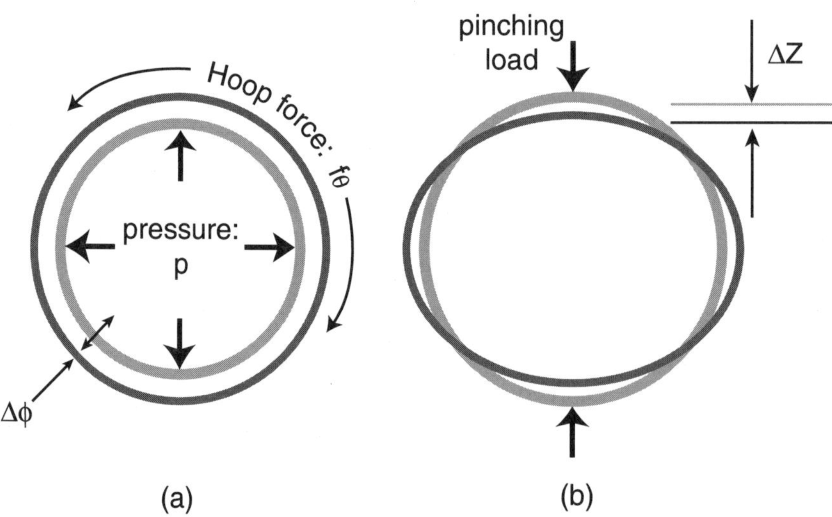

Figure 1. The two most common loading modes for stents are (**a**) radial or hoop, and (**b**) pinching.

(p) and the hoop stress (σ) in a thin-walled cylindrical object such as a vessel or stent are related by:

$$\sigma = p\phi/2t \tag{1}$$

where ϕ is the vessel diameter and t the vessel wall thickness. We can describe the hoop force, F_θ, in a vessel wall as:

$$F_\theta = \sigma \, t \, L = p \, \phi \, L/2 \tag{2}$$

where L is the stent length. In fact, it is more convenient to define hoop force per unit length as:

$$f_\theta = F_\theta/L = \sigma \, t = p \, \phi/2 \tag{3}$$

As an example, a blood pressure of p=100 mm Hg would apply a hoop force (or hoop load) on an 8-mm-diameter vessel of:

$$f_\theta = (100 \text{ mm Hg}) \, [1.33\times10^{-4} \, (\text{N/mm}^2)/\text{mm Hg}] \, (8 \text{ mm})/2 = 0.053 \text{ N/mm} \tag{4}$$

where 1.33×10^{-4} (N /mm^2)/mm Hg is the conversion from mm Hg to N/mm^2 or MPa. Thus, each millimeter of vessel length experiences a tensile load in the hoop direction of 0.053 N.

Hoop or Radial Strength

While hoop stress, total hoop force, and pressure are all equivalent descriptors of vessel forces, we find f_θ to be most convenient because it best correlates to strength, or the maximum hoop load that can be carried without failure. In the case of a vessel or pipe, failure is suitably defined as burst or rupture. Failure would occur when the hoop stress exceeds the ultimate tensile strength of the material used to manufacture the vessel or pipe.

All the same concepts apply to a stent within a vessel. Pressures acting on the vessel result in hoop loading of the stent that is being used to scaffold, or support, the vessel. The concept of 'failure,' however, now becomes illusive. A stent is intended to hold the vessel open, not to prevent rupture. A stent may fail to perform its intended function and still be fully intact, so the concept of fracture as the failure criteria is no longer relevant. Failure is often defined as the onset of permanent, or plastic, deformation (yielding). In balloon-expandable stents there exists some pressure that causes plastic deformation of the stent, thus providing a basis for defining the strength of the stent. (Of course radial strength can and is often used instead of hoop strength, with the two quantities related through equation 3.) In contrast to balloon-expandable stents, however, Nitinol knows no such limitations: it cannot be deformed or broken by clinically relevant external stresses. Therefore, *Nitinol has no physically appropriate hoop or radial strength limit.*

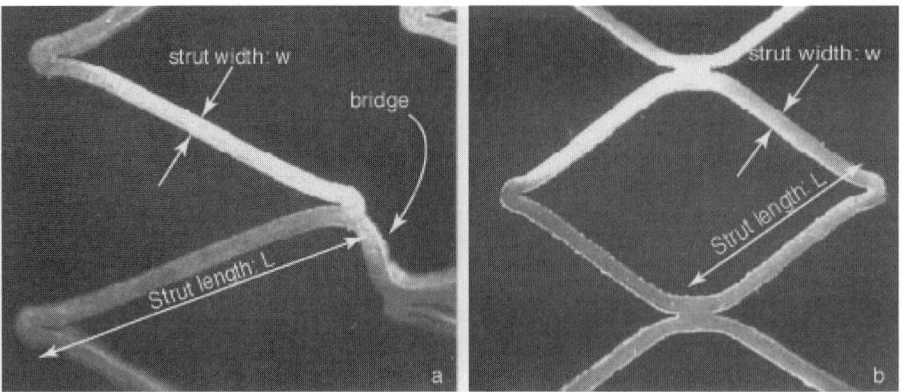

Figure 2. Most stents are variations on either (**a**) z's, or (**b**) diamonds.

Radial or Hoop Stiffness

While we therefore cannot compare the strength of a self-expanding stent to a balloon-expandable stent, we can and should compare their stiffnesses. Stiffness measures the elastic response of a device to an applied load and thus will reflect the effectiveness of the stent in resisting diameter loss due to vessel recoil and other mechanical events. Just as above, the choice of radial or hoop stiffness is only one of terminology, but we prefer the mathematics of hoop stiffness because of its more direct correlation to design. More specifically, we can define the hoop stiffness of a stent or a vessel as the hoop force per unit length required to elastically change its diameter, or:

$$k_\theta = f_\theta/\Delta\phi \qquad (5)$$

Note that stiffness is the inverse of another commonly used term, compliance, or diameter change at a specific applied pressure. Vessel compliance (C_o) is usually reported as the percent diameter change at a given pressure, P_o. Thus, hoop stiffness is related to radial compliance through:

$$k_\theta = P_o/2\,C_o \qquad (6)$$

With the commonly assumed pressure of P_o=100 mm Hg or 0.0133 N/mm^2, we have k_θ=(0.00665 N/mm^2)/$C_{100\ mm\ Hg}$.

Using analytical mechanics,[3] we can estimate the stiffness of a conventional diamond or z-strut (Fig. 2). While we need not concern ourselves with the detailed calculations, it is interesting to summarize trends. The change in stent diameter due to an applied load is related to the stent geometry by:

$$\Delta\phi \propto f_\theta\, n\, L_s^3/E\, w^3\, t \qquad (7)$$

or, substituting equation 3, the change in stent diameter may be related to an applied pressure by:

$$\Delta\phi \propto p\,\phi\,n\,L_s^3/E\,w^3\,t \tag{8}$$

where L_s is the length of a z-strut or half-diamond, w the strut width, t the thickness of the stent, n the number of struts around the circumference, and E the elastic modulus of the material. It follows from equations 3 and 8 that the stiffness per unit length (k_θ) can be determined* by:

$$k_\theta \propto E\,w^3\,t/n\,L_s^3 \tag{9}$$

The stiffness of a stent does have clinical significance in reducing acute recoil and in determining fatigue life (both discussed below).

Pinching Loads and Buckling

Important in equation 9 is the cubic relationship of hoop or radial stiffness to strut width. If instead a stent is squeezed between two fingers or platens, the stent is subjected to a pinching load (Fig. 1b). Pinching loads subject struts to out-of-plane bending, i.e., the struts are not bent around the circumference as in radial compression. The dependence of deflection of a stent on geometry is rather complex and includes tension, torsion, and bending components, but we can approximate the primary bending component as follows:

$$k_{pinching} \propto Et^3\,w/n\,L_s^3 \tag{10}$$

Note that under a pinching load, strut width now demonstrates only a linear contribution, while thickness a cubic dependence, precisely the opposite of hoop strength, for which strut width has the dominate role. Thus *the stiffness of a stent determined by flattening has little to do with the clinically relevant stiffness of the stent.* In fact, design changes aimed at increasing crush resistance may well decrease radial stiffness. Because pinching loads and deflections are far easier to measure than hoop, one must be vigilant not to erroneously use this as a gauge of stent strength or stiffness.

Buckling refers to unstable deformation, meaning that an applied load can be reduced by increasing deformation. Most objects loaded in compression are potentially subject to buckling, such as a walking cane that might bend suddenly if leaned on too hard. Once a structure buckles, its stiffness is generally dramatically reduced. A stent experiences circumferential compression and may, in cases, become unstable and buckle outside the circumferential plane into a half-moon shape. This can be exacerbated if the compression loads are not radially symmetric, as in the 'kissing' stent-grafts shown in Figure 3. Be-

---

*Equations 7 through 10 are only good approximations for small linear deflections within the linear elastic range of the material; larger deformations and more complicated geometry require other techniques such as finite element analysis.

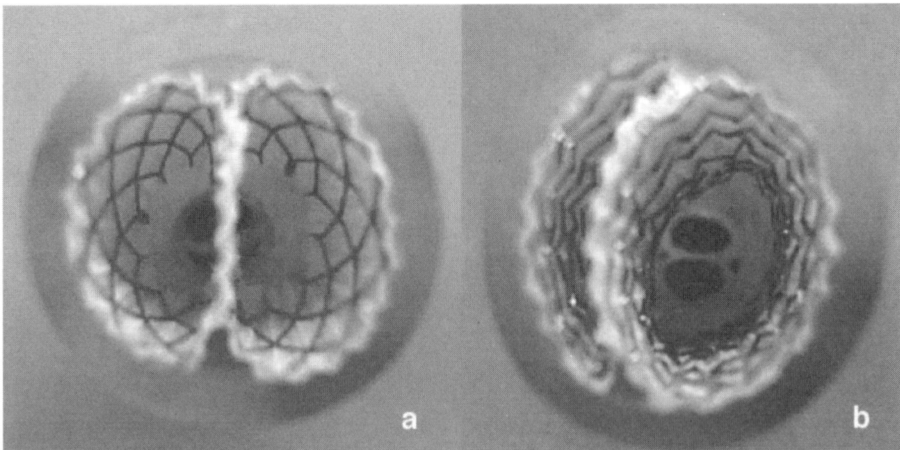

Figure 3. Two "kissing" Nitinol stent-grafts of equivalent radial stiffness, both shape set to the same circular cross section, but with different pinching stiffness. The design on the left can be crushed in any direction and will return to the desired configuration shown. The design on the right prefers to buckle out of plane and return to a half-moon geometry, occluding one of the branches.

ing an out-of-plane deformation, buckling is resisted by the pinching stiffness described in equation 10. Thus, a lower hoop stiffness but more stable shape can be obtained by maximizing thickness and minimizing width. One must be careful to balance the two stiffnesses.

Elastic Modulus and Biased Stiffness

Next we consider the elastic modulus, E, in equations 7 through 10, a simple constant for conventional materials, but an enormously complex concept in Nitinol.[1] The modulus of all stainless steel stents is approximately 200 GPa; variations in device stiffness result only from the geometry variations described in equation 9. Nitinol, however, is a nonlinear, path-dependent, and temperature-dependent material, making E anything but a constant. One certainty, however, is that E is always lower in Nitinol than it is in stainless steel; thus, *a stainless steel stent will always be stiffer, or less compliant, than a Nitinol stent made to the same design*. In fact, a balloon-expandable stent will be at least 3 times as stiff as an identical Nitinol self-expanding stent. Clearly this has important implications to recoil, which is discussed later in this chapter.

The hysteresis or path dependence of Nitinol results in another very important feature termed biased stiffness. This concept is illustrated in Figure 4. Shown in light gray is a typical schematic superelastic stress-strain curve for Nitinol, illustrating both nonlinear response and hysteresis. Superimposed on the curve is the crimping and deployment of a self-expanding stent. The axes have been changed from stress-strain to hoop force-stent diameter. This particular schematic stent has been manufactured with an 8-mm diameter (a in Fig. 4), crimped into a delivery catheter (point b), then packaged, sterilized,

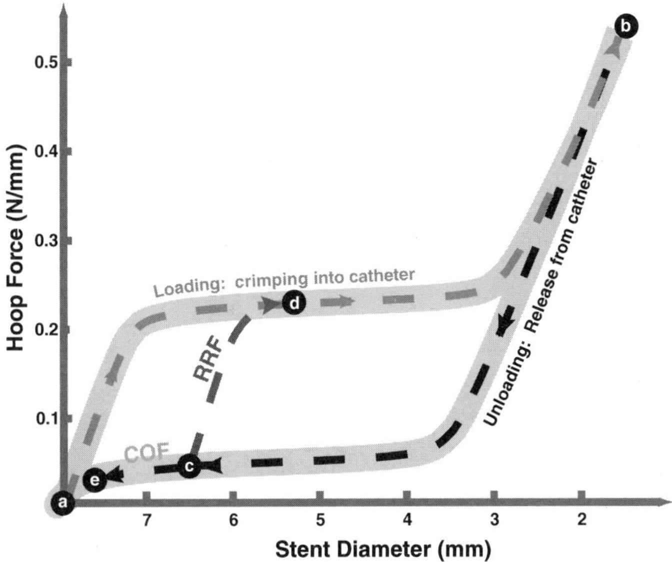

Figure 4. A typical superelastic stress-strain curve is transposed onto a hoop force-diameter diagram, illustrating the concept of biased stiffness. An 8-mm stent is compressed into a catheter (b), then released to a diameter (c). Further deformation forces are resisted by the radial resistive force (d), while the opening chronic outward force remains constant and gentle (e).

and shipped. After insertion to the target site, the stent is released into a vessel, expanding from b until movement is stopped by impingement with the vessel (point c). Having reached equilibrium with the vessel, recoil pressures are resisted by forces dictated by the loading curve (brown trace toward point d), which is substantially steeper (stiffer) than the unloading line (trace from point c to point e).

In the next section we examine this 'impingement' in more detail, but already we can see some of the significance of Nitinol's unusual elastic hysteresis. This biased stiffness means that the continuing opening force of the stent acting on the vessel wall, or chronic outward force (COF) remains very low through large deflections and oversizing. Meanwhile, the forces generated by the stent to resist compression, or radial resistive force (RRF), increase rapidly with deflection until a plateau stress is reached. As a matter of definition, we again find it most convenient to define both RRF and COF as hoop forces per unit length of stent, thus allowing a constant value within a family of stents of varying diameter and length. We discuss the clinical relevance of COF and RRF in later sections of this chapter, but *in general, stent designers should strive for as high an RRF with as low a COF as possible.*

Figure 5 shows actual measurements of hoop force versus diameter for a commercially available 10-mm Nitinol stent.* The device is crimped to 2 mm

*The actual diameter of the stent is closer to 10.5 mm. Self-expanding stents are typically larger than their nominal diameter. Since the consequence of oversizing is substantially less than the consequence of undersizing, a 'one-sided tolerance' is often applied.

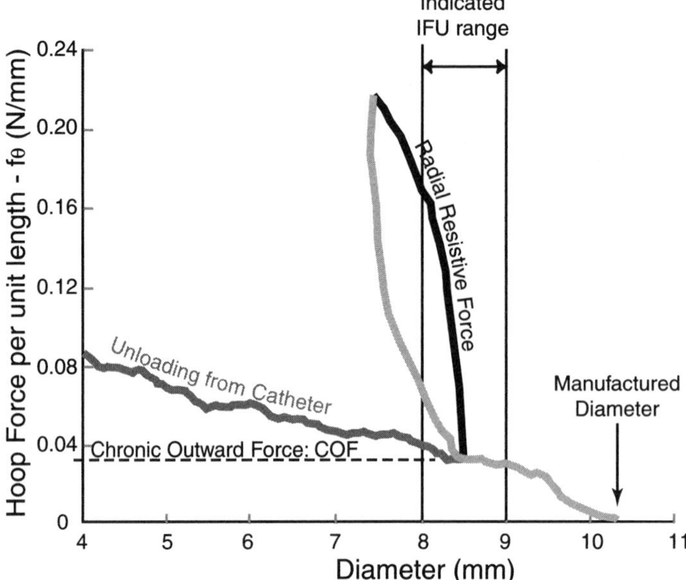

Figure 5. Hoop forces are measured during the release of a commercially available, laser-cut Nitinol self-expanding stent with a nominal 10-mm diameter. The release is halted at the center of the intended diameter range of 8 to 9 mm, at which point the stent is compressed 1 mm in order to demonstrate biased stiffness. After the compression, the stent is again unloaded, quickly returning to the original unloading path but with a small hysteresis.

and is deployed into an emulated 8.5-mm vessel diameter (data at diameters $<$4 mm are not recorded). At 8.5 mm, the RRF is recorded by crimping the stent back to 7.5 mm, then the stent is unloaded entirely to its original diameter. One can see that the COF is quite constant at 0.035 N/mm throughout the indicated diameter range (8 to 9 mm). The RRF increases sharply as the stent is deformed from the equilibrium diameter, reaching 0.22 N/mm after a 1-mm deflection. Continued deformation would indicate a plateau at approximately 0.24 N/mm.

Note that the RRF is not a property of the stent, but must be defined by applying some relevant diameter change, in this case 1 mm. Note that unloading (lightest gray trace) does not follow the same line as loading but instead shows additional hysteresis, rejoining the original unloading line at the point at which loading began. With cycling, this hysteresis will reduce to nearly zero, and the RRF slope will decrease.

Post Dilatation and Acute Recoil

Having described the behavior of a stent alone, we can now examine the "impingement" and interaction of the stent with the vessel during deployment. To illustrate this, Figure 6 follows the same 10-mm stent illustrated in Figure 5 as it contacts a 7-mm vessel with a hoop stiffness of 0.11 N/mm^2 (a compli-

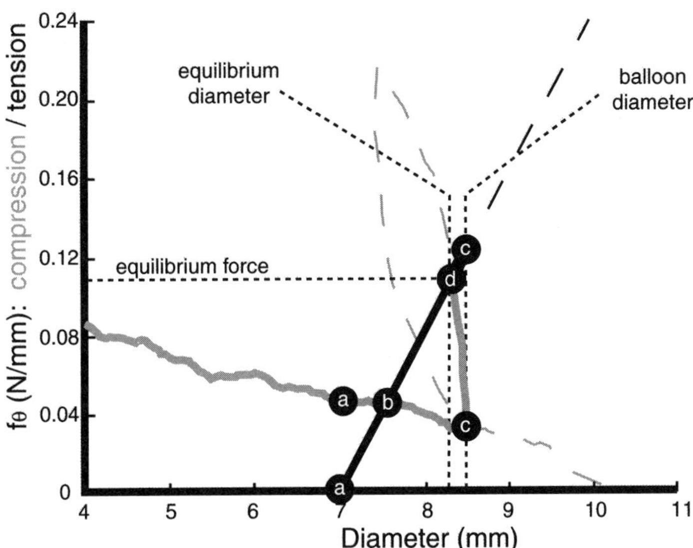

Figure 6. The interaction of a vessel with a typical self-expanding stent is illustrated by examining the delivery process and post dilatation. (Note that the stent forces are compressive, while the vessel forces are tensile.) The stent is released from the delivery system, making vessel contact at point a, then reaching a stress equilibrium at point b. Post dilation further unloads the stent, and stretches the vessel, to points c, and finally deflation of the balloon loads the stent and relaxes the vessel to the final equilibrium point d.

ance of 6% per 100 mm Hg). During this sequence, the vessel will experience tensile hoop forces and the stent will be in compression, though for reasons of convenience they are plotted on the same axis. The stent is released from the delivery catheter and unloads to meet the vessel wall (shown by the dark gray traces). The stent contacts the vessel at point a and reaches an initial equilibrium diameter at point b. Note that this equilibrium diameter is dictated by an equilibrium between the compressive stent COF and the tensile hoop forces in the vessel wall. The stent is then balloon dilated to 8.7 mm, forcing stent and vessel to diameter c. Finally, the balloon is deflated, allowing the vessel to recoil, achieving a new stress equilibrium at point d. During dilation, the stent is unloaded and during recoil it is loaded. Since the stent is now being loaded to the final diameter, equilibrium is now determined by the RRF of the stent rather than the COF.

Except for the biased stiffness of Nitinol, post dilatation of a healthy elastic vessel would be completely ineffective, and would return the original equilibrium diameter at point b. We should note that there is at least one stainless steel self-expanding stent on the market, made of braided wire. While stainless steel does not inherently provide biased stiffness, friction between braided wires can emulate this effect.

It is interesting to compare Figure 6 with the same scenario carried out with a balloon-expandable stent (Fig. 7). The vessel is the same in Figures 6 and 7, but in Figure 7 it is superimposed with the hoop force versus diameter

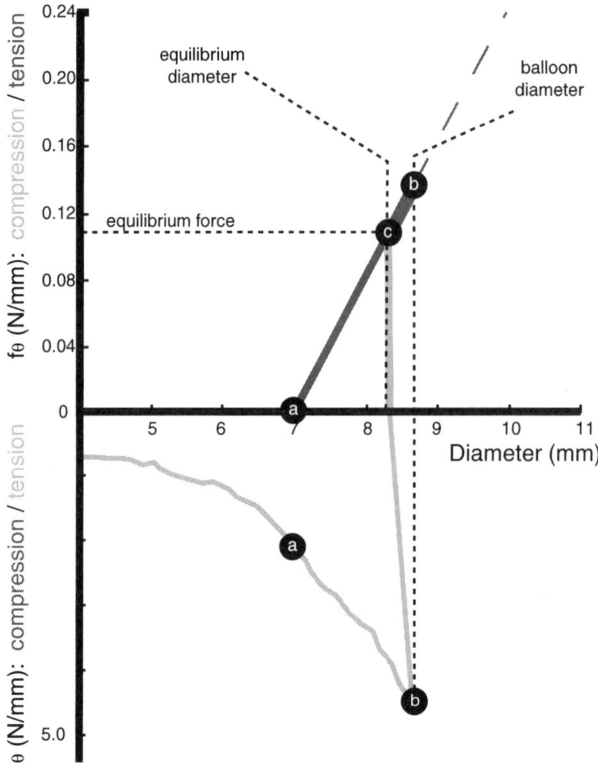

Figure 7. The same vessel as shown in Figure 6 is now stented with a typical stainless steel laser-cut stent rated for use up to 9 mm, and mounted on a noncompliant balloon. Inflation pressures far in excess of those shown in Figure 6 are required to bring balloon and stent to 9 mm (c). Deflation unloads the stent, then loads it in compression to the final equilibrium (points b). (Note that the scale below the axis is much coarser than above.)

characteristics of a typical peripheral balloon-expandable stent. (Note that the sense of the forces for stent and vessel are reversed, just as in Fig. 6, and that the scale below the axis is much coarser than that above.) In this case, the balloon-expandable stent is plastically deformed to 8.0 mm by the balloon pressures. Vessel contact is made in passing point a, after which both vessel and stent are stretched to b. During deflation, the tensile hoop forces in the stent are relieved until a stress equilibrium with the vessel is achieved at point c.

Both balloon-expandable and self-expanding stents recoil to a diameter less than that of the balloon. Scenarios exist in which the balloon-expandable and the self-expanding stent exhibit greater recoil, depending upon geometry, vessel compliance, and oversizing. Similarly, the *equilibrium interference stresses resulting from balloon-expandable and self-expanding stenting are approximately the same*, as is hypotensive risk. The most obvious difference is the enormous difference in balloon pressures used to achieve the final result. While this should cause no damage to a straight vessel, inflation requires stiffer, higher pressure balloons, and this may increase acute damage to vessel, particularly in tortuous anatomy in which high-pressure balloons temporarily straighten the vessel, creating trauma at the balloon ends.

Dynamic Scaffolding and Cyclic Effects

The above analysis shows that there are only minor static and acute differences between the balloon-expandable and self-expanding stents; now we turn our attention to the postimplant dynamics and long-term outcome. Here we see large and important differences. We begin by examining responses to vessel diameter changes. Figure 8 is used to illustrate some important concepts by superimposing the stiffness curves of the balloon-expandable and self-expanding stents of Figures 6 and 7, with both the original nominal vessel as well as an expanded and a contracted native vessel. Such vessel diameter changes can arise from the systolic-diastolic cycle, or from other sources. While somewhat simplistic, this model is a useful way to understand how the intersection points, or equilibrium diameters and stresses, change as the native vessel undergoes change.

On the horizontal axis, one sees that the equilibrium diameter of the self-expanding stented vessel changes far more than that of the balloon-expandable stented vessel; in other words, the balloon-expandable stent is more effective in preventing diameter change. On the other hand, the Nitinol stent dynamically scaffolds or supports the vessel, meaning that if the vessel were to move away from the stent, the stent would follow and continue to apply a

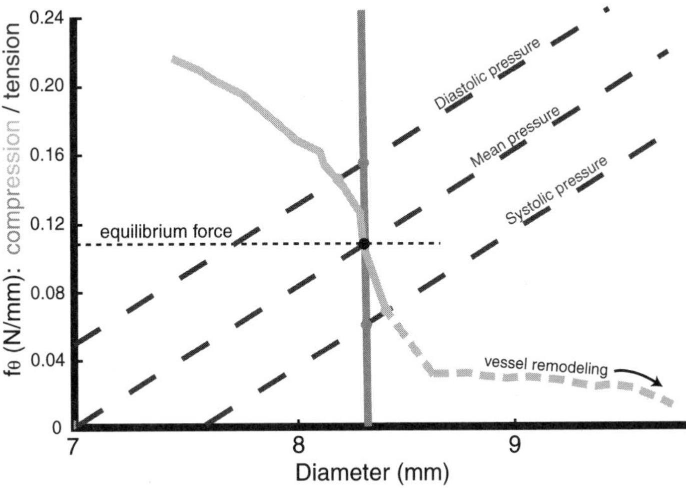

Figure 8. Dynamic effects on the vessel-stent interaction are exemplified by considering the effect of variations in the native vessel diameter on the equilibrium forces and equilibrium stented vessel diameter. The dashed curves represent three native vessel diameters (diastolic, mid cycle, and systolic, for example). The dark gray circles illustrate the stented vessel equilibrium forces and diameters corresponding to a balloon-expandable stent. The light gray circles correspond to a self-expanding stent.

force. Support from the balloon-expandable stent quickly dissipates and the stent could end up in the within the vessel lumen. Dynamic scaffolding may play a particularly important role in drug and radiation therapy where the vessel lumen may actually increase over time. While these differences are marked, it is not clear if the better clinical outcome results from rigid or compliant scaffolding. It is, however, clear that the greater diameter change experienced by the Nitinol device creates a complex and severe fatigue environment (discussed later).

Completing the picture, a look at the changes in equilibrium stress indicates that the balloon-expandable stents experience larger variations in hoop strength and thus contact pressure, which may contribute to pressure necrosis or atrophy of the smooth muscle layer. Thus, while the balloon-expandable stent reduces the compliance of the vessel, it does so be applying high localized pressures. Because of its oversimplistic approach, Figure 8 understates this effect. Again, however, the clinical relevance of this difference is not clear.

Time-Dependent Effects

While the cyclic differences between balloon-expandable and self-expanding stents are significant, the most important differences arise from the time dependency of the vessel-stent equilibrium. The properties of Nitinol itself are not time dependent but those of tissue are. For short times, vessels can be reasonably modeled as elastic tubes, but over longer periods, tissue remodeling occurs in response to the interference stresses. Balloon-expandable interference stresses are applied only over a very short distance, and thus stresses are very quickly dissipated without detectable stent migration. A balloon-expandable stent quickly becomes an inert, stiff prosthesis maintaining a diameter very close to its original diameter. The COF of self-expanding stents, however, acts over a relatively long distance, and thus a self-expanding stent migrates toward the outside of a vessel (see the dashed line in Fig. 8). Angiographic evidence of migration is commonly observed during follow-up (Fig. 9). While no studies of COF versus migration rate have been published, it would seem logical to believe that migration rates are determined by the contact pressure of the stent (the radial force divided by the footprint, or contact area of the stent). While we know of no definitive studies of COF and migration, limited data from animals provide some qualitative insights (D. Wilson et al, unpublished data, 1998). There appear to be times when the stent reaches an equilibrium position at the outside of the vessel wall and other times when the outside diameter of the vessel is barreled out. Further, there appears to be only a weak dependence of stent growth on oversizing, perhaps indicating that a second chronic stress equilibrium is reached once the stent has migrated to the outer layers of the vessel wall. It also appears that the majority of the outward growth occurs during the first 2 weeks of implantation. It is important to note that even this premature evidence is based on 'healthy' animal vessels, and not calcified vessels.

Concerns have been expressed about excessive stent oversizing leading to

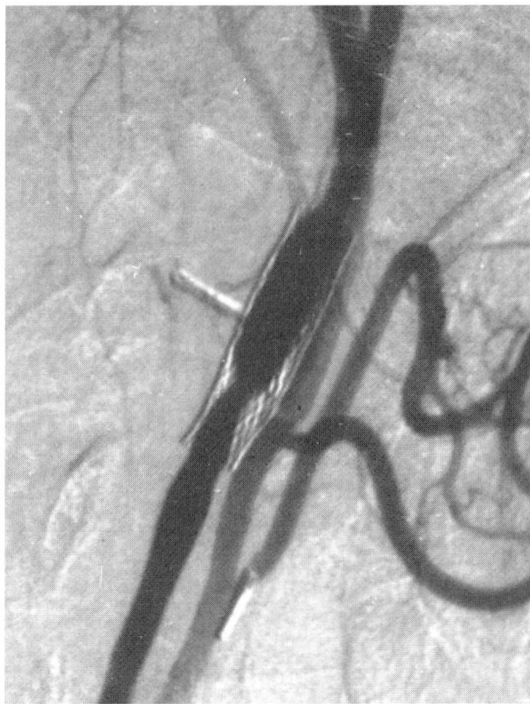

Figure 9. View of a self-expanding stent 4 months after implantation in an internal carotid artery, illustrating that the stent is scaffolding the vessel from the outside of the vessel wall.

vessel perforation, pressure necrosis, or a stress-related complication such as Horner's syndrome. We know of no clinical evidence of this. In fact, animal studies of exaggerated oversizing have demonstrated that the ends of stents can protrude as much as 2 mm outside the adventitia, but remain covered by connective tissue, exhibiting no adverse clinical reaction (Fig. 10). Still, it would seem prudent to limit oversizing and reduce COF. Typically, when a self-expanding stent migrates outward, the lumen does not necessarily follow but instead hyperplasia occurs and the original lumen diameter is maintained.

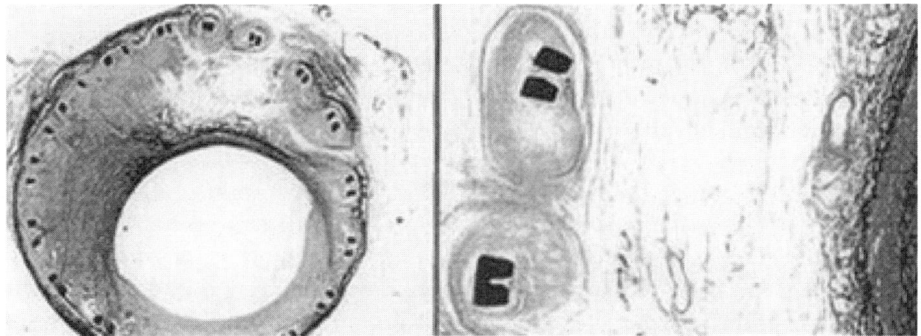

Figure 10. Histology slides 6 months after implantation of a 9-mm self-expanding stent in a 5-mm porcine subclavian artery show that the original lumen is maintained though the stent has migrated well into the vessel wall. The view on the right shows two struts at the end of the stent that have migrated outside the vessel itself.

This contrasts sharply with hyperplasia in balloon-expandable stents, in which hyperplasia represents true lumen loss. Thus, one must be careful in viewing histology slides such as Figure 10: one cannot simply assume that hyperplasia is problematic.

In summary, there are three noteworthy time-dependent differences between balloon-expandable and self-expanding stents:

1. Balloon-expandable stents tend to support from within the lumen, while self-expanding stents support near the outside of the adventitia, imbedded deeply into smooth muscle.
2. Hyperplasia is not indicative of restenosis or lumen loss in a self-expanding stent, as it is in a balloon-expandable stent.
3. Self-expanding stents may exhibit chronic lumen opening, while balloon-expandable stented lumens can only become constricted with time.

Clearly, more research must be done to fully understand the effects of COF and oversizing regimens on stent growth, particularly in diseased vessels. One can envision that perhaps direct stenting will be possible without post dilation, but simply relying on the COF to gently open the vessel over a period. Of course the acute result may not be as aesthetically pleasing as one would obtain with aggressive pre- or post dilation, but certain indications may profit from such gentler treatment. Thus, our earlier assumption that one should minimize COF and maximize RRF is conservatively based on regulatory considerations and the lack of a proper study, and may in fact be incorrect.

Conformability and Wall Apposition

Conformability refers to the ability of a stent to adopt the tortuous path of a vessel rather than forcing the vessel to straighten. Intuitively, one might expect that self-expanding stents conform better to tortuous anatomies. Indeed, many self-expanding stents are very conformable, but there are no technical grounds for this. Conformability depends far more on the design of the stent than on the flexibility of the material from which it is made: segmented, helical, and flexible bridge patterns all tend to provide conformability and can be incorporated equally well into balloon-expandable and self-expanding designs. Of course the far greater balloon pressures experienced during balloon-expandable stenting cause an initial straightening and attendant vessel trauma, but after deflation a well-designed balloon-expandable stent should relax to the vessel morphology.

Wall apposition refers to the ability of a stent to remain in close contact with the wall of the vessel. Separation from the wall can occur if the vessel cross section is eccentric, when the vessel changes diameter along its length, or at a bifurcation. A balloon-expandable stent takes on a rigid cylindrical character during balloon expansion and is quite forceful in dictating a circular vessel cross section—thus, the acute appearance is typically perfect, with good apposition and an excellent lumen. A self-expanding stent, on the other hand, will tend to conform to the native cross section and axial shape and fill the available lumen without forcing acute change—the result is often not as aestheti-

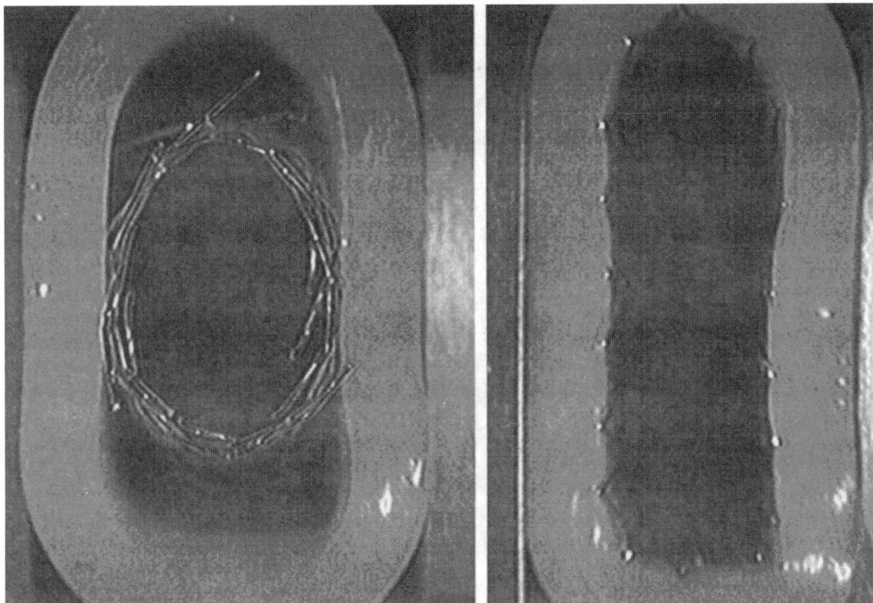

Figure 11. Two commercially available self-expanding stents of the same nominal diameter are deployed into a flattened lumen. The stent on the right exhibits excellent wall apposition while the one on the left does not.

cally pleasing, but less invasive. Moreover, if the vessel morphology changes due to remodeling, flexing, or crushing, a self-expanding stent will move to fill the changing lumen while a balloon-expandable stent will remain static.

While the self-expanding process is generally a gentler and physiologically more correct process, we must be careful not to assume that all self-expanding stents are the same in this regard. Designs with a low pinching stiffness will tend to conform better than very stiff designs (though, as mentioned earlier, buckling can occur if one goes too far). As an extreme example, Figure 11 shows two commercially available self-expanding stents of the same diameter deployed into flattened lumens. Note that the same results are obtained if one deploys the stents into a circular cross section then flattens them; thus, apposition is both a static and dynamic design consideration. The stent on the left has a higher pinching stiffness and a lower radial stiffness than does the stent on the right and, thus, is very insistent in maintaining a circular cross section.

Pulsatile Fatigue

Native vessels undergo diameter changes of approximately 3% to 10% when subjected to 100-mm Hg pulse pressures.[4] A stent placed in these environments is usually expected to remain patent for 10 years, or 40 billion systolic cycles. This is no easy task, and again balloon-expandable and self-expanding stent design philosophies are in juxtaposition.

Stainless steel stents cannot survive such large diameter changes but are sufficiently rigid to prevent the vessel from 'breathing' because of the pulse pressure. Vessels stented with balloon-expandable stents generally pulse less than 0.25% of their diameter, making fatigue essentially a stress-controlled problem. As shown in Figure 8, Nitinol stents are generally similar in compliance to a healthy vessel, and thus undergo much larger pulsatile diameter changes (albeit somewhat reduced from those of the native vessel).* Fortunately, the displacement-controlled fatigue lifetime of Nitinol far exceeds that of ordinary metals, and stents are able to survive this harsh service.

The US Food and Drug Administration currently requires that a statistically relevant number of stents is tested to 400 million cycles at the clinically relevant condition and that no failures are observed. It is rather parochial to think that one can understand and predict life without causing failure. Ideally, one should test to failure and project a safety margin with respect to an endurance limit. This can be done theoretically by using a strain-based Goodman approach, approximating survival by considering a pulsatile strain, $\Delta\epsilon$ (cyclic pulse amplitude due to pulse pressure), and a mean strain,ϵ_m (the strain at mid pulse). Assumptions regarding pulse pressure (Δp) and the stented vessel compliance yield a value for $\Delta\epsilon$, the principal driver for fatigue damage. Mean strains in self-expanding stents can be estimated from assumptions concerning equilibrium diameters, vessel compliance, tortuosity, and oversizing. Such approaches are also used to evaluate the life of balloon-expandable stents, but there are no substantial oversizing strains in balloon-expandable stents; instead, mean strains arise from residual strains from the plastic deformation.

Analyses such as these are complex and beyond the scope of this chapter. Intensive work is under way to better understand the effects of mean strain on fatigue lifetime.[5–8] All studies indicate that the lifetime of Nitinol at high mean strains is far better than one would expect using classic Goodman analysis techniques. This is particularly important in tortuous anatomies, since static bending tends to increase mean strains by have little effect on pulsatile strain. In the end, we cannot say that the pulsatile life of Nitinol stents is better or worse than that of balloon-expandable stents, just that their diametrically opposed approaches may suit individual indications in different ways.

Bending/Crushing Fatigue

Often ignored are a host of other fatigue influences including crushing and bending as one might experience under the inguinal ligament or in the popliteal, as well as tensile and bending fatigue experiences in the coronary vessels as a result of the systolic expansion of the heart. Particularly challenging is the first anatomy that severely flexes and/or buckles a very large number of times and that cannot practically be prevented from doing so by rein-

*Obviously, it is possible to design a self-expanding stent so that it is as stiff as a balloon-expandable stent in which case fatigue can be ignored. It is our assumption here that a high compliance is a desirable feature of a self-expanding stent.

forcement with a stiff balloon-expandable stent. Nitinol performs far better than any other known metal in displacement-controlled environments such as these, but even so, such severe dynamic cycling may exceed even the limitations of existing Nitinol stents. The second type of fatigue condition also warrants some discussion. As the heart expands and contracts, the topology of the surface undergoes large changes exposing vessels to high cycle bending and stretching. First-generation balloon-expandable stents were very rigid, and would locally reinforce to the extent that bending and stretching fatigue was not an issue. The market is demanding more and more flexible stents, however, and even though these later balloon-expandable devices are radially stiff, they are typically very compliant in bending and tension and are thus subject to these fatigue modes. Ultimately this may lead to advantages for the more fatigue-resistant Nitinol.

Thermal Response and A_f Control

The origins of superelasticity were briefly outlined in the introduction of this chapter. While a complete mechanistic description is unnecessary to the task at hand, it is important to note that the transformation from austenite to martensite is driven by temperature as well as by stress. When no stress is applied, we define A_f as the temperature at which martensite is completely transformed to austenite upon heating.* Within a limited range, alloy producers can control the A_f temperatures of Nitinol. The higher the A_f temperature, the lower the stress needed to induce the transformation to martensite. Thus, the difference between body temperature and the A_f temperature dictates the material properties of the material and thus the apparent stiffness of the stent. For each degree that A_f is below body temperature, the tensile loading and unloading stresses of Nitinol increase by approximately 4 N/mm^2. These are very important concepts that can be vividly demonstrated simply by 'feeling' a Nitinol stent at room temperature and body temperature. Figure 12 illustrates the temperature dependence by comparing the unloading-loading-unloading cycle for a 10-mm Nitinol stent at three different temperatures. Note that the *COF is increased by nearly 50% in warming from just 30° to 37°C*!

Choosing and controlling the A_f temperature of a stent is one of the most important tasks facing design engineers. A_f must be below body temperature to assure the stent will fully deploy. The lower A_f is set, the stiffer the stent; but a very low A_f can lead to unacceptably high COF values. Of course a designer can compensate for a low A_f by designing a weaker structure (e.g., reducing strut width). This, however, will severely reduce RRF. In fact, *the most efficient combination of RRF and COF is obtained by using A_f temperatures as close to body temperature as possible* (without running the risk of being above body temperature, of course).

Still another important consideration, illustrated in Figure 13, relates to

*This is a somewhat simplified definition that ignores several complexities that are important but have no bearing on this specific subject.

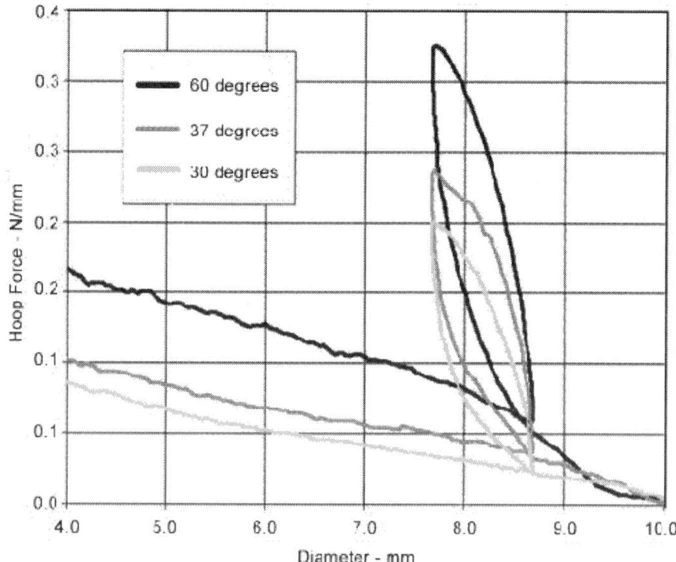

Figure 12. A commercially available 10-mm stent is unloaded in the same cycle as shown in Figure 5, but at three different temperatures. Note that the chronic outward force forces are increased by nearly 50% as the stent is warmed from 30° to 37°C.

elevated temperature exposure during shipping, storage, or sterilization. As ambient temperature is increased, the forces applied by the stent on the delivery system increase. If the temperature becomes too great, either the stent will damage the delivery system or the stent will damage itself and fail to recover fully to its prescribed diameter once released.[9] It is therefore necessary to control both the stent A_f and the temperatures to which it may be exposed after crimping. Some manufacturers have put thermal markers on packaging to assure that the stent system is not exposed to temperatures above tested limits.

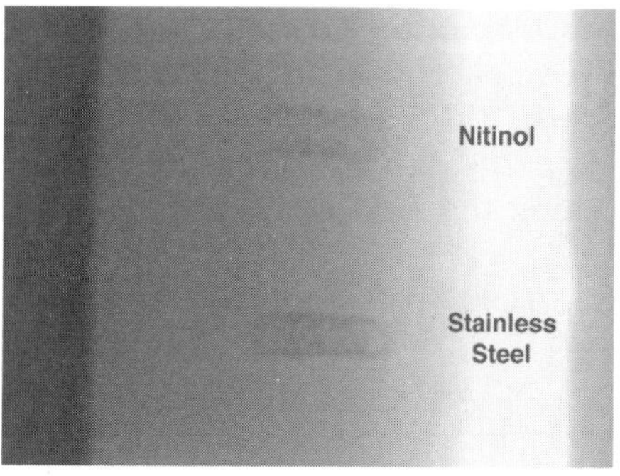

Figure 13. Two geometrically identical stents are viewed radiographically.

Deployment Precision and Foreshortening

Obviously stent performance is critically dependent on getting the stent to the target location and accurately deploying it once there. There are a variety of factors that contribute to accuracy.

- Foreshortening refers to the fact that the opening of the geometry of Figure 1 results in geometric shortening. If there is uncertainty in the direction of the foreshortening, this can lead to large inaccuracies in deployment. In fact, there are a variety of ways to reduce this effect. One can design stents such that strut shortening is compensated by stretching of bridges (see Fig. 1). Other designs exist that use wave designs such that diamonds or struts initially lengthen during expansion, then shorten. Foreshortening can be somewhat more easily eliminated in balloon-expandable stent design, but is clearly a design, not material, issue.
- As the leading end of the stent is begins to emerge from the constraint, there is a natural tendency to spring forward. In the extreme, the stent can jump completely out of the delivery catheter. Several attributes influence this tendency including bridge design, longitudinal stiffness, pinching stiffness, and friction. While it can be managed to a minimum in a self-expanding stent, this potential source of inaccuracy simply does not exist in a balloon-expandable stent.
- Finally, most self-expanding delivery systems consist of an inner and outer member, which are axially stressed during delivery. Since designers strive for flexibility in delivery catheters, these members are generally not rigid and thus they stretch or compress. Experienced deployment and the application of some pre-stress to the delivery system will mitigate these effects, but again this is an issue that is peculiar to self-expanding stents.

In summary, while the accuracy of self-expanding stenting has improved dramatically and will likely continue to improve, it would appear that balloon-expandable stents will continue to be more accurate.

X-Ray and Magnetic Resonance Visibility

The x-ray density of Nitinol is very similar to that of stainless steel (Fig. 13). Differences in perceived opacity are a result of stent design as well as the resolution and energy of the imaging equipment. As stents continue to evolve toward lower mass and finer features, so will imaging equipment need to improve. Some stent manufacturers have resorted to coatings or markers to improve visibility. This is not a straightforward solution: as will be discussed below, dissimilar metal contact can dramatically impact the corrosion resistance of Nitinol. Gold and platinum in particular are ill-advised materials unless insulated from corrosive media.

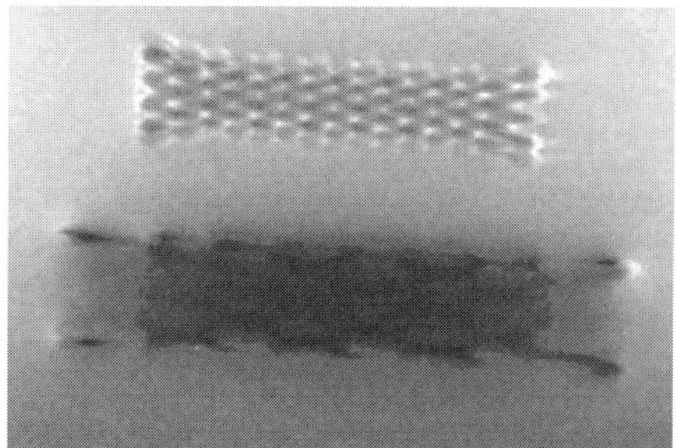

Figure 14. Two different commercially available Nitinol self-expanding stents shown by magnetic resonance imaging, illustrating the importance of surface finish and design on magnetic resonance compatibility.

Magnetic resonance visibility, however, is quite different between stainless steel and Nitinol. Stainless steel interacts strongly with the magnetic resonance field and can create artifacts, making imaging of nearby areas difficult. With appropriate surface treatment, Nitinol exhibits a very low magnetic susceptibility and provides clean detailed images. Interestingly, Nitinol is not universally magnetic resonance compatible because of differences in surface treatment and design (Fig. 14). Certain common surface conditions can be magnetic and can interfere with imaging.

Thrombogenicity and Biocompatibility

These attributes have been discussed in detail in other publications.[10,11] In short, both thrombogenicity and corrosion resistance of Nitinol are superior to that of stainless steel, but it appears unlikely that these differences are of clinical significance—or at least no viable evidence of this sort has been presented. Still, a few questions are often asked and should be summarized:

- There is often concern expressed regarding nickel allergies and the 50% nickel content of Nitinol. Although stainless steel contains less nickel, the nickel is released at a more rapid rate than in Nitinol. The reasons for this relate to the extremely high energy bonds formed between nickel and titanium, and the chemistry of the surface. The surface of properly treated Nitinol is the same, very stable TiO_2 that is formed on pure titanium.[12]
- Dissimilar metal contact has already been mentioned. Theoretically, whenever two dissimilar metals are in contact, there is a galvanic couple causing one of the two metals to corrode at an accelerated rate, the other at a retarded rate. The galvanic potential of stainless steel and Nitinol are very similar, making this effect almost unmeasurable. Tantalum and Elgiloy too are galvanically similar to Nitinol and have been shown to be safe. This does not mean, however, that there is never an issue. Contact with noble metals such as gold or platinum should be avoided unless the coated areas are completely protected from the corrosive media. Stainless steel corrosion performance can also be dramatically deteriorated by contact with gold.

- Concerns have been expressed about scratches. The concern revolves around the fact that both stainless steel and Nitinol resist corrosion through the formation of a passive oxide layer that seals and protects the reactive metal from the corrosive media. When damaged, these passive layers reform and reprotect the base material. The concern is whether the layer can heal itself if no oxygen is present or if the device is immersed in a corrosive environment when damaged. In short, there does not appear to be a significant difference between stainless steel and Nitinol stents. In general, however, any fretting opportunities should be avoided whenever possible, regardless of the stent material; this includes braided wire stents and designs that incorporate interlocking features.
- Finally, various Nitinol stent manufacturers produce different surface finishes, ranging from dark blue oxides to highly polished and bright surfaces. Most recent work indicates that highly polished surfaces with no coloration are preferred.[13]

Martensitic Nitinol

While the vast majority of Nitinol stents are superelastic and self expanding, three other types of Nitinol stents have been proposed: stents that are installed cold then thermally recover their specified shape when exposed to body temperature,[14] stents that recover their desired diameter by heating above body temperature after insertion into the body,[15] and balloon-expandable martensitic stents that can be later heated to cause shrinkage to assist in removal.[16] The last of these is probably the most interesting, but has still not been commercially successful. In addition to removability, these stents offer more uniform expansion, but at a price: martensitic Nitinol is inherently weak and requires large, bulky structures. Moreover, martensitic Nitinol is not superelastic and thus offers none of the typical advantages of Nitinol self-expanding stents.

Conclusions

Self-expanding and balloon-expandable stents differ in many respects, but thematically summarizing, self-expanding stents become part of the anatomy and act in harmony with native vessels while balloon-expandable stents change the geometry and properties of the anatomy. Self-expanding stents assist, balloon-expandable stents dictate. Clearly there is a place for both in radiology suites. Perhaps the most important unknown regarding self-expanding stenting concerns the effect of COF or chronic outward growth of a stent. Physicians are beginning to experiment with eliminating post dilation and relying on COF to slowly remodel the vessel to the desired diameter. While short-term results may not be as good, the lessened trauma may lead to a better long-term outcome.

References

1. Duerig TW, Melton KN, Wayman CM. *Engineering Aspects of Shape Memory Alloys.* Boston: Butterworth-Heinemann; 1990.
2. Lau KW, Sigwart U. Intracoronary Stents. *Indian Heart J* 1991;43:127.
3. Tolomeo DE, Duerig TW. Criteria for fatigue resistant design of superelastic stents. *Proc Shape Memory Superelastic Technol* 2001, in press.
4. Pederson OM, Aslaksen A, Vik-Mo H. Ultrasound measurement of the luminal diameter of the abdominal aorta and iliac arteries in patients without vascular disease. *J Vasc Surg* 1993;17:596–601.
5. Berg B. ICOMAT-99, Barolocia, Argentina. *Mater Sci Eng* 1999;A273-A275.
6. Tolomeo DE, Davidson S, Santinoranont M. Cyclic properties of superelastic Nitinol: Design implications. In Russell SM, Pelton AR (eds): *SMST- 2000: Proceedings of the International Conference on Shape Memory and Superelastic Technologies.* Pacific Grove, CA: International Organization on SMST; 2001:471.
7. Kugler C, Matson D, Perry K. Non-zero mean fatigue test protocol for NiTi. In Russell SM, Pelton AR (eds): *SMST- 2000: Proceedings of the International Conference on Shape Memory and Superelastic Technologies.* Pacific Grove, CA: International Organization on SMST; 2001:409.
8. Harrison W, Lin Z. The study of Nitinol bending fatigue. In Russell SM, Pelton AR (eds): *SMST- 2000: Proceedings of the International Conference on Shape Memory and Superelastic Technologies.* Pacific Grove, CA: International Organization on SMST; 2001:391.
9. Martynov V, Basin F. Effect of constraining temperature on the post-deployment parameters of self-expanding Nitinol Stents. In Russell SM, Pelton AR (eds): *SMST- 2000: Proceedings of the International Conference on Shape Memory and Superelastic Technologies.* Pacific Grove, CA: International Organization on SMST; 2001:649.
10. Venugopalan R, Trepanier C. Corrosion of Nitinol. In Russell SM, Pelton AR (eds): *SMST- 2000: Proceedings of the International Conference on Shape Memory and Superelastic Technologies.* Pacific Grove, CA: International Organization on SMST; 2001:261.
11. Thierry B, et al. Blood compatibility of Nitinol compared to stainless steel. In Russell SM, Pelton AR (eds): *SMST- 2000: Proceedings of the International Conference on Shape Memory and Superelastic Technologies.* Pacific Grove, CA: International Organization on SMST; 2001:285.
12. Chan CM, Trigwell S, Duerig T. Oxidation of an NiTi alloy. *Surf Interface Anal* 1990;15:349.
13. Trepanier C, Tabrizian M, Yahia L'H, et al. Effect of the modification of the oxide layer on NiTi stent corrosion resistance. *J Biomed Material Res* 1998;43:433–440.
14. Balko A, Piasecki GJ, Shah DM, et al. Transfemoral placement of intraluminal polyurethane prosthesis for abdominal aortic aneurysm. *J Surg Res* 1986;40:305.
15. Alfidi RJ, Cross WB, inventor. Vessel implantable appliance and method of implanting it. US patent 3 868 956. 1975.
16. Hess RL, inventor; Advanced Coronary Technology, Inc. assignee. Removable heat-recoverable tissue supporting device. US patent 5 197 978. March 30, 1993.

13

Laparoscopic Techniques in Vascular Surgery

Carlos R. Gracia, MD and Yves-Marie Dion, MD, MSc

Introduction

Minimally invasive surgical techniques have evolved over the past decade with the development of superior optics, video imaging equipment, and design of instrumentation to work remotely. Numerous advances have revolved around gastrointestinal, gynecologic, urologic, and general thoracic procedures. Consequently, laparoscopy has grown predominantly within nonvascular circles, and current minimally invasive surgical instrument technology has centered mostly on gastrointestinal laparoscopy. Advances in minimally invasive surgical technology for cardiovascular disease have centered attention on minimally invasive surgical cardiac surgery and not on peripheral vascular reconstruction, thus limiting vascular surgeons' exposure to laparoscopic technique and technology.

Modern day vascular surgeons have been consumed with primarily pursuing the only other currently available minimally invasive option, endovascular therapies. The current minimally invasive surgical techniques for arterial disease are endoluminal and include angioplasty and stent placement. Experience is also being reported with stent-grafts for not only aneurysmal disease, but also for aortoiliac occlusive disease.[1] These endoluminal modalities have grown due to an investment in the technology to enable their reproducibility and applicability. Confusion exists, however, due to differences in reported early and late results of the various options for the various therapeutic modalities. No one single option for revascularization is ideal or applicable to all cases.

The application of technology for laparoscopic vascular reconstruction has lagged significantly. The fundamentals of vascular surgery (exposure, vascular control, vascular occlusion, anastomosis of vessels and/or grafts, and hemostasis)

From Criado FJ (ed): *Endovascular Intervention: New Tools and Techniques for the 21st Century.* Armonk, NY: Futura Publishing Co., Inc.; ©2002.

are significant technological challenges that are not readily solved without instrumentation dedicated to solving them. However, the field of vascular surgery has begun to unfold a role for new advances. Minimally invasive techniques using scopes and specialized instrumentation have been evolving for saphenous vein harvesting and for subfascial endoscopic perforator vein surgery.[2] Despite these developments, vascular surgeons have been slow to apply minimally invasive surgical techniques to aortoiliac disease, in part due to these items.

For most patients with diffuse aortoiliac occlusive disease, aortobifemoral grafts remain the most durable and functionally effective means of revascularization and should continue to be rightfully regarded as the gold standard or basis of comparison with which other options must be properly compared.[3] Since 1993, applications of laparoscopy to aortic surgery have been reported. Although still early in development, laparoscopy-assisted techniques[4–6] and totally laparoscopic procedures have been reported[7–10] for aortoiliac occlusive lesions. Other recent studies[11–13] have also confirmed that laparoscopic abdominal aortic aneurysm (AAA) repair is a feasible technique. These studies suggest that the benefits of laparoscopy seen in general surgery—decreased use of analgesics, shortened ileus, earlier ambulation, and shortened length of stay—could be translated to aortic surgery for occlusive disease or AAA repair.

This chapter reviews the developmental aspects of laparoscopic techniques in vascular surgery and their current successful application in clinical settings.

Experimental Development

Models for laparoscopic aortic surgery have been described in dogs and piglets.[14–18] A number of animal studies have demonstrated that laparoscopic aortoiliac surgery is feasible for occlusive disease. The earliest experimental work, performed by Dion et al[5] from 1991 to 1992, led to the conclusion that exposure of the aorta by laparoscopy was possible. An original abdominal wall-lifting device (Laborie Surgical Ltd., Longueil, Quebec, Canada) was used because of concerns regarding venous carbon dioxide embolism and the inability to use suction while working on vascular structures under pneumoperitoneum. As early instrumentation was also nonexistent, this model allowed for conventional vascular instrumentation (particularly occlusive clamps and needle drivers) to be used. In this model, these instruments could be inserted through blunt ports without concerns about leakage of pneumoperitoneum.

Experimental work by Dion[19] ensued, demonstrating that the potential concern over venous carbon dioxide embolism was theoretical. Laparoscopic work in this field now also continued under insufflation. Between 1993 and 1994, Dion et al demonstrated the feasibility of a totally laparoscopic technique under pneumoperitoneum to perform aortic surgery. Under pneumoperitoneum, a vascular patch of Dacron was successfully sutured into a 2-cm aortotomy with laparoscopic vascular control using a Satinsky clamp adapted for laparoscopy. This work led to the first application of laparoscopy to aortic surgery in humans, performed by Dion et al[5] in 1993 with a laparoscopically assisted technique for aortobifemoral bypass by a transperitoneal approach.

Effort directed toward a retroperitoneal approach to provide the necessary exposure was first reported by Dion et al[16] in 1995. The anterior retroperitoneal approach of Schumacker[20] was initially used via a right lateral decubitus position. Balloon dissectors aided in retroperitoneal dissection to create a retroperitoneal space, after which visualization of the aorta from the left renal artery and distally was possible. Totally laparoscopic aortoprosthetic anastomoses were performed using abdominal wall suspension (Laparolift, Origin Medsystems, Menlo Park, CA). With this retroperitoneal approach, bowel retraction became less of a problem. In order to complete the aortobifemoral bypass procedure, however, the animals had to be turned to a supine position for exposure of the femoral vessels and tunneling of the prosthetic graft to the groins. To completely translate this model to actual human application would require the undesirable task of turning the patient from a lateral position. Turning the patient would not allow access for proximal control once the patient was repositioned, and could allow for breaks in the sterile technique. Considering the consequences of aortic prosthetic infection and bleeding, it would be important to avoid these risks. This approach would need to be modified in order for the patient to remain in a supine rather than lateral position.

Other investigators were also looking at the challenges of applying laparoscopy to vascular surgery. In 1996, Jones et al[17] reported on evaluation of both transperitoneal and retroperitoneal approaches. Ten aortofemoral procedures were performed with five animals used for each different approach. Unlike in the previous work, the anastomoses were performed via the minilaparotomy, with overall experience demonstrating acceptable clamp times and overall operative times. The laparoscopic technique-related complications in this experience pertained to retraction of small bowel, occurring only in the transperitoneal group. These investigators reported both approaches effective for gasless laparoscopic-assisted exposure of the aorta, but noted that the retroperitoneal approach facilitated bowel retraction by using the intact peritoneal sac.

We[21] described a retroperitoneal anterolateral laparoscopic approach that allowed the patients to remain in a supine position for the entirety of the procedure. Construction of aortobifemoral bypass was consistently performed in less than 4 hours, with blood loss never exceeding 550 cc. The totally laparoscopic aortic anastomosis did not take more than 60 minutes to perform. No operative mortality was encountered in our collective experience, which accounted for 34 consecutive totally laparoscopic aortobifemoral bypasses. The laboratory results demonstrated safe and consistently reproducible completion of totally laparoscopic aortobifemoral bypass; however, the animal models have limitations in translating to humans. The porcine aorta does not contain calcified atheromata, the bulk of an aneurysmal mass, or the commonplace destruction of the posterior wall of the aorta in aneurysmal disease. However, once consistent exposure and anastomosis could be constructed in the laboratory animal model without excessive blood loss, excessive surgery times, or operative mortality, it seemed appropriate to begin to offer patients the option of laparoscopic aortobifemoral bypass.

Clinical Experience

Dion et al[5] completed the first human aortic vascular experience in 1993, as previously noted. A laparoscopically assisted aortobifemoral bypass graft was performed in a 63-year-old male with a history of myocardial infarction. He had developed ischemic rest pain because of aortoiliac occlusive inflow disease. Four additional procedures were performed and reported.[22] The only intraoperative complication was a small bowel perforation resulting from retraction difficulties from the transperitoneal route. Postoperatively, patients felt less pain and were able to cough better and walk more easily. There were no postoperative complications. A second series, with a variety of procedures, was reported in 1995 by Berens and Herde.[4] Their experience included 1 left iliofemoral bypass, 1 aortobifemoral bypass, 1 right iliofemoral bypass, and 1 aortoiliac endarterectomy. The two iliac patients were ambulating early and taking a diet within 24 hours with discharge in 24 hours. The aortic procedure patients were taking a diet at 48 hours postoperatively and discharged on the third postoperative day. There were no complications. A transperitoneal route was used on both these patients, whereas Dion used gas insufflation for the working space and Berens and Herde used an abdominal wall-lift device (Guidant). Both experiences also note the difficulties of retraction of intra-abdominal organs rendering aortic dissection and end-to-side aortoprosthetic anastomosis tedious.

A third experience was reported by Fabiani et al[6] in 1997. A combination of procedures and access were used. Aortobifemoral bypass was completed in 3 patients by a transperitoneal approach, while unilateral aortofemoral bypass was performed by a retroperitoneal approach in 4 patients. Two other patients had been attempted but converted to open laparotomy due to inadequate aortic exposure in one and extensive aortic calcification in the other. The procedures were completed under what was termed video-assistance. Dissection, vascular control, tunneling, and placement of graft were all accomplished under laparoscopic view. A small 3-cm median minilaparotomy allowed for insertion of a Satinsky clamp, at which time the aortotomy and anastomoses were performed through this route with video guidance of the laparoscope. Patient experience was again favorable. Short postoperative ileus was noted with enteral diets started 48 hours postoperatively. Lengths of stay in the hospital ranged from 4 to 7 days. This was again a transperitoneal laparoscopically assisted approach.

These pioneering experiences identified important issues. Experience was obtained with both a gasless and a traditional gas-insufflation technique. Frustrations were present with both of the earliest techniques. Were these difficulties the result of problems intrinsic to either of these techniques or to the transperitoneal route common in these experiences? Is there a solution in a retroperitoneal approach were the peritoneal sac would function as an organ "container" to provide improved exposure to the major vessels? What about the future of working laparoscopically assisted as in the previous series? The early human clinical experience of Dion et al,[5,22] confirmed the difficulties associated with both a transperitoneal route with respect to bowel retraction and working laparoscopically assisted. Laparoscopically assisted surgery is fraught with potential problems. The variability of the thickness of the abdominal wall in patients of different sizes is problematic. With increased abdominal wall thickness, the incisions must increase in size in order to maintain exposure. It is difficult to make small incisions in patients with thick or obese abdominal walls. At some point, any advantages sought by minimizing trauma from the access are lost. Therefore, a completely laparoscopic approach may ultimately be more reproducible and may overcome limitations imposed by small incisions. This would require resolution of further technical challenges, as well as development of appropriate instrumentation for these tasks.

In contrast to the previous reports, which were on laparoscopically assisted procedures, the two first totally laparoscopic aortobifemoral bypasses were offered to humans by Dion and Gracia and colleagues in 1995.[23,24] One case was completed with a gasless technique using an abdominal wall-lift device (Laparolift). This proved long and difficult. An improvement was made in the second case by the use of insufflation. There was an obvious benefit to the exposure by insufflation with its three-dimensional compressing effect; however, other problems surfaced in maintaining the exposure in the retroperitoneum with insufflation. Whether the peritoneal lining was violated or not, competitive insufflation with the peritoneal cavity would work against attempts to maintain exposure as the case continued, with reduction in the size of the retroperitoneal cavity. In addition, the limited size of the contained retroperitoneal space required a very little volume of carbon dioxide to maintain. As a result, it was highly sensitive to suction. With a modest amount of suction and loss of only a small amount of carbon dioxide, the space would collapse. The difficulty and lengthiness of these procedures was in part due to the difficulty in maintaining exposure. The lack of purpose-built laparoscopic vascular instrumentation was also a contributing factor to the difficulties.

A modification to the totally retroperitoneal approach was deemed appropriate to help overcome these limitations. The "apron" technique was developed in the laboratory and applied clinically.[8] This improved working space by removing the problem of competitive insufflation of the peritoneal cavity as a result of time or damage to the peritoneum. In addition, the peritoneal cavity was now completely used as the insufflation space. The much larger volume of carbon dioxide gas insufflated using both cavities as if they were one increased the workspace. As a result, suction no longer collapsed the exposure. It provided superior containment of abdominal contents and removed the troublesome need to constantly retract the intestines.

Technique

Patients are placed in a supine position. General anesthesia is then induced, with hemodynamic monitoring as necessary. A padded gel roll is placed under the patient's left flank to elevate it and provide for adequate access to the lateral abdominal wall (Fig. 1). The right arm is preferentially tucked at the side and the left arm placed out at 90°. The patient is then prepped and draped in the standard fashion to expose the entire abdomen and groin. Carbon dioxide pneumoperitoneum is instituted via an umbilical site to an in-

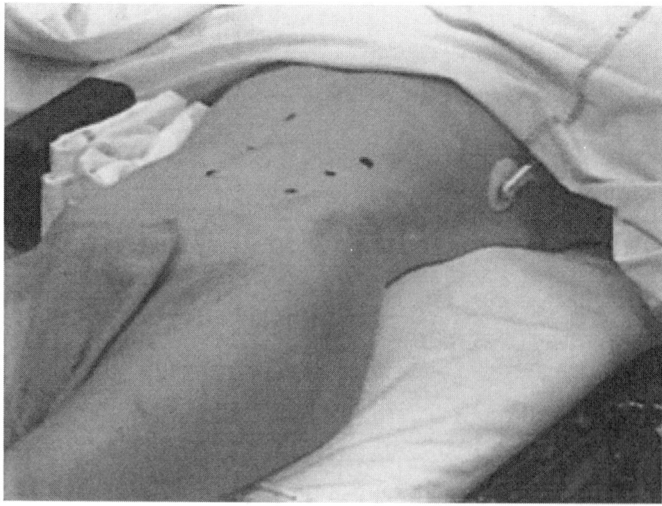

Figure 1. Patient in supine position on the operating room table allowing simultaneous access of the abdomen and groins. A gel roll is placed under the patient's left flank to elevate it and provide for adequate access to the lateral abdominal wall. The positions of the 6 primary trocar sites are marked on the abdominal wall in their typical positions.

traperitoneal pressure of 14 mm Hg. A 10-mm trocar (trocar #1, Fig. 2) is then introduced at this site. A 0° or a 30° laparoscope can be used to inspect the peritoneal cavity. The two additional midline trocars are then inserted under direct vision. One is placed halfway from the umbilicus to the xiphoid process (trocar #2) and the other is placed halfway from the umbilicus to the symphysis pubis

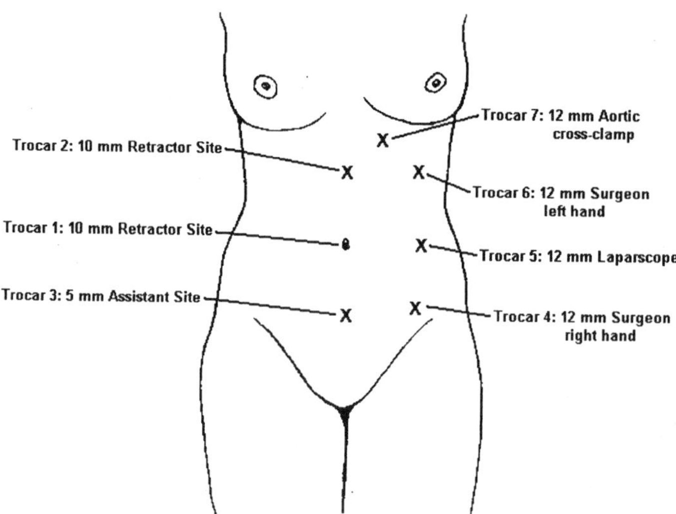

Figure 2. Illustration of trocar sites with the order in which they are inserted and a description of their use.

(trocar #3). The pressure on the insufflator is then decreased to ~7 mm Hg to facilitate the retroperitoneal dissection.

The retroperitoneal dissection is then begun through the site of the intended trocar position #4 (Fig. 2), located 1.5 cm both medial and superior to the anterior-superior iliac crest. A muscle-splitting 1.5-cm opening is made through the various layers of the lateral abdominal wall to identify the preperitoneal space. Gentle blunt dissection is then performed with the index finger to open a small retroperitoneal space directed at the psoas muscle. The left iliac artery is commonly palpated and is a useful landmark. It is useful at this time to monitor this dissection with the intraperitoneal view from the umbilicus to be certain that the peritoneum is not violated. This initial finger dissection of the retroperitoneal space need only be large enough to bluntly insert a 12-mm trocar (trocar #4, Fig. 2). The retroperitoneal space can now be insufflated using a pressure of 14 mm Hg. A 0° laparoscope is used to gently dissect the now crepitant retroperitoneal areolar tissue. As this dissection proceeds, the best landmark is to find the left external iliac artery and follow it up to the common iliac artery and ureter. Effort is now made to dissect on top of the ureter to leave it on the psoas muscle and to not injure it. As this continues medially, the aorta is commonly seen pulsating surrounded by its retroperitoneal connective layers. Dissection is finally carried cephalad and laterally under the lateral aspect of Gerota's fascia to mobilize the kidney. With use of the pneumoretroperitoneum and gentle blunt scope dissection, a very large hemostatic retroperitoneal space can be rapidly created.

The creation of the "apron" now begins approximately 3 cm above the left internal inguinal ring. The midline ports (numbered 1 to 3, Fig. 2) are used in order to place the laparoscope with a grasping forceps and laparoscopic scissors. The appropriate line of incision of the peritoneum is just to the left of the lateral edge of the rectus abdominus muscle. It is important to mobilize the peritoneum not only completely laterally but also cephalad to approximately 6 cm above the left costal margin. This will create the necessary space in order to place trocar #7, in its superiorly located transrectus position, as the best location for application of the aortic cross-clamp. Dissection in the correct plane between the peritoneum and the posterior fascia will proceed quickly and hemostatically. One must be cautious to be in the correct extraperitoneal plane. If the dissection begins by incision through the peritoneum and behind the fascia, the dissection becomes bloody and will stop laterally. Following the successful incision of the peritoneum, the peritoneum is mobilized laterally to connect the intraperitoneal cavity with the previous retroperitoneal dissection. This thereby creates the "apron" that will be used as the internal retractor of the intestines. Once the peritoneum is completely mobilized, connecting the peritoneal cavity and the retroperitoneal dissection, the remaining trocars, numbered 5 and 6 in Figure 2, are inserted along a parallel line from trocar #4.

The peritoneal "apron" must now be suspended in order to function as a retractor. This is a critical part of the technique in order to use the "apron" effectively and hide the abdominal contents from view. It is suspended at its incised upper edge at three sites corresponding to the three midline trocars. This is done by using the lateral trocars for placement of the laparoscope and with the use of needle drivers. A suture of 0-nylon on a straight needle is placed through the abdominal wall behind each of the midline trocars. This needle is grasped and sutured through the upper cut edge of the peritoneum before being passed back through the abdominal wall. This creates a suspension suture that will suspend the peritoneal "apron" behind each midline trocar (Fig. 3). This in effect compartmentalizes the peritoneal cavity, with several advantages. It eliminates the threat of competitive insufflation as the spaces are connected. It also creates a larger working space with a larger volume of insufflated carbon dioxide. Therefore, suctioning can be performed more aggressively before one sees a compromise in the working space. Most importantly, it removes any further concern regarding retraction of the intestines, as they are securely held back gently in their own natural environment without any manipulation. With the "apron" now created, the midline trocars are always directed into the retroperitoneal space.

Two fan retractors are inserted through trocars #1 and #2 behind the apron and opened. The superior retractor (trocar #2) is used to retract more cephalad, bringing the kidney cephalad and toward the midline. The retractor in trocar #1 is used to provide medial retraction, keeping the weight of the abdominal contents off the aorta. These retractors can be held in place for the du-

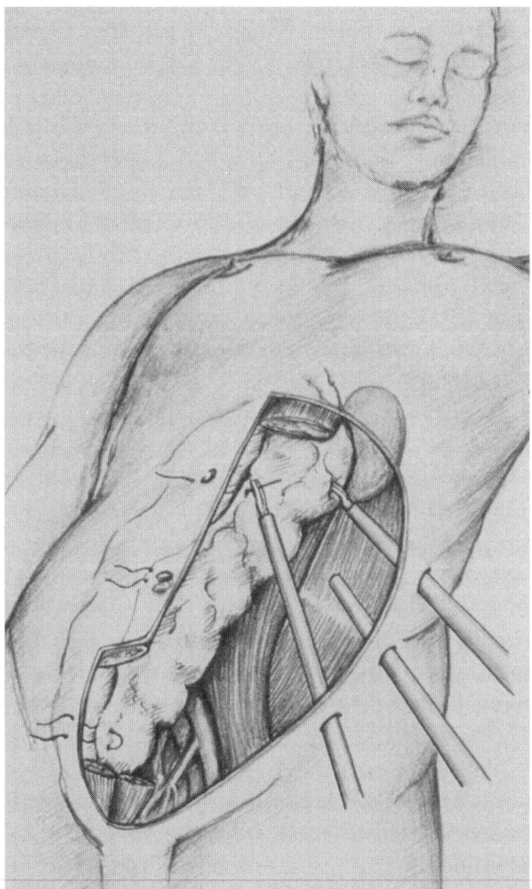

Figure 3. A critical step in the technique in order to use the "apron" effectively and hide the abdominal contents from view. A suture of 0-nylon on a straight needle is placed through and through the abdominal wall behind each of the midline trocars. This needle will be grasped and sutured through the upper cut edge of the peritoneum before being passed back through the abdominal wall. This creates a suspension suture that will suspend the peritoneal "apron" behind each midline trocar.

ration of the case by an external fixation device secured to the rails of the operating table (Omni-Tract, Minnesota Scientific, Minneapolis, MN). Tilting the table right side down and using from 10° to 20° Trendelenburg position is also important to facilitate this retraction process.

The surgeon works from the patient's left via the ports #4 to #6. The assistant works from the inferior midline trocar #3, which provides ready access for suction, adding additional retraction, or assisting in completion of the anastomosis. Dissection now begins by identifying the left common iliac artery and ureter. Dissection follows medially and cephalad to identify the aortic bifurcation and the right common iliac artery. Dissection is continued along the course of the right iliac artery for the intra-abdominal portion of a retroperitoneal tunnel to the right groin. Dissection continues up the aorta to the inferior mesenteric artery. It is divided or left intact based on the patient's arteriogram. If it is occluded, its division will facilitate further exposure. If it is patent or if there is a question regarding dividing it, leaving it intact will not compromise the exposure. Continued cephalad dissection will expose the remaining infrarenal aorta and the left renal vein. Care must be taken to not injure the left gonadal vein, from more aggressive retraction, as it joins the left renal vein.

The proximal site of aortic cross-clamping is carefully dissected. The site for anastomosis is carefully inspected now and palpated to evaluate for calcification. It has proven useful to obtain preoperative computed tomography scans to evaluate for aortic calcifications or venous anomaly. Vigilance for retroaortic renal veins and other venous anomalies is as important here as it is in the standard open exposure (Fig. 4). The infrarenal aorta is now further dissected in a caudal direction, freeing it up posteriorly and carefully inspecting for lumbar arteries. This left anterolateral approach provides excellent visualization of the posterior aorta allowing the lumbar arteries to be clipped and/or divided

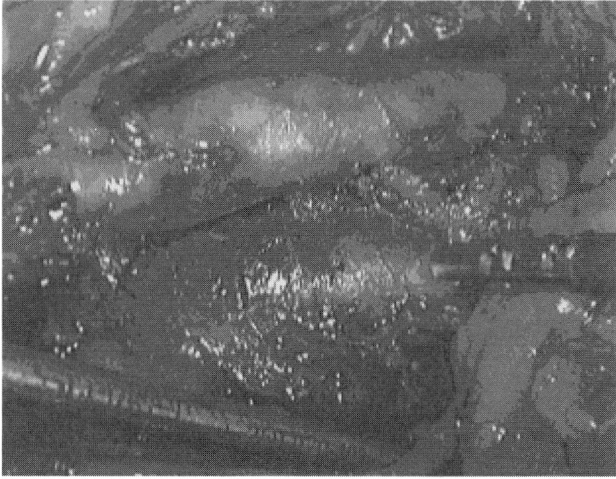

Figure 4. Vigilance for retroaortic renal veins and other venous anomalies is as important here as it is in the standard open exposure. In this case, a duplicate inferior vena cava is seen on the left of the infrarenal aorta. This was known on preoperative computed tomography scan. Failure to identify this sort of anomaly could be catastrophic.

as necessary to mobilize the aorta for the site of anastomosis (Fig. 5). Generally, not more than one or two pairs require clipping and/or division. The preoperative arteriogram is also useful for predicting the location and number of lumbar arteries with which to contend. Also, during this posterior dissection, once must take care to identify lumbar veins, which may be torn or injured if unrecognized. These maneuvers are particularly important for an end-to-end anastomosis. Posterior control of the lumbar arteries is not necessary for end-to-side anastomosis. In the case of an end-to-side anastomosis, only satisfactory mobilization of the right side of the aorta is necessary in order to place a Satinsky clamp on the aorta. Once the posterior aorta is free, it is necessary to dissect the periaortic areolar tissue on the right of the aorta to separate the inferior vena cava. It is important to be certain that the vena cava is free from the lateral wall of the aorta so that it is not injured when the aorta is transected and that it does not interfere during the anastomosis. Satisfactory mobilization of the right side of the aorta is necessary for both end-to-end anastomosis and end-to-side anastomosis. Trocar #7 position is ideally located for an anterior-to-posterior approach to the aorta. The dissecting scissors can be placed through this trocar with visualization via the angled 30° laparoscope to see over the right side of the aorta.

At this point, attention is directed toward the groins. Groin incisions are made bilaterally to perform the appropriate dissection of the femoral vessels. Upon completion of the groin dissection, the aorta is sized and the appropriately sized conventional bifurcated vascular graft (Hemashield, Meadox/ Boston Scientific, Natick, MA) is selected. It can be readily introduced into the abdomen through any of the lateral trocars. In contrast to tunneling in open cases, the surgeon should resist the temptation to make large blunt dissection maneuvers under the inguinal ligament to tunnel into the retroperitoneum.

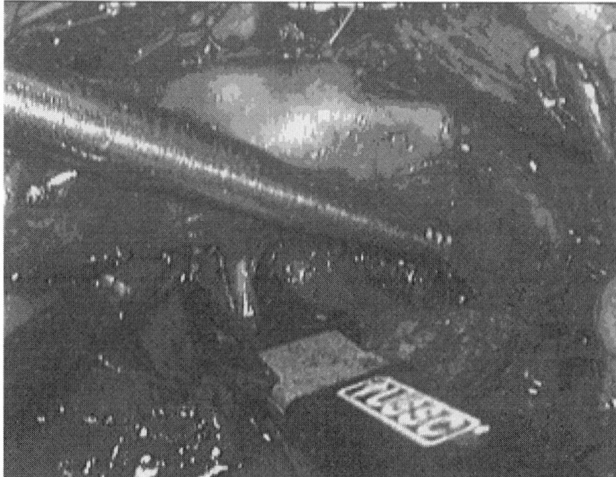

Figure 5. The left anterolateral approach provides excellent visualization of the posterior aorta. Lumbar arteries can be clipped and/or divided as necessary to mobilize the aorta for the site of anastomosis. Generally, not more than one or two pairs require clipping and or division.

These maneuvers may result in bleeding or leakage of the pneumoperitoneum through an excessively patulous tunnel. The tunneling is begun with gentle upward retraction on the inguinal ligament to be certain that no vessels on top of the common femoral artery are injured. A malleable grasper with a blunt tip (Karl Storz Endoscopy of America, Culver City, CA) is designed to tunnel easily and atraumatically. This process is observed from the abdomen with the laparoscope. The right limb of the graft is tunneled first. Laparoscopically, the limbs of the graft are carefully oriented and observed to avoid any rotation while they are delivered into the groins. The limbs are clamped after they are tunneled, to prevent leakage of the pneumoperitoneum. The graft is completely positioned as described before aortic occlusion in order to limit cross-clamp time. The final trocar #7, which is for the aortic cross-clamp, is inserted in its transrectus position (Figs. 2 and 6). This provides for optimal position toward the selected infrarenal clamp site on the aorta. The patient is then systemically heparinized. The aorta is cross-clamped with a laparoscopic DeBakey clamp (Karl Storz Endoscopy of America) inserted through trocar #7. The previously mobilized aorta above the inferior mesenteric artery is transected with a laparoscopic GIA 30 (Tyco-U.S. Surgical, Norwalk, CT) (Fig. 7).

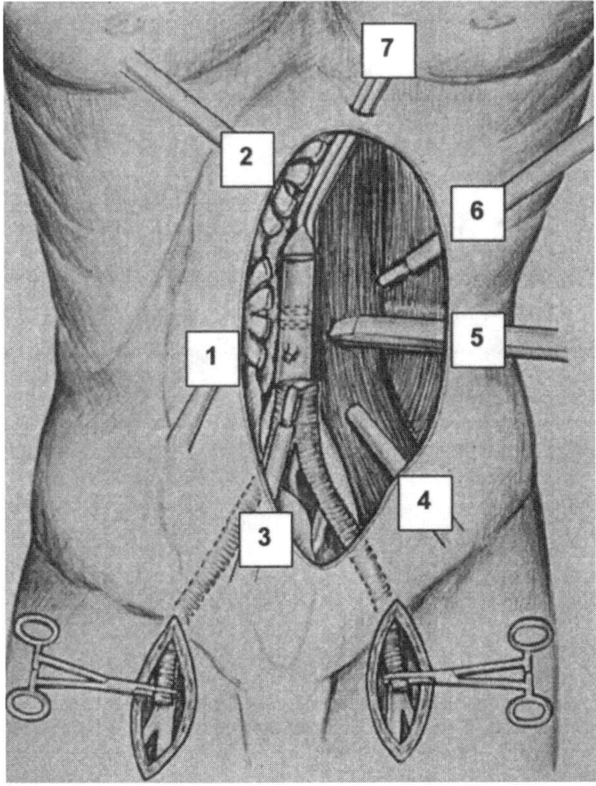

Figure 6. Illustration with everything in place. Retraction is provided by fans behind the "apron" in trocars 1 and 2. The assistant is using port 3. The surgeon is using ports 4, 5, and 6. Through these, the graft is inserted before tunneling into the groins. Here, the graft is tunneled into place. The GIA-30 (Tyco-U.S. Surgical, Norwalk, CT) has been inserted through the laparoscope port 5, after moving the laparoscope to port 4. The advantage of having all lateral 12-mm trocars is that endomechanicals or sutures can be readily inserted via any of these ports depending on what is required. The cross-clamp is seen advancing through port 7, which is transrectus and as close to the midline as possible providing an excellent angle for application in an anteroposterior direction. The DeBakey-style clamp can be advanced directly into the spine, which is readily palpated as in open surgery to ensure clamping completely across the aorta.

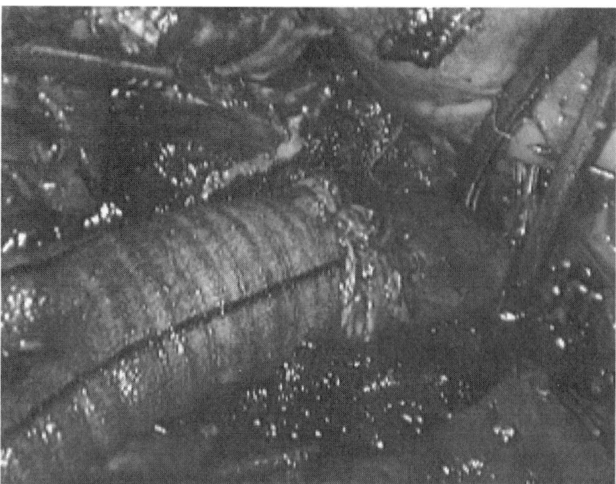

Figure 7. Intraoperative photograph of completed end-to-end anastomosis of a bifurcated Hemashield graft to the infrarenal aorta. The aortic cross-clamp has just been opened following conventional flushing techniques.

In the case of an end-to-end anastomosis, the aorta is now transected at a suitable location between the staple line and the cross-clamp. The transected aorta is evaluated for plaque and thrombus directly. Appropriate instrumentation in the form of DeBakey style grasping forceps and endarterectomy instruments (Karl Storz Endoscopy of America) enable endarterectomy of the aortic cuff as necessary. Previous conversions to minilaparotomy in our earliest experiences were exclusively for difficulties in dealing with aortic plaque and calcifications while constructing the anastomosis. Since appropriate instrumentation is now available, we approach the proximal cuff as we do in open surgery, in order to prepare it for the best possible anastomosis. In the case of an end-to-side anastomosis, a Satinsky clamp is inserted through the lower abdomen to the right of the midline and apron suspension line. A 10-mm trocar puncture is made, allowing the laparoscopic Satinsky clamp to be inserted securely without leakage of pneumoperitoneum.

Anastomosis is now completed with two running 3-0 Prolene (Ethicon, Inc., a Johnson & Johnson Company, Somerville, NJ) sutures. This is done with intracorporeal laparoscopic suturing technique. In the end-to-end anastomosis (Fig. 6), the first suture is started posteriorly at the 7 o'clock position and run up the right side of the anastomosis. Once the anastomosis is half completed, the second suture is placed adjacent to the previous posterior suture. It is now run across the back wall and around the left side of the anastomosis and across the anterior portion. The two sutures are tied anteriorly. In the case of an end-to-side anastomosis (Fig. 8) two similar 3-0 Prolene sutures are used. The first is started at the heel of the aortotomy and runs along the right side of the anastomosis and around the toe. The second suture begins at the heel near the first one and runs toward the toe to complete the anastomosis when the two are tied together. Conventional flushing techniques are used both after the aortic anastomosis is complete and upon completion of the distal anastomoses to the femoral arteries.

Once satisfactory hemostasis is identified throughout, the peritoneal "apron" sutures are removed and the peritoneum is allowed to fall back into place. As the pneumoperitoneum is released, the peritoneum comes to lie back in its normal position and completely covers the prosthetic graft material. Trocar sites are closed either with one layer of 0-Vicryl or with through-and-through strands of 0-Vicryl (Ethicon, Inc., a Johnson & Johnson Company) placed with an EndoClose (Tyco-U.S. Surgical) device. The groin incisions are closed in a conventional manner.

Results

From March 1996 to April 1999, 25 patients (18 men and 7 women) aged between 42 and 76 years (mean 58) received a laparoscopic aortobifemoral bypass according to the previously described transabdominal retroperitoneal technique. The indication for surgery in all 25 patients was incapacitating claudication (ankle-brachial index <0.60) with aortoiliac occlusive disease. Patients were considered to not be ideal candidates for percutaneous interventions for their aortoiliac occlusive disease. Two patients (1 male, 1 female) had had previous failed angioplasty and stent placement in the iliac vasculature. Laparoscopic aortobifemoral bypass was completed in all patients. This "apron" suspension was used in each case. One modification in technique was made in this experience. Starting with patient 6, the ureter was not mobilized but left intact along its place on the psoas muscle.

In the first 21 cases, surgery time decreased from more than 8 hours (510 minutes) to 3 hours and 23 minutes (mean 326 minutes) (Fig. 9). Eighteen

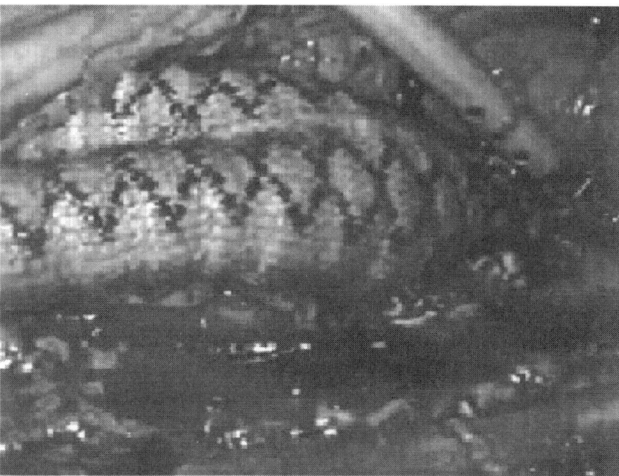

Figure 8. Completed view of an end-to-side anastomosis. In this case, only satisfactory mobilization of the right side of the aorta is necessary in order to place a Satinsky clamp on the aorta. Extensive posterior control of the lumbars is not necessary for end-to-side anastomosis.

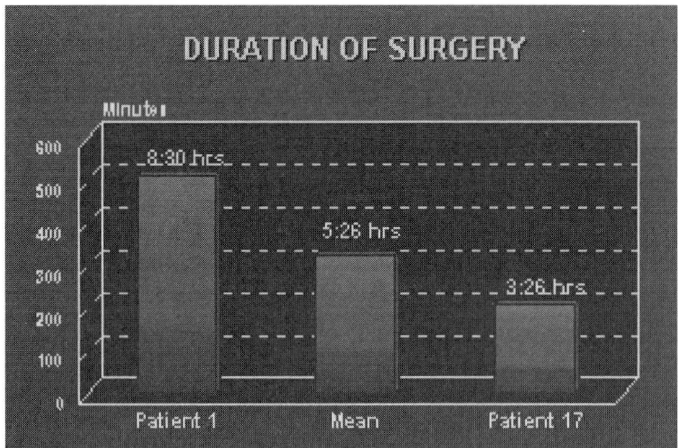

Figure 9. Demonstration of the dramatic improvement in operating times for totally laparoscopic aortic bypass. This shows not only the effect of flattening the learning curve but also of the effect of introducing technology in the form of vascular-specific instrumentation designed for laparoscopy.

anastomoses were performed end-to-end and the remaining three were completed end-to-side. All anastomosis were completed with intracorporeal laparoscopic suturing using continuous running monofilament suture. Mean aortic cross-clamping time was 100 minutes (range 56 to 189 minutes) and mean time to perform the proximal aortic anastomosis was 55 minutes (range 22 to 155 minutes). Average fluid administration was 6080 mL (range 4000 to 8500 mL). Mean blood loss was 820 mL (range 300 to 3050 mL) with four patients receiving homologous transfusions. A retroaortic left renal vein was injured, accounting for the 3050 mL blood loss in the one patient.

Intraoperative complications occurred in three patients requiring conversion. At no time was conversion ever necessary for a life-threatening circumstance. Conversions were all made to minilaparotomy in these three cases by making an incision between trocars #1 and #2. Small renal vein retractors could be inserted behind the retroperitoneal "apron" to readily expose the infrarenal anastomotic area without interference or difficulties in bowel retraction. In 2 of these 3 patients, conversion occurred for anastomotic difficulties related to heavily calcified atheromata at the proximal aorta. The first female developed a disruption of a calcified plaque by the aortic clamp that led to graft occlusion immediately after unclamping. The aortic cuff of the other patient with difficulties from atherosclerotic plaque had been endarterectomized laparoscopically. As this was the first patient to undergo complete endarterectomy of the aortic cuff, conversion to minilaparotomy was deemed prudent. Upon inspection, a satisfactory technical result was confirmed and no revision of the anastomosis necessary. Although the use of the "apron" allowed for excellent exposure in this case as well, cross-clamp time was 189 minutes (the longest of all patients). Conversions in these cases certainly affect the overall times of surgery and cross-clamping. However, this resulted in difficulty only in the previous conversion, with a cross-clamp time of 189 minutes. The patient developed a mild compartment syndrome of the right leg, which did not require intervention. The final patient undergoing conversion did so for two unidentified tears in the graft proximally that were likely caused at the time of graft insertion or manipulation. These were not recognized until after the anastomosis was completed. It was elected to replace the graft. The limbs of the new graft were tied to the cut limbs of the old graft, allowing them to be pulled into correct position via a limited 4- to 5-cm incision. This resulted in a cross-clamp time of 179 minutes.

The most serious postoperative complication occurred in one patient who required reoperation for an acute false aneurysm that eroded into the left ureter. Upon reoperation, this was believed to be related to difficulties in constructing the proximal anastomosis because of aortic calcifications. This experience, combined with our previous three conversions for plaque-related difficulties, strengthened our resolve to deal with the aortic cuff laparoscopically as one does in traditional open surgery. Because of growing experience in handling the proximal aortic disease and the availability of purpose-built instrumentation to handle the vessel wall and atheromata, overall times have consistently improved and should continue to approximate that of open surgery.

There was one mortality in a 71-year-old male who had undergone uneventful completion of his laparoscopic aortobifemoral bypass with an operative time of 4 hours. Despite preoperative cardiac evaluation and clearance, the patient developed ventricular irritability, had a sudden collapse on postoperative day 6, and failed to resuscitate. It was believed that this was likely due to a sudden ventricular arrhythmia, from either myocardial ischemia or pulmonary embolus. Bleeding difficulties occurred in only two cases. The patient with injury to the graft requiring replacement also had a retroaortic left renal vein, which was not recognized on preoperative computed tomography scan. Blood loss in this case (3050 mL) was the highest in this group of patients. The patient did develop postoperative thrombosis of the left renal vein and an edematous left kidney, which had recovered upon follow-up duplex ultrasonography 6 weeks later. A second patient had lost ~2000 mL due to postoperative bleeding from a trocar injury to the superior epigastric artery.

Mean postoperative hospital stay in this group was 7 days (range 4 to 23 days). Review of the postoperative hospital stay in this experience is not, in our opinion, representative of the laparoscopic approach. Two patients with uneventful procedures and hospital courses were in the hospital 9 and 12 days for social reasons. Three patients stayed longer because of geographical issues: they lived more than 300 miles from the hospital. This included the patient with left renal edema (23-day stay), whose status was evaluated while he was an inpatient, also because of the distance of his home from the hospital. The oldest patient was discharged on the seventh day while a younger patient with a mitral valve prosthesis was not discharged until the eighth day because of the need to regulate her anticoagulant therapy for her cardiac prosthesis. Other patients were discharged between 3 and 6 days.

Clinically, patients with successfully completed laparoscopic aortobifemoral bypasses appeared to experience less pain than their counterparts operated through a standard laparotomy. The visual analog pain scale was used. There was very little pain noted by the third postoperative day. It was not uncommon to have patients complain more about their groin incisions than their abdominal trocar sites. It was astonishing to see the vast majority of patients ambulatory with little or no assistance by the second postoperative day. In essence, these patients had the typical postoperative appearance similar to patients undergoing other laparoscopic abdominal operations such as gastric fundoplication or colectomy.

Discussion

Aortofemoral bypasses, iliofemoral bypasses, and aortoiliac endarterectomies have been performed clinically. Two concepts are being investigated. The first considers that laparoscopic vascular procedures are best performed assisted with a minilaparotomy through which the anastomosis can be safely done under direct vision using conventional instrumentation.[4–6] The other concept is to avoid the minilaparotomy, assuming that as more of the abdominal wall is left intact, the patient's recovery will be smoother and faster.[7,8,25] The fate reserved for the minilaparotomy could well resemble what happened in surgery for the gallbladder. Making a short incision to perform major surgery does not necessarily render the procedure easier or safer. Presently, however, performance of a totally laparoscopic aortic bypass procedure is still very challenging.

Frequent criticism of these early results commonly revolves around the operative times. There is much to consider when evaluating these results. Surgery times are difficult to compare overall, due to many variables and lack of documentation in the literature. The early lengthy surgical times should be evaluated in light of learning curve issues and lack of technology. The effects of a flattening learning curve and increased abilities with technology can be seen in the problems revolving around handling of proximal aortic calcifications. Patient 21 presented with a much more heavily calcified aorta than patient 7. They both required endarterectomy for this problem. Patient 7 had an extended operating time and a cross-clamp time of 189 minutes, the longest of all patients. In contrast, with patient 21, experience and purpose-built instrumentation for dealing with the aorta and its plaque resulted in significantly reduced operative and cross-clamp times. Endarterectomy of the aortic stump was performed without difficulty before proceeding on to the end-to-end anastomosis. Patient disease and morphology affect overall operative times as well, for both the experienced and the learning surgeon. In peripheral vascular reconstructions, one must also take into account other difficulties in dealing with these patients intraoperatively. The status of their distal circulation must also be taken into account. For example, in patient 12, a left in situ below-knee bypass and right profundaplasty were necessary because of the poor condition of his peripheral run-off circulation. Patient 13 required completion of a lengthy profundaplasty on the right and a common femoral endarterectomy and profundaplasty on the left for the same reasons.

Many of the early applications of laparoscopy to gastrointestinal procedures commonly took several hours. With flat learning curves and appropriate instrumentation, many laparoscopic operations are now within the normal open operative times of many laparoscopic surgeons. For the application of laparoscopy to be successful in the reproduction of aortobifemoral or iliofemoral bypass grafting, further improvement and evolution of what has been learned would be necessary. Attention must be applied to the technology and instrumentation to not only improve operating times, but also contribute to the reproducibility of the procedure. Needs for specific vascular instrumentation have been recognized and addressed. Technology and experience improves the reproducibility and ability to do laborious tasks in shorter times. As a consequence, one can expect these procedures to become less demanding for the surgeon.

Another component of these procedures to evaluate is the issue of a gasless approach versus the use of insufflation. The initial argument for a gasless approach was the fact that one could use conventional instrumentation for retraction and anastomosis.[4] It would also impart the ability to suction with impunity, as there would be no decrease in insufflation pressure and resultant collapse of the working space, as there is with pneumoperitoneum. This becomes intimately related with a minilaparotomy approach and its ability to allow the insertion of conventional instrumentation; however, variation in body size and morphology of patients could make working under a gasless environment more difficult. There is no clear benefit of a gasless environment over a traditional insufflation approach despite the ability to suction with impunity and to insert a variety of traditional instrumentation. In abdominal laparoscopy at large, insufflation techniques dominate. Although gasless technique would represent an alternative to pneumoperitoneum when surgery is performed in localized regions of the abdomen such as the pelvis or upper abdomen, its application to the peritoneal cavity at large can become problematic. The compressing effect of carbon dioxide under normal working pressures (12 to 15 mm Hg) is not present under a gasless environment. Therefore, the small bowel tends to occupy more space in the abdominal cavity. The three-dimensional compressing effect of working with gas insufflation is known, workable, and desirable.

There is also ongoing debate regarding a transperitoneal versus a retroperitoneal approach. Barbera et al[10] reported on another large series of completely laparoscopic aortobifemoral bypass (11 patients) and aortofemoral bypass (5 patients). They worked with insufflation and by a transperitoneal approach. They comment on the fact that the small bowel had to be repeatedly removed from the operative field. Despite this, they were able to report comparable operating times for aortobifemoral bypass ranging from 450 to 210 minutes, with constant improvement as their experience grew. Comparably improved patient outcomes were also noted, with mobilization and oral feeding started on the day after surgery and generally well tolerated. In our experience, however, the transabdominal approach modified by the "apron" did indeed have advantages over a purely transperitoneal approach.

We feel at this time that laparoscopic aortic surgery is feasible. It has been developed in the laboratory[14–18,21,23,24,26,27] and performed on a few well-selected patients.[4–8,10] The totally laparoscopic approach to the aortoiliac segment, in our experience and evaluation, appears to be more appealing than a laparoscopically assisted method using an 8- to 10-cm incision[4–6] or a purely minilaparotomy approach.[28] Clinical experiences demonstrated that laparoscopic vascular surgery of the infrarenal aortoiliac segment has the potential

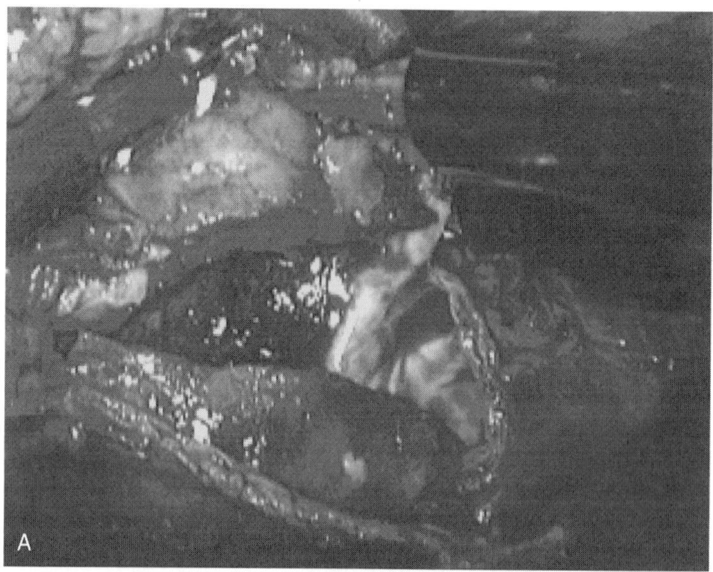

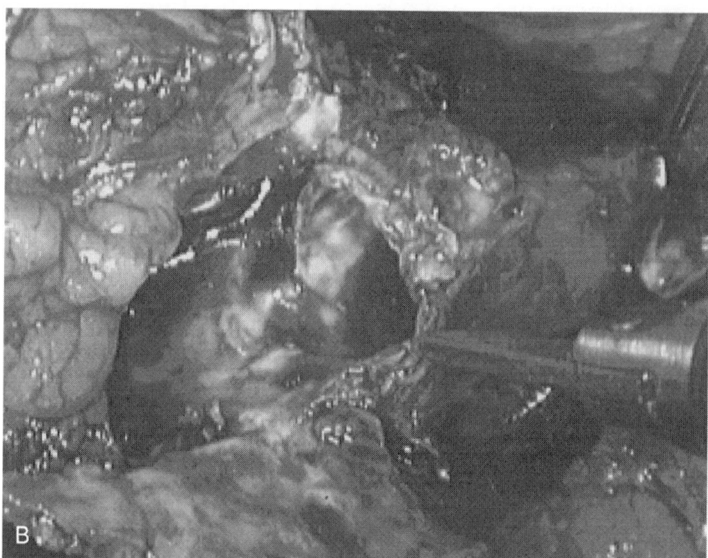

Figure 10. Intraoperative photographs of a totally laparoscopic repair of an aortic aneurysm. The aorta has been cross-clamped proximally. The right iliac system was occluded and the left had a high-grade stenosis. Repair of this clinical problem required an aortofemoral bypass. In **A**, note the mural thrombosis on the aortic wall as the aneurysm has been opened. In **B**, the proximal cuff is being prepared for end-to-end anastomosis in typical fashion.

to benefit the patient. In occlusive disease, it differs only by the approach (laparoscopic versus open). Therefore, the long-term results are expected to be similar. For further application of laparoscopy to aortoiliac surgery, additional developments are necessary. The instrument design is critical. Not only will standard vascular instruments need to be adapted to work laparoscopically, but also new technology and concepts will be required, as with occlusion devices that may be deployed intracorporeally. The anastomosis will require instrumentation that will allow the consistent construction of safe and durable anastomosis.

Performing laparoscopic surgery for occlusive disease is presently easier than attempting to treat AAAs completely laparoscopically. The role of laparoscopy in the ultimate treatment of aortic aneurysm will still require definition and investigation, which will depend on the continued interest in and the fate of endoluminal stent-grafts. Recent studies[11–13] have also confirmed that laparoscopic AAA repair is a feasible technique. The vast majority of this clinical experience is by laparoscopically assisted repair; however, in our recent experience,[29] totally laparoscopic aortic aneurysm repair is feasible (Fig. 10, panels A and B).

Vascular surgeons' exposure to and training in laparoscopy are variable and often limited. Current developments with endoscopic venous techniques offer vascular surgeons the opportunity to become acquainted with nonendoluminal minimally invasive techniques, skills, and instrumentation. Over the next several years, experience should be more uniform as many of tomorrow's vascular surgeons come from training programs having had laparoscopic training and experience. The desired outcome of this work is to improve patient outcomes. No one single option for revascularization is ideal or applicable to all cases. Vascular surgeon exposure and interest must increase to adopt minimally invasive surgical technology and techniques to broaden their modern day armamentarium.

References

1. Marin M, Veith F, Cynamon J. Transfemoral endovascular stented graft treatment of aortoiliac and femoropopliteal occlusive disease for limb salvage. *Am J Surg* 1994;168:156–162.
2. Bergan J, Murray J, Greason K. Subfascial endoscopic perforator vein surgery: A preliminary report. *Ann Vasc Surg* 1996;10:211–219.
3. Brewster DC. Current controversies in the management of aortoiliac occlusive disease. *J Vasc Surg* 1997;25:365–379.
4. Berens ES, Herde JR. Laparoscopic vascular surgery: Four case reports. *J Vasc Surg* 1995;22:73–79.
5. Dion YM, Katkhouda N, Rouleau C, Aucoin A. Laparoscopy-assisted aortobifemoral bypass. *Surg Laparosc Endosc* 1993;3:425–429.
6. Fabiani JN, Mercier F, Carpentier A, et al. Video-assisted aortofemoral bypass. *Ann Vasc Surg* 1997;11:273–277.
7. Ahn SS, Hiyama DT, Rudkin GH, et al. Laparoscopic aortobifemoral bypass. *J Vasc Surg* 1997;26:218–232.
8. Dion YM, Gracia CR. A new technique for laparoscopic aortobifemoral grafting in occlusive aortoiliac disease. *J Vasc Surg* 1997;26:685–692.
9. Dion YM, Gracia CR, Demalcy JC. Laparoscopic aortic surgery [letter to the editors]. *J Vasc Surg* 1995;23:539.

10. Barbera L, Mumme A, Metin S, et al. Operative results and outcome of twenty-four totally laparoscopic vascular procedures for aortoiliac occlusive disease. *J Vasc Surg* 1998;28:136–142.
11. Kline RG, D'Angelo AJ, Chen MH, et al. Laparoscopically assisted abdominal aortic aneurysm repair: First 20 cases. *J Vasc Surg* 1998;27:81–87.
12. Edoga JK, James KV, Resnikoff M, et al. Laparoscopic aortic aneurysm resection. *J Endovasc Surg* 1998;5:335–344.
13. Jobe BA, Duncan W, Swanstrom LL. Totally laparoscopic abdominal aortic aneurysm repair. *Surg Endosc* 1999;13:77–79.
14. Ahn SS, Clem MF, Braithwaite BD, et al. Laparoscopic aortofemoral bypass: Initial experience in an animal model. *Ann Surg* 1995;222:677–683.
15. Byrne J, Hallett JW, Kollmorgen CP, et al. Totally laparoscopic aortobifemoral bypass grafting in an experimental model: Description of technique with initial surgical results. *Ann Vasc Surg* 1996;10:156–165.
16. Dion YM, Chin AK, Thompson A. Experimental laparoscopic aortobifemoral bypass. *Surg Endosc* 1995;9:894–897.
17. Jones DB, Thompson RW, Soper N, et al. Development and comparison of transperitoneal and retroperitoneal approaches to laparoscopic-assisted aortofemoral bypass in a porcine model. *J Vasc Surg* 1996;23:466–471.
18. Said S, Benhidjeb T, Jacobi CA, Muller JM. Videoendoscopic surgery on aortoiliac vessels. An experimental study. *Surg Endosc* 1996;10:1140–1144.
19. Dion YM, Lévesque C, Doillon CJ. Experimental carbon dioxide pulmonary embolization after vena cava laceration under pneumo-peritoneum. *Surg Endosc* 1995;9:1065–1069.
20. Shumacker HB. Midline extraperitoneal exposure of the abdominal aorta and iliac arteries. *Surg Gynecol Obstet* 1972;135:791–792.
21. Dion YM, Gracia CR. Experimental laparoscopic aortic aneurysm resection and aortobifemoral bypass. *Surg Laparosc Endosc* 1996;6:184–190.
22. Dion YM, Rouleau C, Aucoin A. Laparoscopy-assisted aortobifemoral bypass. *Surg Endosc* 1994;8:438.
23. Dion YM, Gaillard F, Demalsy JC, Gracia CR. Experimental laparoscopic aortobifemoral bypass for occlusive aortoiliac disease. *Can J Surg* 1996;39:451–455.
24. Dion YM, Gracia CR, Demalsy JC, Estakhri M. Laparoscopic and laparoscopy-assisted aortoiliac surgery: Animal and clinical evaluation. *J Endovasc Surg* 1996;3:114.
25. Said S, Muller JM. Introduction to video endoscopic vascular surgery of the pelvic area. *Zentralbl Chir* 1997;122:757–761.
26. Dion YM, Gracia CR, Demalsy JC, Estakhri M. Laparoscopic aortic surgery: Animal and human clinical evaluation. *Minim Invasive Ther* 1995;4(suppl 1):40.
27. Dion YM, Gracia CR. A reproducible animal model for laparoscopic retroperitoneal aortobifemoral bypass in aortoiliac occlusive disease. *Surg Endosc* 1996;10:270.
28. Weber G, Jako GJ. Retroperitoneal "mini" approach for aortoiliac reconstructive surgery. *Vasc Surg* 1995;29:387–392.
29. Dion YM, Gracia CR, Ben El Kadi HH. Totally laparoscopic abdominal aortic aneurysm repair. *J Vasc Surg* 2001;33:181–185.

14

Endovascular Intervention:

What Does the Future Hold?

Frank J. Criado, MD

The future of catheter-based vascular intervention is undoubtedly bright. Current trends are likely to continue, as will the pace of innovation in its unrelenting course toward a 'less invasive future' for the care of patients with vascular disease. While it would be pretentious and even unrealistic to attempt to predict the future, I am nonetheless going to delineate probable directions of technology and practice in some of the areas that are presently considered most important. This is what I see happening over the next 5 years:

Enthusiasm for endovascular repair of abdominal aortic aneurysms (AAAs) will not diminish, and several more stent-grafts will receive approval from the US Food and Drug Administration (FDA). I do not foresee anything radically different from a device design perspective any time soon. The emerging emphasis on long-term durability and device integrity will continue and strengthen. A better understanding of procedure- and device-related failures may lead to technological improvements, as well as a better definition of indications for individual patients. Availability of truly percutaneous (<14 F) endograft devices is very likely. Significant developments in endovascular treatment of ruptured and juxtarenal aneurysms can be predicted. Standard surgical repair will retain its role, but will lose ground in cases with "endo-favorable" anatomy.

The role of stent-graft repair in the aortic arch and descending thoracic aorta is likely to expand dramatically. We can expect significant new technologies, with greater resources being put behind the development of devices designed specifically for the thoracic aortic territory. It is safe to state that treatment of thoracic aortic pathology is the most appealing and clinically sound application of stent-graft technology. This view—and technical capabilities—will likely grow rapidly over the next few years.

From Criado FJ (ed): *Endovascular Intervention: New Tools and Techniques for the 21st Century.* Armonk, NY: Futura Publishing Co., Inc.; ©2002.

Carotid intervention (carotid angioplasty-stenting) will consolidate its "vedette" status as increasing number of practitioners embrace it. Continued rapid developments in brain protection technologies and better ("carotid-dedicated") stent devices, together with emerging data from ongoing trials, are going to produce an even greater momentum for this most important area of vascular intervention. A "carotid stenting system" (stent + protection) is likely to receive FDA approval in the first half of 2003, at least for a "high-risk" indication. Universal application (with a greatly diminished role for carotid endarterectomy) is not going to occur for several more years, pending demonstration of long-term efficacy in large randomized clinical trials. But it will take a much shorter time for carotid angioplasty-stenting to achieve carotid endarterectomy-level safety; in fact, this has already occurred in the hands of experienced operators who have access to protection devices!

Infrainguinal intervention is another area of great promise, especially as it relates to drug-eluting stents for endovascular therapy of stenotic and occlusive disease in the superficial femoral artery. These technologies, in fact, may well become "game changers" and spur a truly explosive growth in interventional managements of coronary and peripheral arterial disease. Early data from ongoing trials could not be more encouraging! The Sirolimus-coated stents are quickly emerging as the most promising at this time. The same technologies, if effective, will undoubtedly be used in many if not all vascular territories, especially renal arteries, dialysis access procedures, iliac, and carotid arteries.

Developments with genetic therapy and brachytherapy are of great interest, but the clinical roles of these modalities remain undefined at this time.

On the political side, "turf battles" are likely to continue in the foreseeable future. Vascular centers, various interdisciplinary collaborative arrangements, and "solo" efforts are all worthy of consideration. As always, in the end, what really matters is the local mix of politics and power. We must keep in mind, however, that optimal patient care can only be produced by qualified, highly trained, dedicated operators, regardless of specialty background. The procedure, however, is only a part—sometimes small—of the overall care of a vascular patient. Therefore, whoever accepts responsibility for vascular care, he, she, or they must be willing and prepared to conduct a complete evaluation, understand the indications for intervention (or surgery, or neither), manage postprocedure complications, and provide follow-up care, including risk factor modification and target vessel performance after repair. It is this that matters most, and not so much who does what where!

Index

THE AMERICAN FIRST AMENDMENT IN THE TWENTY-FIRST CENTURY

Cases and Materials

Third Edition

By

WILLIAM W. VAN ALSTYNE
William R. & Thomas S. Perkins Professor of Law
Duke University School of Law

New York, New York
FOUNDATION PRESS
2002

395 Hudson Street
New York, NY 10014
Phone Toll Free 1–877–888–1330
Fax (212) 367–6799
fdpress.com

Printed in the United States of America

ISBN 1–56662–965–9

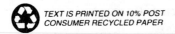

This book is dedicated
to
James Madison, Thomas Jefferson,
and John Stuart Mill

PREFACE TO THE THIRD EDITION

This new edition was completed in late summer of 2001, just following the release of the last case decided by the Supreme Court, June 28th, on the last day of its term that began the preceding October, in 2000. Fittingly, that last case was itself a first amendment case, *Lorillard Tobacco Co. v. Reilly*, in which significant parts of still another act of Congress were found wanting and struck down. It was merely the most recent of nearly a full dozen acts of Congress the Court held to be unconstitutional just during the short interval (less than six years) since the previous edition of this work. A principal objective of undertaking this new edition has been to integrate these significant doctrinal developments, to fit them into the appropriate chapters and sections of the previous edition, and to trace the degree of change and of direction the first amendment has undergone in just this extraordinarily brief interval of time.

A principal objective of the undertaking has been equally to account for and to integrate the decisions of the Court adjudicating the large number and wide range of state laws it reviewed, and likewise passed upon, during this same short interval. This task was equally challenging as the first. For here, as well, the Court rejected as many such laws (actually more) than the number of congressional enactments it determined to be unconstitutional on first amendment grounds. In fact, not to put too fine a point on this development, there has *never* been *any* equivalently brief, six-year period in American history rivaling the immediate past half-decade of dynamic First Amendment judicial activity in which so large a number of congressional acts (as well as a like number of state and local laws) were held void on their face or unenforceable as interpreted and applied, for failure to pay due heed to the first amendment as understood and administered by the Court.

This passage we have just now negotiated into the new, twenty-first century, thus has been both exhilarating and tumultuous, in first amendment terms. Attempting to keep pace in mere annual installments, in an ad hoc supply of yearly supplements to the previous (second) edition of this work, was unsatisfactory. Thus, a more substantial revision of that previous edition, and new integration with the main body of that work, was required.

The need to undertake that substantial revision, however, also provided an opportunity to reconsider and revise a number of chapters, in keeping with suggestions received from a number of teachers and students engaged in using the earlier work. A number of chapters, cases, and topics have been reorganized, partly just the better to account for more recent developments, but also to provide greater doctrinal clarity, and to provide shorter chapters, more topically identified, and more easily divided for ease of more flexible assignment and use. The objective here is to make it easier to adjust one's assignments more flexibly, in keeping with what may be one's own professional tastes of emphasis, as well as in keeping with whatever the length of one's course may happen to allow.

Fourth, however, the intellectual rigor of this work as reflected in the previous editions has not been compromised (at least not by design) merely to make it modern in the sense of reporting and integrating recent developments. The history of the speech-and-press clauses, and likewise of the religion clauses, is given serious attention, fully as much as emphasized in the first and second editions. The earliest, seminal cases laying the foundations of what has brought us into the third century of the American first amendment are all laid out for the teacher and reader to take into account, so far as they may (and should) be inclined to do.

Finally, then, the objective here is not merely to provide a professional training set of materials for law students (which is a major objective). It is to provide any educated person interested in the intellectual history of the first amendment and of its application to this diverse, fractious, religiously riven, ethnically eclectic, churning and boisterous nation, with materials useful to find their own way. Most of all, it is to let one see, whether one is from this country or from some other, how this country has tended so much to use and rely upon its courts to reconcile liberty and (dis)order, for ill or well, under the oldest continuously operating, judicially enforced constitution in the world. –And how it does so under a first amendment at once as old as it surely is–and yet again, in the age of the internet, globalized television, cable, and wireless–utterly vital, always youthful and indeed, for the moment at least, the strongest of any that dominate the world scene today.

Preparing this new edition has been a pleasure, made so by the continuing challenge of the material one struggles to understand and present as best one can. I hope it may give the reader some similar sense of interest and of worthwhile memory as well.

WILLIAM VAN ALSTYNE[1]

Durham, North Carolina
August 20, 2001

---

1. With special thanks to Dawn Blalock for her indispensable assistance in the preparation of this work.

SUMMARY OF CONTENTS

TABLE OF CONTENTS

TABLE OF CASES

References are to pages. Principal cases are in italic type.

THE CONSTITUTION OF THE UNITED STATES OF AMERICA 1787

We the people of the United States, in Order to form a more perfect Union, establish Justice, insure domestic Tranquility, provide for the common defence, promote the general Welfare, and secure the Blessings of Liberty to ourselves and our Posterity, do ordain and establish this Constitution for the United States of America.

Article I

Section. 1. All legislative Powers herein granted shall be vested in a Congress of the United States, which shall consist of a Senate and House of Representatives.

Section. 2. The House of Representatives shall be composed of Members chosen every second Year by the People of the several States, and the Electors in each State shall have the Qualifications requisite for Electors of the most numerous Branch of the State Legislature.

No Person shall be a Representative who shall not have attained to the Age of twenty five Years, and been seven Years a Citizen of the United States, and who shall not, when elected, be an Inhabitant of that State in which he shall be chosen.

[Representatives and direct Taxes shall be apportioned among the several States which may be included within this Union, according to their respective Numbers, which shall be determined by adding to the whole Number of free Persons, including those bound to Service for a Term of Years, and excluding Indians not taxed, three fifths of all other Persons.][1] The actual Enumeration shall be made within three Years after the first Meeting of the Congress of the United States, and within every subsequent Term of ten Years, in such Manner as they shall by Law direct. The Number of Representatives shall not exceed one for every thirty Thousand, but each State shall have at Least one Representative; and until such enumeration shall be made, the State of New Hampshire shall be entitled to chuse three, Massachusetts eight, Rhode-Island and Providence Plantations one, Connecticut five, New-York six, New Jersey four, Pennsylvania eight, Delaware one, Maryland six, Virginia ten, North Carolina five, South Carolina five, and Georgia three.

When vacancies happen in the Representation from any State, the Executive Authority thereof shall issue Writs of Election to fill such Vacancies.

The House of Representatives shall chuse their Speaker and other Officers; and shall have the sole Power of Impeachment.

Section. 3. The Senate of the United States shall be composed of two Senators from each State, [chosen by the Legislature thereof,][2] for six Years; and each Senator shall have one Vote.

Immediately after they shall be assembled in Consequence of the first Election, they shall be divided as equally as may be into three Classes. The Seats of the Senators of the first Class shall be vacated at the Expiration of the second Year, of the second Class at the Expiration of the fourth Year, and of the third Class at the Expiration of the sixth Year, so that one third may be chosen every second Year; [and if Vacancies happen by Resignation, or otherwise, during the Recess of the Legislature of any State, the Executive thereof may make

1. Changed by section 2 of the Fourteenth Amendment.
2. Changed by the Seventeenth Amendment.

temporary Appointments until the next Meeting of the Legislature, which shall then fill such Vacancies.][3]

No Person shall be a Senator who shall not have attained to the Age of thirty Years, and been nine Years a Citizen of the United States, and who shall not, when elected, be an Inhabitant of that State for which he shall be chosen.

The Vice President of the United States shall be President of the Senate, but shall have no Vote, unless they be equally divided.

The Senate shall chuse their other Officers, and also a President pro tempore, in the Absence of the Vice President, or when he shall exercise the Office of President of the United States.

The Senate shall have the sole Power to try all Impeachments. When sitting for that Purpose, they shall be on Oath or Affirmation. When the President of the United States is tried, the Chief Justice shall preside: And no Person shall be convicted without the Concurrence of two thirds of the Members present.

Judgment in Cases of Impeachment shall not extend further than to removal rom Office, and disqualification to hold and enjoy any Office of honor, Trust or Profit under the United States: but the Party convicted shall nevertheless be liable and subject to Indictment, Trial, Judgment and Punishment, according to Law.

Section. 4. The Times, Places and Manner of holding Elections for Senators and Representatives, shall be prescribed in each State by the Legislature thereof; but the Congress may at any time by Law make or alter such Regulations, except as to the Places of chusing Senators.

The Congress shall assemble at least once in every Year, and such Meeting shall be [on the first Monday in December,][4] unless they shall by Law appoint a different Day.

Section. 5. Each House shall be the Judge of the Elections, Returns and Qualifications of its own Members, and a Majority of each shall constitute a Quorum to do Business; but a smaller Number may adjourn from day to day, and may be authorized to compel the Attendance of absent Members, in such Manner, and under such Penalties as each House may provide.

Each House may determine the Rules of its Proceedings, punish its Members for disorderly Behaviour, and, with the Concurrence of two thirds, expel a Member.

Each House shall keep a Journal of its Proceedings, and from time to time publish the same, excepting such Parts as may in their Judgment require Secrecy; and the Yeas and Nays of the Members of either House on any question shall, at the Desire of one fifth of those Present, be entered on the Journal.

Neither House, during the Session of Congress, shall, without the Consent of the other, adjourn for more than three days, nor to any other Place than that in which the two Houses shall be sitting.

Section. 6. The Senators and Representatives shall receive a Compensation for their Services, to be ascertained by Law, and paid out of the Treasury of the United States. They

---

3. Changed by the Seventeenth Amendment.
4. Changed by section 2 of the Twentieth Amendment.

shall in all Cases, except Treason, Felony and Breach of the Peace, be privileged from Arrest during their Attendance at the Session of their respective Houses, and in going to and returning from the same; and for any Speech or Debate in either House, they shall not be questioned in any other Place.

No Senator or Representative shall, during the Time for which he was elected, be appointed to any civil Office under the Authority of the United States, which shall have been created, or the Emoluments whereof shall have been encreased during such time; and no Person holding any Office under the United States, shall be a Member of either House during his Continuance in Office.

Section. 7. All Bills for raising Revenue shall originate in the House of Representatives; but the Senate may propose or concur with Amendments as on other Bills.

Every Bill which shall have passed the House of Representatives and the Senate, shall, before it becomes a Law, be presented to the President of the United States; If he approve he shall sign it, but if not he shall return it, with his Objections to that House in which it shall have originated, who shall enter the Objections at large on their Journal, and proceed to reconsider it. If after such reconsideration two thirds of that House shall agree to pass the Bill, it shall be sent, together with the Objections, to the other House, by which it shall likewise be reconsidered, and if approved by two thirds of that House, it shall become a Law. But in all such Cases the Votes of both Houses shall be determined by Yeas and Nays, and the Names of the Persons voting for and against the Bill shall be entered on the Journal of each House respectively. If any Bill shall not be returned by the President within ten Days (Sundays excepted) after it shall have been presented to him, the Same shall be a Law, in like Manner as if he had signed it, unless the Congress by their Adjournment prevent its Return, in which Case it shall not be a Law.

Every Order, Resolution, or Vote to which the Concurrence of the Senate and House of Representatives may be necessary (except on a question of Adjournment) shall be presented to the President of the United States; and before the Same shall take Effect, shall be approved by him, or being disapproved by him, shall be repassed by two thirds of the Senate and House of Representatives, according to the Rules and Limitations prescribed in the Case of a Bill.

Section. 8. The Congress shall have Power To lay and collect Taxes, Duties, Imposts and Excises, to pay the Debts and provide for the common Defence and general Welfare of the United States; but all Duties, Imposts and Excises shall be uniform throughout the United States;

To borrow Money on the credit of the United States;

To regulate Commerce with foreign Nations, and among the several States, and with the Indian Tribes;

To establish an uniform Rule of Naturalization, and uniform Laws on the subject of Bankruptcies throughout the United States;

To coin Money, regulate the Value thereof, and of foreign Coin, and fix the Standard of Weights and Measures;

To provide for the Punishment of counterfeiting the Securities and current Coin of the United States;

To establish Post Offices and post Roads;

To promote the Progress of Science and useful Arts, by securing for limited Times to Authors and Inventors the exclusive Right to their respective Writings and Discoveries;

To constitute Tribunals inferior to the supreme Court;

To define and punish Piracies and Felonies committed on the high Seas, and Offences against the Law of Nations;

To declare War, grant Letters of Marque and Reprisal, and make Rules concerning Captures on Land and Water;

To raise and support Armies, but no Appropriation of Money to that Use shall be for a longer Term than two Years;

To provide and maintain a Navy;

To make Rules for the Government and Regulation of the land and naval Forces;

To provide for calling forth the Militia to execute the Laws of the Union, suppress Insurrections and repel Invasions;

To provide for organizing, arming, and disciplining, the Militia, and for governing such Part of them as may be employed in the Service of the United States, reserving to the States respectively, the Appointment of the Officers, and the Authority of training the Militia according to the discipline prescribed by Congress;

To exercise exclusive Legislation in all Cases whatsoever, over such District (not exceeding ten Miles square) as may, by Cession of particular States, and the Acceptance of Congress, become the Seat of the Government of the United States, and to exercise like Authority over all Places purchased by the Consent of the Legislature of the State in which the Same shall be, for the Erection of Forts, Magazines, Arsenals, dock-Yards, and other needful Buildings;—And

To make all Laws which shall be necessary and proper for carrying into Execution the foregoing Powers, and all other Powers vested by this Constitution in the Government of the United States, or in any Department or Officer thereof.

Section. 9. The Migration or Importation of such Persons as any of the States now existing shall think proper to admit, shall not be prohibited by the Congress prior to the Year one thousand eight hundred and eight, but a Tax or duty may be imposed on such Importation, not exceeding ten dollars for each Person.

The Privilege of the Writ of Habeas Corpus shall not be suspended, unless when in Cases of Rebellion or Invasion the public Safety may require it.

No Bill of Attainder or ex post facto Law shall be passed.

[No Capitation, or other direct, Tax shall be laid, unless in Proportion to the Census or Enumeration herein before directed to be taken.][5]

No Tax or Duty shall be laid on Articles exported from any State.

No Preference shall be given by any Regulation of Commerce or Revenue to the Ports of one State over those of another; nor shall Vessels bound to, or from, one State, be obliged to enter, clear, or pay Duties in another.

---

5. Changed by the Sixteenth Amendment.

No Money shall be drawn from the Treasury, but in Consequence of Appropriations made by Law; and a regular Statement and Account of the Receipts and Expenditures of all public Money shall be published from time to time.

No Title of Nobility shall be granted by the United States: and no Person holding any Office of Profit or Trust under them, shall, without the Consent of the Congress, accept of any present, Emolument, Office, or Title, of any kind whatever, from any King, Prince, or foreign State.

Section. 10. No State shall enter into any Treaty, Alliance, or Confederation; grant Letters of Marque and Reprisal; coin Money; emit Bills of Credit; make any Thing but gold and silver Coin a Tender in Payment of Debts; pass any Bill of Attainder, ex post facto Law, or Law impairing the Obligation of Contracts, or grant any Title of Nobility.

No State shall, without the Consent of the Congress, lay any Imposts or Duties on Imports or Exports, except what may be absolutely necessary for executing it's inspection Laws: and the net Produce of all Duties and Imposts, laid by any State on Imports or Exports, shall be for the Use of the Treasury of the United States; and all such Laws shall be subject to the Revision and Controul of the Congress.

No State shall, without the Consent of Congress, lay any Duty of Tonnage, keep Troops, or Ships of War in time of Peace, enter into any Agreement or Compact with another State, or with a foreign Power, or engage in War, unless actually invaded, or in such imminent Danger as will not admit of delay.

Article II

Section. 1. The executive Power shall be vested in a President of the United States of America. He shall hold his Office during the Term of four Years, and, together with the Vice President, chosen for the same Term, be elected, as follows

Each State shall appoint, in such Manner as the Legislature thereof may direct, a Number of Electors, equal to the whole Number of Senators and Representatives to which the State may be entitled in the Congress: but no Senator or Representative, or Person holding an Office of Trust or Profit under the United States, shall be appointed an Elector.

[The Electors shall meet in their respective States, and vote by Ballot for two Persons, of whom one at least shall not be an Inhabitant of the same State with themselves. And they shall make a List of all the Persons voted for, and of the Number of Votes for each; which List they shall sign and certify, and transmit sealed to the Seat of the Government of the United States, directed to the President of the Senate. The President of the Senate shall, in the Presence of the Senate and House of Representatives, open all the Certificates, and the Votes shall then be counted. The Person having the greatest Number of Votes shall be the President, if such Number be a Majority of the whole Number of Electors appointed; and if there be more than one who have such Majority, and have an equal Number of Votes, then the House of Representatives shall immediately chuse by Ballot one of them for President; and if no Person have a Majority, then from the five highest on the List the said House shall in like Manner chuse the President. But in chusing the President, the Votes shall be taken by States, the Representative from each State having one Vote; A quorum for this Purpose shall consist of a Member or Members from two thirds of the States, and a Majority of all the

States shall be necessary to a Choice. In every Case, after the Choice of the President, the Person having the greatest Number of Votes of the Electors shall be the Vice President. But if there should remain two or more who have equal Votes, the Senate shall chuse from them by Ballot the Vice President.][6]

The Congress may determine the Time of chusing the Electors, and the Day on which they shall give their Votes; which Day shall be the same throughout the United States.

No Person except a natural born Citizen, or a Citizen of the United States, at the time of the Adoption of this Constitution, shall be eligible to the Office of President; neither shall any Person be eligible to that Office who shall not have attained to the Age of thirty five Years, and been fourteen Years a Resident within the United States.

[In Case of the Removal of the President from Office, or of his Death, Resignation, or Inability to discharge the Powers and Duties of the said Office, the Same shall devolve on the Vice President, and the Congress may by Law provide for the Case of Removal, Death, Resignation or Inability, both of the President and Vice President, declaring what Officer shall then act as President, and such Officer shall act accordingly, until the Disability be removed, or a President shall be elected.][7]

The President shall, at stated Times, receive for his Services, a Compensation, which shall neither be encreased nor diminished during the Period for which he shall have been elected, and he shall not receive within that Period any other Emolument from the United States, or any of them.

Before he enter on the Execution of his Office, he shall take the following Oath or Affirmation:—"I do solemnly swear (or affirm) that I will faithfully execute the Office of President of the United States, and will to the best of my Ability, preserve, protect and defend the Constitution of the United States."

Section. 2. The President shall be Commander in Chief of the Army and Navy of the United States, and of the Militia of the several States, when called into the actual Service of the United States; he may require the Opinion, in writing, of the principal Officer in each of the executive Departments, upon any Subject relating to the Duties of their respective Offices, and he shall have Power to grant Reprieves and Pardons for Offences against the United States, except in Cases of Impeachment.

He shall have Power, by and with the Advice and Consent of the Senate, to make Treaties, provided two thirds of the Senators present concur; and he shall nominate, and by and with the Advice and Consent of the Senate, shall appoint Ambassadors, other public Ministers and Consuls, Judges of the supreme Court, and all other Officers of the United States, whose Appointments are not herein otherwise provided for, and which shall be established by Law: but the Congress may by Law vest the Appointment of such inferior Officers, as they think proper, in the President alone, in the Courts of Law, or in the Heads of Departments.

---

6. Changed by the Twelfth Amendment.
7. Changed by the Twenty-fifth Amendment.

The President shall have Power to fill up all Vacancies that may happen during the Recess of the Senate, by granting Commissions which shall expire at he End of their next Session.

Section. 3. He shall from time to time give to the Congress Information of the State of the Union, and recommend to their Consideration such Measures as he shall judge necessary and expedient; he may, on extraordinary Occasions, convene both Houses, or either of them, and in Case of Disagreement between them, with Respect to the Time of Adjournment, he may adjourn them to such Time as he shall think proper; he shall receive Ambassadors and other public Ministers; he shall take Care that the Laws be faithfully executed, and shall Commission all the Officers of the United States.

Section. 4. The President, Vice President and all civil Officers of the United States, shall be removed from Office on Impeachment for, and Conviction of, Treason, Bribery, or other high Crimes and Misdemeanors.

Article III

Section. 1. The judicial Power of the United States, shall be vested in one supreme Court, and in such inferior Courts as the Congress may from time to time ordain and establish. The Judges, both of the supreme and inferior Courts, shall hold their Offices during good Behaviour, and shall, at stated Times, receive for their Services, a Compensation, which shall not be diminished during their Continuance in Office.

Section. 2. The judicial Power shall extend to all Cases, in Law and Equity, arising under this Constitution, the Laws of the United States, and Treaties made, or which shall be made, under their Authority;—to all Cases affecting Ambassadors, other public Ministers and Consuls;—to all Cases of admiralty and maritime Jurisdiction;—to Controversies to which the United States shall be a Party;—to Controversies between two or more States;—between a State and Citizens of another State;— between Citizens of different States;— between Citizens of the same State claiming Lands under Grants of different States, [and between a State, or the Citizens thereof, and foreign States, Citizens or Subjects.][8]

In all Cases affecting Ambassadors, other public Ministers and Consuls, and those in which a State shall be Party, the supreme Court shall have original Jurisdiction. In all the other Cases before mentioned, the supreme Court shall have appellate Jurisdiction, both as to Law and Fact, with such Exceptions, and under such Regulations as the Congress shall make.

The Trial of all Crimes, except in Cases of Impeachment, shall be by Jury; and such Trial shall be held in the State where the said Crimes shall have been committed; but when not committed within any State, the Trial shall be at such Place or Places as the Congress may by Law have directed.

Section. 3. Treason against the United States, shall consist only in levying War against them, or in adhering to their Enemies, giving them Aid and Comfort. No Person shall be

8. Changed by the Eleventh Amendment.

convicted of Treason unless on the Testimony of two Witnesses to the same overt Act, or on Confession in open Court.

The Congress shall have Power to declare the Punishment of Treason, but no Attainder of Treason shall work Corruption of Blood, or Forfeiture except during the Life of the Person attained.

Article IV

Section. 1. Full Faith and Credit shall be given in each State to the public Acts, Records, and judicial Proceedings of every other State. And the Congress may by general Laws prescribe the Manner in which such Acts, Records and Proceedings shall be proved, and the Effect thereof.

Section. 2. The Citizens of each State shall be entitled to all Privileges and Immunities of Citizens in the several States.

A Person charged in any State with Treason, Felony, or other Crime, who shall flee from Justice, and be found in another State, shall on Demand of the executive Authority of the State from which he fled, be delivered up, to be removed to the State having Jurisdiction of the Crime.

[No Person held to Service or Labour in one State, under the Laws thereof, escaping into another, shall, in Consequence of any Law or Regulation therein, be discharged from such Service or Labour, but shall be delivered up on Claim of the Party to whom such Service or Labour may be due.][9]

Section. 3. New States may be admitted by the Congress into this Union; but no new State shall be formed or erected within the Jurisdiction of any other State; nor any State be formed by the Junction of two or more States, or Parts of States, without the Consent of the Legislatures of the States concerned as well as of the Congress.

The Congress shall have Power to dispose of and make all needful Rules and Regulations respecting the Territory or other Property belonging to the United States; and nothing in this Constitution shall be so construed as to Prejudice any Claims of the United States, or of any particular State.

Section. 4. The United States shall guarantee to every State in this Union a Republican Form of Government, and shall protect each of them against Invasion; and on Application of the Legislature, or of the Executive (when the Legislature cannot be convened) against domestic Violence.

Article V

The Congress, whenever two thirds of both Houses shall deem it necessary, shall propose Amendments to this Constitution, or, on the Application of the Legislatures of two thirds of the several States, shall call a Convention for proposing Amendments, which, in either Case, shall be valid to all Intents and Purposes, as Part of this Constitution, when

9. Changed by the Thirteenth Amendment.

ratified by the Legislatures of three fourths of the several States, or by Conventions in three fourths thereof, as the one or the other Mode of Ratification may be proposed by the Congress; Provided that no Amendment which may be made prior to the Year One thousand eight hundred and eight shall in any Manner affect the first and fourth Clauses in the Ninth Section of the first Article; and that no State, without its Consent, shall be deprived of its equal Suffrage in the Senate.

Article VI

All Debts contracted and Engagements entered into, before the Adoption of this Constitution, shall be as valid against the United States under this Constitution, as under the Confederation.

This Constitution, and the Laws of the United States which shall be made in Pursuance thereof; and all Treaties made, or which shall be made, under the Authority of the United States, shall be the supreme Law of the Land; and the Judges in every State shall be bound thereby, any Thing in the Constitution or Laws of any State to the Contrary notwithstanding.

The Senators and Representatives before mentioned, and the Members of the several State Legislatures, and all executive and judicial Officers, both of the United States and of the several States, shall be bound by Oath or Affirmation, to support this Constitution; but no religious Test shall ever be required as a Qualification to any Office or public Trust under the United States.

Article VII

The Ratification of the Conventions of nine States, shall be sufficient for the Establishment of this Constitution between the States so ratifying the Same.

Done in convention by the Unanimous consent of the States present the Seventeenth Day of September in the Year of our Lord one thousand seven hundred and Eight seven and of the Independence of the United States of America the Twelfth In Witness whereof We have hereunto subscribed our Names.

Amendments to the Constitution of the United States of America

Articles in Addition To, and Amendment Of, the Constitution of the United States of America, Proposed by Congress, and Ratified by the Legislatures of the Several States Pursuant to the Fifth Article of the Original Constitution

Amendment I[10]

Congress shall make no law respecting an establishment of religion, or prohibiting the free exercise thereof; or abridging the freedom of speech, or of the press; or the right of the people peaceably to assemble, and to petition the Government for a redress of grievances.

Amendment II

A well regulated Militia, being necessary to the security of a free State, the right of the people to keep and bear Arms, shall not be infringed.

Amendment III

No Soldier shall, in time of peace be quartered in any house, without the consent of the Owner, nor in time of war, but in a manner to be prescribed by law.

Amendment IV

The right of the people to be secure in their persons, houses, papers, and effects, against unreasonable searches and seizures, shall not be violated, and no Warrants shall issue, but upon probable cause, supported by Oath or affirmation, and particularly describing the place to be searched, and the persons or things to be seized.

Amendment V

No person shall be held to answer for a capital, or otherwise infamous crime, unless on a presentment or indictment of a Grand Jury, except in cases arising in the land or naval forces, or in the Militia, when in actual service in time of War or public danger; nor shall any person be subject for the same offence to be twice put in jeopardy of life or limb; nor shall be compelled in any criminal case to be a witness against himself, nor be deprived of life, liberty, or property, without due process of law; nor shall private property be taken for public use, without just compensation.

Amendment VI

In all criminal prosecutions, the accused shall enjoy the right to a speedy and public trial, by an impartial jury of the State and district wherein the crime shall have been committed, which district shall have been previously ascertained by law, and to be informed of the nature

---

10. The first ten amendments to the Constitution of the United States were proposed to the legislatures of the several States by the First Congress, on the 25th of September 1789. They were ratified by the following States and the notifications of ratification by the governors thereof were successively communicated by the President to Congress: New Jersey, November 20, 1789; Maryland, December 19, 1789; North Carolina, December 22, 1789; South Carolina, January 19, 1790; New Hampshire, January 25, 1790; Delaware, January 28, 1790; Pennsylvania, March 10, 1790; New York, March 27, 1790; Rhode Island, June 15, 1790; Vermont, November 3, 1791, and Virginia, December 15, 1791. The legislatures of Connecticut, Georgia, and Massachusetts ratified them on April 19, 1939, March 18, 1939, and March 2, 1939, respectively.

and cause of the accusation; to be confronted with the witnesses against him; to have compulsory process for obtaining Witnesses in his favor, and to have the Assistance of Counsel for his defence.

Amendment VII

In Suits at common law, where the value in controversy shall exceed twenty dollars, the right of trial by jury shall be preserved, and no fact tried by a jury, shall be otherwise reexamined in any Court of the United States, than according to the rules of the common law.

Amendment VIII

Excessive bail shall not be required, nor excessive fines imposed, nor cruel and unusual punishments inflicted.

Amendment IX

The enumeration in the Constitution, of certain rights, shall not be construed to deny or disparage others retained by the people.

Amendment X

The powers not delegated to the United States by the Constitution, nor prohibited by it to the States, are reserved to the States respectively, or to the people.

Amendment XI[11]

The Judicial power of the United States shall not be construed to extend to any suit in law or equity, commenced or prosecuted against one of the United States by Citizens of another State, or by Citizens or Subjects of any Foreign State.

Amendment XII[12]

The Electors shall meet in their respective states, and vote by ballot for President and Vice-President, one of whom, at least, shall not be an inhabitant of the same state with themselves; they shall name in their ballots the person voted for as President, and in distinct ballots the person voted for as Vice-President, and they shall make distinct lists of all persons voted for as President, and of all persons voted for as Vice-President, and of the number of votes for each, which lists they shall sign and certify, and transmit sealed to the seat of the government of the United States, directed to the President of the Senate;—The President of the Senate shall, in the presence of the Senate and House of Representatives, open all the certificates and the votes shall then be counted;—The person having the greatest number of votes for President, shall be the President, if such number be a majority of the whole number

---

11. The Eleventh Amendment was ratified February 7, 1795.
12. The Twelfth Amendment was ratified June 15, 1804.

of Electors appointed; and if no person have such majority, then from the persons having the highest numbers not exceeding three on the list of those voted for as President, the House of Representatives shall choose immediately, by ballot, the President. But in choosing the President, the votes shall be taken by states, the representation from each state having one vote; a quorum for this purpose shall consist of a member or members from two-thirds of the states, and a majority of all the states shall be necessary to a choice. [And if the House of Representatives shall not choose a President whenever the right of choice shall devolve upon them, before the fourth day of March next following, then the Vice-President shall act as President, as in the case of the death or other constitutional disability of the President.][13] The person having the greatest number of votes as Vice- President, shall be the Vice-President, if such number be a majority of the whole number of Electors appointed, and if no person have a majority, then from the two highest numbers on the list, the Senate shall choose the Vice-President; a quorum for the purpose shall consist of two-thirds of the whole number of Senators, and a majority of the whole number shall be necessary to a choice. But no person constitutionally ineligible to the office of President shall be eligible to that of Vice-President of the United States.

Amendment XIII[14]

Section 1. Neither slavery nor involuntary servitude, except as a punishment for crime whereof the party shall have been duly convicted, shall exist within he United States, or any place subject to their jurisdiction.

Section 2. Congress shall have power to enforce this article by appropriate legislation.

Amendment XIV.[15]

Section 1. All persons born or naturalized in the United States, and subject o the jurisdiction thereof, are citizens of the United States and of the State wherein they reside. No State shall make or enforce any law which shall abridge the privileges or immunities of citizens of the United states; nor shall any State deprive any person of life, liberty, or property, without due process of law; nor deny to any person within its jurisdiction the equal protection of the laws.

Section 2. Representatives shall be appointed among the several States according to their respective numbers, counting the whole number of persons in each State, excluding Indians not taxed. But when the right to vote at any election for the choice of electors for President and Vice President of the United States, Representatives in Congress, the Executive and Judicial officers of a State, or the members of the Legislature thereof, is denied to any of the male inhabitants of such State, being twenty-one years of age, and citizens of the United States, or in any way abridged, except for participation in rebellion, or other crime, the basis

---

13. Superseded by section 3 of the Twentieth Amendment.
14. The Thirteenth Amendment was ratified December 6, 1865.
15. The Fourteenth Amendment was ratified July 9, 1868.

of representation therein shall be reduced in the proportion which the number of such male citizens shall bear to the whole number of male citizens twenty-one years of age in such State.

Section 3. No person shall be a Senator or Representative in Congress, or elector of President and Vice President, or hold any office, civil or military, under the United States, or under any State, who, having previously taken an oath, as a member of Congress, or as an officer of the United States, or as a member of any State legislature, or as an executive or judicial officer of any State, to support the Constitution of the United States, shall have engaged in insurrection or rebellion against the same, or given aid or comfort to the enemies thereof. But Congress may by a vote of two- thirds of each House, remove such disability.

Section 4. The validity of the public debt of the United States, authorized by law, including debts incurred for payment of pensions and bounties for services in suppressing insurrection or rebellion, shall not be questioned. But neither the United States nor any State shall assume or pay any debt or obligation incurred in aid of insurrection or rebellion against the United States, or any claim for the loss or emancipation of any slave; but all such debts, obligations and claims shall be held illegal and void.

Section 5. The Congress shall have power to enforce, by appropriate legislation, the provisions of this article.

Amendment XV[16]

Section 1. The right of citizens of the United States to vote shall not be denied or abridged by the United States or by any State on account of race, color, or previous condition of servitude.

Section 2. The Congress shall have power to enforce this article by appropriate legislation.

Amendment XVI[17]

The Congress shall have power to lay and collect taxes on incomes, from whatever source derived, without apportionment among the several States, and without regard to any census or enumeration.

Amendment XVII[18]

The Senate of the United States shall be composed of two Senators from each state, elected by the people thereof, for six years; and each Senator shall have one vote. The electors in each State shall have the qualifications requisite for electors of the most numerous branch of the State legislatures.

When vacancies happen in the representation of any State in the Senate, the executive authority of such State shall issue writs of election to fill such vacancies: Provided, That the

---

16. The Fifteenth Amendment was ratified February 3, 1870.
17. The Sixteenth Amendment was ratified February 3, 1870.
18. The Seventeenth Amendment was ratified April 8, 1913.

legislature of any State may empower the executive thereof to make temporary appointments until the people fill the vacancies by election as the legislature may direct.

This amendment shall not be so construed as to affect the election or term of any Senator chosen before it becomes valid as part of the Constitution.

Amendment XVIII[19]

Section 1. After one year from the ratification of this article the manufacture, sale, or transportation of intoxicating liquors within, the importation thereof into, or the exportation thereof from the United States and all territory subject to the jurisdiction thereof for beverage purposes is hereby prohibited.

Section 2. The Congress and the several States shall have concurrent power to enforce this article by appropriate legislation.

Section 3. This article shall be inoperative unless it shall have been ratified as an amendment to the Constitution by the legislatures of the several States, as provided in the Constitution, within seven years from the date of the submission hereof to the States by the Congress.

Amendment XIX[20]

The right of citizens of the United States to vote shall not be denied or abridged by the United States or by any State on account of sex.

Congress shall have power to enforce this article by appropriate legislation.

Amendment XX[21]

Section 1. The terms of the President and Vice President shall end at noon on the 20th day of January, and the terms of Senators and Representatives at noon on the 3d day of January, of the years in which such terms would have ended if this article had not been ratified; and the terms of their successors shall then begin.

Section 2. The Congress shall assemble at least once in every year, and such meeting shall begin at noon on the 3d day of January, unless they shall by law appoint a different day.

Section 3. If, at the time fixed for the beginning of the term of the President, the President elect shall have died, the Vice President elect shall become President. If a President shall not have been chosen before the time fixed for the beginning of his term, or if the President elect shall have failed to qualify, then the Vice President elect shall act as President until a President shall have qualified; and the Congress may by law provide for the case wherein neither a President elect nor a Vice President elect shall have qualified, declaring who shall then act as President, or the manner in which one who is to act shall be selected, and such person shall act accordingly until a President or Vice President shall have qualified.

---

19. The Eighteenth Amendment was ratified January 6, 1919. It was repealed by the Twenty-first Amendment, December 5, 1933.

20. The Nineteenth Amendment was ratified August 18, 1920.

21. The Twentieth Amendment was ratified January 23, 1933.

Section 4. The Congress may by law provide for the case of the death of any of the persons from whom the House of Representatives may choose a President whenever the right of choice shall have devolved upon them, and for the case of the death of any of the persons from whom the Senate may choose a Vice President whenever the right of choice shall have devolved upon them.

Section 5. Sections 1 and 2 shall take effect on the 15th day of October following the ratification of this article.

Section 6. This article shall be inoperative unless it shall have been ratified as an amendment to the Constitution by the legislatures of three-fourths of the several States within seven years from the date of its submission.

Amendment XXI[22]

Section 1. The eighteenth article of amendment to the Constitution of the United States is hereby repealed.

Section 2. The transportation or importation into any State, Territory, or possession of the United States for delivery or use therein of intoxicating liquors, in violation of the laws thereof, is hereby prohibited.

Section 3. This article shall be inoperative unless it shall have been ratified as an amendment to the Constitution by conventions in the several States, as provided in the Constitution, within seven years from the date of the submission hereof to the States by the Congress.

Amendment XXII[23]

Section 1. No person shall be elected to the office of the President more than twice, and no person who has held the office of President, or acted as President, for more than two years of a term to which some other person was elected President shall be elected to the office of the President more than once. But this Article shall not apply to any person holding the office of President when this Article was proposed by the Congress, and shall not prevent any person who may be holding the office of President, or acting as President, during the term within which this Article becomes operative from holding the office of President or acting as President during the remainder of such term.

Section 2. This article shall be inoperative unless it shall have been ratified as an amendment to the Constitution by the legislatures of three-fourths of the several States within seven years from the date of its submission to the States by the Congress.

Amendment XXIII[24]

Section 1. The District constituting the seat of Government of the United States shall appoint in such manner as the Congress may direct:

---

22. The Twenty-first Amendment was ratified December 5, 1933.
23. The Twenty-second Amendment was ratified February 27, 1951.
24. The Twenty-third Amendment was ratified March 29, 1961.

A number of electors of President and Vice President equal to the whole number of Senators and Representatives in Congress to which the District would be entitled if it were a State, but in no event more than the least populous State; they shall be in addition to those appointed by the States, but they shall be considered, for the purposes of the election of President and Vice President, to be electors appointed by a State; and they shall meet in the District and perform such duties as provided by the twelfth article of amendment.

Section 2. The Congress shall have power to enforce this article by appropriate legislation.

Amendment XXIV[25]

Section 1. The right of citizens of the United States to vote in any primary or other election for President or Vice President, for electors for President or Vice President, or for Senator or Representative in Congress, shall not be denied or abridged by the United States or any State by reason of failure to pay any poll tax or other tax.

Section 2. The Congress shall have power to enforce this article by appropriate legislation.

Amendment XXV[26]

Section 1. In case of the removal of the President from office or of his death or resignation, the Vice President shall become President.

Section 2. Whenever there is a vacancy in the office of the Vice President, the President shall nominate a Vice President who shall take office upon confirmation by a majority vote of both Houses of Congress.

Section 3. Whenever the President transmits to the President pro tempore of the Senate and the Speaker of the House of Representatives his written declaration that he is unable to discharge the powers and duties of his office, and until he transmits to them a written declaration to the contrary, such powers and duties shall be discharged by the Vice President as Acting President.

Section 4. Whenever the Vice President and a majority of either the principal officers of the executive departments or of such other body as Congress may by law provide, transmit to the President pro tempore of the Senate and the Speaker of the House of Representatives their written declaration that the President is unable to discharge the powers and duties of his office, the Vice President shall immediately assume the powers and duties of the office as Acting President.

Thereafter, when the President transmits to the President pro tempore of the Senate and the Speaker of the House of Representatives his written declaration that no inability exists, he shall resume the powers and duties of his office unless the Vice President and a majority of either the principal officers of the executive department or of such other body as Congress may by law provide, transmit within four days to the President pro tempore of the Senate and

---

25. The Twenty-fourth Amendment was ratified January 23, 1964.
26. The Twenty-fifth Amendment was ratified February 10, 1967.

the Speaker of the House of Representatives their written declaration that the President is unable to discharge the powers and duties of his office. Thereupon Congress shall decide the issue, assembling within forty-eight hours for that purpose if not in session. If the Congress, within twenty-one days after receipt of the latter written declaration, or, if Congress is not in session, within twenty- one days after Congress is required to assemble, determines by two-thirds vote of both Houses that the President is unable to discharge the powers and duties of his office, the Vice President shall continue to discharge the same as Acting President; otherwise, the President shall resume the powers and duties of his office.

Amendment XXVI[27]

Section 1. The right of citizens of the United States, who are eighteen years of age or older, to vote shall not be denied or abridged by the United States or by any State on account of age.

Section 2. The Congress shall have power to enforce this article by appropriate legislation.

Amendment XXVII[28]

No law, varying the compensation for the services of Senators and Representatives, shall take effect, until an election of Representatives shall have intervened.

---

27. The Twenty-sixth Amendment was ratified July 1, 1971.

28. The Twenty-seventh Amendment was ratified by a thirty-eighth state (Michigan), May 7, 1992, more than two centuries following its proposal by Congress, in 1789. On May 21, 1992, it was declared to be "valid *** as part of the Constitution of the United States" by concurrent resolution in Congress. The vote was 99-0 in the Senate and 414-3 in the House. This amendment is the original second amendment of the twelve amendments proposed by Congress in 1789, i.e. it was one of two amendments that failed to achieve ratification as part of the Bill of Rights. [*Query* whether an amendment proposed by Congress in 1789 as part of a larger set, having failed to attract the requisite consensus of state ratifications common to the rest of the set, and never renewed by any later Congress during a time span of two hundred years, can be deemed to survive for purposes of acquiring sufficient ratifications at a time so far removed from its original initiating date. For one suggested answer, *see* Dillon v. Gloss, 256 U.S. 368, 374-75 (1921).]

Part I

THE FREE SPEECH AND FREE PRESS CLAUSES

Chapter 1

AN INTRODUCTION TO THE FIRST AMENDMENT

I

Some of the materials in the basic course on constitutional law were doctrinally related to the first amendment, including some popular cases that provide a natural introduction for starting our work here. Specifically, *Griswold v. Connecticut*[1] and *Roe v. Wade*[2] ought to suggest an orientation to an easy approach to free speech and free press. Accordingly, we begin our brief introductory review with the very suggestion one's work in the first year course would most strongly endorse.

A

Whatever casebook and instructor you may have had as a guide to *Griswold* and *Roe*, you will recall that the starting point was the determination of the proper standard of judicial review. What was different in the Court's treatment of those cases was, most of all, the *strict scrutiny* standard the Supreme Court applied. Beginning with *Griswold*, the Court required that the state demonstrate a *compelling* interest in regulating the birth control practices of married couples. And it required also that the state demonstrate not only a *compelling* interest in regulating what was otherwise regarded as a highly protected subject of intensely personal concern, but that it also show that *no less intrusive* a form of regulation could avoid the social evil or kind of harm that the state sought to avoid.[3] The same generic approach was applied in *Roe*.[4] You will recall, too, that the rationale for demanding

---

1. 381 U.S. 479 (1965).

2. 410 U.S. 113 (1973).

3. So, as you will recall, the state of Connecticut argued that the criminal ban of any device preventing conception would act as a useful additional deterrent to adultery—by putting adulterous persons at personal risk—but the Court held that even assuming the state's interest (in the avoidance of adulterous relations) was "compelling," the complete outlawry of birth control devices was too sweeping and draconian under the circumstances. The state would have to proceed by narrower means of control (e.g., by increasing the criminal penalties for adultery), to avoid unreasonably interfering with the private intimate relations of married couples.

4. Indeed, recall that the case remains highly controversial not because the standard of judicial review was necessarily regarded as improper, but because of disagreement by many with the Court's view that the Texas statute did not meet that standard (namely, disagreement about whether the protection of fetal life from destruction prior to the point of *ex utero* viability, was a sufficiently "compelling" interest to disallow abortion except when necessary to protect the pregnant woman from life-imperiling risks of carrying the fetus to full term). See, e.g., Planned Parenthood v. Casey, 510 U.S. 1309 (1994).

greater justification and *tighter* boundaries on state or national laws affecting the kinds of personal liberties involved in *Griswold* and in *Roe*, than on those affecting other kinds of personal liberties involved in certain other cases,[5] was rooted in a set of observations by the Court regarding "penumbras" and the Bill of Rights.

The Court defended the objectivity of requiring more justification by government for burdening some "rights" (e.g., relations within marriage) than other "rights" (e.g., conditions of conducting one's business enterprise—economic rights) by reference to several clauses, and many cases, arising under the first, fourth, and fifth amendments. Its point was that the Constitution itself expressly singled out certain interests for protection against abridgment, as to which there was simply no question of the Court's duty to see they were upheld (it specifically mentioned "freedom of speech" as an example).[6] It then noted that while related rights might not themselves be as fully protected as these rights were fully protected, still, to the extent that they *were* related (e.g., connected to them in some way), they were to that extent more-of-a-piece with these explicitly guaranteed rights than other kinds of rights claims. Recall that one of Justice Douglas's examples, in *Griswold*, was the "right of association." Justice Douglas noted that the Court had previously struck down certain state laws interfering with political rights of association, applying a stern standard of judicial review, and explaining the use of the standard partly in terms of the relation between being able to associate freely with others for political purposes and the right of free speech and peaceable assembly. So, while "the right of association" as such is not an enumerated first amendment right, by virtue of its "penumbra" status it gained a textual connection to the first amendment itself. And on that basis, even cases predating *Griswold* had applied strict scrutiny review.

The point of this brief recapitulation, of course, is not to revisit Con Law I. It is, rather, simply to suggest that in one sense you have already had an introduction of one sort to the first amendment. Indeed, what that introduction would seem to suggest is this: if even certain rights not in the first amendment are *highly* protected merely on the strength of having some penumbral consanguinity with that amendment,[7] *then presumably the rights that* are *expressly provided for by that amendment*

5. E.g., Nebbia v. New York, 291 U.S. 502 (1934) (sustaining a state price-fixing law forbidding the sale of milk at retail for less than nine cents a quart) (repudiating *Lochner*, and holding generally that economic liberties will receive only *minimal* due process review).

6. See Justice Douglas's elaboration in Griswold v. Connecticut, 381 U.S. 479 (1965).

7. I.e. if they are protected under the very demanding standard of judicial review reflected in cases such as Griswold v. Connecticut, 381 U.S. 479 (1965), and Roe v. Wade, 410 U.S. 113 (1973) (and note how far removed the kinds of interests *actually* involved in both those cases seem to be from anything facially suggested by the first amendment itself).

will be altogether strictly respected by the Supreme Court, i.e. not subject to being balanced away (by the judiciary) or traded off at all.[8]

B

In support of this notion, moreover, consider the following observation as well: that the first amendment to the constitution is more absolute in its terms than are other amendments and other provisions that secure certain other rights even in the Bill of Rights itself. The fourth amendment, for example, secures the right of the people only from "unreasonable" searches and seizures; the fifth amendment provides for "due" process of law; and the eighth amendment prohibits "cruel and unusual" punishments and "excessive" fines or bails. The first amendment, by the way of contrast, acknowledges no overriding conditions that would provide any excuse for any Act of Congress abridging the freedom of speech or of the press.

C

The same conclusion might also seem well warranted on the following grounds as well, namely: a comparison of the first amendment in the Constitution of the United States with the more compromised style of provisions respecting freedom of speech and of the press in other constitutions. (Nearly 200 countries currently operate under written constitutions, incidentally, but the majority of these national constitutions have been adopted only since 1970, and scarcely a half-dozen predate 1900.) Note how they differ from our own:

Norway (1814), Article 100: There shall be liberty of the Press. No person may be punished for any writing, whatever its contents, which he has caused to be printed or published, *unless* he willfully and manifestly has either himself shown, or incited others to, disobedience to the laws, contempt of religion, morality or the constitutional powers, or resistance to their orders, *or* has made false and defamatory accusations against anyone.[9]

---

8. Additionally, one might also take for granted that, given the Court's generous notion of "penumbras" of the first amendment, the amendment's own terms will of course be very generously construed, e.g., be deemed to cover varieties of expression though not themselves literally "speech" in the narrowest dictionary sense (e.g., arm bands, flags, sculptures). Indeed, the usual presumption that dates at least from McCulloch v. Maryland, 17 U.S. (4 Wheat.) 316 (1819) (Marshall's famous dictum that it is a Constitution that is being expounded, one intended to endure and to be equal to circumstances only dimly foreseen, and thus not grudgingly to be construed), ought also apply to the first amendment especially since, freedom of speech and of the press being explicitly mentioned liberties in the Bill of Rights, they are among the "preferred" liberties the Constitution enshrines.

9. The Constitution of Norway is the second oldest in the world; it is antedated only by our own.

The People's Republic of China (1982), Article 35: Citizens of the Peoples Republic of China enjoy freedom of speech, of the press, of assembly, of association, of procession and of demonstration.[10]

The Former Soviet Union (1978), Article 50: *In accordance with the interests of the people and in order to strengthen and develop the socialist system*, citizens of the USSR are guaranteed freedom of speech, of the press, and of assembly, meetings, street processions and demonstrations.[11]

England ( ), Article ( ):[12]

Denmark (1953), Article 77: Any person shall be entitled to publish his thoughts in printing, in writing, and in speech, *provided* that he may be held answerable in a court of justice.[13]

Germany (Federal Republic) (1949), Article V: (1) Everyone shall have the right freely to express and disseminate his opinion by speech, writing and pictures and freely to instruct himself from generally accessible sources *** (2) *These rights are limited by the provisions of the general laws* ***.[14]

The Federal Republic of Nigeria, Sections 38 and 43: [38] Every person shall be entitled to freedom of expression, including freedom to hold opinions and to receive and impart ideas and information without interference. *** [43] Nothing in section *** 38 *** of this Constitution shall invalidate any law that is reasonably justifiable in a democratic society—in the interest of defense, public safety, public order, public morality, or public health ***.

---

10. But see also Article 51 ("The exercise by citizens *** of their freedoms *** may not infringe upon the interests of the state, of society and of the collective ***.").

11. See also Article 59 ("Citizens of the USSR are obliged to *** comply with the standards of socialist conduct ***.).

12. The English have no constitutional provision respecting freedom of speech or of the press—they have no written constitution at all. The English retain the criminal common law of blasphemy (albeit only scandalous and offensive attacks on the religion of the realm are thus punishable, and not equivalently offensive treatment of other religions, e.g., Islam); prior restraints, contempt of court sanctions over the press, and quite strict liability for defamation remain more sweeping in England than in the U.S.; statutory criminal sanctions and civil liability are also substantially broader in England, e.g., under the Official Secrets Act, the Race Relations Act. For a contemporary and comprehensive treatise on limitations on speech and press in England, see Individual Rights and the Law in Britain (McCrudeen & Chambers, eds., 1994).

13. See also Article 79 ("The citizen shall without previous permission be entitled to assemble unarmed [but] open-air meetings may be prohibited when it is feared that they may constitute a danger to the public peace.")

14. See also Article 18 ("Whoever abuses the freedom of expression *** in order to attack the free, democratic basic order, shall forfeit these basic rights."). For a comprehensive comparative treatise on German and U.S. constitutional law, noting the significant areas of difference with respect to freedom of speech and press, see David P. Currie, The Constitution of the Federal Republic of Germany (1994).

Canadian Charter of Rights and Freedoms (1982): §2. Everyone has the following fundamental freedoms:

(a) Freedom of Conscience and Religion

(b) Freedom of thought, belief, opinion and expression, including freedom of the press and other media of communications.

(c) Freedom of Peaceful assembly; and

(d) Freedom of association.

§1. The Canadian Charter of Rights and Freedoms guarantees the rights and freedoms set out in it subject only to such reasonable limits prescribed by law as can be demonstrably justified in a free and democratic society.

The United States (1791), First Amendment: Congress shall make no law abridging the freedom of speech or of the press.[15]

Note that these provisions tend to fall into three or, at most, four, categories. Roughly, they may be described in the following way. **First**, most characteristically, the constitutional protection furnished freedom of speech and of the press from government regulation is *significantly qualified* in some way. Or, **second**, there is just *no* constitutional protection provided at all. The Norwegian, Soviet, and West German provisions all seem on their face to be of the first, substantially qualified sort. As an example of the second sort, the English have no written constitution and thus no clauses protecting free speech and press to apply. Or, **third**, the constitutional provision may seem on its face to be of a sort that is merely assertive, rather than prohibitory against legislative power. The provision from the 1982 Constitution of China seems to be of this sort, i.e. it merely makes a claim that may or may not actually be true.[16] And, as noted in the footnote accompanying the principal provision even in this modern Constitution of The People's Republic of China, that provision is also heavily qualified by other provisions elsewhere found in the same Constitution. Among the three types (precatory, heavily qualified, or nonexistent), the *likely* protection to be furnished in litigation seeking to forestall the application of acts adopted by the national legislature may be pretty limited and uncertain, may it not?

---

15. I.e. Congress shall make NO law abridging the freedom of speech or of the press. "NO LAW" at all.

16. E.g., recall the events in the streets of Beijing, in the summer of 1989, in Tiananmen Square. And see Assoc. Press wire release, dateline Beijing, June 2, 1995 ("Torture, forced labor and detention without trial underpin worsening political repression in China, Amnesty International said in a report today. *** The report's release coincides with the anniversary of the June 4, 1989, crackdown on the pro-democracy movement at Tiananmen Square, in which hundreds of people were slaughtered by Chinese troops. *** Foreign Ministry spokesman, Chen Jian, said Thursday that dwelling on the 1989 "incident" was of no use. *** "Chinese citizens have the right to exercise their democratic rights in accordance with the constitution," Chen said. "The Chinese judicial departments and authorities are also entitled to take actions against those things in violation of Chinese laws.").

Additionally, even in respect to these *qualified* clauses protecting freedom of speech and of the press (note, once again, for instance, the qualifying clause in the Constitution of the German Federal Republic), some may turn out to be even less substantial in practice than one might suppose. Such would be the case, for instance, if the clause in question is *not one the courts are deemed authorized to enforce*. As it happens, this turns out to be the case in respect to the relevant clause in the constitution of China. Indeed it is true of *most* constitutions throughout the world. So, while such constitutional clauses are not necessarily useless (these kinds of express constitutional clauses may provide some sense of self-restraint within the respective national assemblies of those countries that have adopted them), they are not very reassuring on their face.

In contrast, the one uncompromised, stand-alone clause not captured in any of these three categories is the last and also the earliest; i.e. that of the Constitution of the United States, dating, as it does, unchanged, from 1791. To be sure, the first amendment says nothing about what state legislatures or even local city councils may be free to do (a problem we shall need to worry about).[17] But, as to *Congress*, well, it seems to be quite plain and absolutely unequivocal: "Congress shall make NO law abridging the freedom of speech or of the press," i.e. not just "not many laws," not just "laws unreasonably" abridging the freedom of speech, but NO laws at all, absolutely, positively, NONE.[18] So, we start this course on the first amendment with that very notion. For the reasons we have now briefly canvassed, it would seem to be exactly the right place to start.

The "reasons," again, are these. *First*, we already know that some rights merely penumbral to the first amendment are highly protected (*Griswold, Roe*) simply on the strength of that penumbral relationship, and even though those rights are not

17. Note, too, that on its face it also says nothing to restrain either *the courts* or *the executive* from interfering with freedom of speech or of the press (i.e. it is directed solely to Congress). Might this pose some problem also?

18. Justice Hugo L. Black, who served on the Supreme Court during the most active period of the Court's first amendment doctrinal developments (1937-1971), entirely agreed. See, e.g., Barenblatt v. United States, 360 U.S. 109, 141-43 (1959) (dissenting opinion) ("I do not agree that laws *** abridging First Amendment freedoms can be justified by a congressional or judicial balancing process. *** Not only does this violate the genius of our *written* Constitution, but it runs expressly counter to the injunction to Court and Congress made by Madison when he introduced the Bill of Rights.") (emphasis in original.); New York Times v. Sullivan, 376 U.S. 254, 293, 295 (1964) (concurring opinion) ("In my opinion the Federal Constitution *** has grant[ed] the press an *absolute* immunity for criticism of the way public officials do their public duty.") (emphasis added). For a well written defense of Justice Black's textual literalism in matters of constitutional interpretation, see Charles Black, Mr. Justice Black, the Supreme Court and the Bill of Rights, Harper's, Feb. 1961, at 63. See also Tinsley E. Yarbrough, Mr. Justice Black and His Critics 130-150, 164-197 (1988); Hugo L. Black, The Bill of Rights, 35 N.Y.U.L.Rev. 865, 867 (1960); Edmond Cahn, Justice Black and First Amendment "Absolutes": A Public Interview, 37 N.Y.U. L.Rev. 549 (1962); Harry Kalven, Upon Rereading Mr. Justice Black on the First Amendment, 14 U.C.L.A.L.Rev. 428 (1967); Charles A. Reich, Mr. Justice Black and the Living Constitution, 76 Harv.L.Rev. 673 (1963).

expressly protected; presumably, express first amendment rights ("the freedom of speech and of the press") will be protected more fully than such penumbral rights already highly protected though not explicitly enumerated at all. *Second,* the first amendment itself acknowledges no overriding conditions that would provide excuse for any act of Congress abridging the freedom of speech or of the press. *Third,* the first amendment differs in this respect from other amendments that acknowledge some excusing condition in respect to some other express preferred rights (e.g., a search that is not an "unreasonable" search is not forbidden by the terms of the fourth amendment—the first amendment has no equivalently excusing phrase). *Fourth,* the first amendment differs in the same way from "free speech" provisions in other constitutions, too, i.e. unlike them, it does not provide that there are occasions and circumstances when one's freedom of speech must yield to other social interests of a more compelling good. In short, to paraphrase Justice Black, *the framers did all the "balancing" when they adopted the first amendment in the absolute form Madison proposed.*[19] It is, therefore, not for the courts to "interpret" the first amendment to read into it phantom exceptions, qualifications, or limitations. It is, rather, their obligation to apply it, until such time as it may be changed. *Quod Erat Demonstrandum* (Q.E.D.), the first amendment absolutely protects free speech. The following figure may capture this perspective quite well:

Justice Black's First Amendment

[Protected Absolutely]

The Freedom of Speech
and of the Press

19. See n. 18 supra. See also Konigsberg v. California, 366 U.S. 36, 61 (1960) (Black, J. dissenting) ("...I believe that the First Amendment's unequivical command that there shall be no abridgement of the rights of free speech and assembly shows that the men who drafted our Bill of Rights did all the 'balancing' that was to be done in this field. The history of the First Amendment is too well known to require repeating here except to say that it certainly cannot be denied that the very object of adopting the First Amendment, as well as the other provisions of the Bill of Rights, was to put the freedoms protected there completely out of the area of a congressional control that may be attempted through the exercise of precisely those powers that are now being used to 'balance' the Bill of Rights out of existence.")

The following materials, however, show what became of this view, relatively early on.

II (A)
PATTERSON v. COLORADO
205 U.S. 454 (1907)

MR. JUSTICE HOLMES delivered the opinion of the court.

This is a writ of error to review a judgment upon an information for contempt. The contempt alleged was the publication of certain articles and a cartoon, which it was charged, reflected upon the motives and conduct of the Supreme Court of Colorado in cases still pending and were intended to embarrass the court in the impartial administration of justice.* There was a motion to quash on grounds of local law and the state constitution and also of the Fourteenth Amendment to the Constitution of the United States. This was overruled and thereupon an answer was filed, admitting the publication, denying the contempt, also denying that the cases referred to were still pending, except that the time for motions for rehearing had not elapsed, and averring that the motions for rehearing subsequently were overruled, except that in certain cases the orders were amended so that the democratic officeholders concerned could be sooner turned out of their offices. The answer went on to narrate the transactions commented on, at length, intimating that the conduct of the court was unconstitutional and usurping, and alleging that it was in aid of a scheme, fully explained, to seat various republican candidates, including the governor of the State, in place of democrats who had been elected, and that two of the judges of the court got their seats as a part of the scheme. Finally, the answer alleged that the respondent published the articles in pursuance of what he regarded as a public duty, repeated the previous objections to the information, averred the truth of the articles, and set up and

---

*. **[Ed. Note.** Thomas Patterson was a director, officer, and the principal shareholder of the News-Times Publishing Company, which owned The Rocky Mountain News and The Denver Times, and Patterson was manager and editor-in-chief of both newspapers. Colorado had adopted an amendment to the state constitution changing certain political processes, pursuant to which Democrats were elected in Denver. The state supreme court ruled the amendments invalid, in effect restoring the political mechanism as it had been prior to the amendments. In a series of articles, cartoons, and editorials, the News and the Times condemned the decision, suggesting that it was without any proper basis, and in words allegedly implying the judges reached the decision on crass political grounds favoring corporate interests and the Republican Party. (E.g., one early editorial, after lambasting the decision, concluded: "What next? If somebody will let us know what next the utility corporations of Denver and the political machine they control will demand, the question will be answered.") In criminal contempt proceedings brought in the state supreme court by the Attorney General, the court held Patterson guilty of common law criminal contempt as charged in the Attorney General's unverified information, imposed a fine of $1,000, and ordered "a committal until the payment thereof." The full case is reported at 35 Col. 253-461 (1906). See also L. A. Scot Powe, Jr., The Fourth Estate and the Constitution 1-16 (1991) (reviewing the highly partisan political circumstances associated with the *Patterson* case).]

claimed the right to prove the truth under the Constitution of the United States. Upon this answer the court, on motion, ordered judgment fining the plaintiff in error for contempt.

The foregoing proceedings are set forth in a bill of exceptions, and several errors are alleged. The difficulties with those most pressed is that they raise questions of local law, which are not open to reexamination here. The requirement in the Fourteenth Amendment of due process of law does not take up the special provisions of the state constitution and laws into the Fourteenth Amendment for purposes of the case, and in that way subject a state decision that they have been complied with to revision by this court. French v. Taylor, 199 U.S. 274, 278; Rawlins v. Georgia, 201 U.S. 638, 639; Burt v. Smith, 203 U.S. 129, 135. For this reason, if for no other, the objection that the information was not supported by an affidavit until after it was filed cannot be considered. See further Ex parte Wall, 107 U.S. 265. The same is true of the contention that the suits referred to in the article complained of were not pending. Whether a case shall be regarded as pending while it is possible that petition for rehearing may be filed, or, if in an appellate court, until the remittitur is issued, are questions which the local law can settle as it pleases without interference from the Constitution of the United States. It is admitted that this may be true in some other sense, but it is not true, it is said, for the purpose of fixing the limits of possible contempts. But here again the plaintiff in error confounds the argument as to the common law, or as to what it might be wise and humane to hold, with that concerning the State's constitutional power. If a State should see fit to provide in its constitution that conduct otherwise amounting to a contempt should be punishable as such if occurring at any time while the court affected retained authority to modify its judgment, the Fourteenth Amendment would not forbid. The only question for this court is the power of the State. Virginia v. Rives, 100 U.S. 313, 318; Missouri v. Dockery, 191 U.S. 165, 171. ***

It is argued that the articles did not constitute a contempt. In view of the answer, which sets out more plainly and in fuller detail what the articles insinuate and suggest, and in view of the position of the plaintiff in error that he was performing a public duty, the argument for a favorable interpretation of the printed words loses some of its force. However, it is enough for us to say that they are far from showing that innocent conduct has been laid hold of as an arbitrary pretense for an arbitrary punishment. Supposing that such a case would give the plaintiff in error a standing here, anything short of that is for the state court to decide. What constitutes contempt, as well as the time during which it may be committed, is a matter of local law.

The defense upon which the plaintiff in error most relies is raised by the allegation that the articles complained of are true and the claim of the right to prove the truth. He claimed this right under the constitutions both of the State and of the United States, but the latter ground alone comes into consideration here, for reasons already stated. Ex parte Kemmler, 136 U.S. 436. We do not pause to consider whether the claim was sufficient in point of form, although it is easier to refer to the Constitution generally for the supposed right than to point to the clause from which it springs. We leave undecided the question whether there is to be found in the Fourteenth Amendment a prohibition similar to that in the First. But even if we were to assume that freedom of speech and freedom of the press were protected from abridgment on the part not only of the United States but also of the States, still we should be far from the conclusion that the plaintiff in error would have us reach. In the first place, the main purpose of such constitutional provisions is "to prevent all such*previous restraints* upon publications as had been practiced by other governments," and they do not prevent the subsequent punishment of such as may be deemed contrary to the public welfare. Commonwealth v. Blanding, 3 Pick. 304, 313, 314; Respubica v. Oswald, 1 Dallas, 319, 325. The preliminary freedom extends as well to the false as to the true; the subsequent punishment may extend as well to the true as to the false. This was the law of criminal libel apart from statute in most cases, if not in all. Commonwealth v. Blanding, ubi sup.; 4 Bl.Com. 150.

In the next place, the rule applied to criminal libels applies yet more clearly to contempts. A publication likely to reach the eyes of a jury, declaring a witness in a pending cause a perjurer, would be none the less a contempt that it was true. It would tend to obstruct the administration of justice, because even a correct conclusion is not to be reached or helped in that way, if our system of trials is to be maintained. The theory of our system is that the conclusions to be reached in a case will be induced only by evidence and argument in open court, and not by any outside influence, whether of private talk or public print.

What is true with reference to a jury is true also with reference to a court. Cases like the present are more likely to arise, no doubt, when there is a jury and the publication may affect their judgment. Judges generally, perhaps, are less apprehensive that publications impugning their own reasoning or motives will interfere with their administration of the law. But if a court regards, as it may, a publication concerning a matter of law pending before it, as tending toward such an interference, it may punish it as in the instance put. When a case is finished, courts are subject to the same criticism as other people, but the propriety and necessity of preventing interference with the course of justice by premature statement, argument or intimidation hardly can be denied. Ex parte Terry, 128 U.S. 289; Telegram Newspaper Co. v. Commonwealth, 172 Massachusetts, 294; State v. Hart, 24 W. Va. 416; Myers v. State, 46 Ohio St. 473, 491; Hunt v. Clarke, 58 L.J.Q.B. 490, 492; Rex v. Parke [1903], 2 K.B. 432. It is objected that the judges were sitting in their own case. But the grounds upon which contempts are punished are impersonal. United States v. Shipp, 203 U.S. 563, 574. No doubt judges naturally would be slower to punish when the contempt carried with it a personally dishonoring charge, but a man cannot expect to secure immunity from punishment by the proper tribunal, by adding to illegal conduct a personal attack. It only remains to add that the plaintiff in error had his day in court and opportunity to be heard. We have scrutinized the case, but cannot say that it shows an infraction of rights under the Constitution of the United States, or discloses more than the formal appeal to that instrument in the answer to found the jurisdiction of this court.

Writ of error dismissed.

MR. JUSTICE HARLAN, dissenting.

I cannot agree that this writ of error should be dismissed.

By the First Amendment of the Constitution of the United States, it is provided that "Congress shall make no law respecting an establishment of religion, or abridging the freedom of speech, or of the press, or of the right of the people peaceably to assemble and to petition the Government for redress." In the Civil Rights cases, 109 U.S. 1, 20, it was adjudged that the Thirteenth Amendment, although in form prohibitory, had a reflex character in that it established and decreed universal civil and political freedom throughout the United States. In United States v. Cruikshank, 92 U.S. 542, 552, we held that the right of the people peaceably to assemble and to petition the Government for a redress of grievances—one of the rights recognized in and protected by the First Amendment against hostile legislation by Congress—was an attribute of "national citizenship." So the First Amendment, although in form prohibitory, is to be regarded as having a reflex character and as affirmatively recognizing freedom of speech and freedom of the press as rights belonging to citizens of the United States; that is, those rights are to be deemed attributes of national citizenship or citizenship of the United States. No one, I take it, will hesitate to say that a judgment of a Federal court, prior to the adoption of the Fourteenth Amendment, impairing or abridging freedom of speech or of the press, would have been in violation of the rights of "citizens of the United States" as guaranteed by the First Amendment; this, for the reason that the rights of free speech and a free press were, as already said, attributes of national citizenship before the Fourteenth Amendment was made a part of the Constitution.

Now, the Fourteenth Amendment declares, in express words, that "no State shall make or enforce any law which shall abridge the privileges or immunities of citizens of the United States." As the First Amendment guaranteed the rights of free speech and of a free press against hostile action by the United States, it would seem clear that when the Fourteenth Amendment prohibited the States from impairing or abridging the privileges of citizens of the United States it necessarily prohibited the States from impairing or abridging the constitutional rights of such citizens to free speech and a free press. But the court announces that it leaves undecided the specific question whether there is to be found in the Fourteenth Amendment a prohibition as to the rights of free speech and a free press similar to that in the First. It yet proceeds to say that the main purpose of such constitutional provisions was to prevent all such "*previous* restraints" upon publications as had been practiced by other governments, but not to prevent the subsequent punishment of such as may be deemed contrary to the public welfare. I cannot assent to that view, if it be meant that the legislature may impair or abridge the rights of a free press and of free speech whenever it thinks that the public welfare requires that to be done. The public welfare cannot override constitutional privileges, and if the rights of free speech and of a free press are, in their essence, attributes of national citizenship, as I think they are, then neither Congress nor any State since the adoption of the Fourteenth Amendment can, by legislative enactments or by judicial action, impair or abridge them. In my judgment the action of the court below was in violation of the rights of free speech and a free press as guaranteed by the Constitution.

I go further and hold that the privileges of free speech and of a free press, belonging to every citizen of the United States, constitute essential parts of every man's liberty, and are protected against violation by that clause of the Fourteenth Amendment forbidding a State to deprive any person of his liberty without due process of law. It is, I think, impossible to conceive of liberty, as secured by the Constitution against hostile action, whether by the Nation or by the States, which does not embrace the right to enjoy free speech and the right to have a free press. ***

B

In assessing how the view of the first amendment reflected in the majority opinion in *Patterson v. Colorado* differs from the "absolute" view with which we began, consider once again the following excerpt Justice Holmes provided for the Supreme Court in this case. Note, particularly, the citation of authority provided at the end:

> We leave undecided the question whether there is to be found in the Fourteenth Amendment a prohibition similar to that in the First. But even if we were to assume that freedom of speech and freedom of the press were protected from abridgment on the part not only of the United States but also of the States, still we should be far from the conclusion that the plaintiff in error would have us reach. In the first place, the main purpose of such constitutional provisions is "to prevent all such *previous restraints* upon publication as had been practiced by other governments," and they do not prevent the subsequent punishment of such as may be deemed contrary to the public welfare. *** The preliminary freedom extends to the false as to the true; the subsequent punishment may extend as well to the true as to the false. *** 4 Bl.Com.150.

C

The reference at the end (4 Bl.Com. 150) is citation shorthand for volume 4 of William Blackstone's Commentaries on the Laws of England. A reference to that work confirms Justice Holmes' impression. Here is Blackstone's own summary, which follows the page cited by Holmes:

W. Blackstone, IV Commentaries on the Laws of England 151-52 (1769):

In this [review of the form of criminal libel just discussed on page 150, namely, *libelli famosi*], and the other instances which we have lately considered, where blasphemous, immoral, treasonable, schismatical, seditious, or scandalous libels are punished by the English law, some with a greater, others with a less degree of severity, the *liberty of the press*, properly understood, is by no means infringed or violated. The liberty of the press is indeed essential to the nature of a free state: but this consists in laying no *previous* restraints upon publications, and not in freedom from censure for criminal matter when published. Every freeman has an undoubted right to lay what sentiments he pleases before the public; to forbid this, is to destroy the freedom of the press: but if he publishes what is improper, mischievous, or illegal, he must take the consequence of his own temerity. To subject the press to the restrictive power of a licenser, as was formerly done, both before and since the revolution,* is to subject all freedom of sentiment to the prejudices of one man, and make him the arbitrary and infallible judge of all controverted points in learning, religion,

---

*The art of printing, soon after its introduction, was looked upon (as well in England as in other countries) as merely a matter of state, and subject to the coercion of the crown. It was therefore regulated with us by the king's proclamations, prohibitions, charters of privilege and of licence, and finally by the decrees of the court of star chamber; which limited the number of printers, and of presses which each should employ, and prohibited new publications unless previously approved by proper licensers. On the demolition of this odious jurisdiction in 1641, the long parliament of Charles I, after their rupture with that prince, assumed the same powers as the starchamber exercised with respect to the licensing of books; and in 1643, 1647, 1649, and 1652, issued their ordinances for that purpose, founded principally on the starchamber decree of 1637. [These licensings practices and acts were] continued to 1692. It was then continued for two years longer by statute 4 W. & M. c. 24, but though frequent attempts were made by the government to revive it, in the subsequent part of that reign *** yet the parliament resisted it so strongly, that it finally expired, and the press became properly free, in 1694; and has ever since so continued. [Footnote by Blackstone.]

[**Ed. Note.** In 1644, a half-century before Parliament allowed the last press licensing law to expire without renewing it (as Blackstone notes *supra*), John Milton wrote his famous *Areopagitica*. The title is taken from "Areopagus," the council of ancient Athens and the place where petitions were presented to that council—the areopagus stands on a slight hill nearby the agora, the place where popular assemblies met. You may recall from Milton's compelling prose some of his moving passages on freedom of speech and of the press. ("Give me the liberty to know, to utter, and to argue freely according to conscience, above all liberties. *** And though all the winds of doctrine were let loose to play upon the earth, so Truth be in the field, we do injuriously by licencing and prohibiting to misdoubt her strength. Let her and Falsehood grapple; who ever knew Truth put to the wors, in a free and open encounter. Her confuting is the best and surest suppressing.") Milton's essay was addressed to Parliament. It was directed to licensing, and it is thus titled ("For the Liberty of *Unlicenc'd Printing*") (emphasis added). ("I mean not tolerated Popery, and open superstition, which as it extirpates all religions and civil supremacies, so it self should be extirpate *** that also which is impious or evil absolutely either against faith or manners no law can possibly permit, that intends not to unlaw it self ***.").]

and government. But to punish (as the law does at present) any dangerous or offensive writings, which, when published, shall on a fair and impartial trial be adjudged of a pernicious tendency, is necessary for the preservation of peace and good order, of government and religion, the only solid foundations of civil liberty. Thus the will of individuals is still left free; the abuse only of that free will is the object of legal punishment. Neither is any restraint hereby laid upon freedom of thought or enquiry: liberty of private sentiment is still left; the disseminating, or making public, of bad sentiments, destructive of the ends of society, is the crime which society corrects. A man (says a fine writer on this subject) may be allowed to keep poisons in his closet, but not publicly to vend them as cordials. And to this we may add, that the only plausible argument heretofore used for restraining the just freedom of the press, "that it was necessary to prevent the abuse of it," will entirely lose its force, when it is shewn (by a reasonable exertion of the laws) that the press cannot be abused to any bad purpose, without incurring a suitable punishment: whereas it never can be used to any good one, when under the control of an inspector. So true will it be found, that to censure the licentiousness, is to maintain the liberty, of the press.

D

The Court's treatment of the first amendment, in *Patterson v. Colorado*, is surely startling, especially when coupled with the extracts from Blackstone's Commentaries, on which Holmes relied in deciding the case, finding no reversible error in the conviction and fine of Patterson, for criminal contempt.[19] How does the Court understand the first amendment? And how does *Patterson* square with our first, "absolute," view?

Evidently, the answer to both questions is found in a single solution. It is found by taking a more measured view of that amendment, reading it in the following way: "Congress shall make NO law abridging *the* freedom of speech or of the press"—and by suggesting that "the" freedom of speech and "the" freedom of the press is coterminous with that freedom as it was understood as of 1769, which it was

19. Note, among other elements: (1) There was no state criminal law statute Patterson was alleged to have violated. (2) He was subjected to trial though no grand jury had determined suitable cause. (3) He was tried without benefit of jury [a significant matter—in the history of free speech and press, jury nullification played a powerful role]. (4) He was tried and sentenced by persons with a direct interest in the case. (5) The case on which the newspaper published its comments had already been concluded on the merits (only a motion for rehearing following final judgment was still pending). (6) The published statements alleged to constitute criminal contempt were obviously expressions of Patterson's opinion, i.e. an account of what, in his view, explained what had taken place. (7) Factual truth itself was ruled not to matter, i.e. *to be irrelevant as a matter of law.* (8) The court may also have not adhered even to state law. (On which of these issues would a different result be reached today? In England? In the United States? Why?)

the design of the first amendment to give constitutional status, as of 1791.[20]

If this is correct, there is nonetheless very little problem in squaring *Patterson* with the first amendment. Ironically, there is also no problem squaring it with the literalist views of Justice Black. Nor is there any problem squaring it with our preliminary review, comparing the first amendment with other constitutional clauses. Rather, the suggested resolution is simple. It is this. The first amendment *is* unqualified, i.e. it *is* absolute: Congress shall, indeed, make no law abridging the freedom of speech or of the press, whether for a compelling reason or for any other reason. If it does, the Court is quite prepared to strike the law down. But, that which Congress is (unqualifiedly) forbidden to make any law abridging is simply "the" freedom of speech and of the press, i.e. "the" freedom referred to by the amendment. Thus, so long as Congress makes no law abridging "the" freedom of speech or of the press (i.e. the freedom of speech or of the press referred to by the amendment itself), it does nothing to offend the first amendment *at all*. The Court is not called upon to "balance" any interests, moreover, any more than Justice Black supposed. Rather, it is merely to determine objectively, even as Holmes did in *Patterson*, whether there was any congressional trespass on "the" freedom of speech or of the press to which the amendment itself refers.

To be sure, "the" freedom of speech and of the press thus secured by the first amendment may not be known without reference to something lying outside the Constitution itself, but once the proper reference is made (and its content objectively supplied and accordingly filled in), the amendment fully applies. The reference is to the freedom of speech and of the press as it was known to have developed roughly as of the date the first amendment was adopted, *nothing less*, albeit, of course, also *nothing more*.[21]

E

Does this view of the matter effectively trash the amendment? Or does it, for instance, make the first amendment virtually no better than what the English have (namely, no first amendment at all)? Clearly, it does not, in the following sense. The difference is that, lacking our first amendment, the English continue to be dependent upon the sufferance of Parliament *even today* to preserve the enjoyment of such free-

---

20. To be sure, *Patterson* is a case reviewing "the freedom of *the press*" (rather than "the freedom of *speech*"), referring to that freedom (even as Blackstone does) as the absence of prior restraints, not protection from post-publication amercement) (and note Holmes' point—that "[t]he preliminary freedom extends as well to the false as to the true; *the subsequent punishment may extend as well to the true as to the false*."). But there is no reason to suppose the point of reference for determining "the freedom of speech" would be a different one, is there? Presumably it will be the same point of reference: what was protected in English law as of 1769, but not more (for it is *that* freedom of speech which is understood by "the" freedom of speech), is protected by the first amendment.

21. Additional protection for freedom of the press and of speech would be sought in positive legislation, i.e. the first amendment merely establishes the minimum, not the maximum Congress (or each state) might affirmatively provide.

dom of speech and of the press as they had secured as of 1769 (the date of Blackstone's Commentaries). In the United States, the first amendment protects that complement of free speech and free press from congressional interference, albeit, perhaps, nothing more. Presumably Parliament could even now reinstate a requirement of press licensing although it has had no such system since 1694. In the United States, presumably, Congress could do nothing of the sort.[22]

Still, even allowing for this difference, one would agree that the first amendment as thus construed falls far short of providing the absolute bulwark we earlier supposed.

III (A)

Note that the dissent by Justice Harlan, in *Patterson*, was mainly directed to the question of the extent to which the fourteenth amendment did or did not pull over the protections of the first amendment into the privileges and immunities clause of the fourteenth amendment, rather than to the additional question, namely, assuming that it did, what then? If the first amendment would not preclude a federal criminal contempt prosecution in a like set of circumstances as those involved in the *Patterson* case (and where is Justice Harlan's demonstration that it would?), what does his dissent come to, in the end? The equivalency, if there is one, between the fourteenth amendment and the first amendment, is unquestionably highly consequential.[23] Even so, i.e. even under Justice Harlan's view, water does not rise higher than the source from which it flows. Accordingly, the fourteenth amendment will not provide more protection from state court contempt sanctions than the first amendment would provide in like circumstances from federal court sanctions, for the fourteenth amendment does not rise "higher" than the first. If, then, the first amendment would not forbid an equivalent federal criminal contempt prosecution, the dissent fails to show how the fourteenth amendment forbids such a prosecution in a state court even by its own test. So the main issue seems to be the one we have examined here, as the

---

22. Presumably Congress could not do so, moreover, regardless of how "compelling" the circumstances and regardless of how few, or easy, the conditions of securing such a license might be. (**Query**, however: if it is true as a minimum that at least the first amendment flatly forbids any act of Congress from imposing a licensing system on freedom of speech or of the press, how can one square the constitutionality of the Federal Communications Act of 1934, insofar as it makes it a criminal offense to broadcast *without a license* granted by the FCC, subject to grant, renewal, and cancellation, under such standards as are provided for in the act? Is CBS *not* a part of "the press"? Is Dan Rather *less* engaged in free speech than George Will? Isn't the FCA a modern example of exactly the kind of licensing system even a pure "Blackstone" view of the first amendment forbids?)

23. We have already noted that the vast majority of likely abridgments of free speech and of the press will numerically arise as a consequence of state, city, and county laws and practices, rather than from Congress; it is no coincidence that the vast majority of "first amendment" cases decided by the Supreme Court during the past fifty years arise under state or local laws. So of course the so-called "incorporation" debate (i.e. the extent to which the fourteenth amendment pulls across the Bill of Rights for purposes of equal protection against the states) is highly consequential. We shall look at it, again, in due course. See *infra* pages 56-70.

important one, after all. And, treating that issue straightforwardly, as we have now tried to do, fairly and fully, it has brought us to a rather disappointing place.

B

It may seem odd that the conclusion we have reached seems to be what it is. What it suggests is that to understand the first amendment (and also, therefore, to study for this course), what one needs best to do is to "read Blackstone's Commentaries on the Laws of England, principally volume iv of the 1769 edition."

As, according to Blackstone, the criminal contempt prosecution of an editor in Patterson's position was entertainable at common law (and "the *liberty of the press*, properly understood, is by no means [thereby] infringed or violated"[24]), we would proceed in the same fashion in every case, including all cases involving acts of Congress such as the Sedition Act of 1798[25] were it re-enacted even now. If, by the same reference, i.e. to Blackstone, *the* liberty of the press "properly understood" would not have been regarded as thereby infringed by any equivalent criminal prosecution for seditious libel at common law, in England, around 1769, neither would it be objectionable here, pursuant to an act of Congress, so far as the first amendment is concerned. If, but only if, by the same reference, such a prosecution would have been regarded as infringing "the" liberty of the press, according to Blackstone's report, then neither may it be pursued here, and an act of Congress presuming to authorize it would be void. Both ways, evidently, our proposition will hold. *Quod Erat Demonstrandum*: studying Blackstone is the proper, objective

---

24. We are merely quoting here from the passages from Blackstone reproduced earlier. (The italics are in the original.)

25. The Act referred to may be found in 1 Stat. 596. Patterned after the English law of seditious libel, it was adopted in response to the seeming imminence of war with France, just seven years after the first amendment was ratified. It was applied a number of times and sustained against constitutional objection in the lower courts, but the Supreme Court never addressed it (though several of the Supreme Court Justices were involved in the cases in which it was used, in their role as circuit court judges), and it expired by its own terms, in 1801. Shortly after coming to office as President, Jefferson issued unconditional pardons to all those convicted under the act, answering in correspondence to an inquiry by Abigail Adams, John Adams' wife, that he did so because in his view the Sedition Act was unconstitutional and invalid under the first amendment. (The prosecutions and convictions had been obtained during John Adams' administration.) The principal provision was this: "*If any person shall write, print, utter or publish any false and malicious writing against the government of the United States, or either house of congress, or the president, with intent to defame them, or either of them, or to bring them or either of them into contempt, or disrepute; or to excite against them or either of them, the hatred of the good people of the United States, then such person, being thereof convicted before any court of the United States having jurisdiction thereof shall be punished by a fine not exceeding two thousand dollars, and by imprisonment not exceeding two years.*"

measure of the first amendment and of this course.[26]

Moreover, if this proposition does hold, neither should it matter if that study should turn out to yield a rather disappointing content.[27] And neither should it matter if that study would show that the first amendment is a more weakly enacted restriction on national acts of speech and press regulation than the foreign constitutional provisions we were tentatively (and unfavorably) comparing earlier on. So far as either may be true, still, to take Justice Black's own point seriously—that the first amendment is to be respected by the courts until such time as it is altered by amendment—it is obviously not for the courts to "balance" the claims of free speech or press differently than was done by the Constitution. It is, rather, for the courts to apply the Constitution, no more, no less, as it is.[28] One may put the same point more aggressively in the following way: If we were inclined to rally to this view respecting the role and duty of the Supreme Court when we held the view that the first amendment was "actually" very strong and highly protective, what inconsistency now moves us to desert it, merely seeing the mistake we had laid up in our earlier hopes?

C

Yet, before leaving this discussion, as though it were now quite complete, if the Harlan opinion does *not* convincingly show that the amendment meant to repudiate Blackstone,[29] on the other hand, in fairness to Harlan, the Holmes opinion may not

---

26. Just so, Leonard Levy concludes: "If *** a choice must be made between two propositions, first, that the [freedom of speech and press] clause substantially embodied the Blackstonian definition and left the law of seditious libel in force, or repudiated Blackstone and superseded the common law, *the evidence points strongly in support of the former proposition.*" Leonard W. Levy, Emergence of a Free Press 281 (1985) (emphasis added).

27. It would yield "a rather disappointing content," incidentally, even as illustrated by the *Patterson* case itself. If one will take the time to read Blackstone's coverage of the common law and of parliamentary discretion to limit speech and press in England (to avoid all speech and publication of a "pernicious tendency" as noted in one part of the excerpt we have already earlier quoted), as of 1769, one will find not a great deal that could not be done. (Indeed, it raises a fair question of why an amendment doing no more than to enact Blackstone, so to speak, would have been thought worthwhile to bother with at all. Certainly there is no suggestion that there was otherwise such likelihood that Congress might somehow embark on a press licensing system, i.e. that it was proposed to head off some imminent or feared possibility of such a system.)

28. The framers, we might say, did all the balancing when they adopted the first amendment in the Blackstone form, as they did. Such alterations as may come, must come—if at all—solely pursuant to article V.

29. And if to repudiate Blackstone, then, instead, to enact *what*? I.e. if one were to succeed in showing that there is no convincing evidence that the first amendment deliberately used the phrase "the freedom of speech and of the press" with any such limited reference in mind as "the extent of protection generally respected in England and/or among the colonies and states as of 1769 or 1789 protecting freedom of speech and of the press from prior restraints *but not otherwise*" [which, in a nutshell, was Blackstone's view of the law of England], what then? Nothing else follows per se. (E.g., does it follow that therefore an act of Congress, say, forbidding an interstate dealer in pork bellies knowingly to misrepresent the nutritional benefits of pork bellies, on pain of civil sanctions to be imposed by the FTC

be much better to show the opposite, i.e. that the amendment meant merely to shield speech and press from certain kinds of prior restraints it might be feared Congress might be tempted to impose.[30] Rather, Holmes also seemed to take much for granted, didn't he, but he did not pursue the matter as he is clear that, in any event, the fourteenth amendment (which is all that is involved in the*Patterson* case) may not incorporate the first amendment—so the exact field of the first amendment is not important—in *Patterson*—to decide.

Actually, the scholarship otherwise supporting the "Blackstone-enactment" view of the first amendment, including Leonard Levy's own (excellent) work, is quite mixed.[31] What it may show is, principally, that there was very considerable apprehension of what Congress might presume to do once launched under its new, larger set of enumerated powers just then granted in the new Constitution of 1789. And what it may also show is that there was a widespread unwillingness to trust to earlier assurances that the Congress would, even without any first amendment,[32]

(Federal Trade Commission) after a full and fair due process hearing reviewable on appeal, is obviously a violation of the first amendment? Literally, under Justice Black's view, it would seem to be so. Is it arguable, however, that "something in between" Blackstone and Black can logically be worked out? But how will one determine what that "something in between" is?

30. Both of the cases cited by Justice Holmes in *Patterson* were themselves also merely state cases (*Oswald* is a 1788 state criminal contempt case decided by the Pennsylvania supreme court; *Blanding* is an 1825 case from Massachusetts.) *Neither* involve an act of Congress or the first amendment as such. As we will see early on, moreover, Holmes substantially changed his mind about this matter. *See*, e.g., Abrams v. United States, 250 U.S. 616, 630-631 (1919); David S. Bogen, The Free Speech Metamorphosis of Mr. Justice Holmes, 11 Hofstra L.Rev. 97 (1982); David P. Rabban, The Emergence of Modern First Amendment Doctrine, 50 U.Chi.L.Rev. 1205, 1303-20 (1983).

31. For three critical reviews of Levy, see David A. Anderson, The Origins of the Press Clause, 30 U.C.L.A.L.Rev. 455 (1983) (replied to, 32 U.C.L.A.L.Rev. 177 (1984); William T. Mayton, Seditious Libel and the Lost Guarantee of a Freedom of Expression, 84 Colum.L.Rev. 91 (1984) (replied to, 37 Stan.L.Rev. 767 (1875)); David P. Rabban, The Ahistorical Historian: Leonard Levy on Freedom of Expression in Early American History, 37 Stan.L.Rev. 795 (1985). For two of the best historical works on freedom of speech and of the press in England and in early America, see Edward Gerard Hudon, Freedom of Speech and Press in America (1963); Fred Seaton Siebert, Freedom of the Press in England 1476-1776 (1952). The standard work in support of the view that the first amendment repudiated, rather than assimilated, Blackstone and the common law of seditious libel is Zechariah Chafee, Free Speech in the United States (1942).

32. The first amendment, incidentally, was originally the third amendment within the list of twelve amendments Congress submitted for ratification by the states, in 1789. The first two amendments did not achieve a sufficient number of state ratification votes to become part of the Constitution. (The original first amendment would have fixed a certain formula for the number of Representatives. The original second amendment provided that "No law, varying the compensation for the services of Senators and Representatives, shall take effect, until an election for Representatives shall have intervened." The original second amendment was finally ratified by a thirty-eighth state (Michigan) on May 7, 1992, more than two centuries after its proposal by Congress. It is now the twenty-seventh amendment, although a question remains as to whether the drawn out ratification process satisfied Article V. *See supra* page xlii.

simply have no power whatever in respect to speech or press.[33] The several states in fact treated freedom of speech and of the press quite variously. The first amendment may well have reflected a widespread resolve that however much that state of affairs would continue even after the Constitution went into effect, *Congress* (in contradistinction to the several states) should have little or no role to play.[34] And, if

---

33. Alexander Hamilton, in Federalist No. 84, pressed this argument as a reason for not proposing anything resembling the first amendment. He argued that whatever form of words might be used in framing some section of the Constitution, or some amendment to the Constitution, respecting protection of freedom of the press, would be confusing: "For why declare that things shall not be done which there is no power to do? Why, for instance, should it be said, that the liberty of the press shall not be restrained, when no power is given by which restrictions may be imposed?"

The argument was only a partial and temporary success. Others pointed out that Article I, Section 9 of the Constitution already enumerated a short list of positive restrictions on Congress, thus the precedent for taking additional express precautions was already set. The absence of a more elaborate Bill of Rights held up ratification in a number of states including New York and Virginia (both states were considered crucial even if nine other states might ratify); in North Carolina, ratification was delayed until the Bill of Rights was actually introduced. As reflected in St. George Tucker's observations (see note 34 *infra*), the fact that no express power was granted to Congress to regulate speech or press was deemed insufficient; the concern was that the power would be claimed indirectly, e.g., as an incident to regulate commerce among the several states or as an incident of other powers enumerated in Article I.See also L. A. Scot Powe, Jr., *The Fourth Estate and the Constitution* 1-16 (1991) (as a result of controversy associated with the Sedition Act of 1798, "subsequently the Supreme Court, historians, and lawyers would ask of the First Amendment a question it was not intended to answer: what did the First Amendment say about the *scope* of freedom of the press? The First Amendment was not intended to answer that question, because that question was left entirely to the states.")

34. For example, in his appendix to his 1803 edition of Blackstone's Commentaries, St. George Tucker (Professor of Law at William & Mary) distinguished the pertinence of Blackstone in just this way (at 29): "The danger justly apprehended by those states which insisted that the federal government should possess no power, directly or *indirectly*, over the subject, was, that those who were entrusted with the administration might be forward in considering every thing as a crime against the government, which might operate to their own personal disadvantage; it was therefore made a fundamental article of the federal compact, that no such power should be exercised, or claimed by the federal government; leaving it to the state governments to exercise such jurisdiction and control over the subject, as their several constitutions and laws permit." (emphasis added). Levy acknowledges that this was consistently James Madison's view (at 318): ("The amendment, Madison declared, was intended to have the broadest construction on freedom of the press as well as religion. It 'meant a positive denial to Congress of any power whatever on the subject.'")

In proposing the Bill of Rights in the first Congress, Madison also recorded his expectation of judicial enforcement as well. Address by James Madison before the United States House of Representatives, June 8, 1789, reprinted in 5 The Writings of James Madison 389 (G. Hunt ed. 1904) ("If they are incorporated into the constitution, independent tribunals of justice will consider themselves in a peculiar manner the guardians of these rights.") See also William Van Alstyne, Congressional Power and Free Speech: Levy's Legacy Revisited, 99 Harv.L.Rev. 1089 (1986). The concern of the Bill of Rights was a concern to restrict Congress, see Barron v. Mayor and City Council of Baltimore, 32 U.S. (7 Pet.) 243 (1833). ("[I]t is universally understood, it is a part of the history of the day, that the great revolution which established the constitution of the Untied States, was not effected without immense opposition. Serious fears were extensively entertained, that those powers which the patriot statesmen, who then

that were so, then certainly a reference to Blackstone would be a very poor guide in understanding the stringency of the first amendment enacted as a restriction on *Congress*, or on the national government, understanding that it would have no implications for the several states.

D

Between such words as "little" and "no" (i.e. as in the phrase that the first amendment meant that Congress "should have *little or no* role" in regulating free speech or the free press in the United States), however, there is still an equivocation, isn't there, respecting what Congress may or may not be able to do. So, what shall one do about that?[35]

One might simply want to eliminate the weasel word, "little," of course. That would take care of the problem. It would also be consistent with some things we covered in Part I—as well as greatly shorten this course. There are, however, two sorts of problems with this solution: one that perhaps ought not trouble us, intellectually, but the other of which probably will.

The first is merely the practical problem that the courts (including the Supreme Court) have never been willing to read the first amendment as disarming Congress of *all* power to legislate in reference to things spoken or printed. Even worse, despite the review we have attempted here, it is difficult to find an Archimedean point strong enough to insist that the first amendment so demands.[36] Some of the problems that

---

watched over the interests of the country, deemed essential to union, and to the attainment of those invaluable objects for which union was sought, might be exercised in a manner dangerous to liberty. In almost every convention by which the constitution was adopted, amendments to guard against the abuse of power were recommended. These amendments demanded security against the apprehended encroachments of the general government—not against those of the local governments. In compliance with a sentiment thus generally expressed, to quiet fears thus extensively entertained, amendments were proposed by the required majority in congress, and adopted by the states. These amendments contain no expression indicating an intention to apply them to the state governments.")

35. I.e. which is it, "little" or "no" role [for Congress to play]? And if "little" (rather than "no") role, just *how* little, and as determined by *whose* opinion, and by *what* standards?

36. Footnote 29 *supra* provided an example of an act of Congress regulating speech of a sort: (an act authorizing Federal Trade Commission cease and desist orders against false and misleading advertising of commercial goods and services in interstate commerce, after full hearing, with full judicial review. Doubtless such an act may raise substantial first amendment questions. Still, it is difficult to find support for the argument that Congress has *no* power (but, rather, is forbidden by the first amendment) to provide *any* remedies at all for interstate commercial fraud committed by means of oral or printed speech.

Consider also acts of Congress such as these: an act subjecting one to federal criminal prosecution for committing perjury as a sworn witness in a federal court; or an act making it a federal felony to solicit another to kill the President of the United States. Each is an instance of "speech" specifically criminalized by Act of Congress. Does the first amendment invalidate the congressional act? Does it forbid either act from being applied? Would the act punishing criminal solicitation be valid only if the solicitation were actually acted upon? But why should that make any difference, either way?

The book most often credited with presenting the historical case for a strong first amendment (in contrast with the Levy book, previously cited), is Zechariah Chafee, Free Speech in the United States

beset the first amendment are apparently quite genuine. They will not all, easily, just "go away." If that is so, however, then where are we? At worst we are simply better prepared, more intelligently to begin on our work, once again.

Indeed, one struggles with these things, even as you will now do, conscientiously, as a student. It may well be the case that the first amendment did not just enact Blackstone into constitutional status. As we shall see, moreover, the Supreme Court eventually agreed. *Patterson v. Colorado* is not the last word. As to the many other questions we have now raised for purposes of introduction, the cases we shall be studying show a long series of provisional answers, many of which are highly contestable as, indeed, we shall see. Even so, despite its difficulties, this is a serious and worthy subject—there may be none personally more absorbing, or overall more significant,[37] to pursue. We shall have too little time to consider the full subject in every detail. Still, we shall come to terms with most of the basic field.[38] So far as our introductory tour is concerned, we have taken the measure of two very different views of the first amendment, neither of which appears quite to have worked out:

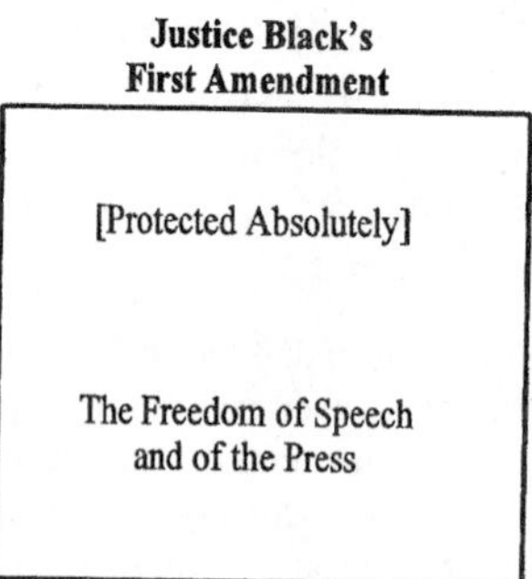

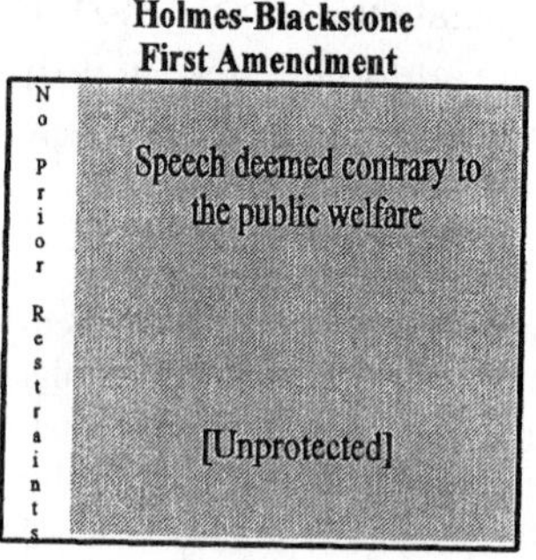

(1942) (also cited in note 31 *supra*). Yet, Professor Chafee's presentation falls very short of adopting the "absolute" form of the first amendment. (Id. at 145, 149-50: "We can all agree that the free speech clauses do not wipe out the common law as to obscenity, profanity, and defamation of individuals. *** [O]bscenity, profanity, and gross libels of individuals *** fall outside the protection of the free speech clauses as I have defined them [as do criminal solicitation or even talking scurrilously about the flag].") Actually, there is good reason to disagree with Professor Chafee on some of these matters, as to Congress, as we shall see in this course. The point remains, however, that Chafee's examples gave him some difficulty nonetheless.

37. It is an idle pastime, a child's game, perhaps, to say which portions of the entire Constitution one might regard as most critical (e.g., the equal protection clause?—the clauses protecting one's right to vote?—that which provides for amendments?—those enabling Congress to act?). Taking the world all in all, however, a good case can be made that even here in the United States, the most vital clauses may be Article I, Section 9's provision for habeas corpus and the first amendment clause on free speech and free press. The first may enable one to be released from prison when one is wrongfully held against one's will by government power. The second enables one freely to speak one's mind. Grant people guarantees such as these to live by and they may be able to move the world.

38. The latter third of these materials takes up the first amendment clauses addressed to religion ("Congress shall make no law respecting an establishment of religion or prohibiting the free exercise

We now begin again, with a somewhat more complex figure that will look more like the following one:

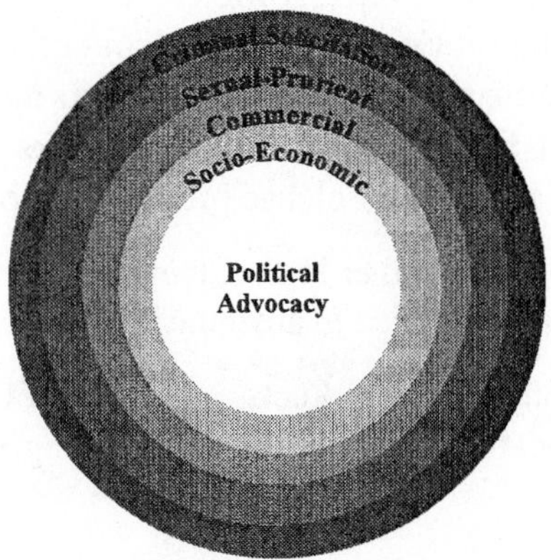

Before embarking on the modern case law of the first amendment, however, it may also be helpful to review the following Coda on other constitutional clauses—clauses related to each other and to the first amendment, in the constitutional history of freedom of speech and of the press, both in England and in the United States.

CODA TO "THE INTRODUCTION TO THE FIRST AMENDMENT": *OTHER* CLAUSES RELATED TO THE FREEDOM OF SPEECH AND OF THE PRESS

The constitutional clauses interpreted in*Patterson v. Colorado* were drawn from the first and fourteenth amendments, of course, just as will routinely be true throughout this course. There are, however, other clauses in the Constitution one should want to know more about because they, too, may bear on the subject in which we are engaged. Because this course does not provide time to deal with these other clauses in any systematic way, and because not all of them are necessarily treated in other courses for their relevance to the subject we are particularly concerned with in this course, it is useful at least to be aware of them, now. There may be times when reference to one or another of these clauses would usefully provide argumentative support buttressing a direct first amendment question as such (i.e. there may be a synergy among several clauses).[39] Thus this very brief additional review.

A

There is in fact a strong free speech clause in the Constitution that predates the first amendment. It is found in article I, section 6. Briefly, this clause enacts for the protection of Congress what in England was Parliament's hard-won freedom from subordination to the monarchy: a freedom not to have its members seized and locked in the Tower of London by crown order, for remarks made in the course of parliamentary debate.[40] The relevant clause provides as follows:[41]

> For any Speech or Debate in either House, they [i.e. the Senators and Representatives] shall not be questioned in any other Place.[42]

The Speech and Debate clause protects a member of Congress from having to answer elsewhere in respect to what he or she says in Congress. Insofar as a member

---

39. For example, to the extent that the fourth amendment (discussed *infra*) has a distinctive history *linked to the development of freedom of the press*, it is worthwhile to bear that connection in mind in considering police practices of search and seizure of newspaper files, in the investigation of crimes. Arguably, the standard fourth amendment requirements for search warrants, sufficient in other circumstances, ought not always be deemed sufficient when the police seek to capture and search through newspaper files when their interest—and application for a search warrant—has been triggered by a published news report of matters of general political and public concern. See, e.g., Zurcher v. Stanford Daily, 436 U.S. 547 (1978) (especially the concurring opinion by Justice Powell and the dissenting opinion by Justice Stevens). An argument in the Supreme Court is an argument about a whole case and not simply an argument addressed to different points of law lined up inside one's brief like dominoes where one pushes on one and then moves freshly to the next, pushing on it in turn. A different way of putting the same proposition is that the strength of one's case is equal to the *sum* of its parts and not just the sum divided all over again by the number of parts. For a useful general review, see Charles Lund Black, Structure and Relationship in Constitutional Law (1969).

40. See, for a brief review and discussion, United States v. Johnson, 383 U.S. 169, 178 (1966); David S. Bogen, Bulwark of Liberty: The Court and The First Amendment 8-10 (1984).

41. Note its close similarity to the provision in the English Bill of Rights, enacted in 1689, "That the freedom of speech and debates in Parliament ought not to be impeached or questioned in any court or place out of Parliament." 1 W. & M. Sess. 2, c. 2.

42. Relatedly, the habeas corpus clause (Article I, Section 9) has a connecting thread. In part, the habeas corpus clause's origin tracks back to the successful effort by Parliament to ensure that persons held in crown custody must be held pursuant to the common law or pursuant to an act of Parliament, and not by executive fiat alone. The Habeas Corpus Act in England was itself a means by which anyone seized for remarks made in Parliament might have special legal process to get released. See, e.g., William F. Duker, A Constitutional History of Habeas Corpus 45, 62 (1980) ("As long as the executive retained authority to imprison arbitrarily, Parliament remained subordinate."); The Constitution of the United States, Analysis and Interpretation 651 (Cong. Research Serv., Johnny H. Killian, ed., 1987) ("At the English common law, *habeas corpus* was available to attack pretrial detention and confinement by executive order; it could not be used to question the conviction of a person pursuant to the judgment of a court with jurisdiction over the person.")

of Congress may repeat the same remarks elsewhere, however, e.g., as in issuing a news release, the absolute immunity may be lost.[43] Additionally, despite the shield furnished by the clause providing that one need not answer for any debate or vote in Congress, the clause does not immunize Members of Congress from criminal prosecution for alleged bribe taking or bribe solicitation.[44]

B

One will note that "treason" is a crime itself defined in the Constitution, and the punishment for treason is also limited, in article III, section 3:

> Treason against the United States, shall consist only in levying War against them, or in adhering to their Enemies, giving them Aid and Comfort. No person shall be convicted of Treason unless on the Testimony of two Witnesses to the same overt Act, or on Confession in open Court.
>
> The Congress shall have Power to declare the Punishment of Treason, but no Attainder of Treason shall work corruption of Blood, or Forfeiture except during the Life of the Person attained.

This narrow, constitutionally-entrenched definition of treason—and the special proof the crime requires and the limitation on punishment—is related to the history of printing and to possible prosecution for what one writes down even as a private record of one's thoughts. According to Blackstone,[45] there was a species of treason in the common law called "constructive treason," namely, compassing or imagining the death of the king. The offense was separate from the offense of seditious libel. Conviction of constructive treason required proof of an overt act, but the act of putting pen to paper, even in an unsent, purely speculative letter, was at one time held to suffice as an overt act. On the other hand, oral discourse disclosing a state of mind of a like character, while punishable as seditious libel, was not per se deemed to be a sufficient overt act for this highly extended definition of treason as such.[46] In one

---

43. See, e.g., Hutchinson v. Proxmire, 443 U.S. 111 (1979) (private civil libel action sustained over demurrer by Senator Proxmire re "Golden Fleece" award identifying plaintiff in news release ridiculing plaintiff's government-funded research, though the same remarks would have been absolutely privileged when made on Senate floor).

44. See United States v. Helstoski, 442 U.S. 477 (1979); United States v. Brewster, 408 U.S. 501 (1972). Cf. United States v. Johnson, 383 U.S. 169 (1966).

45. Vol. 4, pp. 99-104. See also Mayton, *supra* p. 19 note 31, at 98-102.

46. Treason was a most heinous offense, and it was specially punished, by "drawing and quartering" (manacling the condemned person to be dragged through the streets behind horses until nearly dead, and, while alive, disemboweled before his own eyes, his innards burnt, his body then to be hacked into quarters, to be scattered, the head to be put atop a pikestaff along the public way), all goods and estates to be forfeited, all relatives deprived of inheritance and support. The constitutionally narrowed definition of treason, incidentally, was singularly responsible for saving Aaron Burr from conviction for treason during the Jefferson administration. (At trial before John Marshall, presiding as trial judge on circuit, Burr was determined as a matter of law not to have engaged in sufficient overt acts. See United States v. Burr, 8 U.S. (4 Cranch) 469, Appx (1807).) (The *Burr* case is additionally interesting

respect, then, the treason clause reflects its own (albeit limited) concern for a free press.[47]

C

Relatedly, the fourth amendment has a first amendment tie as well. Briefly, it is this. Recall that the fourth amendment provides:

> The right of the people to be secure in their persons, houses, papers, and effects, against unreasonable searches and seizures, shall not be violated, and no Warrants shall issue, but upon probable cause, supported by Oath or affirmation, and particularly describing the place to be searched, and the persons or things to be seized.

General writs of assistance, and general warrants of search, had figured prominently in English history, respecting the licensed press. The licensing system was enforced by ferreting out unlicensed print presses; their discovery and seizure proceeded pursuant to general writs of assistance and general warrants of search. The fourth amendment is, in part, a reaction to such practices; it disallows general warrants of search.[48]

---

because it involved an early use and testing of claims of "executive privilege." Burr claimed that a letter in President Thomas Jefferson's possession would tend to exonerate him; after initially resisting the court's request to submit the letter to the court, Jefferson, reluctantly, complied.)

47. For a stronger view, namely, that the treason clause reflexively restricts seditious libel as a possible alternative crime, see James Willard Hurst, The Law of Treason in the United States 152 (1971). ("[T]he record does suggest that the clause was intended to guarantee nonviolent political processes against prosecution under any theory or charge, the burden of which was the allegedly seditious character of the conduct in question.") See also Mayton, *supra* p. 19 note 31, at 95, 98, 116. ("In the United States we have devised criminal statutes in the nature of constructive treason, but have instead characterized them as sedition or espionage laws, and thereby have avoided one of our own constitutional safeguards—the treason clause—against such laws. *** *The recorded discussion of the treason clause shows a common understanding of the clause as a free speech provision.")* (Emphesis added.)

48. Perhaps the most famous English case is Entick v. Carrington, 19 Howell's State Trials 1029, 95 Eng. 807 (1705), cited and relied upon by our Supreme Court in Boyd v. United States, 116 U.S. 616, 626 (1886). Entick, an associate of John Wilkes, successfully sued state officers who broke into his house and seized a mass of charts and pamphlets owned by Entick (Wilkes had published polemical pamphlets attacking crown policies and the king), pursuant to a general warrant, issued without a record of probable cause. The particularity requirement of the fourth amendment has been given its most stringent application when first amendment protected political materials have been the object of search warrants. See, e.g., Stanford v. Texas, 379 U.S. 476 (1965). Additionally, in respect to seizure of books and films, prior review by the warrant-issuing magistrate of each item may be specially required, seizures incidental to an otherwise lawful arrest may be disallowed (because no magistrate will have made an independent determination re their first amendment status), and an exceedingly prompt post-seizure adversary hearing may have to be provided to test "obscenity" seizures of allegedly criminally contraband materials as against the claim that they are not "obscene" by first amendment standards of law. See, e.g., Marcus v. Search Warrant, 367 U.S. 717 (1961); A Quantity of Books v. Kansas, 378 U.S. 205 (1964); Heller v. New York, 413 U.S. 483 (1973). But see New York v. P.J. Video, Inc., 475 U.S. 868, 875 n.6 (1986) (no higher standard of probable cause required than in other

D

Additionally, there is strong suggestion in the press history literature that the assurances of trial by jury (article III and the sixth amendment) drew partly from freedom of press concerns:

> The Trial of all Crimes, except in Cases of Impeachment, shall be by Jury.
>
> ***
>
> In all criminal prosecutions, the accused shall enjoy the right to a speedy and public trial, by an impartial jury of the State and district wherein the crime shall have been committed.

The assurance of trial by jury might mitigate the rigor of "the law." A jury may decline to apply a law it finds unduly harsh though a judge, in a bench trial, would not.[49] In modern free speech and free press cases, the issue may also arise respecting the extent to which the jury determines whether the first amendment's legal standard (whatever it is) has or has not been met by the prosecutor in a speech or press case, i.e. that that issue is not solely for the judge to decide but, rather, the jury must itself be persuaded that that standard has been met. There is also a related question that can be important, namely, whether the trial jury can be required to return a special

---

cases).

49. In seditious libel cases at common law, incidentally, the jury's role was very narrow; the jury was confined to determining whether the accused was in fact the printer or author of the indicted material, and whether the publication identified the aspersed party, as alleged. On the other hand, whether the material was "libelous" and "malicious" were deemed to be questions of law solely for the judge's determination; nor was a proffer of evidence in behalf of the accused respecting the truth of any factual statement admissible as a matter of law; nor was the jury to determine the law at all. Even so, despite a judge's clear instructions on these several points, juries sometimes acquitted despite the evidence. (They had no "right" to do so, albeit they possessed the "power" to do so, as the distinction was said to be). Several famous trials (e.g., Peter Zenger's trial in 1735) saved printers from serving prison terms solely by force of jury nullification. (For an excellent review of Zenger's case, see Levy, *supra* note 26, at 37- 44.) (Query: how, if at all, would any of this apply to *Patterson*? Was Patterson entitled to trial by jury? In a similar case today, would the fourteenth amendment be construed to entitle someone in Patterson's position to trial by jury?)

[In an earlier footnote, n. 25 at page 19, the critical provisions of the Sedition Act of 1798 were quoted. Section 3 of the Sedition Act, however, did provide for two safeguards that common law trials for seditious libel had lacked: namely, (a) an expanded jury role; and (b) truth as an affirmative defense. Specifically, Section 3 of the Sedition Act provided: "*And be it further enacted and declared*, That if any person shall be prosecuted under this act, for the writing or publishing any libel aforesaid, it shall be lawful for the defendant, upon the trial of the cause, to give in evidence in his defense, the truth of the matter contained in the publication charged as a libel. And the jury who shall try the cause, shall have a right to determine the law and the fact, under the direction of the court, as in other cases."]

verdict (to report on each factual question submitted to it) rather than a general (i.e. overall) verdict.[50]

E

Finally, in completing this circle of other constitutional provisions specially entwined with the first amendment provisions on freedom of speech and of the press, it is fitting to return to the full first amendment itself. That amendment has two linked provisions at its end, each of which may have an independent and a synergistic litigative use:

> Congress shall make no law *** abridging the freedom of speech, or of the press; or *the right of the people peaceably to assemble, and to petition the Government for a redress of grievances.*

The right to petition the government for a redress of grievances dates from 1215, and Magna Carta,[51] which provided (in chapter 61) as follows:

> If we *** offend in any respect against any man, or transgress against any of the articles of the peace *** and the offense is made known to four of the twenty-five barons [who shall be elected to secure the king's continuing compliance with Magna Carta itself], they shall come to us—or in our absence from the kingdom to the chief justice —to declare it and claim immediate redress. If we, or in our absence abroad the chief justice, make no redress within forty days, *** the four barons shall refer the matter to the twenty-five barons, who may *** assail us in every possible way, with the support of the whole community of the land, by seizing our castles [etc.] until they have secured such redress as they have determined upon.

In 1669, the right of petition was confirmed by Parliament as a right vested in every English commoner "in case of grievance" to petition Parliament itself for redress, although Parliament reserved the privilege to determine to its own satis-

---

50. If the jury can be directed by the court to report serially, and only on each of the factual questions submitted to it, and not overall, i.e. not any general verdict (such as, "we find the defendant guilty," or, "we find the defendant not guilty"), the imposition of that procedure might significantly cut down on jury nullification practice. If judgment cannot be passed on the accused by the court unless the jury does find the defendant "guilty," and the jury is willing to find only that the defendant published the material as alleged in the information or indictment (but not that the defendant is "guilty"), again the defendant will effectively have won. The tie-in between the right to jury trial and the first amendment, was, historically, quite important. Arguably, in some settings, it still is.

51. Chapters 39 and 40 of Magna Carta, incidentally, are the familiar source of other portions of our Bill of Rights (e.g., the fifth and sixth amendments). Respectively, they provide:

> "39. No free man shall be seized or imprisoned, or stripped of his rights or possessions, or outlawed or exiled, or deprived of his standing in any other way, nor will we proceed with force against him, or send others to do so, except by the lawful judgment of his equals or by the law of the land.
>
> "40. To no one will we sell, to no one deny or delay right or justice."

faction whether the petition was fit to be received.[52] In 1689, following the Glorious Revolution, the Bill of Rights asserted the right of subjects to petition the King, and "all commitments and prosecutions for such petitioning" were made illegal.[53]

An interesting link between the right to petition the national government as assured by the first amendment, and the privileges and immunities clause of the fourteenth amendment, should be noted. From the beginning, the fourteenth amendment privileges and immunities clause[54] was very narrowly construed by the Supreme Court, in *In re Slaughter-House Cases*.[55] Even so, the privilege of assembling in order to frame a petition for redress of felt grievances *addressed to Congress* or to the national government (e.g., to have a law changed or a law enacted by Congress in response to what citizens of the United States deem to be a just grievance), was regarded as a privilege expressly conferred by the first amendment on all citizens of the United States and, as such, a privilege protected from abridgment by the states.[56] To this extent, freedom of political association, assembly, and speech, do not depend upon the general debate regarding the extent to which the first amendment and/or the whole Bill of Rights is or is not "incorporated" into the fourteenth amendment.

---

52. Additionally, Blackstone's Commentaries (vol. 4, p. 147, 1769 ed.) describes the crime of *tumultuous petitioning*. The crime consisted of appending more than twenty names to any petition to the king or to either house of Parliament, or the delivery of a petition by a company of more than ten persons. The offense applied even when the petition merely sought "any alteration of matters established by law in church or state," i.e. even when the petition sought a change in the substantive law through an act by Parliament itself. (Evidently, the number of names on the petition, or the number of persons involved in delivering the petition, were felt to be unduly threatening or intimidating if they exceeded the specified maximum numbers.)

Similarly, with respect to freedom of peaceable assembly, Blackstone (iv at 142) notes the crime of *riotous assembly*. It consisted of an assembly by twelve or more persons failing to disperse when commanded to do so by proclamation of a peace officer (thus, the origin of the phrase, "to read the riot act"). The offense might arise though the assembly had as its object "to change the laws of the kingdom," and the act providing for the offense also granted immunity from liability to persons who might be called on to help disperse the "mob" once the proclamation was made requiring them to disperse.

53. 12 Encyclopedia of the Social Sciences 98 (1934).

54. "No State shall make or enforce any law which shall abridge the privileges or immunities of citizens of the United States ***."

55. 83 U.S. (16 Wall.) 36 (1872) (distinguishing privileges and immunities of national citizenship from general liberty, infringements of which are not forbidden by this clause). Subsequent cases, identifying selective absorption or incorporation of the Bill of Rights into the fourteenth amendment by way of the "due process" clause rather than the privileges and immunities clause, create the textual awkwardness of using a clause that reads virtually the same as the fifth amendment due process clause to embrace much more than the fifth amendment clause itself.

56. See, e.g., Hague v. CIO, 307 U.S. 496, 515 (1939) ("The privilege of a citizen of the United States to use the streets and parks for communication of views *on national questions* *** must not, in the guise of regulation, be abridged or denied.") (emphasis added); United States v. Cruikshank, 92 U.S. 542, 552-553 (1876) ("The right of the people peaceably to assemble for the purpose of petitioning Congress for a redress of grievances, or for anything else connected with the powers or the duties of the *National Government*, is an attribute of national citizenship ***.") (emphasis added).

Rather, the framing of grievances addressed to powers Congress possesses, or to responsibilities the President possesses under article II (e.g., the responsibility to take care that the laws of the United States be faithfully executed, the power to issue pardons, the qualified power to veto legislative acts, etc.) is a part of the first amendment assembly-and-redress-petition privilege, the exercise of which, by citizens of the United States,[57] the states may not seek to abridge. Additionally, the clause has also been construed to apply to petitions for redress of grievances to be brought in the courts, or federal agencies, of the United States.[58]

The "peaceably to assemble" clause, moreover, may have a distinct significance. In one aspect, it shelters an activity (namely, meeting with others, assembling in numbers) not explicit either in freedom of speech as such, freedom of the press as such, or the right to petition for a redress of grievances as such. And as the clause nestles among its neighbors within the first amendment, it may give them (and take from them) a synergistic effect, i.e. assembling peaceably for the purpose of discussing political matters, framing resolutions seeking redress of felt grievances, and the like.[59] It may also be useful in elaborating a basis for objecting to laws that (unreasonably?) restrict who may meet, how many may meet, the auspices of the meeting, or the place where peaceable assembly is disallowed (i.e. laws that do not on their face restrict what may be said and thus do not, in a strict sense, abridge freedom of speech). The "peaceably to assemble" clause, linked with the petition for a redress of grievances clause, may also have something to say about *public forum* doctrine, i.e. the extent to which streets, parks, auditoriums, etc., may not be disallowed by positive law as rallying places or places for demonstrations. In an extended sense, it may provide some ground also for identifying some sort of first amendment "right" of political association as well.

To be sure, all of this is highly preliminary. But precisely because from now on our sharper focus is nominally on the free speech-and-free-press clause (as well, of course, as the fourteenth amendment's relationship to that clause), it is useful to see how these other clauses may have: (a) a separate significance; and (b) an integrative or synergistic significance, with the free speech and free press clauses, even as we have also noted with reference to several other clauses we have now briefly reviewed.

---

57. Note, therefore, that aliens are not similarly protected according to this view (since they are not citizens of the United States), and probably neither are corporations as such (i.e. the clause is limited to natural persons).

58. See, e.g., Brotherhood of R.R. Trainmen v. Virginia, 377 U.S. 1 (1964); NAACP v. Button, 371 U.S. 415 (1963) (first amendment petition clause relied upon in holding invalid application of state ban on use of lay solicitors by NAACP to secure test cases for desegregation cases to be filed in federal court); California Motor Transport Co. v. Trucking Unlimited, 404 U.S. 508, 510 (1972); Eastern R.R. Presidents Conference v. Noerr Motor Freight, 365 U.S. 127 (1961).

59. See, e.g., De Jonge v. Oregon, 299 U.S. 353, 365 (1937) ("The holding of meetings for peaceable political action cannot be proscribed.")

To the extent that some of these clauses seem intimately concerned with processes of *political* involvement (e.g., the assembly and petition clauses, freedom of debate within Congress itself), and delimitations on *political* crimes (e.g., treason), moreover, they may lend some weight and point to the peculiar diagram featured in the earlier materials placing political speech at the core of the first amendment itself.

SELECTED BIBLIOGRAPHY OF NOTABLE RECENT BOOK-LENGTH TREATMENTS OF THE FREE SPEECH AND FREE PRESS CLAUSES

Abel, Richard, Speech and Respect (1994).

Abel, Richard, Speaking Respect, Respecting Speech (1998).

Abrams, Kathryn, The Limits of Expression in American Intellectual Life (1993).

Baker, C. Edwin, Human Liberty and Freedom of Speech (1989).

Bezanson, Randall P., Taxes on Knowledge in America: Exactions on the Press from Colonial Times to the Present (1994).

Bollinger, Lee C., Images of a Free Press (1991).

Bollinger, Lee, The Tolerant Society: Freedom of Speech and Extremist Speech in America (1986).

Bracken, Harry M., Freedom of Speech: Words Are Not Deeds (1994).

Bunker, Matthew D. Critiquing Free Speech: First Amendment Theory and the Challenge of Interdisciplinarity. (2001).

Butler, Judith, Excitable Speech: A Politics of the Performative (1997).

Calvert, Clay. Voyeur Nation: Media, Privacy and Peering in Modern Culture. (2000).

Corner, Richard C., The Kingfish and the Constitution: Huey Long, the First Amendment, and the Emergence of Modern Press Freedom in America (1996).

Curtis, Michael Kent. Free Speech, "The Peoples' Darling Privilege:" Struggles for Freedom of Expression in American History. (2000).

Davis, Charles N. and Splichal, Sigman L. (eds.) Access Denied: freedom of Information in the Information Age. (2000).

de Grazia, Edward, Girls Lean Back Everywhere (1992).

Dickerson, Donna L., The Course of Tolerance: Freedom of Press in Nineteenth Century America (1990).

Emord, Jonathan, Freedom, Technology, and the First Amendment (1991).

Ferber, Daniel, The First Amendment (1998).

Fish, Stanley E., There's No Such Thing as Free Speech (1994).

Fish, Stanley E., The Trouble with Principle (1999).

Fiss, Owen, Liberalism Divided: Freedom of Speech and the Many Uses of State Power (1996).

Golding, Martin, Free Speech on Campus (2000).

Goldstein, Robert Justin. Flag Burning and Free Speech: The Case of Texas v. Johnson. (2000).

Gurstein, Rochelle, The Repeal of Reticence: A History of America's Cultural and Legal Struggles over Free Speech, Obscenity, Sexual Liberation, and Modern Art (1996).

Gutman, Amy and Thompson, Dennis, Democracy and Disagreement (1996).

Haiman, Franklin, S., "Speech Acts" and the First Amendment (1993).

Hamilton, James T., Channeling Violence: The Economic Market for Violent Television Programming (1998).

Harvey, Philip D. and Strossen, Nadine. The Government vs. Erotica: The Siege of Adam and Eve. (2001).

Kors, A.C., and Silvergate, H.A., The Shadow University: The Betrayal of Liberty on America's Campuses (1998).

Levy, Leonard W., Blasphemy: Verbal Offense Against the Sacred from Moses to Salman Rushdie (1993).

Levy, Leonard W., Emergence of a Free Press (1995).

Lewis, Anthony, Make No Law (1991).

Lowenthal, David, No Liberty for License: The Forgotten Logic of the First Amendment (1997).

MacKinnon, Catherine A., Only Words (1993).

MacKinnon, Catherine and Dworkin, Andrea (eds.), In Harm's Way: The Pornography Civil Rights Hearings (1998).

Matsuda, Mari J. et al., Words that Wound: Critical Race Theory, Assaultive Speech, and the First Amendment (1993).

McWhirter, Darien A., Freedom of Speech, Press, and Assembly (1994).

Menand, Louis (ed.), The Future of Academic Freedom (1996).

O'Neil, Robert M., Free Speech in the College Community (1997).

Post,Robert C., Constitutional Domains: Democracy, Community, Management (1995).

Post, Robert C., ed., Censorship and Silencing: Practices of Cultural Regulation (1998).

Rabban, David, Free Speech in Its Forgotten Years (1997).

Rawls, John, Political Liberalism (1993).

Schuster, Joseph F., The First Amendment in the Balance (1993).

Scot Powe, Jr.L. A., The Fourth Estate and the Constitution (1991).

Shiffrin, Steven H., The First Amendment, Democracy, and Romance (1990).

Shiffrin, Steven H., Dissent, Injustice, and the Meanings of America (1999).

Smith, Bradley A. Unfree Speech: The Folly of Campaign Finance Reform. (2001).

Smolla, Rodney, Free Speech in an Open Society (1992).

Smolla, Rodney A. The First Amendment: Freedom of Expression, regulation of Mass Media, Freedom of Religion. (2000).

Snepp, Frank and Lewis, Anthony. Irreparable Harm: A First Hand Account of How One Agent Took on the CIA in an Epic Battle Over Free Speech. (2001).

Strossen, Nadine, Defending Pornography: Free Speech, Sex and the Fight for Women's Rights (1995).

Strum, Philippa. When the Nazis Came to Skokie: Freedom of Speech We Hate. (1999).

Sunstein, Cass R., Democracy and the Problem of Free Speech (1992).

Tedford, Thomas L., Freedom of Speech in the United States (1993).

Tillinghast, Charles H. American Broadcast Regulation and the First Amendment: Another Look. (2000).

Van Alstyne, William (ed.), Freedom and Tenure in the Academy (1993).

Vanderham, Paul, James Joyce and Censorship: The Trials of Ulysses (1998).

Walker, Samuel , Hate Speech: The History of an American Controversy (1994)

Weinstein, James, Hate Speech, Pornography, and the Radical Attack on Free Speech Doctrine (1999).

Wierenius, John F. First Amendment, First Principles: Verbal Acts and Freedom of Speech. (2000).

Chapter 2

THE FIRST AMENDMENT IN FORMATIVE TRANSITION AND THE CENTRALITY OF UNTRAMMELED SOCIAL ADVOCACY IN THE UNITED STATES

A. "Bad Tendency and Legislative Deference" versus "Clear and Present Danger" with strict case-by-case independent judicial review. An original alternative proposed by Learned Hand. The strengthening addition by Brandeis to the clear and present danger test. A comparison of the first and fourteenth amendments, with differentiating federalism considerations playing a role. The "Gravity of Evil" balancing formula also proposed by Learned Hand. The fusion of the original Hand and Holmes-Brandeis tests in the *Brandenburg* case.

SCHENCK v. UNITED STATES
249 U.S. 47 (1919)

MR. JUSTICE HOLMES delivered the opinion of the Court.

This is an indictment in three counts. The first charges a conspiracy to violate the Espionage Act of June 15, 1917, *** by causing and attempting to cause insubordination, &c., in the military and naval forces of the United States, and to obstruct the recruiting and enlistment service of the United States when the United States was at war with the German empire, to-wit, that the defendants wilfully conspired to have printed and circulated to men who had been called and accepted for military service under the Act of May 18, 1917, a document set forth and alleged to be calculated to cause such insubordination and obstruction. The count alleges overt acts in pursuance of the conspiracy, ending in the distribution of the document set forth. The second count alleges a conspiracy to commit an offence against the United States, to-wit, to use the mails for the transmission of matter declared to be non-mailable by Title XII, § 2 of the Act of June 15, 1917, to-wit, the above mentioned document, with an averment of the same overt acts. The third count charges an unlawful use of the mails for the transmission of the same matter and otherwise as above. The defendants were found guilty on all the counts. They set up the First Amendment to the Constitution forbidding Congress to make any law abridging the freedom of speech, or of the press, and bringing the case here on that ground have argued some other points also of which we must dispose.

It is argued that the evidence, if admissible, was not sufficient to prove that the defendant Schenck was concerned in sending the documents. According to the testimony Schenck said he was general secretary of the Socialist party and had charge of the Socialist headquarters from which the documents were sent. He identified a book found there as the minutes of the Executive Committee of the party. The book showed a resolution of August 13, 1917, that 15,000 leaflets should be printed on the other side of one of them in use, to be mailed to men who has passed exemption boards, and for distribution. Schenck personally attended to the printing. On August 20, the general secretary's report said "Obtained new leaflets from printer and started work addressing envelopes" &c.; and there was a resolve that Comrade Schenck be allowed $125 for sending leaflets through the mail. He said that he had about fifteen or sixteen thousand printed. There were files of the circular in question in the inner office which he said were printed on the other side of the one sided circular and were there for distribution. Other copies were proved to have been sent through the mails to drafted men. Without going into confirmatory details that were proved, no reasonable man could doubt that the defendant Schenck was largely instrumental in sending the circulars about. As to the defendant Baer there was evidence that she was a member of the Executive Board and that the minutes of its transactions were hers. The argument as to the sufficiency of the evidence that the defendants conspired to send the documents only impairs the seriousness of the real defense. ***

The document in question upon its first printed side recited the first section of the Thirteenth Amendment, said that the idea embodied in it was violated by the Conscription Act and that a conscript is little better than a convict. In impassioned language it intimated that conscription was despotism in its worst form and a monstrous wrong against humanity in the interest of Wall Street's chosen few. It said "Do not submit to intimidation," but in form at least confined itself to peaceful measures such as a petition for the repeal of the act. The other and later printed side of the sheet was headed "Assert Your Rights." It stated reasons for alleging that any one violated the Constitution when he refused to recognize "your right to assert your opposition to the draft," and went on "If you do not assert and support your rights, you are helping to deny or disparage rights which it is the solemn duty of all citizens and residents of the United States to retain." It described the arguments on the other side as coming from cunning politicians and a mercenary capitalist press, and even silent consent to the conscription law as helping to support an infamous conspiracy. It denied the power to send our citizens away to foreign shores to shoot up the people of other lands, and added that words could not express the condemnation such cold-blooded ruthlessness deserves, &c., &c., winding up "You must do your share to maintain, support and uphold the rights of the people of this country." Of course the document would not have been sent unless it had been intended to have some effect, and we do not see what effect it could be expected to have upon persons subject to the draft except to influence them to obstruct the carrying of it out. The defendants do not deny that the jury might find against them on this point.

But it is said, suppose that that was the tendency of this circular, it is protected by the First Amendment to the Constitution. Two of the strongest expressions are said to be quoted respectively from well-known public men. It well may be that the prohibition of laws abridging the freedom of speech is not confined to previous restraints, although to prevent them may have been the main purpose, as intimated in Patterson v. Colorado, 205 U. S. 454, 462. We admit that in many places and in ordinary times the defendants in saying all that was said in the circular would have been within their constitutional rights. But the character of every act depends upon the circumstances in which it is done. The most stringent protection of freedom of speech would not protect a man in falsely shouting fire in a theatre and causing a panic. *** The question in every case is whether the words used are used in such circumstances and are of such a nature as to create a clear and present danger that they will bring about the substantive evils that Congress has a right to prevent. It is a question of proximity and degree. When a nation is at war many things that might be said in time of peace are such a hindrance to its effort that their utterance would not be endured so long as men fight and that no Court could regard them as protected by any constitutional right. It seems to be admitted that if an actual obstruction of the recruiting service were proved, liability for words that produced that effect might be enforced. The statute of 1917 in § 4 punishes conspiracies to obstruct as well as actual obstruction. If the act (speaking, or circulating a paper), its tendency and the intent with which it is done are the same, we perceive no ground for saying that success alone warrants making the act a crime. Goldman v. United States, 245 U. S. 474, 477. Indeed that case might be said to dispose of the present contention if the precedent covers all *media concludendi*. But as the right to free speech was not referred to specially, we have thought fit to add a few words. ***

Judgments affirmed.

---

1. The Clear and Present Danger Test: Pitfalls and Problems

1. What alteration, if any, does *Schenck* represent in the common law (un)protection of free speech?—Surely the second part, i.e. the requirement that the "substantive evils" sought to be prevented must be of a kind "that Congress has a right to prevent," merely reiterates the standard requirement of federalism. Whenever Congress legislates, it must do so pursuant to some expressly enumerated or implied power vested in Congress in Article I or elsewhere. So much of *Schenck* is thus simply an ordinary matter of federalism review. In no respect is it peculiar to first amendment cases as such.

On the other hand, the requirement that "the words used [must be] used in such circumstances and [must be] of such a nature as to create a clear and present danger" of such an evil, does seem new. It implies that when a statute punishing criminal conspiracies is applied simply to written or to spoken advocacy, the first amendment forbids the common law standard of intent (to obstruct) plus some material step (mailing the leaflets) to suffice for conviction. Rather, the advocacy must also pose a clear and present danger of actual interference, nothing less. Otherwise the defendant is to go free. But why should this be so?

If one is satisfied beyond reasonable doubt that Schenck (a) mailed his leaflets to persons who had already received draft notices, and (b) did so at least partly to persuade them to refuse to report when called (and not merely to share with them his strong objections to the draft and to the war), why ought this not be enough to convict him of attempting to obstruct the draft?[1] Why, moreover, should the government have to prove that the "danger" to unobstructed military recruitment presented by Schenck's specific mailing was not only a "clear" danger but also a "*present*" danger, i.e. what of significance is provided by this addition to the test?[2]

2. Despite the evident innovation made in *Schenck* ("that the prohibition of laws abridging the freedom of speech is not confined to previous restraints" but extends to social advocacy and to political criticism absent circumstances and words creating a clear and present danger of a preventable wrong akin to the false shouting of fire in a crowded theater causing a panic), does it appear that any actual obstruction to recruitment was in fact proved? Does it appear that there was evidence to support a claim that, at least, such actual obstruction was highly likely in fact?[3]

3. The clear and present danger test is perhaps rightly thought to be relatively more protective of free speech than anything that preceded it. Nevertheless, it has been subject to the (seemingly odd?) criticism that even clear proof of clear and present danger of inducing illegal acts or violent acts by one's speech is not sufficient to meet an appropriate first amendment test. Why might that be so? Consider the following observation by Justice Rutledge:

> It is axiomatic that a democratic state may not deny its citizens the right to criticize existing laws and to urge that they be changed. And yet, in order to succeed in an effort to legalize polygamy [as an example], it is obviously necessary to convince a substantial number of people that such conduct is

---

1. In the ordinary law of criminal attempts, is it usually necessary to prove the likelihood of the attempt to succeed in fact in order to hold the attempt punishable?

2. For partial answers to both sets of questions, see the Holmes and Brandeis opinions *infra* (in Abrams v. United States, 250 U.S. 616 (1919); Gitlow v. New York, 268 U.S. 652 (1925); and Whitney v. California, 274 U.S. 357 (1927)). See also the next opinion by Judge Hand in Masses Publishing Co. v. Patten, 244 Fed. 535 (S.D.N.Y. 1917).

3. Note the accompanying statements in the opinion re the "tendency" of the circular (a tendency to obstruct the draft or a tendency to create a clear and present danger of obstruction?). See also Debs v. United States, 249 U.S. 211 (1919); Frohwerk v. United States, 249 U.S. 204 (1919) (sustaining convictions, opinion by Holmes). For other criticism and comment, see Ernest Freund, The Debs Case and Freedom of Speech, 40 U.Chi.L.Rev. 239 (1973), reprinted from The New Republic, May 3, 1919, p. 13; Harry Kalven, Ernest Freund and the First Amendment Tradition, 40 U.Chi.L.Rev. 235 (1972); David P. Rabban, The First Amendment in Its Forgotten Years, 90 Yale L.J. 514 (1981).

desirable. But conviction that the practice is desirable has a natural tendency to induce the practice itself. Thus, depending on where the circular reasoning is started, the advocacy of polygamy may either be unlawful as inducing a violation of law, or be constitutionally protected as essential to the proper functioning of the democratic process.[4]

Justice Rutledge seems to propound a conundrum, even after adjusting the words of this quoted paragraph to take full account of the "clear and present danger" test, put forth by Holmes in *Schenck v. United States*.[5] So, similar to the case Justice Rutledge put, to the extent that one desires a change in the law such that the preferential hiring of women[6] would be allowed, obviously one must first persuade people that that practice would be—and in fact is—desirable, though contrary to the view reflected in existing law.[7] To the extent that one's advocacy of the practice is persuasive, however, some, on becoming persuaded—seeing no good but rather, only harm in the present law that disallows such preferential hiring—may jump the gun; that is, they will not wait for the change in the law but, rather, they will engage in the practice itself. If one's advocacy of the practice or of its desirability creates a "clear and present danger" of just such third party reaction, may it be prohibited and punished on that account? May it be prohibited and punished at least insofar as the speaker knows or should know of that danger? Why not, assuming the danger can be established as a matter of fact? If the advocacy stops short of specifically

4. Musser v. Utah, 333 U.S. 95, 101-102 (1948) (Rutledge, J., dissenting).

5. I.e. in the quoted paragraph, Rutledge adverts to the "natural tendency" to induce the practice itself, rather than a "clear and present danger" that the practice may be engaged in. We may agree that, according to Holmes, the latter would have to be shown instead, under the *Schenck* test.

6. Alternatively, substitute "men" for the word "women" in this sentence. Alternatively, still, substitute "blacks" or "whites." (In responding to the questions subsequently raised here, will it make any difference to you *which* object of advocacy is being pressed?)

Cf. also the opening footnote to J. S. Mill, On Liberty (1859) (probably the single most influential essay ever written on free speech):

> If the arguments of the present chapter are of any validity, there ought to exist the fullest liberty of professing and discussing, as a matter of ethical conviction, any doctrine, however immoral it may be considered. It would, therefore, be irrelevant and out of place to examine here, whether the doctrine of Tyrannicide deserves that title. I shall content myself with saying that the subject has been at all times one of the open questions of morals; that the act of a private citizen in striking down a criminal, who, by raising himself above the law, has placed himself beyond the reach of legal punishment or control, has been accounted by whole nations, and by some of the best and wisest men, not a crime, but an act of exalted virtue; and that, right or wrong, it is not of the nature of assassination, but of civil war. As such, I hold that the instigation of it, in a specific case, may be a proper subject of punishment, but only if an overt act has followed, and at least a probable connection can be established between the act and the instigation.

7. E.g., contrary to some valid state statute forbidding employment discrimination based on sex, or contrary to the provision in Title VII of the Civil Rights Act of 1964, forbidding employment discrimination based on race, sex, religion, or national origin.

advocating violating the existing law, should it be deemed protected even though it has the effect of foreseeably inducing actual violations?[8] If the advocacy included advocacy of violating the existing law, then, though in fact it did not produce that effect, and, moreover, cannot be shown even to have created a clear and present danger of inducing a violation, how should it fare? Ought it be prohibitable because it sought a forbidden end (e.g., "discrimination") and also urged a forbidden act (e.g., violation of "the law")?

Is there, or ought there be, a constitutional distinction between, say, an essay persuasive to the reader that women ought preferentially to hire other women[9] (such that some then presume to do so regardless of the existing law), and another that indeed urges them to take the law into their own hands? The clear and present "danger" may be as real in the one case as in the other, even as the author may well be aware. So why distinguish the two situations for first amendment purposes? Justice Rutledge's conundrum surely poses a good point.

The following case,[10] though not from the Supreme Court, proposed an answer from a different point of view. The author, Judge Learned Hand, thought the test expressed in his opinion in this case to be a better one than that which Holmes laid down in *Schenck.* Do you agree? Just how would it help, and how would it work? Is it vulnerable to a weakness not found in Holmes's test? Does either one—or even both combined—seem sufficient for the adequate protection of free speech?[11]

MASSES PUBLISHING COMPANY v. PATTEN
244 Fed. 535 (S.D.N.Y. 1917)

In Equity. Suit by the Masses Publishing Company against T. G. Patten, Postmaster of the City of New York. On motion for preliminary injunction. Motion granted.

---

8. Incidentally, what does it mean to "advocate the violation of an existing law," or even to advocate the desirability of a certain practice not now allowed by law, for purposes of first amendment review? What would you say about Marc Anthony's address in Shakespeare's *Julius Caesar*? (Was Marc Anthony advocating that the crowd attack Brutus and the others involved in Caesar's assassination, or was he merely suggesting that Caesar's death ought to be seen as less than a deserved fate?)

9. Or, indeed, that men ought preferentially hire other men, or that members of some racial group ought preferentially to hire those (racially) like themselves.

10. Reversed on appeal, 246 Fed. 24 (2d Cir. 1917). Discussed and compared with Holmes' early standard, in Vincent A. Blasi, Learned Hand and the First Amendment, 61 Colum.L.Rev. 1 (1990); Gerald Gunther, Learned Hand and the Origins of Modern First Amendment Doctrine: Some Fragments of History, 27 Stan.L.Rev. 719 (1975). See also Gerald Gunther, Learned Hand: The Man and the Judge 151-161 (1994).

11. For consideration of still other views strongly advanced during this time, respecting the protection the First Amendment should be deemed to provide for freedom of socially-agitative speech, see David Rabban, Free Speech in its Forgotten Years (1997).

The plaintiff applies for a preliminary injunction against the postmaster of New York to forbid his refusal to accept its magazine in the mails under the following circumstances: The plaintiff is a publishing company in the city of New York engaged in the production of a monthly revolutionary journal called "The Masses," containing both text and cartoons, each issue of which is ready for the mails during the first ten days of the preceding month. In July, 1917, the postmaster of New York, acting upon the direction of the Postmaster General, advised the plaintiff that the August number to which he had had access would be denied the mails under the Espionage Act of June 15, 1917. Though professing willingness to excerpt from the number any particular matter which was objectionable in the opinion of the Postmaster General, the plaintiff was unable to learn any specification of objection, and thereupon filed this bill, and now applies for a preliminary injunction upon a statement of the facts.

Upon return of the rule to show cause the defendant, while objecting generally that the whole purport of the number was in violation of the law, since it tended to produce a violation of the law, to encourage the enemies of the United States, and to hamper the government in the conduct of the war, specified four cartoons and four pieces of text as especially falling within sections 1 and 2 of title 12 of the act and by the reference of section 1 as within section 3 of title 1. These sections are quoted in the margin.[1]

The four cartoons are entitled respectively, "Liberty Bell," "Conscription," "Making the World Safe for Capitalism," "Congress and Big Business." The first is a picture of the Liberty Bell broken in fragments. The obvious implication, taking the cartoon in its context with the number as a whole, is that the origin, purposes, and

---

1. TITLE I. Espionage.

Section. 3. Whoever, when the United States is at war, shall willfully make or convey false reports or false statements with the intent to interfere with the operation or success of the military or naval forces of the United States or to promote the success of its enemies and whoever when the United States is at war, shall willfully cause or attempt to cause insubordination, disloyalty, mutiny, or refusal of duty, in the military or naval forces of the United States, or shall willfully obstruct the recruiting or enlistment service of the United States, to the injury of the service or of the United States, shall be punished by a fine of not more than $10,000 or imprisonment for not more than twenty years, or both.

TITLE XII. Use of Mails.

Section 1. Every letter, writing, circular, postal card, picture, print, engraving, photograph, newspaper, pamphlet, book, or other publication, matter or thing, of any kind, in violation of any of the provisions of this act is hereby declared to be nonmailable matter and shall not be conveyed in the mails or delivered from any post office or by any letter carrier: Provided, that nothing in this act shall be so construed as to authorize any person other than an employé of the dead letter office, duly authorized there to, or other person upon a search warrant authorized by law, to open any letter not addressed to himself.

Section 2. Every letter, writing, circular, postal card, picture, print, engraving, photograph, newspaper, pamphlet, book, or other publication, matter or thing, of any kind, containing any matter advocating or urging treason, insurrection, or forcible resistance to any law of the United States, is hereby declared to be nonmailable.

conduct of the war have already destroyed the liberties of the country. It is a fair inference that the draft law is an especial instance of the violation of the liberty and fundamental rights of any free people. ***

The challenged text, omitting the excerpts just mentioned, total about one page out of a total of 28. Throughout the rest are sprinkled other texts designed to arouse animosity to the draft and to the war, and criticisms of the President's consistency in favoring the declaration of war.

The defendant attaches to its papers as well copies of the June and July numbers of The Masses and a number of Mother Earth, a magazine edited by Emma Goldman and Alexander Berkman, recently convicted in this court for a conspiracy to resist the draft. The earlier copies of The Masses contain inflammatory articles upon the war and conscription in revolutionary vein, some of which go to the extent of counselling those subject to conscription to resist. This case does not concern them except in so far as the defendant's position is correct that in the interpretation of the August number the purpose of the writers may be inferred from what preceded, and that an audience addressed in the earlier numbers would put upon the later number a significance beyond what the contents would naturally bear if it stood alone. ***

LEARNED HAND, DISTRICT JUDGE (after stating the facts as above).

***

Coming to the act itself, it is conceded that the defendant's only direct authority arises from title 12 of the act, §§ 1 and 2. His position is that under section 1 any writing which by its utterance would infringe any of the provisions of other titles in the act becomes nonmailable. I may accept that assumption for the sake of argument and turn directly to section 3 of title 1, which the plaintiff is said to violate. That section contains three provisions. The first is, in substance, that no one shall make any false statements with intent to interfere with the operation or success of the military or naval forces of the United States or to promote the success of its enemies. The defendant says that the cartoons and text of the magazine, constituting, as they certainly do, a virulent attack upon the war and those laws which have been enacted to assist its prosecution, may interfere with the success of the military forces of the United States. That such utterances may have the effect so ascribed to them is unhappily true; publications of this kind enervate public feeling at home which is their chief purpose, and encourage the success of the enemies of the United States abroad, to which they are generally indifferent. Dissension within a country is a high source of comfort and assistance to its enemies; the least intimation of it they seize upon with jubilation. There cannot be the slightest question of the mischievous effects of such agitation upon the success of the national project, or of the correctness of the defendant's position.

All this, however, is beside the question whether such an attack is a willfully false statement. That phrase properly includes only a statement of fact which the utterer knows to be false, and it cannot be maintained that any of these statements are of fact, or that the plaintiff believes them to be false. They are all within the range of opinion and of criticism; they are all certainly believed to be true by the utterer. As such they fall within the scope of that right to criticize either by temperate reasoning, or by immoderate and indecent invective, which is normally the privilege of the individual in countries dependent upon the free expression of opinion as the ultimate source of authority. The argument may be trivial in substance, and violent and perverse in manner, but so long as it is confined to abuse of existing policies or laws, it is impossible to class it as a false statement of facts of the kind here in question. To modify this provision, so clearly intended to prevent the spreading of false rumors which may embarrass the military, into the prohibition of any kind of propaganda, honest or vicious, is to disregard the meaning of the language, established by legal construction and common use, and to raise it into a means of suppressing intemperate and inflammatory public discussion, which was surely not its purpose.

The next phrase relied upon is that which forbids any one from willfully causing insubordination, disloyalty, mutiny, or refusal of duty in the military or naval forces of the United States. The defendant's position is that to arouse discontent and disaffection among the people with the prosecution of the war and with the draft tends to promote a mutinous and insubordinate temper among the troops. This, too, is true; men who become satisfied that they are engaged in an enterprise dictated by the unconscionable selfishness of the rich, and effectuated by a tyrannous disregard for the will of those who must suffer and die, will be more prone to insubordination than those who have faith in the cause and acquiesce in the means. Yet to interpret the word "cause" so broadly would, as before, involve necessarily as a consequence the suppression of all hostile criticism, and of all opinion except what encouraged and supported the existing policies, or which fell within the range of temperate argument. It would contradict the normal assumption of democratic government that the suppression of hostile criticism does not turn upon the justice of its substance or the decency and propriety of its temper. Assuming that the power to repress such opinion may rest in Congress in the throes of a struggle for the very existence of the state, its exercise is so contrary to the use and wont of our people that only the clearest expression of such a power justifies the conclusion that it was intended.

The defendant's position, therefore, in so far as it involves the suppression of the free utterance of abuse and criticism of the existing law, or of the policies of the war, is not, in my judgment, supported by the language of the statute. Yet there has always been a recognized limit to such expressions, incident indeed to the existence of any compulsive power of the state itself. One may not counsel or advise others to violate the law as it stands. Words are not only the keys of persuasion, but the triggers of action, and those which have no purport but to counsel the violation of law cannot by any latitude of interpretation be a part of that public opinion which is the final source of government in a democratic state. The defendant asserts not only that the magazine indirectly through its propaganda leads to a disintegration of loyalty and a disobedience of law, but that in addition it counsels and advises resistance to existing law, especially to the draft. The consideration of this aspect of the case more properly arises under the third phrase of section 3, which forbids any willful obstruction of the recruiting or enlistment service of the United States, but, as the defendant urges that the magazine falls within each phrase, it is as well to take it up now. To counsel or advise a man to an act is to urge upon him either that it is his interest or his duty to do it. While, of course, this may be accomplished as well by indirection as expressly, since words carry the meaning that they impart, the definition is exhaustive, I think, and I shall use it. Political agitation, by the passions it arouses or the convictions it engenders, may in fact stimulate men to the violation of law. Detestation of existing policies is easily transformed into forcible resistance of the authority which puts them in execution, and it would be folly to disregard the causal relation between the two. Yet to assimilate agitation, legitimate as such, with direct incitement to violent resistance, is to disregard the tolerance of all methods of political agitation which in normal times is a safeguard of free government. The distinction is not a scholastic subterfuge, but a hard-bought acquisition in the fight for freedom, and the purpose to disregard it must be evident when the power exists. If one stops short of urging upon others that it is their duty or their interest to resist the law, it seems to me one should not be held to have attempted to cause its violation. If that be not the test, I can see no escape from the conclusion that under this section every political agitation which can be shown to be apt to create a seditious temper is illegal. I am confident that by such language Congress had no such revolutionary purpose in view.

It seems to me, however, quite plain that none of the language and none of the cartoons in this paper can be thought directly to counsel or advise insubordination or mutiny, without a violation of their meaning quite beyond any tolerable understanding. I come, therefore, to the third phrase of the section, which forbids any one from willfully obstructing the recruiting or enlistment service of the United States. I am not prepared to assent to the plaintiff's position that this only refers to acts other than words, nor that the act thus defined must be shown to have been successful. One may obstruct without preventing, and the mere obstruction is an injury to the service; for it throws impediments in its way. Here again, however, since the question is of the expression of opinion, I construe the sentence, so far as it restrains public utterance, as I have construed the other two, and as therefore limited to the direct advocacy of resistance to the recruiting and enlistment service. If so, the inquiry is narrowed to the question whether any of the challenged matter may be said to advocate resistance to the draft, taking the meaning of the words with the utmost latitude which they can bear.

As to the cartoons it seems to me quite clear that they do not fall within such a test. Certainly the nearest is that entitled "Conscription," and the most that can be said of that is that it may breed such animosity to the draft as will promote resistance and strengthen the determination of those disposed to be recalcitrant. There is no intimation that, however hateful the draft may be, one is in duty bound to resist it, certainly not that such resistances is to one's interest. I cannot, therefore, even with the limitations which surround the power of the court, assent to the assertion that any of the cartoons violate the act.

The text offers more embarrassment. The poem to Emma Goldman and Alexander Berkman, at most, goes no further than to say that they are martyrs in the cause of love among nations. Such a sentiment holds them up to admiration, and hence their conduct to possible emulation. The paragraph in which the editor offers to receive funds for their appeal also expresses admiration for them, but goes no further. The paragraphs upon conscientious objectors are of the same kind. They go no further than to express high admiration for those who have held and are holding out for their convictions even to the extent of resisting the law. It is plain enough that the paper has the fullest sympathy for these people, that it admires their courage, and that it presumptively approves their conduct. Indeed, in the earlier numbers and before the draft went into effect the editor urged resistance. Since I must interpret the language in the most hostile sense, it is fair to suppose, therefore, that these passages go as far as to say:

> "These men and women are heroes and worthy of a freeman's admiration. We approve their conduct; we will help to secure them their legal rights. They are working for the betterment of mankind through their obdurate consciences."

Moreover, these passages, it must be remembered, occur in a magazine which attacks with the utmost violence the draft and the war. That such comments have a tendency to arouse emulation in others is clear enough, but that they counsel others to follow these examples is not so plain. Literally at least they do not, and while, as I have said, the words are to be taken, not literally, but according to their full import, the literal meaning is the starting point for interpretation. One may admire and approve the course of a hero without feeling any duty to follow him. There is not the least implied intimation in these words that others are under a duty to follow. The most that can be said is that, if others do follow, they will get the same admiration and the same approval. Now, there is surely an appreciable distance between esteem and emulation; and unless there is here some advocacy of such emulation, I cannot see how the passages can be said to fall within the law. If they do, it would follow that, while one might express admiration and approval for the Quakers or any established sect which is excused from the draft, one could not legally express the same admiration and approval for others who entertain the same conviction, but do not happen to belong to the society of Friends. It cannot be that the law means to curtail such expressions merely, because the convictions of the class within the draft are stronger than their sense of obedience to the law. There is ample evidence in history that the Quaker is as recalcitrant to legal compulsion as any man; his obstinacy has been regarded in the act, but his disposition is as disobedient as that of any other conscientious objector. Surely, if the draft had not excepted Quakers, it would be too strong a doctrine to say that any who openly admire their fortitude or even approved their conduct was willfully obstructing the draft. ***

It follows that the plaintiff is entitled to the usual preliminary injunction.

ABRAMS v. UNITED STATES
250 U.S. 616 (1919).

MR. JUSTICE CLARKE delivered the opinion of the Court.

On a single indictment, containing four counts, the five plaintiffs in error, hereinafter designated the defendants, were convicted of conspiring to violate provisions of the Espionage Act of Congress (§ 3, Title I, of Act approved June 15, 1917, as amended May 16, 1918, 40 Stat. 553).

Each of the first three counts charged the defendants with conspiring, when the United States was at war with the Imperial Government of Germany, to unlawfully utter, print, write and publish: In the first count, "disloyal, scurrilous and abusive language about the form of Government of the United States;" in the second count, language "intended to bring the form of Government of the United States into contempt, scorn, contumely and disrepute;" and in the third count, language "intended to incite, provoke and encourage resistance to the United States in said war." The charge in the fourth count was that the defendants conspired "when the United States was at war with the Imperial German Government, *** unlawfully and wilfully, by utterance, writing, printing and publication, to urge, incite and advocate curtailment of production of things and products, to wit, ordnance and ammunition, necessary and essential to the prosecution of the war." The offenses were charged in the language of the act of Congress.

It was charged in each count of the indictment that it was a part of the conspiracy that the defendants would attempt to accomplish their unlawful purpose by printing, writing and distributing in the City of New York many copies of a leaflet or circular, printed in the English language, and of another printed in the Yiddish language, copies of which, properly identified, were attached to the indictment.

All of the five defendants were born in Russia. They were intelligent, had considerable schooling, and at the time they were arrested they had lived in the United States terms varying from five to ten years, but none of them had applied for naturalization. Four of them testified as witnesses in their own behalf and of these, three frankly avowed that they were "rebels," "revolutionists," "anarchists," that they did not believe in government in any form, and they declared that they had no interest whatever in the Government of the United States. The fourth defendant testified that he was a "socialist" and believed in "a proper kind of government, not capitalistic," but in his classification the Government of the United States was "capitalistic."

It was admitted on the trial that the defendants had united to print and distribute the described circulars and that five thousand of them had been printed and distributed about the 22d day of August, 1918. The group had a meeting place in New York City, in rooms rented by defendant Abrams, under an assumed name, and there the subject of printing the circulars was discussed about two weeks before the defendants were arrested. The defendant Abrams, although not a printer, on July 27, 1918, purchased the printing outfit with which the circulars were printed and installed it in a basement room where the work was done at night. The circulars were distributed some by throwing them from a window of a building where one of the defendants was employed and other secretly, in New York City.

The defendants pleaded "not guilty," and the case of the Government consisted in showing the facts we have stated, and in introducing in evidence copies of the two printed circulars attached to the indictment, a sheet entitled "Revolutionists Unite for Action," written by the defendant Lipman, and found on him when he was arrested, and another paper, found at the headquarters of the group, and for which Abrams assumed responsibility.

Thus the conspiracy and the doing of the overt acts charged were largely admitted and were fully established.

On the record thus described it is argued, somewhat faintly, that the acts charged against the defendants were not unlawful because within the protection of that freedom of speech and of the press which is guaranteed by the first amendment to the Constitution of the United States, and that the entire Espionage Act is unconstitutional because in conflict with that Amendment.

This contention is sufficiently discussed and is definitely negatived in*Schenck v. United States* and Baer v. United States, 239 U.S. 47; and in Frohwerk v. United States, 249 U.S. 204.

The claim chiefly elaborated upon by the defendants in the oral argument and in their brief is that there is no substantial evidence in the record to support the judgment upon the verdict of guilty and that the motion of the defendants for an instructed verdict in their favor was erroneously denied. A question of law is thus presented, which calls for an examination of the record, not for the purpose of weighing conflicting testimony, but only to determine whether there was some evidence, competent and substantial, before the jury, fairly tending to sustain the verdict. *** [S]ince the sentence imposed did not exceed that which might lawfully have been imposed under any single count, the judgment upon the verdict of the jury must be affirmed if the evidence is sufficient to sustain any one of the counts. ***

The first of the two articles attached to the indictment is conspicuously headed, "The Hypocrisy of the United States and her Allies." After denouncing President Wilson as a hypocrite and a coward because troops were sent into Russia, it proceeds to assail our Government in general, saying:

> "His [the President's] shameful, cowardly silence about the intervention in Russia reveals the hypocrisy of the plutocratic gang in Washington and vicinity."

It continues:

> "He [the President] is too much of a coward to come out openly and say: 'We capitalistic nations cannot afford to have a proletarian republic in Russia.'"

Among the capitalistic nations Abrams testified the United States was included. Growing more inflammatory as it proceeds, the circular culminates in:

> "The Russian Revolution cries: Workers of the World! Awake! Rise! Put down your enemy and mine!
>
> Yes! friends, there is only one enemy of the workers of the world and that is CAPITALISM."

This is clearly an appeal to the "workers" of this country to arise and put down by force the Government of the United States which they characterize as their "hypocritical," "cowardly" and "capitalistic" enemy.

It concludes:

> "Awake! Awake, you Workers of the World!
> "REVOLUTIONISTS."

The second of the articles was printed in the Yiddish language and in the translation is headed, "Workers—Wake up." After referring to "his Majesty, Mr. Wilson, and the rest of the gang; dogs of all colors!", it continues:

> "Workers, Russian emigrants, you who had the least belief in the honesty of *our* Government," which defendants admitted referred to the United States Government, "must now throw away all confidence, must spit in the face the false, hypocritic, military propaganda which has fooled you so relentlessly, calling forth your sympathy, your help, to the prosecution of the war." ***

This is not an attempt to bring about a change of administration by candid discussion, for no matter what may have incited the outbreak on the part of the defendant anarchists, the manifest purpose of such a publication was to create an attempt to defeat the war plans of the Government of the United States, by bringing upon the country the paralysis of a general strike, thereby arresting the production of all munitions and other things essential to the conduct of the war.

This purpose is emphasized in the next paragraph, which reads:

> "Do not let the Government scare you with their wild punishment in prisons, hanging and shooting. We must not and will not betray the splendid fighters of Russia. *Workers, up to fight.*"

After more of the same kind, the circular concludes:

> "Woe unto those who will be in the way of progress. Let solidarity live!"

It is signed, "The Rebels."

*** One of these circulars is headed: "Revolutionists! Unite for Action!"

After denouncing the President as "Our Kaiser" and the hypocrisy of the United States and her Allies, this article concludes:

> "Socialists, Anarchists, Industrial Workers of the World, Socialists, Labor party men and other revolutionary organizations *Unite for action* and let us save the Workers' Republic of Russia!
>
> *Know you lovers of freedom that in order to save the Russian revolution, we must keep the armies of the allied countries busy at home.*"

Thus was again avowed the purpose to throw the county into a state of revolution if possible and to thereby frustrate the military program of the Government. ***

These excerpts sufficiently show, that while the immediate occasion for this particular outbreak of lawlessness, on the part of the defendant alien anarchists, may have been resentment caused by our Government sending troops into Russia as a strategic operation against the Germans on the eastern battle front, yet the plain purpose of their propaganda was to excite, at the supreme crisis of the war, disaffection, sedition, riots, and, as they hoped, revolution, in this country for the purpose of embarrassing and if possible defeating the military plans of the Government in Europe. *** Thus it is clear not only that some evidence but that much persuasive evidence was before the jury tending to prove that the defendants were guilty as charged in both the third and fourth counts of the indictment and under the long established rule of law hereinbefore stated the judgment of the District Court must be affirmed.

MR. JUSTICE HOLMES dissenting.

This indictment is founded wholly upon the publication of two leaflets which I shall describe in a moment. The first count charges a conspiracy pending the war with Germany to publish abusive language about the form of government of the United States, laying the preparation and publishing of the first leaflet as overt acts. The second count charges a conspiracy pending the war to publish language intended to bring the form of government into contempt, laying the preparation and publishing of the two leaflets as overt acts. The third count alleges a conspiracy to encourage resistance to the United States in the same war and to attempt to effectuate the purpose by publishing the same leaflets. The fourth count lays a conspiracy to incite curtailment of production of things necessary to the prosecution of the war and to attempt to accomplish it by publishing the second leaflet to which I have referred. ***

No argument seems to me necessary to show that these pronunciamentos in no way attack the form of government of the United States, or that they do not support either of the first two counts. What little I have to say about the third count may be postponed until I have considered the fourth. With regard to that it seems too plain to be denied that the suggestion to workers in the ammunition factories that they are producing bullets to murder their dearest, and the further advocacy of a general strike, both in the second leaflet, do urge curtailment of production of things necessary to the prosecution of the war within the meaning of the Act of May 16, 1918, c. 75, 40 Stat. 553, amending § 3 of the earlier Act of 1917. But to make the conduct criminal that statute requires that it should be "with intent by such curtailment to cripple or hinder the United States in the prosecution of the war." It seems to me that no such intent is proved.

I am aware of course that the word intent as vaguely used in ordinary legal discussion means no more than knowledge at the time of the act that the consequences said to be intended will ensue. Even less than that will satisfy the general principal of civil and criminal liability. A man may have to pay damages, may be sent to prison, at common law might be hanged, if at the time of his act he knew facts from which common experience showed that the consequences would follow, whether he individually could foresee them or not. But, when words are used exactly, a deed is not done with intent to produce a consequence unless that consequence is the aim of the deed. It may be obvious, and obvious to the actor, that the consequence will follow, and he may be liable for it even if he regrets it, but he does not do the act with intent to produce it unless the aim to produce it is the proximate motive of the specific act, although there may be some deeper motive behind.

It seems to me that this statute must be taken to use its words in a strict and accurate sense. They would be absurd in any other. A patriot might think that we were wasting money on aeroplanes, or making more cannon of a certain kind than we needed, and might advocate curtailment with success, yet even if it turned out that the curtailment hindered and was thought by other minds to have been obviously likely to hinder the United States in the prosecution of the war, no one would hold such conduct a crime. I admit that my illustration does not answer all that might be said but it is enough to show what I think and to let me pass to a more important aspect of the case. I refer to the First Amendment to the Constitution that Congress shall make no law abridging the freedom of speech.

I never have seen any reason to doubt that the questions of law that alone were before this Court in the cases of *Schenck, Frohwerk* and *Debs*, 249 U. S. 47, 204, 211, were rightly decided. I do not doubt for a moment that by the same reasoning that would justify punishing persuasion to murder, the United States constitutionally may punish speech that produces or is intended to produce a clear and imminent danger that it will bring about forthwith certain substantive evils that the United States constitutionally may seek to prevent. The power undoubtedly is greater in time of war than in time of peace because war opens dangers that do not exist at other times.

But as against dangers peculiar to war, as against others, the principle of the right to free speech is always the same. It is only the present danger of immediate evil or an intent to bring it about that warrants Congress in setting a limit to the expression of opinion where private rights are not concerned. Congress certainly cannot forbid all effort to change the mind of the country. Now nobody can suppose that the surreptitious publishing of a silly leaflet by an unknown man, without more, would present any immediate danger that its opinions would hinder the success of the government arms or have any appreciable tendency to do so. Publishing those opinions for the very purpose of obstructing however, might indicate a greater danger and at any rate would have the quality of an attempt. So I assume that the second leaflet if published for the purposes alleged in the fourth count might be punishable. But it seems pretty clear to me that nothing less than that would bring these papers within the scope of this law. ***

I do not see how anyone can find the intent required by the statute in any of the defendants' words. The second leaflet is the only one that affords even a foundation for the charge, and there, without invoking the hatred of German militarism expressed in the former one, it is evident from the beginning to the end that the only object of the paper is to help Russia and stop American intervention there against the popular government—not to impede the United States in the war that it was carrying on. To say that two phrases taken literally might import a suggestion of conduct that would have interference with the war as an indirect and probably undesired effect seems to me by no means enough to show an attempt to produce that effect. ***

In this case sentences of twenty years imprisonment have been imposed for the publishing of two leaflets that I believe the defendants had as much right to publish as the Government has to publish the Constitution of the United States now vainly invoked by them. Even if I am technically wrong and enough can be squeezed from these poor and puny anonymities to turn the color of legal litmus paper; I will add, even if what I think the necessary intent were shown; the most nominal punishment seems to me all that possibly could be inflicted, unless the defendants are to be made to suffer not for what the indictment alleges but for the creed that they avow—a creed that I believe to be the creed of ignorance and immaturity when honestly held, as I see no reason to doubt that it was held here, but which although made the subject of examination at the trial, no one has a right even to consider in dealing with the charges before the Court.

Persecution for the expression of opinions seems to me perfectly logical. If you have no doubt of your premises or your power and want a certain result with all your heart you naturally express your wishes in law and sweep away all opposition. To allow opposition by speech seems to indicate that you think the speech impotent, as when a man says that he has squared the circle, or that you do not care whole-heartedly for the result, or that you doubt either your power or your premises. But when men have realized that time has upset many fighting faiths, they may come to believe even more than they believe the very foundations of their own conduct that the ultimate good desired is better reached by free trade in ideas—that the best test of truth is the power of the thought to get itself accepted in the competition of the market, and that truth is the only ground upon which their wishes safely can be carried out. That at any rate is the theory of our Constitution. It is an experiment, as all life is an experiment. Every year if not every day we have to wager our salvation upon some prophecy based upon imperfect knowledge. While that experiment is part of our system I think that we should be eternally vigilant against attempts to check the expression of opinions that we loathe and believe to be fraught with death, unless they so imminently threaten immediate interference with the lawful and pressing purposes of the law that an immediate check is required to save the country. I wholly disagree with the argument of the Government that the First Amendment left the common law as to seditious libel in force. History seems to me against the notion. I had conceived that the United States through many years had shown its repentance for the Sedition Act of 1798, by repaying fines that it imposed. Only the emergency that makes it immediately dangerous to leave the correction of evil counsels to time warrants making any exception to the sweeping command, "Congress shall make no law *** abridging the freedom of speech." Of course I am speaking only of expressions of opinion and exhortations, which were all that were uttered here, but I regret that I cannot put into more impressive words my belief that in their conviction upon this indictment the defendants were deprived of their rights under the Constitution of the United States.

MR. JUSTICE BRANDEIS concurs with the foregoing opinion.

NOTE

Justice Holmes' dissent in *Abrams* is among the most frequently quoted statements expounding the freedom of speech as the freedom to win adherents regardless of ideology. It dates the identification of "the centrality of untrammeled social advocacy" in first amendment doctrine and it is thought to mark a fundamental change in Holmes's own thinking as well. Perhaps no stronger statement on freedom of speech since John Stuart Mill's *Essay on Liberty* (1859) (Pt. II, Of Liberty of Thought and Discussion) can be found in any prior opinion within the Supreme Court. (For a more recent suggestion that *Abrams* did not in fact mark any break from his earlier opinions, however, see Sheldon M. Novick, The Unrevised Holmes and Freedom of Expression, 1991 Sup. Ct. Rev. 303.) Note also Holmes' additional suggestion that even where the facts are sufficient to clear the first amendment to find the defendants guilty, and the sentence (here, twenty years imprisonment) does not exceed the statute's provisions, insofar as the sentence lacks adequate explanation apart from a desire to express disapproval of "the creed"—the ideology —the defendants avow, it cannot be reconciled with the first amendment (*not* the eighth amendment's prohibition on "cruel and unusual punishment," but the *first* amendment's prohibition on punishment for political beliefs and/or for protected speech).

GITLOW v. PEOPLE OF NEW YORK

268 U.S. 652 (1925)

MR. JUSTICE SANFORD delivered the opinion of the Court.

Benjamin Gitlow was indicted in the Supreme Court of New York, with three others, for the statutory crime of criminal anarchy. New York Penal Laws, §§ 160, 161. He was separately tried, convicted, and sentenced to imprisonment. The judgment was affirmed by the Appellate Division and by the Court of Appeals. ***

The contention here is that the statute, by its terms and as applied in this case, is repugnant to the due process clause of the Fourteenth Amendment. Its material provisions are:

"§ 160. *Criminal anarchy defined.* Criminal anarchy is the doctrine that organized government should be overthrown by force or violence, or by assassination of the executive head or of any of the executive officials of government, or by any unlawful means. The advocacy of such doctrine either by word of mouth or writing is a felony."

"§ 161. *Advocacy of criminal anarchy.* Any person who:

"1. By word of mouth or writing advocates, advises or teaches the duty, necessity or propriety of overthrowing or overturning organized government by force or violence, or by assassination of the executive head or of any of the executive officials of government, or by any unlawful means; or,

"2. Prints, publishes, edits, issues or knowingly circulates, sells, distributes or publicly displays any book, paper, document, or written or printed matter in any form, containing or advocating, advising or teaching the doctrine that organized government should be overthrown by force, violence, or any unlawful means ***."

***

The following facts were established on the trial by undisputed evidence and admissions: The defendant is a member of the Left Wing Section of the Socialist Party, a dissenting branch or faction of that party formed in opposition to its dominant policy of "moderate Socialism." Membership in both is open to aliens as well as citizens. The Left Wing Section was organized nationally at a conference in New York City in June, 1919, attended by ninety delegates from twenty different States. The conference elected a National Council, of which the defendant was a member, and left to it the adoption of a "Manifesto." This was published in The Revolutionary Age, the official organ of the Left Wing. The defendant was on the board of managers of the paper and was its business manager. He arranged for the printing of the paper and took to the printer the manuscript of the first issue which contained the left Wing Manifesto, and also a Communist Program and a Program of the Left Wing that had been adopted by the conference. Sixteen thousand copies were printed, which were delivered at the premises in New York City used as the office of the Revolutionary Age and the headquarters of the Left Wing, and occupied by the defendant and other officials. These copies were paid for by the defendant, as business manager of the paper. Employees at this office wrapped and mailed out copies of the paper under the defendant's direction; and copies were sold from this office. ***

There was no evidence of any effect resulting from the publication and circulation of the Manifesto.

No witnesses were offered in behalf of the defendant.

*** Coupled with a review of the rise of Socialism, [the Manifesto] condemned the dominant "moderate Socialism" for its recognition of the necessity of the democratic parliamentary state; repudiated its policy of introducing Socialism by legislative measures; and advocated, in plain and unequivocal language, the necessity of accomplishing the "Communist Revolution" by a militant and "revolutionary Socialism," based on "the class struggle" and mobilizing the "power of the proletariat in action," through mass industrial revolts developing into mass political strikes and "revolutionary mass action," for the purpose of conquering and destroying the parliamentary state and establishing in its place, through a "revolutionary dictatorship of the proletariat," the system of Communist Socialism. The then recent strikes in Seattle and Winnipeg[3] were cited as instances of a development already verging on revolutionary action and suggestive of proletarian dictatorship, in which the strike-workers were "trying to usurp the functions of municipal government;" and revolutionary Socialism, it was urged, must use these mass industrial revolts to broaden the strike, make it general and militant, and develop it into mass political strikes and revolutionary mass action for the annihilation of the parliamentary state. ***

The Court of Appeals held that the Manifesto "advocated the overthrow of this government by violence, or by unlawful means."

*** The sole contention here is, essentially, that as there was no evidence of any concrete result flowing from the publication of the Manifesto or of circumstances showing the likelihood of such result, the statute as construed and applied by the trial court penalizes the mere utterance, as such, of "doctrine" having no quality of incitement, without regard either to the circumstances of its utterance or to the likelihood of unlawful sequences; and that, as the exercise of the right of free expression with relation to government is only punishable "in circumstances involving likelihood of substantive evil," the statute contravenes the due process clause of the Fourteenth Amendment. The argument in support of this contention rests primarily upon the

3. There was testimony at the trial that "there was an extended strike at Winnipeg commencing May 15, 1919, during which the production and supply of necessities, transportation, postal and telegraphic communication and fire and sanitary protection were suspended or seriously curtailed."

following propositions: 1st, That the "liberty" protected by the Fourteenth Amendment includes the liberty of speech and of the press; and 2nd, That while liberty of expression "is not absolute," it may be restrained "only in circumstances where its exercise bears a causal relation with some substantive evil, consummated, attempted or likely," and as the statute "takes no account of circumstances," it unduly restrains this liberty and is therefore unconstitutional.

The precise question presented, and the only question which we can consider under this writ of error, then is, whether the statute, as construed and applied in this case by the state courts, deprived the defendant of his liberty of expression in violation of the due process clause of the Fourteenth Amendment.***

For present purposes we may and do assume that freedom of speech and of the press—which are protected by the First Amendment from abridgment by Congress—are among the fundamental personal rights and "liberties" protected by the due process clause of the Fourteenth Amendment from impairment by the States. ***

It is a fundamental principle, long established, that the freedom of speech and of the press which is secured by the Constitution, does not confer an absolute right to speak or publish, without responsibility, whatever one may choose, or an unrestricted and unbridled license that gives immunity for every possible use of language and prevents the punishment of those who abuse this freedom. *** That a State in the exercise of its police power may punish those who abuse this freedom by utterances inimical to the public welfare, tending to corrupt public morals, incite to crime, or disturb the public peace, is not open to question.*** And, for yet more imperative reasons, a State may punish utterances endangering the foundations of organized government and threatening its overthrow by unlawful means. These imperil its own existence as a constitutional State. Freedom of speech and press, said Story *** does not protect disturbances to the public peace or the attempt to subvert the government. ***

By enacting the present statute the State has determined, through its legislative body, that utterances advocating the overthrow of organized government by force, violence and unlawful means, are so inimical to the general welfare and involve such danger of substantive evil that they may be penalized in the exercise of its police power. That determination must be given great weight. Every presumption is to be indulged in favor of the validity of the statute. Mugler v. Kansas, 123 U.S. 623, 661. And the case is to be considered "in the light of the principle that the State is primarily the judge of regulations required in the interest of public safety and welfare;" and that its police "statutes may only be declared unconstitutional where they are arbitrary or unreasonable attempts to exercise authority vested in the State in the public interest." Great Northern Ry. v. Clara City, 246 U.S. 434, 439. That utterances inciting to the overthrow of organized government by unlawful means, present a sufficient danger of substantive evil to bring their punishment within the range of legislative discretion, is clear. Such utterances, by their very nature, involve danger to the public peace and to the security of the State. They threaten breaches of the peace and ultimate revolution. And the immediate danger is none the less real and substantial, because the effect of a given utterance cannot be accurately foreseen. The State cannot reasonably be required to measure the danger from every such utterance in the nice balance of a jeweler's scale. A single revolutionary spark may kindle a fire that, smouldering for a time, may burst into a sweeping and destructive conflagration. *** If the State were compelled to wait until the apprehended danger became certain, then its right to protect itself would come into being simultaneously with the overthrow of the government, when there would be neither prosecuting officers nor courts for the enforcement of the law.

We cannot hold that the present statute is an arbitrary or unreasonable exercise of the police power of the State unwarrantably infringing the freedom of speech or press; and we must and do sustain its constitutionality.

This being so it may be applied to every utterance—not too trivial to be beneath the notice of the law—which is of such a character and used with such intent and purpose as to bring it within the prohibition of the statute. ***

And finding, for the reasons stated, that the statute is not in itself unconstitutional, and that it has not been applied in the present case in derogation of any constitutional right, the judgment of the Court of Appeals is affirmed.

MR. JUSTICE HOLMES, dissenting.

MR. JUSTICE BRANDEIS and I are of opinion that this judgment should be reversed. The general principle of free speech, it seems to me, must be taken to be included in the Fourteenth Amendment, in view of the scope that has been given to the word "liberty" as there used, although perhaps it may be accepted with a somewhat larger latitude of interpretation than is allowed to Congress by the sweeping language that governs or ought to govern the laws of the United States. If I am right, then I think that the criterion sanctioned by the full Court in Schenck v. United States, 249 U.S. 47, 52, applies. "The question in every case is whether the words used are used in such circumstances and are of such a nature as to create a clear and present danger that they will bring about the substantive evils that [the State] has a right to prevent." It is true that in my opinion this criterion was departed from in Abrams v. United States, 250 U.S. 616, but the convictions that I expressed in that case are too deep for it to be possible for me as yet to believe that it and Schaefer v. United States, 251 U.S. 466, have settled the law. If what I think the correct test is applied, it is manifest that there was no present danger of an attempt to overthrow the government by force on the part of the admittedly small minority who shared the defendant's views. It is said that this manifesto was more than a theory, that it was an incitement. Every idea is an incitement. It offers itself for belief and if believed it is acted on unless some other belief outweighs it or some failure of energy stifles the movement at its birth. The only difference between the expression of an opinion and an incitement in the narrower sense is the speaker's enthusiasm for the result. Eloquence may set fire to reason. But whatever may be thought of the redundant discourse before us it had no chance of starting a present conflagration. If in the long run the beliefs expressed in proletarian dictatorship are destined to be accepted by the dominant forces of the community, the only meaning of free speech is that they should be given their chance and have their way.

If the publication of this document had been laid as an attempt to induce an uprising against government at once and not at some indefinite time in the future it would have presented a different question. The object would have been one with which the law might deal, subject to the doubt whether there was any danger that the publication could produce any result, or in other words, whether it was not futile and too remote from possible consequences. But the indictment alleges the publication and nothing more.

NOTES ON THE ANSWER PROVIDED BY *GITLOW V. NEW YORK* TO THE UNADDRESSED QUESTION IN *PATTERSON V. COLORADO*: THE RELEVANCE OF THE FIRST AMENDMENT TO THE STATES

The question the Court left unaddressed in *Patterson v. Colorado* was whether (or to what extent, if any) the fourteenth amendment applies the first amendment to the states. The answer provided by *Gitlow*, in the majority Opinion, is that the fourteenth amendment fully applies the free speech and free press clause of the first amendment to the states, by force of the due process clause contained in §1.

This feature of *Gitlow v. New York* has continued to be cited and to be relied upon by the Supreme Court, ever since 1925. Indeed, *Gitlow* is probably more frequently cited for the proposition "that the first amendment applies equally to the states by force of the due process clause of the fourteenth amendment," than for anything else,[11] and more frequently than any other case is similarly cited for the same proposition. *Gitlow* also is frequently[12] cited as the first case "incorporating" some express clause in the Bill of Rights into the due process clause of the fourteenth amendment. For this reason especially (i.e. its prominence in more general disputes respecting the alleged relationship between the Bill of Rights and the fourteenth amendment), it is very much at the heart of one of the major, enduring controversies respecting the Supreme Court's entire jurisprudence in respect to the fourteenth amendment: the identification of the due process clause as an "incorporation" clause of the Bill of Rights. Here is a brief review of several different, strongly held views.

I

Between the incorporation of the Fourteenth Amendment into the Constitution and the beginning of the present membership of the Court—a period

---

11. Indeed, as we shall see, its substantive holding was subsequently undermined and abandoned, i.e. later cases adopt the Holmes-Brandeis dissent, respecting the application of the first amendment to the facts of the case.

12. But mistakenly (see discussion *infra*).

> of seventy years—the scope of that Amendment was passed upon by forty-three judges. Of all these judges, *only one*, who may respectfully be called an eccentric exception, *ever indicated the belief that the Fourteenth Amendment was a shorthand summary of the first eight Amendments theretofore limiting only the Federal Government, and that due process incorporated those eight Amendments as restrictions upon the powers of the States.*** It ought not to require argument to reject the notion that 'due process of law' meant one thing in the Fifth Amendment and another in the Fourteenth.*

This blunt paragraph written by Justice Felix Frankfurter, appears in *Adamson v. California*,[13] the single most elaborate judicial examination and most emphatic rejection of the thesis that the fourteenth amendment incorporates the Bill of Rights. It also raises a fair question whether the turn taken in *Gitlow* was in error. The *Adamson* case itself was not one concerning free speech. But it did yield a discussion that raises the question of finding anything more in the due process clause of the fourteenth amendment, applicable to the states, than one is prepared to find in the due process clause of the fifth amendment, applicable to the United States.

In *Adamson*, the Supreme Court rejected a claim that the clause in the fifth amendment that immediately precedes the fifth amendment due process clause, namely, the clause that "*no person shall be compelled in any criminal case to be a witness against himself*," was also applicable to the states via the fourteenth amendment. Frankfurter's point, in concurring in that decision, was, obviously, that the fourteenth amendment does track and, indeed, does repeat that part of the fifth amendment providing for due process. But the fourteenth amendment does not track, indeed, it does not repeat, any other part of the fifth amendment. Much less does it track or repeat any other portion of the Bill of Rights.

Accordingly, he suggested, while fourteenth amendment "due process" might very well provide protection from physically coerced confessions (e.g., confessions extracted by torture, beatings, prolonged isolation, sensory privations, etc.),[14] it does not excuse one from being compelled by judicial process to take the stand in an open, public courtroom to give evidence in one's own case. That different kind of protection arises in federal court from the special provision in the fifth amendment. The fourteenth amendment does not copy that special provision, that no person shall be compelled in any criminal case to be a witness against himself, but, rather, copies

13. 332 U.S. 46, 62 (1947) (emphasis added).

14. See, e.g, Rochin v. California, 342 U.S. 165 (1952) (convicting a person on the strength of evidence physically coerced from the accused is not due process of law).

only the provision respecting due process. The latter, not the former, was made binding upon the states.[15]

---

15. *Adamson* was a first degree murder, death penalty case from California. Reversal of Adamson's conviction was sought (unsuccessfully) on the ground that the prosecutor was permitted by state law to comment in the course of the trial on the failure of the defendant to explain or to deny evidence against him, a procedure the majority of the Court assumed the fifth amendment disallowed "if this were a trial in a court of the United States under a similar law," which it was not. The Court disposed of Adamson's claim of alleged constitutional error in the following way.

First, relying upon an earlier decision (Twining v. New Jersey, 211 U.S. 78 (1908)), the Court rejected Adamson's claim that the privilege against self-incrimination was a privilege of national citizenship states were forbidden to abridge under the fourteenth amendment privileges and immunities clause (*Twining* is, on this point, an elaboration of the *Slaughterhouse Cases*, a holding that remains undisturbed even today). Second, the Court held that the privilege was as such not subsumed, either, within the due process clause of the fourteenth amendment. Justice Frankfurter's point (quoted earlier) was expressly addressed to Adamson's due process claim. Accordingly, the Court held there was no error in the state procedure, and the judgment of the California Supreme Court, affirming the conviction and death penalty, was affirmed.

Despite the outcome in *Adamson v. California*, however, seventeen years later, in Malloy v. Hogan, 378 U.S. 1 (1964), a majority of the Supreme Court concluded that the privilege against self-incrimination is applicable to the states under the due process clause as part-and-parcel of a fair trial. In so holding, moreover, it also declared that the scope of the privilege would be measured by "the *same* standards that [are used to measure that scope] against federal encroachment" (id. at 10) (emphasis added). Effectively, then, in *Malloy v. Hogan*, the Supreme Court announced two kinds of change. It now regarded the fourteenth amendment's due process clause as absorbing a fifth amendment privilege against self-incrimination. And it regarded that privilege as fully fungible with (i.e. as equally broad as) the express fifth amendment privilege itself. Justice Brennan's clinching statement was this: "The Court thus has rejected the notion that the Fourteenth Amendment applies to the States only a 'watered-down subjective version of the individual guarantees of the Bill of Rights'" (id. at 10-11). Thus the notion that insofar as the fourteenth amendment absorbs some provision within the Bill of Rights albeit incidental to its own due process clause, when it does so, it does so literally "jot-for-jot" and "tittle for tittle." In passing also, Justice Brennan noted that as of the date of *Malloy*, 1964, the number of Justices expressing themselves as supporting the view that the fourteenth amendment incorporates *all* of the first eight amendments, had risen to ten (id. at 4). (Cf. Frankfurter's number, quotation in text *supra*).

Shortly after *Malloy v. Hogan*, in Griffin v. California, 380 U.S. 609 (1965), the Court dealt with the same aspect of the privilege against self-incrimination as had been involved in the *Adamson* case (namely, the permissibility of prosecutorial comment to the jury on the failure of the accused to explain or to deny evidence against him, as would not be permitted in a federal proceeding consistent with long-standing interpretations of the fifth amendment self-incrimination clause). The Court applied the new view announced in the *Malloy* case. On the basis of fungible equivalence between fourteenth amendment due process and the express fifth amendment self-incrimination privilege, it reversed Griffin's conviction because of the permitted prosecutorial comment. It also expressly overruled *Adamson* itself.

Even as of 1964 Justice Brennan was referring to ten Justices overall, not ten *at any one time*. In fact, at no one time has the total number of Justices holding this view ever constituted a majority of the Court. Specifically, neither the second amendment, the third, the seventh, nor even one part of the fifth amendment itself (namely, the very first part requiring any trial of a capital or other infamous offense to be preceded by grand jury indictment), has yet been held applicable to the states. Moreover, despite the general statement in *Malloy* and its application in *Griffin*, it is not true that whenever a provision

If Justice Frankfurter's position makes good sense to you, in this brief excerpt from *Adamson*, then how does one account for the position the Supreme Court took in *Gitlow v. New York*? There, the majority of the Court, even while sustaining Gitlow's state law conviction, nevertheless also wrote:

> For present purposes we may and do assume that freedom of speech and of the press—which are protected by the First Amendment from abridgment by Congress—are among the fundamental personal rights and 'liberties' *protected by the due process clause* of the Fourteenth Amendment from impairment by the States ***

And Holmes (writing for himself and for Justice Brandeis), while dissenting on the outcome, concurred albeit in the following qualified way:

> The general principle of free speech, it seems to me, must be taken to be included in the Fourteenth Amendment, in view of the scope that has been given to the word 'liberty' as there used, although perhaps it may be accepted with a somewhat larger latitude of interpretation than is allowed to Congress by the sweeping language that governs or ought to govern the laws of the United States.

Gitlow thus answers the question the Court found unnecessary to decide in *Patterson v. Colorado*. But how satisfactory is that answer?

In *Adamson v. California*, Justice Frankfurter says that it seems very odd to read the first of these next-quoted clauses as equivalent to the second, five-part provision of which it repeats only one part:

> Nor shall any State *deprive any person of life, liberty, or property, without due process of law*
>
> (fourteenth amendment)
>
> *No person shall be* held to answer for a capital, or otherwise infamous crime, unless on a presentment or indictment of a Grand Jury [etc.]; nor shall any person be subject for the same offence to be twice put in jeopardy of life or limb, nor shall be compelled in any criminal case to be a witness against

---

from the Bill of Rights has been deemed applicable to the states via the due process clause of the fourteenth amendment, the scope of the particular provision in the Bill of Rights has been applied coextensively to the state. See, e.g., Apodaca v. Oregon, 406 U.S. 404 (1972), the sixth amendment may require unanimous jury verdicts (as part of the express sixth amendment right to trial by jury), but the fourteenth amendment, although interpreted as assimilating a right to trial by jury in serious cases as a requirement of due process (Duncan v. Louisiana, 391 U.S. 145 (1968)), permits a state to provide for jury verdict by less than unanimous vote (nine-of-twelve). The sixth amendment and fourteenth amendment trial-by-jury standards are thus not necessarily coextensive nor is the sixth amendment necessarily carried over jot- for-jot and tittle-for-tittle into the due process clause of the fourteenth amendment. Might that possibility also apply as between the first amendment and the fourteenth amendment?

> himself, nor be *deprived of life, liberty, or property, without due process of law*; nor shall private property be taken for public use without just compensation.
>
> (fifth amendment)

If reading even any one or more of the other four provisions of the fifth amendment into the one look-alike provision (the due process provision) of the fourteenth amendment would seem strange, doesn't the Court's even bolder approach in *Gitlow* seem more strange by far? The fifth amendment "due process" clause might, conceivably, be thought of as itself embracing some of the other, explicitly-enumerated fifth amendment rights, since their particular enumeration within the fifth amendment might be thought of as precautionary enumerations of due process, i.e. as examples of due process of law.[16] But even with that sort of stretching of fifth amendment interpretation, it hardly seems sufficient also to go beyond the boundaries of the fifth amendment, i.e. to absorb the first amendment—or the second amendment, or the third amendment—as well. And, indeed, as Justice Frankfurter suggests in *Adamson*, it would be a most remarkable fact of the Constitution if the mere due process clause of the fifth amendment were somehow understood to be, miraculously, a compact sort of shorthand for everything else in the Bill of Rights! Yet, unless the fifth amendment due process clause somehow does this (or unless it at least picks up the first amendment), how can it possibly be argued that the mere due process clause of the fourteenth amendment nonetheless does that task in respect to the states?

Consider the matter in the following way. "Water," we have previously observed in these materials, "does not naturally rise higher than its source." If the antecedent referent of the post Civil War fourteenth amendment due process clause is the fifth amendment due process clause,[17] how, then, can the fourteenth amendment due process clause absorb the first amendment *when the fifth amendment due process clause obviously does no such thing*? Frankfurter's acerbic observations

---

16. One might try to argue that protection from double jeopardy, protection from trial without indictment by grand jury, and protection from compelled self-incrimination, are themselves merely examples of "due" process of law. (But in that case, probably one would also expect the notion to be reflected in the fifth amendment itself, i.e. that the due process clause would say "nor be otherwise deprived of life, liberty, or property, without due process of law," etc., rather than to read as it does.) (Moreover, as already observed in a previous footnote, in fact the Supreme Court has *not* regarded indictment by grand jury to be a feature of fourteenth amendment due process, *even now*. Yet, if the prerequisite of indictment by grand jury is to be seen as merely a specified example of due process, rather than as a separate fifth amendment requirement apart from due process as such, this approach by the Court seems very odd. A clause closely neighboring on the due process clause itself within the fifth amendment — the grand jury clause—is not deemed to be absorbed within the counterpart fourteenth amendment due process clause binding upon the states, but a clause found four amendments away, namely the speech and press clause in the first amendment, though having nothing to do with process as such, is deemed, in *Gitlow*, to be thus absorbed. Why?)

17. And if it is not, despite its identity of language, then to what does it refer for the content of the protection it supplies?

in *Adamson* thus surely do provide an occasion for pause. And once the issue has been raised in this fashion, how does one propose to work it out? Here is an alternative, proposed by Justice Hugo Black.

II

> My study of the historical events that culminated in the Fourteenth Amendment, and the expressions of those who sponsored and favored, as well as those who opposed its submission and passage, persuades me that one of the chief objects that the provisions of the Amendment's *first section*, separately, and *as a whole*, were intended to accomplish *was to make the Bill of Rights, applicable to the states.*[5] With full knowledge of the import of the *Barron* decision,[18] the framers and backers of the Fourteenth Amendment proclaimed its purpose to be to overturn the constitutional rule that case had announced. This historical purpose has never received full consideration or exposition in any opinion of this Court interpreting the Amendment.

These sentences appear in Justice Black's lengthy dissenting opinion in *Adamson.*[19] Among other sources reviewed in the Appendix to that opinion, Justice Black quoted elaborately from the record of debates in Congress on the proposed fourteenth amendment, in 1866. Here is one of his more telling references:[20]

> On May 23, 1866, Senator Howard introduced the proposed amendment to the Senate in the absence of Senator Fessenden who was sick. Senator Howard prefaced his remarks by stating:
> "I *** present to the Senate *** the views and the motives [of the Reconstruction Committee].
> "The first section of the amendment *** submitted for the consideration of the two Houses relates to the privileges and immunities of citizens of the several States, and to the rights and privileges of all persons, whether citizens or others, under the laws of the United States ***

---

5. [Footnote in Justice Black's opinion.] Another prime purpose was to make colored people citizens entitled to full equal rights as citizens despite what this Court decided in the *Dred Scott* case. Scott v. Sandford, 19 How. 393.

A comprehensive analysis of the historical origins of the Fourteenth Amendment, Flack, The Adoption of the Fourteenth Amendment (1908) 94, concludes that "Congress, the House and the Senate, had the following objects and motives in view for submitting the first section of the Fourteenth Amendment to the States for ratification:

"1.To make the Bill of Rights (the first eight Amendments) binding upon, or applicable to, the States.

"2. To give validity to the Civil Rights Bill.

"3. To declare who were citizens of the United States.

18. (Justice Black refers here is to Barron v. Baltimore, 7 Pet. 243, the 1833 decision holding that the Bill of Rights was a set of limitations only on the new national government and not on the states.)

19. 332 U.S. 68-123 (the quoted sentences appear at pp. 71-72) (emphasis added).

20. Id. at 104-107 (emphasis added).

"It will be observed that *this is a general prohibition upon all the States, as such, from abridging the privileges and immunities of the citizens of the United States. That is its first clause, and I regard it as very important.* It also prohibits each one of the States from depriving any person of life, liberty, or property without due process of law, or denying to any person within the jurisdiction of the State the equal protection of its laws. ***

"It would be a curious question to solve what are the privileges and immunities of citizens of each of the States in the Several States *** I am not aware that the Supreme Court has ever undertaken to define either the nature or extent of the privileges and immunities thus guaranteed. *** But we may gather some intimation of what probably will be the opinion of the judiciary by referring to Corfield v. Coryell [Here Senator Howard quoted at length from that opinion].

"Such is the character of the privileges and immunities spoken of in the second section of the fourth article of the Constitution. *To these privileges and immunities* whatever they may be—for they are not and cannot be fully defined in their entire extent and precise nature—to these *should be added the personal rights guarantied and secured by the first eight amendments of the Constitution; such as the freedom of speech and of the press; the right of the people peaceably to assemble and petition the Government for a redress of grievances, a right appertaining to each and all the people*; the right to keep and to bear arms; the right to be exempted from the quartering of soldiers in a house without the consent of the owner; the right to be exempt from unreasonable searches and seizures, and from any search or seizure except by virtue of a warrant issued upon a formal oath or affidavit; the right of an accused person to be informed of the nature of the accusation against him, and his right to be tried by an impartial jury of the vicinage; and also the right to be secure against excessive bail and against cruel and unusual punishments.

"Now, sir, here is a mass of privileges, immunities, and rights, some of them secured by the second section of the fourth article of the Constitution, which I have recited, *some by the first eight amendments of the Constitution*; and it is a fact worthy of attention that the course of decision in our courts and the present settled doctrine is, that all these immunities, privileges, rights, thus guarantied by the Constitution or recognized by it, are secured to the citizens solely as a citizen of the United States and as a party in their courts. They do not operate in the slightest degree as a restraint or prohibition upon State legislation. States are not affected by them, and it has been repeatedly held that the restriction contained in the Constitution against the taking of private property for public used without just compensation is not a restriction upon State legislation, but applies only to the legislation of Congress.

"Now, sir, there is no power given in the Constitution to enforce and to carry out any of these guaranties. They are not powers granted by the Constitution to Congress, and of course do not come within the sweeping clause of the Constitution authorizing Congress to pass all laws necessary and proper for carrying out the foregoing or granted powers, but they stand simply as a bill of rights in the Constitution, without power on the part of Congress to give them full effect; while at the same time the States are not restrained from violating the principles embraced in them except by their local constitutions, which may be altered from year to year. *The great object of the first section of this amendment is, therefore, to restrain the power of the States and compel them at all times to respect these fundamental guarantees.*"

In agreement with these rather emphatic expressions by Senator Howard, as Justice Black indicated in his footnote, was an early work by Horace Flack, written in 1908. In agreement also is a strongly argued, re-researched modern work by Michael Curtis, exactly to the same effect.[21] The latter, moreover, provides several examples in which the privileges and immunities clause was referred to during the state-by-state ratification process as prospectively protecting free speech, free press, and peaceable assembly, in particular, from state abridgments.[22] In contrast, a much-relied upon article by Charles Fairman, written after the *Adamson* case, argued strongly that Justice Black was mistaken.[23] And Raoul Berger, responding further

---

21. Michael K. Curtis, No State Shall Abridge: The Fourteenth Amendment and the Bill of Rights (2d printing 1987, Duke University Press). See also Henry J. Abraham & Barbara Perry, Freedom and the Court: Civil Rights and Civil Liberties in the United States 30-91 (6th ed. 1994); 2 William Winslow Crosskey, Politics and the Constitution chs. xxxi, xxxii (1953); William Dameron Guthrie, The Fourteenth Article of Amendment to the Constitution of the United States (1898); Harold M. Hyman & William M. Wiecek, Equal Justice Under Law 386-438 (1982); Joseph B. James, The Framing of the Fourteenth Amendment (1956); Alfred Avins, Incorporation of the Bill of Rights: The Crosskey-Fairman Debates Revisited, 6 Harv.J. on Legis. 1 (1968); Louis B. Boudin, Truth and Fiction about the Fourteenth Amendment, 16 N.Y.U.L.Q.Rev. 19 (1938); William Winslow Crosskey & Charles Fairman, "Legislative History," and the Constitutional Limitations on State Authority, 22 U.Chi.L.Rev. 1 (1954).

22. Curtis, *supra* p. 63 note 21, at 138-140, 148-49. (The examples are from pro-ratification speeches deploring the manner in which abolitionist speech was suppressed in the secessionist states, a condition the speaker insisted would end once the fourteenth amendment was approved.) See also Joseph B. James, The Ratification of the Fourteenth Amendment 46, 162 (1984).

23. Charles Fairman, Does the Fourteenth Amendment Incorporate the Bill of Rights?, 2 Stan. L. Rev. 5 (1949). See also Richard G. Stevens, Frankfurter and Due Process (1987). In 1968, however, Justice Black expressed himself as underwhelmed by the Fairman article Justice Harlan had relied on. Duncan v. Louisiana, 391 U.S. 145, 164-65 (1968) (Black, J., dissenting). ("My Brother Harlan's objections to my *Adamson* dissent history, like that of most of the objectors, relies most heavily on a criticism written by Professor Charles Fairman ***. I have read and studied this article extensively, including the historical references, but am compelled to add that in my view it has completely failed to refute the inferences and arguments that I suggested. *** The historical appendix to my *Adamson* dissent leaves no doubt in my mind that both its sponsors and those who opposed it believed the Fourteenth Amendment made the first eight Amendments of the Constitution (the Bill of Rights) applicable to the States.") (Id. at 165.) And, further to avoid the trap of being accused of discovering all of the Bill of Rights in only that part of the fourteenth amendment worded the same as but one part of the fifth amendment (i.e. the due process clause), Justice Black added the following footnote: "My view has been and is that the Fourteenth Amendment, *as a whole*, makes the Bill of

to this seemingly endless debate, has insisted that Curtis is equally mistaken as was Justice Black.[24]

Still, however one may consider the matter, it is surely plain that resolution of the first amendment-fourteenth amendment relationship question does not in fact require that one hinge the scope of first amendment protection from state law abridgments merely, or even importantly, to the "due" process clause, as the Court in *Gitlow* presumed to do, isn't it? And on that basis, criticism aimed against applying the fourteenth amendment to free speech cases would seem seriously misspent, because one's freedom of speech need not be seen as an aspect of "liberty" not to be taken away without "due process," but, rather, as a protected privilege and immunity of national citizenship no state may make or enforce any law to abridge—a privilege and immunity as strongly protected against state action as the first amendment protects it against acts of Congress, at least if one believes Justice Black's view.

But alas, for our immediate purposes, this embarrassment, so far as it undercuts Justice Frankfurter's point, cuts both ways in view of *Gitlow v. New York* itself. The embarrassment cuts *both* ways because, to return to *Gitlow v. New York*, it was on the pedigree of the due process clause (i.e. the due process clause alone rather than the privileges-and-immunities clause, or rather than the first section of the fourteenth amendment "as a whole") upon which the majority of the Court as well as Justices Holmes and Brandeis did rely in *Gitlow v. New York*. And seemingly, that reliance, for the reasons canvassed incidental to our review of Frankfurter's opinion in *Adamson v. California*, seems to be rather shaky.[25] Indeed, except for the Supreme Court, few have been willing to read the fourteenth amendment's due process clause as, all by itself, a *per se* shorthand for the Bill of Rights.[26]

Rights applicable to the States. This would certainly include the language of the Privileges and Immunities Clauses, as well as the Due Process Clause." (Id. at 166.)

24. Raoul Berger, The Fourteenth Amendment and the Bill of Rights (1989). In Mr. Berger's view, the fourteenth amendment was limited to the constitutionalizing of the Civil Rights Act of 1866. See Raoul Berger, Government by Judiciary: The Transformation of the Fourteenth Amendment (1977).

25. Indeed, as we have seen, Justice Black did not himself embrace it (and note the title to the Michael Curtis book—an obvious reference to the privileges and immunities clause and not to the due process clause).

26. Moreover, as we saw in an earlier footnote, even the Supreme Court does not now treat all of the first eight amendments as thus absorbed through the due process clause of the fourteenth amendment and thus made applicable to the states; some are not even yet deemed to apply, and other parts of other amendments may not apply wholly. Rather, the Court majority's position has been one of so-called selective absorption or partial incorporation of some but not all of the provisions of the first nine amendments through the due process clause of the fourteenth amendment. The rationale, according to which the selection of some but not all is required, appears in its best known form in an opinion by Justice Cardozo, in Palko v. Connecticut, 302 U.S. 319 (1937). Such rights or privileges as seem so essential to be "ranked as fundamental" in "the very essence of a scheme of ordered liberty" are identified also to the fourteenth amendment and limit the state governments as they limit the national government, but not all rights or privileges found in the first nine amendments are necessarily deemed

As we already observed elsewhere in these materials, moreover, it could make some real difference which clause—if any—in the fourteenth amendment is regarded as the proper anchor for the protection of free speech. The one clause, the privileges and immunities clause, shields those who are "citizens of the United States," a limited class defined in the opening sentence of the fourteenth amendment itself. The other, the due process clause, shields all who are "persons," whether or not they are citizens as well. By no means, then, is it a small matter to say which clause is to do what kind of work.[27] The tie the *Gitlow* case makes, between the first amendment and the due process clause (rather than between the first amendment and the privileges and immunities clause), is not a mere technician's or aesthetician's cavil on which nothing turns.[28]

Indeed, to pursue the distinction we have been examining within the fourteenth amendment, it may be thought that it would be eminently logical to regard certain enumerated substantive rights as rights of citizenship protected from state abridgment by the privileges and immunities clause of the fourteenth amendment, but certain procedural rights (e.g., to a fair trial) as rights shared more generally, by all persons within a state's jurisdiction, whether or not all such persons are also citizens of the United States. Consider the particular free speech cases thus far reviewed in this course in light of such a possible distinction. These have been speech cases, each involving some kind of political agitation including open public advocacy urging resistance to the law itself. That prerogative of complaining about the laws might be found suitable for citizens of the polity, i.e. a protected prerogative of one's citizenship status. Would it necessarily belong to those not citizens? Consider the obvious comparison of finding oneself a visitor or a resident alien in France or in England.

One might not be greatly surprised if one were not regarded as a sufficient member of the French national polity to have the same latitude of political agitation freedom while within France as French citizens within France might be constitu-

---

to be of this kind. The rationale continues to sit uncomfortably astride the bench. For two recent additional perspectives of addressing the relationship between the fourteenth amendment and the Bill of Rights, see Akhil R. Amar, The Bill of Rights and the Fourteenth Amendment, 101 Yale L.J. 1193 (1992); John Harrison, Reconstructing the Privileges and Immunities Clause, 101 Yale L.J. 1385 (1992).

27. Nor, because of the difference in respect to the different classes respectively protected by the privileges and immunities clause vis-à-vis the due process clause, may one avoid making a specific selection of the proper clause by saying merely that freedom of speech, press, assembly, and petition are protected by the first section of the fourteenth amendment "as a whole."

28. Notice that the location of free speech protection to the privileges and immunities clause rather than to the due process clause might also affect the first amendment standing of corporations—they are not "citizens of the United States" within the meaning of the relevant clause of the fourteenth amendment. (Regarded as "persons," corporations have been sheltered as having rights of free speech. See, e.g., First National Bank of Boston v. Bellotti, 435 U.S. 765 (1978) (state restriction on commercial corporate expenditures to influence ballot referendum struck down).)

tionally guaranteed. As an alien assigned, say, to the Paris office of an American law firm even for three, four, five years, or indefinitely, for instance, one might also lack the right to vote. Yet, one might still expect that insofar as one were charged with committing a crime while within France, or even were one sued civilly in France, the kind of trial one received would be conducted unexceptionably, i.e. with the same due process the French provide their own citizens in any like case. In brief, one might not be surprised were one's freedom to participate substantively in French politics (by voting or by speech) deemed to be more circumscribed substantively by French law, consistent with a Constitution written even in the same terms as our own Constitution, even while one might still receive equal protection in the French courts of all due process French courts are otherwise constitutionally expected to observe under provisions like those expressly found in our fifth and fourteenth amendments—providing a uniform standard of due process for persons (whether or not "citizens"). Providing a uniformity of due process would be quite consistent, jurisprudentially speaking, with wholly distinguishing privileges and immunities of citizenship as such. Perhaps that is just what the fourteenth amendment provides in separating the privileges and immunities clause from the due process clause, and, in doing so, moreover, carries over a like distinction between the first and fifth amendment themselves.[29]

III

All of the above having been considered, however, it is not sufficient to leave the *Gitlow* answer to the *Patterson* question behind us without some few paragraphs more. The linkage of one's substantive freedom of speech to the due process clause of the fourteenth amendment (rather than, if at all, to the privileges and immunities clause of the same amendment) does seem tenuous,[30] and it is consequential. Still, despite all that, it is not without its own history that gives it a certain quasi-support. Here is just a bit of that history.

In two cases arising under the fifth amendment prior to the Civil War (and thus prior also to the fourteenth amendment), the Supreme Court had already declared that an Act of Congress adversely affecting private property as a virtual taking or depri-

---

29. But see Bridges v. California, 314 U.S. 252, 257 (1941). (Harry Bridges was a citizen of Australia and not a citizen of the United States.)

30. Despite one's impatience with worrying about such matters once Supreme Court precedent appears to entrench a certain point of view so that its original constitutional integrity no longer seems to matter as a practical concern, moreover, there is the sense that, eventually, others may scratch the itch of even entrenched error until it is no longer bearable. There is a resentment that stubborn truth harbors against falsehood. (The Court has overruled its own constitutional decisions on more than 180 occasions.) Despite the special place of precedent (*stare decisis*) in Anglo-American law, moreover, the Court has itself asserted that the force of *stare decisis* is less, rather than more, compelling in constitutional cases. See, e.g., United States v. Scott, 437 U.S. 82, 101 (1978); Burnet v. Coronado Oil & Gas Co., 285 U.S. 393, 406-08 (1932) (Brandeis, J., dissenting). But see H. Monaghan, Stare Decisis and Constitutional Adjudication, 88 Colum.L.Rev. 723 (1988).

vation of an identifiable person's property was subject to judicial check and nullification in the Supreme Court according to the terms of the fifth amendment due process clause rather than the "takings" clause as such.[31] In 1896, following these precedents, the Court applied those fifth amendment, substantive "due process" clause restrictions to the states via the parallel due process clause of the fourteenth amendment.[32] Indeed, in a critical follow-up case that did so, the Court treated the fourteenth amendment due process clause as doing even more than foreclosing any substantively arbitrary restrictions on private property as such; rather, it held that due consideration of the owner's interests also implied a duty of compensation insofar as some appropriative public use (or third party use) was involved, to satisfy the imperatives of due process as such.[33] So, the fourteenth amendment, though having

---

31. Den v. Hoboken Land & Improvement Co., 59 U.S. (18 How.) 272, 276 (1856); Dred Scott v. Sandford, 60 U.S. (19 How.) 393, 450 (1857) ("[A]n Act of Congress which deprives a citizen of the United States of his liberty or property, merely because he came himself or brought his property into a particular Territory of the United States, and who had committed no offense against the laws, *could hardly be dignified with the name of due process of law.*") (emphasis added). (Thus, the Court suggested in *Dred Scott,* an Act of Congress that would work a divestiture of a slave owner's property in his slave merely by crossing over into a state with his slave for a short time and then exiting again, would affront the fifth amendment due process clause and would be held unconstitutional.) Additionally, certain pre-fourteenth amendment state supreme court cases applied state constitutional due process clauses as furnishing substantive limitations on state legislative power. The leading example is Wynehamer v. People, 13 N.Y. 378 (1856). A recent and comprehensive tracing of substantive due process in American legal history is provided in Frank R. Strong, Substantive Due Process (1986). See also Edward D. Corwin, The Doctrine of Due Process of Law Before the Civil War, 24 Harv.L.Rev. 366 (1911).

32. The transition is commonly associated with dicta in Davidson v. New Orleans, 96 U.S. 97 (1878). The Court discussed the jurisprudence of due process from Magna Carta forward, concluding: "It seems to us that a statute which declared in terms, and without more, that the full and exclusive title of a described piece of land, which is now in A, shall be and is hereby vested in B, would, if effectual, deprive A of his property without due process of law, within the meaning of the constitutional provision [of the fourteenth amendment]." Missouri Pac. Ry. v. Nebraska, 164 U.S. 403, 417 (1896), applied Justice Miller's dictum in this way, and did so for a unanimous court. ("The taking by a state of the private property of one person or corporation, without the owner's consent, for the private use of another, is not due process of law, and is a violation of the fourteenth article of amendment of the constitution of the United States.") Chicago, B. & Q. R.R. v. Chicago, 166 U.S. 226, 235 (1897) treats the dictum in *Davidson* in just this way, too.

33. Chicago, B. & Q. R.R. v. Chicago, 166 U.S. 226, 235, 239, 241 (1897). ("In our opinion, a judgment of a state court, even if it be authorized by statute, whereby private property is taken for the State or under its direction for public use, without compensation made or secured to the owner, is, upon principle and authority, wanting in the due process of law required by the Fourteenth Amendment of the Constitution of the United States ***.") (The Court then went forward to determine whether the compensation paid the railroad in the case satisfied the "just compensation" demanded by consistency with its view of the imperatives of substantive due process, finally concluding that it was.) See also First English Evangelical Lutheran Church of Glendale v. County of Los Angeles, 482 U.S. 304 (1987) (requiring compensation for a temporary taking by twinning the fifth amendment takings clause with the fourteenth amendment due process clause, i.e. treating them as fungible, suggesting no distinction between the two).

no just compensation clause like that expressly found in the fifth amendment, was deemed to absorb such a clause as of 1897, as a feature of (substantive) due process of law.

Chicago, Burlington and Quincy Railroad Co. v. Chicago, this 1897 decision by the Court, rather than *Gitlow v. New York*, is actually the first example of substantive due process absorption from a technically distinct part of the Bill of Rights (specifically, the takings clause of the fifth amendment) into the due process clause of the fourteenth amendment. Yet, the roots of that decision do seem to extend in some logical and traceable manner from sources located in the Court's own pre-fourteenth amendment substantive due process case law, namely, fifth amendment "substantive" due process case law. To this extent, then, the association of some cognate fourteenth amendment substantive due process rights separately identified within the Bill of Rights (e.g., the takings clause that adjoins the fifth amendment due process clause), has an integrated logic that antedates *Gitlow* by nearly thirty years, and a pre-fourteenth amendment due process history as well, linked into the fifth amendment due process clause itself.

These were, of course, property cases. But, as with "property" and substantive due process constraints upon legislative powers, so also with "liberty" and substantive due process constraints. The two are of a piece, so far as the due process clause is concerned. So, in *Lochner v. New York*,[35] insofar as the due process clause of the fourteenth amendment had already been applied to enforce its limits on legislative invasions of private property, the same clause, on its face equally protecting "liberty" as much as "property," was applied to liberty of a kind.[36] And so, in this fashion, the circle of our discussion begins to close. It is obviously this larger framework of substantive due process legal history the majority accepts in *Gitlow v. New York*, when it says:

> For present purposes we may and do assume that freedom of speech and of the press—which are protected by the First Amendment from abridgment by Congress—are among the fundamental personal rights and "liberties" protected by the due process clause of the Fourteenth Amendment from impairment by the States.[37]

---

35. 198 U.S. 45 (1905). See also Allgeyer v. Louisiana, 165 U.S. 578 (1897).

36. The "liberty" involved in *Lochner* was one's liberty to make contracts. The question treated in the Supreme Court was the question of the extent to which a state legislature might substantively restrict that liberty. The majority thought the answer was "not much," while Holmes, dissenting, thought the answer was "pretty much as the legislature prefers."

37. (*Applied in* Near v. Minnesota, 283 U.S. 697 (1931), holding a state statute invalid as interpreted to authorize an injunction against future publication of scandalous or defamatory matter, and declaring that "[i]t is no longer open to doubt that the liberty of the press and of speech is within the liberty safeguarded by the due process clause of the Fourteenth Amendment from invasion by state action")

And it is that same legal history Holmes (with Brandeis) also took into account concurringly,[38] saying:

> The general principle of free speech, it seems to me, must be taken to be included in the Fourteenth Amendment, in view of the scope that has been given to the word "liberty" as there used, although perhaps it may be accepted with a somewhat larger latitude of interpretation than is allowed to Congress by the sweeping language that governs or ought to govern the laws of the United States.

The original, robust controversy, therefore, became attenuated and virtually mooted in practice. The due process clause (rather than the privileges and immunities clause abandoned in the *Slaughterhouse Cases*), absorbed the chief work of fourteenth amendment, free speech review.[39] In turn, the first amendment, while not usually spoken of as literally "incorporated," is regarded as informing that review, and, indeed, as setting its basic standards in the Supreme Court.[40] In that sense, Justice Black has, more-or-less, won out for his own views.

Even so, not every member of the Court has regarded first and fourteenth amendment cases interchangeably, and not all of them find a complete equivalency between the first amendment and the fourteenth amendment. For some quite distinguished judges, the concrete facts of a case may make a real difference, including such "facts" as which level of government presumed to author the objectionable law, and what is the range of its effects. You will doubtless have noted, moreover, that both Holmes and Brandeis likewise reserved some leeway for first and fourteenth amendment distinctions to be drawn, though both were strongly

---

38. Note also that Justice Harlan, dissenting in *Patterson v. Colorado* in 1907, declined to rely wholly upon the privileges and immunities clause although that clause was for him (as later on, for Justice Black) the principally relevant text. Still, he added: "It is, I think, impossible to conceive of liberty, as secured by the Constitution against hostile action, whether by the Nation or by the States, which does not embrace the right to enjoy free speech and the right to have a free press," and referred expressly to the fourteenth amendment clause "forbidding a State to deprive any person of his liberty without due process of law." 205 U.S. at 465.

39. In Whitney v. California, 274 U.S. 357, 373 (1927), Justice Brandeis mused for one last time on the general problem we have addressed, in the setting of a free speech case. ("Despite arguments to the contrary which had seemed to me persuasive, it is settled that the due process clause of the Fourteenth Amendment applies to matters of substantive law as well as to matters of procedure.")

40. In West Va. Bd. of Educ. v. Barnette, 319 U.S. 624, 639 (1944), Justice Jackson expressed the matter in the following way: "The test of legislation which collides with the Fourteenth Amendment, because it also collides with the principles of the First, is much more definite than the test when only the Fourteenth is involved. Much of the vagueness of the due process clause disappears when the specific prohibitions of the First become its standard. *** It is important to note that while it is the Fourteenth Amendment which bears directly upon the State it is the more specific limiting principles of the First Amendment that finally govern this case."

committed to the political imperatives of free speech.[41] But we have concluded about as much as we can on the questions that first raised this inquiry, at least for the moment, and it is time to resume where we left off.

WHITNEY v. CALIFORNIA
274 U.S. 357 (1927)

MR. JUSTICE SANFORD delivered the opinion of the Court.

By a criminal information filed in the Superior Court of Alameda County, California, the plaintiff in error was charged, in five counts, with violations of the Criminal Syndicalism Act of that State. She was tried, convicted on the first count, and sentenced to imprisonment. The judgment was affirmed by the District Court of Appeal. ***

The pertinent provisions of the Criminal Syndicalism Act are:

> "Section 1. The term 'criminal syndicalism' as used in this act is hereby defined as any doctrine or precept advocating, teaching or aiding and abetting the commission of crime, sabotage (which word is hereby defined as meaning wilful and malicious physical damage or injury to physical property), or unlawful acts of force and violence or unlawful methods of terrorism as a means of accomplishing a change in industrial ownership or control, or effecting any political change.
>
> "Sec. 2. Any person who: *** 4. Organizes or assists in organizing, or is or knowingly becomes a member of, any organization, society, group or assemblage of persons organized or assembled to advocate, teach or aid and abet criminal syndicalism ***
>
> "Is guilty of a felony and punishable by imprisonment."

The first count of the information, on which the conviction was had, charged that on or about November 28, 1919, in Alameda County, the defendant, in violation of the Criminal Syndicalism Act, "did then and there unlawfully, wilfully, wrongfully, deliberately and feloniously organize and assist in organizing, and was, is, and knowingly became a member of an organization, society, group and assemblage of

---

41. I.e. note the manner in which Holmes cast his language in the case, and the distinction he also drew: "The general principle of free speech, it seems to me, must be taken to be included in the Fourteenth Amendment, in view of the scope that has been given to the word 'liberty' as there used, although perhaps it may be accepted with a somewhat larger latitude of interpretation than is allowed to Congress by the sweeping language that governs or ought to govern the laws of the United States." Note, also, however, that it was Holmes and Brandeis (rather than the majority of the Court), who voted to hold the state statute invalid in *Gitlow v. New York* itself; their test, even under the fourteenth amendment, was far more stringent than the majority used and, indeed, the same as Holmes employed in *Abrams v. United States*.

persons organized and assembled to advocate, teach, aid and abet criminal syndicalism." ***

Nor is the Syndicalism Act as applied in this case repugnant to the due process clause as a restraint of the rights of free speech, assembly, and association.

That the freedom of speech which is secured by the Constitution does not confer an absolute right to speak, without responsibility, whatever one may choose, or an unrestricted and unbridled license giving immunity for every possible use of language and preventing the punishment of those who abuse this freedom; and that a State in the exercise of its police power may punish those who abuse this freedom by utterances inimical to the public welfare, tending to incite to crime, disturb the public peace, or endanger the foundations of organized government and threaten its overthrow by unlawful means, is not open to question. Gitlow v. New York, 268 U.S. 652, 666-668, and cases cited.

By enacting the provisions of the Syndicalism Act the State has declared, through its legislative body, that to knowingly be or become a member of or assist in organizing an association to advocate, teach or aid and abet the commission of crimes or unlawful acts of force, violence or terrorism as a means of accomplishing industrial or political changes, involves such danger to the public peace and the security of the State, that these acts should be penalized in the exercise of its police power. *** The essence of the offense denounced by the Act is the combining with others in an association for the accomplishment of the desired ends through the advocacy and use of criminal and unlawful methods. It partakes of the nature of a criminal conspiracy. ***

The order dismissing the writ of error will be vacated and set aside, and the judgment of the Court of Appeal [a]ffirmed.

MR. JUSTICE BRANDEIS, concurring.

Miss Whitney was convicted of the felony of assisting in organizing, in the year 1919, the Communist Labor Party of California, of being a member of it, and of assembling with it. These acts are held to constitute a crime, because the party was formed to teach criminal syndicalism. The statute which made these acts a crime restricted the right of free speech and of assembly theretofore existing. The claim is that the statute, as applied, denied to Miss Whitney the liberty guaranteed by the Fourteenth Amendment.

The felony which the statute created is a crime very unlike the old felony of conspiracy or the old misdemeanor of unlawful assembly. The mere act of assisting in forming a society for teaching syndicalism, of becoming a member of it, or of assembling with others for that purpose is given the dynamic quality of crime. There is guilt although the society may not contemplate immediate promulgation of the doctrine. Thus the accused is to be punished, not for contempt, incitement or conspiracy, but for a step in preparation, which, if it threatens the public order at all, does so only remotely. The novelty in the prohibition introduced is that the statute aims, not at the practice of criminal syndicalism, nor even directly at the preaching of it, but at association with those who propose to preach it.

Despite arguments to the contrary which had seemed to me persuasive, it is settled that the due process clause of the Fourteenth Amendment applies to matters of substantive law as well as to matters of procedure. Thus all fundamental rights comprised within the term liberty are protected by the Federal Constitution from invasion by the States. The right of free speech, the right to teach and the right of assembly are, of course, fundamental rights. See Meyer v. Nebraska, 262 U.S. 390; Pierce v. Society of Sisters, 268 U.S. 510; Gitlow v. New York, 268 U.S. 652, 666; Farrington v. Tokushige, 273 U.S. 284. These may not be denied or abridged. But, although the rights of free speech and assembly are fundamental, they are not in their nature absolute. Their exercise is subject to restriction, if the particular restriction proposed is required in order to protect the State from destruction or from serious injury, political, economic or moral. That the necessity which is essential to a valid restriction does not exist unless speech would produce, or is intended to produce, a clear and imminent danger of some substantive evil which the State constitutionally may seek to prevent has been settled. See Schenck v. United States, 249 U.S. 47, 52.

The legislature must obviously decide, in the first instance, whether a danger exists which calls for a particular protective measure. But where a statute is valid only in case certain conditions exist, the enactment of the statute cannot alone establish the facts which are essential to its validity. Prohibitory legislation has repeatedly been held invalid, because unnecessary, where the denial of liberty involved was that of engaging in a particular business. The power of the courts to strike down an offending law is no less when the interests involved are not property rights, but the fundamental personal rights of free speech and assembly.

This Court has not yet fixed the standard by which to determine when a danger shall be deemed clear; how remote the danger may be and yet be deemed present; and what degree of evil shall be deemed sufficiently substantial to justify resort to abridgement of free speech and assembly as the means of protection. To reach sound conclusions on these matters, we must bear in mind why a State is, ordinarily, denied the power to prohibit dissemination of social, economic and political doctrine which a vast majority of its citizens believes to be false and fraught with evil consequence.

Fear of serious injury cannot alone justify suppression of free speech and assembly. Men feared witches and burnt women. It is the function of speech to free men from the bondage of irrational fears. To justify suppression of free speech there must be reasonable ground to fear that serious evil will result if free speech is practiced. There must be reasonable ground to believe that the danger apprehended is imminent. There must be reasonable ground to believe that the evil to be prevented is a serious one. Every denunciation of existing law tends in some measure to increase the probability that there will be a violation of it.[1] Condonation of a breach enhances the probability. Expressions of approval add to the probability. Propagation of the criminal state of mind by teaching syndicalism increases it. Advocacy of law-breaking heightens it still further. But even advocacy of violation, however reprehensible morally, is not a justification for denying free speech where the advocacy falls short of incitement and there is nothing to indicate that the advocacy would be immediately acted on. The wide difference between the advocacy and incitement, between preparation and attempt, between assembling and conspiracy, must be borne in mind. In order to support a finding of clear and present danger it must be shown either that immediate serious violence was to be expected or was advocated, or that the past conduct furnished reason to believe that such advocacy was then contemplated.

Those who won our independence by revolution were not cowards. They did not fear political change. They did not exalt order at the cost of liberty. To courageous self-reliant men, with confidence in the power of free and fearless reasoning applied through the processes of popular government, no danger flowing from speech can be deemed clear and present, unless the incidence of the evil apprehended is so imminent that it may befall before there is opportunity for full discussion. If there be time to expose through discussion the falsehood and fallacies, to avert the evil by the processes of education, the remedy to be applied is more speech, not enforced silence. Only an emergency can justify repression. Such must be the rule if authority is to be reconciled with freedom.[2] Such, in my opinion, is the command of the Constitution. It is therefore always open to Americans to challenge a law abridging free speech and assembly by showing that there was no emergency justifying it.

Moreover, even imminent danger cannot justify resort to prohibition of these functions essential to effective democracy, unless the evil apprehended is relatively serious. Prohibition of free speech and assembly is a measure so stringent that it would be inappropriate as the means for averting a relatively trivial harm to society. A police measure may be unconstitutional merely because the remedy, although effective as means of protection, is unduly harsh or oppressive. Thus, a State might, in the exercise of its police power, make any trespass upon the land of another a crime, regardless of the results or of the intent or purpose of the trespasser. It might, also, punish an attempt, a conspiracy, or an incitement to commit the trespass. But it is hardly conceivable that this Court would hold constitutional a statute which

---

1. Compare Judge Learned Hand in Masses Publishing Co. v. Patten, 244 Fed. 535, 540.

2. Compare Thomas Jefferson: "We have nothing to fear from the demoralizing reasonings of some, if others are left free to demonstrate their errors and especially when the law stands ready to punish the first criminal act produced by the false reasonings; these are safer corrections than the conscience of the judge." Quoted by Charles A. Beard, The Nation, July 7, 1926, vol. 123, p. 8. Also in first Inaugural Address: "If there be any among us who would wish to dissolve this union or change its republican form, let them stand undisturbed as monuments of the safety with which error of opinion may be tolerated where reason is left to combat it."

punished as a felony the mere voluntary assembly with a society formed to teach that pedestrians had the moral right to cross unenclosed, unposted, waste lands and to advocate their doing so, even if there was imminent danger that advocacy would lead to a trespass. The fact that speech is likely to result in some violence or in destruction of property is not enough to justify its suppression. There must be the probability of serious injury to the State. Among free men, the deterrents ordinarily to be applied to prevent crime are education and punishment for violations of the law, not abridgment of the rights of free speech and assembly. ***

Whether in 1919, when Miss Whitney did the things complained of, there was in California such clear and present danger of serious evil, might have been made the important issue in the case. She might have required that the issue be determined either by the court or the jury. She claimed below that the statute as applied to her violated the Federal Constitution; but she did not claim that it was void because there was no clear and present danger of serious evil, nor did she request that the existence of these conditions of a valid measure thus restricting the rights of free speech and assembly be passed upon by the court or a jury. *** Under these circumstances the judgment of the state court cannot be disturbed.* ***

MR. JUSTICE HOLMES joins in this opinion.

BRIDGES v. CALIFORNIA

314 U. S. 252 (1941)

MR. JUSTICE BLACK delivered the opinion of the Court.

*** All of the petitioners were adjudged guilty and fined for contempt of court by the Superior Court of Los Angeles County. Their conviction rested upon comments pertaining to pending litigation which were published in newspapers. ***

I

It is to be noted at once that we have no direction by the legislature of California that publications outside the court room which comment upon a pending case in a specified manner should be punishable. *** The judgments below, therefore, do not come to us encased in the armor wrought by prior legislative deliberation. Under such circumstances, this Court has said that "it must necessarily be found, as an original question," that the specified publications involved created "such likelihood of bringing about the substantive evil as to deprive [them] of the constitutional protection." Gitlow v. New York, 268 U.S. 652, 671.

---

*. **[Ed. Note**. For a careful and excellent review of *Whitney*, see Vincent A. Blasi, The First Amendment and the Ideal of Civil Courage: The Brandeis Opinion in Whitney v. California, 29 Wm. & Mary L. Rev. 653 (1988).]

How much "likelihood" is another question, "a question of proximity and degree"[4] that cannot be completely captured in a formula. In *Schenck v. United States*, however, this Court said that there must be a determination of whether or not "the words used are used in such circumstances and are of such a nature as to create a clear and present danger that they will bring about the substantive evils." We recognize that this statement, however helpful, does not comprehend the whole problem. As Mr. Justice Brandeis said in his concurring opinion in Whitney v. California, 274 U.S. 357, 374: "This Court has not yet fixed the standard by which to determine when a danger shall be deemed clear; how remote the danger may be and yet be deemed present." Nevertheless, the "clear and present danger" language[5] of the *Schenck* case has afforded practical guidance in a great variety of cases in which the scope of constitutional protections of freedom of expression was in issue.

*** Moreover, the likelihood, however great, that a substantive evil will result cannot alone justify a restriction upon freedom of speech or the press. The evil itself must be "substantial," Brandeis, J., concurring in *Whitney v. California, supra*, 374; it must be "serious," *id.* 376. And even the expression of "legislative preferences or beliefs" cannot transform minor matters of public inconvenience or annoyance into substantive evils of sufficient weight to warrant the curtailment of liberty of expression. Schneider v. State, 308 U.S. 147, 161.

What finally emerges from the "clear and present danger" cases is a working principle that the substantive evil must be extremely serious and the degree of imminence extremely high before utterances can be punished. Those cases do not purport to mark the furthermost constitutional boundaries of protected expression, nor do we here. They do no more than recognize a minimum compulsion of the Bill of Rights. For the First Amendment does not speak equivocally. It prohibits any law "abridging the freedom of speech, or of the press." It must be taken as a command of the broadest scope that explicit language, read in the context of a liberty-loving society, will allow.

---

4. Schenck v. United States, 249 U. S. 47, 52.

5. Restatement of the phrase "clear and present danger" in other terms has been infrequent. Compare, however: "*** the test to be applied *** *is not the remote or possible effect*." Brandeis, J., dissenting in Schaefer v. United States, 251 U.S. 466, 486; "*** we should be eternally vigilant against attempts to check the expression of opinions that we loathe and believe to be fraught with death, *unless they so imminently threaten immediate interference with the lawful and pressing purposes of the law that an immediate check is required to save the country*." Holmes, J., dissenting in Abrams v. United States, 250 U.S. 616, 630; "To justify suppression of free speech *there must be reasonable ground to fear that serious evil will result* if free speech is practiced. *There must be reasonable ground to believe that the danger apprehended is imminent*." Brandeis, J., concurring in Whitney v. California, 274 U.S. 357, 376. The italics are ours.

II

Before analyzing the punished utterances and the circumstances surrounding their publication, we must consider an argument which, if valid, would destroy the relevance of the foregoing discussion to this case. In brief, this argument is that the publications here in question belong to a special category marked off by history,—a category to which the criteria of constitutional immunity from punishment used where other types of utterances are concerned are not applicable. For, the argument runs, the power of judges to punish by contempt out-of-court publications tending to obstruct the orderly and fair administration of justice in a pending case was deeply rooted in English common law at the time the Constitution was adopted. That this historical contention is dubious has been persuasively argued elsewhere. Fox, *Contempt of Court, passim, e.g.*, 207. See also Stansbury, *Trial of James H. Peck*, 430. ***

More specifically, it is to forget the environment in which the First Amendment was ratified. In presenting the proposals which were later embodied in the Bill of Rights, James Madison, the leader in the preparation of the First Amendment, said: "Although I know whenever the great rights, the trial by jury, freedom of the press, or liberty of conscience, come in question in that body [Parliament], the invasion of them is resisted by able advocates, yet their Magna Charta does not contain any one provision for the security of those rights, respecting which the people of America are most alarmed. The freedom of the press and rights of conscience, those choicest privileges of the people, are unguarded in the British Constitution." 1 Annals of Congress 1789-1790, 434. And Madison elsewhere wrote that "the state of the press *** under the common law, cannot *** be the standard of its freedom in the United States." VI Writings of James Madison 1790-1802, 387.

There are no contrary implications in any part of the history of the period in which the First Amendment was framed and adopted. No purpose in ratifying the Bill of Rights was clearer than that of securing for the people of the United States much greater freedom of religion, expression, assembly, and petition than the people of Great Britain had ever enjoyed. ***

We are aware that although some states have by statute or decision expressly repudiated the power of judges to punish publications as contempts on a finding of mere tendency to interfere with the orderly administration of justice in a pending case, other states have sanctioned the exercise of such a power. But state power in this field was not tested in this Court for more than a century.[13] Not until 1925, with the decision in Gitlow v. New York, *supra*, 268 U.S. 652, did this Court recognize in the Fourteenth Amendment the application to the states of the same standards of

---

13. Patterson v. Colorado, 205 U.S. 454, the only case before this Court during that period in which a state court's power to punish out-of-court publications by contempt was in issue, cannot be taken as a decision squarely on this point. Cf.: "We leave undecided the question whether there is to be found in the Fourteenth Amendment a prohibition similar to that in the First." *Id.* 462.

freedom of expression as, under the First Amendment, are applicable to the federal government. And this is the first time since 1925 that we have been called upon to determine the constitutionality of a state's exercise of the contempt power in this kind of situation. Now that such a case is before us, we cannot allow the mere existence of other untested state decisions to destroy the historic constitutional meaning of freedom of speech and of the press.

History affords no support for the contention that the criteria applicable under the Constitution to other types of utterances are not applicable, in contempt proceedings, to out-of-court publications pertaining to a pending case.

III

***

No suggestion can be found in the Constitution that the freedom there guaranteed for speech and the press bears an inverse ratio to the timeliness and importance of the ideas seeking expression. Yet, it would follow as a practical result of the decisions below that anyone who might wish to give public expression to his views on a pending case involving no matter what problem of public interest, just at the time his audience would be most receptive, would be as effectively discouraged as if a deliberate statutory scheme of censorship had been adopted. ***

*** An endless series of moratoria on public discussion, even if each were very short, could hardly be dismissed as an insignificant abridgement of freedom of expression. And to assume that each would be short is to overlook the fact that the "pendency" of a case is frequently a matter of months or even years rather than days or weeks.

For these reasons we are convinced that the judgments below result in a curtailment of expression that cannot be dismissed as insignificant. If they can be justified at all, it must be in terms of some serious substantive evil which they are designed to avert. The substantive evil here sought to be averted has been variously described below.[15] It appears to be double: disrespect for the judiciary; and disorderly and unfair administration of justice. The assumption that respect for the judiciary can be won by shielding judges from published criticism wrongly appraises the character of American public opinion. For it is a prized American privilege to speak one's mind, although not always with perfect good taste,[16] on all public insti

---

15. Cf.: "*** said telegram *** had an inherent tendency *** *to embarrass and influence the actions and decisions of the judge* before whom said action was pending." Bridges v. Superior Court, supra, 14 Cal.2d at p. 471; "The published statement was not only *a criticism of the decision of the court* in an action then pending before said court, but was *a threat* that if an attempt was made to enforce the decision, the ports of the entire Pacific Coast would be tied up." *Id.* 488; "*** the test *** is whether it had a reasonable tendency *to interfere with the orderly administration of justice.*" *Id.* 110. The italics are ours.

16. Compare the following statements from letters of Thomas Jefferson as set out in Padover, Democracy, 150-151: "I deplore *** the putrid state into which our newspapers have passed, and the malignity, the vulgarity, and mendacious spirit of those who write them. *** These ordures are rapidly

tutions. And an enforced silence, however limited, solely in the name of preserving the dignity of the bench, would probably engender resentment, suspicion, and contempt much more than it would enhance respect.

The other evil feared, disorderly and unfair administration of justice, is more plausibly associated with restricting publications which touch upon pending litigation. The very word "trial" connotes decisions on the evidence and arguments properly advanced in open court. Legal trials are not like elections, to be won through the use of the meeting-hall, the radio, and the newspaper. But we cannot start with the assumption that publications of the kind here involved actually do threaten to change the nature of legal trials, and that to preserve judicial impartiality, it is necessary for judges to have a contempt power by which they can close all channels of public expression to all matters which touch upon pending cases. We must therefore turn to the particular utterances here in question and the circumstances of their publication to determine to what extent the substantive evil of unfair administration of justice was a likely consequence, and whether the degree of likelihood was sufficient to justify summary punishment.

The Los Angeles Times Editorials. The Times-Mirror Company, publisher of the Los Angeles Times, and L. D. Hotchkiss, its managing editor, were cited for contempt for the publication of three editorials. *** [The most critical editorial] thus distinguished was entitled "Probation for Gorillas?" After vigorously denouncing two members of a labor union who had previously been found guilty of assaulting non-union truck drivers, it closes with the observation: "Judge A. A. Scott will make a serious mistake if he grants probation to Matthew Shannon and Kennan Holmes. This community needs the example of their assignment to the jute mill." Judge Scott had previously set a day (about a month after the publication) for passing upon the application of Shannon and Holmes for probation and for pronouncing sentence.

The basis for punishing the publication as contempt was by the trial court said to be its "inherent tendency" and by the Supreme Court as its "reasonable tendency" to interfere with the orderly administration of justice in an action then before a court for consideration. In accordance with what we have said on the "clear and present danger" cases, neither "inherent tendency" nor "reasonable tendency" is enough to justify a restriction of free expression. But even if they were appropriate measures, we should find exaggeration in the use of those phrases to describe the facts here.

From the indications in the record of the position taken by the Los Angeles Times on labor controversies in the past, there could have been little doubt of its attitude toward the probation of Shannon and Holmes. In view of the paper's long-continued militancy in this field, it is inconceivable that any judge in Los Angeles would expect anything but adverse criticism from it in the event probation were

---

depraving the public taste.

It is however an evil for which there is no remedy, our liberty depends on the freedom of the press, and that cannot be limited without being lost."

granted. Yet such criticism after final disposition of the proceedings would clearly have been privileged. Hence, this editorial, given the most intimidating construction it will bear, did no more than threaten future adverse criticism which was reasonably to be expected anyway in the event of a lenient disposition of the pending case. To regard it, therefore, as in itself of substantial influence upon the course of justice would be to impute to judges a lack of firmness, wisdom, or honor,—which we cannot accept as a major premise. ***

The Bridges Telegram. While a motion for a new trial was pending in a case involving a dispute between an A. F. of L. union and a C. I. O. union of which Bridges was an officer, he either caused to be published or acquiesced in the publication of a telegram which he had sent to the Secretary of Labor. The telegram referred to the judge's decision as "outrageous"; said that attempted enforcement of it would tie up the port of Los Angeles and involve the entire Pacific Coast; and concluded with the announcement that the C. I. O. union, representing some twelve thousand members, did "not intend to allow state courts to override the majority vote of members in choosing its officers and representatives and to override the National Labor Relations Board." ***

In looking at the reason advanced in support of the judgment of contempt, we find that here, too, the possibility of causing unfair disposition of a pending case is the major justification asserted. And here again the gist of the offense, according to the court below, is intimidation.

Let us assume that the telegram could be construed as an announcement of Bridges' intention to call a strike, something which, it is admitted, neither the general law of California nor the court's decree prohibited. With an eye on the realities of the situation, we cannot assume that Judge Schmidt was unaware of the possibility of a strike as a consequence of his decision. If he was not intimidated by the facts themselves, we do not believe that the most explicit statement of them could have sidetracked the course of justice. Again, we find exaggeration in the conclusion that the utterance even "tended" to interfere with justice. If there was electricity in the atmosphere, it was generated by the facts; the charge added by the Bridges telegram can be dismissed as negligible. The words of Mr. Justice Holmes, spoken in reference to very different facts, seem entirely applicable here: "I confess that I cannot find in all this or in the evidence in the case anything that would have affected a mind of reasonable fortitude, and still less can I find there anything that obstructed the administration of justice in any sense that I possibly can give to those words." Toledo Newspaper Co. v. United States, *supra*, 247 U.S. at 425.

Reversed.

MR. JUSTICE FRANKFURTER, with whom concurred the CHIEF JUSTICE, MR. JUSTICE ROBERTS and MR. JUSTICE BYRNES, dissenting.

***

While the immediate question is that of determining the power of the courts of California to deal with attempts to coerce their judgments in litigation immediately before them, the consequence of the Court's ruling today is a denial to the people of the forty-eight states of a right which they have always regarded as essential for the effective exercise of the judicial process, as well as a denial to the Congress of powers which were exercised from the very beginning even by the framers of the Constitution themselves. To be sure, the majority do not in so many words hold that trial by newspapers has constitutional sanctity. But the atmosphere of their opinion and several of its phrases mean that or they mean nothing. Certainly, the opinion is devoid of any frank recognition of the right of courts to deal with utterances calculated to intimidate the fair course of justice—a right which hitherto all the states have from time to time seen fit to confer upon their courts and which Congress conferred upon the federal courts in the Judiciary Act of 1789. ***

We are not even vouchsafed reference to the specific provision of the Constitution which renders states powerless to insist upon trial by courts rather than trial by newspapers. So far as the Congress of the United States is concerned, we are referred to the First Amendment. That is specific. But we are here dealing with limitations upon California—with restraints upon the states. To say that the protection of freedom of speech of the First Amendment is absorbed by the Fourteenth does not say enough. Which one of the various limitations upon state power introduced by the Fourteenth Amendment absorbs the First? Some provisions of the Fourteenth Amendment apply only to citizens and one of the petitioners here is an alien; some of its provisions apply only to natural persons, and another petitioner here is a corporation. *** The majority opinion is strangely silent in failing to avow the specific constitutional provision upon which its decision rests. ***

The administration of justice by an impartial judiciary has been basic to our conception of freedom ever since Magna Carta. *** A trial is not a "free trade in ideas," nor is the best test of truth in a courtroom "the power of the thought to get itself accepted in the competition of the market." Compare Mr. Justice Holmes in Abrams v. United States, 250 U.S. 616, 630. A court is a forum with strictly defined limits for discussion. It is circumscribed in the range of its inquiry and in its methods by the Constitution, by laws, and by age-old traditions. Its judges are restrained in their freedom of expression by historic compulsions resting on no other officials of government. They are so circumscribed precisely because judges have in their keeping the enforcement of rights and the protection of liberties which, according to the wisdom of the ages, can only be enforced and protected by observing such methods and traditions. ***

Of course freedom of speech and of the press are essential to the enlightenment of a free people and in restraining those who wield power. Particularly should this freedom be employed in comment upon the work of courts, who are without many influences ordinarily making for humor and humility, twin antidotes to the corrosion of power. But the Bill of Rights is not self-destructive. Freedom of expression can hardly carry implications that nullify the guarantees of impartial trials. And since courts are the ultimate resorts for vindicating the Bill of Rights, a state may surely authorize appropriate historic means to assure that the process for such vindication be not wrenched from its rational tracks into the more primitive mêlée of passion and pressure. The need is great that courts be criticized, but just as great that they be allowed to do their duty. ***

*** A publication intended to teach the judge a lesson, or to vent spleen, or to discredit him, or to influence him in his future conduct, would not justify exercise of the contempt power. Compare Judge Learned Hand in Ex parte Craig, 282 F. 138, 160-61. It must refer to a matter under consideration and constitute in effect a threat to its impartial disposition. It must be calculated to create an atmospheric pressure incompatible with rational, impartial adjudication. But to interfere with justice it need not succeed. As with other offenses, the state should be able to proscribe attempts that fail because of the danger that attempts may succeed. The purpose, it will do no harm to repeat, is not to protect the court as a mystical entity or the judges as individuals or as anointed priests set apart from the community and spared the criticism to which in a democracy other public servants are exposed. The purpose is to protect immediate litigants and the public from the mischievous danger of an unfree or coerced tribunal. ***

The rule of law applied in these cases by the California court forbade publications having "a reasonable tendency to interfere with the orderly administration of justice in pending actions." To deny that this age-old formulation of the prohibition against interference with dispassionate adjudication is properly confined to the substantive evil is not only to turn one's back on history but also to indulge in an idle play on words, unworthy of constitutional adjudication. It was urged before us that the words "reasonable tendency" had a fatal pervasiveness, and that their replacement by "clear and present danger" was required to state a constitutionally permissible rule of law. The Constitution, as we have recently had occasion to remark, is not a formulary. *** Nor does it require displacement of an historic test by a phrase which first gained currency on March 3, 1919. Schenck v. United States, 249 U.S. 47. Our duty is not ended with the recitation of phrases that are the short-hand of a complicated historic process. The phrase "clear and present danger" is merely a justification for curbing utterance where that is warranted by the substantive evil to be prevented. The phrase itself is an expression of tendency and not of accomplishment, and the literary difference between it and "reasonable tendency" is not of constitutional dimension. ***

No objections were made before us to the procedure by which the charges of contempt were tried. But it is proper to point out that neither case was tried by a judge who had participated in the trials to which the publications referred. Compare Cooke v. United States, 267 U.S. 517, 539. So it is clear that a disinterested tribunal was furnished, and since the Constitution does not require a state to furnish jury trials, Maxwell v. Dow, 176 U.S. 581; Palko v. Connecticut, 302 U.S. 319, 324, and states have discretion in fashioning criminal remedies, Tigner v. Texas, 310 U.S. 141, the situation here is the same as though a state had made it a crime to publish utterance having a "reasonable tendency to interfere with the orderly administration of justice in pending actions," and not dissimilar from what the United States has done in § 135 of the Criminal Code.

A BRIEF SUMMARY ON *BRIDGES V. CALIFORNIA*

Bridges v. California marks a suitable point for pause. Note it is the first case since *Patterson v. Colorado* that actually concerns the same problem dealt with in *Patterson*, i.e. newspaper contempt of court, alleged threat to fair trial, libel of judges, intimidation of judicial process, etc. "versus" freedom of the press, and in that respect draws a neat circle around the changes in first amendment doctrine since the *Patterson* decision, in 1907. It may warrant a convenient comparison, therefore, with *Patterson*, in marking the course of modern first amendment doctrine.[42] Second, *Bridges* is also a case that applies, through the majority opinion, the rigorized Holmes-Brandeis standard of substantive judicial review derived from the cases we have previously examined (e.g.,*Abrams, Gitlow, Whitney*), but in which that standard appeared principally in dissents. For that reason as well, it provides a convenient way of comparing a newer sort of first amendment "figure" graphically, with the two originally introduced in these materials: the "absolute" view first suggested in the Introduction (sometimes identified to Justice Hugo Black), and the "no licensing" view, identified with Blackstone, and with Holmes in 1907.

Beginning with *Schenck*, Holmes repudiated the mere bad tendency test at least in cases involving political advocacy and criticism, substituting a case-specific, judicially reviewable, "clear and present danger" proof. Beginning with *Gitlow*, Brandeis advanced the stronger position (in which Holmes concurred), that even the actual eventuality of certain "harms" as a foreseen effect of social advocacy speech must be borne by the polity, as a necessary social cost of protecting social advocacy. In this sense, the Holmes-Brandeis view is that the strong form of the first amendment disallows the internalizing of some negative free speech effects by holding the speaker responsible for them (namely, minor harms, moderate inconveniences, etc.) though they are harms otherwise within the police power of the state to avoid, but not when they are the inevitable byproduct of highly protected freedoms of social advocacy or criticism. In a manner of speaking, in Brandeis' view, the first amendment disallows government from putting a higher premium on the avoidance of certain minor harms than on freedom of speech.

---

42. The next several assigned cases are meant principally to furnish a coherent, brief review of "free press-prior restraint" cases, in related settings, with no basic doctrinal changes but, rather, with a few refinements on the analysis provided in the *Bridges* case.

Roughly speaking, the comparisons yield four figures, the last three being the practically significant ones: the second (Blackstone) reflecting a very small area of first amendment operative force, the fourth, represented in the analysis and holding of *Bridges*, extending the field of first amendment preemption in two additional ways:

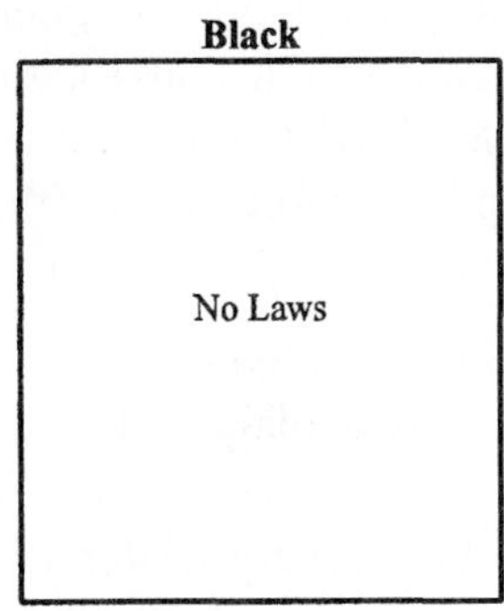

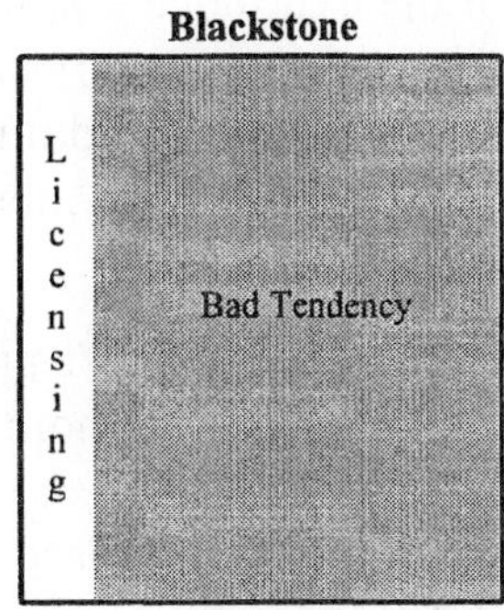

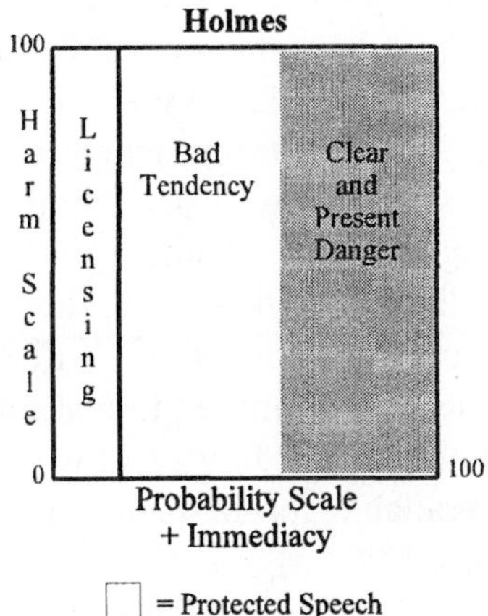

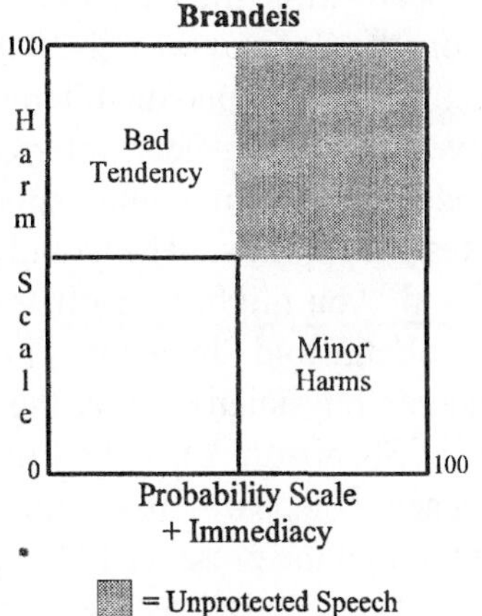

= Protected Speech

= Unprotected Speech

VARIATIONS ON *BRIDGES v. CALIFORNIA*: FREE PRESS, FAIR TRIAL, AND PRIOR RESTRAINTS

SHEPPARD v. MAXWELL
384 U.S. 333 (1966)

MR. JUSTICE CLARK delivered the opinion of the Court.

This federal habeas corpus application involves the question whether Sheppard was deprived of a fair trial in his state conviction for the second-degree murder of his wife because of the trial judge's failure to protect Sheppard sufficiently from the massive, pervasive and prejudicial publicity that attended his prosecution. *** We have concluded that Sheppard did not receive a fair trial consistent with the Due Process Clause of the Fourteenth Amendment and, therefore, reverse the judgment.

I

Marilyn Sheppard, petitioner's pregnant wife, was bludgeoned to death in the upstairs bedroom of their lakeshore home in Bay Village, Ohio, a suburb of Cleveland. ***

From the outset officials focused suspicion on Sheppard. After a search of the house and the premises on the morning of the tragedy, Dr. Gerber, the Coroner, is reported—and it is undenied—to have told his men, "Well, it is evident the doctor did this, so let's go get the confession out of him." He proceeded to interrogate and examine Sheppard while the latter was under sedation in his hospital room. On the same occasion, the Coroner was given the clothes Sheppard wore at the time of the tragedy together with the personal items in them. Later that afternoon Chief Eaton and two Cleveland police officers interrogated Sheppard at some length, confronting him with evidence and demanding explanations. Asked by Officer Shotke to take a lie detector test, Sheppard said he would if it were reliable. Shotke replied that it was "infallible" and "you might as well tell us all about it now." At the end of the interrogation Shotke told Sheppard: "I think you killed your wife." Still later in the same afternoon a physician sent by the Coroner was permitted to make a detailed examination of Sheppard. Until the Coroner's inquest on July 22, at which time he was subpoenaed, Sheppard made himself available for frequent and extended questioning without the presence of an attorney. ***

Throughout this period the newspapers emphasized evidence that tended to incriminate Sheppard and pointed out discrepancies in his statements to authorities. *** The newspapers also delved into Sheppard's personal life. Articles stressed his extramarital love affairs as a motive for the crime. The newspapers portrayed Sheppard as a Lothario, fully explored his relationship with Susan Hayes, and named a number of other women who were allegedly involved with him. The testimony at trial never showed that Sheppard had any illicit relationships besides the one with Susan Hayes.

On July 28, an editorial entitled "Why Don't Police Quiz Top Suspect" demanded that Sheppard be taken to police headquarters. It described him in the following language:

> "Now proved under oath to be a liar, still free to go about his business, shielded by his family, protected by a smart lawyer who has made monkeys of the police and authorities, carrying a gun part of the time, left free to do whatever he pleases *** ."

A front-page editorial on July 30 asked: "Why Isn't Sam Sheppard in Jail?" It was later titled "Quit Stalling—Bring Him In." After calling Sheppard "the most unusual murder suspect ever seen around these parts" the article said that "[e]xcept for some superficial questioning during Coroner Sam Gerber's inquest he has been scot-free of any official grilling ***." It asserted that he was "surrounded by an iron curtain of protection [and] concealment." ***

*** We do not detail the coverage further. There are five volumes filled with similar clippings from each of the three Cleveland newspapers covering the period from the murder until Sheppard's conviction in December 1954. The record includes no excerpts from newscasts on radio and television but since space was reserved in the courtroom for these media we assume that their coverage was equally large.

II

With this background the case came on for trial two weeks before the November general election at which the chief prosecutor was a candidate for common pleas judge and the trial judge, Judge Blythin, was a candidate to succeed himself. Twenty-five days before the case was set, 75 veniremen were called as prospective jurors. All three Cleveland newspapers published the names and addresses of the veniremen. As a consequence, anonymous letters and telephone calls, as well as calls from friends, regarding the impending prosecution were received by all of the prospective jurors. The selection of the jury began on October 18, 1954.

*** Private telephone lines and telegraphic equipment were installed *** so that reports from the trial could be speeded to the papers. Station WSRS was permitted to set up broadcasting facilities on the third floor of the courthouse next door to the jury room, where the jury rested during recesses in the trial and deliberated. Newscasts were made from this room throughout the trial, and while the jury reached its verdict.

On the sidewalk and steps in front of the courthouse, television and newsreel cameras were occasionally used to take motion pictures of the participants in the trial, including the jury and the judge. Indeed, one television broadcast carried a staged interview of the judge as he entered the courthouse. In the corridors outside the courtroom there was a host of photographers and television personnel with flash cameras, portable lights and motion picture cameras. This group photographed the prospective jurors during selection of the jury. After the trial opened, the witnesses, counsel, and jurors were photographed and televised whenever they entered or left the courtroom. Sheppard was brought to the courtroom about 10 minutes before each session began; he was surrounded by reporters and extensively photographed for the newspapers and television. A rule of court prohibited picture-taking in the courtroom during the actual sessions of the court, but no restraints were put on photographers during recesses, which were taken once each morning and afternoon, with a longer period for lunch.

All of these arrangements with the news media and their massive coverage of the trial continued during the entire nine weeks of the trial. ***

The jurors themselves were constantly exposed to the news media. Every juror, except one, testified at *voir dire* to reading about the case in the Cleveland papers or to having heard broadcasts about it. Seven of the 12 jurors who rendered the verdict had one or more Cleveland papers delivered in their home; the remaining jurors were not interrogated on the point. Nor were there questions as to radios or television sets in the jurors' homes, but we must assume that most of them owned such conveniences. As the selection of the jury progressed, individual pictures of prospective members appeared daily. During the trial, pictures of the jury appeared over 40 times in the Cleveland papers alone. The court permitted photographers to take pictures of the jury in the box, and individual pictures of the members in the jury room. One newspaper ran pictures of the jurors at the Sheppard home when they went there to view the scene of the murder. The day before the verdict was rendered—while the jurors were at lunch and sequestered by two bailiffs—the jury was separated into two groups to pose for photographs which appeared in the newspapers.

III

***

While the jury was being selected, a two-inch headline asked: "But Who Will Speak for Marilyn?" The front-page story spoke of the "perfect face" of the accused. "Study that face as long as you want. Never will you get from it a hint of what might be the answer. ***" The two brothers of the accused were described as "Prosperous, poised. His two sisters-in-law. Smart, chic, well-groomed. His elderly father. Courtly, reserved. A perfect type for the patriarch of a staunch clan." The author then noted Marilyn Sheppard was "still off stage," and that she was an only child whose mother died when she was very young and whose father had no interest in the case. But the author—through quotes from Detective Chief James McArthur—assured readers that the prosecution's exhibits would speak for Marilyn. "Her story," McArthur stated, "will come into this courtroom through our witnesses." The article ends:

> "Then you realize how what and who is missing from the perfect setting will be supplied.
>
> "How in the Big Case justice will be done.
>
> "Justice to Sam Sheppard.

"And to Marilyn Sheppard."

As has been mentioned, the jury viewed the scene of the murder on the first day of the trial. Hundreds of reporters, cameramen and onlookers were there, and one representative of the news media was permitted to accompany the jury while it inspected the Sheppard home. The time of the jury's visit was revealed so far in advance that one of the newspapers was able to rent a helicopter and fly over the house taking pictures of the jurors on their tour.

On November 19, a Cleveland police officer gave testimony that tended to contradict details in the written statement Sheppard made to the Cleveland police. Two days later, in a broadcast heard over Station WHK in Cleveland, Robert Considine likened Sheppard to a perjurer and compared the episode to Alger Hiss' confrontation with Whittaker Chambers. Though defense counsel asked the judge to question the jury to ascertain how many heard the broadcast, the court refused to do so. The judge also overruled the motion for continuance based on the same ground, saying:

> "Well, I don't know, we can't stop people, in any event, listening to it. It is a matter of free speech, and the court can't control everybody. *** We are not going to harass the jury every morning. *** It is getting to the point where if we do it every morning, we are suspecting the jury. I have confidence in this jury . ***"

On November 24, a story appeared under an eight-column headline: "Sam Called A 'Jekyll-Hyde' By Marilyn, Cousin To Testify." It was related that Marilyn had recently told friends that Sheppard was a "Dr. Jekyll and Mr. Hyde" character. No such testimony was ever produced at the trial. The story went on to announce: "The prosecution has a 'bombshell witness' on tap who will testify to Dr. Sam's display of fiery temper—countering the defense claim that the defendant is a gentle physician with an even disposition." Defense counsel made motions for change of venue, continuance and mistrial, but they were denied. No action was taken by the court. ***

IV

The principle that justice cannot survive behind walls of silence has long been reflected in the "Anglo-American distrust for secret trials." In re Oliver, 333 U.S. 257, 268 (1948). A responsible press has always been regarded as the handmaiden of effective judicial administration, especially in the criminal field. Its function in this regard is documented by an impressive record of service over several centuries. The press does not simply publish information about trials but guards against the miscarriage of justice by subjecting the police, prosecutors, and judicial processes to extensive public scrutiny and criticism. This Court has, therefore, been unwilling to place any direct limitations on the freedom traditionally exercised by the news media for "[w]hat transpires in the court room is public property." Craig v. Harney, 331 U.S. 367, 374 (1947). The "unqualified prohibitions laid down by the framers were intended to give to liberty of the press *** the broadest scope that could be countenanced in an orderly society." Bridges v. California, 314 U.S. 252, 265 (1941). And where there was "no threat or menace to the integrity of the trial," Craig v. Harney, *supra*, at 377, we have consistently required that the press have a free hand, even though we sometimes deplored its sensationalism.

But the Court has also pointed out that "[l]egal trials are not like elections, to be won through the use of the meeting-hall, the radio, and the newspaper." Bridges v. California, *supra*, at 271. And the Court has insisted that no one be punished for a crime without "a charge fairly made and fairly tried in a public tribunal free of prejudice, passion, excitement, and tyrannical power." Chambers v. Florida, 309 U.S. 227, 236-237 (1940). "Freedom of discussion should be given the widest range compatible with the essential requirement of the fair and orderly administration of justice." ***

The undeviating rule of this Court was expressed by Mr. Justice Holmes over half a century ago in Patterson v. Colorado, 205 U.S. 454, 462 (1907):

> "The theory of our system is that the conclusions to be reached in a case will be induced only by evidence and argument in open court, and not by any outside influence, whether of private talk or public print."

VII

*** [T]he judge never considered other means that are often utilized to reduce the appearance of prejudicial material and to protect the jury from outside influence. We conclude that these procedures would have been sufficient to guarantee Sheppard a fair trial and so do not consider what sanctions might be available against a recalcitrant press nor the charges of bias now made against the state trial judge.

The carnival atmosphere at trial could easily have been avoided since the courtroom and courthouse premises are subject to the control of the court. As we stressed in *Estes*, the presence of the press at judicial proceedings must be limited when it is apparent that the accused might otherwise be prejudiced or disadvantaged.[12] Bearing in mind the massive pretrial publicity, the judge should have adopted stricter rules governing the use of the courtroom by newsmen, as Sheppard's counsel requested. ***

*** And it is obvious that the judge should have further sought to alleviate this problem by imposing control over the statements made to the news media by counsel, witnesses, and especially the Coroner and police officers. ***

More specifically, the trial court might well have proscribed extrajudicial statements by any lawyer, party, witness, or court official which divulged prejudicial matters, such as the refusal of Sheppard to submit to interrogation or take any lie detector

---

12. The judge's awareness of his power in this respect is manifest from his assignment of seats to the press.

tests; any statement made by Sheppard to officials; the identity of prospective witnesses or their probable testimony; any belief in guilt or innocence; or like statements concerning the merits of the case. ***

From the cases coming here we note that unfair and prejudicial news comment on pending trials has become increasingly prevalent. Due process requires that the accused receive a trial by an impartial jury free from outside influences. Given the pervasiveness of modern communications and the difficulty of effacing prejudicial publicity from the minds of the jurors, the trial courts must take strong measures to ensure that the balance is never weighed against the accused. And appellate tribunals have the duty to make an independent evaluation of the circumstances. Of course, there is nothing that proscribes the press from reporting events that transpire in the courtroom. But where there is a reasonable likelihood that prejudicial news prior to trial will prevent a fair trial, the judge should continue the case until the threat abates, or transfer it to another county not so permeated with publicity. In addition, sequestration of the jury was something the judge should have raised *sua sponte* with counsel. If publicity during the proceedings threatens the fairness of the trial, a new trial should be ordered. But we must remember that reversals are but palliatives; the cure lies in those remedial measures that will prevent the prejudice at its inception. The courts must take such steps by rule and regulation that will protect their processes from prejudicial outside interferences. ***

Since the state trial judge did not fulfill his duty to protect Sheppard from the inherently prejudicial publicity which saturated the community and to control disruptive influences in the courtroom, we must reverse the denial of the habeas petition. The case is remanded to the District Court with instructions to issue the writ and order that Sheppard be released from custody unless the State puts him to its charges again within a reasonable time.

It is so ordered.

MR. JUSTICE BLACK dissents.

NEBRASKA PRESS ASSOCIATION v. STUART
427 U S. 539 (1976)

MR. CHIEF JUSTICE BURGER delivered the opinion of the Court.

The respondent State District Judge entered an order restraining the petitioners from publishing or broadcasting accounts of confessions or admissions made by the accused or facts "strongly implicative" of the accused in a widely reported murder of six persons. We granted certiorari to decide whether the entry of such an order on the showing made before the state court violated the constitutional guarantee of freedom of the press.

I

On the evening of October 18, 1975, local police found the six members of the Henry Kellie family murdered in their home in Sutherland, Neb., a town of about 850 people. Police released the description of a suspect, Erwin Charles Simants, to the reporters who had hastened to the scene of the crime. Simants was arrested and arraigned in Lincoln County Court the following morning, ending a tense night for this small rural community.

The crime immediately attracted widespread news coverage, by local, regional, and national newspapers, radio and television stations. Three days after the crime, the County Attorney and Simants' attorney joined in asking the County Court to enter a restrictive order relating to "matters that may or may not be publicly reported or disclosed to the public," because of the "mass coverage by news media" and the "reasonable likelihood of prejudicial news which would make difficult, if not impossible, the impaneling of an impartial jury and tend to prevent a fair trial." The County Court heard oral argument but took no evidence; no attorney for members of the press appeared at this stage. The County Court granted the prosecutor's motion for a restrictive order and entered it the next day, October 22. The order prohibited everyone in attendance from "releas[ing] or authoriz[ing] the release for public dissemination in any form or manner whatsoever any testimony given or evidence adduced"; the order also required members of the press to observe the Nebraska Bar-Press Guidelines.[1]

Simants' preliminary hearing was held the same day, open to the public but subject to the order. The County Court bound over the defendant for trial to the State District Court. The charges, as amended to reflect the autopsy findings, were that Simants had committed the murders in the course of a sexual assault.

Petitioners—several press and broadcast associations, publishers, and individual reporters—moved on October 23 for leave to intervene in the District Court, asking that the restrictive order imposed by the County Court be vacated. The District Court conducted a hearing, at which the County Judge testified and newspaper articles about the *Simants* case were admitted in evidence. The District Judge granted petitioners' motion to intervene and, on October 27, entered his own restrictive order. The judge found "because of the nature of the crimes charged in the complaint that there is a clear and present danger that pre-trial publicity could impinge upon the

1. These Guidelines are voluntary standards adopted by members of the state bar and news media to deal with the reporting of crimes and criminal trials. They outline the matters of fact that may appropriately be reported, and also list what items are not generally appropriate for reporting, including confessions, opinions on guilt or innocence, statements that would influence the outcome of a trial, the results of tests or examinations, comments on the credibility of witnesses, and evidence presented in the jury's absence. The publication of an accused's criminal record should, under the Guidelines, be "considered very carefully." The Guidelines also set out standards for taking and publishing photographs, and set up a joint bar-press committee to foster cooperation in resolving particular problems that emerge.

defendant's right to a fair trial." The order applied only until the jury was impaneled, and specifically prohibited petitioners from reporting five subjects: (1) the existence or contents of a confession Simants had made to law enforcement officers, which had been introduced in open court at the arraignment; (2) the fact or nature of statements Simants had made to other persons; (3) the contents of a note he had written the night of the crime; (4) certain aspects of the medical testimony at the preliminary hearing; and (5) the identity of the victims of the alleged sexual assault and the nature of the assault. It also prohibited reporting the exact nature of the restrictive order itself. Like the County Court's order, this order incorporated the Nebraska Bar-Press Guidelines. ***

The Nebraska Supreme Court balanced the "heavy presumption against [the] onstitutional validity" that an order restraining publication bears, New York Times Co. v. United States, 403 U.S. 713, 714 (1971), against the importance of the defendant's right to trial by an impartial jury. Because of the publicity surrounding the crime, the court determined that this right was in jeopardy. The court noted that Nebraska statutes required the District Court to try Simants within six months of his arrest, and that a change of venue could move the trial only to adjoining counties, which had been subject to essentially the same publicity as Lincoln County. The Nebraska Supreme Court held that "[u]nless the absolutist position of the relators was constitutionally correct, it would appear that the District Court acted properly." 194 Neb., at 797, 236 N.W. 2d, at 803.

The Nebraska Supreme Court rejected that "absolutist position," but modified the District Court's order to accommodate the defendant's right to a fair trial and the petitioners' interest in reporting pretrial events. The order as modified prohibited reporting of only three matters: (a) the existence and nature of any confessions or admissions made by the defendant to law enforcement officers, (b) any confessions or admissions made to any third parties, except members of the press, and (c) other facts "strongly implicative" of the accused. *** We granted certiorari to address the important issues raised by the District Court order as modified by the Nebraska Supreme Court. ***

III

The problems presented by this case are almost as old as the Republic. Neither in the Constitution nor in contemporaneous writings do we find that the conflict between these two important rights was anticipated, yet it is inconceivable that the authors of the Constitution were unaware of the potential conflicts between the right to an unbiased jury and the guarantee of freedom of the press. ***

IV

The Sixth Amendment in terms guarantees "trial, by an impartial jury ***" in federal criminal prosecutions. Because "trial by jury in criminal cases is fundamental to the American scheme of justice," the Due Process Clause of the Fourteenth

Amendment guarantees the same right in state criminal prosecutions. Duncan v. Louisiana, 391 U.S. 145, 149 (1968). ***

The costs of failure to afford a fair trial are high. In the most extreme cases, like *Sheppard* ***, the risk of injustice was avoided when the convictions were reversed. But a reversal means that justice has been delayed for both the defendant and the State; in some cases, because of lapse of time retrial is impossible or further prosecution is gravely handicapped. Moreover, in borderline cases in which the conviction is not reversed, there is some possibility of an injustice unredressed. The "strong measures" outlined in *Sheppard v. Maxwell* are means by which a trial judge can try to avoid exacting these costs from society or from the accused.

The state trial judge in the case before us acted responsibly, out of a legitimate concern, in an effort to protect the defendant's right to a fair trial.[4] What we must decide is not simply whether the Nebraska courts erred in seeing the possibility of real danger to the defendant's rights, but whether in the circumstances of this case the means employed were foreclosed by another provision of the Constitution.

V

*** None of our decided cases on prior restraints involved restrictive orders entered to protect a defendant's right to a fair and impartial jury, but the opinions on prior restraint have a common thread relevant to this case. ***

The thread running through all these cases is that prior restraints on speech and publication are the most serious and the least tolerable infringement on First Amendment rights. A criminal penalty or a judgment in a defamation case is subject to the whole panoply of protections afforded by deferring the impact of the judgement until all avenues of appellate review have been exhausted. Only after judgment has become final, correct or otherwise, does the law's sanction become fully operative.

A prior restraint, by contrast and definition, has an immediate and irreversible sanction. If it can be said that a threat of criminal or civil sanctions after publication "chills" speech, prior restraint "freezes" it at least for the time. ***

VI

We turn now to the record in this case to determine whether, as Learned Hand put it, "the gravity of the 'evil,' discounted by its probability, justifies such invasion of free speech as is necessary to avoid the danger." United States v. Dennis, 183 F.2d 201, 212 (CA2 1950), aff'd, 341 U.S. 494 (1951); see also L. Hand, The Bill of Rights 58-61 (1958). To do so, we must examine the evidence before the trial judge when the order was entered to determine (a) the nature and extent of pretrial news

---

4. The record also reveals that counsel for both sides acted responsibly in this case, and there is no suggestion that either sought to use pretrial news coverage for partisan advantage. A few days after the crime, newspaper accounts indicated that the prosecutor had announced the existence of a confession; we learned at oral argument that these accounts were false, although in fact a confession had been made.

coverage; (b) whether other measures would be likely to mitigate the effects of unrestrained pretrial publicity; and (c) how effectively a restraining order would operate to prevent the threatened danger. The precise terms of the restraining order are also important. We must then consider whether the record supports the entry of a prior restraint on publication, one of the most extraordinary remedies known to our jurisprudence.

In assessing the probable extent of publicity, the trial judge had before him newspapers demonstrating that the crime had already drawn intensive news coverage, and the testimony of the County Judge, who had entered the initial restraining order based on the local and national attention the case had attracted. The District Judge was required to assess the probable publicity that would be given these shocking crimes prior to the time a jury was selected and sequestered. He then had to examine the probable nature of the publicity and determine how it would affect prospective jurors.

Our review of the pretrial record persuades us that the trial judge was justified in concluding that there would be intense and pervasive pretrial publicity concerning this case. He could also reasonably conclude, based on common human experience, that publicity might impair the defendant's right to a fair trial. He did not purport to say more, for he found only "a clear and present danger that pre-trial publicity *could* impinge upon the defendant's right to a fair trial." (Emphasis added.) His conclusion as to the impact of such publicity on prospective jurors was of necessity speculative, dealing as he was with factors unknown and unknowable.

We find little in the record that goes to another aspect of our task, determining whether measures short of an order restraining all publication would have insured the defendant a fair trial. *** Most of the alternatives to prior restraint of publication in these circumstances were discussed with obvious approval in Sheppard v. Maxwell, 384 U.S., at 357-362: (a) change of trial venue to a place less exposed to the intense publicity that seemed imminent in Lincoln County;[7] (b) postponement of the trial to allow public attention to subside; (c) searching questioning of prospective jurors, as Mr. Chief Justice Marshall used in the *Burr* case, to screen out those with fixed opinions as to guilt or innocence; (d) the use of emphatic and clear instructions on the sworn duty of each juror to decide the issues only on evidence presented in open court. Sequestration of jurors is, of course, always available. Although that measure insulates jurors only after they are sworn, it also enhances the likelihood of

---

7. The respondent and intervenors argue here that a change of venue would not have helped, since Nebraska law permits a change only to adjacent counties, which had been as exposed to pretrial publicity in this case as Lincoln County. We have held that state laws restricting venue must on occasion yield to the constitutional requirement that the State afford a fair trial. Groppi v. Wisconsin, 400 U.S. 505 (1971). We note also that the combined population of Lincoln County and the adjacent counties is over 80,000 providing a substantial pool of prospective jurors.

dissipating the impact of pretrial publicity and emphasizes the elements of the jurors' oaths.

*** There is no finding that alternative measures would not have protected Simants' rights, and the Nebraska Supreme Court did no more than imply that such measures might not be adequate. Moreover, the record is lacking in evidence to support such a finding. ***

Finally, another feature of this case leads us to conclude that the restrictive order entered here is not supportable. At the outset the County Court entered a very broad restrictive order, the terms of which are not before us; it then held a preliminary hearing open to the public and the press. There was testimony concerning at least two incriminating statements made by Simants to private persons; the statement —evidently a confession—that he gave to law enforcement officials was also introduced. The State District Court's later order was entered after this public hearing and, as modified by the Nebraska Supreme Court, enjoined reporting of (1) "[c]onfessions or admissions against interest made by the accused to law enforcement officials"; (2) "[c]onfessions or admissions against interest, oral or written, if any, made by the accused to third parties, excepting any statements, if any, made by the accused to representatives of the news media"; and (3) all "[o]ther information strongly implicative of the accused as the perpetrator of the slayings." 194 Neb., at 801, 236 N.W.2d, at 805.

To the extent that this order prohibited the reporting of evidence adduced at the open preliminary hearing, it plainly violated settled principles: "[T]here is nothing that proscribes the press from reporting events that transpire in the courtroom." Sheppard v. Maxwell, 384 U.S., at 362-363. *** The County Court could not know that closure of the preliminary hearing was an alternative open to it until the Nebraska Supreme Court so construed state law; but once a public hearing had been held, what transpired there could not be subject to prior restraint.

The third prohibition of the order was defective in another respect as well. As part of a final order, entered after plenary review, this prohibition regarding "implicative" information is too vague and too broad to survive the scrutiny we have given to restraints on First Amendment rights. *** Reversed.

MR. JUSTICE POWELL, concurring.

Although I join the opinion of the Court, in view of the importance of the case I write to emphasize the unique burden that rests upon the party, whether it be the State or a defendant, who undertakes to show the necessity for prior restraint on pretrial publicity.*

* In Times-Picayune Pub. Corp. v. Schulingkamp, 419 U.S. 1301, 1307 (1974), an in-chambers opinion, I noted that there is a heavy presumption against the constitutional validity of a court order restraining pretrial publicity.

In my judgment a prior restraint properly may issue only when it is shown to be necessary to prevent the dissemination of prejudicial publicity that otherwise poses a high likelihood of preventing, directly and irreparably, the impaneling of a jury meeting the Sixth Amendment requirement of impartiality. This requires a showing that (i) there is a clear threat to the fairness of trial, (ii) such a threat is posed by the actual publicity to be restrained, and (iii) no less restrictive alternatives are available. Notwithstanding such a showing, a restraint may not issue unless it also is shown that previous publicity or publicity from unrestrained sources will not render the restraint inefficacious. The threat to the fairness of the trial is to be evaluated in the context of Sixth Amendment law on impartiality, and any restraint must comply with the standards of specificity always required in the First Amendment context.

MR. JUSTICE BRENNAN, with whom MR. JUSTICE STEWART and MR. JUSTICE MARSHALL join, concurring in the judgment.

The question presented in this case is whether, consistently with the First Amendment, a court may enjoin the press, in advance of publication,[1] from reporting or commenting on information acquired from public court proceedings, public court records, or other sources about pending judicial proceedings. The Nebraska Supreme Court upheld such a direct prior restraint on the press, issued by the judge presiding over a sensational state murder trial, on the ground that there existed a "clear and present danger that pretrial publicity could substantially impair the right of the defendant [in the murder trial] to a trial by an impartial jury unless restraints were imposed." The right to a fair trial by a jury of one's peers is unquestionably one of the most precious and sacred safeguards enshrined in the Bill of Rights. I would hold, however, that resort to prior restraints on the freedom of the press is a constitutionally impermissible method for enforcing that right; judges have at their disposal a broad spectrum of devices for ensuring that fundamental fairness is accorded the accused without necessitating so drastic an incursion on the equally fundamental and salutary constitutional mandate that discussion of public affairs in a free society cannot depend on the preliminary grace of judicial censors.

SEATTLE TIMES COMPANY v. RHINEHART
467 U.S. 20 (1984)

JUSTICE POWELL delivered the opinion of the Court.

This case presents the issue whether parties to civil litigation have a First Amendment right to disseminate, in advance of trial, information gained through the pretrial discovery process.

---

1. In referring to the "press" and to "publication" in this opinion, I of course use those words as terms of art that encompass broadcasting by the electronic media as well.

I

Respondent Rhinehart is the spiritual leader of a religious group, the Aquarian Foundation. The Foundation has fewer than 1,000 members, most of whom live in the State of Washington. Aquarian beliefs include life after death and the ability to communicate with the dead through a medium. Rhinehart is the primary Aquarian medium.

In recent years, the Seattle Times and the Walla Walla Union-Bulletin have published stories about Rhinehart and the Foundation. Altogether 11 articles appeared in the newspapers during the years 1973, 1978, and 1979. The five articles that appeared in 1973 focused on Rhinehart and the manner in which he operated the Foundation. They described seances conducted by Rhinehart in which people paid him to put them in touch with deceased relatives and friends. The articles also stated that Rhinehart had sold magical "stones" that had been "expelled" from his body. One article referred to Rhinehart's conviction, later vacated, for sodomy. ***

II

Rhinehart brought this action in the Washington Superior Court on behalf of himself and the Foundation against the Seattle Times, the Walla Walla Union-Bulletin, the authors of the articles, and the spouses of the authors. *** The complaint alleges that the articles contained statements that were "fictional and untrue," and that the defendants—petitioners here—knew, or should have known, they were false. ***

Petitioners filed an answer, denying many of the allegations of the complaint and asserting affirmative defenses.[3] Petitioners promptly initiated extensive discovery. They deposed Rhinehart, requested production of documents pertaining to the financial affairs of Rhinehart and the Foundation, and served extensive interrogatories on Rhinehart and the other respondents. Respondents turned over a number of financial documents, including several of Rhinehart's income tax returns. Respondents refused, however, to disclose certain financial information, the identity of the Foundation's donors during the preceding 10 years, and a list of its members during that period.

Petitioners filed a motion under the State's Civil Rule 37 requesting an order compelling discovery. *** Respondents opposed the motion, arguing in particular that compelled production of the identities of the Foundation's donors and members would violate the First Amendment rights of members and donors to privacy, freedom of religion, and freedom of association. Respondents also moved for a protective order preventing petitioners from disseminating any information gained through discovery. Respondents noted that petitioners had stated their intention to

3. Affirmative defenses included contentions that the articles were substantially true and accurate, that they were privileged under the First and Fourteenth Amendments, that the statute of limitations had run as to the 1973 articles, that the individual respondents had consented to any invasions of privacy, and that respondents had no reasonable expectation of privacy when performing before 1,100 prisoners.

continue publishing articles about respondents and this litigation, and their intent to use information gained through discovery in future articles.

*** [T]he trial court issued a protective order covering all information obtained through the discovery process that pertained to "the financial affairs of the various plaintiffs, the names and addresses of Aquarian Foundation members, contributors, or clients, and the names and addresses of those who have been contributors, clients, or donors to any of the various plaintiffs." The order prohibited petitioners from publishing, disseminating, or using the information in any way except where necessary to prepare for and try the case. By its terms, the order did not apply to information gained by means other than the discovery process. ***

III

Most States, including Washington, have adopted discovery provisions modeled on Rules 26 through 37 of the Federal Rules of Civil Procedure. *** Rule 26(b)(1) provides that a party "may obtain discovery regarding any matter, not privileged, which is relevant to the subject matter involved in the pending action." It further provides that discovery is not limited to matters that will be admissible at trial so long as the information sought "appears reasonably calculated to lead to the discovery of admissible evidence." *** Under the Rules, the only express limitations are that the information sought is not privileged, and is relevant to the subject matter of the pending action. Thus, the Rules often allow extensive intrusion into the affairs of both litigants and third parties. If a litigant fails to comply with a request for discovery, the court may issue an order directing compliance that is enforceable by the court's contempt powers. ***

IV (A)

At the outset, it is important to recognize the extent of the impairment of First Amendment rights that a protective order, such as the one at issue here, may cause. As in all civil litigation, petitioners gained the information they wish to disseminate only by virtue of the trial court's discovery processes. As the Rules authorizing discovery were adopted by the state legislature, the processes thereunder are a matter of legislative grace. A litigant has no First Amendment right of access to information made available only for purposes of trying his suit. ***

Moreover, pretrial depositions and interrogatories are not public components of a civil trial. Such proceedings were not open to the public at common law, Gannett Co. v. DePasquale, 443 U.S. 368, 389 (1979), and, in general, they are conducted in private as a matter of modern practice. See *id.*, at 396 (BURGER, C. J., concurring); Marcus, Myth and Reality in Protective Order Litigation, 69 Cornell L. Rev. 1 (1983). Much of the information that surfaces during pretrial discovery may be unrelated, or only tangentially related, to the underlying cause of action. Therefore, restraints placed on discovered, but not yet admitted, information are not a restriction on a traditionally public source of information.

Finally, it is significant to note that an order prohibiting dissemination of discovered information before trial is not the kind of classic prior restraint that requires exacting First Amendment scrutiny. See *Gannett Co. v. DePasquale*, *supra*, at 399 (POWELL, J., concurring). As in this case, such a protective order prevents a party from disseminating only that information obtained through use of the discovery process. Thus, the party may disseminate the identical information covered by the protective order as long as the information is gained through means independent of the court's processes. ***

B

Rule 26 furthers a substantial governmental interest unrelated to the suppression of expression. *** The Washington Civil Rules enable parties to litigation to obtain information "relevant to the subject matter involved" that they believe will be helpful in the preparation and trial of the case. Rule 26, however, must be viewed in its entirety. Liberal discovery is provided for the sole purpose of assisting in the preparation and trial, or the settlement, of litigated disputes. Because of the liberality of pretrial discovery permitted by Rule 26(b)(1), it is necessary for the trial court to have the authority to issue protective orders conferred by Rule 26(c). It is clear from experience that pretrial discovery by depositions and interrogatories has a significant potential for abuse.[20] This abuse is not limited to matters of delay and expense; discovery also may seriously implicate privacy interests of litigants and third parties.[21] The Rules do not distinguish between public and private information. Nor do they apply only to parties to the litigation, as relevant information in the hands of third parties may be subject to discovery.

There is an opportunity, therefore, for litigants to obtain—incidentally or purposefully—information that not only is irrelevant but if publicly released could be damaging to reputation and privacy. ***

C

We also find that the provision for protective orders in the Washington Rules requires, in itself, no heightened First Amendment scrutiny. To be sure, Rule 26(c) confers broad discretion on the trial court to decide when a protective order is appro-

---

20. See Comments of the Advisory Committee on the 1983 Amendments to Fed. Rule Civ. Proc. 26 U.S.C. App., pp. 729-730 (1982 ed., Supp. I). In *Herbert v. Lando*, 441 U.S. 153 (1979), the Court observed: "There have been repeated expressions of concern about undue and uncontrolled discovery, and voices from this Court have joined the chorus. But until and unless there are major changes in the present Rules of Civil Procedure, reliance must be had on what in fact and in law are ample powers of the district judge to prevent abuse." *Id.*, at 176-177 (footnote omitted); see also *id.*, at 179 (POWELL, J., concurring). But abuses of the Rules by litigants, and sometimes the inadequate oversight of discovery by trial courts, do not in any respect lessen the importance of discovery in civil litigation and the government's substantial interest in protecting the integrity of the discovery process.

21. Cf. Whalen v. Roe, 429 U.S. 589, 599 (1977); Cox Broadcasting Corp. v. Cohn, 420 U.S. 469, 488-491 (1975). Rule 26 includes among its express purposes the protection of a "party or person from annoyance, embarrassment, oppression or undue burden or expense." Although the Rule contains no specific reference to privacy or to other rights or interests that may be implicated, such matters are implicit in the broad purpose and language of the Rule.

priate and what degree of protection is required. The Legislature of the State of Washington, following the example of the Congress in its approval of the Federal Rules of Civil Procedure, has determined that such discretion is necessary, and we find no reason to disagree. The trial court is in the best position to weigh fairly the competing needs and interests of parties affected by discovery.[23] The unique character of the discovery process requires that the trial court have substantial latitude to fashion protective orders.

V

*** We therefore hold that where, as in this case, a protective order is entered on a showing of good cause as required by Rule 26(c), is limited to the context of pretrial civil discovery, and does not restrict the dissemination of the information if gained from other sources, it does not offend the First Amendment. The judgment accordingly is affirmed.

JUSTICE BRENNAN, with whom JUSTICE MARSHALL joins, concurring.

The Court today recognizes that pretrial protective orders, designed to limit the dissemination of information gained through the civil discovery process, are subject to scrutiny under the First Amendment. As the Court acknowledges, before approving such protective orders, "it is necessary to consider whether the 'practice in question [furthers] an important or substantial governmental interest unrelated to the suppression of expression' and whether 'the limitation of First Amendment freedoms [is] no greater than is necessary or essential to the protection of the particular governmental interest involved.'" ***

*** I agree that the respondents' interests in privacy and religious freedom are sufficient to justify this protective order and to overcome the protections afforded free expression by the First Amendment. I therefore join the Court's opinion.

NOTE

Despite *Bridges*, and *Nebraska Press*, in *Gentile v. State Bar of Nevada* the Supreme Court has also declined to apply the clear and present danger test to state bar sanctions imposed under authority of state law on criminal defense counsel for press comments made in reference to a pending criminal trial. Four justices (Kennedy, Marshall, Blackmun and Stevens) believed that the *Bridges* standard was required by the first amendment. But five justices (Rhenquist, Scalia, O'Connor,

---

23. In addition, heightened First Amendment scrutiny of each request for a protective order would necessitate burdensome evidentiary findings and could lead to time-consuming interlocutory appeals, as this case illustrates. See, *e.g.*, Zenith Radio Corp. v. Matsushita Electric Industrial Co., 529 F. Supp. 866 (ED Pa. 1981).

Souter and White) accepted a significantly lesser standard both as framed in professional rules of conduct and as applied in fact.

GENTILE v. STATE BAR OF NEVADA

501 U.S. 1030 (1991)

Justice KENNEDY announced the judgment of the Court and delivered the opinion of the Court with respect to Parts III and VI, and an opinion with respect to Parts I, II, IV, and V in which JUSTICE MARSHALL, JUSTICE BLACKMUN, and JUSTICE STEVENS join.

Hours after his client was indicted on criminal charges, petitioner Gentile, who is a member of the Bar of the State of Nevada, held a press conference. He made a prepared statement, *** and then he responded to questions. ***

Some six months later, the criminal case was tried to a jury and the client was acquitted on all counts. The State Bar of Nevada then filed a complaint against petitioner alleging a violation of Nevada Supreme Court Rule 177, a rule governing pretrial publicity almost identical to ABA Model Rule of Professional Conduct 3.6. *** Rule 177(1) prohibits an attorney from making "an extrajudicial statement that a reasonable person would expect to be disseminated by means of public communication if the lawyer knows or reasonably should know that it will have a substantial likelihood of materially prejudicing an adjudicative proceeding." ***

Following a hearing, the Southern Nevada Disciplinary Board of the State Bar found that Gentile had made the statements in question and concluded that he violated Rule 177. The board recommended a private reprimand. Petitioner appealed to the Nevada Supreme Court, waiving the confidentiality of the disciplinary proceeding, and the Nevada court affirmed the decision of the Board. ***

I

The matter before us does not call into question the constitutionality of other States' prohibitions upon an attorney's speech that will have a "substantial likelihood of materially prejudicing an adjudicative proceeding," but is limited to Nevada's interpretation of that standard. On the other hand, one central point must dominate the analysis: this case involves classic political speech. The State Bar of Nevada reprimanded petitioner for his assertion, supported by a brief sketch of his client's defense, that the State sought the indictment and conviction of an innocent man as a "scapegoat," and had not "been honest enough to indict the people who did it; the police department, crooked cops." *** At issue here is the constitutionality of a ban on political speech critical of the government and its officials. ***

Public awareness and criticism have even greater importance where, as here, they concern allegations of police corruption, see *Nebraska Press Assn. v. Stuart*, *** (Brennan, J., concurring in judgment) ("commentary on the fact that there is strong evidence implicating a government official in criminal activity goes to the very core of matters of public concern"), or where, as is also the present circumstance, the criticism questions the judgment of an elected public prosecutor.***

We are not called upon to determine the constitutionality of the ABA Model Rule of Professional Conduct 3.6 (1981), but only Rule 177 as it has been interpreted and applied by the State of Nevada. Model Rule 3.6's requirement of substantial likelihood of material prejudice is not necessarily flawed. Interpreted in a proper and narrow manner, for instance, to prevent an attorney of record from releasing information of grave prejudice on the eve of jury selection, the phrase substantial likelihood of material prejudice might punish only speech that creates a danger of imminent and substantial harm. A rule governing speech, even speech entitled to full constitutional protection, need not use the words "clear and present danger" in order to pass constitutional muster. ***

The difference between the requirement of serious and imminent threat found in the disciplinary rules of some States and the more common formulation of substantial likelihood of material prejudice could prove mere semantics. Each standard requires an assessment of proximity and degree of harm. Each may be capable of valid application. Under those principles, nothing inherent in Nevada's formulation fails First Amendment review; but as this case demonstrates, Rule 177 has not been interpreted in conformance with those principles by the Nevada Supreme Court.

II

Even if one were to accept respondent's argument that lawyers participating in judicial proceedings may be subjected, consistent with the First Amendment, to speech restrictions that could not be imposed on the press or general public, the judgment should not be upheld. The record does not support the conclusion that petitioner knew or reasonably should have known his remarks created a substantial likelihood of material prejudice, if the Rule's terms are given any meaningful content. ***

Upon return of the indictment, the court set a trial date for August 1988, some six months in the future. Petitioner knew, at the time of his statement, that a jury would not be empaneled for six months at the earliest, if ever. *** Petitioner was disciplined for statements to the effect that (1) the evidence demonstrated his client's innocence, (2) the likely thief was a police detective, Steve Scholl, and (3) the other victims were not credible, as most were drug dealers or convicted money launderers, all but one of whom had only accused Sanders in response to police pressure, in the process of "trying to work themselves out of something." *** He also strongly implied that Steve Scholl could be observed in a videotape suffering from symptoms of cocaine use. Of course, only a small fraction of petitioner's remarks were disseminated to the public, in two newspaper stories and two television news broadcasts.

The trial took place on schedule in August 1988, with no request by either party for a venue change or continuance. The jury was empaneled with no apparent difficulty. The trial judge questioned the jury venire about publicity. Although many had vague recollections of reports that cocaine stored at Western Vault had been stolen from a police undercover operation, and, as petitioner had feared, one remembered that the police had been cleared of suspicion, not a single juror indicated any recollection of petitioner or his press conference. ***

*** There is no support for the conclusion that petitioner's statement created a likelihood of material prejudice, or indeed of any harm of sufficient magnitude or imminence to support a punishment for speech. ***

IV

The analysis to this point resolves the case, and in the usual order of things the discussion should end here. Five Members of the Court, however, endorse an extended discussion which concludes that Nevada may interpret its requirement of substantial likelihood of material prejudice under a standard more deferential than is the usual rule where speech is concerned. It appears necessary, therefore, to set forth my objections to that conclusion and to the reasoning which underlies it.

Respondent argues speech by an attorney is subject to greater regulation than speech by others, and restrictions on an attorney's speech should be assessed under a balancing test that weighs the State's interest in the regulation of a specialized profession against the lawyer's First Amendment interest in the kind of speech that was at issue. ***

This case involves no speech subject to a restriction under the rationale of *Seattle Times*. Petitioner could not have learned what he revealed at the press conference through the discovery process or other special access afforded to attorneys, for he spoke to the press on the day of indictment, at the outset of his formal participation in the criminal proceeding. We have before us no complaint from the prosecutors, police, or presiding judge that petitioner misused information to which he had special access. *** At the very least, our cases recognize that disciplinary rules governing the legal profession cannot punish activity protected by the First Amendment, and that First Amendment protection survives even when the attorney violates a disciplinary rule he swore to obey when admitted to the practice of law. ***

V

Even if respondent is correct, and as in *Seattle Times* we must balance "whether the 'practice in question [furthers] an important or substantial governmental interest unrelated to the suppression of expression' and whether 'the limitation of First Amendment freedoms [is] no greater than is necessary or essential to the protection of the particular governmental interest involved,'"*** the Rule as interpreted by Nevada fails the searching inquiry required by those precedents.

Only the occasional case presents a danger of prejudice from pre-trial publicity. Empirical research suggests that in the few instances when jurors have been exposed to extensive and prejudicial publicity, they are able to disregard it and base their verdict upon the evidence presented in court. See generally Simon, Does the Court's

Decision in *Nebraska Press Association* Fit the Research Evidence on the Impact on Jurors of News Coverage?, 29 Stan.L.Rev. 515 (1977) *** *Voir dire* can play an important role in reminding jurors to set aside out-of-court information, and to decide the case upon the evidence presented at trial. All of these factors weigh in favor of affording an attorney's speech about ongoing proceedings our traditional First Amendment protections. Our colleagues' historical survey notwithstanding, respondent has not demonstrated any sufficient state interest in restricting the speech of attorneys to justify a lower standard of First Amendment scrutiny.

Still less justification exists for a lower standard of scrutiny here, as this speech involved not the prosecutor or police, but a criminal defense attorney. ***

*** The police, the prosecution, other government officials, and the community at large hold innumerable avenues for the dissemination of information adverse to a criminal defendant, many of which are not within the scope of Rule 177 or any other regulation. By contrast, a defendant cannot speak without fear of incriminating himself and prejudicing his defense, and most criminal defendants have insufficient means to retain a public relations team apart from defense counsel for the sole purpose of countering prosecution statements. These factors underscore my conclusion that blanket rules restricting speech of defense attorneys should not be accepted without careful First Amendment scrutiny. ***

VI

The judgment of the Supreme Court of Nevada is reversed.

CHIEF JUSTICE REHNQUIST delivered the opinion of the Court with respect to Parts I and II, and delivered a dissenting opinion with respect to Part III in which JUSTICE WHITE, JUSTICE SCALIA, and JUSTICE SOUTER joined.

***

I

Petitioner maintains that the First Amendment to the United States Constitution requires a State, such as Nevada in this case, to demonstrate a "clear and present danger" of "actual prejudice or an imminent threat" before any discipline may be imposed on a lawyer who initiates a press conference such as occurred here. He relies on decisions such as Nebraska Press Assn. v. Stuart, 427 U.S. 539 (1976), Bridges v. California, 314 U.S. 252 (1941), Pennekamp v. Florida, 328 U.S. 331 (1946), and Craig v. Harney, 331 U.S. 367 (1947), to support his position.

*** The First Amendment protections of speech and press have been held, in the cases cited above, to require a showing of "clear and present danger" that a malfunction in the criminal justice system will be caused before a State may prohibit media speech or publication about a particular pending trial. The question we must answer in this case is whether a lawyer who represents a defendant involved with the criminal justice system may insist on the same standard before he is disciplined for public pronouncements about the case, or whether the State instead may penalize that sort of speech upon a lesser showing.[5] ***

We think *** that the speech of lawyers representing clients in pending cases may be regulated under a less demanding standard than that established for regulation of the press in Nebraska Press Assn. v. Stuart, 427 U.S. 539 (1976), and the cases which preceded it. *** As noted by Justice Brennan in his concurring opinion in *Nebraska Press*, which was joined by Justices Stewart and Marshall, "[a]s officers of the court, court personnel and attorneys have a fiduciary responsibility not to engage in public debate that will redound to the detriment of the accused or that will obstruct the fair administration of justice." *** We agree with the majority of the States that the "substantial likelihood of material prejudice" standard constitutes a constitutionally permissible balance between the First Amendment rights of attorneys in pending cases and the state's interest in fair trials. ***

The restraint on speech is narrowly tailored to achieve those objectives. The regulation of attorneys' speech is limited—it applies only to speech that is substantially likely to have a materially prejudicial effect; it is neutral as to points of view, applying equally to all attorneys participating in a pending case; and it merely postpones the attorney's comments until after the trial. While supported by the substantial state interest in preventing prejudice to an adjudicative proceeding by those who have a duty to protect its integrity, the Rule is limited on its face to preventing only speech having a substantial likelihood of materially prejudicing that proceeding.

II

***

Petitioner's strongest arguments are that the statement was made well in advance of trial, and that the statements did not in fact taint the jury panel. But the Supreme Court of Nevada pointed out that petitioner's statements were not only highly inflammatory—they portrayed prospective government witnesses as drug users and dealers, and as money launderers-but the statements were timed to have maximum impact, when public interest in the case was at its height immediately after Sanders was indicted. Reviewing independently the entire record, we are convinced that petitioner's statements were "substantially likely to cause material prejudice" to the proceedings. ***

Several *amici* argue that the First Amendment requires the state to show actual prejudice to a judicial proceeding before an attorney may be disciplined for extrajudicial statements, and since the board and the Nevada Supreme Court found no actual prejudice, petitioner should not have been disciplined. But this is simply another way of stating that the stringent standard of *Nebraska Press* should be applied to the

5. The Nevada Supreme Court has consistently read all parts of Rule 177 as applying only to lawyers in pending cases, and not to other lawyers or nonlawyers. We express no opinion on the constitutionality of a rule regulating the statements of a lawyer who is not participating in the pending case about which the statements are made.

speech of a lawyer in a pending case, and for the reasons heretofore given we decline to adopt it. ***

JUSTICE O'CONNOR, concurring.

I agree with much of THE CHIEF JUSTICE's opinion. In particular, I agree that a State may regulate speech by lawyers representing clients in pending cases more readily than it may regulate the press. Lawyers are officers of the court and, as such, may legitimately be subject to ethical precepts that keep them from engaging in what otherwise might be constitutionally protected speech. See *In re* Sawyer, 360 U.S. 622, 646-647 (1959) (Stewart, J., concurring in the result). *

NEW YORK TIMES COMPANY v. UNITED STATES

403 U.S. 713 (1971)

Per Curiam.

We granted certiorari in these cases in which the United States seeks to enjoin the New York Times and the Washington Post from publishing the contents of a classified study entitled "History of U.S. Decision-Making Process on Viet Nam Policy." ***

"Any system of prior restraints of expression comes to this Court bearing a heavy presumption against its constitutional validity." Bantam Books, Inc. v. Sullivan, 372 U.S. 58, 70 (1963); see also Near v. Minnesota, 283 U.S. 697 (1931). The Government "thus carries a heavy burden of showing justification for the imposition of such a restraint." Organization for a Better Austin v. Keefe, 402 U.S. 415, 419 (1971). The District Court for the Southern District of New York in the *New York Times* case and the District Court for the District of Columbia and the Court of Appeals for the District of Columbia Circuit in the *Washington Post* case held that the Government had not met that burden. We agree. The stays entered June 25, 1971, by the Court are vacated. The judgments shall issue forthwith.

So ordered.

MR. JUSTICE BLACK, with whom MR. JUSTICE DOUGLAS joins, concurring.

I adhere to the view that the Government's case against the Washington Post should have been dismissed and that the injunction against the New York Times should have been vacated without oral argument when the cases were first presented

---

*. **[Ed. Note**. For a comprehensive review of managing sensational trials, see Gerald Wetherington, Hansen Lawton & Donald I. Pollock, *Preparing for the High Profile Case: An Omnibus Treatment for Judges & Lawyers,* 51 Fla. L.Rev. 425 (1999). See also United States v. Brown, 250 F.3d 907 (5th Cir. 2001).

to this Court. I believe that every moment's continuance of the injunctions against these newspapers amounts to a flagrant, indefensible, and continuing violation of the First Amendment.

*** Both the history and language of the First Amendment support the view that the press must be left free to publish news, whatever the source, without censorship, injunctions, or prior restraints. *** The Government's power to censor the press was abolished so that the press would remain forever free to censure the Government. The press was protected so that it could bare the secrets of government and inform the people. Only a free and unrestrained press can effectively expose deception in government. ***

The Government's case here is based on premises entirely different from those that guided the Framers of the First Amendment. The Solicitor General has carefully and emphatically stated:

> "Now, Mr. Justice [BLACK], your construction of *** [the First Amendment] is well known, and I certainly respect it. You say that no law means no law, and that should be obvious. I can only say, Mr. Justice, that to me it is equally obvious that 'no law' does not mean 'no law', and I would seek to persuade the Court that that is true. *** [T]here are other parts of the Constitution that grant powers and responsibilities to the Executive, and *** the First Amendment was not intended to make it impossible for the Executive to function or to protect the security of the United States."

And the Government argues in its brief that in spite of the First Amendment, "[t]he authority of the Executive Department to protect the nation against publication of information whose disclosure would endanger the national security stems from two interrelated sources: the constitutional power of the President over the conduct of foreign affairs and his authority as Commander-in-Chief."

In other words, we are asked to hold that despite the First Amendment's emphatic command, the Executive Branch, the Congress, and the Judiciary can make laws enjoining publication of current news and abridging freedom of the press in the name of "national security." The Government does not even attempt to rely on any act of Congress. Instead it makes the bold and dangerously far-reaching contention that the courts should take it upon themselves to "make" a law abridging freedom of the press in the name of equity, presidential power, and national security, even when the representatives of the people in Congress have adhered to the command of the First Amendment and refused to make such a law. See concurring opinion of MR. JUSTICE DOUGLAS. To find that the President has "inherent power" to halt the publication of news by resort to the courts would wipe out the First Amendment and destroy the fundamental liberty and security of the very people the Government hopes to make "secure." No one can read the history of the adoption of the First Amendment without being convinced beyond any doubt that it was injunctions like those sought here that Madison and his collaborators intended to outlaw in this Nation for all time.

The word "security" is a broad, vague generality whose contours should not be invoked to abrogate the fundamental law embodied in the First Amendment. The guarding of military and diplomatic secrets at the expense of informed representative government provides no real security for our Republic. The Framers of the First Amendment, fully aware of both the need to defend a new nation and the abuses of the English and Colonial governments, sought to give this new society strength and security by providing that freedom of speech, press, religion, and assembly should not be abridged. This thought was eloquently expressed in 1937 by Mr. Chief Justice Hughes—great man and great Chief Justice that he was—when the Court held a man could not be punished for attending a meeting run by Communists.

> "The greater the importance of safeguarding the community from incitements to the overthrow of our institutions by force and violence, the more imperative is the need to preserve inviolate the constitutional rights of free speech, free press and free assembly in order to maintain the opportunity for free political discussion, to the end that government may be responsive to the will of the people and that changes, if desired, may be obtained by peaceful means. Therein lies the security of the Republic, the very foundation of constitutional government."

MR. JUSTICE DOUGLAS, with whom MR. JUSTICE BLACK joins, concurring.

It should be noted at the outset that the First Amendment provides that "Congress shall make no law *** abridging the freedom of speech, or of the press." That leaves, in my view, no room for governmental restraint on the press.[1]

There is, moreover, no statute barring the publication by the press of the material which the Times and the Post seek to use. Title 18 U.S.C. § 793 (e) provides that "[w]hoever having unauthorized possession of, access to, or control over any document, writing *** or information relating to the national defense which information the possessor has reason to believe could be used to the injury of the United States or to the advantage of any foreign nation, willfully communicates *** the same to any person not entitled to receive it *** [s]hall be fined not more than $10,000 or imprisoned not more than ten years, or both."

The Government suggests that the word "communicates" is broad enough to encompass publication. There are eight sections in the chapter on espionage and

---

1. See Beauharnais v. Illinois, 343 U.S. 250, 267 (dissenting opinion of MR. JUSTICE BLACK), 284 (my dissenting opinion); Roth v. United States, 354 U.S. 476 508 (my dissenting opinion which MR. JUSTICE BLACK joined); Yates v. United States, 354 U.S. 298, 339 (separate opinion of MR. JUSTICE BLACK which I joined); New York Times Co. v. Sullivan, 376 U.S. 254, 293 (concurring opinion of MR. JUSTICE BLACK which I joined); Garrison v. Louisiana, 379 U.S. 64, 80 (my concurring opinion which MR. JUSTICE BLACK joined).

censorship, §§ 792-799. In three of those eight "publish" is specifically mentioned: *** Thus it is apparent that Congress was capable of and did distinguish between publishing and communication in the various sections of the Espionage Act.

The other evidence that § 793 does not apply to the press is a rejected version of § 793. That version read: "During any national emergency resulting from a war to which the United States is a party, or from threat of such a war, the President may, by proclamation, declare the existence of such emergency and, by proclamation, prohibit the publishing or communicating of, or the attempting to publish or communicate any information relating to the national defense which, in his judgment, is of such character that it is or might be useful to the enemy." During the debates in the Senate the First Amendment was specifically cited and that provision was defeated.

Judge Gurfein's holding in the *Times* case that this Act does not apply to this case was therefore preeminently sound. Moreover, the Act of September 23, 1950, in amending 18 U.S.C. § 793 states in § 1 (b) that:

> "Nothing in this Act shall be construed to authorize, require, or establish military or civilian censorship or in any way to limit or infringe upon freedom of the press or of speech as guaranteed by the Constitution of the United States and no regulation shall be promulgated hereunder having that effect." 64 Stat. 987.

Thus Congress has been faithful to the command of the First Amendment in this area.

So any power that the Government possesses must come from its "inherent power."

The power to wage war is "the power to wage war successfully." See Hirabayashi v. United States, 320 U.S. 81, 93. But the war power stems from a declaration of war. The Constitution by Art. I, § 8, gives Congress, not the President, power "[t]o declare War." Nowhere are presidential wars authorized. We need not decide therefore what leveling effect the war power of Congress might have.

These disclosures[2] may have a serious impact. But that is no basis for sanctioning a previous restraint on the press. ***

MR. JUSTICE BRENNAN, concurring.

***

II

The error that has pervaded these cases from the outset was the granting of any injunctive relief whatsoever, interim or otherwise. The entire thrust of the Govern-

---

2. There are numerous sets of this material in existence and they apparently are not under any controlled custody. Moreover, the President has sent a set to the Congress. We start then with a case where there already is rather wide distribution of the material that is destined for publicity, not secrecy. I have gone over the material listed in the *in camera* brief of the United States. It is all history, not future events. None of it is more recent than 1968.

ment's claim throughout these cases has been that publication of the material sought to be enjoined "could," or "might," or "may" prejudice the national interest in various ways. But the First Amendment tolerates absolutely no prior judicial restraints of the press predicated upon surmise or conjecture that untoward consequences may result. Our cases, it is true, have indicated that there is a single, extremely narrow class of cases in which the First Amendment's ban on prior judicial restraint may be overridden. Our cases have thus far indicated that such cases may arise only when the Nation "is at war," Schenck v. United States, 249 U.S. 47, 52 (1919), during which times "[n]o one would question that a government might prevent actual obstruction to its recruiting service or the publication of the sailing dates of transports or the number and locations of troops." Near v. Minnesota, 283 U.S. 697, 716 (1931). Even if the present world situation were assumed to be tantamount to a time of war, or if the power of presently available armaments would justify even in peacetime the suppression of information that would set in motion a nuclear holocaust, in neither of these actions has the Government presented or even alleged that publication of items from or based upon the material at issue would cause the happening of any event of that nature. *** [O]nly governmental allegation and proof that publication must inevitably, directly, and immediately cause the occurrence of an event kindred to imperiling the safety of a transport already at sea can support even the issuance of an interim restraining order. In no event may mere conclusions be sufficient: for if the Executive Branch seeks judicial aid in preventing publication, it must inevitably submit the basis upon which that aid is sought to scrutiny by the judiciary. And therefore, every restraint issued in this case, whatever its form, has violated the First Amendment—and not less so because that restraint was justified as necessary to afford the courts an opportunity to examine the claim more thoroughly. Unless and until the Government has clearly made out its case, the First Amendment commands that no injunction may issue.

MR. JUSTICE STEWART, with whom MR. JUSTICE WHITE joins, concurring.

In the governmental structure created by our Constitution, the Executive is endowed with enormous power in the two related areas of national defense and international relations. This power, largely unchecked by the Legislative and Judicial branches, has been pressed to the very hilt since the advent of the nuclear missile age. For better or for worse, the simple fact is that a President of the United States possesses vastly greater constitutional independence in these two vital areas of power than does, say, a prime minister of a country with a parliamentary form of government.

In the absence of the governmental checks and balances present in other areas of our national life, the only effective restraint upon executive policy and power in the areas of national defense and international affairs may lie in an enlightened citizenry —in an informed and critical public opinion which alone can here protect the values of democratic government. For this reason, it is perhaps here that a press that is alert, aware, and free most vitally serves the basic purpose of the First Amendment. For without an informed and free press there cannot be an enlightened people.

Yet it is elementary that the successful conduct of international diplomacy and the maintenance of an effective national defense require both confidentiality and secrecy. Other nations can hardly deal with this Nation in an atmosphere of mutual trust unless they can be assured that their confidences will be kept. And within our own executive departments, the development of considered and intelligent international policies would be impossible if those charged with their formulation could not communicate with each other freely, frankly, and in confidence. In the area of basic national defense the frequent need for absolute secrecy is, of course, self-evident.

I think there can be but one answer to this dilemma, if dilemma it be. The responsibility must be where the power is. If the Constitution gives the Executive a large degree of unshared power in the conduct of foreign affairs and the maintenance of our national defense, then under the Constitution the Executive must have the largely unshared duty to determine and preserve the degree of internal security necessary to exercise that power successfully. [I]t is clear to me that it is the constitutional duty of the Executive—as a matter of sovereign prerogative and not as a matter of law as the courts know law— through the promulgation and enforcement of executive regulations, to protect the confidentiality necessary to carry out its responsibilities in the fields of international relations and national defense.

This is not to say that Congress and the courts have no role to play. Undoubtedly Congress has the power to enact specific and appropriate criminal laws to protect government property and preserve government secrets. Congress has passed such laws, and several of them are of very colorable relevance to the apparent circumstances of these cases. And if a criminal prosecution is instituted, it will be the responsibility of the courts to decide the applicability of the criminal law under which the charge is brought. Moreover, if Congress should pass a specific law authorizing civil proceedings in this field, the courts would likewise have the duty to decide the constitutionality of such a law as well as its applicability to the facts proved.

But in the cases before us we are asked neither to construe specific regulations nor to apply specific laws. We are asked, instead, to perform a function that the Constitution gave to the Executive, not the Judiciary. We are asked, quite simply, to prevent the publication by two newspapers of material that the Executive Branch insists should not, in the national interest, be published. I am convinced that the Executive is correct with respect to some of the documents involved. But I cannot say that disclosure of any of them will surely result in direct, immediate, and irreparable damage to our Nation or its people. That being so, there can under the First Amendment be but one judicial resolution of the issues before us. I join the judgments of the Court.

MR. JUSTICE WHITE, with whom MR. JUSTICE STEWART joins, concurring.

I concur in today's judgments, but only because of the concededly extraordinary protection against prior restraints enjoyed by the press under our constitutional system. I do not say that in no circumstances would the First Amendment permit an injunction against publishing information about government plans or operations. Nor, after examining the materials the Government characterizes as the most sensitive and destructive, can I deny that revelation of these documents will do substantial damage to public interests. Indeed, I am confident that their disclosure will have that result. But I nevertheless agree that the United States has not satisfied the very heavy burden that it must meet to warrant an injunction against publication in these cases, at least in the absence of express and appropriately limited congressional authorization for prior restraints in circumstances such as these. ***

The Criminal Code contains numerous provisions potentially relevant to these cases. Section 797 makes it a crime to publish certain photographs or drawings of military installations. Section 798, also in precise language, proscribes knowing and willful publication of any classified information concerning the cryptographic systems or communication intelligence activities of the United States as well as any information obtained from communication intelligence operations. If any of the material here at issue is of this nature, the newspapers are presumably now on full notice of the position of the United States and must face the consequences if they publish. I would have no difficulty in sustaining convictions under these sections on facts that would not justify the intervention of equity and the imposition of a prior restraint. ***

MR. CHIEF JUSTICE BURGER, dissenting.

So clear are the constitutional limitations on prior restraint against expression, that from the time of Near v. Minnesota, 283 U.S. 697 (1931), we have had little occasion to be concerned with cases involving prior restraints against news reporting on matters of public interest. Adherence to this basic constitutional principle, however, does not make these cases simple. *** Only those who view the First Amendment as an absolute in all circumstances—a view I respect, but reject—can find such cases as these to be simple or easy.

These cases are not simple for another and more immediate reason. We do not know the facts of the cases. No District Judge knew all the facts. No Court of Appeals judge knew all the facts. No member of this Court knows all the facts.

Why are we in this posture, in which only those judges to whom the First Amendment is absolute and permits of no restraint in any circumstances or for any reason, are really in a position to act?

I suggest we are in this posture because these cases have been conducted in unseemly haste. MR. JUSTICE HARLAN covers the chronology of events demonstrating the hectic pressures under which these cases have been processed and I need not restate them. *** Here, moreover, the frenetic haste is due in large part to the manner in which the Times proceeded from the date it obtained the purloined documents. It seems reasonably clear now that the haste precluded reasonable and deliberate judicial treatment of these cases and was not warranted. *** An issue of this importance should be tried and heard in a judicial atmosphere conducive to thoughtful, reflective deliberation, especially when haste, in terms of hours, is unwarranted in light of the long period the Times, by its own choice, deferred publication.[1]

It is not disputed that the Times has had unauthorized possession of the documents for three to four months, during which it has had its expert analysts studying them, presumably digesting them and preparing the material for publication. During all of this time, the Times, presumably in its capacity as trustee of the public's "right to know," has held up publication for purposes it considered proper and thus public knowledge was delayed. No doubt this was for a good reason; the analysis of 7,000 pages of complex material drawn from a vastly greater volume of material would inevitably take time and the writing of good news stories takes time. But why should the United States Government, from whom this information was illegally acquired by someone, along with all the counsel, trial judges, and appellate judges be placed under needless pressure? After these months of deferral, the alleged "right to know" has somehow and suddenly become a right that must be vindicated instanter. ***

I would affirm the Court of Appeals for the Second Circuit and allow the District Court to complete the trial aborted by our grant of certiorari, meanwhile preserving the status quo in the *Post* case. I would direct that the District Court on remand give priority to the *Times* case to the exclusion of all other business of that court but I would not set arbitrary deadlines.

I should add that I am in general agreement with much of what Mr. Justice White has expressed with respect to penal sanctions concerning communication or retention of documents or information relating to the national defense.

We all crave speedier judicial processes but when judges are pressured as in these cases the result is a parody of the judicial function.

MR. JUSTICE HARLAN, with whom THE CHIEF JUSTICE and MR. JUSTICE BLACKMUN join, dissenting.

These cases forcefully call to mind the wise admonition of Mr. Justice Holmes, dissenting in Northern Securities Co. v. United States, 193 U.S. 197, 400-401 (1904):

---

1. As noted elsewhere the Times conducted its analysis of the 47 volumes of Government documents over a period of several months and did so with a degree of security that a government might envy. Such security was essential, of course, to protect the enterprise from others. Meanwhile the Times has copyrighted its material and there were strong intimations in the oral argument that the Times contemplated enjoining its use by any other publisher in violation of its copyright. Paradoxically this would afford it a protection, analogous to prior restraint, against all others—a protection the Times denies the Government of the United States.

> "Great cases like hard cases make bad law. For great cases are called great, not by reason of their real importance in shaping the law of the future, but because of some accident of immediate overwhelming interest which appeals to the feelings and distorts the judgment. These immediate interests exercise a kind of hydraulic pressure which makes what previously was clear seem doubtful, and before which even well settled principles of law will bend."

With all respect, I consider that the Court has been almost irresponsibly feverish in dealing with these cases. ***

These are difficult questions of fact, of law, and of judgment; the potential consequences of erroneous decision are enormous. *** Forced as I am to reach the merits of these cases, I dissent from the opinion and judgments of the Court. Within the severe limitations imposed by the time constraints under which I have been required to operate, I can only state my reasons in telescoped form, even though in different circumstances I would have felt constrained to deal with the cases in the fuller sweep indicated above.

It is a sufficient basis for affirming the Court of Appeals of the Second Circuit in the *Times* litigation to observe that its order must rest on the conclusion that because of the time elements the Government had not been given an adequate opportunity to present its case to the District Court. At the least this conclusion was not an abuse of discretion.

NOTE

The preceding cases (*Sheppard* through *The Pentagon Papers Case*) principally traced the working standards of first amendment prior restraint law as applied to the press. They are doctrinal derivatives from *Bridges v. California*, tracking that case (so to speak) and its general principles, to illustrate the Supreme Court's application of those principles in several ways, even to the current time. In proceeding in this fashion, however, we have in some measure departed from the previous main theme of our work, namely, the more general first amendment problem of social and political advocacy speech.

This central issue of first amendment controversy did not suddenly cease with cases of the sort we were last concerned with, such as *Gitlow v. New York* and *Whitney v. California*. To the contrary. *Dennis v. United States*, the next principal case, resumes virtually where we left off with the supposition—unsupported by example—that the rigorized Holmes-Brandeis standard (as reflected in *Bridges*) would control. Does it? And if it does, in what manner and degree? Just how is it to be applied?

DENNIS v. UNITED STATES
341 U.S. 494 (1951)

MR. CHIEF JUSTICE VINSON announced the judgment of the Court and an opinion in which MR. JUSTICE REED, MR. JUSTICE BURTON and MR. JUSTICE MINTON join.

Petitioners were indicted July, 1948, for violation of the conspiracy provisions of the Smith Act. A verdict of guilty as to all the petitioners was returned by the jury on October 14, 1949. The Court of Appeals affirmed the convictions. We granted certiorari limited to the following two questions: (1) Whether either § 2 or § 3 of the Smith Act, inherently or as construed and applied in the instant case, violates the First Amendment and other provisions of the Bill of Rights; (2) whether either § 2 or § 3 of the Act, inherently or as construed and applied in the instant case, violates the First and Fifth Amendments because of indefiniteness.

Sections 2 and 3 of the Smith Act provide as follows:

> "SEC. 2. (a) It shall be unlawful for any person—
>
> "(1) to knowingly or willfully advocate, abet, advise, or teach the duty, necessity, desirability, or propriety of overthrowing or destroying any government in the United States by force or violence, or by the assassination of any officer of any such government;
>
> "(2) with intent to cause the overthrow or destruction of any government in the United States, to print, publish, edit, issue, circulate, sell, distribute, or publicly display any written or printed matter advocating, advising, or teaching the duty, necessity, desirability, or propriety of overthrowing or destroying any government in the United States by force or violence;
>
> "(3) to organize or help to organize any society, group, or assembly of persons who teach, advocate, or encourage the overthrow or destruction of any government in the United States by force or violence; or to be or become a member of, or affiliate with, any such society, group, or assembly of persons, knowing the purposes thereof.
>
> "(b) For the purposes of this section, the term 'government in the United States' means the Government of the United States, the government of any State, Territory, or possession of the United States, the government of the District of Columbia, or the government of any political subdivision of any of them.
>
> "SEC. 3. It shall be unlawful for any person to attempt to commit, or to conspire to commit, any of the acts prohibited by the provisions of this title."

The indictment charged the petitioners with wilfully and knowingly conspiring (1) to organize as the Communist Party of the United States of America a society, group and assembly of persons who teach and advocate the overthrow and destruction of the Government of the United States by force and violence, and (2) knowingly and wilfully to advocate and teach the duty and necessity of overthrowing and destroying the Government of the United States by force and violence. The indictment further alleged that § 2 of the Smith Act proscribes these acts and that any conspiracy to take such action is a violation of § 3 of the Act.

The trial of the case extended over nine months, six of which were devoted to the taking of evidence, resulting in a record of 16,000 pages. *** [T]he Court of Appeals held that the record supports the following broad conclusions: By virtue of their control over the political apparatus of the Communist Political Association,[1] petitioners were able to transform that organization into the Communist Party; that the policies of the Association were changed from peaceful cooperation with the United States and its economic and political structure to a policy which had existed before the United States and the Soviet Union were fighting a common enemy, namely, a policy which worked for the overthrow of the Government by force and violence; that the Communist Party is a highly disciplined organization, adept at infiltration into strategic positions, use of aliases, and double-meaning language; that the Party is rigidly controlled; that Communists, unlike other political parties, tolerate no dissension from the policy laid down by the guiding forces, but that the approved program is slavishly followed by the members of the Party; that the literature of the Party and the statement and activities of its leaders, petitioners here, advocate, and the general goal of the Party was, during the period in question, to achieve a successful overthrow of the existing order by force and violence. ***

I

The obvious purpose of the statute is to protect existing Government, not from change by peaceable, lawful and constitutional means, but from change by violence, revolution and terrorism. That it is within the *power* of the Congress to protect the Government of the United States from armed rebellion is a proposition which requires little discussion. Whatever theoretical merit there may be to the argument that there is a "right" to rebellion against dictatorial governments is without force where the existing structure of the government provides for peaceful and orderly change. We reject any principle of governmental helplessness in the face of preparation for revolution, which principle, carried to its logical conclusion, must lead to anarchy. No one could conceive that it is not within the power of Congress to prohibit acts intended to overthrow the Government by force and violence. The question with which we are concerned here is not whether Congress has such *power*, but whether the *means* which it has employed conflict with the First and Fifth Amendments to the Constitution.

One of the bases for the contention that the means which Congress has employed are invalid takes the form of an attack on the face of the statute on the grounds that

---

1. Following the dissolution of the Communist International in 1943, the Communist Party of the United States dissolved and was reconstituted as Communist Political Association. The program of this Association was one of cooperation between labor and management, and, in general, one designed to achieve national unity and peace and prosperity in the post-war period.

by its terms it prohibits academic discussion of the merits of Marxism-Leninism, that it stifles ideas and is contrary to all concepts of a free speech and a free press. Although we do not agree that the language itself has that significance, we must bear in mind that it is the duty of the federal courts to interpret federal legislation in a manner not inconsistent with the demands of the Constitution. ***

The very language of the Smith Act negates the interpretation which petitioners would have us impose on that Act. It is directed at advocacy, not discussion. Thus, the trial judge properly charged the jury that they could not convict if they found that petitioners did "no more than pursue peaceful studies and discussions or teaching and advocacy in the realm of ideas." He further charged that it was not unlawful "to conduct in an American college or university a course explaining the philosophical theories set forth in the books which have been placed in evidence." Such a charge is in strict accord with the statutory language, and illustrates the meaning to be placed on those words. Congress did not intend to eradicate the free discussion of political theories, to destroy the traditional rights of Americans to discuss and evaluate ideas without fear of governmental sanction. Rather Congress was concerned with the very kind of activity in which the evidence showed these petitioners engaged.

II

***

Although no case subsequent to *Whitney* and *Gitlow* has expressly overruled the majority opinions in those cases, there is little doubt that subsequent opinions have inclined toward the Holmes-Brandeis rationale.*** But *** neither Justice Holmes nor Justice Brandeis ever envisioned that a shorthand phrase should be crystallized into a rigid rule to be applied inflexibly without regard to the circumstances of each case. Speech is not an absolute, above and beyond control by the legislature when its judgment, subject to review here, is that certain kinds of speech are so undesirable as to warrant criminal sanction. Nothing is more certain in modern society than the principle that there are no absolutes, that a name, a phrase, a standard has meaning only when associated with the considerations which gave birth to the nomenclature. ***

The situation with which Justices Holmes and Brandeis were concerned in *Gitlow* was a comparatively isolated event, bearing little relation in their minds to any substantial threat to the safety of the community. *** They were not confronted with any situation comparable to the instant one—the development of an apparatus designed and dedicated to the overthrow of the Government, in the context of world crisis after crisis.

Chief Judge Learned Hand, writing for the majority below, interpreted the phrase as follows: "In each case [courts] must ask whether the gravity of the 'evil,' discounted by its improbability, justifies such invasion of free speech as is necessary to avoid the danger." 183 F.2d 212. We adopt this statement of the rule. As articulated by Chief Judge Hand, it is as succinct and inclusive as any other we might devise at this time. It takes into consideration those factors which we deem relevant, and relates their significances. More we cannot expect from words.

Likewise, we are in accord with the court below, which affirmed the trial court's finding that the requisite danger existed. The mere fact that from the period 1945 to 1948 petitioners' activities did not result in an attempt to overthrow the Government by force and violence is of course no answer to the fact that there was a group that was ready to make the attempt. The formation by petitioners of such a highly organized conspiracy, with rigidly disciplined members subject to call when the leaders, these petitioners, felt that the time had come for action, coupled with the inflammable nature of world conditions, similar uprisings in other countries, and the touch-and-go nature of our relations with countries with whom petitioners were in the very least ideologically attuned, convince us that their convictions were justified on this score. And this analysis disposes of the contention that a conspiracy to advocate, as distinguished from the advocacy itself, cannot be constitutionally restrained, because it comprises only the preparation. It is the existence of the conspiracy which creates the danger. If the ingredients of the reaction are present, we cannot bind the Government to wait until the catalyst is added.

III

Although we have concluded that the finding that there was a sufficient danger to warrant the application of the statute was justified on the merits, there remains the problem of whether the trial judge's treatment of the issue was correct. He charged the jury, in relevant part, as follows:

> "In further construction and interpretation of the statute I charge you that it is not the abstract doctrine of overthrowing or destroying organized government by unlawful means which is denounced by this law, but the teaching and advocacy of action for the accomplishment of that purpose, by language reasonably and ordinarily calculated to incite persons to such action. Accordingly, you cannot find the defendants or any of them guilty of the crime charged unless you are satisfied beyond a reasonable doubt that they conspired to organize a society, group and assembly of persons who teach and advocate the overthrow or destruction of the Government of the United States by force and violence and to advocate and teach the duty and necessity of overthrowing or destroying the Government of the United States by force and violence, with the intent that such teaching and advocacy be of a rule or principle of action and by language reasonably and ordinarily calculated to incite persons to such action, all with the intent to cause the overthrow or destruction of the Government of the United States by force and violence as speedily as circumstances would permit.
>
> ***
>
> "If you are satisfied that the evidence establishes beyond a reasonable doubt that the defendants, or any of them, are guilty of a violation of the statute, as I have interpreted it to you, I find as matter of law that there is sufficient

danger of a substantive evil that the Congress has a right to prevent to justify the application of the statute under the First Amendment of the Constitution. ***"

It is thus clear that he reserved the question of the existence of the danger for his own determination, and the question becomes whether the issue is of such a nature that it should have been submitted to the jury.

*** The argument that the action of the trial court is erroneous, in declaring as a matter of law that such violation shows sufficient danger to justify the punishment despite the First Amendment, rests on the theory that a jury must decide a question of the application of the First Amendment. We do not agree.

When facts are found that establish the violation of a statute, the protection against conviction afforded by the First Amendment is a matter of law. The doctrine that there must be a clear and present danger of a substantive evil that Congress has a right to prevent is a judicial rule to be applied as a matter of law by the courts. The guilt is established by proof of facts. Whether the First Amendment protects the activity which constitutes the violation of the statute must depend upon a judicial determination of the scope of the First Amendment applied to the circumstances of the case.

Petitioners' reliance upon Justice Brandeis' language in his concurrence in *Whitney, supra*, is misplaced. In that case Justice Brandeis pointed out that the defendant could have made the existence of the requisite danger the important issue at her trial, but that she had not done so. In discussing this failure, he stated that the defendant could have had the issue determined by the court *or* the jury.[6] No realistic construction of this disjunctive language could arrive at the conclusion that he intended to state that the question was *only* determinable by a jury. ***

The question in this case is whether the statute which the legislature has enacted may be constitutionally applied. In other words, the Court must examine judicially the application of the statute to the particular situation, to ascertain if the Constitution prohibits the conviction. We hold that the statute may be applied where there is a "clear and present danger" of the substantive evil which the legislature had the right to prevent. Bearing, as it does, the marks of a "question of law," the issue is properly one for the judge to decide.***

Affirmed.

---

6. "Whether in 1919, when Miss Whitney did the things complained of, there was in California such clear and present danger of serious evil, might have been made the important issue in the case. She might have required that the issue be determined either by the *court or the jury*. She claimed below that the statute as applied to her violated the Federal Constitution; but she did not claim that it was void because there was no clear and present danger of serious evil, nor did she request that the existence of these conditions of a valid measure thus restricting the rights of free speech and assembly be passed upon by *the court or a jury*. On the other hand, there was evidence which *the court or jury* might have found that such danger existed." (Emphasis added.) 274 U.S. at 379.

MR. JUSTICE CLARK took no part in the consideration or decision of this case.

MR. JUSTICE FRANKFURTER, concurring in affirmance of the judgment.

The First Amendment categorically demands that "Congress shall make no law *** abridging the freedom of speech, or of the press; or the right of the people peaceably to assemble, and to petition the Government for a redress of grievances." The right of a man to think what he pleases, to write what he thinks, and to have his thoughts made available for others to hear or read has an engaging ring of universality. The Smith Act and this conviction under it no doubt restrict the exercise of free speech and assembly. Does that, without more, dispose of the matter? ***

*** Absolute rules would inevitably lead to absolute exceptions, and such exceptions would eventually corrode the rules.[5] The demands of free speech in a democratic society as well as the interest in national security are better served by candid and informed weighing of the competing interests, within the confines of the judicial process, than by announcing dogmas too inflexible for the non-Euclidian problems to be solved.

But how are competing interests to be assumed? Since they are not subject to quantitative ascertainment, the issue necessarily resolves itself into asking, who is to make the adjustment?—who is to balance the relevant factors and ascertain which interest is in the circumstances to prevail? ***

Primary responsibility for adjusting the interests which compete in the situation before us of necessity belongs to the Congress. The nature of the power to be exercised by this Court has been delineated in decisions not charged with the emotional appeal of situations such as that now before us. We are to set aside the judgment of those whose duty it is to legislate only if there is no reasonable basis for it. ***

Free-speech cases are not an exception to the principle that we are not legislators, that direct policy-making is not our province. How best to reconcile competing interests is the business of legislatures, and the balance they strike is a judgment not to be displaced by ours, but to be respected unless outside the pale of fair judgment.

One of the judges below rested his affirmance on the *Gitlow* decision, and the defendants do not attempt to distinguish the case. They place their argument

---

5. Professor Alexander Meiklejohn is a leading exponent of the absolutist interpretation of the First Amendment. Recognizing that certain forms of speech require regulation, he excludes those forms of expression entirely from the protection accorded by the Amendment. "The constitutional status of a merchant advertising his wares, of a paid lobbyist fighting for the advantage of his client, is utterly different from that of a citizen who is planning for the general welfare." Meiklejohn, Free Speech, 39. "The radio as it now operates among us is not free. Nor is it entitled to the protection of the First Amendment. It is not engaged in the task of enlarging and enriching human communication. It is engaged in making money." *Id.* at 104. Professor Meiklejohn even suggests that scholarship may now require such subvention and control that it no longer is entitled to protection by the First Amendment. See *id.* at 99-100. Professor Chafee in his review of the Meiklejohn book, 62 Harv. L. Rev. 894, has subjected this position to trenchant comment.

squarely on the ground that the case has been overruled by subsequent decisions. It has not been explicitly overruled. But it would be disingenuous to deny that the dissent in *Gitlow* has been treated with the respect usually accorded to a decision.

The result of the *Gitlow* decision was to send a left-wing Socialist to jail for publishing a Manifesto expressing Marxist exhortations. It requires excessive tolerance of the legislative judgment to suppose that the *Gitlow* publication in the circumstances could justify serious concern.

In contrast, there is ample justification for a legislative judgment that the conspiracy now before us is a substantial threat to national order and security. If the Smith Act is justified at all, it is justified precisely because it may serve to prohibit the type of conspiracy for which these defendants were convicted. The court below properly held that as a matter of separability the Smith Act may be limited to those situations to which it can constitutionally be applied. Our decision today certainly does not mean that the Smith Act can constitutionally be applied to facts like those in *Gitlow v. New York*. While reliance may properly be placed on the attitude of judicial self-restraint which the *Gitlow* decision reflects, it is not necessary to depend on the facts or the full extent of the theory of that case in order to find that the judgment of Congress, as applied to the facts of the case now before us, is not in conflict with the First Amendment. ***

It is true that there is no divining rod by which we may locate "advocacy." Exposition of ideas readily merges into advocacy. The same Justice who gave currency to application of the incitement doctrine in this field dissented four times from what he thought was its misapplication. As he said in the *Gitlow* dissent, "Every idea is an incitement." 268 U.S. at 673. Even though advocacy of overthrow deserves little protection, we should hesitate to prohibit it if we thereby inhibit the interchange of rational ideas so essential to representative government and free society.

But there is underlying validity in the distinction between advocacy and the interchange of ideas, and we do not discard a useful tool because it may be misused. That such a distinction could be used unreasonably by those in power against hostile or unorthodox views does not negate the fact that it may be used reasonably against an organization wielding the power of the centrally controlled international Communist movement. The object of the conspiracy before us is so clear that the chance of error in saying that the defendants conspired to advocate rather than to express ideas is slight. MR. JUSTICE DOUGLAS quite properly points out that the conspiracy before us is not a conspiracy to overthrow the Government. But it would be equally wrong to treat it as a seminar in political theory.

Of course no government can recognize a "right" of revolution, or a "right" to incite revolution if the incitement has no other purpose or effect. But speech is seldom restricted to a single purpose, and its effects may be manifold. A public interest is not wanting in granting freedom to speak their minds even to those who advocate the overthrow of the Government by force. For, as the evidence in this case abundantly illustrates, coupled with such advocacy is criticism of defects in our society. *** It is a commonplace that there may be a grain of truth in the most uncouth doctrine, however false and repellent the balance may be. Suppressing advocates of overthrow inevitably will also silence critics who do not advocate overthrow but fear that their criticism may be so construed. No matter how clear we may be that the defendants now before us are preparing to overthrow our Government at the propitious moment, it is self- delusion to think that we can punish them for their advocacy without adding to the risks run by loyal citizens who honestly believe in some of the reforms these defendants advance. It is a sobering fact that in sustaining the convictions before us we can hardly escape restriction on the interchange of ideas. ***

It is not for us to decide how we would adjust the clash of interests which this case presents were the primary responsibility for reconciling it ours. Congress has determined that the danger created by advocacy of overthrow justifies the ensuing restriction on freedom of speech. The determination was made after due deliberation, and the seriousness of the congressional purpose is attested by the volume of legislation passed to effectuate the same ends. ***

*** All the Court says is that Congress was not forbidden by the Constitution to pass this enactment and that a prosecution under it may be brought against a conspiracy such as the one before us. ***

MR. JUSTICE JACKSON, concurring. ***

Activity here charged to be criminal is conspiracy—that defendants conspired to teach and advocate, and to organize the Communist Party to teach and advocate, overthrow and destruction of the Government by force and violence. There is no charge of actual violence or attempt at overthrow. ***

The "clear and present danger" test was an innovation by Mr. Justice Holmes in the *Schenck* case, reiterated and refined by him and Mr. Justice Brandeis in later cases, all arising before the era of World War II revealed the subtlety and efficacy of modernized revolutionary techniques used by totalitarian parties. ***

I would save it, unmodified, for application as a "rule of reason" in the kind of case for which it was devised. When the issue is criminality of a hot-headed speech on a street corner, or circulation of a few incendiary pamphlets, or parading by some zealots behind a red flag, or refusal of a handful of school children to salute our flag, it is not beyond the capacity of the judicial process to gather, comprehend, and weigh the necessary materials for decision whether it is a clear and present danger of substantive evil or a harmless letting off of steam. ***

In more recent times these problems have been complicated by the intervention between the state and the citizen of permanently organized, well-financed, semisecret and highly disciplined political organizations. Totalitarian groups here and abroad perfected the technique of creating private paramilitary organizations to coerce both the public government and its citizens. These organizations assert as against our Government all of the constitutional rights and immunities of individuals and at the same time exercise over their followers much of the authority which they deny to the Government. The Communist Party realistically is a state within a state, an authoritarian dictatorship within a republic. It demands these freedoms, not for its members, but for the organized party. It denies to its own members at the same time the freedom to dissent, to debate, to deviate from the party line, and enforces its authoritarian rule by crude purges, if nothing more violent.

The law of conspiracy has been the chief means at the Government's disposal to deal with the growing problems created by such organizations. I happen to think it is an awkward and inept remedy, but I find no constitutional authority for taking this weapon from the Government. There is no constitutional right to "gang up" on the Government.

While I think there was power in Congress to enact this statute and that, as applied in this case, it cannot be held unconstitutional,[15] I add that I have little faith in the long-range effectiveness of this conviction to stop the rise of the Communist movement. ***

MR. JUSTICE BLACK, dissenting. [Omitted.]

MR. JUSTICE DOUGLAS, dissenting.

If this were a case where those who claimed protection under the First Amendment were teaching the techniques of sabotage, the assassination of the President, the filching of documents from public files, the planting of bombs, the art of street warfare, and the like, I would have no doubts. The freedom to speak is not absolute; the teaching of methods of terror and other seditious conduct should be beyond the pale along with obscenity and immorality. This case was argued as if those were the facts. The argument imported much seditious conduct into the record. That is easy and it has popular appeal for the activities of Communists in plotting and scheming against the free world are common knowledge. But the fact is that no such evidence was introduced at the trial. *** It may well be that indoctrination in the techniques of terror to destroy the Government would be indictable under either statute. But the teaching which is condemned here is of a different character.

So far as the present record is concerned, what petitioners did was to organize people to teach and themselves teach the Marxist-Leninist doctrine contained chiefly in four books:[3] Stalin, Foundations of Leninism (1924); Marx and Engels, Manifest of the Communist Party (1848); Lenin, The State and Revolution (1917); History of the Communist Party of the Soviet Union (B.) (1939).

---

15. The defendants have had the benefit so far in this case of all the doubts and confusions afforded by attempts to apply the "clear and present danger" doctrine. While I think it has no proper application to the case, these efforts have been in response to their own contentions and favored rather than prejudiced them. There is no call for reversal on account of it.

3. Other books taught were Stalin, Problems of Leninism, Strategy and Facts of World Communism (H. R. Doc. No. 619, 80th Cong., 2d Sess.), and Program of the Communist International.

Those books are to Soviet Communism what Mein Kampf was to Nazism. If they are understood, the ugliness of Communism is revealed, its deceit and cunning are exposed, the nature of its activities becomes apparent, and the chances of its success less likely. That is not, of course, the reason why petitioners chose these books for their classrooms. They are fervent Communists to whom these volumes are gospel. They preached the creed with the hope that some day it would be acted upon.

The opinion of the Court does not outlaw these texts nor condemn them to the fire, as the Communists do literature offensive to their creed. But if the books themselves are not outlawed, if they can lawfully remain on library shelves, by what reasoning does their use in a classroom become a crime? It would not be a crime under the Act to introduce these books to a class, though that would be teaching what the creed of violent overthrow of the Government is. The Act, as construed, requires the element of intent—that those who teach the creed believe in it. The crime then depends not on what is taught but on who the teacher is. That is to make freedom of speech turn not on *what is said*, but on the *intent* with which it is said. Once we start down that road we enter territory dangerous to the liberties of every citizen.

There was a time in England when the concept of constructive treason flourished. Men were punished not for raising a hand against the king but for thinking murderous thoughts about him. The Framers of the Constitution were alive to that abuse and took steps to see that the practice would not flourish here. Treason was defined to require overt acts—the evolution of a plot against the country into an actual project. The present case is not one of treason. But the analogy is close when the illegality is made to turn on intent, not on the nature of the act. ***

There comes a time when even speech loses its constitutional immunity. Speech innocuous one year may at another time fan such destructive flames that it must be halted in the interests of the safety of the Republic. That is the meaning of the clear and present danger test. When conditions are so critical that there will be no time to avoid the evil that the speech threatens, it is time to call a halt. Otherwise, free speech which is the strength of the Nation will be the cause of its destruction. ***

I had assumed that the question of the clear and present danger, being so critical an issue in the case, would be a matter for submission to the jury. *** Yet whether the question is one for the Court or the jury, there should be evidence of record on the issue. This record, however, contains no evidence whatsoever showing that the acts charged, *viz*., the teaching of the Soviet theory of revolution with the hope that it will be realized, have created any clear and present danger to the Nation. The Court, however, rules to the contrary. It says, "The formation by petitioners of such a highly organized conspiracy, with rigidly disciplined members subject to call when the leaders, these petitioners, felt that the time had come for action, coupled with the inflammable nature of world conditions, similar uprisings in other countries, and the touch-and-go nature of our relations with countries with whom petitioners were in the very least ideologically attuned, convince us that their convictions were justified on this score."

That ruling is in my view not responsive to the issue in the case. *** The nature of Communism as a force on the world scene would, of course, be relevant to the issue of clear and present danger of petitioners' advocacy within the United States. But the primary consideration is the strength and tactical position of petitioners and their converts in this country. On that there is no evidence in the record. *** Communism in the world scene is no bogeyman; but Communism as a political faction or party in this country plainly is. Communism has been so thoroughly exposed in this country that it has been crippled as a political force. Free speech has destroyed it as an effective political party. It is inconceivable that those who went up and down this country preaching the doctrine of revolution which petitioners espouse would have any success. In days of trouble and confusion, when bread lines were long, when the unemployed walked the streets, when people were starving, the advocates of a short-cut by revolution might have a chance to gain adherents. But today there are no such conditions. The country is not in despair; the people know Soviet Communism; the doctrine of Soviet revolution is exposed in all of its ugliness and the American people want none of it.

How it can be said that there is a clear and present danger that this advocacy will succeed is, therefore, a mystery. ***

Vishinsky wrote in 1938 in The Law of the Soviet State, "In our state, naturally, there is and can be no place for freedom of speech, press, and so on for the foes of socialism." *** Our concern should be that we accept no such standard for the United States.

A BRIEF NOTE ON THE *DENNIS* CASE

Dennis v. United States marked the return of serious "sedition" cases to the Supreme Court.[43] The formula for first amendment judicial review, adopted and utilized in the majority opinion, obviously reflects some modification in the "clear and present" danger test as previously understood and applied in a variety of different factual settings during the previous decade-and-a-half, e.g., in *Bridges v. California*. There are, moreover, additional features of the opinion well worth some separate attention and discussion.[44]

---

43. And correspondingly yielded a very wide range of critical academic reflections at the time. See, e.g., John A. Gorfinkel & Julian W. Mack, II, Dennis v. United States and the Clear and Present Danger Rule, 39 Cal.L.Rev. 475 (1951); Louis L. Jaffe, Foreword, 65 Harv.L.Rev. 107 (1951); Nathaniel L. Nathanson, The Communist Trial and the Clear-and-Present-Danger Test, 63 Harv.L.Rev. 1167 (1950). The Smith Act provisions involved in *Dennis* were substantially narrowed, by statutory interpretation, in Yates v. Unites States, 354 U.S. 298 (1957). Cf. Scales v. United States, 367 U.S. 302 (1961); Noto v. United States, 367 U.S. 290 (1961).

44. E.g., the extent to which the Court deferred to congressional "findings" respecting the extent of the threat to national security posed by militant international communism, the linkage between the American Communist Party and external communist movements, the nexus between its program of

The recast form of the first amendment standard against which courts are to test the constitutional permissibility of the prosecution was supplied by Judge Learned Hand, in the court of appeals. It is this recast form that Chief Justice Vinson accepts in the Supreme Court, that in each case the question[45] is

> **Whether the gravity of the evil, discounted by its improbability, justifies such invasion of free speech as is necessary to avoid the danger.**

This would appear to suggest a revised figure of first amendment review, perhaps of the following sort:

Learned Hand's *Dennis* Test

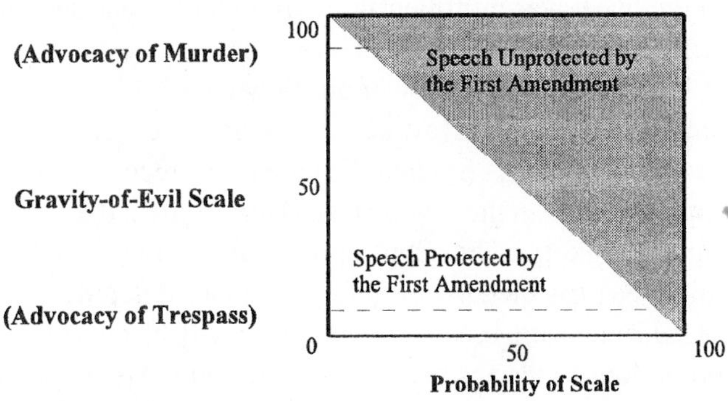

Judge Hand's formula is generally understood as a "sliding scale," trading off a greater latitude of constitutionally protected speech as against risks of bearable harms, while permitting more stringent measures against speech that threatens greater harms, the avoidance of which justifies interventions much more in advance of the threatened putsch. Yet, Hand's test may not be quite this simple. Note that the test is posed in the form of a *question* (i.e. the question in each case is *whether* the gravity

---

domestic advocacy and preparation for violent action pursuant to Soviet direction, etc. Presumably the domestic advocacy program of the Party would have been differently assessed had these connections not been assumed or deemed relevant in light of the specific charges brought under the Smith Act (cf. the opinion of Justice Douglas).

45. For whom? Is "the question" principally or solely for *the legislature* that enacted the applicable criminal statute (to take the measure of the gravity of the harm felt sufficient to warrant the restriction on speech as the resulting statute does); or for *the trial judge* independently to determine (as an incident of the particular prosecution)? Or is it, rather, principally *a jury* question, to be determined in response to an instruction by the trial judge (re what the prosecution must prove to the jury's satisfaction beyond reasonable doubt, such that if the jury does not find the evidence in the case sufficient, it is to acquit)? Or is it, rather, a first amendment requirement-of-law (constitutional law), determinable de novo such that unless the record on the appeal clearly proves the elements of the test, the court of appeals is to reverse?

of the evil, discounted by its improbability, justifies such invasion of free speech as is necessary to avoid the danger). It leaves open the possibility that in some instances, the answer is "no," perhaps just because the kind or degree of harm sought to be avoided does *not* justify such invasion of free speech as concededly may be necessary to avoid the danger, given the kind of speech at stake. In the protection of social advocacy or political speech, in other words, some kinds or some degree of "harm" may have to be accepted as the price of freedom of speech—a price the first amendment exacts.[46]

Social advocacy speech urging others to disregard trespass restrictions the speaker believes to be unfair and unworthy of respect, threaten only a relatively commonplace and, at that, a not very weighty social harm. Such specific advocacy of law violation may be subject to successful prosecution, but only if it actually induced such action or, at the least, was imminently likely to have done so at the moment of the speaker's arrest. Otherwise, the speech is protected by the first amendment, whether or not it involved the advocacy of an illegal act.[47]

Advocacy speech urging others to take violent measures (e.g., arson, killing), on the other hand, is virtually always beyond the pale of protected speech, according to the figure seemingly implicit in the*Dennis* test. Thus, only in the instance where the advocacy was highly unlikely to be acted upon, considering all of the relevant circumstances, would it be protected under the first amendment properly applied. This appears to be Judge Hand's suggestion in explaining why he concurred in sustaining the Smith Act convictions of the accused—for organizing to plan for and to advocate violence, to overthrow the government by force, despite the lack of evidence that there was imminent danger of either. Judge Hand's test is reminiscent of his approach in the field of torts.[48] Here, the trade off is between the gravity of the evil to be avoided, discounted by its improbability despite the speaker's advocacy aimed at bringing it to pass.[49]

---

46. See, e.g., Cohen v. California, 403 U.S. 15 (1971); Texas v. Johnson, 491 U.S. 397 (1989); see also Brandeis' statements in Whitney v. California, 274 U.S. 357 (1927)). Cf. Richard A. Posner, Free Speech in an Economic Perspective, 20 Suffolk L.Rev. 1, 8-9, 36-37 (1986).

47. Notice this change from the earlier Hand formulation, in *The Masses* case.

48. See, e.g., United States v. Carroll Towing Co., 159 F.2d 169, 173 (2d Cir. 1947).

49. So, on the graphic diagram, even the direct advocacy of trespass remains protected by the first amendment except in the instance where, locating the particular case on the horizontal probability axis, the advocacy will almost certainly produce the law violation (rather than merely "have a tendency" or even have been "reasonably likely to have done so"), such that it falls into the grey (unprotected) zone rather than the white (protected) zone under the circumstances (e.g., it appears roughly at the "97%" point on the probability scale). Oppositely, the direct advocacy of someone's murder (or some group's killing) is validly subject to prosecution though there were but a bare possibility of action (e.g., a "3%" chance on the probability axis is enough to clear any first amendment defense), even fully assuming the advocacy is also part of a political movement or protest. Correspondingly, intermediately scaled kinds and degrees of "harm" are located appropriately on the vertical 0 to 100 (least to greatest) "gravity of evil" scale, with the first amendment defense failing at the point where, on the horizontal probability

In what respect(s) does this differ from the Holmes-Brandeis formulation? What would you say are the comparative strengths or weaknesses, as between the two? What other sorts of questions might one want to have answered in deciding these matters? What is your view of the decision in *Dennis* itself?

BRANDENBURG v. OHIO

395 U.S. 444 (1969)

PER CURIAM.

The appellant, a leader of a Ku Klux Klan group, was convicted under the Ohio Criminal Syndicalism statute for "advocat[ing] *** the duty, necessity, or propriety of crime, sabotage, violence, or unlawful methods of terrorism as a means of accomplishing industrial or political reform" and for "voluntarily assembl[ing] with any society, group, or assemblage of persons formed to teach or advocate the doctrines of criminal syndicalism." He was fined $1,000 and sentenced to one to 10 years' imprisonment. The appellant challenged the constitutionality of the criminal syndicalism statute under the First and Fourteenth Amendments to the United States Constitution, but the intermediate appellate court of Ohio affirmed his conviction without opinion. The Supreme Court of Ohio dismissed his appeal, *sua sponte*, "for the reason that no substantial constitutional question exists herein." It did not file an opinion or explain its conclusions. Appeal was taken to this Court, and we noted probable jurisdiction. We reverse.

The record shows that a man identified at trial as the appellant, telephoned an announcer-reporter on the staff of a Cincinnati television station and invited him to come to a Ku Klux Klan "rally" to be held at a farm in Hamilton County. With the cooperation of the organizers, the reporter and a cameraman attended the meeting and filmed the events. Portions of the films were later broadcast on the local station and on a national network.

The prosecution's case rested on the films and on testimony identifying the appellant as the person who communicated with the reporter and who spoke at the rally. The State also introduced into evidence several articles appearing in the film, including a pistol, a rifle, a shotgun, ammunition, a Bible, and a red hood worn by the speaker in the films.

One film showed 12 hooded figures, some of whom carried firearms. They gathered around a large wooden cross, which they burned. No one was present other than the participants and the newsmen who made the film. Most of the words uttered during the scene were incomprehensible when the film was projected, but scattered phrases could be understood that were derogatory of Negroes and, in one instance,

---

axis, the facts of the particular case would place the case in the grey (unprotected) area rather than the white (protected) area.

of Jews. Another scene on the same film showed the appellant, in Klan regalia, making a speech. The speech, in full, was as follows:

> "This is an organizers' meeting. We have had quite a few members here today which are—we have hundreds, hundreds of members throughout the State of Ohio. I can quote from a newspaper clipping from the Columbus, Ohio Dispatch, five weeks ago Sunday morning. The Klan has more members in the State of Ohio than does any other organization. We're not a revengent organization, but if our President, our Congress, our Supreme Court, continues to suppress the white, Caucasian race, it's possible that there might have to be some revengeance taken.
>
> We are marching on Congress July the Fourth, four hundred thousand strong. From there we are dividing into two groups, one group to march on St. Augustine, Florida, the other group to march into Mississippi. Thank you."

The second film showed six hooded figures one of whom, later identified as the appellant, repeated a speech very similar to that recorded on the first film. The reference to the possibility of "revengeance" was omitted, and one sentence was added: "Personally, I believe the nigger should be returned to Africa, the Jew returned to Israel." Though some of the figures in the films carried weapons, the speaker did not.

The Ohio Criminal Syndicalism Statute was enacted in 1919. From 1917 to 1920, identical or similar laws were adopted by 20 States and two territories. In 1927, this Court sustained the constitutionality of California's Criminal Syndicalism Act, *** the text of which is quite similar to that of the laws of Ohio. Whitney v. California, 274 U.S. 357 (1927). The Court upheld the statute on the ground that, without more, "advocating" violent means to effect political and economic change involves such danger to the security of the State that the State may outlaw it. *** But *Whitney* has been thoroughly discredited by later decisions. See Dennis v. United States, 341 U.S. 494, at 507 (1951).

These later decisions have fashioned the principle that the constitutional guarantees of free speech and free press do not permit a State to forbid or proscribe advocacy of the use of force or of law violation except where such advocacy is directed to inciting or producing imminent lawless action and is likely to incite or produce such action.[2] As we said in Noto v. United States, 367 U.S. 290, 297-298 (1961), "the mere abstract teaching *** of the moral propriety or even moral

---

2. It was on the theory that the Smith Act, 54 Stat. 670, 18 U.S.C. § 2385, embodied such a principle and that it had been applied only in conformity with it that this Court sustained the Act's constitutionality. Dennis v. United States, 341 U.S. 494 (1951). That this was the basis for *Dennis* was emphasized in Yates v. United States, 354 U.S. 298, 320-324 (1957), in which the Court overturned convictions for advocacy of the forcible overthrow of the Government under the Smith Act, because the trial judge's instructions had allowed conviction for mere advocacy, unrelated to its tendency to produce forcible action.

necessity for a resort to force and violence, is not the same as preparing a group for violent action and steeling it to such action." See also Herndon v. Lowry, 301 U.S. 242, 259-261 (1937); Bond v. Floyd, 385 U.S. 116, 134 (1966). A statute which fails to draw this distinction impermissibly intrudes upon the freedoms guaranteed by the First and Fourteenth Amendments. It sweeps within its condemnation speech which our Constitution has immunized from governmental control. Cf. Yates v. United States, 354 U.S. 298 (1957); De Jonge v. Oregon, 299 U.S. 353 (1937); Stromberg v. California, 283 U.S. 359 (1931). See also United States v. Robel, 389 U. S. 258 (1967); Keyishian v. Board of Regents, 385 U.S. 589 (1967); Elfbrandt v. Russell, 384 U.S. 11 (1966); Aptheker v. Secretary of State, 378 U.S. 500 (1964); Baggett v. Bullitt, 377 U.S. 360 (1964).

Measured by this test, Ohio's Criminal Syndicalism Act cannot be sustained. The Act punishes persons who "advocate or teach the duty, necessity, or propriety" of violence "as a means of accomplishing industrial or political reform"; or who publish or circulate or display any book or paper containing such advocacy; or who "justify" the commission of violent acts "with intent to exemplify, spread or advocate the propriety of the doctrines of criminal syndicalism" or who "voluntarily assemble" with a group formed "to teach or advocate the doctrines of criminal syndicalism." Neither the indictment nor the trial judge's instructions to the jury in any way refined the statute's bald definition of the crime in terms of mere advocacy not distinguished from incitement to imminent lawless action.

Accordingly, we are here confronted with a statute which, by its own words and as applied, purports to punish mere advocacy and to forbid, on pain of criminal punishment, assembly with others merely to advocate the described type of action. Such a statute falls within the condemnation of the First and Fourteenth Amendments. The contrary teaching of *Whitney v. California, supra,* cannot be supported, and that decision is therefore overruled.

MR. JUSTICE BLACK, concurring.

I agree with the views expressed by MR. JUSTICE DOUGLAS in his concurring opinion in this case that the "clear and present danger" doctrine should have no place in the interpretation of the First Amendment. I join the Court's opinion, which, as I understand it, simply cites Dennis v. United States, 341 U.S. 494 (1951), but does not indicate any agreement on the Court's part with the "clear and present danger" doctrine on which *Dennis* purported to rely.

MR. JUSTICE DOUGLAS, concurring.

*** The dissents in *Abrams, Schaefer,* and *Pierce* show how easily "clear and present danger" is manipulated to crush what Brandeis called "[t]he fundamental right of free men to strive for better conditions through new legislation and new institutions" by argument and discourse (*Pierce v. United States, supra,* at 273) even in time of war. Though I doubt if the "clear and present danger" test is congenial to the First Amendment in time of a declared war, I am certain it is not reconcilable with the First Amendment in days of peace. ***

*** In Bridges v. California, 314 U.S. 252, 261-263, we approved the "clear and present danger" test in an elaborate dictum that tightened it and confined it to a narrow category. But in Dennis v. United States, 341 U.S. 494, we opened wide the door, distorting the "clear and present danger" test beyond recognition.

In that case the prosecution dubbed an agreement to teach the Marxist creed a "conspiracy." The case was submitted to a jury on a charge that the jury could not convict unless it found that the defendants "intended to overthrow the Government 'as speedily as circumstances would permit.'" *** The Court sustained convictions under that charge, construing it to mean a determination of "'whether the gravity of the "evil," discounted by its improbability, justifies such invasion of free speech as is necessary to avoid the danger.'"

Judge Learned Hand, who wrote for the Court of Appeals in affirming the judgment in *Dennis*, coined the "not improbable" test, 183 F.2d 201, 214, which this Court adopted and which Judge Hand preferred over the "clear and present danger" test. Indeed, in his book, The Bill of Rights 59 (1985), in referring to Holmes' creation of the "clear and present danger" test, he said, "I cannot help thinking that for once Homer nodded."

My own view is quite different. I see no place in the regime of the First Amendment for any "clear and present danger" test, whether strict and tight as some would make it, or free-wheeling as the Court in *Dennis* rephrased it.

When one reads the opinions closely and sees when and how the "clear and present danger" test has been applied, great misgivings are aroused. First, the threats were often loud but always puny and made serious only by judges so wedded to the *status quo* that critical analysis made them nervous. Second, the test was so twisted and perverted in *Dennis* as to make the trial of those teachers of Marxism an all-out political trial which was part and parcel of the cold war that has eroded substantial parts of the First Amendment. ***

The line between what is permissible and not subject to control and what may be made impermissible and subject to regulation is the line between ideas and overt acts.

The example usually given by those who would punish speech is the case of one who falsely shouts fire in a crowded theatre.

This is, however, a classic case where speech is brigaded with action. See Speiser v. Randall, 357 U.S. 513, 536-537 (DOUGLAS, J., concurring). They are indeed inseparable and a prosecution can be launched for the overt acts actually caused. Apart from rare instances of that kind, speech is, I think, immune from prosecution.

COHEN v. CALIFORNIA
403 U.S. 15 (1971)

MR. JUSTICE HARLAN delivered the opinion of the Court.

This case may seem at first blush too inconsequential to find its way into our books, but the issue it presents is of no small constitutional significance.

Appellant Paul Robert Cohen was convicted in the Los Angeles Municipal Court of violating that part of California Penal Code § 415 which prohibits "maliciously and willfully disturb[ing] the peace or quiet of any neighborhood or person *** by *** offensive conduct ***." He was given 30 days' imprisonment. The facts upon which his conviction rests are detailed in the opinion of the Court of Appeal of California, Second Appellate District, as follows:

> "On April 26, 1968, the defendant was observed in the Los Angeles County Courthouse in the corridor outside of division 20 of the municipal court wearing a jacket bearing the words 'Fuck the Draft' which were plainly visible. There were women and children present in the corridor. The defendant was arrested. The defendant testified that he wore the jacket knowing that the words were on the jacket as a means of informing the public of the depth of his feelings against the Vietnam War and the draft.
>
> The defendant did not engage in, nor threaten to engage in, nor did anyone as the result of his conduct in fact commit or threaten to commit any act of violence. The defendant did not make any loud or unusual noise, nor was there any evidence that he uttered any sound prior to his arrest." ***

In affirming the conviction the Court of Appeal held that "offensive conduct" means "behavior which has a tendency to provoke *others* to acts of violence or to in turn disturb the peace," and that the State had proved this element because, on the facts of this case, "[i]t was certainly reasonably foreseeable that such conduct might cause others to rise up to commit a violent act against the person of the defendant or attempt to forcibly remove his jacket." *** The California Supreme Court declined review by a divided vote. *** We now reverse. ***

I

In order to lay hands on the precise issue which this case involves, it is useful first to canvass various matters which this record does *not* present.

The conviction quite clearly rests upon the asserted offensiveness of the *words* Cohen used to convey his message to the public. The only "conduct" which the State sought to punish is the fact of communication. Thus, we deal here with a conviction resting solely upon "speech," not upon any separately identifiable conduct which allegedly was intended by Cohen to be perceived by others as expressive of particular views but which, on its face, does not necessarily convey any message and hence arguably could be regulated without effectively repressing Cohen's ability to express himself. Further, the State certainly lacks power to punish Cohen for the underlying content of the message the inscription conveyed. At least so long as there is no showing of an intent to incite disobedience to or disruption of the draft, Cohen could not, consistently with the First and Fourteenth Amendments, be punished for asserting the evident position on the inutility or immorality of the draft his jacket reflected. Yates v. United States, 354 U.S. 298 (1957).

Appellant's conviction, then, rests squarely upon his exercise of the "freedom of speech" protected from arbitrary governmental interference by the Constitution and can be justified, if at all, only as a valid regulation of the manner in which he exercised that freedom, not as a permissible prohibition on the substantive message it conveys. This does not end the inquiry, of course, for the First and Fourteenth Amendments have never been thought to give absolute protection to every individual to speak whenever or wherever he pleases or to use any form of address in any circumstances that he chooses. In this vein, too, however, we think it important to note that several issues typically associated with such problems are not presented here.

In the first place, Cohen was tried under a statute applicable throughout the entire State. Any attempt to support this conviction on the ground that the statute seeks to preserve an appropriately decorous atmosphere in the courthouse where Cohen was arrested must fail in the absence of any language in the statute that would have put appellant on notice that certain kinds of otherwise permissible speech or conduct would nevertheless, under California law, not be tolerated in certain places. ***

In the second place, as it comes to us, this case cannot be said to fall within those relatively few categories of instances where prior decisions have established the power of government to deal more comprehensively with certain forms of individual expression simply upon a showing that such a form was employed. This is not, for example, an obscenity case. Whatever else may be necessary to give rise to the States' broader power to prohibit obscene expression, such expression must be, in some significant way, erotic. Roth v. United States, 354 U.S. 476 (1957). It cannot plausibly be maintained that this vulgar allusion to the Selective Service System would conjure up such psychic stimulation in anyone likely to be confronted with Cohen's crudely defaced jacket.

This Court has also held that the States are free to ban the simple use, without a demonstration of additional justifying circumstances, of so-called "fighting words," those personally abusive epithets which, when addressed to the ordinary citizen, are, as a matter of common knowledge, inherently likely to provoke violent reaction. Chaplinsky v. New Hampshire, 315 U.S. 568 (1942). While the four-letter word displayed by Cohen in relation to the draft is not uncommonly employed in a personally provocative fashion, in this instance it was clearly not "directed to the person of the hearer." Cantwell v. Connecticut, 310 U.S. 296, 309 (1940). No individual actually or likely to be present could reasonably have regarded the words on appellant's jacket as a direct personal insult. Nor do we have here an instance of the exercise of the State's police power to prevent a speaker from intentionally provoking a given group to hostile reaction. Cf. Feiner v. New York, 340 U.S. 315 (1951); Terminiello v. Chicago, 337 U.S. 1 (1949). There is, as noted above, no showing that anyone who saw Cohen was in fact violently aroused or that appellant intended such a result.

Finally, in arguments before this Court, much has been made of the claim that Cohen's distasteful mode of expression was thrust upon unwilling or unsuspecting viewers, and that the State might therefore legitimately act as it did in order to protect the sensitive from otherwise unavoidable exposure to appellant's crude form of protest. *** While this Court has recognized that government may properly act in many situations to prohibit intrusion into the privacy of the home of unwelcome views and ideas which cannot be totally banned from the public dialogue, e.g., Rowan v. Postmaster General, 397 U.S. 728 (1970), we have at the same time consistently stressed that "we are often 'captives' outside the sanctuary of the home and subject to objectionable speech." Id., at 738. The ability of government, consonant with the Constitution, to shut off discourse solely to protect others from hearing it is, in other words, dependent upon a showing that substantial privacy interests are being invaded in an essentially intolerable manner. Any broader view of this authority would effectively empower a majority to silence dissidents simply as a matter of personal predilections.

In this regard, persons confronted with Cohen's jacket were in a quite different posture than, say, those subjected to the raucous emissions of sound trucks blaring outside their residences. Those in the Los Angeles courthouse could effectively avoid further bombardment of their sensibilities simply by averting their eyes. And while it may be that one has a more substantial claim to a recognizable privacy interest when walking through a courthouse corridor than, for example, strolling through Central Park, surely it is nothing like the interest in being free from unwanted expression in the confines of one's own home. Given the subtlety and complexity of the factors involved, if Cohen's "speech" was otherwise entitled to constitutional protection, we do not think the fact that some unwilling "listeners" in a public building may have been briefly exposed to it can serve to justify this breach of the peace conviction where, as here, there was no evidence that persons powerless to avoid appellant's conduct did in fact object to it, and where that portion of the statute upon which Cohen's conviction rests evinces no concern, either on its face or as construed by the California courts, with the special plight of the captive audience, but, instead, indiscriminately sweeps within its prohibitions all "offensive conduct" that disturbs "any neighborhood or person."

II

Against this background, the issue flushed by this case stands out in bold relief. It is whether California can excise, as "offensive conduct," one particular scurrilous epithet from the public discourse, either upon the theory of the court below that its use is inherently likely to cause violent reaction or upon a more general assertion that the States, acting as guardians of public morality, may properly remove this offensive word from the public vocabulary.

The rationale of the California court is plainly untenable. At most it reflects an "undifferentiated fear or apprehension of disturbance [which] is not enough to overcome the right to freedom of expression." Tinker v. Des Moines Indep. Community School Dist., 393 U.S. 503, 508 (1969). We have been shown no evidence that substantial numbers of citizens are standing ready to strike out physically at whoever may assault their sensibilities with execrations like that uttered by Cohen. There may be some persons about with such lawless and violent proclivities, but that is an insufficient base upon which to erect, consistently with constitutional values, a governmental power to force persons who wish to ventilate their dissident views into avoiding particular forms of expression. The argument amounts to little more than the self- defeating proposition that to avoid physical censorship of one who has not sought to provoke such a response by a hypothetical coterie of the violent and lawless, the States may more appropriately effectuate that censorship themselves. ***

Admittedly, it is not so obvious that the First and Fourteenth Amendments must be taken to disable the States from punishing public utterance of this unseemly expletive in order to maintain what they regard as a suitable level of discourse within the body politic.[5] We think, however, that examination and reflection will reveal the shortcomings of a contrary viewpoint.

At the outset, we cannot overemphasize that, in our judgment, most situations where the State has a justifiable interest in regulating speech will fall within one or more of the various established exceptions, discussed above but not applicable here, to the usual rule that governmental bodies may not prescribe the form or content of individual expression. Equally important to our conclusion is the constitutional backdrop against which our decision must be made. The constitutional right of free expression is powerful medicine in a society as diverse and populous as ours. It is designed and intended to remove governmental restraints from the arena of public discussion, putting the decision as to what views shall be voiced largely into the hands of each of us, in the hope that use of such freedom will ultimately produce a more capable citizenry and more perfect polity and in the belief that no other approach would comport with the premise of individual dignity and choice upon

5. The *amicus* urges, with some force, that this issue is not properly before us since the statute, as construed, punishes only conduct that might cause others to react violently. However, because the opinion below appears to erect a virtually irrebuttable presumption that use of this word will produce such results, the statute as thus construed appears to impose, in effect, a flat ban on the public utterance of this word. With the case in this posture, it does not seem inappropriate to inquire whether any other rationale might properly support this result. While we think it clear, for the reasons expressed above, that no statute which merely proscribes "offensive conduct" and has been construed as broadly as this one was below can subsequently be justified in this Court as discriminating between conduct that occurs in different places or that offends only certain persons, it is not so unreasonable to seek to justify its full broad sweep on an alternate rationale such as this. Because it is not so patently clear that acceptance of the justification presently under consideration would render the statute overbroad or unconstitutionally vague, and because the answer to appellee's argument seems quite clear, we do not pass on the contention that this claim is not presented on this record.

which our political system rests. See Whitney v. California, 274 U.S. 357, 375-377 (1927) (Brandeis, J., concurring).

To many, the immediate consequence of this freedom may often appear to be only verbal tumult, discord, and even offensive utterance. These are, however, within established limits, in truth necessary side effects of the broader enduring values which the process of open debate permits us to achieve. That the air may at times seem filled with verbal cacophony is, in this sense not a sign of weakness but of strength. We cannot lose sight of the fact that, in what otherwise might seem a trifling and annoying instance of individual distasteful abuse of a privilege, these fundamental societal values are truly implicated. That is why "[w]holly neutral futilities *** come under the protection of free speech as fully as do Keats' poems or Donne's sermons," Winters v. New York, 333 U.S. 507 (1948) (Frankfurter, J., dissenting), and why "so long as the means are peaceful, the communication need not meet standards of acceptability." Organization for a Better Austin v. Keefe, 402 U.S. 415 (1971).

Against this perception of the constitutional policies involved, we discern certain more particularized considerations that peculiarly call for reversal of this conviction. First, the principle contended for by the State seems inherently boundless. How is one to distinguish this from any other offensive word? *** For, while the particular four-letter word being litigated here is perhaps more distasteful than most others of its genre, it is nevertheless often true that one man's vulgarity is another's lyric. Indeed, we think it is largely because governmental officials cannot make principled distinctions in this area that the Constitution leaves matters of taste and style so largely to the individual.

Additionally, we cannot overlook the fact, because it is well illustrated by the episode involved here, that much linguistic expression serves a dual communicative function: it conveys not only ideas capable of relatively precise, detached explication, but otherwise inexpressible emotions as well. In fact, words are often chosen as much for their emotive as their cognitive force. We cannot sanction the view that the Constitution, while solicitous of the cognitive content of individual speech has little or no regard for that emotive function which practically speaking, may often be the more important element of the overall message sought to be communicated. Indeed, as Mr. Justice Frankfurter has said, "[o]ne of the prerogatives of American citizenship is the right to criticize public men and measures—and that means not only informed and responsible criticism but the freedom to speak foolishly and without moderation." Baumgartner v. United States, 322 U.S. 665, 673-674 (1944).

Finally, and in the same vein, we cannot indulge the facile assumption that one can forbid particular words without also running a substantial risk of suppressing ideas in the process. Indeed, governments might soon seize upon the censorship of particular words as a convenient guise for banning the expression of unpopular views. We have been able, as noted above, to discern little social benefit that might result from running the risk of opening the door to such grave results.

It is, in sum, our judgment that, absent a more particularized and compelling reason for its actions, the State may not, consistently with the First and Fourteenth Amendments, make the simple public display here involved of this single four-letter expletive a criminal offense. Because that is the only arguably sustainable rationale for the conviction here at issue, the judgment below must be reversed.

Reversed.

MR. JUSTICE BLACKMUN, with whom THE CHIEF JUSTICE and MR. JUSTICE BLACK join.

I dissent, and I do so for two reasons:

1. Cohen's absurd and immature antic, in my view, was mainly conduct and little speech. *** The California Court of Appeal appears so to have described it, and I cannot characterize it otherwise. Further, the case appears to me to be well within the sphere of Chaplinsky v. New Hampshire, 315 U.S. 568 (1942), where Mr. Justice Murphy, a known champion of First Amendment freedoms, wrote for a unanimous bench. As a consequence, this Court's agonizing over First Amendment values seem misplaced and unnecessary.

2. I am not at all certain that the California Court of Appeal's construction of § 415 is now the authoritative California construction. The Court of Appeal filed its opinion on October 22, 1969. The Supreme Court of California declined review by a four-to-three vote on December 17. See 1 Cal.App.3d at 104, 81 Cal.Rptr., at 503. A month later on January 27, 1970, the State Supreme Court in another case construed § 415, evidently for the first time. In re Bushman, 1 Cal.3d 767, 83 Cal. Rptr. 375, 463 P.2d 727. *** Inasmuch as this Court does not dismiss this case, it ought to be remanded to the California Court of Appeal for reconsideration in the light of the subsequently rendered decision by the State's highest tribunal in *Bushman*.

MR. JUSTICE WHITE concurs in Paragraph 2 of MR. JUSTICE BLACKMUN's dissenting opinion.

HESS v. INDIANA

414 U.S. 105 (1973)

PER CURIAM.

Gregory Hess appeals from his conviction in the Indiana courts for violating the State's disorderly conduct statute.[1] ***

---

1. "Whoever shall act in a loud, boisterous or disorderly manner so as to disturb the peace and quiet of any neighborhood or family, by loud or unusual noise, or by tumultuous or offensive behavior, threatening, traducing, quarreling, challenging to fight or fighting, shall be deemed guilty of disorderly

The events leading to Hess' conviction began with an antiwar demonstration on the campus of Indiana University. In the course of the demonstration, approximately 100 to 150 of the demonstrators moved into a public street and blocked the passage of vehicles. When the demonstrators did not respond to verbal directions from the sheriff to clear the street, the sheriff and his deputies began walking up the street, and the demonstrators in their path moved to the curbs on either side, joining a large number of spectators who had gathered. Hess was standing off the street as the sheriff passed him. The sheriff heard Hess utter the word "fuck" in what he later described as a loud voice and immediately arrested him on the disorderly conduct charge. It was later stipulated that what appellant had said was "We'll take the fucking street later," or "We'll take the fucking street again." Two witnesses who were in the immediate vicinity testified, apparently without contradiction, that they heard Hess' words and witnessed his arrest. They indicated that Hess did not appear to be exhorting the crowd to go back into the street, that he was facing the crowd and not the street when he uttered the statement, that his statement did not appear to be addressed to any particular person or group, and that his tone, although loud, was no louder than that of the other people in the area.

Indiana's disorderly conduct statute was applied in this case to punish only spoken words. It hardly needs repeating that "[t]he constitutional guarantees of freedom of speech forbid the States to punish the use of words or language not within 'narrowly limited classes of speech.'" Gooding v. Wilson, [405 U.S. 518,] 521-522 [(1972)]. The words here did not fall within any of these "limited classes." In the first place, it is clear that the Indiana courts specifically abjured any suggestion that Hess' words could be punished as obscene under Roth v. United States, 354 U.S. 476 (1957), and its progeny. Indeed, after Cohen v. California, 403 U.S. 15 (1971), such a contention with regard to the language at issue would not be tenable. By the same token, any suggestion that Hess' speech amounted to "fighting words," Chaplinsky v. New Hampshire, 315 U.S. 568 (1942), could not withstand scrutiny. Even if under other circumstances this language could be regarded as a personal insult, the evidence is undisputed that Hess' statement was not directed to any person or group in particular. Although the sheriff testified that he was offended by the language, he also stated that he did not interpret the expression as being directed personally at him, and the evidence is clear that appellant had his back to the sheriff at the time. Thus, under our decisions, the State could not punish this speech as "fighting words." Cantwell v. Connecticut, 310 U.S. 296, 309 (1940); *Cohen v. California, supra*, at 20.

---

conduct, and upon conviction, shall be fined in any sum not exceeding five hundred dollars [$500] to which may be added imprisonment for not to exceed one hundred eighty [180] days." ***

In addition, there was no evidence to indicate that Hess' speech amounted to a public nuisance in that privacy interests were being invaded. "The ability of government, consonant with the Constitution, to shut off discourse solely to protect others from hearing it is *** dependent upon a showing that substantial privacy interests are being invaded in an essentially intolerable manner." *Cohen v. California, supra*, at 21. The prosecution made no such showing in this case.

The Indiana Supreme Court placed primary reliance on the trial court's finding that Hess' statement "was intended to incite further lawless action on the part of the crowd in the vicinity of appellant and was likely to produce such action." *** At best, however, the statement could be taken as counsel for present moderation; at worst, it amounted to nothing more than advocacy of illegal action at some indefinite future time. This is not sufficient to permit the State to punish Hess' speech. Under our decisions, "the constitutional guarantees of free speech and free press do not permit a State to forbid or proscribe advocacy of the use of force or of law violation except where such advocacy is directed to inciting or producing *imminent* lawless action and is likely to incite or produce such action." Brandenburg v. Ohio, 395 U.S. 444, 447 (1969). (Emphasis added.) *** Since the uncontroverted evidence showed that Hess' statement was not directed to any person or group of persons, it cannot be said that he was advocating, in the normal sense, any action. And since there was no evidence, or rational inference from the import of the language, that his words were intended to produce, and likely to produce, *imminent* disorder, those words could not be punished by the State on the ground that they had "a 'tendency to lead to violence.'" ***

Accordingly, *** the judgment of the Supreme Court of Indiana is reversed.

MR. JUSTICE REHNQUIST, with whom THE CHIEF JUSTICE and MR. JUSTICE BLACKMUN join, dissenting.

***

The simple explanation for the result in this case is that the majority has interpreted the evidence differently from the courts below. In doing so, however, I believe the Court has exceeded the proper scope of our review. Rather than considering the "evidence" in the light most favorable to the appellee and resolving credibility questions against the appellant, as many of our cases have required, the Court has instead fashioned its own version of events from a paper record, some "uncontroverted evidence," and a large measure of conjecture. Since this is not the traditional function of any appellate court, and is surely not a wise or proper use of the authority of this Court, I dissent.

B. POWERS OF TAXATION AS APPLIED TO "THE PRESS"

"The Power to tax involves the power to destroy."

Chief Justice John Marshall[50]

"The Power to tax is not the power to destroy *while this Court sits*."

Justice Oliver Wendell Holmes, Jr.[51]

INTRODUCTION

The question is not whether taxes *can* destroy a given activity, for so much is obvious. Assuredly they can, sometimes deliberately,[52] sometimes not. Rather the question is the extent to which, "*while this Court sits*," the first amendment will be brought to bear to head off that tendency or that effect. If the first amendment is to be brought to bear, in what way, by what analysis, and by means of what particular standards of judicial review? The more salient Supreme Court cases addressed to these questions are presented in this chapter to enable the reader to make that assessment as best can be done given the limited materials we have.

In this brief introduction, however, it is useful to have drawn on Justice Holmes, even as we did in early chapters, beginning with Chapter 1. It is useful because, once again, his observations may help us with a relevant history. In Chapter 1, the inquiry was into licensing and other forms of prior restraint, a subject Holmes believed to be especially informed by history and the origins of the first amendment.[53] Here, to be

---

50. McCulloch v. Maryland, 17 U.S. (4 Wheat.) 316, 431 (1819).

51. Panhandle Oil Co. v. Mississippi ex rel. Knox, 277 U.S. 218, 223 (1928) (emphasis added). But see also Holmes' equally famous aphorism on taxes, in Compania de Tabacos de Filipinas v. Collector of Internal Revenue, 275 U.S. 87, 100 (1927) ("Taxes are what we pay for civilized society."). (Somewhat self-servingly, perhaps, these words are also carved into the stone frieze above the entrance to the I.R.S. offices in Washington, D.C.).

52. See, e.g., Bailey v. Drexel Furniture Co., 259 U.S. 20 (1922) (striking scheme which imposed federal excise tax of 10% of annual net profits on employers employing anyone younger than a specified minimum age, but imposed no such tax, in any amount, on employers who would refuse employment to such persons. Speaking to the point of the tax—to put an end to an activity Congress disapproved—the Court observed: "All others can see and understand this. How can we properly shut our minds to it?") *Bailey*, however, marks the exceptional case in federalism cases involving the power of Congress to levy taxes; more often, the Court sustains even deliberately "activity destroying" federal taxes, so long as the activity thus impaired or destroyed receives no special constitutional protection. For useful examples, see, e.g., United States v. Kahriger, 345 U.S. 22 (1953); Minor v. United States, 396 U.S. 87 (1969).

53. Patterson v. Colorado, 205 U.S. 454, 462 (1908) ("[T]he main purpose of [the constitutional provisions addressed to the freedom of the press] is 'to prevent all such *previous restraints* upon publications as had been practiced by other governments' ***.") (Holmes, J.) (relying on William Blackstone, Commentaries, vol. iv, 150-52, retracing the history of licensing, and concluding that "the press became properly free" only in 1694 with the expiration of the last acts of Parliament for licensing and regulating the press). See also Bantum Books. v. Sullivan, 372 U.S. 58, 70 (1963) ("Any system of prior restraints of expression comes to this Court bearing a heavy presumption against its

sure, the inquiry is into taxes and the press. These two subjects, first, licensing, and second, taxes, however, do not merely share a common history in some general sense. To the contrary, the connection between them, historically, is considerably more interesting and more intimate than that. As one may see from the following excerpts from Frederick S. Siebert's impressive volume on Freedom of the Press in England,[54] the second—press taxes—followed almost at once where the first—licensing and prior restraints—left off. So, as Siebert gives us his own account of the time when William Blackstone concluded the press "became properly free,"[55] in 1694, not all were inclined to take so sublime a view:

> Following the expiration of the last licensing act in [1694], the eighteenth-century statesmen saw no reason to revive such obviously unsavory methods of control as state licensing and printing-trade regulation. There were other methods, more subtle, more indirect, and therefore less dangerous. Taxation, subsidization, and prosecution under due process of law—these were the methods employed by the state to control and regulate the press during the period between the death of Anne and the Declaration of American Independence.
>
> ***
>
> The principal impetus in the search for a substitute for the Regulation of Printing Act [the licensing system permitted to expire in 1694, which the Commons refused to renew] came from the government. The queen, the ministry, and the clergy were continuously scandalized by the flood of pamphlets and newspapers. *** The eventual method of control devised by Anne's ministers and adopted by Parliament was neither precipitous nor accidental. The revenue act of 1710 *** for the first time imposed a tax on printed matter [one penny per copy].
>
> ***
>
> Henry St. John, Viscount Bolingbroke, is credited with the discovery that a tax on publications would serve the double purpose of providing revenue and at the same time serve as a substitute for the Regulation of Printing Act. Which motive was uppermost in the minds of the ministers or the members of Parliament is almost impossible to tell, but it appears that the principal objective of the first Stamp tax (10 Anne, cap. 19, 1712) was the control of "licentious, schismatical, and scandalous" publications. Defoe had warned the

---

constitutional validity.").

54. Frederick S. Siebert, Freedom of the Press in England 1476-1776 305-45 (1965) ("Control Through Taxation"). See also Randall P. Bezanson, Taxes on Knowledge in America: Exactions on the Press from Colonial Times to the Present (1994); Dobson Collett, History of the Taxes on Knowledge: Their Origin and Repeal (1933); F. Knight Hunt, The Fourth Estate: Contributions Towards a History of Newspapers, and of the Liberty of the Press (1850).

55. See note 53 *supra* (and the longer excerpt in chap. 1, *supra* p. 14-16).

government *** that the tax would not suppress criticism of the government but would drive it underground. The ministers, however, felt that they could not lose. If the Stamp tax produced revenue, well and good; if it discouraged periodical publications, so much the better.

***

On 16 May 1712 the first tax on newspapers was passed. The Act contained four general provisions affecting the press: (1) the tax on newspapers and pamphlets, (2) the tax on advertisements, (3) the tax on paper, and (4) registration and enforcement provisions. *** [T]hat printed books larger than six sheets were exempted entirely from the tax indicates that the principal objective of the government was the suppression of the small ephemeral publications which were sniping at the policies of the ministry. *** Swift wrote *** : "Do you know that all Grub-street is dead and gone last week? *** The *Observator* is fallen; *** the *Spectator* keeps up and doubles it price. I know not how long it will last."

THE PRINCIPAL CASES

The first significant case in the Supreme Court challenging a tax as applied to the press in this country involved a state tax strikingly similar to one of the newspaper taxes enacted in England in the reign of Queen Anne: a tax (albeit not in a very great amount) on gross receipts from advertisement sales of large newspapers, exempting those smaller in circulation. We begin our brief review with this case, *Grosjean v. American Press Co.*, from 1936.[56]

GROSJEAN v. AMERICAN PRESS CO.

297 U.S. 233 (1936)

MR. JUSTICE SUTHERLAND delivered the opinion of the Court.

This suit was brought by appellees, nine publishers of newspapers in the state of Louisiana, to enjoin the enforcement against them of the provisions of section 1 of the act of the Legislature of Louisiana known as Act No. 23, passed and approved July 12, 1934, as follows:

> "That every person, firm, association or corporation, *** engaged in the business of selling, or making any charge for, advertising or for advertisements *** to be printed or published, in any newspaper, magazine, periodical or

---

56. For a fuller description of *Grosjean*, see the recent book by Richard C. Corner, The Kingfish and the Constitution: Huey Long, The First Amendment, and the Emergence of Modern Press Freedom in America (1996).

> publication whatever having a circulation of more than 20,000 copies per week, *** shall, in addition to all other taxes and licenses levied and assessed in this State, pay a license tax for the privilege of engaging in such business in this State of two per cent. (2%) of the gross receipts of such business."

The nine publishers who brought the suit publish thirteen newspapers; and these thirteen publications are the only ones within the state of Louisiana having each a circulation of more than 20,000 copies per week, although the lower court finds there are four other daily newspapers each having a circulation of "slightly less than 20,000 copies per week" which are in competition with those published by appellees both as to circulation and as to advertising. In addition, there are 120 weekly newspapers published in the state, also in competition, to a greater or less degree, with the newspapers of appellees. The revenue derived from appellees' newspapers comes almost entirely from regular subscribers or purchasers thereof and from payments received for the insertion of advertisements therein.

*** The validity of the act is assailed as violating the Federal Constitution in two particulars: (1) That it abridges the freedom of the press in contravention of the due process clause contained in section 1 of the Fourteenth Amendment; (2) that it denies appellees the equal protection of the laws in contravention of the same amendment.

1. The first point presents a question of the utmost gravity and importance; for, if well made, it goes to the heart of the natural right of the members of an organized society, united for their common good, to impart and acquire information about their common interests.*** While [the first amendment] is not a restraint upon the powers of the states, the states are precluded from abridging the freedom of speech or of the press by force of the due process clause of the Fourteenth Amendment. ***

The tax imposed is designated a "license tax for the privilege of engaging in such business," that is to say, the business of selling, or making any charge for, advertising. As applied to appellees, it is a tax of 2 per cent. on the gross receipts derived from advertisements carried in their newspapers when, and only when, the newspapers of each enjoy a circulation of more than 20,000 copies per week. It thus operates as a restraint in a double sense. First, its effect is to curtail the amount of revenue realized from advertising; and, second, its direct tendency is to restrict circulation. This is plain enough when we consider that, if it were increased to a high degree, as it could be if valid, it well might result in destroying both advertising and circulation.

A determination of the question whether the tax is valid in respect of the point now under review requires an examination of the history and circumstances which antedated and attended the adoption of the abridgement clause of the First Amendment. *** The history is a long one; but for present purposes it may be greatly abbreviated.

For more than a century prior to the adoption of the amendment—and, indeed, for many years thereafter—history discloses a persistent effort on the part of the

British government to prevent or abridge the free expression of any opinion which seemed to criticize or exhibit in an unfavorable light, however truly, the agencies and operations of the government. ***

In 1712, in response to a message from Queen Anne (Hansard's Parliamentary History of England, vol. 6, p. 1063), Parliament imposed a tax upon all newspapers and upon advertisements. ***

These duties were quite commonly characterized as "taxes on knowledge," a phrase used for the purpose of describing the effect of the exactions and at the same time condemning them. That the taxes had, and were intended to have, the effect of curtailing the circulation of newspapers, and particularly the cheaper ones whose readers were generally found among the masses of the people, went almost without question, even on the part of those who defended the act. ***

*** It is idle to suppose that so many of the best men of England would for a century of time have waged, as they did, stubborn and often precarious warfare against these taxes if a mere matter of taxation had been involved. The aim of the struggle was not to relieve taxpayers from a burden, but to establish and preserve the right of the English people to full information in respect of the doings or misdoings of their government. ***

In 1785, only four years before Congress had proposed the First Amendment, the Massachusetts Legislature, following the English example, imposed a stamp tax on all newspapers and magazines. The following year an advertisement tax was imposed. Both taxes met with such violent opposition that the former was repealed in 1786, and the latter in 1788. Duniway, Freedom of the Press in Massachusetts, pp. 136, 137.

The framers of the First Amendment were familiar with the English struggle, which then had continued for nearly eighty years and was destined to go on for another sixty-five years, at the end of which time it culminated in a lasting abandonment of the obnoxious taxes. The framers were likewise familiar with the then recent Massachusetts episode. *** It is impossible to concede that by the words "freedom of the press" the framers of the amendment intended to adopt merely the narrow view then reflected by the law of England that such freedom consisted only in immunity from previous censorship; for this abuse had then permanently disappeared from English practice. It is equally impossible to believe that it was not intended to bring within the reach of these words such modes of restraint as were embodied in the two forms of taxation already described. ***

In the light of all that has now been said, it is evident that the restricted rules of the English law in respect of the freedom of the press in force when the Constitution was adopted were never accepted by the American colonists, and that by the First Amendment it was meant to preclude the national government, and by the Fourteenth Amendment to preclude the states, from adopting any form of previous restraint upon printed publications, or their circulation, including that which had theretofore been effected by these two well known and odious methods. ***

It is not intended by anything we have said to suggest that the owners of newspapers are immune from any of the ordinary forms of taxation for support of the government. But this is not an ordinary form of tax, but one single in kind, with a long history of hostile misuse against the freedom of the press.

The predominant purpose of the grant of immunity here invoked was to preserve an untrammeled press as a vital source of public information. *** The tax here involved is bad not because it takes money from the pockets of the appellees. If that were all, a wholly different question would be presented. It is bad because, in the light of its history and of its present setting, it is seen to be a deliberate and calculated device in the guise of a tax to limit the circulation of information to which the public is entitled in virtue of the constitutional guaranties. A free press stands as one of the great interpreters between the government and the people. To allow it to be fettered is to fetter ourselves.

In view of the persistent search for new subjects of taxation, it is not without significance that, with the single exception of the Louisiana statute, so far as we can discover, no state during the one hundred fifty years of our national existence has undertaken to impose a tax like that now in question.

The form in which the tax is imposed is in itself suspicious. It is not measured or limited by the volume of advertisements. It is measured alone by the extent of the circulation of the publication in which the advertisements are carried, with the plain purpose of penalizing the publishers and curtailing the circulation of a selected group of newspapers.

2. Having reached the conclusion that the act imposing the tax in question is unconstitutional under the due process of law clause because it abridges the freedom of the press, we deem it unnecessary to consider the further ground assigned, that it also constitutes a denial of the equal protection of the laws.

Decree affirmed.

QUESTIONS AND NOTES

Justice Harlan, dissenting in a case in which he was unable to see exactly what it was that persuaded his colleagues to find a constitutional violation, expressed his frustration in the following bemused way:[57]

> The Court's opinion, by a process of first undiscriminatingly throwing together various factual bits and pieces and then undermining the resulting structure by an equally vague disclaimer, seems to me to leave completely at sea just what it is in this record that [satisfactorily explains the result].

57. Burton v. Wilmington Parking Authority, 365 U.S. 715, 862-63 (1961).

May something of the same sort apply also to the Court's opinion in *Grosjean*? Here, too, the Court has an undermining disclaimer, for it goes out of its way to say near the end:

> It is not intended by anything we have said to suggest that the owners of newspapers are immune from any of the ordinary forms of taxation for support of the government.

Granted that so much is true, what was it, then, specifically, about *this* particular tax that led to its being held to run afoul of the first amendment, while more "ordinary" taxes imposed on (or inclusive of) newspapers and other publishers would not have been? Consider the following points.

1. Early in the opinion, the Court notes that "[t]he tax imposed is designated a 'license tax for the privilege of engaging in [the business of selling advertisement space].'" May this suggest that the first amendment vice inhered in the presumption of the state to "license" (or not) a newspaper, depending upon its payment of a particular tax? *Was tying the tax to a license—as a form of prior restraint—the key?*[58]

2. The Court also notes that the tax, though only of two per cent of gross receipts[59] from advertising revenue (and even then only of publications enjoying a circulation in excess of 20,000 weekly copies), "operate[d] as a restraint in a *double* sense:"[60]

> First, its effect is to curtail the amount of revenue realized from advertising, and, second, its direct tendency is to restrict circulation.

While this may be true, wouldn't both effects also be felt insofar as retail sales of newspapers and magazines may be subject to "ordinary" state sales taxes (for example, an ordinary 6% state or local sales tax)? As a direct tax burden on sales, such a tax may likewise adversely affect sales (by adding 6% to what the consumer must pay) and, to that extent, likewise reduce circulation and sales revenue. So how does the Louisiana tax significantly differ in either of these ways?[61]

---

58. But is there any reason to think the result would be different—or should be different—had the state made no such claim (about licensing), i.e. had it labeled the tax simply as an excise tax on gross receipts derived from advertising revenue of any publication having a circulation of more than 20,000 copies per week, enforceable by the usual means?

59. Would it (should it) make a difference if the tax were merely on *net* receipts (i.e. receipts in excess of expenses or costs) rather than *gross* receipts? If so, why might that be? Note that the Court expressly disclaims a critical interest in the actual extent to which the tax did or did not curtail either advertising revenue or circulation. It is evidently not the actual burden a tax may impose that matters, rather, it appears to be that certain *kinds* of taxes are thought to be the problem (taxes of the kind identified to the era of Queen Anne and the successor "taxes on knowledge" in England).

60. 297 U.S. at 244 (emphasis added).

61. May it follow from *Grosjean* that state sales taxes may have to provide an exemption for "first amendment products" (e.g., for newspapers, books, magazines, videotapes, cassettes)? May it imply at least that any differential (i.e., higher) rate applicable to such sales might be void?

3. Was it, rather, that the tax did not apply to *all* publishers who solicited and sold advertising space in their publications—it applied only to *some* publishers? Quite apart from the equal protection claim the Court found it unnecessary to address,[62] was *this* the first amendment vice of the law, favoritism of some publishers (by exemption), so as to deny a level playing field to "tax-disfavored" publishers?

But tax exemption, and tax rate differences, are *frequently* provided for *smaller* businesses, are they not?[63] Where the difference in tax treatment is measured by this ordinary distinction of size (rather than by content or by point of view), does the first amendment ordinarily disallow distinctions of this sort? If not, why did it seem to matter here?

4. Near the end of the opinion, however, note how the Court takes a different turn, hinting (but not insisting) that this tax may have been enacted less to raise revenue than to strike at nine particular publishers[64] the legislature and governor may have wanted to reach, much in the manner noted by crown ministers in 1712.[65] See again this puzzling passage:

> The tax here involved is bad not because it takes money from the pockets of the appellees. If that were all, a wholly different question would be presented. It is bad because, in the light of its history and of its present setting, it is seen as a deliberate and calculated device in the guise of a tax to limit the circulation of information to which the public is entitled in virtue of the constitutional guaranties.

Why does the Court describe this as a something that is in "*the guise*[66] of a tax," unless it means to imply some misgivings of its own that the Louisiana measure is somehow "not genuinely a tax," or not merely a tax, or something more than a tax? But if it— this particular tax—is (or is also) "something more," what is it, and what makes it "bad" on *that* account?

We have already noticed that all taxes burden those who pay them, and all (or virtually all) taxes also implicitly represent some conscious modicum of express

---

62. 297 U.S. at 251 ("[W]e deem it unnecessary to consider the further ground assigned that it also constitutes a denial of the equal protection of the laws.").

63. Smaller enterprises are often favored through tax breaks or tax exemptions, in the belief that they are less able to absorb the tax burden than larger enterprises, and also that they are socially desirable as such. (Accordingly, equal protection arguments complaining of differential tax treatment more burdensome to large enterprises than to small enterprises very seldom succeed—the distinction is nearly always sustained under mere "rationality review.")

64. I.e. the only publishers of publications with a weekly circulation in excess of 20,000 copies.

65. See Siebert, *supra* page 141 ("The ministers *** felt that they could not lose. If the *** tax produced revenue, well and good; if it discouraged periodical publications, so much the better.").

66. "guise *n.* 1. Outward appearance; aspect. 2. *False appearance; pretence.*" Amer. Heritage Dictionary 586 (1971) (emphasis added).

social choice.[67] Does the Court mean to say merely that the first amendment operates to forbid a tax *where the "social choice" represented by the tax is one that disvalues the circulation of newspapers or periodical publications vis-à-vis other services or goods*? That insofar as a state may seek to raise revenue, it must at least steer clear of raising it by means implicitly reflecting a lesser concern for the costs of publishing and distributing information and news, than, say, the costs of producing and distributing cars, paper clips, or food? If this is the true holding of *Grosjean* (though the Court never quite declares it), the case would be important just on that account.[68] Still, if that was the issue, it confuses the point for the Court to have described the measure as something in *"the guise of"* a tax rather than simply as "a tax of a kind the first amendment forbids."[69]

5. In the end, however, the Court's opinion hints at something else: the darker idea that a reduction in net advertising revenue the affected publishers might experience because of the tax (and such loss in circulation the publishers might experience consequential to the tax) was not simply something the legislature was prepared to accept as a foreseeable (even probable) effect of the tax—rather, that *that* effect was an equal objective—perhaps even a *principal* objective—of the tax. That the gross receipts advertising revenue tax was a mere "cellophane wrapper,"[70] enacted not to raise revenue or to distinguish between large and small publishing houses. That it

---

67. That is, taxes are seldom "economically neutral" in the sense of leaving unaffected the supply or demand for the goods, services, or activities to which they attach.

68. As the subsequent case law (*infra*) suggests, this idea does become more centrally a feature of how the first amendment applies to this general field. The later cases also carry through the suggestion that the first amendment limits social choices regarding taxes and the media, that it disallows taxes reflecting a lesser concern for the economic health of one kind of media than another (as though the general content characteristic of one media were "less worthy" than what another commercial medium tends to present).

69. That is, the first amendment would "forbid" such a measure, because it reflects a particular social preference in the adjustment of taxes forbidden by the first amendment (namely, a willingness to burden first amendment products and first amendment services more than other goods and other services, in order to meet either general or specific revenue needs).

70. The phrase is famously identified to a dissenting opinion by Justice Felix Frankfurter, in United States v. Kahriger, 345 U.S. 22, 38 (1953). *Kahriger*, too, was a tax case. It involved an act of Congress which imposed an excise tax on all wagering transactions, with provisions requiring detailed records including the names and addresses of all those placing wagers, accessible to state and local law enforcement agencies in jurisdictions with anti-wagering laws. In form a tax, it was sustained in the Supreme Court since Congress is given an express power to levy excise taxes. In purpose and in effect (in Frankfurter's view), it was an effort by Congress to stamp out wagering practices, a subject not committed by the Constitution to Congress. Though a New Deal appointee by President Franklin Roosevelt (and thus expected to vote to sustain such acts of Congress as would seem to Congress to be in the best national interest), Frankfurter dissented, penning the following complaint: "[W]hen oblique use is made of the taxing power as to matters which substantively are not within the powers delegated to Congress, the Court cannot shut its eyes to what is obviously, because designedly, at attempt to control conduct which the Constitution left to the responsibility of the States, merely because Congress wrapped the legislation in the verbal cellophane of a revenue measure." His colleagues disagreed.

was, rather, a tax adopted with a certain malice aforethought, i.e., adopted with *no* particular concern one way or the other as to its *revenue* consequences, but adopted to discourage particular publications. That the legislature would be content if *this* were the *chief* effect of the law. Indeed, the Court finally tended to characterize the Louisiana statute virtually in these terms. In the end it wrote of "*the plain purpose* [of the act] of *penalizing* the publishers *and curtailing* the circulation of a *selected* group of newspapers."[71]

If this were true, then doubtless the Act may well run afoul of the first amendment and protection of a free press. Selecting designated publishers to tax in order to "penalize" them and "curtail" the circulation of what they publish is precisely one of the principal government tendencies the first amendment was enacted to forbid. The conscientious reader's problem, however, is that the Court nowhere seems to offer anything more than its own conclusionary statements for this demonizing description of the Act (as having a "plain purpose" of "*penalizing*" certain publishers as such). Why this description? Certainly nothing on the face of the Act, and nothing detailed in the Court's opinion, seems sufficient to support this description of the tax statute as having been adopted "with the plain purpose of penalizing" certain publishers, rather than as a good faith measure to tap an additional source of needed revenue from a plausible source, exempting smaller publishers regarded by the legislature as less able to bear the cost.

What is thus missing from the opinion (doesn't it matter?) is any kind of "smoking gun" evidence establishing the ultimate claim that the legislature was indeed "enacting a penalty" rather than "enacting a (valid) tax."[72] Because that is so, many who have read *Grosjean* closely find the case somewhat unsatisfactory in the end. Having made the same kind of attentive review we have tried to undertake here, they know the result—but they are not sure why or what it means.[73]

Subsequent to *Grosjean*, there were two very different ways of viewing the decision, one narrow, and one quite broad. The narrow view (the predominant view) was that the legislature may not seek to do indirectly (by taxation) that which the first

---

71. 297 U.S. at 251 (emphasis added).

72. As we have already twice observed, the fact that only a small number of publishers would turn out to be affected by the tax does not *per se* indicate any "punitive" design by the legislature. (Of the 13 affected publications—the largest in the state—it just happened (!) that 12 of the 13 editorially espoused views critical of the most formidable political figure by far in Louisiana, Senator Huey Long. A circular distributed by Long and the Governor to each member of the state legislature described the tax as "a tax on lying. ***" (Brief for Appellees, Grosjean v. American Press Co., O. T. 1936, No. 303, at 9).

73. I.e. just as Justice Harlan said of the Court's opinion in Burton v Wilmington Parking Authority, 365 U.S. at 863), the Court's opinion leaves "at sea just what it is in this record that [satisfactorily explains the result]."

amendment forbids it to do directly (by licensing, regulation, or criminal law). From this perspective, *Grosjean* is best understood simply as a useful and vivid example of judicial diligence in the application of "purpose and effect" review.[74] The broader view was that the first amendment may protect publishers ("the press") in an additional fashion, not unlike the judicial doctrine of the "negative voice" of the commerce clause as historically invoked in the courts: first, that taxes singling out ("discriminating" against) first amendment properties, products, raw material, or activity (for example, a special sales tax, inventory tax, or employment tax imposed upon newspapers) are presumptively invalid;[75] second, that taxes "unduly burdening" the press may be forbidden as well.[76]

Nearly a half century was to elapse before the uncertainty was resolved. Just since 1982, it has been resolved in favor of the latter view. The case law in which this general position is elaborated, however, has generated its own new problems of application as one will readily see.[77]

MINNEAPOLIS STAR AND TRIBUNE COMPANY v. MINNESOTA COMMISSIONER OF REVENUE
460 U.S. 575 (1983)

Justice O'CONNOR delivered the opinion of the Court.

This case presents the question of a State's power to impose a special tax on the press and, by enacting exemptions, to limit its effect to only a few newspapers.

I

Since 1967, Minnesota has imposed a sales tax on most sales of goods for a price in excess of a nominal sum.[1] An exemption for industrial and agricultural users shields from the tax sales of components to be used in the production of goods that will themselves be sold at retail. As part of this general system of taxation and in support of the sales tax, Minnesota also enacted a tax on the "privilege of using,

---

74. See, e.g., Note, 46 Okla. L. Rev. 713, 714 (1993) ("The Court in *Grosjean* declared the tax unconstitutional because it was deliberately directed at stifling particular ideas.") (On this accounting, but for this fact, the tax would have been sustained. So, too, an identical tax, not harboring such a purpose, would have been sustained—though it applied in just the same way and affected the same publishers' revenues and circulation figures in precisely the same way.) The doctrine as applied here is merely the same doctrine one reviews in constitutional law and the equal protection clause, e.g., in Washington v. Davis, 426 U.S. 229 (1976), and Personnel Administrator of Massachusetts v. Feeney, 442 U.S. 256 (1979).

75. (Just as a prior restraint is presumptively invalid.)

76. (It being a principal responsibility of the courts to say what such an "undue burden" is, presumably by some sort of overall balancing test.)

77. For an effort to reconcile the doctrines in this trilogy of cases, see Randall P. Bezanson, Taxes on Knowledge in America: Exactions on the Press from Colonial Times to the Present 252-85 (1994).

1. Currently the tax applies to sales of items for more than 9¢.

storing or consuming in Minnesota tangible personal property." This use tax applies to any nonexempt tangible personal property unless the sales tax was paid on the sales price. Like the classic use tax, this use tax protects the State's sales tax by eliminating the residents' incentive to travel to States with lower sales taxes to buy goods rather than buying them in Minnesota.

The appellant, Minneapolis Star and Tribune Company "Star Tribune," is the publisher of a morning newspaper and an evening newspaper in Minneapolis. From 1967 until 1971, it enjoyed an exemption from the sales and use tax provided by Minnesota for periodic publications. In 1971, however, while leaving the exemption from the sales tax in place, the legislature amended the scheme to impose a "use tax" on the cost of paper and ink products consumed in the production of a publication. Ink and paper used in publications became the only items subject to the use tax that were components of goods to be sold at retail. In 1974, the legislature again amended the statute, this time to exempt the first $100,000 worth of ink and paper consumed by a publication in any calendar year, in effect giving each publication an annual tax credit of $4,000. Publications remained exempt from the sales tax.

After the enactment of the $100,000 exemption, 11 publishers, producing 14 of the 388 paid circulation newspapers in the State, incurred a tax liability in 1974. Star Tribune was one of the 11, and, of the $893,355 collected, it paid $608,634, or roughly two-thirds of the total revenue raised by the tax.

Star Tribune instituted this action to seek a refund of the use taxes it paid from January 1, 1974 to May 31, 1975. The Minnesota Supreme Court upheld the tax against the federal constitutional challenge. We now reverse.

II

Star Tribune argues that we must strike this tax on the authority of *Grosjean v. American Press Co., Inc.*, 297 U.S. 233 (1936). Although there are similarities between the two cases, we agree with the State that *Grosjean* is not controlling. ***

We think that the result in *Grosjean* may have been attributable in part to the perception on the part of the Court that the state imposed the tax with an intent to penalize a selected group of newspapers. In the case currently before us, however, there is no *** indication, apart from the structure of the tax itself, of any impermissible or censorial motive on the part of the legislature. We cannot resolve the case by simple citation to *Grosjean*. Instead, we must analyze the problem anew under the general principles of the First Amendment.

III

Clearly, the First Amendment does not prohibit all regulation of the press. It is beyond dispute that the States and the Federal Government can subject newspapers to generally applicable economic regulations without creating constitutional problems. See, *e.g.*, *Citizens Publishing Co. v. United States*, 394 U.S. 131, 139 (1969) (antitrust laws); *Associated Press v. NLRB*, 301 U.S. 103 (1937) (NLRA); see also *Branzburg v. Hayes*, 408 U.S. 665 (1972) (enforcement of subpoenas).

Minnesota, however, has not chosen to apply its general sales and use tax to newspapers. Instead, it has created a special tax that applies only to certain publications protected by the First Amendment. Although the State argues now that the tax on paper and ink is part of the general scheme of taxation, the use tax provision is facially discriminatory, singling out publications for treatment that is, to our knowledge, unique in Minnesota tax law.

Minnesota's treatment of publications differs from that of other enterprises in at least two important respects: it imposes a use tax that does not serve the function of protecting the sales tax, and it taxes an intermediate transaction rather than the ultimate retail sale. A use tax ordinarily serves to complement the sales tax by eliminating the incentive to make major purchases in States with lower sales taxes; it requires the resident who shops out-of-state to pay a use tax equal to the sales tax savings. Thus, in general, items exempt from the sales tax are not subject to the use tax, for, in the event of a sales tax exemption, there is no "complementary function" for a use tax to serve. But the use tax on ink and paper serves no such complementary function; it applies to all uses, whether or not the taxpayer purchased the ink and paper in-state, and it applies to items exempt from the sales tax.

Further, the ordinary rule in Minnesota, as discussed above, is to tax only the ultimate, or retail, sale rather than the use of components like ink and paper. *** Publishers, however, are taxed on their purchase of components, even though they will eventually sell their publications at retail.

By creating this special use tax, which, to our knowledge, is without parallel in the State's tax scheme, Minnesota has singled out the press for special treatment. We then must determine whether the First Amendment permits such special taxation. A tax that burdens rights protected by the First Amendment cannot stand unless the burden is necessary to achieve an overriding governmental interest. Any tax that the press must pay, of course, imposes some "burden." But, as we have observed, this Court has long upheld economic regulation of the press. The cases approving such economic regulation, however, emphasized the general applicability of the challenged regulation to all businesses, suggesting that a regulation that singled out the press might place a heavier burden of justification on the State, and we now conclude that the special problems created by differential treatment do indeed impose such a burden.

There is substantial evidence that differential taxation of the press would have troubled the Framers of the First Amendment.[6] The role of the press in mobilizing

---

6. It is true that our opinions rarely speculate on precisely how the Framers would have analyzed a given regulation of expression. In general, though, we have only limited evidence of exactly how the Framers intended the First Amendment to apply. *** Consequently, we ordinarily simply apply those general principles, requiring the government to justify any burdens on First Amendment rights by showing that they are necessary to achieve a legitimate overriding governmental interest, see note 7, *infra*. But when we do have evidence that a particular law would have offended the Framers, we have not hesitated to invalidate it on that ground alone. Prior restraints, for instance, clearly strike to the core

sentiment in favor of independence was critical to the Revolution. When the Constitution was proposed without an explicit guarantee of freedom of the press, the Antifederalists objected. Proponents of the Constitution, relying on the principle of enumerated powers, responded that such a guarantee was unnecessary because the Constitution granted Congress no power to control the press. The remarks of Richard Henry Lee are typical of the rejoinders of the Antifederalists:

> "I confess I do not see in what cases the congress can, with any pretence of right, make a law to suppress the freedom of the press; though I am not clear, that congress is restrained from laying any duties whatever on printing, and from laying duties particularly heavy on certain pieces printed."

The fears of the Antifederalists were well-founded. A power to tax differentially, as opposed to a power to tax generally, gives a government a powerful weapon against the taxpayer selected. When the State imposes a generally applicable tax, there is little cause for concern. We need not fear that a government will destroy a selected group of taxpayers by burdensome taxation if it must impose the same burden on the rest of its constituency. When the State singles out the press, though, the political constraints that prevent a legislature from passing crippling taxes of general applicability are weakened, and the threat of burdensome taxes becomes acute. ***

Further, differential treatment, unless justified by some special characteristic of the press, suggests that the goal of the regulation is not unrelated to suppression of expression, and such a goal is presumptively unconstitutional. Differential taxation of the press, then, places such a burden on the interests protected by the First Amendment that we cannot countenance such treatment unless the State asserts a counterbalancing interest of compelling importance that it cannot achieve without differential taxation.[7]

IV

Addressing the concern with differential treatment, Minnesota invites us to look beyond the form of the tax to its substance. The tax is, according to the State, merely a substitute for the sales tax, which, as a generally applicable tax, would be constitutional as applied to the press. There are two fatal flaws in this reasoning. First, the State has offered no explanation of why it chose to use a substitute for the sales

---

of the Framers' concerns, leading this Court to treat them as particularly suspect.

7. JUSTICE REHNQUIST's dissent analyzes this case solely as a problem of equal protection, applying the familiar tiers of scrutiny. We, however, view the problem as one arising directly under the First Amendment, for, as our discussion shows, the Framers perceived singling out the press for taxation as a means of abridging the freedom of the press, see note 6, *supra*. The appropriate method of analysis thus is to balance the burden implicit in singling out the press against the interest asserted by the State. Under a long line of precedent, the regulation can survive only if the governmental interest outweighs the burden and cannot be achieved by means that do not infringe First Amendment rights as significantly.

tax rather than the sales tax itself. The court below speculated that the State might have been concerned that collection of a tax on such small transactions would be impractical. That suggestion is unpersuasive, for sales of other low-priced goods are not exempt, see n. 1, *supra.*[10] If the real goal of this tax is to duplicate the sales tax, it is difficult to see why the State did not achieve that goal by the obvious and effective expedient of applying the sales tax.

Further, even assuming that the legislature did have valid reasons for substituting another tax for the sales tax, we are not persuaded that this tax does serve as a substitute. The State asserts that this scheme actually *favors* the press over other businesses, because the same rate of tax is applied, but, for the press, the rate applies to the cost of components rather than to the sales price. We would be hesitant to fashion a rule that automatically allowed the State to single out the press for a different method of taxation as long as the effective burden was no different from that on other taxpayers or the burden on the press was lighter than that on other businesses. One reason for this reluctance is that the very selection of the press for special treatment threatens the press not only with the current *differential* treatment, but with the possibility of subsequent differentially *more burdensome* treatment. ***

A second reason to avoid the proposed rule is that courts as institutions are poorly equipped to evaluate with precision the relative burdens of various methods of taxation. [T]he possibility of error inherent in the proposed rule poses too great a threat to concerns at the heart of the First Amendment, and we cannot tolerate that possibility.[13] Minnesota, therefore, has offered no adequate justification for the special treatment of newspapers.[14]

---

10. JUSTICE REHNQUIST's dissent explains that collecting sales taxes on newspapers entails special problems because of the unusual marketing practices for newspapers—sales from vending machines and at newstands, for instance. The dissent does not, however, explain why the State cannot resolve these problems by using the same methods used for items like chewing gum and candy, marketed in these same unusual ways and subject to the sales tax, see Minn.Stat. § 297A.01(3)(c)(vi), (viii) (defining the sale of food from vending machines as a sale); see also § 297A.04 (dealing with vending machine operators). ***

13. If a State employed the same *method* of taxation but applied a lower rate to the press, so that there could be no doubt that the legislature was not singling out the press to bear a more burdensome tax, we would, of course, be in a position to evaluate the relative burdens. *** Thus, our decision does not, as the dissent suggests, require Minnesota to impose a greater tax burden on publications.

14. Disparaging our concern with the complexities of economic proof, JUSTICE REHNQUIST's dissent undertakes to calculate a hypothetical sales tax liability for Star Tribune for the years 1974 and 1975. That undertaking, we think, illustrates some of the problems that inhere in any such inquiry, see generally R. Musgrave and P. Musgrave, Public Finance in Theory and Practice 461 (2d ed. 1976) (detailing some of the complexities of calculating the burden of a tax). *** Since newspapers receive a substantial portion of their revenues from advertising, see generally Newsprint Information Committee, Newspaper and Newsprint Facts at a Glance 12 (24th ed. 1982), it is not necessarily true even for profitable newspapers that the price of the finished product will exceed the cost of inputs. Consequently, it is not necessary that a tax imposed on components is less burdensome than a tax at the

V

Minnesota's ink and paper tax violates the First Amendment not only because it singles out the press, but also because it targets a small group of newspapers. The effect of the $100,000 exemption enacted in 1974 is that only a handful of publishers pay any tax at all, and even fewer pay any significant amount of tax. The State explains this exemption as part of a policy favoring an "equitable" tax system, although there are no comparable exemptions for small enterprises outside the press. *** Whatever the motive of the legislature in this case, we think that recognizing a power in the State not only to single out the press but also to tailor the tax so that it singles out a few members of the press presents such a potential for abuse that no interest suggested by Minnesota can justify the scheme. *** The current system, it explains, promotes equity because it places the burden on large publications that impose more social costs than do smaller publications and that are more likely to be able to bear the burden of the tax. Even if we were willing to accept the premise that large businesses are more profitable and therefore better able to bear the burden of the tax, the State's commitment to this "equity" is questionable, for the concern has not led the State to grant benefits to small businesses in general.[15] And when the exemption selects such a narrowly defined group to bear the full burden of the tax, the tax begins to resemble more a penalty for a few of the largest newspapers than an attempt to favor struggling smaller enterprises.

VI

We need not and do not impugn the motives of the Minnesota legislature in passing the ink and paper tax. Illicit legislative intent is not the sine qua non of a violation of the First Amendment. *** A tax that singles out the press, or that targets individual publications within the press, places a heavy burden on the State to justify its action. Since Minnesota has offered no satisfactory justification for its tax on the use of ink and paper, the tax violates the First Amendment, and the judgment below is [r]eversed.

JUSTICE WHITE, concurring in part and dissenting in part.

---

same rate imposed on the price of the product. ***

Second, if, as the dissent assumes elsewhere, the sales tax increases the price, that price increase presumably will cause a decrease in demand. The decrease in demand may lead to lower total revenues and, therefore, to a lower total sales tax burden than that calculated by the dissent. See generally P. Samuelson, Economics 381-383, 389-390 (10th ed. 1976); R. Musgrave and P. Musgrave, Public Finance in Theory and Practice 21 (3d ed. 1980) ("[I]t is necessary, in designing fiscal policies, to allow for how the private setor will respond."). The dissent's calculations, then, can only be characterized as hypothetical. Taking the chance that these calculations or others like them are erroneous is a risk that the First Amendment forbids.

15. Cf. *Mabee v. White Plains Publishing Co.*, 327 U.S. 178, 183, 184 (1946) (upholding exemption from Fair Labor Standards Act of small weekly and semi-weekly newspapers where the purpose of the exemption "was to put those papers more on a parity with other small town enterprises.")

This case is not difficult. The exemption for the first $100,000 of paper and ink limits the burden of the Minnesota tax to only a few papers. This feature alone is sufficient reason to invalidate the Minnesota tax and reverse the judgment of the Minnesota Supreme Court. The Court recognizes that Minnesota's tax violates the First Amendment for this reason, and I subscribe to Part V of the Court's opinion and concur in the judgment.

JUSTICE REHNQUIST, dissenting.

I agree with the Court that the First Amendment does not per se prevent the State of Minnesota from regulating the press even though such regulation imposes an economic burden. I further agree with the Court that application of general sales and use taxes to the press would be sanctioned under this line of cases. The Court recognizes in several parts of its opinion that the State of Minnesota could avoid constitutional problems by imposing on newspapers the 4% sales tax that it imposes on other retailers.

The record reveals that in 1974 the Minneapolis Star & Tribune had an average daily circulation of 489,345 copies. The Sunday circulation for 1974 was 640,756. Had a 4% sales tax been imposed, the Minneapolis Star & Tribune would have been liable for $1,859,950 in 1974. *** [H]ad the sales tax been imposed, as the Court agrees would have been permissible, the Minneapolis Star & Tribune's liability for 1974 and 1975 would have been $3,685,092.

The record further indicates that the Minneapolis Star & Tribune paid $608,634 in use taxes in 1974 and $636,113 in 1975—a total liability of $1,244,747. We need no expert testimony from modern day Euclids or Einsteins to determine that the $1,224,747 paid in use taxes is significantly less burdensome than the $3,685,092 that could have been levied by a sales tax. A fortiori, the Minnesota taxing scheme which singles out newspapers for "differential treatment" has benefitted, not burdened, the "freedom of speech, [and] of the press." ***

Wisely not relying solely on its inability to weigh the burdens of the Minnesota tax scheme, the Court also says that even if the resultant burden on the press is lighter than on others

> "the very selection of the press for special treatment threatens the press not only with the current *differential* treatment, but with the possibility of subsequent differentially *more burdensome* treatment. Thus, even without actually imposing an extra burden on the press, the government might be able to achieve censorial effects, for '[t]he threat of sanctions may deter [the] exercise of [First Amendment] rights almost as potently as the actual application of sanctions.'"

Surely the Court does not mean what it seems to say. *** [T]he Court itself intimates that if the State had employed "the same *method* of taxation but applied a lower *rate* to the press, so that there could be no doubt that the legislature was not singling out the press to bear a more burdensome tax" the taxing scheme would be constitutionally permissible. This obviously has the same potential for "the threat of sanctions," because the legislature could at any time raise the taxes to the higher rate. Likewise, the newspapers' absolute exemption from the sales tax, which the Court acknowledges is used by many other States, would be subject to the same attack; the exemption could be taken away.

The Court finds in very summary fashion that the exemption newspapers receive for the first $100,000 of ink and paper used also violates the First Amendment because the result is that only a few of the newspapers actually pay a use tax. I cannot agree. As explained by the Minnesota Supreme Court, the exemption is in effect a $4,000 credit which benefits all newspapers. Minneapolis Star & Tribune was benefitted to the amount of *** $4,000 each year for its morning paper and $4,000 each year for its evening paper. Absent any improper motive on the part of the Minnesota legislature in drawing the limits of this exemption, it cannot be construed as violating the First Amendment. *** There is no reason to conclude that the State, in drafting the $4,000 credit, acted other than reasonably and rationally to fit its sales and use tax scheme to its own local needs and usages.

To collect from newspapers their fair share of taxes under the sales and use tax scheme and at the same time avoid abridging the freedoms of speech and press, the Court holds today that Minnesota must subject newspapers to millions of additional dollars in sales tax liability. Certainly this is a hollow victory for the newspapers and I seriously doubt the Court's conclusion that this result would have been intended by the "Framers of the First Amendment."

For the reasons set forth above, I would affirm the judgment of the Minnesota Supreme Court.

ARKANSAS WRITERS' PROJECT, INC. v. RAGLAND

481 U.S. 221 (1987)

JUSTICE MARSHALL delivered the opinion of the Court.

The question presented in this case is whether a state sales tax scheme that taxes general interest magazines, but exempts newspapers and religious, professional, trade, and sports journals, violates the First Amendment's guarantee of freedom of the press.

I

Since 1935, Arkansas has imposed a tax on receipts from sales of tangible personal property. The rate of tax is currently four percent of gross receipts. Numerous items are exempt from the state sales tax, however. These include "[g]ross receipts or gross proceeds derived from the sale of newspapers," (newspaper exemption), and "religious, professional, trade and sports journals and/or publications printed and published within this State *** when sold through regular subscriptions."

Appellant Arkansas Writers' Project, Inc. publishes Arkansas Times, a general interest monthly magazine with a circulation of approximately 28,000. The magazine includes articles on a variety of subjects, including religion and sports. It is printed and published in Arkansas, and is sold through mail subscriptions, coin-operated stands, and over-the-counter sales. ***

The Arkansas Supreme Court construed § 84-1904(j) as creating a single exemption and held that, in order to qualify for this exemption, a magazine had to be a "religious, professional, trade, or sports periodical." *** As to appellant's First Amendment objections, the court noted that this Court has held that "the owners of newspapers are not immune from any of the 'ordinary forms of taxation' for support of the government." In contrast to *Minneapolis Star* and *Grosjean*, the Arkansas Supreme Court concluded that the *Arkansas* sales tax was a permissible "ordinary form of taxation."

We noted probable jurisdiction, and we now reverse.

III

***

On the facts of this case, the fundamental question is not whether the tax singles out the press as a whole, but whether it targets a small group within the press. While we indicated in *Minneapolis Star* that a genuinely nondiscriminatory tax on the receipts of newspapers would be constitutionally permissible, the Arkansas sales tax cannot be characterized as nondiscriminatory, because it is not evenly applied to all magazines. To the contrary, the magazine exemption means that only a few Arkansas magazines pay any sales tax;[4] in that respect, it operates in much the same way as did the $100,000 exemption to the Minnesota use tax. Because the Arkansas sales tax scheme treats some magazines less favorably than others, it suffers from the second type of discrimination identified in *Minneapolis Star*.

Indeed, this case involves a more disturbing use of selective taxation than *Minneapolis Star*, because the basis on which Arkansas differentiates between magazines is particularly repugnant to First Amendment principles: a magazine's tax status depends entirely on its *content*. ***

If articles in Arkansas Times were uniformly devoted to religion or sports, the magaziner would be exempt from the sales tax under § 84-1904(j). However, because the articles deal with a variety of subjects (sometimes including religion and sports), the Commissioner has determined that the magazine's sales may be taxed. *** Arkansas' system of selective taxation does not evade the strictures of the First Amendment merely because it does not burden the expression of particular views by specific magazines. ***

---

4. Appellant maintains that Arkansas Times is the only Arkansas publication that pays sales tax. The Commissioner contends that there are two periodicals, in addition to Arkansas Times, that pay tax. Whether there are three Arkansas magazines paying tax or only one, the burden of the tax clearly falls on a limited group of publishers.

Nor are the requirements of the First Amendment avoided by the fact that Arkansas grants an exemption to other members of the media that might publish discussions of the various subjects contained in Arkansas Times. For example, exempting newspapers from the tax, see § 84-1904(f), does not change the fact that the State discriminates in determining the tax status of *magazines* published in Arkansas. ***

Arkansas faces a heavy burden in attempting to defend its content-based approach to taxation of magazines. In order to justify such differential taxation, the State must show that its regulation is necessary to serve a compelling state interest and is narrowly drawn to achieve that end. See *Minneapolis Star*, 460 U.S., at 591-592.

The Commissioner asserts the State's general interest in raising revenue. While we have recognized that this interest is an important one, it does not explain selective imposition of the sales tax on some magazines and not others, based solely on their content.

The Commissioner also suggests that the exemption of religious, professional, trade, and sports journals was intended to encourage "fledgling" publishers, who have only limited audiences and therefore do not have access to the same volume of advertising revenues as general interest magazines such as Arkansas Times. Even assuming that an interest in encouraging fledgling publications might be a compelling one, we do not find the exemption in § 84-1904(j) of religious, professional, trade, and sports journals narrowly tailored to achieve that end. To the contrary, the exemption is both overinclusive and underinclusive. The types of magazines enumerated in §84- 1904(j) are exempt, regardless of whether they are "fledgling"; even the most lucrative and well-established religious, professional, trade, and sports journals do not pay sales tax. By contrast, struggling general interest magazines and struggling specialty magazines on subjects other than those specified in § 84-1904(j) are ineligible for favorable tax treatment.

Appellant [also] argues that the Arkansas tax scheme violates the First Amendment because it exempts all newspapers from the tax, but only some magazines. *** Because we hold today that the State's selective application of its sales tax to magazines is unconstitutional and therefore invalid, our ruling eliminates the differential treatment of newspapers and magazines. Accordingly, we need not decide whether a distinction between different types of periodicals presents an additional basis for invalidating the sales tax, as applied to the press. *** [W]e reverse the judgment of the Arkansas Supreme Court and remand for proceedings not inconsistent with this opinion.

JUSTICE STEVENS, concurring in the judgment. [Omitted.]

JUSTICE SCALIA, with whom THE CHIEF JUSTICE joins, dissenting.

*** I dissent from today's decision because it provides no rational basis for distinguishing the subsidy scheme here under challenge from many others that are common and unquestionably lawful. It thereby introduces into First Amendment law an element of arbitrariness that ultimately erodes rather than fosters the important freedoms at issue. ***

Here, as in the Court's earlier decision in *Minneapolis Star & Tribune Co. v. Minnesota Comm'r of Revenue*, 460 U.S. 575 (1983), application of the "strict scrutiny" test rests upon the premise that for First Amendment purposes denial of exemption from taxation is equivalent to regulation. That premise is demonstrably erroneous and cannot be consistently applied. Our opinions have long recognized—in First Amendment contexts as elsewhere—the reality that tax exemptions, credits, and deductions are "a form of subsidy that is administered through the tax system," and the general rule that "a legislature's decision not to subsidize the exercise of a fundamental right does not infringe the right, and thus is not subject to strict scrutiny." *Regan v. Taxation With Representation of Washington*, 461 U.S. 540, 544, 549 (1983) (upholding denial of tax exemption for organization engaged in lobbying even though veterans' organizations received exemption regardless of lobbying activities).

The reason that denial of participation in a tax exemption or other subsidy scheme does not necessarily "infringe" a fundamental right is that—unlike direct restriction or prohibition—such a denial does not, as a general rule, have any significant coercive effect. ***

Perhaps a more stringent, prophylactic rule is appropriate, and can consistently be applied, when the subsidy pertains to the expression of a particular viewpoint on a matter of political concern—a tax exemption, for example, that is expressly available only to publications that take a particular point of view on a controversial issue of foreign policy. Political speech has been accorded special protection elsewhere. There is no need, however, and it is realistically quite impossible, to extend to all speech the same degree of protection against exclusion from a subsidy that one might think appropriate for opposing shades of political expression.

By seeking to do so, the majority casts doubt upon a wide variety of tax preferences and subsidies that draw distinctions based upon subject matter. The United States Postal Service, for example, grants a special bulk rate to written material disseminated by certain nonprofit organizations—religious, educational, scientific, philanthropic, agricultural, labor, veterans', and fraternal organizations. See Domestic Mail Manual § 623 (1985). Must this preference be justified by a "compelling governmental need" because a nonprofit organization devoted to some other purpose— dissemination of information about boxing, for example--does not receive the special rate? The Kennedy Center, which is subsidized by the Federal Government in the amount of up to $23 million per year, is authorized by statute to "present classical and contemporary music, opera, drama, dance, and poetry." Is this subsidy subject to strict scrutiny because other kinds of expressive activity, such as learned lectures and political speeches, are excluded? ***

Because there is no principled basis to distinguish the subsidization of speech in these areas—which we would surely uphold—from the subsidization that we strike down here, our decision today places the granting or denial of protection within our own idiosyncratic discretion. In my view, that threatens First Amendment rights infinitely more than the tax exemption at issue. I dissent.

LEATHERS v. MEDLOCK

499 U.S. 439 (1991)

JUSTICE O'CONNOR delivered the opinion of the Court.

These consolidated cases require us to consider the constitutionality of a state sales tax that excludes or exempts certain segments of the media but not others.

I

Arkansas' Gross Receipts Act imposes a 4% tax on receipts from the sale of all tangible personal property and specified services. *** The Act expressly exempts receipts from subscription and over- the-counter newspaper sales and subscription magazine sales. In 1987, Arkansas amended the Gross Receipts Act to impose the sales tax on cable television.

Daniel L. Medlock, a cable television subscriber, and the Arkansas Cable Television Association, Inc., a trade organization composed of approximately 80 cable operators with systems throughout the State (cable petitioners), brought this class action in the Arkansas Chancery Court to challenge the extension of the sales tax to cable television services. They argued that Arkansas' sales taxation of cable services, and exemption or exclusion from the tax of newspapers, magazines, and satellite broadcast services, violated their constitutional rights under the First Amendment and under the Equal Protection Clause of the Fourteenth Amendment. ***

In 1989 Arkansas extended the sales tax to "all other distribution of television, video or radio services with or without the use of wires provided to subscribers or paying customers or users." The [Arkansas] Supreme Court rejected the claim that the tax was invalid after the passage of Act 769, holding that the Constitution does not prohibit the differential taxation of different media. The court believed, however, that the First Amendment prohibits discriminatory taxation among members of the same medium. It therefore held that Arkansas' sales tax was unconstitutional under the First Amendment for the period during which cable television, but not satellite broadcast services, were subject to the tax.

II

Cable television provides to its subscribers news, information, and entertainment. It is engaged in "speech" under the First Amendment, and is, in much of its operation, part of the "press." That it is taxed differently from other media does not by itself, however, raise First Amendment concerns. Our cases have held that a tax that discriminates among speakers is constitutionally suspect only in certain circumstances. ***

*** [In *Minneapolis Star & Tribune Co. v. Minnesota Comm'r of Revenue*,] [w]e found no evidence of impermissible legislative motive in the case apart from the structure of the tax itself. We nevertheless held the Minnesota tax unconstitutional for two reasons. ***

Beyond singling out the press, the Minnesota tax targeted a small group of newspapers—those so large that they remained subject to the tax despite its exemption for the first $100,000 of ink and paper consumed annually. The tax thus resembled a penalty for certain newspapers. *** Absent a compelling justification, the government may not exercise its taxing power to single out the press. The press plays a unique role as a check on government abuse, and a tax limited to the press raises concerns about censorship of critical information and opinion. A tax is also suspect if it targets a small group of speakers. Again, the fear is censorship of particular ideas or viewpoints. Finally, for reasons that are obvious, a tax will trigger heightened scrutiny under the First Amendment if it discriminates on the basis of the content of taxpayer speech.

The Arkansas tax at issue here presents none of these types of discrimination. The Arkansas sales tax is a tax of general applicability. It applies to receipts from the sale of all tangible personal property and a broad range of services, unless within a group of specific exemptions. *** The tax does not single out the press and does not therefore threaten to hinder the press as a watchdog of government activity. We have said repeatedly that a State may impose on the press a generally applicable tax.

Furthermore, there is no indication in this case that Arkansas has targeted cable television in a purposeful attempt to interfere with its First Amendment activities. Nor is the tax one that is structured so as to raise suspicion that it was intended to do so.

The tax is also structurally dissimilar to the tax involved in *Arkansas Writers'*. In that case, only "a few" Arkansas magazines paid the State's sales tax. *** In contrast, Act 188 extended Arkansas' sales tax uniformly to the approximately 100 cable systems then operating in the State. While none of the seven scrambled satellite broadcast services then available in Arkansas was taxed until Act 769 became effective, Arkansas' extension of its sales tax to cable television hardly resembles a "penalty for a few." *** That the Arkansas Supreme Court found cable and satellite television to be the same medium does not change this conclusion. Even if we accept this finding, the fact remains that the tax affected approximately 100 suppliers of cable television services. This is not a tax structure that resembles a penalty for particular speakers or particular ideas.

Finally, Arkansas' sales tax is not content based. There is nothing in the language of the statute that refers to the content of mass media communications. Moreover, the record establishes that cable television offers subscribers a variety of programming that presents a mixture of news, information, and entertainment. ***

Because the Arkansas sales tax presents none of the First Amendment difficulties that have led us to strike down differential taxation in the past, cable petitioners can prevail only if the Arkansas tax scheme presents "an additional basis" for concluding that the State has violated petitioners First Amendment rights. Petitioners argue that such a basis exists here: Arkansas' tax discriminates among media and, if the Arkansas Supreme Court's conclusion regarding cable and satellite television is accepted, discriminated for a time within a medium. Petitioners argue that such intermedia and intramedia discrimination, even in the absence of any evidence of intent to suppress speech or of any effect on the expression of particular ideas, violates the First Amendment. Our cases do not support such a rule.

Regan v. Taxation with Representation of Wash. stands for the proposition that a tax scheme that discriminates among speakers does not implicate the First Amendment unless it discriminates on the basis of ideas. In that case, we considered provisions of the Internal Revenue Code that discriminated between contributions to lobbying organizations. One section of the Code conferred tax-exempt status on certain nonprofit organizations that did not engage in lobbying activities. Contributions to those organizations were deductible. Another section of the Code conferred tax-exempt status on certain other nonprofit organizations that did lobby, but contributions to them were not deductible. Taxpayers contributing to veterans' organizations were, however, permitted to deduct their contributions regardless of those organizations' lobbying activities.

The tax distinction between these lobbying organizations did not trigger heightened scrutiny under the First Amendment. We explained that a legislature is not required to subsidize First Amendment rights through a tax exemption or tax deduction.[3] ***

That a differential burden on speakers is insufficient by itself to raise First Amendment concerns is evident as well from *Mabee v. White Plains Publishing Co.*, 327 U.S. 178 (1946), and *Oklahoma Press Publishing Co. v. Walling*, 327 U.S. 186 (1946). Those cases do not involve taxation, but they do involve government action that places differential burdens on members of the press. The Fair Labor Standards Act of 1938 applies generally to newspapers as to other businesses, but it exempts from its requirements certain small papers. Publishers of larger daily newspapers argued that the differential burden thereby placed on them violates the First Amendment. The Court upheld the exemption because there was no indication that the government had singled out the press for special treatment, or that the exemption was a "'"deliberate and calculated device"'" to penalize a certain group of newspapers, *Mabee, supra*, 327 U.S., at 184, quoting *Grosjean*, 297 U.S., at 250.

3. Certain *amici* in support of cable petitioners argue that *Regan* is distinguishable from this case because the petitioners in Regan were complaining that their contributions to lobbying organizations should be tax deductible, while cable petitioners complain that sales of their services should be tax *exempt*. This is a distinction without a difference. As we explained in *Regan*, "[b]oth tax exemptions and tax deductibility are a form of subsidy that is administered through the tax system."

Taken together, *Regan*, *Mabee*, and *Oklahoma Press* establish that differential taxation of speakers, even members of the press, does not implicate the First Amendment unless the tax is directed at, or presents the danger of suppressing, particular ideas. That was the case in *Grosjean*, *Minneapolis Star*, and *Arkansas Writers'*, but it is not the case here. *** We conclude that the State's extension of its generally applicable sales tax to cable television services alone, or to cable and satellite services, while exempting the print media, does not violate the First Amendment. ***

For the foregoing reasons, the judgment of the Arkansas Supreme Court is affirmed in part and reversed in part, and the cases are remanded for further proceedings not inconsistent with this opinion.

JUSTICE MARSHALL, with whom JUSTICE BLACKMUN joins, dissenting.

This case squarely presents the question whether the State may discriminate between distinct information media, for under Arkansas' general sales tax scheme, cable operators pay a sales tax on their subscription fees that is not paid by newspaper or magazine companies on their subscription fees or by television or radio broadcasters on their advertising revenues. In my view, the principles that animate our selective-taxation cases clearly condemn this form of discrimination. ***

Because cable competes with members of the print and electronic media in the larger information market, the power to discriminate between these media triggers the central concern underlying the nondiscrimination principle: the risk of covert censorship. The nondiscrimination principle protects the press from censorship prophylactically, condemning any selective-taxation scheme that presents the "potential for abuse" by the State, *Minneapolis Star*, 460 U.S., at 592 (emphasis added), independent of any actual "evidence of an improper censorial motive," *Arkansas Writers' Project, supra*, 481 U.S., at 228; see *Minneapolis Star, supra*, 460 U.S., at 592 ("Illicit legislative intent is not the *sine qua non* of a violation of the First Amendment"). ***

Because the power selectively to tax cable operators triggers the concerns that underlie the nondiscrimination principle, the State bears the burden of demonstrating that "differential treatment" of cable television is justified by some "special characteristic" of that particular information medium or by some other "counterbalancing interest of compelling importance that [the State] cannot achieve without differential taxation." *Minneapolis Star, supra*, 460 U.S., at 585. The State has failed to make such a showing in this case. The only justification that the State asserts for taxing cable operators more heavily than newspapers, magazines, television broadcasters and radio stations is its interest in raising revenue. This interest is not sufficiently compelling to overcome the presumption of unconstitutionality under the nondiscrimination principle.

The majority dismisses the risk of governmental abuse under the Arkansas tax scheme on the ground that the number of media actors exposed to the tax is "large." ***

To start, the majority's approach provides no meaningful guidance on the inter-media scope of the nondiscrimination principle. From the majority's discussion, we can infer that three is a sufficiently "small" number of affected actors to trigger First Amendment problems and that one hundred is too "large" to do so. But the majority fails to pinpoint the magic number *between* three and one hundred actors above which discriminatory taxation can be accomplished with impunity. Would the result in this case be different if Arkansas had only 50 cable-service providers? Or 25? ***

In addition, the majority's focus on absolute numbers fails to reflect the concerns that inform the nondiscrimination principle. *** The record in this case furnishes ample support for the conclusion that the State's cable operators make unique contributions to the information market. See, *e.g.*, App. 82 (testimony of cable operator that he offers "certain religious programming" that "people demand *** because they otherwise could not have access to it"); *id.*, at 138 (cable offers Spanish-language information network); *id.*, at 150 (cable broadcast of local city council meetings). The majority offers no reason to believe that programs like these are duplicated by other media. Thus, to the extent that selective taxation makes it harder for Arkansas' 100 cable operators to compete with Arkansas' 500 newspapers, magazines, and broadcast television and radio stations, see 1 Gale Directory of Publications and Broadcast Media 67-68 (123d ed. 1991), Arkansas' discriminatory tax does "risk *** affecting only a limited range of views," and may well "distort the market for ideas" in a manner akin to direct "content- based regulation." ***

Indeed, the facts of this case highlight the potential for governmental abuse inherent in the power to discriminate among like-situated media based on their identities. *** [F]or all we know, the legislature's initial decision selectively to tax cable may have been prompted by a similar plea from traditional broadcast media to curtail competition from the emerging cable industry. If the legislature did indeed respond to such importunings, the tax would implicate government censorship as surely as if the government itself disapproved of the new competitors. *** If *Minneapolis Star, Arkansas Writers' Project,* and *Grosjean* stand for anything, it is that the "power to tax" does not include "the power to discriminate" when the press is involved. ***

Because they distort the competitive forces that animate this institution, tax differentials that fail to correspond to the social cost associated with different information media, and that are justified by nothing more than the State's desire for revenue, violate government's obligation of evenhandedness. Clearly, this is true of disproportionate taxation of cable television. Under the First Amendment, government simply has no business interfering with the process by which citizens' preferences for information formats evolve.

Today's decision unwisely discards these teachings. I dissent.

C. POLITICS, PRIVACY, LIBEL[77] AND TORT LAW

First amendment revisions of the common law and a comparison of the complexity of modern views.

> "The concept of seditious libel strikes at the very heart of democracy. Political freedom ends when government can use its powers and its courts to silence its critics. My point is not the tepid one that there should be leeway for criticism of the government. It is rather that defamation of the government is an impossible notion for a democracy. In brief, I suggest, that the presence or absence in the law of the concept of seditious libel defines the society. A society may or may not treat obscenity or contempt by publication as legal offenses without altering its basic nature. If, however, it makes seditious libel an offense, it is not a free society no matter what its other characteristics."[78]

The figure of the first amendment we have been examining in the development of free speech-free press doctrine is one of concentric circles. At its core—where the greatest protection is provided—is "political process" speech: criticism of government policy; dissent from the political status quo; direct social advocacy of alternative policies; sharply offensive attacks on prevailing conventions; denunciations of the law itself.

In the general realm of social or political advocacy, we have seen several case examples that the modern first amendment is given considerable force. The nature

---

77. "Libel" is from Latin, "libellus," the diminutive of "liber"—meaning "a book" (as in "library"—a place for books.) Generally, it is anything in print or pictures that disparages a readily identifiable person or group of persons, tending to subject them to obloquy in the community at large, or diminishing their personal standing and reputation, or subjecting them to ridicule—anything likely to cause third parties to think ill of them and on that account to draw away. Libel is the cousin of slander, from Old French "esclandre," a variant of "escandle," from Latin "scandalum," meaning scandal. (To slander a person is thus to utter something scandalous about them.) Together libel and slander comprise the core of the private law of defamation. See, e.g., cases and discussion in George C. Christie, Cases and Materials on Torts 1065-1132 (3d ed. 1997); Richard A. Epstein, Cases and Materials on Torts 1029-1115 (7th ed. 2000). See also Shakespeare (Othello, act III, sc. III (London 1622)):

Who steals my purse steals trash; 'tis something, nothing;
'Twas mine, 'tis his, and has been slave to thousands;
But he that filches from me my good name
Robs me of that which not enriches him,
And makes me poor indeed.

78. Harry Kalven, The New York Times Case: A Note on "The Central Meaning" of the First Amendment, 1964 Sup.Ct.Rev. 191, 205. See also Harry Kalven, A Worthy Tradition (1988); Alexander M. Meiklejohn, Free Speech and Its Relation to Self-Government (1948); Vincent A. Blasi, The Pathological Perspective and the First Amendment, 85 Colum.L.Rev. 449 (1985); Vincent A. Blasi, The Checking Value in First Amendment Theory, 1977 Am.B.Found.Res.J. 521; Alexander M. Meiklejohn, The First Amendment Is an Absolute, 1961 Sup.Ct.Rev. 245.

of the public interest must be highly substantial to trench upon such speech by means of prior restraints or criminal prosecutions brought by government. A certain amount of public disturbance and of unwelcome affront in public places may have to be endured (e.g., *Cohen*). A certain level of public anxiety and of possible real danger will have to be accepted as well. A wide range of ideological expression, exhortation and of advocacy—even advocacy of law-breaking and of violence—may be protected (e.g., under the *Brandenburg* test).[79] Consider Holmes' strong proposition still again:

> Only the emergency that makes it immediately dangerous to leave the correction of evil counsel to time warrants making any exception to the sweeping command, 'Congress shall make no law *** abridging the freedom of speech.' *** That at any rate is the theory of our Constitution. It is an experiment, as all life is an experiment. Every year if not every day we have to wager our salvation upon some prophecy based upon imperfect knowledge. While that experiment is part of our system I think that we should be eternally vigilant against attempts to check the expression of opinions that we loathe and believe to be fraught with death, unless they so imminently threaten immediate interference with the lawful and pressing purposes of the law that an immediate check is required to save the country.[80]

In synthesizing these twentieth century case law developments, a keen student of the first amendment also saw them in a larger sense as a synecdoche for the repudiation of "seditious libel" as a possible public offense. Liability for defamation of government (i.e. preserving confidence in government) is an "impossible notion" in a democratic country. It cannot serve as a trigger of liability for political speech,

---

79. For endorsing reviews of *Brandenburg* (as framing a strong general standard combining the case specific, judicially reviewable, clear-and-present danger requirement of Holmes-Brandeis plus the direct advocacy requirement of Hand in *The Masses*), see Lillian R. BeVier, The First Amendment and Political Speech: An Inquiry into the Substance and Limit of Principle, 30 Stan.L.Rev. 299 (1978); Gerald Gunther, Learned Hand and the Origins of Modern First Amendment Doctrine: Some Fragments of History, 27 Stan.L.Rev. 719 (1975); Frank R. Strong, Fifty Years of "Clear and Present Danger": From *Schenck* to *Brandenburg*—and Beyond, 1969 Sup.Ct.Rev. 41; Comment, *Brandenburg v. Ohio*: A Speech Test for All Seasons?, 43 U.Chi.L.Rev. 151 (1975). See also, Jed Rubenfeld, The First Ammendment's Purpose, 53 Stan. L. Rev. 767, 826-830 (2001).For criticisms, see Thomas L. Emerson, First Amendment Doctrine and the Burger Court, 68 Cal.L.Rev. 422 (1980); Hans A. Linde, "Clear and Present Danger" Reexamined: Dissonance in the *Brandenburg* Concerto, 22 Stan.L.Rev. 1163 (1970).

80. The familiar quotation is from his dissent in *Abrams*. (And recall the Brandeis dictum, in *Whitney v. California*, that even "[t]he fact that speech is likely to result in some violence or in destruction of property is not enough to justify its suppression. There must be the probability of serious injury to the State. Among free men, the deterrents ordinarily to be applied to prevent crime are education and punishment for violation of the law, not abridgement of the rights of free speech and assembly.")

Harry Kalven suggested. It is irreconcilable with a strong view of the first amendment itself. Thus the quotation *supra*, with which this subsection begins.[81]

At some general level of suitable abstraction, it is likely that nearly everyone will agree with this view—if merely because the point is kept quite abstract. The difficulty comes in the usual way, in trying to get more down to earth. We have seen this strong view of the first amendment at work in specific cases involving *prior restraints* and *criminal* statutes in a broad range of settings, to be sure, but just how far does this general notion repudiating "seditious libel" extend? Does it extend not just to the complete protection of defaming characterizations of government incidental to political and politicized speech, and not just to the expression of polemics that may—in the opinion of many—flagrantly mischaracterize government policy or totally misstate the reasons for that policy, but also to defamatory falsehoods of those involved in public service as part of government? Are all those who give up their privacy to seek public service to pay a bitter price? Are those who step into, or are drawn into, public controversy inviting their own destruction as some sort of constitutional price-to-be-paid?

Anticipating such questions as these even in his dissent in *Abrams*, Justice Holmes drew a cautionary distinction between "seditious libel"—statements about government that may not only be critical but also false-in-fact and yet cannot on that account be made the object of prosecution[82]—and cases in which "private rights" seek more ordinary *civil* protection through legal process. May the more ordinary, civil tort law of libel and of slander re-enter the picture at this point?[83]

To what extent, then, may the civil law of defamation and of privacy survive the first (and fourteenth) amendment intact?[84] The following cases—opening with *New*

81. Again, the origin of the idea is in *Abrams*, where Holmes broke from his previous views in this regard. ("I wholly disagree with the argument that the First Amendment left the common law of seditious libel in force. History seems to me against the notion. I had conceived that the United States through many years had shown its repentance for the Sedition Act of 1798, by repaying fines it imposed.")

82. (Only *false* defamatory statements about government were punishable under the Sedition Act of 1798, yet Holmes suggested that the history—of repaying fines levied under the Act—had repudiated the Sedition Act as being inconsistent with the first amendment.)

83. Zachariah Chafee, whose work strongly supported the Holmes-Brandeis view (that the first amendment did not leave "the common law as to *seditious* libel in force"), also suggested that the first amendment left the general tort law of *personal civil* libel actions unimpaired: "We can all agree that the free speech clauses do not wipe out the common law as to *** defamation of individuals." Zachariah Chafee, Free Speech in the United States 150 (1942).

84. Or, more generally, as Kalven put the question sharply: "At what point does the First Amendment no longer permit the states to afford *tort* remedies for harms [actually] caused by speech?" Harry Kalven, The Reasonable Man and the First Amendment: Hill, Butts, and Walker, 1967 Sup.Ct.Rev. 267, 278 (emphasis added).

York Times Company v. Sullivan—provide some rough guide to the Supreme Court's uneven response. The tort law of defamation has become extremely complex.[85]

NEW YORK TIMES COMPANY v. SULLIVAN
376 U.S. 254 (1964)

MR. JUSTICE BRENNAN delivered the opinion of the Court.

We are required in this case to determine for the first time the extent to which the constitutional protections for speech and press limit a State's power to award damages in a libel action brought by a public official against critics of his official conduct.

Respondent L. B. Sullivan is one of the three elected Commissioners of the City of Montgomery, Alabama. He testified that he was "Commissioner of Public Affairs and the duties are supervision of the Police Department, Fire Department, Department of Cemetery and Department of Scales." He brought this civil libel action against the four individual petitioners, who are Negroes and Alabama clergymen, and against petitioner the New York Times Company, a New York corporation which publishes the New York Times, a daily newspaper. A jury in the Circuit Court of Montgomery County awarded him damages of $500,000, the full amount claimed, against all the petitioners, and the Supreme Court of Alabama affirmed.

Respondent's complaint alleged that he had been libeled by statements in a full-page advertisement that was carried in the New York Times on March 29, 1960. Entitled "Heed Their Rising Voices," the advertisement began by stating that "As the whole world knows by now, thousands of Southern Negro students are engaged in widespread non-violent demonstrations in positive affirmation of the right to live in human dignity as guaranteed by the U.S. Constitution and the Bill of Rights." It went on to charge that "in their efforts to uphold these guarantees, they are being met by an unprecedented wave of terror by those who would deny and negate that document which the whole world looks upon as setting the pattern for modern freedom. ***" Succeeding paragraphs purported to illustrate the "wave of terror" by describing certain alleged events. The text concluded with an appeal for funds for three purposes: support of the student movement, "the struggle for the right- to-vote," and the legal defense of Dr. Martin Luther King, Jr., leader of the movement, against a perjury indictment then pending in Montgomery.

---

85. See generally Rodney A. Smolla, Law of Defamation (1989), and chart at § 3.05; Rodney A. Smolla, Let the Author Beware: The Rejuvenation of the American Law of Libel, 132 U.Pa.L.Rev. 1 (1983). For a good overall review of the complexities merely through 1972, see Joel D. Eaton, The American Law of Defamation Through Gertz v. Robert Welch, Inc. and Beyond: An Analytical Primer, 61 Va.L.Rev. 1349 (1975).

The text appeared over the names of 64 persons, many widely known for their activities in public affairs, religion, trade unions, and the performing arts. Below these names, and under a line reading "We in the south who are struggling daily for dignity and of freedom warmly endorse this appeal," appeared the names of the four individual petitioners and 16 other persons, all but two of whom were identified as clergymen in various Southern cities. The advertisement was signed at the bottom of the page by a "Committee to Defend Martin Luther King and the Struggle for Freedom in the South," and the officers of the Committee were listed.

Of the 10 paragraphs of text in the advertisement, the third and a portion of the sixth were the basis of respondent's claim of libel. They read as follows:

> "In Montgomery, Alabama, after students sang 'My Country, 'Tis of Thee' on the State Capitol steps, their leaders were expelled from school, and truckloads of police armed with shotguns and tear-gas ringed the Alabama State College Campus. When the entire student body protested to state authorities by refusing to re-register, their dining hall was padlocked in an attempt to starve them into submission."

> "Again and again the Southern violators have answered Dr. King's peaceful protests with intimidation and violence. They have bombed his home almost killing his wife and child. They have assaulted his person. They have arrested him seven times—for 'speeding,' 'loitering' and similar 'offenses.' And now they have charged him with 'perjury'—a *felony* under which they could imprison him for *ten years*. ***"

Although neither of these statements mentions respondent by name, he contended that the word "police" in the third paragraph referred to him as the Montgomery Commissioner who supervised the Police Department, so that he was being accused of "ringing" the campus with police. He further claimed that the paragraph would be read as imputing to the police, and hence to him, the padlocking of the dining hall in order to starve the students into submission. As to the sixth paragraph, he contended that since arrests are ordinarily made by the police, the statement "They have arrested [Dr. King] seven times" would read as referring to him; he further contended that the "They" who did the arresting would be equated with the "They" who committed the other described acts and with the "Southern violators." Thus, he argued, the paragraph would be read as accusing the Montgomery police, and hence him, of answering Dr. King's protests with "intimidation and violence," bombing his home, assaulting his person, and charging him with perjury. Respondent and six other Montgomery residents testified that they read some or all of the statements as referring to him in his capacity as Commissioner.

It is uncontroverted that some of the statements contained in the two paragraphs were not accurate descriptions of events which occurred in Montgomery. *** The campus dining hall was not padlocked on any occasion, and the only students who may have been barred from eating there were the few who had neither signed a pre-registration application nor requested temporary meal tickets. Although the police were deployed near the campus in large numbers on three occasions, they did not at any time "ring" the campus, and they were not called to the campus in connection with the demonstration on the State Capitol steps, as the third paragraph implied. Dr. King had not been arrested seven times, but only four; and although he claimed to have been assaulted some years earlier in connection with his arrest for loitering outside a courtroom, one of the officers who made the arrest denied that there was such an assault.

On the premise that the charges in the sixth paragraph could be read as referring to him, respondent was allowed to prove that he had not participated in the events described. ***

Respondent made no effort to prove that he suffered actual pecuniary loss as a result of the alleged libel.[3] One of his witnesses, a former employer, testified that if he had believed the statements, he doubted whether he "would want to be associated with anybody who would be a party to such things that are stated in that ad," and that he would not re-employ respondent if he believed "that he allowed the Police Department to do the things that the paper say he did." But neither this witness nor any of the others testified that he had actually believed the statements in their supposed reference to respondent.

The cost of the advertisement was approximately $4800, and it was published by the Times upon an order from a New York advertising agency acting for the signatory Committee. The agency submitted the advertisement with a letter from A. Philip Randolph, Chairman of the Committee, certifying that the persons whose names appeared on the advertisement had given their permission. Mr. Randolph was known to the Times' Advertising Acceptability Department as a responsible person, and in accepting the letter as sufficient proof of authorization it followed its established practice. There was testimony that the copy of the advertisement which accompanied the letter listed only the 64 names appearing under the text, and that the statement, "We in the south *** warmly endorse this appeal," and the list of names thereunder, which included those of the individual petitioners, were subsequently added when the first proof of the advertisement was received. Each of the individual petitioners testified that he had not authorized use of his name, and that he had been unaware of its use until receipt of respondent's demand for a retraction. The manager of the Advertising Acceptability Department testified that he had approved the advertisement for publication because he knew nothing to cause him to believe that anything in it was false, and because it bore the endorsement of "a number of people who are well known and whose reputation" he "had no reason to question." Neither he nor anyone else at the Times made an effort to confirm the accuracy of

---

3. Approximately 394 copies of the edition of the Times containing the advertisement were circulated in Alabama. Of these, about 35 copies were distributed in Montgomery County. The total circulation of the Times for that day was approximately 650,000 copies.

the advertisement, either by checking it against recent Times news stories relating to some of the described events or by any other means.

The trial judge submitted the case to the jury under instructions that the statements in the advertisement were "libelous per se" and were not privileged, so that petitioners might be held liable if the jury found that they had published the advertisement and that the statements were made "of and concerning" respondent. The jury was instructed that, because the statements were libelous*per se*, "the law *** implies legal injury from the bare fact of publication itself," "falsity and malice are presumed," "general damages need not be alleged or proved but are presumed," and "punitive damages may be awarded by the jury even though the amount of actual damages is neither found nor shown." An award of punitive damages—as distinguished from "general" damages, which are compensatory in nature—apparently requires proof of actual malice under Alabama law, and the judge charged that "mere negligence or carelessness is not evidence of actual malice or malice in fact, and does not justify an award of exemplary or punitive damages." He refused to charge, however, that the jury must be "convinced" of malice, in the sense of "actual intent" to harm or "gross negligence and recklessness," to make such an award, and he also refused to require that a verdict for respondent differentiate between compensatory and punitive damages. *** In affirming the judgment, the Supreme Court of Alabama sustained the trial judge's rulings and instructions in all respects. ***

We reverse the judgment. We hold that the rule of law applied by the Alabama courts is constitutionally deficient for failure to provide the safeguards for freedom of speech and of the press that are required by the First and Fourteenth Amendments in a libel action brought by a public official against critics of his conduct. We further hold that under the proper safeguards the evidence presented in this case is constitutionally insufficient to support the judgment for respondent.

I

We may dispose at the outset of two grounds asserted to insulate the judgment of the Alabama courts from constitutional scrutiny. The first is the proposition relied on by the State Supreme Court—that "The Fourteenth Amendment is directed against State action and not private action." That proposition has no application to this case. Although this is a civil lawsuit between private parties, the Alabama courts have applied a state rule of law which petitioners claim to impose invalid restrictions on their constitutional freedoms of speech and press. It matters not that the law has been applied in a civil action and that it is common law only, though supplemented by statute. ***

The second contention is that the constitutional guarantees of freedom of speech and of the press are inapplicable here, at least so far as the Times is concerned, because the allegedly libelous statements were published as part of a paid, "commercial" advertisement. The argument relies on Valentine v. Chrestensen, 316 U.S. 52. *** The reliance is wholly misplaced. The Court in *Chrestensen* reaffirmed the constitutional protection for "the freedom of communicating information and disseminating opinion;" its holding was based upon the factual conclusions that the handbill was "purely commercial advertising" and that the protest against official action had been added only to evade the ordinance.

The publication here was not a "commercial" advertisement in the sense in which the word was used in *Chrestensen.* It communicated information, expressed opinion, recited grievances, protested claimed abuses, and sought financial support on behalf of a movement whose existence and objectives are matters of the highest public interest and concern. *** That the Times was paid for publishing the advertisement is as immaterial in this connection as is the fact that newspapers and books are sold. [W]e hold that if the allegedly libelous statements would otherwise be constitutionally protected from the present judgment, they do not forfeit that protection because they were published in the form of a paid advertisement.

II

Under Alabama law as applied in this case, a publication is "libelous per se" if the words "tend to injure a person *** in his reputation" or to "bring [him] into public contempt"; the trial court stated that the standard was met if the words are such as to "injure him in his public office, or impute misconduct to him in his office or want of official integrity, or want of fidelity to a public trust ." Once "libel per se" has been established, the defendant has no defense as to stated facts unless he can persuade the jury that they were true in all their particulars. ***

Respondent relies heavily, as did the Alabama courts, on statements of this Court to the effect that the Constitution does not protect libelous publications. Those statements do not foreclose our inquiry here. None of the cases sustained the use of libel laws to impose sanctions upon expression critical of the official conduct of public officials. The dictum in Pennekamp v. Florida, 328 U.S. 331, 348-349, that "when the statements amount to defamation, a judge has such remedy, in damages for libel as do other public servants," implied no view as to what remedy might constitutionally be afforded to public officials. *** [L]ibel can claim no talismanic immunity from constitutional limitations. It must be measured by standards that satisfy the First Amendment.

*** [W]e consider this case against the background of a profound national commitment to the principle that debate on public issues should be uninhibited, robust, and wide-open, and that it may well include vehement, caustic and sometimes unpleasantly sharp attacks on government and public officials. *** The present advertisement, as an expression of grievance and protest on one of the major public issues of our time, would seem clearly to qualify for the constitutional protection. The question is whether it forfeits that protection by the falsity of some of its factual statements and by its alleged defamation of respondent.

Authoritative interpretations of the First Amendment guarantees have consistently refused to recognize an exception for any test of truth—whether administered by judges, juries, or administrative officials—and especially one that puts the burden of proving truth on the speaker. *** As Madison said, "Some degree of abuse is inseparable from the proper use of every thing; and in no instance is this more true than in that of the press." 4 Elliot's Debates on the Federal Constitution (1876), p. 571. In Cantwell v. Connecticut, 310 U.S. 296, 310, the Court declared:

> "In the realm of religious faith, and in that of political belief, sharp differences arise. In both fields the tenets of one man may seem the rankest error to his neighbor. To persuade others to his own point of view, the pleader, as we know, at times, resorts to exaggeration, to vilification of men who have been, or are, prominent in church or state, and even to false statement. But the people of this nation have ordained in the light of history, that, in spite of the probability of excesses and abuses, these liberties are, in the long view, essential to enlightened opinion and right conduct on the part of the citizens of a democracy."

***

Injury to official reputation affords no more warrant for repressing speech that would otherwise be free than does factual error. Where judicial officers are involved, this Court has held that concern for the dignity and reputation of the courts does not justify the punishment as criminal contempt of criticism of the judge or his decision. Bridges v. California, 314 U.S. 252. This is true even though the utterance contains "half-truths" and "misinformation." *** Such repression can be justified, if at all, only by a clear and present danger of the obstruction of justice. ***

If neither factual error nor defamatory content suffices to remove the constitutional shield from criticism of official conduct, the combination of the two elements is no less inadequate. This is the lesson to be drawn from the great controversy over the Sedition Act of 1798, 1 Stat. 596, which first crystallized a national awareness of the central meaning of the First Amendment. *** The Act allowed the defendant the defense of truth, and provided that the jury were to be judges both of the law and the facts. Despite these qualifications, the Act was vigorously condemned as unconstitutional in an attack joined in by Jefferson and Madison. ***

What a State may not constitutionally bring about by means of a criminal statute is likewise beyond the reach of its civil law of libel. The fear of damage awards under a rule such as that invoked by the Alabama courts here may be markedly more inhibiting than the fear of prosecution under a criminal statute. *** The judgment awarded in this case—without the need for any proof of actual pecuniary loss—was one thousand times greater than the maximum fine provided by the Alabama criminal statute, and one hundred times greater than that provided by the Sedition Act. And since there is no double-jeopardy limitation applicable to civil lawsuits, this is not the only judgment that may be awarded against petitioners for the same publication.

The state rule of law is not saved by its allowance of the defense of truth. *** A rule compelling the critic of official conduct to guarantee the truth of all his factual assertions—and to do so on pain of libel judgments virtually unlimited in amount —leads to a comparable "self-censorship." Allowance of the defense of truth, with the burden of proving it on the defendant, does not mean that only false speech will be deterred.[19] *** Under such a rule, would-be critics of official conduct may be deterred from voicing their criticism, even though it is believed to be true and even though it is in fact true, because of doubt whether it can be proved in court or fear of the expense of having to do so. They tend to make only statements which "steer far wider of the unlawful zone." *** The rule thus dampens the vigor and limits the variety of public debate. It is inconsistent with the First and Fourteenth Amendments.

The constitutional guarantees require, we think, a federal rule that prohibits a public official from recovering damages for a defamatory falsehood relating to his official conduct unless he proves that the statement was made with "actual malice"—that is, with knowledge that it was false or with reckless disregard of whether it was false or not. ***

Such a privilege for criticism of official conduct is appropriately analogous to the protection accorded a public official when *he* is sued for libel by a private citizen. In Barr v. Mateo, 360 U.S. 564, 575, this Court held the utterance of a federal official to be absolutely privileged if made "within the outer perimeter" of his duties. *** It would give public servants an unjustified preference over the public they serve, if critics of official conduct did not have a fair equivalent of the immunity granted to the officials themselves.

We conclude that such a privilege is required by the First and Fourteenth Amendments.

III

We hold today that the Constitution delimits a State's power to award damages for libel in actions brought by public officials against critics of their official conduct. Since this is such an action, the rule requiring proof of actual malice is applicable. While Alabama law apparently requires proof of actual malice for an award of punitive damages, where general damages are concerned malice is "presumed." Such a presumption is inconsistent with federal rule. Since the trial judge did not instruct the jury to differentiate between general and punitive damages, it may be that the verdict was wholly an award of one or the other. But it is impossible to know, in view of the general verdict returned. Because of this uncertainty, the judgment must be reversed and the case remanded.

Since respondent may seek a new trial, we deem that considerations of effective judicial administration require us to review the evidence in the present record to determine whether it could constitutionally support a judgment for respondent. *** [W]e consider that the proof presented to show actual malice lacks the convincing clarity which the constitutional standard demands, and hence that it would not

19. Even a false statement may be deemed to make a valuable contribution to public debate, since it brings about "the clearer perception and livelier impression of truth, produced by its collision with error." Mill, On Liberty (Oxford: Blackwell, 1947), at 15; see also Milton, Areopagitica, in Prose Works (Yale, 1959), Vol. II, at 561.

constitutionally sustain the judgment for respondent under the proper rule of law. The case of the individual petitioners requires little discussion. ***

As to the Times, we similarly conclude that the facts do not support a finding of malice. ***

[T]here is evidence that the Times published the advertisement without checking its accuracy against the news stories in the Times' own files. The mere presence of the stories in the files does not, of course, establish that the Times "knew" the advertisement was false, since the state of mind required for actual malice would have to be brought home to the persons in the Times' organization having responsibility for the publication of the advertisement. With respect to the failure of those persons to make the check, the record shows that they relied upon their knowledge of the good reputation of many of whose names were listed as sponsors of the advertisement, *** We think the evidence against the Times supports at most a finding of negligence in failing to discover the misstatements, and is constitutionally insufficient to show the recklessness that is required for a finding of actual malice. ***

We also think the evidence was constitutionally defective in another respect: it was incapable of supporting the jury's finding that the allegedly libelous statements were made "of and concerning" respondent. *** There was no reference to respondent in the advertisement, either by name or official position. [T]o the extent that some of the witnesses thought respondent to have been charged with ordering or approving the conduct or otherwise being personally involved in it, they based this notion not on any statements in the advertisement, and not on any evidence that he had in fact been so involved, but solely on the unsupported assumption that, because of his official position, he must have been. ***

We hold that such a proposition may not constitutionally be utilized to establish that an otherwise impersonal attack on governmental operations was a libel of an official responsible for those operations. Since it was relied on exclusively here, and there was no other evidence to connect the statements with respondent, the evidence was constitutionally insufficient to support a finding that the statements referred to respondent.

The judgment of the Supreme Court of Alabama is reversed and the case is remanded to that court for further proceedings not inconsistent with this opinion.

MR. JUSTICE BLACK, with whom MR. JUSTICE DOUGLAS joins, concurring.

*** I base my vote to reverse on the belief that the First and Fourteenth Amendments not merely "delimit" a State's power to award damages to "public officials against critics of their official conduct" but completely prohibit a State from exercising such a power. "Malice," even as defined by the Court, is an elusive, abstract concept, hard to prove and hard to disprove. The requirement that malice be proved provides at best an evanescent protection for the right critically to discuss public affairs and certainly does not measure up to the sturdy safeguard embodied in the First Amendment. Unlike the Court, therefore, I vote to reverse exclusively on the ground that the Times and the individual defendants had an absolute, unconditional constitutional right to publish in the Times advertisement their criticisms of the Montgomery agencies and officials. *** We would, I think, more faithfully interpret the First Amendment by holding that at the very least it leaves the people and the press free to criticize officials and discuss public affairs with impunity. *** An unconditional right to say what one pleases about public affairs is what I consider to be the minimum guarantee of the First Amendment.

I regret that the Court has stopped short of this holding indispensable to preserve our free press from destruction.

MR. JUSTICE GOLDBERG, with whom MR. JUSTICE DOUGLAS joins, concurring in the result.

*** In my view, the First and Fourteenth Amendments to the Constitution afford to the citizen and to the press an absolute, unconditional privilege to criticize official conduct despite the harm which may flow from excesses and abuses. ***

It may be urged that deliberately and maliciously false statements have no conceivable value as free speech. That argument, however is not responsive to the real issue presented by this case, which is whether that freedom of speech which all agree is constitutionally protected can be effectively safeguarded by a rule allowing the imposition of liability upon a jury's evaluation of the speaker's state of mind. ***

This is not to say that the Constitution protects defamatory statements directed against the private conduct of a public official or private citizen. Freedom of press and of speech insures that government will respond to the will of the people and that changes may be obtained by peaceful means. Purely private defamation has little to do with the political ends of a self-governing society. The imposition of liability for private defamation does not abridge the freedom of public speech or any other freedom protected by the First Amendment.[4]

For these reasons, I strongly believe that the Constitution accords citizens and press an unconditional freedom to criticize official conduct. It necessarily follows that in a case such as this, where all agree that the allegedly defamatory statements related to official conduct, the judgments for libel cannot constitutionally be sustained.

---

4. In most cases, as in the case at bar, there will be little difficulty in distinguishing defamatory speech relating to private conduct from that relating to official conduct. I recognize, of course, that there will be a gray area. The difficulties of applying a public-private standard are, however, certainly a different genre from those attending the differentiation between a malicious and nonmalicious state of mind. If the constitutional standard is to be shaped by a concept of malice, the speaker takes the risk not only that the jury will inaccurately determine his state of mind but also that the jury will fail properly to apply the constitutional standard set by the elusive concept of malice. ***

NOTE

In *New York Times v. Sullivan*,[86] doubtless the noteworthy point is the direct comparison the Court drew between a particular category of civil libel actions and the general category of classic seditious libel actions, such that the two should be treated alike. A particular private libel action—one "brought by public officials against critics of their official conduct," carries with it virtually all the dampening effects historically associated with criminal seditious libel prosecutions—prosecutions also based on charges of false claims, albeit false claims about the government itself. The chilling prospect of having to answer in damages to the first kind of case (albeit a case privately brought in a civil proceeding by a public official at his or her own expense) is, by the Court, likened to the chilling prospect of having to answer to a seditious libel prosecution similarly based on a claim of false facts. Accordingly, if nonreckless factual inaccuracy would not sustain a successful prosecution of the latter sort despite the public damage such as it may be from the broadcast of the false statements thus made, then such nonreckless factual inaccuracy cannot be an occasion to be made to answer in a private civil action brought by the public official, albeit an action brought separately as a private, civil action for libel, for damages, in tort. The correction of error in each instance must rest with such resources of countervailing speech as the government (in the one case) and the public official (in the other case) can command, absent "malice."[87] Insofar as that effort may not succeed in correcting the error, the residue of loss is to be treated by the courts as *damnum absque injuria*. The imperatives of the first amendment are said to require no less.[88]

---

86. See Anthony Lewis, Make No Law: The Sullivan Case and the First Amendment (1991). See also Garrison v. Louisiana, 379 U.S. 64 (1964) (defamation of state court judges by local prosecutor protected by *Sullivan* from criminal defamation prosecution absent "malice" as defined in *Sullivan*).

87. "Malice" is defined specially as a minimum level of scienter: proof by evidence of convincing clarity that the statements were not merely false in fact but made under circumstances demonstrating a reckless disregard and indifference to truth or falsity—"that the defendant in fact entertained serious doubts as to the truth of his publication." St. Amant v. Thompson, 390 U.S. 727, 731 (1968). It does not go to motive such as profit or self-interest in office, etc.; this does not satisfy the *Sullivan* standard. See also Hustler Magazine v. Falwell, 485 U.S. 46 (1988); Beckley Newspapers Corp. v. Hanks, 389 U.S. 81, 82 (1967).

88. Is it arguable, however, that the first amendment should not be interpreted in this manner, at least not insofar as the plaintiff may not seek damages *but only correction or retraction* of the false statements? Cf. a modified libel remedy furnished by state law that (a) does not require proof of "malice" to compel a published retraction but (b) disallows money damages absent proof of malice. Wherein is the undue "chilling effect" on the publisher obliged simply to correct the original error by court order, after a full adversary hearing in which the plaintiff has shown the statements made were untrue? Even supposing the "government" as such might not be deemed entitled to any such remedy, why not the injured person, pursuant to a personal civil suit, recovering merely his costs and attorneys' fees? Cf. Franklyn Saul Haiman, Speech and Law in a Free Society 48-51 (1981); Reforming Libel Law (John Soloski & Randall P. Bezanson eds., 1992); David A. Anderson, Is Libel Law Worth Reforming?, 140 U.Pa.L.Rev. 487 (1991); Marc A. Franklin, Good Names and Bad Law: A Critique of Libel Law and a Proposal, 18 U.S.F.L.Rev. 1, 10 (1983); Stanley Ingber, Defamation: A Conflict

On the other hand, the more removed a private party may be from having any effective means at his disposal to counter what has been falsely said of him, the less effective the Court's suggestion may seem to be. In that circumstance perhaps the first amendment ought not be regarded as erecting so severe a barrier to an ordinary tort action in defamation. And accordingly one might suppose that the first amendment ratio deciendi of *New York Times v. Sullivan* will not erect the same barriers against more ordinary defamation suits, i.e. those not involving public officials or their official conduct.[89] Perhaps the suggestion of concentric circles may itself be serviceable still again in describing these sorts of distinctions—of different first amendment standards in respect to different kinds of libel cases—depending upon who has brought the particular tort action, the subject of the claim, and the nature of the defendant. The case law refinements since *New York Times v. Sullivan* represent four decades of drawing the lines.

TIME, INC. v. HILL
385 U.S. 374 (1966)

MR. JUSTICE BRENNAN delivered the opinion of the Court.

The question in this case is whether appellant, publisher of Life Magazine, was denied constitutional protections of speech and press by the application by the New York courts of §§ 50-51 of the New York Civil Rights Law to award appellee damages on allegations that Life falsely reported that a new play portrayed an experience suffered by appellee and his family.

Between Reason and Decency, 65 Va.L.Rev. 785 (1979); Kathryn Dix Sowle, A Matter of Opinion: *Milkovich* Four Years Later, 3 Wm. & Mary Bill of Rights J. 467 (1994); Note, Vindication of the Reputation of a Public Official, 80 Harv.L.Rev. 1730 (1967). Aside from defense fees with which publishers might still be concerned when defending against such suits—a matter that might be addressed through fee-shifting provisions—is there a possible additional problem for publishers who might find themselves sued in a hostile forum? Note, for example, where the New York Times was sued, in the *Sullivan* case. Also consider this problem in light of Keeton v. Hustler Magazine, Inc., 465 U.S. 770 (1984) (personal jurisdiction over defendant publisher under state long arm statute sustained in private libel action; *held*, the first amendment requires no special contacts to secure personal jurisdiction over libel defendant, i.e. publisher is suable in any place in which plaintiff can meet minimum fourteenth amendment ordinary due process standards). Cf. Miami Herald Pub. Co. v. Tornillo, 418 U.S. 241 (1974).

89. So the majority reads the first amendment requirement of proof of "malice" in a libel action only in respect to "a State's power to award damages for libel in actions brought by public officials against critics of their official conduct." Even the Black-Goldberg-Douglas position that would furnish an absolute immunity for defamation "related to official conduct" offers no such immunity unless the defamation does relate to "official conduct." And, they insist, the line will not be difficult to draw. ("In most cases *** there will be little difficulty in distinguishing defamatory speech relating to private conduct from that relating to official conduct.")

The article appeared in Life in February 1955. It was entitled "True Crime Inspires Tense Play," with the subtitle, "The ordeal of a family trapped by convicts gives Broadway a new thriller, 'The Desperate Hours.'" The text of the article reads as follows:

> "Three years ago Americans all over the country read about the desperate ordeal of the James Hill family, who were held prisoners in their home outside Philadelphia by three escaped convicts. Later they read about it in Joseph Hayes's novel, *The Desperate Hours*, inspired by the family's experience. Now they can see the story re-enacted in Hayes's Broadway play based on the book, and next year will see it in his movie, which has been filmed but is being held up until the play has a chance to pay off.
>
> "The play, directed by Robert Montgomery and expertly acted, is a heart-stopping account of how a family rose to heroism in a crisis. LIFE photographed the play during its Philadelphia tryout, transported some of the actors to the actual house where the Hills were besieged. On the next page scenes from the play are re-enacted on the site of the crime."

The pictures on the ensuing two pages included an enactment of the son being "roughed up" by one of the convicts, entitled "brutish convict," a picture of the daughter biting the hand of a convict to make him drop a gun, entitled "daring daughter," and one of the father throwing his gun through the door after a "brave try" to save his family is foiled.

The James Hill referred to in the article is the appellee. He and his wife and five children involuntarily became the subjects of a front-page news story after being held hostage by three escaped convicts in their suburban, Whitemarsh, Pennsylvania, home for 19 hours on September 11-12, 1952. The family was released unharmed. In an interview with newsmen after the convicts departed, appellee stressed that the convicts had treated the family courteously, had not molested them, and had not been at all violent. The convicts were thereafter apprehended in a widely publicized encounter with the police which resulted in the killing of two of the convicts. Shortly thereafter the family moved to Connecticut. The appellee discouraged all efforts to keep them in the public spotlight through magazine articles or appearances on television.

In the spring of 1953, Joseph Hayes' novel, The Desperate Hours, was published. The story depicted the experience of a family of four held hostage by three escaped convicts in the family's suburban home. But, unlike Hill's experience, the family of the story suffer violence at the hands of the convicts; the father and son are beaten and the daughter subjected to a verbal sexual insult.

The book was made into a play, also entitled The Desperate Hours, and it is Life's article about the play which is the subject of appellee's action. The complaint sought damages under §§ 50-51 on allegations that the Life article was intended to, and did, give the impression that the play mirrored the Hill family's experience, which, to the knowledge of defendant " *** was false and untrue." Appellant's defense was that the article was "a subject of legitimate news interest," "a subject of general interest and of value and concern to the public" at the time of publication, and that it was "published in good faith without any malice whatsoever ***." A motion to dismiss the complaint for substantially these reasons was made at the close of the case and was denied by the trial judge on the ground that the proofs presented a jury question as to the truth of the article.

The jury awarded appellee $50,000 compensatory and $25,000 punitive damages. On appeal the Appellate Division of the Supreme Court ordered a new trial as to damages but sustained the jury verdict of liability. The court said as to liability:

> "Although the play was fictionalized, *Life*'s article portrayed it as a re- enactment of the Hills' experience. It is an inescapable conclusion that this was done to advertise and attract further attention to the play, and to increase present and future magazine circulation as well. It is evident that the article cannot be characterized as a mere dissemination of news, nor even an effort to supply legitimate newsworthy information in which the public had, or might have a proper interest."

At the new trial on damages, a jury was waived and the court awarded $30,000 compensatory damages without punitive damages.

*** We reverse and remand the case to the Court of Appeals for further proceedings not inconsistent with this opinion.

Since the reargument, we have had the advantage of an opinion of the Court of Appeals of New York which has materially aided us in our understanding of that court's construction of the statute. *** The statute was enacted in 1903 following the decision of the Court of Appeals in 1902 in Roberson v. Rochester Folding Box Co., 171 N.Y. 538, 64 N.E. 442. *Roberson* was an action against defendants for adorning their flour bags with plaintiff's picture without her consent. It was grounded upon an alleged invasion of a "right of privacy," defined by the Court of Appeals to be "the claim that a man has the right to pass through this world, if he wills, without having his picture published *** or his eccentricities commented upon either in handbills, circulars, catalogues, periodicals or newspapers." The Court of Appeals traced the theory to the celebrated article of Warren and Brandeis, entitled The Right to Privacy, published in 1890. 4 Harv. L. Rev. 193. The Court of Appeals, however, denied the existence of such a right at common law but observed that "[t]he legislative body could very well interfere and arbitrarily provide that no one should be permitted for his own selfish purpose to use the picture or the name of another for advertising purposes without his consent." The legislature enacted §§ 50-51 in response to that observation.

Although "Right of Privacy" is the caption of §§ 50-51, the term nowhere appears in the text of the statute itself. The text of the statute appears to proscribe only conduct of the kind involved in Roberson, that is, the appropriation and use in advertising or to promote the sale of goods, of another's name, portrait or picture without his consent. An application of that limited scope would present different questions of violation of the constitutional protections for speech and press.

The New York courts have, however, construed the statute to operate much more broadly. In *Spahn* the Court of Appeals stated that "Over the years since the statute's enactment in 1903, its social desirability and remedial nature have led to its being given a liberal construction consonant with its over-all purpose." 221 N.E. 2d, at 544. Specifically, it has been held in some circumstances to authorize a remedy against the press and other communications media which publish the names, pictures, or portraits of people without their consent. Reflecting the fact, however, that such applications may raise serious questions of conflict with the constitutional protections for speech and press, decisions under the statute have tended to limit the statute's application.

*** [I]t is particularly relevant that the Court of Appeals made crystal clear in the *Spahn* opinion that truth is a complete defense in actions under the statute based upon reports of newsworthy people or events. ***

If this is meant to imply that proof of knowing or reckless falsity is not essential to a constitutional application of the statute in these cases, we disagree with the Court of Appeals. We hold that the constitutional protections for speech and press preclude the application of the New York statute to redress false reports of matters of public interest in the absence of proof that the defendant published the report with knowledge of its falsity or in reckless disregard of the truth.

The guarantees for speech and press are not the preserve of political expression or comment upon public affairs, essential as those are to healthy government. We have no doubt that the subject of the Life article, the opening of a new play linked to an actual incident, is a matter of public interest. "The line between the informing and the entertaining is too elusive for the protection of [freedom of the press]." Winters v. New York, 333 U.S. 507, 510. Erroneous statement is no less inevitable in such a case than in the case of comment upon public affairs, and in both, if innocent or merely negligent, "it must be protected if the freedoms of expression are to have the 'breathing space' that they 'need to survive.'" *New York Times Co. v. Sullivan, supra*, at 271-272. ***

We find applicable here the standard of knowing or reckless falsehood, not through blind application of *New York Times Co. v. Sullivan*, relating solely to libel actions by public officials, but only upon consideration of the factors which arise in the particular context of the application of the New York statute in cases involving private individuals. This is neither a libel action by a private individual nor a statutory action by a public official. Therefore, although the First Amendment principles pronounced in *New York Times* guide our conclusion, we reach that conclusion only by applying these principles in this discrete context. It therefore serves no purpose to distinguish the facts here from those in *New York Times*. Were this a libel action, the distinction which has been suggested between the relative opportunities of the public official and the private individual to rebut defamatory charges might be germane. And the additional state interest in the protection of the individual against damage to his reputation would be involved. Moreover, a different test might be required in a statutory action by a public official, as opposed to a libel action by a public official or a statutory action by a private individual. Different considerations might arise concerning the degree of "waiver" of the protection the State might afford. But the question whether the same standard should be applicable both to persons voluntarily and involuntarily thrust into the public limelight is not here before us.

Turning to the facts of the present case, the proofs reasonably would support either a jury finding of innocent or merely negligent misstatement by Life, or a finding that Life portrayed the play as a re-enactment of the Hill family's experience reckless of the truth or with actual knowledge that the portrayal was false. We do not think, however, that the instructions confined the jury to a verdict of liability based on a finding that the statements in the article were made with knowledge of their falsity or in reckless disregard of the truth.***

The requirement that the jury also find that the article was published "for trade purposes," as defined in the charge, cannot save the charge from constitutional infirmity. "That books, newspapers, and magazines are published and sold for profit does not prevent them from being a form of expression whose liberty is safeguarded by the First Amendment." Joseph Burstyn, Inc. v. Wilson, 343 U.S. 495, 501-502.

The judgment of the Court of Appeals is set aside and the case is remanded for further proceedings not inconsistent with this opinion.

MR. JUSTICE BLACK, with whom MR. JUSTICE DOUGLAS joins, concurring. [Omitted.]

MR. JUSTICE DOUGLAS, concurring. [Omitted.]

MR. JUSTICE HARLAN, concurring in part and dissenting in part.

While I find much with which I agree in the opinion of the Court, I am constrained to express my disagreement with its view of the proper standard of liability to be applied on remand. Were the jury on retrial to find negligent rather than, as the Court requires, reckless or knowing "fictionalization," I think that federal constitutional requirements would be met.

*** [T]here is a vast difference in the state interest in protecting individuals like Mr. Hill from irresponsibly prepared publicity and the state interest in similar protection for a public official. In *New York Times* we acknowledged public officials to be a breed from whom hardiness to exposure to charges, innuendoes, and criticisms might be demanded and who voluntarily assumed the risk of such things by entry into the public arena. But Mr. Hill came to public attention through an unfortunate circumstance not of his making rather than his voluntary actions and he can in no sense be considered to have "waived" any protection the State might justifiably afford him from irresponsible publicity. Not being inured to the vicissitudes of journalistic scrutiny such an individual is more easily injured and his means of self-defense are more limited. The public is less likely to view with normal skepticism what is written about him because it is not accustomed to seeing his name in the press and expects only a disinterested report.

The coincidence of these factors in this situation leads me to the view that a State should be free to hold the press to a duty of making a reasonable investigation of the underlying facts and limiting itself to "fair comment"[6] on the materials so gathered. Theoretically, of course, such a rule might slightly limit press discussion of matters touching individuals like Mr. Hill. But, from a pragmatic standpoint, until now the press, at least in New York, labored under the more exacting handicap of the existing New York privacy law and has certainly remained robust. ***

MR. JUSTICE FORTAS, with whom THE CHIEF JUSTICE and MR. JUSTICE CLARK join, dissenting. ***

The Court today does not repeat the ringing words of so many of its members on so many occasions in exaltation of the right of privacy. Instead, it reverses a decision under the New York "Right of Privacy" statute because of the "failure of the trial judge to instruct the jury that a verdict of liability could be predicated only on a finding of knowing or reckless falsity in the publication of the Life article." In my opinion, the jury instructions, although they were not a textbook model, satisfied this standard.

NOTE

1. The Hill family, unlike Sullivan, were assuredly not public officials. Nor were they seeking public influence or office.[90] Nor was the exaggerated portrayal of their experience in any sense part of any claim about official conduct, the actions of government, or the like. Accordingly their case may seem to be quite far removed from seditious libel and justified concerns regarding inhibitions on reportage of alleged government wrongdoing or alleged abuses by public figures or of large, well-financed private organizations wielding influence, power, or authority. Why, then,

---

6. A negligence standard has been applied in libel actions both where the underlying facts are alleged to be libelous, Layne v. Tribune Co., 146 So. 234, and where comment is the subject of the action, Clancy v. Daily News Corp., 277 N.W. 264. Similarly the press should not be constitutionally insulated from privacy actions brought by parties in the position of Mr. Hill when reasonable care has not been taken in ascertaining or communicating the underlying facts or where the publisher has not kept within the traditional boundaries of "fair comment" with relation to underlying facts and honest opinion. ***

90. Cf., e.g., Monitor Patriot Co. v. Roy, 401 U.S. 265 (1971) (*Sullivan* applied to protect newspaper charge against senatorial candidate defaming him (as having a bootlegging background), *held*, "a charge of criminal conduct, no matter how remote in time or place, can never be irrelevant to an official's or a candidate's fitness for office for purposes of the 'knowing falsehood or reckless disregard' rule of *New York Times v. Sullivan*.")

the extension of the *Sullivan* "malice" standard to this kind of case, i.e. why did the Court make it as difficult in this case as in *Sullivan*, to recover any damages at all?

2. In *Hill*, on the other hand, what *was* the harm for which the Hill family sought redress from *Life* magazine's larger-than-life references to their circumstances and actions during the time they were visited by the three convicts on the run? (a) Injury to their standing in the community (i.e. reputation)?[91] (b) The simple right not to be known *falsely,* albeit not necessarily defamingly?[92] (c) The right "to be left alone?"[93] (d) The right to bury the past?[94] A combination of (b), (c) and (d)? Granted that none of these need be dismissed as a frivolous interest, nonetheless some tension remains: how substantially can they weigh against a freedom of the press generally to report on various events in public or in private life? More fundamentally, to what extent can one frame a suitable set of highly particularized liability rules that do not also merely serve to entrench the status quo as to what shall be deemed fit to print?

3. Suppose, as a test of that problem, that New York law protected privacy very generally, even as Warren and Brandeis implied might be done; suppose that absent demonstrable newsworthy interest and public information value in the disclosure of

---

91. Consider the Court's following statements: "This is [not] a libel action brought by a private individual. *** Were this a libel action, the distinction which has been suggested between the relative opportunities of the public official and the private individual to rebut defamatory charges might be germane. And the additional state interest in the protection of the individual against damage to his reputation would be involved." (Had the story been regarded as "defamatory," i.e. as damaging to Hill's reputation, the Court thus implies that he might have recovered damages (including damages for mental suffering), without need to prove "malice in fact.") Cf. Gertz v. Robert Welch, Inc., 418 U.S. 323 (1974).

92. Cf. Cantrell v. Forest City Pub. Co., 419 U.S. 145 (1974) (reinstating jury award of compensation damages for false light privacy claim for factual exaggerations by newspaper of wife's circumstances as more pitiful than the reporter knew to be true). As illustrated by *Cantrell* and *Hill*, while false light privacy claims may be distinguishable from ordinary libel claims—the "libelous" misportrayal causes (or is presumed to cause) shunning and disapproval rather than pity, sympathy, or adulation—they have the strong common feature of misrepresentations of persons as such. Not every jurisdiction permits recovery for false light claims, however, even assuming the *Sullivan* standard can be met. See, e.g., Renwick v. News and Observer Pub. Co., 312 S.E.2d 405 (N.C. 1984). See also Harry Kalven, Privacy in Tort Law—Were Warren and Brandeis Wrong?, 31 Law & Contemp. Probs. 326 (1966); Harvey L. Zuckman, Invasion of Privacy—Some Communicative Torts Whose Time Has Gone, 47 Wash. & Lee L.Rev. 253 (1990). For a discussion of the history of the protection of opinion, see Robert D. Sack, *Protection of Opinion Under the First Amendment: Reflections on Alfred Hill, "Defamation & Privacy Under the First Amendment,"* 100 Colum. L. Rev. 294 (2000).

93. See Samuel D. Warren & Louis D. Brandeis, The Right to Privacy, 4 Harv.L.Rev. 193 (1890).

94. Cf. Briscoe v. Reader's Digest Ass'n, 483 P.2d 34 (1971) (Eleven years after the event, plaintiff was mentioned by name in a Reader's Digest review of truck hijackings; meantime he had become an exemplary citizen in a community unaware of his past. Publication brought the matter to light and to local attention—including that of his eleven year old daughter whom he had never told. Held, on demurrer, that the first amendment would not bar action for publishing in alleged reckless disregard of personal privacy, though the report was unchallenged for accuracy. The court distinguished *Time v. Hill*. But query whether one would agree.)

any person's particular activities, name, or personal address, no commercial publication might publish such information without first securing his or her consent. The exemption would of course cover a wide swath of ordinary political coverage easily inclusive of allegations of misconduct by public officials or by many private parties, including all those who are public figures with an admitted impact on public affairs. On the other hand, consider in light of such a possible law the practice of a newspaper to include the identification of crime victims (e.g., of murder, or burglary, or rape) as part of its general reporting, without securing each such person's consent. Must the newspaper be prepared to demonstrate the "newsworthy interest" and "public information value" of *each* mention, in *each* case, or face damages for failure to censor its own reports? (Who is to say that there is no such value in information of this sort?)[95]

---

95. See, e.g., Robert C. Post, The Constitutional Concept of Public Discourse: Outrageous Opinion, Democratic Deliberation, and Hustler Magazine v. Falwell, 103 Harv.L.Rev. 601, 681 (1990) ("all speech is potentially relevant to democratic self-governance ***"). See also Florida Star v. B.J.F., 491 U.S. 524 (1989) and Cox Broadcasting Corp. v. Cohn, 420 U.S. 469 (1975) (name of rape victim secured from public record, suit for damages by the named person under a state statute forbidding the practice); see also State v. Globe Comm. Corp., 648 So.2d 110 (Fla. 1994) (re Florida statute mandating criminal sanctions for identifying sex offense victim in instrument of mass communications). It is strongly argued that publication of a rape victim's name gratuitously adds to the victim's anguish, that it may further discourage what is already regarded to be an underreported crime, and that it puts the victim at further risk of harassment and humiliation, e.g., by obscene telephone calls.

It is also argued, however, that the fact of singling out rape for mandatory press censorship is itself a disservice that contributes to the status quo attitude toward rape—that it is somehow not the same as assault, attempted murder, or any other serious crime, and that state laws and press custom prohibiting its full and frank reporting are part of the problem and not any part of the answer. Suppose, moreover, a given newspaper strongly agrees with this latter view. So, consistent with the first amendment, who is to decide?

At the same time, and under just such a general statute as posited in the text, consider a newspaper which accurately identifies crime arrestees, i.e. the names of persons arrested for and charged with (but not yet either tried or convicted of crimes). How should one feel about this? Is the one (publication of alleged crime victims' names) prohibitable? Is the other (publication of the accused person's name) nonetheless all right? Why? Because there is a more legitimate public interest in knowing the one rather than the other? How so? Because the resulting harm or prejudice or anguish is manifestly greater in the one instance than in the other instance? Who says? What, then, is the difference to be, if any, in saying which may be forbidden and which not? (Cf. the Supreme Court's defense of editorial choice in Miami Herald Pub. Co. v. Tornillo, 418 U.S. 241 (1974).

Had there been no Broadway play production to which the Life magazine photo-journalism story was deemed sufficiently pertinent at the time of its publication (to render it appropriately newsworthy as part of the play's actual origin and background), *then* should the civil action in *Hill* have prevailed? Even if (changing the facts still again) it were an accurate and not a "false light" sensationalized account? Why? Because even as a wholly accurate account of what had occurred in fact, its reporting is too peripheral to "political process" values of free speech to warrant any significant constitutional protection (such as the negligent and false reporting of misconduct by public figures receives under *New York Times v. Sullivan*)? Who decides whether that is so?

Suppose there were no statutory restriction of the full and accurate reporting of crimes, and a newspaper accurately reported a particular crime. Suppose, however, the crime victim subsequently

4. Alternatively, suppose (contrary to the actual facts), that the Hill family had been negotiating with *Look* magazine, pursuant to a proposed agreement that *Look* would have exclusive rights to publish a photo-journalism story of their adventure in exchange for $10,000—an arrangement that collapsed once *Life* published its own coverage as it did. On what legal theory might the Hill family attempt to recover

---

sued the newspaper for damages after being terrorized by the culprit who learned of her name and address from reading the local newspaper. May the victim recover on a theory of negligence, i.e. that the newspaper knew or ought to have known of the risk their publication thus engendered? Will the first amendment provide defense? Some courts believe it does not. See, e.g., Hyde v. City of Columbia, 637 S.W.2d 251 (Mo.Ct.App. 1982), cert. denied sub nom. Tribune Pub. Co. v. Hyde, 459 U.S. 1226 (1983). For comments, see Douglas O. Linder, When Names Are not News, They're Negligence: Media Liability for Personal Injuries Resulting from the Publication of Accurate Information, 52 UMKC L.Rev. (1984); Note, Liability for Nonlibelous Negligent Statements: First Amendment Considerations, 93 Yale L.J. 744 (1984).

A similar issue arises when magazine publishers are sued in tort for printing ambiguous personal service advertisements (for example, a person offering to be a "gun for hire," or offering to do "dirty work") that result in a "murder for hire" (or another violent crime "for hire"). See Braun v. Soldier of Fortune Magazine, Inc., 968 F.2d 1110 (11th Cir. 1992), cert. denied, 506 U.S. 1071 (1993); Eimann v. Soldier of Fortune Magazine, Inc., 880 F.2d 830 (5th Cir. 1989), cert. denied, 493 U.S. 1024 (1990); Stephen T. Raptis, Note, Guns for Hire: Commercial Speech and Tort Liability: Making a Case for Preserving First Amendment Free Speech Rights, 97 W.Va.L.Rev. 215 (1994). *See also Rice v. Paladin Enterprises*, 128 F.3d 233 (4th Cir. 1997), *cert. denied*, 523 U.S. 1074 (1998) (commercial publisher of a book ("Hit Man"), in which the author detailed methods of how to succeed as a hired killer, held liable to relatives in wrongful death action and for civil damages for "aiding and abetting" murder of victim slain by killer who, attracted by book title and publisher's representations, followed instructions provided in the book, where publisher stipulated "it not only knew [the book's] instructions might be used by murderers, but...intended to provide assistance to murderers and would-be murderers;" dicta approving the viability of such tort claims without such a stipulation).

For a critical commentary on negligence tort actions for press and media reportage or dramatizations inspiring imitative conduct harmful to others, see John Charles Kunich, *Natural Born Copycat Killers and the Law of Shock Torts*, 78 Wash, U.L.Q. 1157, (2000); Mike Quinlan & Jim Persels, It's not My Fault, the Devil Made Me Do It: Attempting to Impose Tort Liability on Publishers, Producers, and Artists for Injuries Allegedly "Inspired" by Media Speech, 18 So.Ill.U.L.J. 417 (1994); Laura W. Brill, Note, The First Amendment and the Power of Suggestion: Protecting Negligent Speakers in Cases of Imitative Harm, 94 Colum.L.Rev. 984 (1994). *See also* Sandra Davidson, *Blood Money: When Media Expose Others to Risk of Bodily Harm*, 19 Hastings Comm./Ent. L.J. 225 (1997); David Anderson, *Torts, Speech and Contracts*, 75 Texas L.Rev. 1499, 1504-1513 (1997); Keith C. Buell, *Start Spreading the News: Why Republishing Material from "Disreputable" News Reports Must Be Constitutionally Protected*, N.Y.U. L.Rev. 96 (2000); Randall P. *Bezanson, The Developing Law of Editorial Judgment*, 78 Neb. L.Rev. 754 (1999); Loris S. Bakken, *Providing the Recipe for Destruction: Protected or Unprotected Speech*, 32 McGeorge L.Rev. 289 (2000).

$10,000 from *Life*?[96] And why, on perfectly straightforward first amendment grounds, might the action nonetheless fail?

5. Consider, as a variation on *Time, Inc. v. Hill*, a different sort of false light privacy claim, namely, a journalist's false rendering of quoted statements, presenting the plaintiff as saying words other than or different from those he or she actually used. Of course any alteration of a verbatim quote, reported as an actual quote, is a false report of the interviewee's actual words. If the journalist*consciously* made the alterations (i.e. did not merely carelessly omit a word or mistranscribe something but knowingly altered the words to put them in the form then to be quoted in the published story), is the "malice" element of*Hill* and of *Sullivan* satisfied, or must something more also be shown? If something more, then what (e.g., that the alterations were "material" or "substantial" or also were of a sort a reasonable person would also regard as representing a "substantial" rather than an "insubstantial" change)?[97]

Suppose the change were of a substantial sort (whatever that may mean), but yet not a change the reader would regard as reflecting badly on the person thus quoted (to the contrary—the altered quote is *impressive* to readers). Then may the action for defamation fail on that account? Even if it would fail as a "defamation" action,

---

96. Cf. Zacchini v. Scripps-Howard Pub. Co., 433 U.S. 562 (1977). In *Zacchini*, a freelance reporter for Scripps-Howard video-taped a fifteen second human cannonball act by the plaintiff at a commercial performance, despite the plaintiff's request that he not do so. The tape was shown with favorable comment on the nightly news. Plaintiff did not seek an injunction; rather, he sought damages for appropriation of commercial value. The Court held, five to four in an opinion by Justice White, that the first amendment did not bar the action for "unlawful appropriation of plaintiff's professional property." Cf. Campbell v. Acuff-Rose Music, Inc., 510 U.S. 569 (1994).

Acuff was a suit for copyright infringement for the substantial (and obvious) copying of Roy Orbison's "Pretty Woman" by 2-Live Crew in an unlicensed parody. Plaintiff sought an injunction plus damages (namely, all proceeds from the sales of the unlicensed original). The Court held the parody "protected fair use" under the Copyright Act, reasoning that: (a) the parody is itself original; (b) there is no possible confusion of the parody with the original; and (c) there is no claim or intimation that there was any authorization by the copyright holder; even though (d) there was substantial borrowing and imitation (as there must be, in order for a parody to be recognizable as such); and (e) the parody might undermine the market for the original (by puncturing the dignity of the original).

The case was decided solely under the fair use exception of the Copyright Act of 1976. See 17 U.S.C. § 107 (1988 ed. & Supp. IV). The Court's opinion is, nevertheless, indistinguishable from an opinion the Court might have written had the fair use provision not been deemed applicable, and had the first amendment instead applied as a limitation on copyright. See also Hustler Magazine v. Falwell, 485 U.S. 46 1 (1988) (parody as a nearly absolutely protected form of comment on public figures, groups, and institutions). See Kenneth E. Spahn, The Right of Publicity: A Matter of Privacy, Property, or Public Domain, 19 Nova L.Rev. 1013, 1038-43 (1995). For a variation in the trademark infringement and trademark dilution context, see *Mattel Inc. v. MCA Records*, 28 F. Supp. 2d 1120 (C.D. Cal. 1998) (release of song entitled "Barbie Girl" with the singers referring to Barbie as a "blond bimbo girl" who loves to party and whose "life is plastic"). See also Symposium, Cyberspace & Privacy: A New Legal Paradigm, 52 Stan. L.Rev. 987 (2000).

97. For the Supreme Court's (divided) disposition of just this question, see Masson v. New Yorker Magazine, Inc., 501 U.S. 496 (1991).

might it succeed as a "false light privacy" claim, or would this claim fail as well? What of a third possibility—plaintiff seeks damages for misappropriation of personal likeness (the falsely attributed quotes). Or consider a consumer's action (for commercial deception by the publisher for falsely representing what the person purportedly quoted actually said)?

The issues raised in these variations on *Hill* (i.e. torts *other than* defamation and persons *other than* public officials or political figures) have momentarily taken us out of the post-*Sullivan* refinements on defamation as such. To gain some surer grasp on that particular subject, however, it may be well to turn to some further defamation cases again.

GERTZ v. ROBERT WELCH, INC.

418 U.S. 323 (1974)

MR. JUSTICE POWELL delivered the opinion of the Court.

This Court has struggled for nearly a decade to define the proper accommodation between the law of defamation and the freedoms of speech and press protected by the First Amendment. With this decision we return to that effort. We granted certiorari to reconsider the extent of a publisher's constitutional privilege against liability for defamation of a private citizen.

I

In 1968 a Chicago policeman named Nuccio shot and killed a youth named Nelson. The state authorities prosecuted Nuccio for the homicide and ultimately obtained a conviction for murder in the second degree. The Nelson family retained petitioner Elmer Gertz, a reputable attorney, to represent them in civil litigation against Nuccio.

Respondent publishes American Opinion, a monthly outlet for the views of the John Birch Society. Early in the 1960s the magazine began to warn of a nationwide conspiracy to discredit local law enforcement agencies and create in their stead a national police force capable of supporting a Communist dictatorship. As part of the continuing effort to alert the public to this assumed danger, the managing editor of American Opinion commissioned an article on the murder trial of Officer Nuccio. For this purpose he engaged a regular contributor to the magazine. In March 1969 respondent published the resulting article under the title "FRAME-UP: Richard Nuccio And The War On Police." The article purports to demonstrate that the testimony against Nuccio at his criminal trial was false and that his prosecution was part of the Communist campaign against the police.

In his capacity as counsel for the Nelson family in the civil litigation, petitioner attended the coroner's inquest into the boy's death and initiated actions for damages, but he neither discussed Officer Nuccio with the press nor played any part in the crimnal proceeding. Notwithstanding petitioner's remote connection with the prosecution of Nuccio, respondent's magazine portrayed him as an architect of the "frame-up." According to the article, the police file on petitioner took "a big, Irish cop to lift." The article stated that petitioner had been an official of the "Marxist League for Industrial Democracy, originally known as the Intercollegiate Socialist Society, which has advocated the violent seizure of our government." It labeled Gertz a "Leninist" and a "Communist-fronter." It also stated that Gertz had been an officer of the National Lawyers Guild, described as a Communist organization that "probably did more than any other outfit to plan the Communist attack on the Chicago police during the 1968 Democratic Convention."

These statements contained serious inaccuracies. The implication that petitioner had a criminal record was false. Petitioner had been a member and officer of the National Lawyers Guild some 15 years earlier, but there was no evidence that he or that organization had taken any part in planning the 1968 demonstrations in Chicago. There was also no basis for the charge that petitioner was a "Leninist" or a "Communist- fronter." And he had never been a member of the "Marxist League for Industrial Democracy" or the "Intercollegiate Socialist Society."

The managing editor of American Opinion made no effort to verify or substantiate the charges against petitioner. Instead, he appended an editorial introduction stating that the author had "conducted extensive research into the Richard Nuccio Case." And he included in the article a photograph of petitioner and wrote the caption that appeared under it: "Elmer Gertz of Red Guild harasses Nuccio." Respondent placed the issue of American Opinion containing the article on sale at newsstands throughout the country and distributed reprints of the article on the streets of Chicago.

Petitioner filed a diversity action for libel in the United States District Court for the Northern District of Illinois. He claimed that the falsehoods published by respondent injured his reputation as a lawyer and a citizen. *** After answering the complaint, respondent filed a pretrial motion for summary judgment, claiming a constitutional privilege against liability for defamation. It asserted that petitioner was a public official or a public figure and that the article concerned an issue of public interest and concern. For those reasons, respondent argued, it was entitled to invoke the privilege enunciated in New York Times Co. v. Sullivan, 376 U.S. 254 (1964). ***

Following the jury verdict and on further reflection, the District Court concluded that the *New York Times* standard should govern this case even though petitioner was not a public official or public figure. It accepted respondent's contention that that privilege protected discussion of any public issue without regard to the status of a person defamed therein. Accordingly, the court entered judgment for respondent notwithstanding the jury's verdict. This conclusion anticipated the reasoning of a plurality of this Court in Rosenbloom v. Metromedia, Inc., 403 U.S. 29 (1971).

Petitioner appealed to contest the applicability of the *New York Times* standard to this case. Although the Court of Appeals for the Seventh Circuit doubted the correctness of the District Court's determination that petitioner was not a public figure, it did not overturn that finding.[3] It agreed with the District Court that respondent could assert the constitutional privilege because the article concerned a matter of public interest, citing this Court's intervening decision in *Rosenbloom v. Metromedia, Inc., supra.* The Court of Appeals read *Rosenbloom* to require application of the *New York Times* standard to any publication or broadcast about an issue of significant public interest, without regard to the position, fame, or anonymity of the person defamed, and it concluded that respondent's statements concerned such an issue. *** The Court of Appeals therefore affirmed. For the reasons stated below, we reverse. ***

III

We begin with the common ground. Under the First Amendment there is no such thing as a false idea. However pernicious an opinion may seem, we depend for its correction not on the conscience of judges and juries but on competition of other ideas.[8] But there is no constitutional value in false statements of fact. Neither the intentional lie nor the careless error materially advances society's interest in "uninhibited, robust, and wide-open" debate on public issues. New York Times v. Sullivan, 376 U.S., at 270. They belong to that category of utterances which "are no essential part of any exposition of ideas, and are of such slight social value as a step to truth that any benefit that may be derived from them is clearly outweighed by the social interest in order and morality." Chaplinsky v. New Hampshire, 315 U.S. 568, 572 (1942).

Although the erroneous statement of fact is not worthy of constitutional protection, it is nevertheless inevitable in free debate. *** Our decisions recognize that a rule of strict liability that compels a publisher or broadcaster to guarantee the accuracy of his factual assertions may lead to intolerable self- censorship. Allowing the media to avoid liability only by proving the truth of all injurious statements does not accord adequate protection to First Amendment liberties. As the Court stated in *New York Times Co. v. Sullivan, supra,* at 279: "Allowance of the defense of truth with the burden of proving it on the defendant, does not mean that only false speech will be deterred." The First Amendment requires that we protect some falsehood in order to protect speech that matters.

The need to avoid self-censorship by the news media is, however, not the only societal value at issue. *** The legitimate state interest underlying the law of libel

---

3. The court stated:

"[Petitioner's] considerable stature as a lawyer, author, lecturer, and participant in matters of public import undermine[s] the validity of the assumption that he is not a "public figure" as that term has been used by the progeny of *New York Times*. Nevertheless, for purposes of decision we make that assumption and test the availability of the claim of privilege by the subject matter of the article."

8. As Thomas Jefferson made the point in his first Inaugural Address: "If there be any among us who would wish to dissolve this Union or change its republican form, let them stand undisturbed as monuments of the safety with which error of opinion may be tolerated where reason is left free to combat it."

is the compensation of individuals for the harm inflicted on them by defamatory falsehood. We would not lightly require the State to abandon this purpose, for, as MR. JUSTICE STEWART has reminded us, the individual's right to the protection of his own good name

> "reflects no more than our basic concept of the essential dignity and worth of every human being—a concept at the root of any decent system of ordered liberty. The protection of private personality, like the protection of life itself, is left primarily to the individual States under the Ninth and Tenth Amendments. But this does not mean that the right is entitled to any less recognition by this Court as a basic of our constitutional system." Rosenblatt v. Baer, 383 U.S. 75, 92 (1966) (concurring opinion).

***

The *New York Times* standard defines the level of constitutional protection appropriate to the context of defamation of a public person. Those who, by reason of the notoriety of their achievements or the vigor and success with which they seek the public's attention, are properly classed as public figures and those who hold governmental office may recover for injury to reputation only on clear and convincing proof that the defamatory falsehood was made with knowledge of its falsity or with reckless disregard for the truth. This standard administers an extremely powerful antidote to the inducement to media self-censorship of the common-law rule of strict liability for libel and slander. And it exacts a correspondingly high price from the victims of defamatory falsehood. Plainly many deserving plaintiffs, including some intentionally subjected to injury, will be unable to surmount the barrier of the*New York Times* test. Despite this substantial abridgement of the state law right to compensation for wrongful hurt to one's reputation, the Court has concluded that the protection of the *New York Times* privilege should be available to publishers and broadcasters of defamatory falsehood concerning public officials and public figures. *** For the reasons stated below, we conclude that the state interest in compensating injury to the reputation of private individuals requires that a different rule obtain with respect to them.

Theoretically, of course, the balance between the needs of the press and the individual's claim to compensation for wrongful injury might be struck on a case-by-case basis. As Mr. Justice Harlan hypothesized, "it might seem, purely as an abstract matter, that the most utilitarian approach would be to scrutinize carefully every jury verdict in every libel case, in order to ascertain whether the final judgment leaves fully protected whatever First Amendment values transcend the legitimate state interest in protecting the particular plaintiff who prevailed." Rosenbloom v. Metromedia, Inc., 403 U.S., at 63 (footnote omitted). But this approach would lead to unpredictable results and uncertain expectations, and it could render our duty to supervise the lower courts unmanageable. Because an *ad hoc* resolution of the competing interests at stake in each particular case is not feasible, we must lay down broad rules of general application. Such rules necessarily treat alike various cases involving differences as well as similarities. Thus it is often true that not all of the considerations which justify adoption of a given rule will obtain in each particular case decided under its authority.

With that caveat we have no difficulty in distinguishing among defamation plaintiffs. The first remedy of any victim of defamation is self-help—using available opportunities to contradict the lie or correct the error and thereby to minimize its adverse impact on reputation. Public officials and public figures usually enjoy significantly greater access to the channels of effective communication and hence have a more realistic opportunity to counteract false statements than private individuals normally enjoy.[9] Private individuals are therefore more vulnerable to injury, and the state interest in protecting them is correspondingly greater.

More important than the likelihood that private individuals will lack effective opportunities for rebuttal, there is a compelling normative consideration underlying the distinction between public and private defamation plaintiffs. An individual who decides to seek governmental office must accept certain necessary consequences of that involvement in public affairs. He runs the risk of closer public scrutiny than might otherwise be the case. And society's interest in the officers of government is not strictly limited to the formal discharge of official duties. As the Court pointed out in Garrison v. Louisiana, 379 U. S., at 77, the public's interest extends to "anything which might touch on an official's fitness for office ***. Few personal attributes are more germane to fitness for office than dishonesty, malfeasance, or improper motivation, even though these characteristics may also affect the official's private character."

Those classed as public figures stand in a similar position. Hypothetically, it may be possible for someone to become a public figure through no purposeful action of his own, but the instances of truly involuntary public figures must be exceedingly rare. For the most part those who attain this status have assumed roles of especial prominence in the affairs of society. Some occupy positions of such persuasive power and influence that they are deemed public figures for all purposes. More commonly, those classed as public figures have thrust themselves to the forefront of particular public controversies in order to influence the resolution of the issues involved. In either event, they invite attention and comment.

Even if the foregoing generalities do not obtain in every instance, the communications media are entitled to act on the assumption that public officials and public figures have voluntarily exposed themselves to increased risk of injury from defamatory falsehood concerning them. No such assumption is justified with respect to a private individual. He has not accepted public office or assumed an "influential role in ordering society." Curtis Publishing Co. v. Butts, 388 U.S., at 164 (Warren, C. J.,

---

9. Of course, an opportunity for rebuttal seldom suffices to undo harm of defamatory falsehood. Indeed, the law of defamation is rooted in our experience that the truth rarely catches up with a lie. But the fact that the self-help remedy of rebuttal, standing alone, is inadequate to its task does not mean that it is irrelevant to our inquiry.

concurring in result). He has relinquished no part of his interest in the protection of his own good name, and consequently he has a more compelling call on the courts for redress of injury inflicted by defamatory falsehood. Thus, private individuals are not only more vulnerable to injury than public officials and public figures; they are also more deserving of recovery.

For those reasons we conclude that the States should retain substantial latitude in their efforts to enforce a legal remedy for defamatory falsehood injurious to the reputation of a private individual. ***

We hold that, so long as they do not impose liability without fault, the States may define for themselves the appropriate standard of liability for a publisher or broadcaster of defamatory falsehood injurious to a private individual. *** At least this conclusion obtains where as here, the substance of the defamatory statement "makes substantial danger to reputation apparent." This phrase places in perspective the conclusion we announce today. Our inquiry would involve considerations somewhat different from those discussed above if a State purported to condition civil liability on a factual misstatement whose content did not warn a reasonably prudent editor or broadcaster of its defamatory potential. Cf. Time, Inc. v. Hill, 385 U.S. 374 (1967). Such a case is not now before us, and we intimate no view as to its proper resolution.

IV

Our accommodation of the competing values at stake in defamation suits by private individuals allows the States to impose liability on the publisher or broadcaster of defamatory falsehood on a less demanding showing than that required by *New York Times*. This conclusion is not based on a belief that the considerations which prompted the adoption of the *New York Times* privilege for defamation of public officials and its extension to public figures are wholly inapplicable to the context of private individuals. Rather, we endorse this approach in recognition of the strong and legitimate state interest in compensating private individuals for injury to reputation. But this countervailing state interest extends no further than compensation for actual injury. *** It is therefore appropriate to require that state remedies for defamatory falsehood reach no farther than is necessary to protect the legitimate interest involved. It is necessary to restrict defamation plaintiffs who do not prove knowledge of falsity or reckless disregard for the truth to compensation for actual injury. [A]ctual injury is not limited to out-of-pocket loss. Indeed, the more customary types of actual harm inflicted by defamatory falsehood include impairment of reputation and standing in the community, personal humiliation, and mental anguish and suffering. Of course, juries must be limited by appropriate instructions, and all awards must be supported by competent evidence concerning the injury, although there need be no evidence which assigns an actual dollar value to the injury.

*** Like the doctrine of presumed damages, jury discretion to award punitive damages unnecessarily exacerbates the danger of media self-censorship, but, unlike the former rule, punitive damages are wholly irrelevant to the state interest that justifies a negligence standard for private defamation actions. They are not compensation for injury. Instead, they are private fines levied by civil juries to punish reprehensible conduct and to deter its future occurrence. In short, the private defamation plaintiff who establishes liability under a less demanding standard than that stated by *New York Times* may recover only such damages as are sufficient to compensate him for actual injury.

V

***

Respondent's characterization of petitioner as a public figure raises a different question. That designation may rest on either of two alternative bases. In some instances an individual may achieve such pervasive fame or notoriety that he becomes a public figure for all purposes and in all contexts. More commonly, an individual voluntarily injects himself or is drawn into a particular public controversy and thereby becomes a public figure for a limited range of issues. In either case such persons assume special prominence in the resolution of public questions.

*** We would not lightly assume that a citizen's participation in community and professional affairs rendered him a public figure for all purposes. Absent clear evidence of general fame or notoriety in the community, and pervasive involvement in the affairs of society, an individual should not be deemed a public personality for all aspects of his life. It is preferable to reduce the public-figure question to a more meaningful context by looking to the nature and extent of an individual's participation in the particular controversy giving rise to the defamation.

In this context it is plain that petitioner was not a public figure. He played a minimal role at the coroner's inquest, and his participation related solely to his representation of a private client. He took no part in the criminal prosecution of Officer Nuccio. Moreover, he never discussed either the criminal or civil litigation with the press and was never quoted as having done so. He plainly did not thrust himself into the vortex of this public issue, nor did he engage the public's attention in an attempt to influence its outcome. We are persuaded that the trial court did not err in refusing to characterize petitioner as a public figure for the purpose of this litigation.

We therefore conclude that the *New York Times* standard is inapplicable to this case and that the trial court erred in entering judgment for respondent. ***

MR. CHIEF JUSTICE BURGER, dissenting. [Omitted.]

MR. JUSTICE DOUGLAS, dissenting. [Omitted.]

MR. JUSTICE BRENNAN, dissenting.

*** I adhere to my view expressed in *Rosenbloom v. Metromedia, Inc, supra,* that we strike the proper accommodation between avoidance of media self-censorship and protection of individual reputations only when we require States to apply the New York Times Co. v. Sullivan, 376 U.S. 254 (1964), knowing-or-recklessness-falsity standard in civil libel actions concerning media reports of the involvement of private individuals in events of public or general interest.

MR. JUSTICE WHITE, dissenting.

The Court evinces a deep-seated antipathy to "liability without fault." But this catch-phrase has no talismanic significance and is almost meaningless in this context where the Court appears to be addressing those libels and slanders that are defamatory on their face and where the publisher is no doubt aware from the nature of the material that it would be inherently damaging to reputation. He publishes notwithstanding, knowing that he will inflict injury. With this knowledge, he must intend to inflict that injury, his excuse being that he is privileged to do so—that he has published the truth. But as it turns out, what he has circulated to the public is a very damaging falsehood. Is he nevertheless "faultless"? Perhaps it can be said that the mistake about his defense was made in good faith, but the fact remains that it is he who launched the publication knowing that it could ruin a reputation.

In these circumstances, the law has heretofore put the risk of falsehood on the publisher where the victim is a private citizen and no grounds of special privilege are invoked. The Court would now shift this risk to the victim, even though he has done nothing to invite the calumny, is wholly innocent of fault, and is helpless to avoid his injury. *** I find it unacceptable to distribute the risk in this manner and force the wholly innocent victim to bear the injury; for, as between the two, the defamer is the only culpable party. *** The owners of the press and the stockholders of the communications enterprises can much better bear the burden. And if they cannot, the public at large should somehow pay for what is essentially a public benefit derived at private expense.

DUN & BRADSTREET, INC. v. GREENMOSS BUILDERS, INC.
472 U.S. 749 (1985)

JUSTICE POWELL announced the judgment of the Court and delivered an opinion, in which JUSTICE REHNQUIST and JUSTICE O'CONNOR joined.

In Gertz v. Robert Welch, Inc., 418 U.S. 323 (1974), we held that the First Amendment restricted damages that a private individual could obtain from a publisher for a libel that involved a matter of public concern. More specifically, we held that in these circumstances the First Amendment prohibited awards of presumed and punitive damages for false and defamatory statements unless the plaintiff shows "actual malice," that is, knowledge of falsity or reckless disregard for the truth. The question presented in this case is whether this rule of *Gertz* applies when the false and defamatory statements do not involve matters of public concern.

I

Petitioner Dun & Bradstreet, a credit reporting agency, provides subscribers with financial and related information about businesses. All the information is confidential; under the terms of the subscription agreement the subscribers may not reveal it to anyone else. On July 26, 1976, petitioner sent a report to five subscribers indicating that respondent, a construction contractor, had filed a voluntary petition for bankruptcy. This report was false and grossly misrepresented respondent's assets and liabilities. That same day, while discussing the possibility of future financing with its bank, respondent's president was told that the bank had received the defamatory report. He immediately called petitioner's regional office, explained the error, and asked for a correction. In addition, he requested the names of the firms that had received the false report in order to assure them that the company was solvent. Petitioner promised to look into the matter but refused to divulge the names of those who had received the report.

After determining that its report was indeed false, petitioner issued a corrective notice on or about August 3, 1976, to the five subscribers who had received the initial report. The notice stated that one of respondent's former employees, not respondent itself, had filed for bankruptcy and that respondent "continued in business as usual." Respondent told petitioner that it was dissatisfied with the notice, and it again asked for a list of subscribers who had seen the initial report. Again petitioner refused to divulge their names.

Respondent then brought this defamation action in Vermont state court. It alleged that the false report had injured its reputation and sought both compensatory and punitive damages. The trial established that the error in petitioner's report had been caused when one of its employees, a 17-year-old high school student paid to review Vermont bankruptcy pleadings, had inadvertently attributed to respondent a bankruptcy petition filed by one of respondent's former employees. Although petitioner's representative testified that it was routine practice to check the accuracy of such reports with the businesses themselves, it did not try to verify the information about respondent before reporting it.

After trial, the jury returned a verdict in favor of respondent and awarded $50,000 in compensatory or presumed damages and $300,000 in punitive damages. Petitioner moved for a new trial. It argued that in *Gertz v. Robert Welch, Inc.*, this Court had ruled broadly that "the States may not permit recovery of presumed or punitive damages, at least when liability is not based on a showing of knowledge of falsity or reckless disregard for the truth," and it argued that the judge's instructions in this case permitted the jury to award such damages on a lesser showing.*** [The Vermont Supreme Court] held "that as a matter of federal constitutional law, the media protections outlined in *Gertz* are inapplicable to nonmedia defamation actions."

Recognizing disagreement among the lower courts about when the protections of *Gertz* apply, we granted certiorari. We now affirm, although for reasons different from those relied upon by the Vermont Supreme Court.

III-V

***

In Gertz v. Robert Welch, Inc., 418 U.S. 323 (1974), we held that the protections of *New York Times* did not extend as far as *Rosenbloom* suggested. *Gertz* concerned a libelous article appearing in a magazine called American Opinion, the monthly outlet of the John Birch Society. The article in question discussed whether the prosecution of a policeman in Chicago was part of a Communist campaign to discredit local law enforcement agencies. The plaintiff, Gertz, neither a public official nor a public figure, was a lawyer tangentially involved in the prosecution. The magazine alleged that he was the chief architect of the "frame-up" of the police officer and linked him to Communist activity. Like every other case in which this Court has found constitutional limits to state defamation laws, *Gertz* involved expression on a matter of undoubted public concern. ***

*** The First Amendment interest[here], on the other hand, is less important than the one weighed in *Gertz*. We have long recognized that not all speech is of equal First Amendment importance. It is speech on "'matters of public concern'" that is "at the heart of the First Amendment's protection." In contrast, speech on matters of purely private concern is of less First Amendment concern. As a number of state courts, including the court below, have recognized, the role of the Constitution in regulating state libel law is far more limited when the concerns that activated *New Times* and *Gertz* are absent. In such a case,

> "[t]here is no threat to the free and robust debate of public issues; there is no potential interference with a meaningful dialogue of ideas concerning self-government; and there is no threat of liability causing a reaction of self-censorship by the press."

*** In *Gertz,* we found that the state interest in awarding presumed and punitive damages was not "substantial" in view of their effect on speech at the core of First Amendment concern. This interest, however, *is* "substantial" relative to the incidental effect these remedies may have on speech of significantly less constitutional interest. The rationale of the common-law rules has been the experience and judgment of history that "proof of actual damage will be impossible in a great many cases where, from the character of the defamatory words and the circumstances of publication, it is all but certain that serious harm has resulted in fact." W. Prosser, Law of Torts § 112, p. 765 (4th ed. 1971). This rule furthers the state interest in providing remedies for defamation by ensuring that those remedies are effective. In light of the reduced constitutional value of speech involving no matters of public concern, we hold that the state interest adequately supports awards of presumed and punitive damages—even absent a showing of "actual malice."

The only remaining issue is whether petitioner's credit report involved a matter of public concern. In a related context, we have held that "[w]hether *** speech addresses a matter of public concern must be determined by [the expression's] content, form, and context *** as revealed by the whole record." These factors indicate that petitioner's credit report concerns no public issue.[7] It was speech solely in the individual interest of the speaker and its specific business audience. ***

VI

We conclude that permitting recovery of presumed and punitive damages in defamation cases absent a showing of "actual malice" does not violate the First Amendment when the defamatory statements do not involve matters of public concern. Accordingly, we affirm the judgment of the Vermont Supreme Court.

CHIEF JUSTICE BURGER, concurring in the judgment. [Omitted.]

JUSTICE WHITE, concurring in the judgment.

***

*** I remain convinced that *Gertz* was erroneously decided. I have also become convinced that the Court struck an improvident balance in the *New York Times* case between the public's interest in being fully informed about public officials and public affairs and the competing interest of those who have been defamed in vindicating their reputation.

In a country like ours, where the people purport to be able to govern themselves through their elected representatives, adequate information about their government is of transcendent importance. That flow of intelligence deserves full First Amendment protection. Criticism and assessment of the performance of public officials and of government in general are not subject to penalties imposed by law. But these First Amendment values are not at all served by circulating false statements of fact about public officials. On the contrary, erroneous information frustrates these values. *** Yet in *New York Times* cases, the public official's complaint will be dismissed unless he alleges and makes out a jury case of a knowing or reckless falsehood. Absent such proof, there will be no jury verdict or judgment of any kind in his favor, even if the challenged publication is admittedly false. The lie will stand, and the public continue to be misinformed about public matters. This will recurringly happen because the putative plaintiff's burden is so exceedingly difficult to satisfy and can be discharged only by expensive litigation. Even if the plaintiff sues, he frequently loses on summary judgment or never gets to the jury because of insufficient proof of malice. ***

---

7. The dissent suggests that our holding today leaves all credit reporting subject to reduced First Amendment protection. This is incorrect. The protection to be accorded a particular credit report depends on whether the report's "content, form, and context" indicate that it concerns a public matter. ***

The *New York Times* rule thus countenances two evils: first, the stream of information about public officials and public affairs is polluted and often remains polluted by false information; and second, the reputation and professional life of the defeated plaintiff may be destroyed by falsehoods that might have been avoided with a reasonable effort to investigate the facts. In terms of the First Amendment and reputational interests at stake, these seem grossly perverse results. ***

We are not talking in these cases about mere criticism or opinion, but about misstatements of fact that seriously harm the reputation of another, by lowering him in the estimation of the community or to deter third persons from associating or dealing with him. The necessary breathing room for speakers can be ensured by limitations on recoverable damages; it does not also require depriving many public figures of any room to vindicate their reputations sullied by false statements of fact. ***

The question before us is whether *Gertz* is to be applied in this case. For either of two reasons, I believe that it should not. First, I am unreconciled to the *Gertz* holding and believe that it should be overruled. Second, as Justice Powell indicates, the defamatory publication in this case does not deal with a matter of public importance. Consequently, I concur in the Court's judgment.

JUSTICE BRENNAN, with whom JUSTICE MARSHALL, JUSTICE BLACKMUN, and JUSTICE STEVENS join, dissenting.

This case involves a difficult question of the proper application of Gertz v. Robert Welch, Inc., 418 U.S. 323 (1974), to credit reporting—a type of speech at some remove from that which first gave rise to explicit First Amendment restrictions on state defamation law—and has produced a diversity of considered opinions, none of which speaks for the Court. ***

The question presented here is narrow. Neither the parties nor the courts below have suggested that respondent Greenmoss Builders should be required to show actual malice to obtain a judgment and actual compensatory damages. Nor do the parties question the requirement of *Gertz* that respondent must show fault to obtain a judgment and actual damages. The only question presented is whether a jury award of presumed and punitive damages based on less than a showing of actual malice is constitutionally permissible. *Gertz* provides a forthright negative answer. To preserve the jury verdict in this case, therefore, the opinions of JUSTICE POWELL and JUSTICE WHITE have cut away the protective mantle of *Gertz*. ***

*** The special harms caused by inaccurate credit reports, the lack of public sophistication about or access to such reports, and the fact that such reports by and large contain statements that are fairly readily susceptible of verification, all may justify appropriate regulation designed to prevent the social losses caused by false credit reports. And in the libel context, the States' regulatory interest in protecting reputation is served by rules permitting recovery for actual compensatory damages upon a showing of fault. Any further interest in deterring potential defamation through case-by-case judicial imposition of presumed and punitive damages awards on less than a showing of actual malice simply exacts too high a toll on First Amendment values. Accordingly, Greenmoss Builders should be permitted to recover for any actual damage it can show resulted from Dun & Bradstreet's negligently false credit report, but should be required to show actual malice to receive presumed or punitive damages. Because the jury was not instructed in accordance with these principles, we would reverse and remand for further proceedings not inconsistent with this opinion.

MIAMI HERALD PUBLISHING COMPANY v. TORNILLO
418 U.S. 241 (1974)

MR. CHIEF JUSTICE BURGER delivered the opinion of the Court.

The issue in this case is whether a state statute granting a political candidate a right to equal space to reply to criticism and attacks on his record by a newspaper violates the guarantees of a free press.

I-III

In the fall of 1972, appellee, Executive Director of the Classroom Teachers Association, apparently a teachers' collective-bargaining agent, was a candidate for the Florida House of Representatives. On September 20, 1972, and again on September 29, 1972, appellant printed editorials critical of appellee's candidacy. In response to these editorials appellee demanded that appellant print verbatim his replies, defending the role of the Classroom Teachers Association and the organization's accomplishments for the citizens of Dade County. Appellant declined to print the appellee's replies, and appellee brought suit in Circuit Court, Dade County, seeking declaratory and injunctive relief and actual and punitive damages in excess of $5,000. The action was premised on Florida Statute § 104.38 (1973), a "right of reply" statute which provides that if a candidate for nomination or election is assailed regarding his personal character or official record by any newspaper, the candidate has the right to demand that the newspaper print, free of cost to the candidate, any reply the candidate may make to the newspaper's charges. The reply must appear in as conspicuous a place and in the same kind of type as the charges which prompted the reply, provided it does not take up more space than the charges. Failure to comply with the statute constitutes a first-degree misdemeanor.

Appellant sought a declaration that § 104.38 was unconstitutional. *** On direct appeal, the Florida Supreme Court. *** It held that free speech was enhanced and not abridged by the Florida right-of-reply statute, which in that court's view, furthered the "broad social interest in the free flow of information to the public." *** It also held that the statute is not impermissibly vague; the statute informs "those who are subject to it as to what conduct on their part will render them liable to its penalties."[4] Civil remedies, including damages, were held to be available under this statute; the case was remanded to the trial court for further proceedings not inconsistent with the Florida Supreme Court's opinion.

***

The appellee and supporting advocates of an enforceable right of access to the press vigorously argue that government has an obligation to ensure that a wide variety of views reach the public. The contentions of access proponents will be set out in some detail. It is urged that at the time the First Amendment to the Constitution was ratified in 1791 as part of our Bill of Rights the press was broadly representative of the people it was serving. While many of the newspapers were intensely partisan and narrow in their views, the press collectively presented a broad range of opinions to readers. Entry into publishing was inexpensive; pamphlets and books provided meaningful alternatives to the organized press for the expression of unpopular ideas and often treated events and expressed views not covered by conventional newspapers. A true marketplace of ideas existed in which there was relatively easy access to the channels of communication.

Access advocates submit that although newspapers of the present are superficially similar to those of 1791 the press of today is in reality very different from that known in the early years of our national existence. In the past half century a communications revolution has seen the introduction of radio and television into our lives, the promise of a global community through the use of communications satellites, and the specter of a "wired" nation by means of an expanding cable television network with two-way capabilities. The printed press, it is said, has not escaped the effects of this revolution. Newspapers have become big business and there are far fewer of them to serve a larger literate population. Chains of newspapers, national newspapers, national wire and news services, and one-newspaper towns, are the dominant features of a press that has become noncompetitive and enormously powerful and influential in its capacity to manipulate popular opinion and change the course of events. ***

The obvious solution, which was available to dissidents at an earlier time when entry into publishing was relatively inexpensive, today would be to have additional newspapers. But the same economic factors which have caused the disappearance of vast numbers of metropolitan newspapers, have made entry into the marketplace of ideas served by the print media almost impossible. It is urged that the claim of newspapers to be "surrogates for the public" carries with it a concomitant fiduciary obligation to account for that stewardship. From this premise it is reasoned that the only effective way to insure fairness and accuracy and to provide for some accountability is for government to take affirmative action. The First Amendment

4. The Supreme Court placed the following limiting construction on the statute:

"[W]e hold that the mandate of the statute refers to 'any reply' which is wholly responsive to the charge made in the editorial or other article in a newspaper being replied to and further that such reply will be neither libelous nor slanderous of the publication not anyone else, nor vulgar nor profane."

interest of the public in being informed is said to be in peril because the "marketplace of ideas" is today a monopoly controlled by the owners of the market. ***

IV

However much validity may be found in these arguments, at each point the implementation of a remedy such as an enforceable right of access necessarily calls for some mechanism, either governmental or consensual. If it is governmental coercion, this at once brings about a confrontation with the express provisions of the First Amendment and the judicial gloss on that Amendment developed over the years.

*** In Columbia Broadcasting System, Inc. v. Democratic National Committee, 412 U.S. 94, 117 (1973), the plurality opinion as to Part III noted:

> "The power of a privately owned newspaper to advance its own political, social, and economic views is bounded by only two factors: first, the acceptance of a sufficient number of readers—and hence advertisers —to assure financial success; and, second, the journalistic integrity of its editors and publishers."

***

Appellee's argument that the Florida statute does not amount to a restriction of appellant's right to speak because "the statute in question here has not prevented the Miami Herald from saying anything it wished" begs the core question. Compelling editors or publishers to publish that which "'reason' tells them should not be published" is what is at issue in this case. The Florida statute operates as a command in the same sense as a statute or regulation forbidding appellant to publish specified matter. Governmental restraint on publishing need not fall into familiar or traditional patterns to be subject to constitutional limitations governmental powers. Grosjean v. American Press Co., 297 U.S. 233, 244-245 (1936). The Florida statute exacts a penalty on the basis of the content of a newspaper. The first phase of the penalty resulting from the compelled printing of a reply is exacted in terms of the cost in printing and composing time and materials and in taking up space that could be devoted to other material the newspaper may have preferred to print. ***

Faced with the penalties that would accrue to any newspaper that published news or commentary arguably within the reach of the right-of-access statute, editors might well conclude that the safe course is to avoid controversy. Therefore, under the operation of the Florida statute, political and electoral coverage would be blunted or reduced. Government-enforced right of access inescapably "dampens the vigor and limits the variety of public debate,"*New York Times Co. v. Sullivan*, 376 U.S., at 279. ***

Even if a newspaper would face no additional costs to comply with a compulsory access law and would not be forced to forego publication of news or opinion by the inclusion of a reply, the Florida statute fails to clear the barriers of the

First Amendment because of its intrusion into the function of editors. A newspaper is more than a passive receptacle or conduit for news, comment, and advertising. The choice of material to go into a newspaper, and the decisions made as to limitations on the size and content of the paper, and treatment of public issues and public officials—whether fair or unfair—constitute the exercise of editorial control and judgment. It has yet to be demonstrated how governmental regulation of this crucial process can be exercised consistent with the First Amendment guarantees of a free press as they have evolved to this time. Accordingly, the judgment of the Supreme Court of Florida is reversed.

MR. JUSTICE BRENNAN, with whom MR. JUSTICE REHNQUIST joins, concurring.

I join the Court's opinion which, as I understand it, addresses only "right of reply" statutes and implies no view upon the constitutionality of "retraction" statutes affording plaintiffs able to prove defamatory falsehoods a statutory action to require publication of a retraction. ***

NOTES

1. *Tornillo* is surely a very strong case insofar as it interprets the first amendment to reserve to each privately owned publication an editorial autonomy to decide what it will and will not publish. Only if Tornillo can meet the rigorous libel standards of *New York Times v. Sullivan*, then though still unable to dictate to the paper what it shall print, he may be able to recover damages.[97] Short of linking reply-access as a remedy incidental to such a suit, one's access into another's publication is virtually solely for the other to decide.[98]

2. Notwithstanding *Tornillo*, however, we have already noticed some circumstances in which a newspaper's freedom to publish what it deems newsworthy and appropriate may nonetheless sometimes be restricted. And sometimes this was so merely as a result of some kind of condition that the newspaper was required to accept in order to secure the information in the first place. Such was the case, for example, in *Seattle Times v. Rhinehart*.[99] There, the Court upheld a state trial court protective order forbidding a newspaper from publishing information it acquired under limitations of civil discovery incidental to the very libel action in which it was

---

97. And perhaps, but merely as part of the libel remedy, a compelled statement of retraction (see concurring opinion in *Tornillo* by Brennan and Rhenquist).

98. See also Pacific Gas & Elec. Co. v. Public Util. Comm'n, 475 U.S. 1 (1986) (extending *Tornillo*); L. A. Scot Powe, Jr., The Fourth Estate and the Constitution 260-87 (1991) (elaborating on *Tornillo*); Benno C. Schmidt, Jr., Freedom of the Press vs. Public Access (1976); William W. Van Alstyne, Interpretations of the First Amendment 64-67, 76-77 (1984) (elaborating on *Tornillo*); Floyd Abrams, In Defense of Tornillo, 86 Yale L.J. 361 (1976) (reviewing Benno C. Schmidt, Jr., Freedom of the Press vs. Public Access (1976)). For strong critical views, see Jerome A. Barron, Freedom of the Press for Whom? (1973).

99. 467 U.S. 20 (1984).

engaged. The order was upheld despite the newspaper's claim of a first amendment right to publish facts pertinent to a public figure already identified in several previous stories it had run. Are there other circumstances in which a newspaper may be similarly held to some restriction it was made to accept in order to secure information that it might not otherwise have secured?

Suppose a newspaper acquires information only by expressly promising source confidentiality but then decides that identification of the source is appropriately part of the story, and so reveals the source despite the promise it made. Suppose a state law, though not specifically addressed to newspapers, presumes to expose the newspaper to an action for damages in this kind of case. Consider the following argument on behalf of the newspaper that draws squarely from the *Tornillo* case:

> The determination of whether to keep a source confidential, as may have been promised, or, despite that promise, to include it as part of the published story, goes as much to the heart of editorial autonomy as any other decision a newspaper may make. The extent to which its judgment on such matters may or may not be regarded as fair to the informant does not make it any less a decision for the newspaper to decide, nor different in kind from what was involved in the *Tornillo* case. There, too, one may agree or (as is more likely) disagree with the newspaper's decision on the merits which the Court unanimously sustained as part of the freedom of the press. In *Rhinehart*, the information was available due solely to a *court order* enabling the defendant to secure information it might legitimately need merely in preparing for trial, and accordingly within the court's authority to limit exclusively to that use. Here, however, when *private parties* deal with newspapers on their own initiative, they must necessarily understand that the risks they incur in doing so are ultimately risks to be resolved in the editorial room and not in the courts.[100]

But does the Supreme Court agree?

COHEN v. COWLES MEDIA COMPANY

501 U.S. 663 (1991)

Justice WHITE delivered the opinion of the Court.

The question before us is whether the First Amendment prohibits a plaintiff from recovering damages, under state promissory estoppel law, for a newspaper's breach of a promise of confidentiality given to the plaintiff in exchange for information. We hold that it does not.

---

100. For an elaborate review and analysis of the general problem, see Lili Levi, Dangerous Liaisons: Seductions and Betrayal in Confidential Press-Source Relations, 43 Rutgers L.Rev. 609 (1991). For an analysis of *Cowles Media*, see The Supreme Court, 1990 Term—Leading Cases, 105 Harv.L.Rev. 277 (1991).

During the closing days of the 1982 Minnesota gubernatorial race, Dan Cohen, an active Republican associated with Wheelock Whitney's Independent-Republican gubernatorial campaign, approached reporters from the St. Paul Pioneer Press Dispatch (Pioneer Press) and the Minneapolis Star and Tribune (Star Tribune) and offered to provide documents relating to a candidate in the upcoming election. Cohen made clear to the reporters that he would provide the information only if he was given a promise of confidentiality. Reporters from both papers promised to keep Cohen's identity anonymous and Cohen turned over copies of two public court records concerning Marlene Johnson, the Democratic-Farmer-Labor candidate for Lieutenant Governor. The first record indicated that Johnson had been charged in 1969 with three counts of unlawful assembly, and the second that she had been convicted in 1970 of petit theft. Both newspapers interviewed Johnson for her explanation and one reporter tracked down the person who had found the records for Cohen. As it turned out, the unlawful assembly charges arose out of Johnson's participation in a protest of an alleged failure to hire minority workers on municipal construction projects and the charges were eventually dismissed. The petit theft conviction was for leaving a store without paying for $6.00 worth of sewing materials. The incident apparently occurred at a time during which Johnson was emotionally distraught, and the conviction was later vacated.

After consultation and debate, the editorial staffs of the two newspapers independently decided to publish Cohen's name as part of their stories concerning Johnson. In their stories, both papers identified Cohen as the source of the court records, indicated his connection to the Whitney campaign, and included denials by Whitney campaign officials of any role in the matter. The same day the stories appeared, Cohen was fired by his employer.

Cohen sued respondents, the publishers of the Pioneer Press and Star Tribune, in Minnesota state court, alleging fraudulent misrepresentation and breach of contract. The trial court rejected respondents' argument that the First Amendment barred Cohen's lawsuit. A jury returned a verdict in Cohen's favor, awarding him $200,000 in compensatory damages and $500,000 in punitive damages. The Minnesota Court of Appeals, reversed the award of punitive damages after concluding that Cohen had failed to establish a fraud claim, the only claim which would support such an award. A divided Minnesota Supreme Court reversed the compensatory damages award. [T]he court concluded that "in this case enforcement of the promise of confidentiality under a promissory estoppel theory would violate defendants' First Amendment rights." ***

Respondents rely on the proposition that "if a newspaper lawfully obtains truthful information about a matter of public significance then state officials may not constitutionally punish publication of the information, absent a need to further a state interest of the highest order." That proposition is unexceptionable, and it has been applied in various cases that have found insufficient the asserted state interests in preventing publication of truthful, lawfully obtained information. ***

This case, however, is not controlled by this line of cases, but rather, by the equally well-established line of decisions holding that generally applicable laws do not offend the First Amendment simply because their enforcement against the press has incidental effects on its ability to gather and report the news. The press may not with impunity break and enter an office or dwelling to gather news. The press, like others interested in publishing, may not publish copyrighted material without obeying the copyright laws.

There can be little doubt that the Minnesota doctrine of promissory estoppel is a law of general applicability. It does not target or single out the press. Rather, insofar as we are advised, the doctrine is generally applicable to the daily transactions of all the citizens of Minnesota. The First Amendment does not forbid its application to the press.

Nor is Cohen attempting to use a promissory estoppel cause of action to avoid the strict requirements for establishing a libel or defamation claim. As the Minnesota Supreme Court observed here, "Cohen could not sue for defamation because the information disclosed [his name] was true." Cohen is not seeking damages for injury to his reputation or his state of mind. He sought damages in excess of $50,000 for a breach of a promise that caused him to lose his job and lowered his earning capacity.

Respondents and *amici* argue that permitting Cohen to maintain a cause of action for promissory estoppel will inhibit truthful reporting because news organizations will have legal incentives not to disclose a confidential source's identity even when that person's identity is itself newsworthy. JUSTICE SOUTER makes a similar argument. But if this is the case, it is no more than the incidental, and constitutionally insignificant, consequence of applying to the press a generally applicable law that requires those who make certain kinds of promises to keep them.

The Minnesota Supreme Court's incorrect conclusion that the First Amendment barred Cohen's claim may well have truncated its consideration of whether a promissory estoppel claim had otherwise been established under Minnesota law and whether Cohen's jury verdict could be upheld on a promissory estoppel basis. *** Accordingly, the judgment of the Minnesota Supreme Court is reversed, and the case is remanded for further proceedings not inconsistent with this opinion.

JUSTICE BLACKMUN, with whom JUSTICE MARSHALL and JUSTICE SOUTER join, dissenting. [Omitted.]

Justice SOUTER, with whom Justice MARSHALL, Justice BLACKMUN and Justice O'CONNOR join, dissenting.

I agree with JUSTICE BLACKMUN that this case does not fall within the line of authority holding the press to laws of general applicability where commercial activities and relationships, not the content of publication, are at issue. *** Even such general laws as do entail effects on the content of speech, like the one in question, may of course be found constitutional, but only, as Justice Harlan observed,

> "when [such effects] have been justified by subordinating valid governmental interests, a prerequisite to constitutionality which has necessarily involved a weighing of the governmental interest involved. *** Whenever, in such a context, these constitutional protections are asserted against the exercise of valid governmental powers a reconciliation must be effected, and that perforce requires an appropriate weighing of the respective interests involved." ***

Because I do not believe the fact of general applicability to be dispositive, I find it necessary to articulate, measure, and compare the competing interests involved in any given case to determine the legitimacy of burdening constitutional interests, and such has been the Court's recent practice in publication cases.

The importance of this public interest is integral to the balance that should be struck in this case. There can be no doubt that the fact of Cohen's identity expanded the universe of information relevant to the choice faced by Minnesota voters in that State's 1982 gubernatorial election, the publication of which was thus of the sort quintessentially subject to strict First Amendment protection. The propriety of his leak to respondents could be taken to reflect on his character, which in turn could be taken to reflect on the character of the candidate who had retained him as an adviser. An election could turn on just such a factor; if it should, I am ready to assume that it would be to the greater public good, at least over the long run.

This is not to say that the breach of such a promise of confidentiality could never give rise to liability. One can conceive of situations in which the injured party is a private individual, whose identity is of less public concern than that of the petitioner; liability there might not be constitutionally prohibited.

Because I believe the State's interest in enforcing a newspaper's promise of confidentiality insufficient to outweigh the interest in unfettered publication of the information revealed in this case, I respectfully dissent.

NOTE

It is clear from the majority and minority opinions in *Cohen v. Cowles Media* that a newspaper may not, on the basis of *Miami Herald v. Tornillo*, claim an absolute immunity from civil suit for any unkept promises of source confidentiality. That is, Cohen will be able to pursue his promissory estoppel claim.

Similarly, in *New York Times v. Sullivan* the first amendment did not afford the New York Times absolute immunity from suit for defamation. Nevertheless, first amendment considerations *were* held to affect the elements of the common law defamation claim. Might the newspaper in *Cohen v. Cowles Media* argue by analogy that its reasons for not fulfilling its promise must still be given substantial weight *within* the language of Section 90 of the Restatement of Contracts? The Restatement permits damages for promissory estoppel to be limited according to the requirements of "justice."[101] In short, might the newspaper argue that failure to consider its reasons would be inconsistent with the first amendment's concerns for the informing function of a free press?[102]

GLORIA BARTNICKI v. FREDERICK W. VOPPER,
121 S. Ct. 1753 (2001)

Justice STEVENS delivered the opinion of the Court.

The suit at hand involves the repeated intentional disclosure of an illegally intercepted cellular telephone conversation about a public issue. The persons who made the disclosures did not participate in the interception, but they did know--or at least had reason to know--that the interception was unlawful. Accordingly, these cases present a conflict between interests of the highest order--on the one hand, the interest in the full and free dissemination of information concerning public issues, and, on the other hand, the interest in individual privacy and, more specifically, in fostering private speech. ***

I

During 1992 and most of 1993, the Pennsylvania State Education Association, a union representing the teachers at the Wyoming Valley West High School, engaged in collective-bargaining negotiations with the school board. Petitioner Kane, then the president of the local union, testified that the negotiations were "contentious" and received "a lot of media attention." In May 1993, petitioner Bartnicki, who was acting as the union's "chief negotiator," used the cellular phone in her car to call Kane and engage in a lengthy conversation about the status of the negotiations. An unidentified person intercepted and recorded that call. *** At one point, Kane said: "If they're not gonna move for three percent, we're gonna have to go to their, their homes ... To blow off their front porches, we'll have to do some work on some of those guys. Really, uh, really and truthfully because this is, you know, this is bad news."

In the early fall of 1993, the parties accepted a non-binding arbitration proposal that was generally favorable to the teachers. In connection with news reports about the settlement, respondent Vopper, a radio commentator who had been critical of the union in the past, played a tape of the intercepted conversation on his public affairs talk show. Another station also broadcast the tape, and local newspapers published

---

101. See Restatement (Second) of Contracts § 90 ("A promise which the promisor should reasonably expect to induce such action or forbearance on the part of the promisee *** and which does induce such action or forbearance is binding *if injustice can be avoided only by enforcement of the promise*. The remedy granted for the breach may be *limited as justice requires*.") (emphasis added).

102. For the Minnesota Supreme Court's disposition of the case on remand, see Cohen v. Cowles Media Co., 479 N.W.2d 387 (Minn. 1992). See also Note, Damages for a Reporter's Breach of Confidence: *Cohen v. Cowles Media Co.*, 105 Harv.L.Rev. 277 (1991).

its contents. After filing suit against Vopper and other representatives of the media, Bartnicki and Kane learned through discovery that Vopper had obtained the tape from Jack Yocum, the head of a local taxpayers' organization that had opposed the union's demands throughout the negotiations. Yocum, who was added as a defendant, testified that he had found the tape in his mailbox shortly after the interception and recognized the voices of Bartnicki and Kane. Yocum played the tape for some members of the school board, and later delivered the tape itself to Vopper.

II

In their amended complaint, petitioners alleged that their telephone conversation had been surreptitiously intercepted by an unknown person using an electronic device, that Yocum had obtained a tape of that conversation, and that he intentionally disclosed it to Vopper, as well as other individuals and media representatives. Thereafter, Vopper and other members of the media repeatedly published the contents of that conversation. The amended complaint alleged that each of the defendants "knew or had reason to know" that the recording of the private telephone conversation had been obtained by means of an illegal interception. Relying on both federal and Pennsylvania statutory provisions, petitioners sought actual damages, statutory damages, punitive damages, and attorney's fees and costs.[103]

***

The provision most directly at issue in this case, applied to any person who "willfully discloses, or endeavors to disclose, to any other person the contents of any wire or oral communication, knowing or having reason to know that the information was obtained through the interception of a wire or oral communication in violation of this subsection." The constitutional question before us concerns the validity of the statute as applied to the specific facts of this case.

We accept petitioners' submission that the interception was intentional, and therefore unlawful, and that, at a minimum, respondents "had reason to know" that it was unlawful. Accordingly, the disclosure of the contents of the intercepted conversation by Yocum to school board members and to representatives of the media, as well as the subsequent disclosures by the media defendants to the public, violated the federal and state statutes. Under the provisions of the federal statute, as well as its Pennsylvania analog, petitioners are thus entitled to recover damages from each of the respondents. The only question is whether the application of these statutes in such circumstances violates the First Amendment.[8]

---

103. Either actual damages, or "statutory damages of whichever is the greater of $100 a day for each day of violation or $10,000" may be recovered under 18 U.S.C. §2520(c)(2); under the Pennsylvania Act, the amount is the greater of $100 a day or $1,000, but the plaintiff may also recover punitive damages and reasonable attorney's fees. 18 Pa. Cons.Stat. § 5725(a) (2000). **

8. In answering this question, we draw no distinction between the media respondents and Yocum. See, e.g., New York Times Co. v. Sullivan, 376 U.S. 254, 265-266, (1978).

In answering that question, we accept respondents' submission on three factual matters that serve to distinguish most of the cases that have arisen under §2511. First, respondents played no part in the illegal interception. Rather, they found out about the interception only after it occurred, and in fact never learned the identity of the person or persons who made the interception. Second, their access to the information on the tapes was obtained lawfully, even though the information itself was intercepted unlawfully by someone else. Third, the subject matter of the conversation was a matter of public concern. If the statements about the labor negotiations had been made in a public arena--during a bargaining session, for example--they would have been newsworthy. ***

V

We agree with petitioners that §2511(1)(c), as well as its Pennsylvania analog, is in fact a content-neutral law of general applicability. The statute does not distinguish based on the content of the intercepted conversations, nor is it justified by reference to the content of those conversations. Rather, the communications at issue are singled out by virtue of the fact that they were illegally intercepted--by virtue of the source, rather than the subject matter.

On the other hand, the naked prohibition against disclosures is fairly characterized as a regulation of pure speech. *** It is true that the delivery of a tape recording might be regarded as conduct, but given that the purpose of such a delivery is to provide the recipient with the text of recorded statements, it is like the delivery of a handbill or a pamphlet, and as such, it is the kind of "speech" that the First Amendment protects. ***

VI

In New York Times Co. v. United States, 403 U.S. 713, (1971) (per curiam), the Court upheld the right of the press to publish information of great public concern obtained from documents stolen by a third party. In so doing, that decision resolved a conflict between the basic rule against prior restraints on publication and the interest in preserving the secrecy of information that, if disclosed, might seriously impair the security of the Nation. ***

However, New York Times v. United States raised, but did not resolve the question "whether, in cases where information has been acquired unlawfully by a newspaper or by a source, government may ever punish not only the unlawful acquisition, but the ensuing publication as well." Florida Star, 491 U.S., at 535, n. 8, The question here, however, is a narrower version of that still-open question. Simply put, the issue here is this: "Where the punished publisher of information has obtained the information in question in a manner lawful in itself but from a source who has obtained it unlawfully, may the government punish the ensuing publication of that information based on the defect in a chain?"

Our refusal to construe the issue presented more broadly is consistent with this Court's repeated refusal to answer categorically whether truthful publication may ever be punished consistent with the First Amendment. Accordingly, we consider whether, given the facts of this case, the interests served by §2511(1)(c) can justify its restrictions on speech.

The Government identifies two interests served by the statute--first, the interest in removing an incentive for parties to intercept private conversations, and second, the interest in minimizing the harm to persons whose conversations have been illegally intercepted. We assume that those interests adequately justify the prohibition in §2511(1)(d) against the interceptor's own use of information that he or she acquired by violating §2511(1)(a), but it by no means follows that punishing disclosures of lawfully obtained information of public interest by one not involved in the initial illegality is an acceptable means of serving those ends.

The normal method of deterring unlawful conduct is to impose an appropriate punishment on the person who engages in it. If the sanctions that presently attach to a violation of §2511(1)(a) do not provide sufficient deterrence, perhaps those sanctions should be made more severe. But it would be quite remarkable to hold that speech by a law-abiding possessor of information can be suppressed in order to deter conduct by a non-law-abiding third party. Although there are some rare occasions in which a law suppressing one party's speech may be justified by an interest in deterring criminal conduct by another, see, e.g., New York v. Ferber, 458 U.S. 747 (1982), this is not such a case.

With only a handful of exceptions, the violations of §2511(1)(a) that have been described in litigated cases have been motivated by either financial gain or domestic disputes. In virtually all of those cases, the identity of the person or persons intercepting the communication has been known. Moreover, petitioners cite no evidence that Congress viewed the prohibition against disclosures as a response to the difficulty of identifying persons making improper use of scanners and other surveillance devices and accordingly of deterring such conduct, and there is no empirical evidence to support the assumption that the prohibition against disclosures reduces the number of illegal interceptions.

Accordingly, the Government's first suggested justification for applying §2511(1)(c) to an otherwise innocent disclosure of public information is plainly insufficient.[19]

The Government's second argument, however, is considerably stronger. Privacy of communication is an important interest, and Title III's restrictions are intended to

---

19. Our holding, of course, does not apply to punishing parties for obtaining the relevant information unlawfully. "It would be frivolous to assert--and no one does in these cases--that the First Amendment, in the interest of securing news or otherwise, confers a license on either the reporter or his news sources to violate valid criminal laws. Although stealing documents or private wiretapping could provide newsworthy information, neither reporter nor source is immune from conviction for such conduct, whatever the impact on the flow of news." Branzburg v. Hayes, 408 U.S. 665, 691 (1972).

protect that interest, thereby "encouraging the uninhibited exchange of ideas and information among private parties...." Brief for United States 27. Moreover, the fear of public disclosure of private conversations might well have a chilling effect on private speech.

Accordingly, it seems to us that there are important interests to be considered on both sides of the constitutional calculus. In considering that balance, we acknowledge that some intrusions on privacy are more offensive than others, and that the disclosure of the contents of a private conversation can be an even greater intrusion on privacy than the interception itself. As a result, there is a valid independent justification for prohibiting such disclosures by persons who lawfully obtained access to the contents of an illegally intercepted message, even if that prohibition does not play a significant role in preventing such interceptions from occurring in the first place.

We need not decide whether that interest is strong enough to justify the application of §2511(c) to disclosures of trade secrets or domestic gossip or other information of purely private concern. In other words, the outcome of the case does not turn on whether §2511(1)(c) may be enforced with respect to most violations of the statute without offending the First Amendment. The enforcement of that provision in this case, however, implicates the core purposes of the First Amendment because it imposes sanctions on the publication of truthful information of public concern.

Our opinion in New York Times Co. v. Sullivan, reviewed many of the decisions that settled the "general proposition that freedom of expression upon public questions is secured by the First Amendment." We think it clear that parallel reasoning requires the conclusion that a stranger's illegal conduct does not suffice to remove the First Amendment shield from speech about a matter of public concern. The months of negotiations over the proper level of compensation for teachers at the Wyoming Valley West High School were unquestionably a matter of public concern, and respondents were clearly engaged in debate about that concern. That debate may be more mundane than the Communist rhetoric that inspired Justice Brandeis' classic opinion in Whitney v. California, 274 U.S., at 372, but it is no less worthy of constitutional protection.

The judgment is affirmed.

Justice BREYER, with whom Justice O'CONNOR joins, concurring.

I join the Court's opinion because I agree with its "narrow" holding, limited to the special circumstances present here: (1) the radio broadcasters acted lawfully (up to the time of final public disclosure); and (2) the information publicized involved a matter of unusual public concern, namely a threat of potential physical harm to others. I write separately to explain why, in my view, the Court's holding does not imply a significantly broader constitutional immunity for the media.

The statutory restrictions before us directly enhance private speech. The statutes ensure the privacy of telephone conversations much as a trespass statute ensures privacy within the home. That assurance of privacy helps to overcome our natural reluctance to discuss private matters when we fear that our private conversations may become public. And the statutory restrictions consequently encourage conversations that otherwise might not take place.

As a general matter, despite the statutes' direct restrictions on speech, the Federal Constitution must tolerate laws of this kind because of the importance of these privacy and speech-related objectives. Nonetheless, looked at more specifically, the statutes, as applied in these circumstances, do not reasonably reconcile the competing constitutional objectives. Rather, they disproportionately interfere with media freedom. For one thing, the broadcasters here engaged in no unlawful activity other than the ultimate publication of the information another had previously obtained. No one claims that they ordered, counseled, encouraged, or otherwise aided or abetted the interception, the later delivery of the tape by the interceptor to an intermediary, or the tape's still later delivery by the intermediary to the media. And, as the Court points out, the statutes do not forbid the receipt of the tape itself. The Court adds that its holding "does not apply to punishing parties for obtaining the relevant information unlawfully."

For another thing, the speakers had little or no legitimate interest in maintaining the privacy of the particular conversation. That conversation involved a suggestion about "blow[ing] off ... front porches" and "do[ing] some work on some of these guys," thereby raising a significant concern for the safety of others. Where publication of private information constitutes a wrongful act, the law recognizes a privilege allowing the reporting of threats to public safety. Even where the danger may have passed by the time of publication, that fact cannot legitimize the speaker's earlier privacy expectation. Nor should editors, who must make a publication decision quickly, have to determine present or continued danger before publishing this kind of threat.

Further, the speakers themselves, the president of a teacher's union and the union's chief negotiator, were "limited public figures," for they voluntarily engaged in a public controversy. They thereby subjected themselves to somewhat greater public scrutiny and had a lesser interest in privacy than an individual engaged in purely private affairs.

This is not to say that the Constitution requires anyone, including public figures, to give up entirely the right to private communication, i.e., communication free from telephone taps or interceptions. But the subject matter of the conversation at issue here is far removed from that in situations where the media publicizes truly private matters.

Thus, in finding a constitutional privilege to publish unlawfully intercepted conversations of the kind here at issue, the Court does not create a "public interest" exception that swallows up the statutes' privacy-protecting general rule. Rather, it finds constitutional protection for publication of intercepted information of a special kind. Here, the speakers' legitimate privacy expectations are unusually low, and the public interest in defeating those expectations is unusually high. Given these circumstances, along with the lawful nature of respondents' behavior, the statutes' enforcement would disproportionately harm media freedom.

I consequently agree with the Court's holding that the statutes as applied here violate the Constitution, but I would not extend that holding beyond these present circumstances.

Chief Justice REHNQUIST, with whom Justice SCALIA and Justice THOMAS join, dissenting.

Technology now permits millions of important and confidential conversations to occur through a vast system of electronic networks. These advances, however, raise significant privacy concerns. We are placed in the uncomfortable position of not knowing who might have access to our personal and business e- mails, our medical and financial records, or our cordless and cellular telephone conversations. In an attempt to prevent some of the most egregious violations of privacy, the United States, the District of Columbia, and 40 States have enacted laws prohibiting the intentional interception and knowing disclosure of electronic communications. The Court holds that all of these statutes violate the First Amendment insofar as the illegally intercepted conversation touches upon a matter of "public concern," an amorphous concept that the Court does not even attempt to define. But the Court's decision diminishes, rather than enhances, the purposes of the First Amendment: chilling the speech of the millions of Americans who rely upon electronic technology to communicate each day.

The Court correctly observes that these are "content-neutral law[s] of general applicability" which serve recognized interests of the "highest order": "the interest in individual privacy and ... in fostering private speech." It nonetheless subjects these laws to the strict scrutiny normally reserved for governmental attempts to censor different viewpoints or ideas. There is scant support, either in precedent or in reason, for the Court's tacit application of strict scrutiny.

These laws are content neutral; they only regulate information that was illegally obtained; they do not restrict republication of what is already in the public domain; they impose no special burdens upon the media; they have a scienter requirement to provide fair warning; and they promote the privacy and free speech of those using cellular telephones. It is hard to imagine a more narrowly tailored prohibition of the disclosure of illegally intercepted communications, and it distorts our precedents to review these statutes under the often fatal standard of strict scrutiny. These laws therefore should be upheld if they further a substantial governmental interest unrelated to the suppression of free speech, and they do.

———

HUSTLER MAGAZINE v. FALWELL
485 U.S. 46 (1988)

CHIEF JUSTICE REHNQUIST delivered the opinion of the Court.

Petitioner Hustler Magazine, Inc., is a magazine of nationwide circulation. Respondent Jerry Falwell, a nationally known minister who has been active as a commentator on politics and public affairs, sued petitioner and its publisher, petitioner Larry Flynt, to recover damages for invasion of privacy, libel, and intentional infliction of emotional distress. The District Court directed a verdict against respondent on the privacy claim, and submitted the other two claims to a jury. The jury found for petitioners on the defamation claim, but found for respondent on the claim for intentional infliction of emotional distress and awarded damages. We now consider whether this award is consistent with the First and Fourteenth Amendments of the United States Constitution.

The inside front cover of the November 1983 issue of Hustler Magazine featured a "parody" of an advertisement for Campari Liqueur that contained the name and picture of respondent and was entitled "Jerry Falwell talks about his first time." This parody was modeled after actual Campari ads that included interviews with various celebrities about their "first times." Although it was apparent by the end of each interview that this meant the first time they sampled Campari, the ads clearly played on the sexual double entendre of the general subject of "first times." Copying the form and layout of these Campari ads, Hustler's editors chose respondent as the featured celebrity and drafted an alleged "interview" with him in which he states that his "first time" was during a drunken incestuous rendezvous with his mother in an outhouse. The Hustler parody portrays respondent and his mother as drunk and immoral, and suggests that respondent is a hypocrite who preaches only when he is drunk. In small print at the bottom of the page, the ad contains the disclaimer, "ad parody—not to be taken seriously." The magazine's table of contents also lists the ad as "Fiction; Ad and Personality Parody."

Soon after the November issue of Hustler became available to the public, respondent brought this diversity action in the United States District Court for the Western District of Virginia against Hustler Magazine, Inc., Larry C. Flynt, and Flynt Distributing Co., Inc. Respondent stated in his complaint that publication of the ad parody in Hustler entitled him to recover damages for libel, invasion of privacy, and intentional infliction of emotional distress. The case proceeded to trial.[1] At the close of the evidence, the District Court granted a directed verdict for petitioners on the invasion of privacy claim. The jury then found against respondent on the libel claim, specifically finding that the ad parody could not "reasonably be understood as describing actual facts about [respondent] or actual events in which [he] participated."

---

1. While this case was pending, the ad parody was published in Hustler magazine a second time.

The jury ruled for respondent on the intentional infliction of emotional distress claim, however, and stated that he should be awarded $100,000 in compensatory damages, as well as $50,000 each in punitive damages as well as $50,000 each in punitive damages from petitioners.[2] Petitioners' motion for judgment notwithstanding the verdict was denied.

On appeal, the United States Court of Appeals for the Fourth Circuit affirmed the judgment against petitioners. The court rejected petitioners' argument that the "actual malice" standard of New York Times Co. v. Sullivan, 376 U.S. 254 (1964), must be met before respondent can recover for emotional distress. *** In the court's view, the *New York Times* decision emphasized the constitutional importance not of falsity of the statement or the defendant's disregard for the truth, but of the heightened level of culpability embodied in the requirement of "knowing *** or reckless" conduct. Here, the *New York Times* standard is satisfied by the state-law requirement, and the jury's finding, that the defendants have acted intentionally or recklessly.[3] The Court of Appeals then went on to reject the contention that because the jury found that the ad parody did not describe actual facts about respondent, the ad was an opinion that is protected by the First Amendment. As the court put it, this was "irrelevant," as the issue is "whether [the ad's] publication was sufficiently outrageous to constitute intentional infliction of emotional distress." Petitioners then filed a petition for rehearing en banc, but this was denied by a divided court. Given the importance of the constitutional issues involved, we granted certiorari. ***

This case presents us with a novel question involving First Amendment limitations upon a State's authority to protect its citizens from the intentional infliction of emotional distress. We must decide whether a public figure may recover damages for emotional harm caused by the publication of an ad parody offensive to him, and doubtless gross and repugnant in the eyes of most. Respondent would have us find that a State's interest in protecting public figures from emotional distress is sufficient to deny First Amendment protection to speech that is patently offensive and is intended to inflict emotional injury, even when that speech could not reasonably have been interpreted as stating actual facts about the public figure involved. This we decline to do. ***

The sort of robust political debate encouraged by the First Amendment is bound to produce speech that is critical of those who hold public office or those public figures who are "intimately involved in the resolution of important public questions or, by reason of their fame, shape events in areas of concern to society at large."

---

2. The jury found no liability on the part of Flynt Distributing Co., Inc. It is consequently not a party to this appeal.

3. Under Virginia law, in an action for intentional infliction of emotional distress a plaintiff must show that the defendant's conduct (1) is intentional or reckless; (2) offends generally accepted standards of decency or morality; (3) is causally connected with the plaintiff's emotional distress; and (4) caused emotional distress that was severe.

Associated Press v. Walker, decided with Curtis Publishing Co. v. Butts, 388 U.S. 130, 164 (1967) (Warren, C.J., concurring in result). Justice Frankfurter put it succinctly in Baumgartner v. United States, 322 U.S. 665, 673-674 (1944), when he said that "[o]ne of the prerogatives of American citizenship is the right to criticize public men and measures." Such criticism, inevitably, will not always be reasoned or moderate; public figures as well as public officials will be subject to "vehement, caustic, and sometimes unpleasantly sharp attacks," *New York Times*, 376 U.S., at 270. ***

Of course, this does not mean that *any* speech about a public figure is immune from sanction in the form of damages. Since *New York Times Co. v. Sullivan*, we have consistently ruled that a public figure may hold a speaker liable for the damage to reputation caused by publication of a defamatory falsehood, but only if the statement was made "with knowledge that it was false or with reckless disregard of whether it was false or not." False statements of fact are particularly valueless; they interfere with the truth-seeking function of the marketplace of ideas, and they cause damage to an individual's reputation that cannot easily be repaired by counterspeech, however, persuasive or effective. See *Gertz*, 418 U.S. at 340, 344. But even though falsehoods have little value in and of themselves, they are "nevertheless inevitable in free debate," *id.*, at 340, and a rule that would impose strict liability on a publisher for false factual assertions would have an undoubted "chilling" effect on speech relating to public figures that does have constitutional value. "Freedoms of expression require 'breathing space.'" This breathing space is provided by a constitutional rule that allows public figures to recover for libel or defamation only when they can prove *both* that the statement was false and that the statement was made with the requisite level of culpability.

Respondent argues, however, that a different standard should apply in this case because here the State seeks to prevent not reputational damage, but the severe emotional distress suffered by the person who is the subject of an offensive publication. In respondent's view, and in the view of the Court of Appeals, so long as the utterance was intended to inflict emotional distress, was outrageous, and did in fact inflict serious emotional distress, it is of no constitutional import whether the statement was a fact or an opinion, or whether it was true or false. It is the intent to cause injury that is the gravamen of the tort, and the State's interest in preventing emotional harm simply outweighs whatever interest a speaker may have in speech of this type.

Generally speaking the law does not regard the intent to inflict emotional distress as one which should receive much solicitude, and it is quite understandable that most if not all jurisdictions have chosen to make it civilly culpable where the conduct in question is sufficiently "outrageous." But in the world of debate about public affairs, many things done with motives that are less than admirable are protected by the First Amendment. In Garrison v. Louisiana, 379 U.S. 64 (1964), we held that even when a speaker or writer is motivated by hatred or ill-will his expression was protected by the First Amendment:

> "Debate on public issues will not be uninhibited if the speaker must run the risk that it will be proved in court that he spoke out of hatred; even if he did speak out of hatred, utterances honestly believed contribute to the free interchange."

Thus while such a bad motive may be deemed controlling for purposes of tort liability in other areas of the law, we think the First Amendment prohibits such a result in the area of public debate about public figures.

Were we to hold otherwise, there can be little doubt that political cartoonists and satirists would be subjected to damages awards without any showing that their work falsely defamed its subject. Webster's defines a caricature as "the deliberately distorted picturing or imitating of a person, literary style, etc. by exaggerating features or mannerisms for satirical effect." Webster's New Unabridged Twentieth Century Dictionary of the English Language 275 (2d ed. 1979). The appeal of the political cartoon or caricature is often based on exploration of unfortunate physical traits or politically embarrassing events—an exploitation often calculated to injure the feelings of the subject of the portrayal. The art of the cartoonist is often not reasoned or evenhanded, but slashing and one-sided. One cartoonist expressed the nature of the art in these words:

> "The political cartoon is a weapon of attack, of scorn and ridicule and satire; it is least effective when it tries to pat some politician on the back. It is usually as welcome as a bee sting and is always controversial in some quarters." Long, The Political Cartoon: Journalism's Strongest Weapon, The Quill, 56, 67 (Nov. 1962).

Despite their sometimes caustic nature, from the early cartoon portraying George Washington as an ass down to the present day, graphic depictions and satirical cartoons have played a prominent role in public and political debate. Nast's castigation of the Tweed Ring, Walt McDougall's characterization of presidential candidate James G. Blaine's banquet with the millionaires at Delmonico's as "The Royal Feast of Belshazzar," and numerous other efforts have undoubtedly had an effect on the course and outcome of contemporaneous debate. Lincoln's tall, gangling posture, Teddy Roosevelt's glasses and teeth, and Franklin D. Roosevelt's jutting jaw and cigarette holder have been memorialized by political cartoons with an effect that could not have been obtained by the photographer or the portrait artist. From the viewpoint of history it is clear that our political discourse would have been considerably poorer without them.

Respondent contends, however, that the caricature in question here was so "outrageous" as to distinguish it from more traditional political cartoons. There is no doubt that the caricature of respondent and his mother published in Hustler is at best a distant cousin of the political cartoons described above, and a rather poor relation at that. If it were possible by laying down a principled standard to separate the one from the other, public discourse would probably suffer little or no harm. But we doubt that there is any such standard, and we are quite sure that the pejorative description "outrageous" does not supply one. "Outrageousness" in the area of political and social discourse has an inherent subjectiveness about it which would allow a jury to impose liability on the basis of the jurors' tastes or views, or perhaps on the basis of their dislike of a particular expression. ***

We conclude that public figures and public officials may not recover for the tort of intentional infliction of emotional distress by reason of publications such as the one here at issue without showing in addition that the publication contains a false statement of fact which was made with "actual malice" i.e. with knowledge that the statement was false or with reckless disregard as to whether or not it was true. This is not merely a "blind application," of the *New York Times* standard, see Time, Inc. v. Hill, 385 U.S. 374, 390 (1967), it reflects our considered judgment that such a standard is necessary to give adequate "breathing space" to the freedoms protected by the First Amendment.

Here it is clear that respondent Falwell is a "public figure" for purposes of First Amendment law.[5] The jury found against respondent on his libel claim when it decided that the Hustler ad parody could not "reasonably be understood as describing actual facts about [respondent] or actual events in which [he] participated." The Court of Appeals interpreted the jury's finding to be that the ad parody "was not reasonably believable," and in accordance with our custom we accept this finding. Respondent is thus relegated to his claim for damages awarded by the jury for the intentional infliction of emotional distress by "outrageous" conduct. But for reasons heretofore stated this claim cannot, consistently with the First Amendment, form a basis for the award of damages when the conduct in question is the publication of a caricature such as the ad parody involved here. The judgment of the Court of Appeals is accordingly reversed.

Mr. JUSTICE KENNEDY took no part in the consideration or decision of this case.

Mr. JUSTICE WHITE, concurring in the judgment.

As I see it, the decision in New York Times Co. v. Sullivan, 376 U.S. 254 (1964), has little to do with this case, for here the jury found that the ad contained no assertion of fact. But I agree with the Court that the judgment below, which penalized the publication of the parody, cannot be squared with the First Amendment.

---

5. Neither party disputes this conclusion. Respondent is the host of a nationally syndicated television show and was the founder and president of a political organization formerly known as the Moral Majority. He is also the founder of Liberty University in Lynchburg, Virginia, and is the author of several books and publications. Who's Who in America 849 (44th ed. 1986-1987).

NOTES

The lower court opinion reproduced a portion of the deposition of Larry Flynt,[103] including the following:

> Q. Did you want to upset Reverend Falwell?
>
> A. Yes ***.
>
> Q. Do you recognize that in having published what you did in this ad, *you were attempting to convey to the people who read it that Reverend Falwell was just as you characterized him, a liar*?
>
> A. *Yeah. He's a liar, too.*
>
> Q. *How about a hypocrite*?
>
> A. *Yeah.*
>
> Q. *That's what you wanted to convey*?
>
> A. *Yeah.*
>
> Q. Did you appreciate, at the time that you wrote 'okay' or approved this publication, that for Reverend Falwell to function in his livelihood, and in his commitment and career, he has to have an integrity that people believe in? Did you not appreciate that?
>
> A. Yeah.
>
> Q. And wasn't one of your objectives to destroy that integrity, or harm it, if you could?
>
> A. To assassinate it.

The immediate depiction of Falwell in the *Hustler* feature—a feature in turn parodying advertisements for Campari—was, as the Court notes, not presented as an actual interview. Because the jury found that the ad content could not "reasonably be understood as describing [any] actual facts," the libel branch of the plaintiff's cause of action was deemed to self-destruct.

But even assuming that an action in libel requires evidence that defendant published some assertion of a defamatory character in clear reference to the plaintiff— which assertion the plaintiff must prove to be false in fact,[104] in light of the deposition transcript itself might one argue that Falwell could still satisfy this minimum test? Why ought he not be allowed to establish by evidence of convincing clarity to the satisfaction of a jury that in fact he has been viciously maligned, i.e. that he is not in fact anything like the kind of person he has been depicted as being[105]—and that he has plainly, therefore, been libeled by *Hustler*? What bars him

---

103. Falwell v. Flynt, 797 F.2d 1270, 1273 (4th Cir. 1986) (emphasis added).

104. But see Burton v. Crowell Publishing Co., 82 F.2d 154 (2d Cir. 1936) (Learned Hand, J.) (recovery in libel allowed for damage to reputation consequential to publication of unretouched, not false-in-fact photograph).

105. Namely, as prurient and lecherous, a sensualist and hypocrite, etc.

from recovering for defamation, even if he cannot recover for the intentional infliction of emotional distress?

Suppose Flynt had not libeled Falwell in the manner he employed but simply more directly, i.e. by simple assertion such as this: "This man Falwell is a liar and a hypocrite." Assuming Falwell can establish that he is neither, may he now be able to recover defamation damages from Flynt? If he could, at least if he could also meet the *Sullivan* requirement, could he recover not only for a statement published by Flynt of exactly that sort, but possibly even for this one as well: "In my opinion, Falwell is a liar and a hypocrite?"[106]

The case assuredly seems to leave open the possibility that in either of these other kinds of cases, some sort of action for libel might be brought. Perhaps nothing in the material we have already reviewed precludes such an action. Yet, surely the calculated harm arising from either of these forms of defamation may be no greater in fact (and may in some ways be considerably less, may it not?) than the calculated harm inflicted by the device Flynt actually chose. And the degree of real falsehood may be no greater, as well, may it not? Why, then, should the first amendment be deemed to bar one but allow the other, i.e. to make actionability depend upon the mere form in which the libel appears?[107]

Both the purpose and effect of allowing redress in defamation actions may appear to be quite consistent with characteristics of one genre of personal or of group libel, a genre one might call "libel by vicious fiction." Vicious fiction may—and arguably did in this instance—describe the *Hustler* technique.[108] More generally, one might describe "vicious fiction" as "material willfully contrived to induce false, deeply negative, repugnant impressions of the person or the group who are thus made the object of the maligner's art." If such material is nonetheless to be deemed protected by the first amendment from actions in defamation (and *Hustler Magazine v. Falwell* provides a very strong indication that it will be—at least with respect to

---

106. For a recent significant case holding that the recasting of a given statement into the form of an opinion does not automatically convert it from actionable to inactionable, see Milkovich v. Lorain Journal Co., 497 U.S. 1 (1990) (Where the published opinion implies to the reader the existence of facts as presumably known to the publisher and not furnished in the story, recovery may be based on the opinion's implicit claim of actual facts.).

107. Note that the vulgar Hustler parody portrayed Falwell and *his mother* as drunk and immoral, and described Falwell's having engaged in "a drunken incestuous rendezvous *with his mother* in an outhouse." Suppose Mr. Falwell's mother, an elderly and very private person, has her attention brought to this feature in Hustler by a neighbor. Suppose also that she sustains such a sense of humiliation and profound shame that she feels unable even to leave her own home in the small town where she lives. May *she* have a valid cause of action—for the libel? for negligent (or intentional) infliction of emotional distress? for negligence? for invasion of privacy (or "false light" privacy)?

108. For an additional example that makes the treatment of Falwell pale in comparison, see Dworkin v. Hustler Magazine, Inc., 867 F.2d 1188 (9th Cir. 1989).

public figures and political events[109]), it ought to be fairly easy to say why. What does the Court say, in *Hustler Magazine, Inc. v. Falwell*?[110]

This issue is joined strongly still again, in the following case on "false" statements and civil rights claims in a newer setting: a case of the first amendment and the feminist critique. Although it is but a court of appeals decision (summarily affirmed by the Supreme Court), it is a useful bookend on the immediate subject of our review. It also provides one of the strongest statements in American case law on the meaning of freedom of speech.

AMERICAN BOOKSELLERS v. HUDNUT

771 F.2d 323 (7th Cir. 1985), (*summarily aff'd*, 475 U.S. 1001 (1986))

EASTERBROOK, Circuit Judge.

Indianapolis enacted an ordinance defining "pornography" as a practice that discriminates against women. "Pornography" is to be redressed through the administrative and judicial methods used for other discrimination. *** "Pornography" under the ordinance is "the graphic sexually explicit subordination of women, whether in pictures or in words, that also includes one or more of the following:

(1) Women are presented as sexual objects who enjoy pain or humiliation; or

(2) Women are presented as sexual objects who experience sexual pleasure in being raped; or

***

---

109. Indeed, *Hustler Magazine* would appear to limit one's hope for redress to that which can be gotten solely by one's efforts to falsify the critical perspective created by the defaming fiction,—to do so by the way one actually lives one's life and actually conducts oneself.

110. Consider the following conundrum: If (a) something is meant to and does defame; If (b) it also contains no "true" statement (but only a "false" statement insofar as it contains any statement at all); then (c) of what social good can it be such that it should nonetheless be protected by the first amendment? —Or is this a "conundrum" that would, if it were taken seriously, threaten a great deal of fiction indeed, e.g., from Shakespeare through Dickens, Mark Twain, Joseph Heller, and Tom Wolfe, and from Hogarth and Daumier through Nast, Herblock, Oliphant and Larry Flynt. (Moreover, quite depending on your own point of view, might it also potentially threaten an uncertain number of other works as well, e.g., *Das Kapital*, or *Mein Kampf*, or for that matter portions of the *New* or *Old Testament* or the *Qur'an*.)

For a thoughtful review of *Hustler Magazine v. Falwell* in probing such matters more generally, see Post, *supra* note 95 at p. 173. For an attempt to suggest that "[t]he advertisement [in *Hustler Magazine v. Falwell*] was no more worthy of legal protection than a spite fence constructed to inflict harm for its own sake," however, see Bruce Fein, Hustler Magazine v. Falwell: A Mislitigated and Misreasoned Case, 30 Wm. & Mary L.Rev. 905 (1989) (reviewing Rodney A. Smolla, Jerry Falwell v. Larry Flynt: The First Amendment on Trial (1988)). See also Debora Shuger, *Civility and Censorship in Early Modern England*, in Censorship and Silencing: Practices of Cultural Regulation (Post, ed., 1998) (useful discussion of efforts in Tudor and Stuart England to suppress "satire").

(6) Women are presented as sexual objects for domination, conquest, violation, exploitation, possession, or use, or through postures or positions of servility or submission or display.

***

The Indianapolis ordinance does not refer to the prurient interest, to offensiveness, or to the standards of the community. It demands attention to particular depictions, not to the work judged as a whole. It is irrelevant under the ordinance whether the work has literary, artistic, political, or scientific value. The City and many amici point to these omissions as virtues. They maintain that pornography influences attitudes, and the statute is a way to alter the socialization of men and women rather than to vindicate community standards of offensiveness. And as one of the principal drafters of the ordinance has asserted, "if a woman is subjected, why should it matter that the work has other value?" Catharine A. MacKinnon, Pornography, Civil Rights, and Speech, 20 Harv.Civ.Rts.—Civ.Lib.L.Rev. 1, 21 (1985).

Civil rights groups and feminists have entered this case as amici on both sides. Those supporting the ordinance say that it will play an important role in reducing the tendency of men to view women as sexual objects, a tendency that leads to both unacceptable attitudes and discrimination in the workplace and violence away from it. Those opposing the ordinance point out that much radical feminist literature is explicit and depicts women in ways forbidden by the ordinance and that the ordinance would reopen old battles. It is unclear how Indianapolis would treat works from James Joyce's *Ulysses* to Homer's *Iliad*; both depict women as submissive objects for conquest and domination.

We do not try to balance the arguments for and against an ordinance such as this. The ordinance discriminates on the ground of the content of the speech. Speech treating women in the approved way—in sexual encounters "premised on equality" (MacKinnon, *supra*, at 22)—is lawful no matter how sexually explicit. Speech treating women in the disapproved way—as submissive in matters sexual or as enjoying humiliation—is unlawful no matter how significant the literary, artistic, or political qualities of the work taken as a whole. The state may not ordain preferred viewpoints in this way. The Constitution forbids the state to declare one perspective right and silence opponents.

I

***

Trafficking is defined in § 16-3(g)(4) as the "production, sale, exhibition, or distribution of pornography." The offense excludes exhibition in a public or educational library, but a "special display" in a library may be sex discrimination. Section 16-3(g)(4)(C) provides that the trafficking paragraph "shall not be construed to make isolated passages or isolated parts actionable." A woman aggrieved by trafficking in pornography may file a complaint "as a woman acting against the subordination of women" with the office of equal opportunity.

The office investigates and within 30 days makes a recommendation to a panel of the equal opportunity advisory board. The panel then decides whether there is reasonable cause to proceed (§16-24(2)) and may refer the dispute to a conciliation conference or to a complaint adjudication committee for a hearing (§§ 16-24(3), 16-26(a)). The committee uses the same procedures ordinarily associated with civil rights litigation. It may make findings and enter orders, including both orders to cease and desist and orders to "take further affirmative action including but not limited to the power to restore complainant's losses." Either party may appeal the committee's decision to the board, which reviews the record before the committee and may modify its decision. ***

II

The plaintiffs are a congeries of distributors and readers of books, magazines, and films. The American Booksellers Association comprises about 5,200 bookstores and chains. The Association for American Publishers includes most of the country's publishers. Video Shack, Inc., sells and rents video cassettes in Indianapolis. Kelly Bentley, a resident of Indianapolis, reads books and watches films. There are many more plaintiffs. Collectively the plaintiffs (or their members, whose interests they represent) make, sell, or read just about every kind of material that could be affected by the ordinance, from hard-core films to W. B. Yeats's poem "Leda and the Swan" (from the myth of Zeus in the form of a swan impregnating an apparently subordinate Leda) to the collected works of James Joyce, D. H. Lawrence and John Cleland. ***

The district court prevented the ordinance from taking effect. *** [The court concluded that the ordinance regulates speech rather than the conduct involved in making pornography. The regulation of speech could be justified, the court thought, only by a compelling interest in reducing sex discrimination, an interest Indianapolis had not established. The ordinance is also vague and overbroad, the court believed, and establishes a prior restraint of speech.]

III

"If there is any fixed star in our constitutional constellation, it is that no official, high or petty, can prescribe what shall be orthodox in politics, nationalism, religion, or other matters of opinion or force citizens to confess by word or act their faith therein." West Virginia State Board of Education v. Barnette, 319 U.S. 624, 642 (1943). Under the First Amendment the government must leave to the people the evaluation of ideas. Bald or subtle, an idea is as powerful as the audience allows it to be. A belief may be pernicious—the beliefs of Nazis led to the death of millions, those of the Klan to the repression of millions. A pernicious belief may prevail. Totalitarian governments today rule much of the planet, practicing suppression of billions and spreading dogma that may enslave others. One of the things that separates our society from theirs is our absolute right to propagate opinions that the government finds wrong or even hateful.

The ideas of the Klan may be propagated. Brandenburg v. Ohio, 395 U.S. 444 (1969). Communists may speak freely and run for office. DeJonge v. Oregon, 199 U.S. 353 (1937). The Nazi Party may march through a city with a large Jewish population. Collin v. Smith, 578 F.2d 1197 (7th Cir.), cert. denied, 439 U.S. 916 (1978).

People may criticize the President by misrepresenting his positions, and they have a right to post their misrepresentations on public property. Lebron v. Washington Metropolitan Transit Authority, 749 F.2d 893 (D.C.Cir. 1984)(Bork, J.). People may teach religions that others despise. People may seek to repeal laws guaranteeing equal opportunity in employment or to revoke the constitutional amendments granting the vote to blacks and women. They may do this because "above all else, the First Amendment means that government has no power to restrict expression because of its message [or] its ideas. ***" Police Department v. Mosley, 408 U.S. 92, 95 (1972). ***

Under the ordinance graphic sexually explicit speech is "pornography" or not depending on the perspective the author adopts. Speech that "subordinates" women and also, for example, presents women as enjoying pain, humiliation, or rape, or even simply presents women in "positions of servility or submission or display" is forbidden, no matter how great the literary or political value of the work taken as a whole. Speech that portrays women in positions of equality is lawful, no matter how graphic the sexual content. This is thought control. It establishes an "approved" view of women, of how they may react to sexual encounters, of how the sexes may relate to each other. Those who espouse the approved view may use sexual images; those who do not, may not.

Indianapolis justifies the ordinance on the ground that pornography affects thoughts. Men who see women depicted as subordinate are more likely to treat them so. Pornography is an aspect of dominance. It does not persuade people so much as change them. It works by socializing, by establishing the expected and the permissible. In this view pornography is not an idea; pornography is the injury.

There is much to this perspective. Beliefs are also facts. People often act in accordance with the images and patterns they find around them. People raised in a religion tend to accept the tenets of that religion, often without independent examination. People taught from birth that black people are fit only for slavery rarely rebelled against that creed; beliefs coupled with the self-interest of the masters established a social structure that inflicted great harm while enduring for centuries. Words and images act at the level of the subconscious before they persuade at the level of the conscious. Even the truth has little chance unless a statement fits within the framework of beliefs that may never have been subjected to rational study. *** Therefore we accept the premises of this legislation.

Yet this simply demonstrates the power of pornography as speech. All of these unhappy effects depend on mental intermediation. Pornography affects how people see the world, their fellows, and social relations. If pornography is what pornography does, so is other speech. Hitler's orations affected how some Germans saw Jews. Communism is a world view, not simply a *Manifesto* by Marx and Engels or a set of speeches. Efforts to suppress communist speech in the United States were based on the belief that the public acceptability of such ideas would increase the likelihood of totalitarian government. Religions affect socialization in the most pervasive way. *** Many people believe that the existence of television, apart from the content of specific programs, leads to intellectual laziness, to a penchant for violence, to many other ills. The Alien and Sedition Acts passed during the administration of John Adams rested on a sincerely held belief that disrespect for the government leads to social collapse and revolution—a belief with support in the history of many nations. Most governments of the world act on this empirical regularity, suppressing critical speech. In the United States, however, the strength of the support for this belief is irrelevant. ***

Racial bigotry, anti-semitism, violence on television, reporters' biases—these and many more influence the culture and shape our socialization. None is directly answerable by more speech, unless that speech too finds its place in the popular culture. Yet all is protected as speech, however insidious. Any other answer leaves the government in control of all of the institutions of culture, the great censor and director of which thoughts are good for us.

Sexual responses often are unthinking responses, and the association of sexual arousal with the subordination of women therefore may have a substantial effect. But almost all cultural stimuli provoke unconscious responses. Religious ceremonies condition their participants. Teachers convey messages by selecting what not to cover; the implicit message about what is off limits or unthinkable may be more powerful than the messages for which they present rational argument. Television scripts contain unarticulated assumptions. People may be conditioned in subtle ways. If the fact that speech plays a role in a process of conditioning were enough to permit governmental regulation, that would be the end of freedom of speech. ***

Much of Indianapolis's argument rests on the belief that when speech is "unanswerable," and the metaphor that there is a "marketplace of ideas" does not apply, the First Amendment does not apply either. The metaphor is honored; Milton's *Aeropagitica* and John Stewart Mill's *On Liberty* defend freedom of speech on the ground that the truth will prevail and many of the most important cases under the First Amendment recite this position. The Framers undoubtedly believed it. As a general matter it is true. But the Constitution does not make the dominance of truth a necessary condition of freedom of speech. To say that it does would be to confuse an outcome of free speech with a necessary condition for the application of the amendment.

A power to limit speech on the ground that truth has not yet prevailed and is not likely to prevail implies the power to declare truth. At some point the government must be able to say (as Indianapolis has said): "We know what the truth is, yet a free exchange of speech has not driven out falsity, so that we must now prohibit falsity." If the government may declare the truth, why wait for the failure of speech? ***

At any time, some speech is ahead in the game; the more numerous speakers prevail. Supporters of minority candidates may be forever "excluded" from the political process because their candidates never win, because few people believe their positions. This does not mean that freedom of speech has failed. ***

We come finally to the argument that pornography is "low value" speech, that it is enough like obscenity that Indianapolis may prohibit it. Some cases hold that speech far removed from politics and other subjects at the core of the Framers' concerns may be subjected to special regulation. ***

At all events, "pornography"[as defined in the Indianapolis Ordinance] is not low value speech within the meaning of these cases. Indianapolis seeks to prohibit certain speech because it believes this speech influences social relations and politics on a grand scale, that it controls attitudes at home and in the legislature. This precludes a characterization of the speech as low value. True, pornography and obscenity have sex in common. But Indianapolis left out of its definition any reference to literary, artistic, political or scientific value. The ordinance applies to graphic sexually explicit subordination in works great and small.[3] The Court sometimes balances the value of speech against the costs of its restriction, but it does this by category of speech and not by the content of particular works. *** Indianapolis has created an approved point of view and so loses the support of these cases.

Any rationale we could imagine in support of this ordinance could not be limited to sex discrimination. Free speech has been on balance an ally of those seeking change. Governments that want stasis start by restricting speech. Culture is a powerful force of continuity; Indianapolis paints pornography as part of the culture of power. Change in any complex system ultimately depends on the ability of outsiders to challenge accepted views and the reigning institutions. Without a strong guarantee of freedom of speech, there is no effective right to challenge what is.

IV

The definition of "pornography" is unconstitutional. No construction or excision of particular terms could save it. *** No amount of struggle with particular words and phrases in this ordinance can leave anything in effect. The district court came to the same conclusion. Its judgment is therefore *** [a]ffirmed.

SWYGERT, Senior Circuit Judge, concurring. [Omitted.]

---

3. Indianapolis briefly argues that Beauharnais v. Illinois, 343 U.S. 250 (1952), which allowed a state to penalize "group libel," supports the ordinance. In Collin v. Smith, 578 F.2d at 1205, we concluded that cases such as *New York Times v. Sullivan* had so washed away the foundations of *Beauharnais* that it could not be considered authoritative. If we are wrong in this, however, the case still does not support the ordinance. It is not clear that depicting women as subordinate in sexually explicit ways, even combined with a depiction of pleasure in rape, would fit within the definition of a group libel. The well received film *Swept Away* used explicit sex, plus taking pleasure in rape, to make a political statement, not to defame. Work must be an insult or slur for its own sake to come within the ambit of *Beauharnais*, and a work need not be scurrilous at all to be "pornography" under the ordinance.

NOTE

In a case involving a criminal statute similar to the ordinance held invalid in *Hudnut*, the Supreme Court of Canada reached a conclusion opposite to the conclusion in *Hudnut*. See Regina v. Butler, [1992] 1 S.C.R. 452. (See also its decision in Regina v. Keegstra, [1990] 3 S.C.R. 697, sustaining a criminal ban on certain kinds of "hate speech.")

The Canadian Supreme Court acknowledged that sexually explicit material degrading to women was, notwithstanding its content, fully within the protection of the Canadian Constitution provision on freedom of speech (namely, Section 2 of the Canadian Charter of Rights and Freedoms guaranteeing "freedom of thought, belief, opinion, and expression"). It nonetheless held that such material could be forbidden pursuant to a distinct clause also provided in Canada's Constitution, an override clause not found in the Constitution of the United States. The separate clause (Section 1 of the Charter of Rights and Freedoms) expressly subjects any otherwise protected freedom "to such limits prescribed by law as can be demonstrably justified in a free and democratic society," a standard the Court concluded that the Canadian criminal statute met. In *Butler* (and in *Keegstra*), moreover, the Canadian Court accepted (1) the harmful ideology allegedly purveyed by the objected-to material, (2) the harmful acts perhaps encouraged by the material, and (3) harmful acts others fear might be encouraged by the material as satisfying this criterion—that is, as constituting harms the avoidance of which would be "demonstrably justified in free and democratic society." Without doubt, the case is very sharply at odds with *Hudnut,* and several decisions of the U.S. Supreme Court.[111]

More recently, a variation on the question dealt with in *Hudnut* has been addressed in the U.S. Supreme Court, this time, however, in a much more confrontational and physical setting than merely determining what kinds of magazines, films, or books may or may not be prohibited because of the "message" they purvey or the attitude or idea they encourage or tend to reinforce. The case is *R.A.V. v. City of St. Paul.*[112]

---

111. For one (of many) discussions strongly defending the approach adopted in *Regina v. Butler*, however, see Kathleen Mahoney, The Canadian Constitutional Approach to Freedom of Expression in Hate Propaganda and Pornography, 55 Law & Contemp.Probs. 77 (Winter 1992).

112. *R.A.V. v. City of St. Paul*, while very much related to the issues reviewed in *Hudnut*, is complicated by facts raising additional questions about "symbolic" speech (in this instance, burning a cross). It might for that reason be more appropriately considered at p. 326 of the casebook rather than here (pp. 246-292 deal directly with issues of symbolic speech). It also deals with issues of regulations of "time, place, and manner" (p. 387), as well as the doctrine pursuant to which so-called "fighting words" are sometimes said to be excluded from first amendment review (p. 726).

R.A.V. v. CITY OF ST. PAUL
505 U.S. 377 (1992)

JUSTICE SCALIA delivered the opinion of the Court.

In the predawn hours of June 21, 1990, petitioner and several other teenagers allegedly assembled a crudely-made cross by taping together broken chair legs. They then allegedly burned the cross inside the fenced yard of a black family that lived across the street from the house where petitioner was staying. Although this conduct could have been punished under any of a number of laws,[1] one of the two provisions under which respondent city of St. Paul chose to charge petitioner (then a juvenile) was the St. Paul Bias-Motivated Crime Ordinance, which provides:

> Whoever places on public or private property a symbol, object, appellation, characterization or graffiti, including, but not limited to, a burning cross or Nazi swastika, which one knows or has reasonable grounds to know arouses anger, alarm or resentment in others on the basis of race, color, creed, religion or gender commits disorderly conduct and shall be guilty of a misdemeanor.

Petitioner moved to dismiss this count on the ground that the ordinance was substantially overbroad and impermissibly content-based and therefore facially invalid under the First Amendment. The Minnesota Supreme Court rejected petitioner's overbreadth claim because, the modifying phrase "arouses anger, alarm or resentment in others" limited the reach of the ordinance to conduct that amounts to "fighting words," *i.e.*, "conduct that itself inflicts injury or tends to incite immediate violence," and therefore the ordinance reached only expression "that the first amendment does not protect." We granted certiorari.

I

In construing the St. Paul ordinance, we are bound by the construction given to it by the Minnesota court. [W]e accept the Minnesota Supreme Court's authoritative statement that the ordinance reaches only those expressions that constitute "fighting words" within the meaning of *Chaplinsky*. Petitioner and his *amici* urge us to modify the scope of the *Chaplinsky* formulation, thereby invalidating the ordinance as "substantially overbroad," Broadrick v. Oklahoma, 413 U.S. 601, 610 (1973). We find it unnecessary to consider this issue. Assuming, *arguendo*, that all of the expression reached by the ordinance is proscribable under the "fighting words" doctrine, we nonetheless conclude that the ordinance is facially unconstitutional in

---

1. The conduct might have violated Minnesota statutes carrying significant penalties. See, e.g., Minn. Stat. § 609.713(1) (1987) (providing for up to five years in prison for terroristic threats); § 609.563 (arson) (providing for up to five years and a $10,000 fine, depending on the value of the property intended to be damaged); § 606.595 (Supp. 1992) (criminal damage to property) (providing for up to one year and a $3,000 fine, depending upon the extent of the damage to the property).

that it prohibits otherwise permitted speech solely on the basis of the subjects the speech addresses.

The First Amendment generally prevents government from proscribing speech, see, *e.g.*, Cantwell v. Connecticut, 310 U.S. 296, 309-311 (1940), or even expressive conduct, see, *e.g.*, Texas v. Johnson, 491 U.S. 397, 406 (1989), because of disapproval of the ideas expressed. Content-based regulations are presumptively invalid. From 1791 to the present, however, our society, like other free but civilized societies, has permitted restrictions upon the content of speech in a few limited areas, which are "of such slight social value as a step to truth that any benefit that may be derived from them is clearly outweighed by the social interest in order and morality." *** See, *e.g.*, Roth v. United States, 354 U.S. 476 (1957) (obscenity); Beauharnais v. Illinois, 343 U.S. 250 (1952) (defamation); *Chaplinsky v. New Hampshire*, *supra*, ("fighting words"). Our decisions since the 1960's have narrowed the scope of the traditional categorical exceptions for defamation, see New York Times Co. v. Sullivan, 376 U.S. 254 (1964) and for obscenity, see Miller v. California, 413 U.S. 15 (1973), but a limited categorical approach has remained an important part of our First Amendment jurisprudence.

We have sometimes said that these categories of expression are "not within the area of constitutionally protected speech," or that the "protection of the First Amendment does not extend" to them. Such statements must be taken in context, however, and are no more literally true than is the occasionally repeated shorthand characterizing obscenity "as not being speech at all," Sunstein, Pornography and the First Amendment, 1986 Duke L.J. 589, 615, n.146. What they mean is that these areas of speech can, consistently with the First Amendment, be regulated because of their constitutionally proscribable content (obscenity, defamation, etc.)—not that they are categories of speech entirely invisible to the Constitution, so that they may be made the vehicles for content discrimination unrelated to their distinctively proscribable content. Thus, the government may proscribe libel; but it may not make the further content discrimination of proscribing only libel critical of the government. ***

Our cases surely do not establish the proposition that the First Amendment imposes no obstacle whatsoever to regulation of particular instances of such proscribable expression, so that the government "may regulate [them] freely" *** (WHITE, J., concurring in judgment [*infra*]). That would mean that a city council could enact an ordinance prohibiting only those legally obscene works that contain criticism of the city government or, indeed, that do not include endorsement of the city government. Such a simplistic, all-or-nothing-at-all approach to First Amendment protection is at odds with common sense and with our jurisprudence as well.[4]

---

4. JUSTICE WHITE concedes that a city council cannot prohibit only those legally obscene works that contain criticism of the city government *** but asserts that to be the consequence, not of the First Amendment, but of the Equal Protection Clause. Such content-based discrimination would not, he asserts, "be rationally related to a legitimate government interest." But of course the only *reason* that

It is not true that "fighting words" have at most a "*de minimis*" expressive content, or that their content is in all respects "worthless and undeserving of constitutional protection." [S]ometimes they are quite expressive indeed. We have not said that they constitute "no part of the expression of ideas," but only that they constitute "no *essential* part of any exposition of ideas." *Chaplinsky*, 315 U.S., at 572 (emphasis added).

The concurrences describe us as setting forth a new First Amendment principle that prohibition of constitutionally proscribable speech cannot be "underinclusiv[e]" (WHITE, J., concurring in judgment), a First Amendment "absolutism" whereby "within a particular 'proscribable' category of expression, a government must either proscribe *all* speech or no speech at all" (STEVENS, J., concurring in judgment). That easy target is of the concurrences' own invention. In our view, the First Amendment imposes not an "underinclusiveness" limitation but a "content discrimination" limitation upon a State's prohibition of proscribable speech. There is no problem whatever, for example, with a State's prohibiting obscenity (and other forms of proscribable expression) only in certain media or markets, for although that prohibition would be "underinclusive," it would not discriminate on the basis of content. *** A State might choose to prohibit only that obscenity which is the most patently offensive *in its prurience*—i.e., that which involves the most lascivious displays of sexual activity. But it may not prohibit, for example, only that obscenity which includes offensive *political* messages. ***

Another valid basis for according differential treatment to even a content-defined subclass of proscribable speech is that the subclass happens to be associated with particular "secondary effects" of the speech, so that the regulation is "*justified* without reference to the content of the speech," Renton v. Playtime Theatres, Inc., 475 U.S. 41, 48 (1986). A State could, for example, permit all obscene live performances except those involving minors. Moreover, since words can in some circumstances violate laws directed not against speech but against conduct (a law against treason, for example, is violated by telling the enemy the nation's defense secrets),

---

government interest is not a "legitimate" one is that it violates the First Amendment. This Court itself has occasionally fused the First Amendment into the Equal Protection Clause in this fashion, but at least with the acknowledgment (which JUSTICE WHITE cannot afford to make) that the First Amendment underlies its analysis. See Police Dept. of Chicago v. Mosley, 408 U.S. 92, 95 (1972) (ordinance prohibiting only nonlabor picketing violated the Equal Protection Clause because there was no "appropriate governmental interest" supporting the distinction inasmuch as "the First Amendment means that government has no power to restrict expression because of its message, its ideas, its subject matter, or its content") ***.

JUSTICE STEVENS seeks to avoid the point by dismissing the notion of obscene anti-government speech as "fantastical," *** apparently believing that any reference to politics prevents a finding of obscenity. Unfortunately for the purveyors of obscenity, that is obviously false. A shockingly hard core pornographic movie that contains a model sporting a political tattoo can be found, "*taken as* a *whole* [to] lac[k] *serious* literary, artistic, political, or scientific value," Miller v. California, 413 U.S. 15, 24 (1973) (emphasis added). *** And of course the concept of racist fighting words is, unfortunately, anything but a "highly speculative hypothetica[l]" ***.

a particular content-based subcategory of a proscribable class of speech can be swept up incidentally within the reach of a statute directed at conduct rather than speech. Thus, for example, sexually derogatory "fighting words," among other words, may produce a violation of Title VII's general prohibition against sexual discrimination in employment practices. ***

II

Applying these principles to the St. Paul ordinance, we conclude that, even as narrowly construed by the Minnesota Supreme Court, the ordinance is facially unconstitutional. Those who wish to use "fighting words" in connection with other ideas —to express hostility, for example, on the basis of political affiliation, union membership, or homosexuality—are not covered. The First Amendment does not permit St. Paul to impose special prohibitions on those speakers who express views on disfavored subjects.

In its practical operation, moreover, the ordinance goes even beyond mere content discrimination, to actual viewpoint discrimination. Displays containing some words—odious racial epithets, for example—would be prohibited to proponents of all views. But "fighting words" that do not themselves invoke race, color, creed, religion, or gender—aspersions upon a person's mother, for example—would seemingly be usable *ad libitum* in the placards of those arguing *in favor of* racial, color, etc. tolerance and equality, but could not be used by that speaker's opponents. One could hold up a sign saying, for example, that all "anti-Catholic bigots" are misbegotten; but not that all "papists" are, for that would insult and provoke violence "on the basis of religion." St. Paul has no such authority to license one side of a debate to fight freestyle, while requiring the other to follow Marquis of Queensbury Rules.

What we have here, it must be emphasized, is not a prohibition of fighting words that are directed at certain persons or groups (which would be *facially* valid if it met the requirements of the Equal Protection Clause); but rather, a prohibition of fighting words that contain (as the Minnesota Supreme Court repeatedly emphasized) messages of "bias-motivated" hatred and in particular, as applied to this case, messages "based on virulent notions of racial supremacy." One must wholeheartedly agree with the Minnesota Supreme Court that "[i]t is the responsibility, even the obligation, of diverse communities to confront such notions in whatever form they appear," but the manner of that confrontation cannot consist of selective limitations upon speech. St. Paul's brief asserts that a general "fighting words" law would not meet the city's needs because only a content-specific measure can communicate to minority groups that the "group hatred" aspect of such speech "is not condoned by the majority." *** The point of the First Amendment is that majority preferences must be expressed in some fashion other than silencing speech on the basis of its content.

Despite the fact that the Minnesota Supreme Court and St. Paul acknowledge that the ordinance is directed at expression of group hatred, JUSTICE STEVENS suggests that this "fundamentally misreads" the ordinance. *** It is directed, he claims, not to speech of a particular content, but to particular "injur[ies]" that are "qualitatively different" from other injuries. This is word-play. What makes the anger, fear, sense of dishonor, etc. produced by violation of this ordinance distinct from the anger, fear, sense of dishonor, etc. produced by other fighting words is nothing other than the fact that it is caused by a distinctive idea, conveyed by a distinctive message. Indeed, St. Paul argued in the Juvenile Court that "[t]he burning of a cross does express a message and it is, in fact, the content of that message which the St. Paul Ordinance attempts to legislate." ***

The content-based discrimination reflected in the St. Paul ordinance comes within neither any of the specific exceptions to the First Amendment prohibition we discussed earlier, nor within a more general exception for content discrimination that does not threaten censorship of ideas. It assuredly does not fall within the exception for content discrimination based on the very reasons why the particular class of speech at issue (here, fighting words) is proscribable. As explained earlier *** the reason why fighting words are categorically excluded from the protection of the First Amendment is not that their content communicates any particular idea, but that their content embodies a particularly intolerable (and socially unnecessary) *mode* of expressing *whatever* idea the speaker wishes to convey. St. Paul has not singled out an especially offensive mode of expression—it has not, for example, selected for prohibition only those fighting words that communicate ideas in a threatening (as opposed to a merely obnoxious) manner. Rather, it has proscribed fighting words of whatever manner that communicate messages of racial, gender, or religious intolerance. Selectivity of this sort creates the possibility that the city is seeking to handicap the expression of particular ideas. That possibility would alone be enough to render the ordinance presumptively invalid, but St. Paul's comments and concessions in this case elevate the possibility to a certainty. ***

Finally, St. Paul and its *amici* assert that the ordinance helps to ensure the basic human rights of members of groups that have historically been subjected to discrimination, including the right of such group members to live in peace where they wish. The existence of adequate content-neutral alternatives "undercut[s] significantly" any defense of such a statute, [and] cast[s] considerable doubt on the government's protestations that "the asserted justification is in fact an accurate description of the purpose and effect of the law." In fact the only interest distinctively served by the content limitation is that of displaying the city council's special hostility towards the particular biases thus singled out. That is precisely what the First Amendment forbids. The politicians of St. Paul are entitled to express that hostility-but not through the means of imposing unique limitations upon speakers who (however benightedly) disagree. ***

The judgment of the Minnesota Supreme Court is reversed, and the case is remanded for proceedings not inconsistent with this opinion.

JUSTICE WHITE, with whom JUSTICE BLACKMUN and JUSTICE O'CONNOR join, and with whom JUSTICE STEVENS joins except as to Part I(A), concurring in the judgment.

I agree with the majority that the judgment of the Minnesota Supreme Court should be reversed. However, our agreement ends there.

This case could easily be decided within the contours of established First Amendment law by holding, as petitioner argues, that the St. Paul ordinance is fatally overbroad because it criminalizes not only unprotected expression but expression protected by the First Amendment. *** Instead, the Court holds the ordinance facially unconstitutional on a ground that was never presented to the Minnesota Supreme Court. This is hardly a judicious way of proceeding, and the Court's reasoning in reaching its result is transparently wrong.

I (A)

This Court's decisions have plainly stated that expression falling within certain limited categories so lacks the values the First Amendment was designed to protect that the Constitution affords no protection to that expression.

*** Nevertheless, the majority holds that the First Amendment protects those narrow categories of expression long held to be undeserving of First Amendment protection—at least to the extent that lawmakers may not regulate some fighting words more strictly than others because of their content. The Court announces that such content-based distinctions violate the First Amendment because "the government may not regulate use based on hostility—or favoritism—towards the underlying message expressed." Should the government want to criminalize certain fighting words, the Court now requires it to criminalize all fighting words. ***

The majority's observation that fighting words are "quite expressive indeed" is no answer. Fighting words are not a means of exchanging views, rallying supporters, or registering a protest; they are directed against individuals to provoke violence or to inflict injury. *Chaplinsky*, 315 U.S., at 572. Therefore, a ban on all fighting words or on a subset of the fighting words category would restrict only the social evil of hate speech, without creating the danger of driving viewpoints from the marketplace. ***

Therefore, the Court's insistence on inventing its brand of First Amendment underinclusiveness puzzles me. *** Instead, it permits, indeed invites, the continuation of expressive conduct that in this case is evil and worthless in First Amendment terms until the city of St. Paul cures the underbreadth by adding to its ordinance a catch-all phrase such as "and all other fighting words that may constitutionally be subject to this ordinance." *** By placing fighting words, which the Court has long held to be valueless, on at least equal constitutional footing with political discourse and other forms of speech that we have deemed to have the greatest social value, the majority devalues the latter category.***

B

***

Although the First Amendment does not apply to categories of unprotected speech, such as fighting words, the Equal Protection Clause requires that the regulation of unprotected speech be rationally related to a legitimate government interest. A defamation statute that drew distinctions on the basis of political affiliation or "an ordinance prohibiting only those legally obscene works that contain criticism of the city government" *** would unquestionably fail rational basis review.[9]

Turning to the St. Paul ordinance and assuming *arguendo*, as the majority does, that the ordinance is not constitutionally overbroad (but see Part II, *infra*), there is no question that it would pass equal protection review. The ordinance proscribes a subset of "fighting words," those that injure "on the basis of race, color, creed, religion or gender." This selective regulation reflects the City's judgment that harms based on race, color, creed, religion, or gender are more pressing public concerns than the harms caused by other fighting words. In light of our Nation's long and painful experience with discrimination, this determination is plainly reasonable. Indeed, as the majority concedes, the interest is compelling. ***

II

Although I disagree with the Court's analysis, I do agree with its conclusion: The St. Paul ordinance is unconstitutional. However, I would decide the case on overbreadth grounds.

In construing the St. Paul ordinance, the Minnesota Supreme Court drew upon the definition of fighting words that appears in *Chaplinsky*—words "which by their very utterance inflict injury or tend to incite an immediate breach of the peace." However, the Minnesota court was far from clear in identifying the "injur[ies]" inflicted by the expression that St. Paul sought to regulate. Indeed, the Minnesota court emphasized (tracking the language of the ordinance) that "the ordinance censors only those displays that one knows or should know will create anger, alarm or resentment based on racial, ethnic, gender or religious bias." I therefore understand the court to have ruled that St. Paul may constitutionally prohibit expression that "by its very utterance" causes "anger, alarm or resentment."

Our fighting words cases have made clear, however, that such generalized reactions are not sufficient to strip expression of its constitutional protection. The mere fact that expressive activity causes hurt feelings, offense, or resentment does not render the expression unprotected.***

---

9. The majority is mistaken in stating that a ban on obscene works critical of government would fail equal protection review only because the ban would violate the First Amendment. While such decisions as *Police of Chicago v. Mosley*, 408 U.S. 92 (1972), recognize that First Amendment principles may be relevant to an equal protection claim challenging distinctions that impact on protected expression, there is no basis for linking First and Fourteenth Amendment analysis in a case involving unprotected expression. Certainly, one need not resort to First Amendment principles to conclude that the sort of improbable legislation the majority hypothesizes is based on senseless distinctions.

In the First Amendment context, "[c]riminal statutes must be scrutinized with particular care; those that make unlawful a substantial amount of constitutionally protected conduct may be held facially invalid even if they also have legitimate application." Houston v. Hill, 482 U.S. 451, 459 (1987). The St. Paul antibias ordinance is such a law. Although the ordinance reaches conduct that is unprotected, it also makes criminal expressive conduct that causes only hurt feelings, offense, or resentment, and is protected by the First Amendment.[13] The ordinance is therefore fatally overbroad and invalid on its face.

JUSTICE BLACKMUN, concurring in the judgment. [Omitted.]

JUSTICE STEVENS, with whom JUSTICE WHITE and JUSTICE BLACKMUN join as to Part I, concurring in the judgment.

*** [W]hile I agree that the St. Paul ordinance is unconstitutionally overbroad for the reasons stated in Part II of JUSTICE WHITE's opinion, I write separately to suggest how the allure of absolute principles has skewed the analysis of both the majority and concurring opinions.

I

***

Although the Court has, on occasion, declared that content-based regulations of speech are "never permitted," Police Dept. of Chicago v. Mosley, 408 U.S. 92, 99 (1972), such claims are overstated. Indeed, in *Mosley* itself, the Court indicated that Chicago's selective proscription of nonlabor picketing was not *per se* unconstitutional, but rather could be upheld if the City demonstrated that nonlabor picketing was "clearly more disruptive than [labor] picketing." *** Precisely this same reasoning, however, compels the conclusion that St. Paul's ordinance is constitutional. Just as Congress may determine that threats against the President entail more severe consequences than other threats, so St. Paul's City Council may determine that threats based on the target's race, religion, or gender cause more severe harm to both the target and to society than other threats. This latter judgment—that harms caused by racial, religious, and gender-based invective are qualitatively different from that caused by other fighting words—seems to me eminently reasonable and realistic.***

---

13. Although the First Amendment protects offensive speech, *Johnson v. Texas*, 491 U.S., at 414, it does not require us to be subjected to such expression at all times, in all settings. We have held that such expression may be proscribed when it intrudes upon a "captive audience." Frisby v. Schultz, 487 U.S. 474, 484-485 (1988); FCC v. Pacifica Foundation, 438 U.S. 726, 748-749 (1978). And expression may be limited when it merges into conduct. United States v. O'Brien, 391 U.S. 367 (1968); cf. Meritor Savings Bank v. Vinson, 477 U.S. 57, 65 (1986). However, because of the manner in which the Minnesota Supreme Court construed the St. Paul ordinance, those issues are not before us in this case.

II

Although I agree with much of JUSTICE WHITE's analysis, I do not join Part I-A of his opinion because I have reservations about the "categorical approach" to the First Amendment. Admittedly, the categorical approach to the First Amendment has some appeal: either expression is protected or it is not—the categories create safe harbors for governments and speakers alike. But this approach sacrifices subtlety for clarity and is, I am convinced, ultimately unsound. As an initial matter, the concept of "categories" fits poorly with the complex reality of expression. Few dividing lines in First Amendment law are straight and unwavering, and efforts at categorization inevitably give rise only to fuzzy boundaries. The quest for doctrinal certainty through the definition of categories and subcategories is, in my opinion, destined to fail. [T]he categorical approach does not take seriously the importance of *context.* The meaning of any expression and the legitimacy of its regulation can only be determined in context. Whether, for example, a picture or a sentence is obscene cannot be judged in the abstract, but rather only in the context of its setting, its use, and its audience. ***

III

***

Looking to the context of the regulated activity, it is again significant that the statute (by hypothesis) regulates *only* fighting words. Whether words are fighting words is determined in part by their context. Fighting words are not words that merely cause offense; fighting words must be directed at individuals so as to "by their very utterance inflict injury." By hypothesis, then, the St. Paul ordinance restricts speech in confrontational and potentially violent situations. The case at hand is illustrative. The cross-burning in this case—directed as it was to a single African-American family trapped in their home—was nothing more than a crude form of physical intimidation.

The St. Paul ordinance is evenhanded. In a battle between advocates of tolerance and advocates of intolerance, the ordinance does not prevent either side from hurling fighting words at the other on the basis of their conflicting ideas, but it does bar *both* sides from hurling such words on the basis of the target's "race, color, creed, religion or gender." *** It does not, therefore, favor one side of any debate.

Finally, it is noteworthy that the St. Paul ordinance is, as construed by the Court today, quite narrow. The St. Paul ordinance does not ban all "hate speech," nor does it ban, say, all cross-burnings or all swastika displays. Rather it only bans a subcategory of the already narrow category of fighting words. Such a limited ordinance leaves open and protected a vast range of expression on the subjects of racial, religious, and gender equality. As construed by the Court today, the ordinance certainly does not "'raise the specter that the Government may effectively drive certain ideas or viewpoints from the marketplace.'" *** Petitioner is free to burn a cross to announce a rally or to express his views about racial supremacy, he may do so on private property or public land, at day or at night, so long as the burning is not so threatening and so directed at an individual as to "by its very [execution] inflict injury." Such a limited proscription scarcely offends the First Amendment. *** Thus, were the ordinance not overbroad, I would vote to uphold it.

WISCONSIN v. MITCHELL

508 U.S. 476 (1993)

CHIEF JUSTICE REHNQUIST delivered the opinion of the Court.

Respondent Todd Mitchell's sentence for aggravated battery was enhanced because he intentionally selected his victim on account of the victim's race. The question presented in this case is whether this penalty enhancement is prohibited by the First and Fourteenth Amendments. We hold that it is not.

On the evening of October 7, 1989, a group of young black men and boys, including Mitchell, gathered at an apartment complex in Kenosha, Wisconsin. Several members of the group discussed a scene from the motion picture "Mississippi Burning," in which a white man beat a young black boy who was praying. The group moved outside and Mitchell asked them: "'Do you all feel hyped up to move on some white people?'" *** Shortly thereafter, a young white boy approached the group on the opposite side of the street where they were standing. As the boy walked by, Mitchell said: "'You all want to fuck somebody up? There goes a white boy; go get him.'" *** Mitchell counted to three and pointed in the boy's direction. The group ran towards the boy, beat him severely, and stole his tennis shoes. The boy was rendered unconscious and remained in a coma for four days.

After a jury trial in the Circuit Court for Kenosha County, Mitchell was convicted of aggravated battery. That offense ordinarily carries a maximum sentence of two years' imprisonment. But because the jury found that Mitchell had intentionally selected his victim because of the boy's race, the maximum sentence for Mitchell's offense was increased to seven years under § 939.645. That provision enhances the maximum penalty for an offense whenever the defendant "[i]ntentionally selects the person against whom the crime is committed because of the race, religion, color, disability, sexual orientation, national origin or ancestry of that person. ***" The Circuit Court sentenced Mitchell to four years' imprisonment for the aggravated battery.

Mitchell unsuccessfully sought postconviction relief in the Circuit Court. Then he appealed his conviction and sentence, challenging the constitutionality of Wisconsin's penalty-enhancement provision on First Amendment grounds.[2] The Wisconsin

---

2. Mitchell also challenged the statute on Fourteenth Amendment equal protection and vagueness grounds. The Wisconsin Court of Appeals held that Mitchell waived his equal protection claim and rejected his vagueness challenge outright. The Wisconsin Supreme Court declined to address both claims. Mitchell renews his Fourteenth Amendment claims in this Court. But since they were not developed below and plainly fall outside of the question on which we granted

Court of Appeals rejected Mitchell's challenge, but the Wisconsin Supreme Court reversed. The Supreme Court held that the statute "violates the First Amendment directly by punishing what the legislature has deemed to be offensive thought." According to the court, "[t]he statute punishes the 'because of' aspect of the defendant's selection, the *reason* the defendant selected the *victim*, the motive behind the selection." And under R. A. V. v. St. Paul, 505 U.S. [377] (1992), "the Wisconsin legislature cannot criminalize bigoted thought with which it disagrees."

The Supreme Court also held that the penalty-enhancement statute was unconstitutionally overbroad. It reasoned that, in order to prove that a defendant intentionally selected his victim because of the victim's protected status, the State would often have to introduce evidence of the defendant's prior speech, such as racial epithets he may have uttered before the commission of the offense. This evidentiary use of protected speech, the court thought, would have a "chilling effect" on those who feared the possibility of prosecution for offenses subject to penalty enhancement. Finally, the court distinguished antidiscrimination laws, which have long been held constitutional, on the ground that the Wisconsin statute punishes the "subjective mental process" of selecting a victim because of his protected status, whereas antidiscrimination laws prohibit "objective acts of discrimination."

***

The State argues that the statute does not punish bigoted thought, as the Supreme Court of Wisconsin said, but instead punishes only conduct. While this argument is literally correct, it does not dispose of Mitchell's First Amendment challenge. To be sure, our cases reject the "view that an apparently limitless variety of conduct can be labeled 'speech' whenever the person engaging in the conduct intends thereby to express an idea." United States v. O'Brien, 391 U.S. 367, 376 (1968). Thus, a physical assault is not by any stretch of the imagination expressive conduct protected by the First Amendment.***

But the fact remains that under the Wisconsin statute the same criminal conduct may be more heavily punished if the victim is selected because of his race or other protected status than if no such motive obtained. Thus, although the statute punishes criminal conduct, it enhances the maximum penalty for conduct motivated by a discriminatory point of view more severely than the same conduct engaged in for some other reason or for no reason at all. Because the only reason for the enhancement is the defendant's discriminatory motive for selecting his victim, Mitchell argues (and the Wisconsin Supreme Court held) that the statute violates the First Amendment by punishing offenders' bigoted beliefs.

Traditionally, sentencing judges have considered a wide variety of factors in addition to evidence bearing on guilt in determining what sentence to impose on a convicted defendant. The defendant's motive for committing the offense is one important factor. See 1 W. LeFave & A. Scott, Substantive Criminal Law § 3.6(b),

---

certiorari, we do not reach them either.

p. 324 (1986) ("Motives are most relevant when the trial judge sets the defendant's sentence, and it is not uncommon for a defendant to receive a minimum sentence because he was acting with good motives, or a rather high sentence because of his bad motives"). Thus, in many States the commission of a murder, or other capital offense, for pecuniary gain is a separate aggravating circumstance under the capital-sentencing statute.

But it is equally true that a defendant's abstract beliefs, however obnoxious to most people, may not be taken into consideration by a sentencing judge. Dawson v. Delaware, 503 U.S. 159 (1992). In *Dawson*, the State introduced evidence at a capital-sentencing hearing that the defendant was a member of a white supremacist prison gang. Because "the evidence proved nothing more than [the defendant's] abstract beliefs," we held that its admission violated the defendant's First Amendment rights. In so holding, however, we emphasized that "the Constitution does not erect a *per se* barrier to the admission of evidence concerning one's beliefs and associations at sentencing simply because those beliefs and associations are protected by the First Amendment." Thus, in Barclay v. Florida, 463 U.S. 939 (1983) (plurality opinion), we allowed the sentencing judge to take into account the defendant's racial animus towards his victim. The evidence in that case showed that the defendant's membership in the Black Liberation Army and desire to provoke a "race war" were related to the murder of a white man for which he was convicted. Because "the elements of racial hatred in [the] murder" were relevant to several aggravating factors, we held that the trial judge permissibly took this evidence into account in sentencing the defendant to death.***

Mitchell suggests that *Dawson* and *Barclay* are inapposite because they did not involve application of a penalty-enhancement provision. But in *Barclay* we held that it was permissible for the sentencing court to consider the defendant's racial animus in determining whether he should be sentenced to death, surely the most severe "enhancement" of all. And the fact that the Wisconsin Legislature has decided, as a general matter, that bias-motivated offenses warrant greater maximum penalties across the board does not alter the result here. For the primary responsibility for fixing criminal penalties lies with the legislature. ***

Mitchell argues that the Wisconsin penalty-enhancement statute is invalid because it punishes the defendant's discriminatory motive, or reason, for acting. But motive plays the same role under the Wisconsin statute as it does under federal and state antidiscrimination laws, which we have previously upheld against constitutional challenge. Title VII, for example, makes it unlawful for an employer to discriminate against an employee "*because of* such individual's race, color, religion, sex, or national origin." And more recently, in *R.A.V. v. St. Paul*, 505 U.S., at 377 (1992), we cited Title VII (as well as 18 U.S.C. § 242 and 42 U.S.C. §§ 1981 and 1982) as an example of a permissible content- neutral regulation of conduct.

Nothing in our decision last Term in *R.A.V.* compels a different result here. [W]hereas the ordinance struck down in *R.A.V.* was explicitly directed at expression (*i.e.*, "speech" or "messages)," the statute in this case is aimed at conduct unprotected by the First Amendment.

Moreover, the Wisconsin statute singles out for enhancement bias-inspired conduct because this conduct is thought to inflict greater individual and societal harm. For example, according to the State and its *amici*, bias-motivated crimes are more likely to provoke retaliatory crimes, inflict distinct emotional harms on their victims, and incite community unrest. The State's desire to redress these perceived harms provides an adequate explanation for its penalty-enhancement provision over and above mere disagreement with offenders' beliefs or biases.

Finally, there remains to be considered Mitchell's argument that the Wisconsin statute is unconstitutionally overbroad because of its "chilling effect" on free speech. Mitchell argues (and the Wisconsin Supreme Court agreed) that the statute is "overbroad" because evidence of the defendant's prior speech or associations may be used to prove that the defendant intentionally selected his victim on account of the victim's protected status. Consequently, the argument goes, the statute impermissibly chills free expression with respect to such matters by those concerned about the possibility of enhanced sentences if they should in the future commit a criminal offense covered by the statute. We find no merit in this contention.

The First Amendment, does not prohibit the evidentiary use of speech to establish the elements of a crime or to prove motive or intent. Evidence of a defendant's previous declarations or statements is commonly admitted in criminal trials subject to evidentiary rules dealing with relevancy, reliability, and the like. Nearly half a century ago, in Haupt v. United States, 330 U.S. 631 (1947), we rejected a contention similar to that advanced by Mitchell here. Haupt was tried for the offense of treason, which, as defined by the Constitution (Art. III, § 3), may depend very much on proof of motive. To prove that the acts in question were committed out of "adherence to the enemy" rather than "parental solicitude," the Government introduced evidence of conversations that had taken place long prior to the indictment, some of which consisted of statements showing Haupt's sympathy with Germany and Hitler and hostility towards the United States. ***

For the foregoing reasons, we hold that Mitchell's First Amendment rights were not violated by the application of the Wisconsin penalty-enhancement provision in sentencing him. The judgment of the Supreme Court of Wisconsin is therefore reversed, and the case is remanded for further proceedings not inconsistent with this opinion.

It is so ordered.

NOTES ON *MITCHELL* AND *R.A.V.*

1. In *Mitchell*, the Court distinguished the Wisconsin statute from the St. Paul Ordinance in *R.A.V.* as a special penalty enhancement statute for certain standard criminal offenses. In this respect it may merely resemble other penalty enhancement provisions attached to standard criminal offenses—such as for using a gun. And, just as in this example, as the Court notes, *unlike* the St. Paul ordinance—an ordinance on its face directed to the punishment of "symbol[s], appellation[s], characterization[s] or graffiti, including, but not limited to, a burning cross or Nazi swastika"[113]—the Wisconsin enhanced-penalty statute applied not to speech *at all*.[114] Rather it applied strictly to criminal activity of a common *non-speech* sort (pure physical assault).

2. And insofar as the penalty enhancement provision does indeed apply only when a given criminal offense was pursued in a particular way,[115] it evidently raises no first amendment problem. It has an adequate justification quite akin to other provisions of a like sort. Just as the legislature could treat assaults committed with a gun as more serious than other assaults, so, too, it could reasonably regard racially-targeted assaults as a special problem. In the case of racially-targeted assaults, there is an added dimension appropriate for heightened community concern —a fear that even one or two such incidents may trigger retaliatory assaults of a like sort, setting off a ripple effect, or even a wave. In contrast, even the most serious sort of "ordinary" street mugging, while doubtless an occasion for serious concern, will not ordinarily carry potential for this kind of polarization and calamity. The special hazard to the community, the very kind of hazard historically associated with racially-targeted assaults, may reasonably impress the legislature with the need to deal with them with special measures, which is exactly—and [allegedly] all—that the Wisconsin legislature has presumed to do. There is no denial of equal protection in

---

113. All of which are forms of speech (including even a "burning cross" as a "symbol").

114. Note—as confirming evidence—that whether the statute applies or does not apply does *not* turn on whether the defendants did or did not address *any* "hate words," or *any* "fighting words," or *any* other opprobrious epithets to the person whom they assaulted (so in this regard the "plus" part of the sentence imposed on them is in *no* respect a "plus" punishment for any aggravating speech of a certain kind). Note in *Mitchell* itself, the report of the case by the Court does not say whether the defendants even spoke to the boy whom they assaulted, but clearly the statute applied to them, whether they did or did not declare to him why he was singled out. Note, likewise, that had the youngster whom the defendants beat so badly *not* been singled out on racial grounds, moreover, the defendants' punishment could not have exceeded two years, no matter how vile, or how additionally devastating, the character of racial epithets they may have expressed at the time, and no matter what they thought about "whites." See also Florida v. Stalder, 630 So.2d 1072 (Fla. 1994) (if A beats B savagely because of jealousy, in the course of which he calls B a racially derogatory name—held, a "hate crime" penalty-enhancement statute would not *apply*).

115. Namely, when pursued by "intentionally select[ing] the person against whom the crime is [to be] committed *** because of [that person's] race, religion, color, disability, sexual orientation, national origin or ancestry."

the provision made by the statute.[116] Neither does it direct itself in any way to what one says as such (rather it deals solely with what one does).[117] Accordingly, application of the statute turns solely on what the defendant did (intentionally selecting the person to be assaulted because of his race, and assaulting him) and nothing more.[118]

---

116. It does not, for instance, presume to make a racially-targeted assault specially punishable only when committed against a white person, but not specially punishable otherwise (e.g., when it is a racial minority person who is singled out for attack). Likewise, it does not make a racially-targeted assault specially punishable only when committed by a white person against a (racial) minority person, while yet not treating racially-targeted assaults of white persons as a matter of any equal concern. In this regard, it takes no "ideological sides," in the sense of favoring some persons (by race) for special protection, leaving others to file complaints only under the general statute addressed to criminal assaults.

117. See *supra* p. 242 note 115. See also Jed Rubenfeld, The First Amendment's Purpose, 53 Stan. L. Rev. 767, 784 (2001); Eric J. Grannis, Fighting Words and Fighting Freestyle: The Constitutionality of Penalty Enhancement for Bias Crimes, 93 Colum.L.Rev. 178, 179, 194-98 (1993); *id.* at 184 (noting that "Wisconsin takes the unique approach of addressing not the motivation of the crime [the motive is irrelevant as such under the Wisconsin statute] but the [basis of] selection of the victim"—that what the statute reaches is intentional selection of the victim because of the victim's race—exactly as in ordinary Title VII cases). See also the Court's discussion on this point, 113 S.Ct. at 2196, 2200-02 (defendant's motive plays the same role under the Wisconsin statute as it does under federal anti-discrimination statutes).

118. Contrast with *Mitchell*, New Jersey v. Vawter, 642 A.2d 349 (N.J. 1994). In this case the New Jersey Supreme Court reviewed a conviction and sentence imposed pursuant to a variation on a widely-enacted Anti-Defamation League Model "Hate Crime" Law. As in *Mitchell*, the law provided a harsher punishment for certain property crimes including "vandalism," when committed in a certain way. Here, however, the statute mandated an automatic increased punishment when such vandalism (which ordinarily consists of any malicious acts of damage to private property) involved "defacing or damaging private property *** by placing thereon a symbol *** that exposed another to threats of violence, contempt or hatred on the basis of race, color, creed or religion, including but not limited to a burning cross or Nazi swastika." Here, in contrast to the Wisconsin statute, the New Jersey court observed, the statute mandating the enhanced penalty was triggered by some kind of expression accompanying, or made a part of, the (enhanced) offense. The New Jersey Supreme Court held these special add-on penalties were subject to *R.A.V.* (i.e. they were both subject-matter specific and viewpoint specific as well). Tracking *R.A.V.*, the New Jersey Court observed that "Displays containing abusive invective, no matter how vicious or severe, are permissible [i.e. trigger no special penalties] unless they are addressed to one of the specified disfavored topics [race, color, creed, religion, or gender]." The statute was held void on its face.

Other statutes may of course raise similar problems, including even Title VII as applied to speech as such (as distinct from acts). To the extent that Title VII requires employers to forbid speech "having the *** effect of creating an offensive environment" to others by race, sex, national origin, or ancestry, it may well raise first amendment questions under *Hudnut*, *Cohen*, and *Falwell*, as well as under *R.A.V.*. See, e.g., discussions in Kingsley Browne, Title VII as Censorship: Hostile-Environment Harassment and the First Amendment, 52 Ohio St.L.J. 481 (1991); James H. Fowles, III, Note, Hostile Environments and the First Amendment: What Now After *Harris* and *St. Paul*?, 46 S.C.L.Rev. 471, 486-304 (1995); Marcy Stauss, Sexist Speech in the Workplace, 25 Harv. C.R.-C.L.L. Rev. 1 (1990); Eugene Volokh, Freedom of Speech and Workplace Harassment, 39 U.C.L.A. L.Rev. 1791 (1992).

May campus speech codes, including those closely modeled on the EEOC guidelines (originally adopted in reference to employers but currently applicable also under Titles VI and IX of the same act

3. May *Mitchell* nonetheless be less easy than it would seem? It is true that the defendant is not punished on account of what he says—whether to, or about, the person he assaults (and whether in scurrilous rather than nonscurrilous terms),[119] but is it true that he is not being punished for his beliefs (or, if he is, that it is not a matter of any first amendment concern)?[120]

4. That question to one side, moreover, may the explanation we have briefly reviewed (so to sustain the Wisconsin statute as but an interesting but constitutionally unproblematic variation of an otherwise standard "mere nondiscrimination" law) seem a bit incomplete (or facile) in light of *R.A.V.*? May the law seem oddly preferential in its concerns, such as they are alleged to be, even in terms of its own rationale? Note the categories of victim selection not covered by the statute (as well as those that are). How does the selection fit the overall alleged rationale?[121]

---

to universities receiving any federal assistance) likewise do so? For some preliminary (suggestive but inconclusive) lower federal court responses, see Dambrot v. Central Mich. Univ., 839 F.Supp. 477 (E.D. Mich. 1993), aff'd 1995 WL 328470 (6th Cir., June 5, 1995); Doe v. University of Mich. 721 F.Supp. 852 (E.D. Mich. 1989). For further reading, compare Richard Delgado, Campus Antiracism Rules: Constitutional Narratives in Collision, 85 Nw. U. L. Rev. 343 (1991); Charles Lawrence, If He Hollers Let Him Go: On Regulating Racist Speech on Campus, 1990 Duke L.J. 431; Mari Matsuda, Public Response to Racist Speech: Considering the Victim's Story, 87 Mich.L. Rev. 2320 (1989); and Steven H. Shiffrin, Racist Speech, Outsider Jurisprudence and the Meaning of America, 80 Cornell L.Rev. 43 (1994), with Gerald Gunther, Good Speech, Bad Speech—Should Universities Restrict Expression That Is Racist or Otherwise Denigrating? No, 24 Stan.L.Rev. 7 (Spring 1990); Nadine Strossen, Regulating Racist Speech on Campus: A Modest Proposal? 1990 Duke L.J. 484; and William Van Alstyne, The University in the Manner of Tiananmen Square, 21 Hastings Const. L.Q. 1 (1993).)

119. It is true, as the Court says, of course, that what he says may be serviceable against him in court (so that in this sense, he is indeed made to "pay" for what he said). But if so, it is so merely because it is relevant to the question, such as it may be, as to why he happened to assault this person rather than some other. Admitting such evidence as may shed light on that question for this purpose is no different than to admit a statement by X to Y as to why X decided not to hire Z (namely, on account of Z's race). The Court's review of the point seems more than adequate to cover any first amendment ground, if this is all. Is it?

120. Note that within the range of sentences available under the ordinary criminal assault, arson, trespass, or other statute applicable to the defendant, the law already takes into account the supposed worst cases—the case warranting an upper range (rather than a middle range or lower range) sentence. How shall the judge treat the defendant's conduct under that statute, before adding on whatever the "enhancement" provision requires? For a useful review of this and other problems with variations on the Wisconsin statute, see Marc Fleisher, Down the Passage Which We Should Not Take: The Folly of Hate Crime Legislation, 2 J.L. & Pol'y 1 (1994).

121. Note that *no* special punishment is to be imposed by this statute when the defendant merely intentionally selects the assault victim "because of" the *sex* of the victim ("sex" is not included, though "sexual orientation" is). Why is that? Likewise note that *no* special punishment is to be added if the defendant merely intentionally selects the person to be assaulted "because of the *age*" of the victim, and so too with "political belief or affiliation." So, in Wisconsin (and other states having a similar law), a man beating a woman unconscious, putting her into the same four day coma as in this case, having targeted her simply as a woman, picked randomly to vent his rage against women, would receive no more than two years in jail, *not* four (as in this case), and *not* seven (as could have been imposed in the case). Similarly, had the defendant randomly selected an elderly person to beat senseless—so to vent

5. As to *R.A.V.* itself, if the Wisconsin Supreme Court had more narrowly confined the statute exactly to mere "fighting words,"[122] why could not the statute, like that in *Mitchell*, also be reasoned as merely reflecting a similar rationale and similarly permissible, legislative choice?

6. Following the Supreme Court's reversal of defendant's conviction under the St. Paul ordinance in *R.A.V.*, suppose the defendant and the other teenagers with whom he acted in concert were indicted for the same acts under the combination of 18 U.S.C. § 241[123] and 42 U.S.C. § 3631.[124] Are they subject to these statutes? Assuming they may be, would the first amendment issues raised in *R.A.V.* be equally applicable here, or are there critical distinctions? If so, what are they? (After considering the matter, see, for this very sequel to *R.A.V.*, United States v. J.H.H., 22 F.3d 821 (8th Cir. 1994).)

7. For a review of recent, widely varying statutes loosely lumped together as "hate crime laws," see Terry Maroney, *The Struggle Against Hate Crimes: Movement at a Crossroads*, 73 N.Y.U. L. Rev. 564, 589-95 (1998). They continue to reflect some of the same problematic qualities previously reviewed in the **NOTES**. Characteristically, they make a special offense, or attach an automatic sentence enhancement to a pre-existing offense, when the defendant commits some act against the person or property of another "because of," or "on account of," some characteristic (or perceived characteristic) of that person, e.g., his or her race, religion, gender, or disability. Typically, the label of these laws suggests the statute proceeds from an intention to deter crimes based on "animus" or "bias" or "prejudice." But the actual link of these statutes as requiring actions taken from "animus" or "bias" or "prejudice" or "hatred" is frequently unclear. Indeed, it may

---

his hatred and contempt of the elderly, two years is also the most he would have received for aggravated assault. (In *Mitchell* itself, therefore, note that had the young boy been picked out and beaten into unconsciousness "just because" defendants found special satisfaction in picking random *children* to kick into unconsciousness, the offense likewise would have been punishable by not more than two years (rather than up to seven). Likewise, persons identified as preferred targets of aggravated assault by force of their political beliefs or affiliation—pacifists, Communists, Neo-Nazis, etc.—trigger no special concern of the Wisconsin law.

122. Evidently it had not succeeded in doing so (in what respect did it fall short?).

123. 18 U.S.C. § 241 provides: "If two or more persons conspire to injure, oppress, threaten, or intimidate any inhabitant of any State *** in the free exercise or enjoyment of any right or privilege secured to him by the Constitution or laws of the United States, or because of his having so exercised the same *** [they shall be guilty of an offense against the United States]."

124. 42 U.S.C. § 3631 provides: "Whoever *** by force or threat of force willfully injures, intimidates or interferes with, or attempts to injure, intimidate or interfere with—(a) any person because of his race, color, religion, sex, handicap *** familial status *** or national origin because he is *** occupying any dwelling *** [shall be guilty of an offense against the United States]."

be nonexistent. For example, § 3A1.1 of the U.S. Sentencing Commission Guidelines Manual now authorizes a three-level sentence increase if the "finder of fact at trial . . . determines beyond a reasonable doubt that the defendant *intentionally selected any victim* or any property . . . *because of* the actual or perceived race, color, religion, national origin, ethnicity, gender, disability, or sexual orientation of that person." (Notice on the face of the guidelines, it is the basis for selecting the "victim" that evidently matters, not why, i.e., evidently, there need be no animus involved — no "hatred" or hostility of any kind.)[126]

D. POLITICS AND "SYMBOLIC" DISSENT

The putative distinction between standard first amendment review and the different applications under *United States v. O'Brien.*

TINKER v. DES MOINES SCHOOL DISTRICT
393 U.S. 503 (1969)

MR. JUSTICE FORTAS delivered the opinion of the Court.

Petitioner John F. Tinker, 15 years old, and petitioner Christopher Eckhardt, 16 years old, attended high schools in Des Moines, Iowa. Petitioner Mary Beth Tinker, John's sister, was a 13-year-old student in junior high school.

In December 1965, a group of adults and students in Des Moines held a meeting at the Eckhardt home. The group determined to publicize their objections to the hostilities in Vietnam and their support for a truce by wearing black armbands during the holiday season and by fasting on December 16 and New Year's Eve. Petitioners and their parents had previously engaged in similar activities, and they decided to participate in the program.

The principals of the Des Moines schools became aware of the plan to wear armbands. On December 14, 1965, they met and adopted a policy that any student wearing an armband to school would be asked to remove it, and if he refused he

126. For example, a well-informed African American man may principally select white victims as preferred "victims" for ordinary street crimes (e.g., muggings), if he knows from experience what studies also confirm: that, in what is but a very brief encounter, such persons may later not be as readily able to recall any special identifying features of their assailants, at least not as well as another black person might be able to do. (Is this a "hate" crime?) For a discussion of problems with federal hate crimes, see Christopher Chorba, *The Danger of Federalizing Hate Crimes: Congressional Misconceptions and the Unintended Consequences of the Hate Crimes Prevention Act*, 87 Va. L.R. 319 (2001); see also Robert J. Corry, Jr., *Burn This Article: It is Evidence in Your Thought Crime Prosecution*, 4 Tex. Rev. L. & Pol. 460 (2000); *Special Issue: Hate Crimes Legislation*, Christopher Heath Wellman (ed.), 20 Law & Phil. 115 (2001); Nadine Strossen, *Incitement to Hatred: Should There Be a Limit*, 25 S. Ill. U.L.V. 243 (2001).

would be suspended until he returned without the armband. Petitioners were aware of the regulation that the school authorities adopted.

On December 16, Mary Beth and Christopher wore black armbands to their schools. John Tinker wore his armband the next day. They were all sent home and suspended from school until they would come back without their armbands. They did not return to school until after the planned period for wearing armbands had expired—that is, until after New Year's Day.

This complaint was filed in the United States District Court by petitioners, through their fathers, under § 1983 of Title 42 of the United States Code. It prayed for an injunction restraining the respondent school officials and the respondent members of the board of directors of the school district from disciplining the petitioners, and it sought nominal damages. After an evidentiary hearing the District Court dismissed the complaint. It upheld the constitutionality of the school authorities' action on the ground that it was reasonable in order to prevent disturbance of school discipline. The court referred to but expressly declined to follow the Fifth Circuit's holding in a similar case that the wearing of symbols like the armbands cannot be prohibited unless it "materially and substantially interfere[s] with the requirements of appropriate discipline in the operation of the school." Burnside v. Byars, 363 F.2d 744, 749 (1966).[1]

On appeal, the Court of Appeals for the Eighth Circuit considered the case *en banc*. The court was equally divided, and the District Court's decision was accordingly affirmed, without opinion. We granted certiorari.

I

The District Court recognized that the wearing of an armband for the purpose of expressing certain views is the type of symbolic act that is within the Free Speech Clause of the First Amendment. See West Virginia v. Barnette, 319 U.S. 624 (1943); Stromberg v. California, 283 U.S. 359 (1931). Cf. Thornhill v. Alabama, 310 U.S. 88 (1940); Edwards v. South Carolina, 372 U.S. 229 (1963); Brown v. Louisiana, 383 U.S. 131 (1966). As we shall discuss, the wearing of armbands in the circumstances of this case was entirely divorced from actually or potentially disruptive conduct by those participating in it. It was closely akin to "pure speech" which, we have repeatedly held, is entitled to comprehensive protection under the First Amendment. ***

First Amendment rights, applied in light of the special characteristics of the school environment, are available to teachers and students. It can hardly be argued

---

1. In *Burnside*, the Fifth Circuit ordered that high school authorities be enjoined from enforcing a regulation forbidding students to wear "freedom buttons." It is instructive that in Blackwell v. Issaquena County Board of Education, 363 F.2d 749 (1966), the same panel on the same day reached the opposite result on different facts. It declined to enjoin enforcement of such a regulation in another high school where the students wearing freedom buttons harassed students who did not wear them and created much disturbance.

that either students or teachers shed their constitutional rights to freedom of speech or expression at the schoolhouse gate. This has been the unmistakable holding of this Court for almost 50 years. ***

II

The problem posed by the present case does not relate to regulation of the length of skirts or the type of clothing, to hair style or deportment. *** It does not concern aggressive, disruptive action or even group demonstrations. Our problem involves direct, primary First Amendment rights akin to "pure speech."

The school officials banned and sought to punish petitioners for a silent, passive, expression of opinion, unaccompanied by any disorder or disturbance on the part of petitioners. There is here no evidence whatever of petitioners' interference, actual or nascent, with the school's work or of collision with the rights of other students to be secure and to be let alone. Accordingly, this case does not concern speech or action that intrudes upon the work of the school or the rights of other students. ***

The District Court concluded that the action of the school authorities was reasonable because it was based upon their fear of a disturbance from the wearing of the armbands. But, in our system, undifferentiated fear or apprehension of disturbance [the District Court's basis for sustaining the school authorities' action] is not enough to overcome the right to freedom of expression. Any departure from absolute regimentation may cause trouble. Any variation from the majority's opinion may inspire fear. Any words spoken in class, in the lunchroom or on the campus, that deviates from the views of another person, may start an argument or cause a disturbance. But our Constitution says we must take this risk, Terminiello v. Chicago, 337 U.S. 1 (1949); and our history says that it is this sort of hazardous freedom—this kind of openness—that is the basis of our national strength and of the independence and vigor of Americans who grow up and live in this relatively permissive, often disputatious society.

In order for the State in the person of school officials to justify prohibition of a particular expression of opinion, it must be able to show that its action was caused by something more than a mere desire to avoid the discomfort and unpleasantness that always accompany an unpopular viewpoint. Certainly where there is no finding and no showing that the exercise of the forbidden right would "materially and substantially interfere with the requirements of appropriate discipline in the operation of the school," the prohibition cannot be suspended. *Burnside v. Byars*, at 749.

In the present case, the District Court made no such finding, and our independent examination of the record fails to yield evidence that the school authorities had reason to anticipate that the wearing of the armbands would substantially interfere with the work of the school or impinge upon the rights of other students. Even an official memorandum prepared after the suspension that listed the reasons for the ban on wearing the armbands made no reference to the anticipation of such disruption.[3]

On the contrary, the action of the school authorities appears to have been based upon an urgent wish to avoid the controversy which might result from the expression, even by the silent symbol of armbands, of opposition to this Nation's part in the conflagration in Vietnam.[4] It is revealing, in this respect, that the meeting at which the school principals decided to issue the contested regulation was called in response to a student's statement to the journalism teacher in one of the schools that he wanted to write an article on Vietnam and have it published in the school paper. (The student was dissuaded.[5])

It is also relevant that the school authorities did not purport to prohibit the wearing of all symbols of political or controversial significance. The record shows that students in some of the schools wore buttons relating to national political campaigns, and some even wore the Iron Cross, traditionally a symbol of Nazism. The order prohibiting the wearing of armbands did not extend to these. Instead, a particular symbol—black armbands worn to exhibit opposition to this Nation's involvement in Vietnam—was singled out for prohibition. Clearly, the prohibition of expression of one particular opinion, at least without evidence that it is necessary to avoid material and substantial interference with school work or discipline, is not constitutionally permissible.

In our system, state-operated schools may not be enclaves of totalitarianism. School officials do not possess absolute authority over their students. Students in

---

3. The only suggestions of fear of disorder in the report are these:

"A former student of one of our high schools was killed in Viet Nam. Some of his friends are still in school and it was felt that if any kind of a demonstration existed, it might evolve into something which would be difficult to control."

"Students at one of the high schools were heard to say they would wear armbands of other colors if the black bands prevailed."

Moreover, the testimony of school authorities at trial indicates that it was not fear of disruption that motivated the regulation prohibiting the armbands; the regulation was directed against "the principle of the demonstration" itself. School authorities simply felt that "the schools are no place for demonstrations," and if the students "didn't like the way our elected officials were handling things, it should be handled with the ballot box and not in the halls of our public schools."

4. The District Court found that the school authorities, in prohibiting black armbands, were influenced by the fact that "[t]he Viet Nam war and the involvement of the United States therein has been the subject of a major controversy for some time. When the arm band regulation involved herein was promulgated, debate over the Viet Nam war had become vehement in many localities. A protest march against the war had been recently held in Washington, D. C. A wave of draft card burning incidents protesting the war swept the country. At that time two highly publicized draft card burning cases were pending in this Court. Both individuals supporting the war and those opposing it were quite vocal in expressing their views."

5. After the principals' meeting, the director of secondary education and the principal of the high school informed the student that the principals were opposed to publication of his article. They reported that "we felt that it was a very friendly conversation, although we did not feel that we had convinced the student that our decision was a just one."

school as well as out of school are "persons" under our Constitution. They are possessed of fundamental rights which the State must respect, just as they themselves must respect their obligations to the State. In our system, students may not be regarded as closed circuit recipients of only that which the State chooses to communicate. They may not be confined to the expression of those sentiments that are officially approved. In the absence of a specific showing of constitutionally valid reasons to regulate their speech, students are entitled to freedom of expression of their views. ***

The principle of these cases is not confined to the supervised and ordained discussion which takes place in the classroom. The principal use to which the schools are dedicated is to accommodate students during prescribed hours for the purpose of certain types of activities. Among those activities is personal intercommunication among the students.[6] This is not only an inevitable part of the process of attending school; it is also an important part of the educational process. A student's rights therefore, do not embrace merely the classroom hours. When he is in the cafeteria, or on the playing field, or on the campus during the authorized hours, he may express his opinions, even on controversial subjects like the conflict in Vietnam, if he does so without "materially and substantially interfer[ing] with the requirements of appropriate discipline in the operation of the school" and without colliding with the rights of others. *Burnside v. Byars*, at 749. But conduct by the student, in class or out of it, which for any reason—whether it stems from time, place, or type of behavior— materially disrupts classwork or involves substantial disorder or invasion of the rights of others is, of course, not immunized by the constitutional guarantee of freedom of speech. Cf. Blackwell v. Issaquena County Board of Education, 363 F.2d 749 (C.A. 5th Cir. 1966).

Under our Constitution, free speech is not a right that is given only to be so circumscribed that it exists in principle but not in fact. Freedom of expression would not truly exist if the right could be exercised only in an area that a benevolent government was provided as a safe haven for crackpots. The Constitution says that Congress (and the States) may not abridge the right to free speech. This provision means what it says. We properly read it to permit reasonable regulation of speech-connected activities in carefully restricted circumstances. But we do not confine the permissible exercise of First Amendment rights to a telephone booth or the four corners of a pamphlet, or to supervised and ordained discussion in a school classroom.

---

6. In Hammond v. South Carolina State College, 272 F.Supp. 947 (D.C.S.C. 1957), District Judge Hemphill had before him a case involving a meeting on campus of 300 students to express their views on school practices. He pointed out that a school is not like a hospital or a jail enclosure. Cf. Cox v. Louisiana, 379 U.S. 536 (1965); Adderley v. Florida, 385 U.S. 39 (1966). It is a public place, and its dedication to specific uses does not imply that the constitutional rights of persons entitled to be there are to be gauged as if the premises were purely private property. Cf. Edwards v. South Carolina, 372 U.S. 229 (1963); Brown v. Louisiana, 383 U.S. 131 (1966).

If a regulation were adopted by school officials forbidding discussion of the Vietnam conflict, or the expression by any student of opposition to it anywhere on school property except as part of a prescribed classroom exercise, it would be obvious that the regulation would violate the constitutional rights of students, at least if it could not be justified by a showing that the students' activities would materially and substantially disrupt the work and discipline of the school. Cf. Hammond v. South Carolina State College, 272 F. Supp. 947 (D.C.S.C. 1967) (orderly protest meeting on state college campus); Dickey v. Alabama State Board of Education, 273 F. Supp. 613 (D.C.M.D.Ala. 1967) (expulsion of student editor of college newspaper). In the circumstances of the present case, the prohibition of the silent, passive "witness of the armbands," as one of the children called it, is no less offensive to the Constitution's guarantees.

As we have discussed, the record does not demonstrate any facts which might reasonably have led school authorities to forecast substantial disruption of or material interference with school activities, and no disturbances or disorders on the school premises in fact occurred. These petitioners merely went about their ordained rounds in school. Their deviation consisted only in wearing on their sleeve a band of black cloth, not more than two inches wide. They wore it to exhibit their disapproval of the Vietnam hostilities and their advocacy of a truce, to make their views known, and, by their example, to influence others to adopt them. They neither interrupted school activities nor sought to intrude in the school affairs or the lives of others. They caused discussion outside of the classrooms, but no interference with work and no disorder. In the circumstances, our Constitution does not permit officials of the State to deny their form of expression.

We express no opinion as to the form of relief which should be granted, this being a matter for the lower courts to determine. We reverse and remand for further proceedings consistent with this opinion.

MR. JUSTICE STEWART, concurring. [Omitted.]

MR. JUSTICE WHITE, concurring. [Omitted.]

MR. JUSTICE BLACK, dissenting.

The Court's holding in this case ushers in what I deem to be an entirely new era in which the power to control pupils by the elected "officials of state supported public schools ***" in the United States is in ultimate effect transferred to the Supreme Court.[1] The Court brought this particular case here on a petition for certiorari urging that the First and Fourteenth Amendments protect the right of school pupils to express their political views all the way "from kindergarten through high

1. The petition for certiorari here presented this single question:

"Whether the First and Fourteenth Amendments permit officials of state supported public schools to prohibit students from wearing symbols of political views within school premises where the symbols are not disruptive of school discipline or decorum."

school." Here the constitutional right to "political expression" asserted was a right to wear black armbands during school hours and at classes in order to demonstrate to the other students that petitioners were mourning because of the death of United States soldiers in Vietnam and to protest that war which they were against. Ordered to refrain from wearing the armbands in school by the elected school officials and teachers vested with state authority to do so, apparently only seven out of the school system's 18,000 pupils deliberately refused to obey the order. One defying pupil was Paul Tinker, 8 years old, who was in the second grade; another, Hope Tinker, was 11 years old and in the fifth grade; a third member of the Tinker family was 13, in the eighth grade; and a fourth member of the same family was John Tinker, 15 years old, an 11th grade high school pupil. Their father, a Methodist minister without a church, is paid a salary by the American Friends Service Committee. Another student who defied the school order and insisted on wearing an armband in the school was Christopher Eckhardt, an 11th grade pupil and a petitioner in this case. His mother is an official in the Women's International League for Peace and Freedom.

As I read the Court's opinion it relies upon the following grounds for holding unconstitutional the judgment of the Des Moines school officials and the two courts below. First, the Court concludes that the wearing of armbands is "symbolic speech" which is "akin to 'pure speech'" and therefore protected by the First and Fourteenth Amendments. Secondly, the Court decides that the public schools are an appropriate place to exercise "symbolic speech" as long as normal school functions are not "unreasonably" disrupted. Finally, the Court arrogates to itself, rather than to the State's elected officials charged with running the schools, the decision as to which school disciplinary regulations are "reasonable." ***

While the record does not show that any of these armband students shouted, used profane language, or were violent in any manner, detailed testimony by some of them shows their armbands caused comments, warnings by other students, the poking of fun at them, and a warning by an older football player that other, non-protesting students had better let them alone. There is also evidence that a teacher of mathematics had his lesson period practically "wrecked" chiefly by disputes with Mary Beth Tinker, who wore her armband for her "demonstration." Even a casual reading of the record shows that this armband did divert students' minds from their regular lessons, and that talk, comments, etc., made John Tinker "self-conscious" in attending school with his armband. While the absence of obscene remarks or boisterous and loud disorder perhaps justifies the Court's statement that the few armband students did not actually "disrupt" the classwork, I think the record overwhelmingly shows that the armbands did exactly what the elected school officials and principals foresaw they would, that is, took the students' minds off their classwork and diverted them to thoughts about the highly emotional subject of the Vietnam war. And I repeat that if the time has come when pupils of state-supported schools, kindergartens, grammar schools, or high schools, can defy and flout orders of school officials to keep their minds on their own schoolwork, it is the beginning of a new revolutionary era of permissiveness in this country fostered by the judiciary. The next logical step, it appears to me, would be to hold unconstitutional laws that bar pupils under 21 or 18 from voting, or from being elected members of the boards of education. ***

One does not need to be a prophet or the son of a prophet to know that after the Court's holding today some students in Iowa schools and indeed in all schools will be ready, able, and willing to defy their teachers on practically all orders. *** It is no answer to say that the particular students here have not yet reached such high points in their demands to attend classes in order to exercise their political pressures. Turned loose with lawsuits for damages and injunctions against their teachers as they are here, it is nothing but wishful thinking to imagine that young, immature students will not soon believe it is their right to control the schools rather than the right of the States that collect taxes to hire teachers for the benefit of the pupils. This case, therefore, wholly without constitutional reasons in my judgment, subjects all the public schools in the country to the whims and caprices of their loudest-mouthed, but maybe not their brightest, students. *** I dissent.

MR. JUSTICE HARLAN, dissenting.

I certainly agree that state public school authorities in the discharge of their responsibilities are not wholly exempt from the requirements of the Fourteenth Amendment respecting the freedoms of expression and association. At the same time I am reluctant to believe that there is any disagreement between the majority and myself on the proposition that school officials should be accorded the widest authority in maintaining discipline and good order in their institutions. To translate that proposition into a workable constitutional rule, I would, in cases like this, cast upon those complaining the burden of showing that a particular school measure was motivated by other than legitimate school concerns—for example, a desire to prohibit the expression of an unpopular point of view, while permitting expression of the dominant opinion.

Finding nothing in this record which impugns the good faith of respondents in promulgating the arm band regulation, I would affirm the judgement below.

UNITED STATES v. O'BRIEN

391 U.S. 367 (1968)

MR. CHIEF JUSTICE WARREN delivered the opinion of the Court.

On the morning of March 31, 1966, David Paul O'Brien and three companions burned their Selective Service registration certificates on the steps of the South Boston Courthouse. A sizable crowd, including several agents of the Federal Bureau of Investigation, witnessed the event.[1] Immediately after the burning, members of the crowd began attacking O'Brien and his companions. An FBI agent ushered O'Brien to safety inside the courthouse. After he was advised of his right to counsel and to silence, O'Brien stated to FBI agents that he had burned his registration certificate because of his beliefs, knowing that he was violating federal law. He produced the charred remains of the certificate, which, with his consent, were photographed.

For this act, O'Brien was indicted, tried, convicted, and sentenced in the United States District Court for the District of Massachusetts.[2] He did not contest the fact that he had burned the certificate. He stated in argument to the jury that he burned the certificate publicly to influence others to adopt his antiwar beliefs, as he put it, "so that other people would reevaluate their positions with Selective Service, with the armed forces, and reevaluate their place in the culture of today, to hopefully consider my position."

The indictment upon which he was tried charged that he "willfully and knowingly did mutilate, destroy, and change by burning [his] Registration Certificate; in violation of Title 50, App., United States Code, Section 462(b)." Section 462 (b) is part of the Universal Military Training and Service Act of 1948. Section 462(b)(3), one of six numbered subdivisions of § 462(b), was amended by Congress in 1965, 79 Stat. 586 (adding the words italicized below), so that at the time O'Brien burned his certificate an offense was committed by any person,

> "who forges, alters, *knowingly destroys, knowingly mutilates*, or in any manner changes any such certificate. ***" (Italics supplied.)

In the District Court, O'Brien argued that the 1965 Amendment prohibiting the knowing destruction or mutilation of certificates was unconstitutional because it was enacted to abridge free speech, and because it served no legitimate legislative purpose. The District Court rejected these arguments, holding that the statute on its face did not abridge First Amendment rights, that the court was not competent to inquire into the motives of Congress in enacting the 1965 Amendment, and that the Amendment was a reasonable exercise of the power of Congress to raise armies.

On appeal, the Court of Appeals for the First Circuit held the 1965 Amendment unconstitutional as a law abridging freedom of speech. *** We hold that the 1965 Amendment is constitutional both as enacted and as applied. We therefore vacate the

1. At the time of the burning, the agents knew only that O'Brien and his three companions had burned small white cards. They later discovered that the card O'Brien had burned was his registration certificate, and the undisputed assumption is that the same is true of his companions.

2. He was sentenced under the Youth Corrections Act, 18 U.S.C. § 5010(b), to the custody of the Attorney General for a maximum period of six years for supervision and treatment.

judgment of the Court of Appeals and reinstate the judgment and sentence of the District Court *** .

I

***

We note at the outset that the 1965 Amendment plainly does not abridge free speech on its face, and we do not understand O'Brien to argue otherwise. Amended § 12(b)(3) on its face deals with conduct having no connection with speech. It prohibits the knowing destruction of certificates issued by the Selective Service System, and there is nothing necessarily expressive about such conduct. The Amendment does not distinguish between public and private destruction, and it does not punish only destruction engaged in for the purpose of expressing views. Compare Stromberg v. People of State of California, 283 U.S. 359 (1931). A law prohibiting destruction of Selective Service certificates no more abridges free speech on its face than a motor vehicle law prohibiting the destruction of drivers' licenses, or a tax law prohibiting the destruction of books and records.

O'Brien nonetheless argues that the 1965 Amendment is unconstitutional in its application to him, and is unconstitutional as enacted because what he calls the "purpose" of Congress was "to suppress freedom of speech." We consider these arguments separately.

II

O'Brien first argues that the 1965 Amendment is unconstitutional as applied to him because his act of burning his registration certificate was protected "symbolic speech" within the First Amendment. His argument is that the freedom of expression which the First Amendment guarantees includes all modes of "communication of ideas by conduct," and that his conduct is within this definition because he did it in "demonstration against the war and against the draft."

We cannot accept the view that an apparently limitless variety of conduct can be labeled "speech" whenever the person engaging in the conduct intends thereby to express an idea. However, even on the assumption that the alleged communicative element in O'Brien's conduct is sufficient to bring into play the First Amendment, it does not necessarily follow that the destruction of a registration certificate is constitutionally protected activity. This Court has held that when "speech" and "nonspeech" elements are combined in the same course of conduct, a sufficiently important governmental interest in regulating the nonspeech element can justify incidental limitations on First Amendment freedoms. To characterize the quality of the governmental interest which must appear, the Court has employed a variety of descriptive terms: compelling; substantial; subordinating; paramount; cogent; strong. Whatever imprecision inheres in these terms, we think it clear that a government regulation is sufficiently justified if it is within the constitutional power of the Government; if it furthers an important or substantial governmental interest; if the governmental interest is unrelated to the suppression of free expression; and if the incidental restriction on alleged First Amendment freedoms is no greater than is essential to the furtherance of that interest. We find that the 1965 Amendment to

§ 12(b)(3) of the Universal Military Training and Service Act meets all of these requirements, and consequently that O'Brien can be constitutionally convicted for violating it.

The constitutional power of Congress to raise and support armies and to make all laws necessary and proper to that end is broad and sweeping. *** Pursuant to this power, Congress may establish a system of registration for individuals liable for training and service, and may require such individuals within reason to cooperate in the registration system. The issuance of certificates indicting the registration and eligibility classification of individuals is a legitimate and substantial administrative aid in the functioning of this system. And legislation to insure the continuing availability of issued certificates serves a legitimate and substantial purpose in the system's administration.

*** Many of these purposes would be defeated by the certificates' destruction or mutilation. Among these are:

1. The registration certificate serves as proof that the individual described thereon has registered for the draft. The classification certificate shows the eligibility classification of a named but undescribed individual. *** Correspondingly, the availability of the certificates for such display relieves the Selective Service System of the administrative burden it would otherwise have in verifying the registration and classification of all suspected delinquents. Further, since both certificates are in the nature of "receipts" attesting that the registrant has done what the law requires, it is in the interest of the just and efficient administration of the system that they be continually available, in the event, for example, of a mix-up in the registrant's file. Additionally, in a time of national crisis, reasonable availability of each registrant of the two small cards assures a rapid and uncomplicated means for determining his fitness for immediate induction, no matter how distant in our mobile society he may be from his local board.

2. The information supplied on the certificates facilitates communication between registrants and local boards, simplifying the system and benefitting all concerned. To begin with, each certificate bears the address of the registrant's local board, an item unlikely to be committed to memory. Further, each card bears the registrant's Selective Service number, and a registrant who has his number readily available so that he can communicate it to his local board when he supplies or requests information can make simpler the board's task in locating his file. ***

We think it apparent that the continuing availability to each registrant of his Selective Service certificates substantially furthers the smooth and proper functioning of the system that Congress has established to raise armies. We think it also apparent that the Nation has a vital interest in having a system for raising armies that functions with maximum efficiency and is capable of easily and quickly responding to continually changing circumstances. For these reasons, the Government has a substantial interest in assuring the continuing availability of issued Selective Service certificates.

It is equally clear that the 1965 Amendment specifically protects this substantial governmental interest. We perceive no alternative means that would more precisely and narrowly assure the continuing availability of issued Selective Service certificates than a law which prohibits their wilful mutilation or destruction. The 1965 Amendment prohibits such conduct and does nothing more. In other words, both the governmental interest and the operation of the 1965 Amendment are limited to the noncommunicative aspect of O'Brien's conduct. The governmental interest and the scope of the 1965 Amendment are limited to preventing harm to the smooth and efficient functioning of the Selective Service System. When O'Brien deliberately rendered unavailable his registration certificate, he wilfully frustrated this governmental interest. For this noncommunicative impact of his conduct, and for nothing else, he was convicted.

The case at bar is therefore unlike one where the alleged governmental interest in regulating conduct arises in some measure because the communication allegedly integral to the conduct is itself thought to be harmful. In Stromberg v. People of State of California, 283 U.S. 359 (1931), for example, this Court struck down a statutory phrase which punished people who expressed their "opposition to organized government" by displaying "any flag, badge, banner, or device." Since the statute there was aimed at suppressing communication it could not be sustained as a regulation of noncommunicative conduct. ***

III

O'Brien finally argues that the 1965 Amendment is unconstitutional as enacted because what he calls the "purpose" of Congress was "to suppress freedom of speech." We reject this argument because under settled principles the purpose of Congress, as O'Brien uses that term, is not a basis for declaring this legislation unconstitutional.

It is a familiar principle of constitutional law that this Court will not strike down an otherwise constitutional statute on the basis of an alleged illicit legislative motive. As the Court long ago stated:

> "The decisions of this court from the beginning lend no support whatever to the assumption that the judiciary may restrain the exercise of lawful power on the assumption that a wrongful purpose or motive has caused the power to be exerted." McCray v. United States, 195 U.S. 27, 56 (1904).

Inquiries into congressional motives or purposes are a hazardous matter. When the issue is simply the interpretation of legislation, the Court will look to statements by legislators for guidance as to the purpose of the legislature,[30] because the benefit

30. The Court may make the same assumption in a very limited and well-defined class of cases where the very nature of the constitutional question requires an inquiry into legislative purpose. The principal class of cases is readily apparent—those in which statutes have been challenged as bills of attainder. This Court's decisions have defined a bill of attainder as a legislative Act which inflicts punishment on named individuals or members of an easily ascertainable group without a judicial trial.

to sound decision-making in this circumstance is thought sufficient to risk the possibility of misreading Congress' purpose. It is entirely a different matter when we are asked to void a statute that is, under well-settled criteria, constitutional on its face, on the basis of what fewer than a handful of Congressmen said about it. What motivates one legislator to make a speech about a statute is not necessarily what motivates scores of others to enact it, and the stakes are sufficiently high for us to eschew guesswork. We decline to void essentially on the ground that it is unwise legislation which Congress had the undoubted power to enact and which could be reenacted in its exact form if the same or another legislator made a "wiser" speech about it.

*** There was little floor debate on this legislation in either House. Only Senator Thurmond commented on its substantive features in the Senate. After his brief statement, and without any additional substantive comments, the bill, H.R. 10306, passed the Senate. In the House debate only two Congressmen addressed themselves to the Amendment—Congressmen Rivers and Bray. The bill was passed after their statements without any further debate by a vote of 393 to 1. It is principally on the basis of the statements by these three Congressmen that O'Brien makes his congressional-"purpose" argument. We note that if we were to examine legislative purpose in the instant case, we would be obliged to consider not only these statements but also the more authoritative reports of the Senate and House Armed Services Committees. The portions of those reports explaining the purpose of the Amendment are reproduced in the Appendix in their entirety. While both reports make clear a concern with the "defiant" destruction of so-called "draft cards" and with "open" encouragement to others to destroy their cards, both reports also indicate that this concern stemmed from an apprehension that unrestrained destruction of cards would disrupt the smooth functioning of the Selective Service System.

*** [T]he Court of Appeals should have affirmed the judgment of conviction entered by the District Court.

MR. JUSTICE MARSHALL took no part in the consideration or decision of these cases.

In determining whether a particular statute is a bill of attainder, the analysis necessarily requires an inquiry into whether the three definitional elements—specificity in identification, punishment, and lack of a judicial trial—are contained in the statute. The inquiry into whether the challenged statute contains the necessary element of punishment has on occasion led the Court to examine the legislative motive in enacting the statute. See, e.g., United States v. Lovett, 328 U.S. 303 (1946). Two other decisions not involving a bill of attainder analysis contain an inquiry into legislative purpose or motive of the type that O'Brien suggests we engage in in this case. Kennedy v. Mendoza-Martinez, 372 U.S. 144, 169-184 (1963); Trop v. Dulles, 356 U.S. 86, 79-97 (1958). The inquiry into legislative purpose or motive in *Kennedy* and *Trop*, however, was for the same limited purpose as in the bill of attainder decisions—i.e. to determine whether the statutes under review were punitive in nature. We face no such inquiry in this case. The 1965 Amendment to § 462(b) was clearly penal in nature, designed to impose criminal punishment for designated acts.

MR. JUSTICE HARLAN, concurring.

The crux of the Court's opinion, which I join, is of course its general statement that:

> "a government regulation is sufficiently justified if it is within the constitutional power of the Government; if it furthers an important or substantial governmental interest; if the governmental interest is unrelated to the suppression of free expression; and if the incidental restriction on alleged First Amendment freedoms is no greater than is essential to the furtherance of that interest."

I wish to make explicit my understanding that this passage does not foreclose consideration of First Amendment claims in those rare instances when an "incidental" restriction upon expression, imposed by a regulation which furthers an "important or substantial" governmental interest and satisfies the Court's other criteria, in practice has the effect of entirely preventing a "speaker" from reaching a significant audience with whom he could not otherwise lawfully communicate. This is not such a case, since O'Brien manifestly could have conveyed his message in many ways other than by burning his draft card.

MR. JUSTICE DOUGLAS, dissenting. [Omitted.]

CLARK v. COMMUNITY FOR CREATIVE NON-VIOLENCE
468 U.S. 288 (1984)

JUSTICE WHITE delivered the opinion of the Court.

The issue in this case is whether a National Park Service regulation prohibiting camping in certain parks violates the First Amendment when applied to prohibit demonstrators from sleeping in Lafayette Park and the Mall in connection with a demonstration to call attention to the plight of the homeless. We hold that it does not and reverse the contrary judgment of the Court of Appeals.

I

The Interior Department, through the National Park Service, is charged with responsibility for the management and maintenance of the National Parks and is authorized to promulgate rules and regulations for the use of the parks in accordance with the purposes for which they were established. *** Lafayette Park is a roughly 7-acre square located across Pennsylvania Avenue from the White House. Although originally part of the White House grounds, President Jefferson set it aside as a park for the use of residents and visitors. It is a "garden park with a *** formal land scaping of flowers and trees, with fountains, walks and benches." *** The Mall is a stretch of land running westward from the Capitol to the Lincoln Memorial some two miles away. It includes the Washington Monument, a series of reflecting pools, trees, lawns, and other greenery. It is bordered by, *inter alia*, the Smithsonian Institution and the National Gallery of Art. Both the Park and the Mall were included in Major Pierre L'Enfant's original plan for the Capital. Both are visited by vast numbers of visitors from around the country, as well as by large numbers of residents of the Washington metropolitan area.

Under the regulations involved in this case, camping in National Parks is permitted only in campgrounds designated for that purpose. No such campgrounds have ever been designated in Lafayette Park or the Mall. Demonstrations for the airing of views or grievances are permitted in the Memorial-core parks, but for the most part only by Park Service permits. Temporary structures may be erected for demonstration purposes but may not be used for camping. 36 CFR § 50.19(e)(8) (1983).

In 1982, the Park Service issued a renewable permit to respondent Community for Creative Non-Violence (CCNV) to conduct a wintertime demonstration in Lafayette Park and the Mall for the purpose of demonstrating the plight of the homeless. The permit authorized the erection of two symbolic tent cities: 20 tents in Lafayette Park that would accommodate 50 people and 40 tents in the Mall with a capacity of up to 100. The Park Service, however, relying on the above regulations, specifically denied CCNV's request that demonstrators be permitted to sleep in the symbolic tents.

*** The District Court granted summary judgment in favor of the Park Service. The Court of Appeals, sitting en banc, reversed. ***

II

We need not differ with the view of the Court of Appeals that overnight sleeping in connection with the demonstration is expressive conduct protected to some extent by the First Amendment.[5] We assume for present purposes, but do not decide, that such is the case, cf. United States v. O'Brien, 391 U.S. 367, 376 (1968), but this assumption only begins the inquiry. *** Symbolic expression of this kind may be forbidden or regulated if the conduct itself may constitutionally be regulated, if the regulation is narrowly drawn to further a substantial governmental interest, and if the interest is unrelated to the suppression of free speech. *United States v. O'Brien*.

---

5. We reject the suggestion of the plurality below, however, that the burden on the demonstrators is limited to "the advancement of a plausible contention" that their conduct is expressive. Although it is common to place the burden upon the Government to justify impingements on First Amendment interests, it is the obligation of the person desiring to engage in assertedly expressive conduct to demonstrate that the First Amendment even applies. To hold otherwise would be to create a rule that all conduct is presumptively expressive. In the absence of a showing that such a rule is necessary to protect vital First Amendment interests, we decline to deviate from the general rule that one seeking relief bears the burden of demonstrating that he is entitled to it.

Petitioners submit, as they did in the Court of Appeals, that the regulation forbidding sleeping is defensible either as a time, place, or manner restriction or as a regulation of symbolic conduct. We agree with that assessment. The permit that was issued authorized the demonstration but required compliance with 36 CFR § 50.19 (1983), which prohibits "camping" on park lands, that is, the use of park lands for living accommodations, such as sleeping, storing personal belongings, making fires, digging, or cooking. These provisions, including the ban on sleeping are clearly limitations on the manner in which the demonstration could be carried out. ***

[I]t is not disputed here that the prohibition on camping, and on sleeping specifically, is content-neutral and is not being applied because of disagreement with the message presented. Neither was the regulation faulted, nor could it be, on the ground that without overnight sleeping the plight of the homeless could not be communicated in other ways. The regulation otherwise left the demonstration intact, with its symbolic city, signs, and the presence of those who were willing to take their turns in a day-and-night vigil. Respondents do not suggest that there was, or is, any barrier to delivering to the media, or to the public by other means, the intended message concerning the plight of the homeless.

It is also apparent to us that the regulation narrowly focuses on the Government's substantial interest in maintaining the parks in the heart of our Capital in an attractive and intact condition, readily available to the millions of people who wish to see and enjoy them by their presence. To permit camping—using these areas as living accommodations—would be totally inimical to these purposes, as would be readily understood by those who have frequented the National Parks across the country and observed the unfortunate consequences of the activities of those who refuse to confine their camping to designated areas. ***

Contrary to the conclusion of the Court of Appeals, the foregoing analysis demonstrates that the Park Service regulation is sustainable under the four-factor standard of United States v. O'Brien, 391 U.S. 367 (1968), for validating a regulation of expressive conduct, which, in the last analysis is little, if any, different from the standard applied to time, place, or manner restrictions.[8] No one contends that aside from its impact on speech a rule against camping or overnight sleeping in public parks is beyond the constitutional power of the Government to enforce. And for the reasons we have discussed above, there is a substantial Government interest in conserving park property, an interest that is plainly served by, and requires for its

---

8. Reasonable time, place, or manner restrictions are valid even though they directly limit oral or written expression. It would be odd to insist on a higher standard for limitations aimed at regulable conduct and having only an incidental impact on speech. Thus, if the time, place, or manner restriction on expressive sleeping, if that is what is involved in this case, sufficiently and narrowly serves a substantial enough governmental interest to escape First Amendment condemnation, it is untenable to invalidate it under *O'Brien* on the ground that the governmental interest is insufficient to warrant the intrusion on First Amendment concerns or that there is an inadequate nexus between the regulation and the interest sought to be served. ***

implementation, measures such as the proscription of sleeping that are designed to limit the wear and tear on park properties. That interest is unrelated to suppression of expression.

We are unmoved by the Court of Appeals' view that the challenged regulation is unnecessary, and hence invalid, because there are less speech-restrictive alternatives that could have satisfied the Government interest in preserving park lands. There is no gainsaying that preventing overnight sleeping will avoid a measure of actual or threatened damage to Lafayette Park and the Mall. The Court of Appeals' suggestions that the Park Service minimize the possible injury by reducing the size, duration, or frequency of demonstrations would still curtail the total allowable expression in which demonstrators could engage, whether by sleeping or otherwise, and these suggestions represent no more than a disagreement with the Park Service over how much protection the core parks require or how an acceptable level of preservation is to be attained. We do not believe, however, that either *United States v. O'Brien* or the time, place, or manner decisions assign to the judiciary the authority to replace the Park Service as the manager of the Nation's parks or endow the judiciary with the competence to judge how much protection of park lands is wise and how that level of conservation is to be attained.

Accordingly, the judgment of the Court of Appeals is *** reversed.

CHIEF JUSTICE BURGER, concurring. [Omitted.]

JUSTICE MARSHALL with whom JUSTICE BRENNAN joins, dissenting.

I

*** Missing from the majority's description is any inkling that Lafayette Park and the Mall have served as the sites for some of the most rousing political demonstrations in the Nation's history. ***

The primary purpose for making *sleep* an integral part of the demonstration was "to re-enact the central reality of homelessness," and to impress upon public consciousness, in as dramatic a way as possible, that homelessness is a widespread problem, often ignored, that confronts its victims with life-threatening deprivations. *** By using sleep as an integral part of their mode of protest, respondents "can express with their bodies the poignancy of their plight. They can physically demonstrate the neglect from which they suffer with an articulateness even Dickens could not match." Community for Creative Non-Violence v. Watt, 703 F.2d 586, 601 (1983) (Edwards, J. concurring).

The Government contends that a foreseeable difficulty of administration counsels against recognizing sleep as a mode of expression protected by the First Amendment. The predicament the Government envisions can be termed "the imposter problem": the problem of distinguishing bona fide protesters from imposters whose requests for permission to sleep in Lafayette Park or the Mall on First Amendment grounds would mask ulterior designs—the simple desire, for example, to avoid the expense of hotel lodgings. The Government maintains that such distinctions cannot be made without inquiring into the sincerity of demonstrators and that such an inquiry would itself pose dangers to First Amendment values because it would necessarily be content-sensitive. I find this argument unpersuasive. *** If permitting sleep to be used as a form of protected First Amendment activity actually created the administrative problems the Government now envisions, there would emerge a clear factual basis upon which to establish the necessity for the limitation the Government advocates.

*** The Government's argument would pose a difficult problem were the determination whether an act constitutes "speech" the end of First Amendment analysis. But such a determination is not the end. If an act is defined as speech, it must still be balanced against countervailing government interests. The balancing which the First Amendment requires would doom any argument seeking to protect antisocial acts such as assassination or destruction of government property from government interference because compelling interests would outweigh the expressive value of such conduct.

II

Although sleep in the context of this case is symbolic speech protected by the First Amendment, it is nonetheless subject to reasonable time, place, and manner restrictions. I agree with the standard enunciated by the majority: "[R]estrictions of this kind are valid provided that they are justified without reference to the content of the regulated speech, that they are narrowly tailored to serve a significant governmental interest, and that they leave open ample alternative channels for communication of the information."[6] I conclude, however, that the regulations at issue in this case, as applied to respondents, fail to satisfy this standard. ***

III

The disposition of this case impels me to make two additional observations. First, in this case, as in some others involving time, place, and manner restrictions,[11] the Court has dramatically lowered its scrutiny of governmental regulations once it has determined that such regulations are content-neutral. The result has been the creation of a two-tiered approach to First Amendment cases: while regulations that turn on the content of the expression are subjected to a strict form of judicial review, regulations that are aimed at matters other than expression receive only a minimal

---

6. I also agree with the majority that no substantial difference distinguishes the test applicable to time, place, and manner restrictions and the test articulated in United States v. O'Brien, 391 U.S. 367 (1968).

11. See, e.g., City Council of Los Angeles v. Taxpayers for Vincent, 466 U.S. 789 (1984); Heffron v. International Society for Krishna Consciousness, Inc., 452 U.S. 640 (1981). But see United States v. Grace, 461 U.S. 171 (1983); Tinker v. Des Moines School Dist., 393 U.S. 503 (1969); Brown v. Louisiana, 383 U.S. 131 (1966).

level of scrutiny. *** To be sure, the general prohibition against content-based regulations is an essential tool of First Amendment analysis. It helps to put into operation the well- established principle that "government may not grant the use of a forum to people whose views it finds acceptable, but deny use to those wishing to express less favored or more controversial views". Police Department of Chicago v. Mosley, 408 U.S. 92, 95-96 (1972). The Court, however, has transformed the ban against content distinctions from a floor that offers all persons at least equal liberty under the First Amendment into a ceiling that restricts persons to the protection of First Amendment equality —but nothing more.[14] The consistent imposition of silence upon all may fulfill the dictates of an evenhanded content-neutrality. But it offends our "profound national commitment to the principle that debate on public issues should be uninhibited, robust, and wide-open." *New York Times Co. v. Sullivan*, 376 U. S., at 270.

Second, the disposition of this case reveals a mistaken assumption regarding the motives and behavior of Government officials who create and administer content-neutral regulations. *** The Court evidently assumes that the balance struck by officials is deserving of deference so long as it does not appear to be tainted by content discrimination. What the Court fails to recognize is that public officials have strong incentives to overregulate even in the absence of an intent to censor particular views. This incentive stems from the fact that of the two groups whose interests officials must accommodate—on the one hand, the interests of the general public and, on the other, the interests of those who seek to use a particular forum for First Amendment activity —the political power of the former is likely to be far greater than that of the latter.[16]

---

14. Furthermore, a content-neutral regulation does not necessarily fall with random or equal force upon different groups or different points of view. A content-neutral regulation that restricts an inexpensive mode of communication will fall most heavily upon relatively poor speakers and the points of view that such speakers typically espouse. This sort of latent inequality is very much in evidence in this case for respondents lack the financial means necessary to buy access to more conventional modes of persuasion.

A disquieting feature about the disposition of this case is that it lends credence to the charge that judicial administration of the First Amendment, in conjunction with a social order marked by large disparities in wealth and other sources of power, tends systematically to discriminate against efforts by the relatively disadvantaged to convey their political ideas. In the past, this Court has taken such considerations into account in adjudicating the First Amendment rights of those among us who are financially deprived. See, e.g., Martin v. Struthers, 319 U.S. 141, 146 (1943) (striking down ban on door-to-door distribution of circulars in part because this mode of distribution is "essential to the poorly financed causes of little people"). Such solicitude is noticeably absent from the majority's opinion, continuing a trend that has not escaped the attention of commentators. See, e.g., Dorsen & Gora, Free Speech, Property, and The Burger Court: Old Values, New Balances, 1982 S.Ct.Rev. 195; Van Alstyne, The Recrudescence of Property Rights as the Foremost Principle of Civil Liberties: The First Decade of the Burger Court, 43 Law & Contemp. Prob. 66 (summer 1980).

16. See Goldberger, Judicial Scrutiny in Public Forum Cases: Misplaced Trust in the Judgment of Public Officials, 32 Buffalo L.Rev. 175, 208 (1983).

***

For the foregoing reasons, I respectfully dissent.

A NOTE ON "SYMBOLIC EXPRESSION" AND THE "*O'BRIEN* TEST"

Suppose an ordinary jaywalking ordinance, i.e. a city ordinance making it a misdemeanor to "cross city streets other than at intersections and otherwise as designated, within marked lines." Suppose also that X and Y are each in turn arrested for jaywalking. Suppose in respect to X (but not Y), however, that X's very act of jaywalking was itself an obvious part of his remonstrance in protest of the (un)wisdom of the ordinance itself.

> ***Query***: Does X have any invokable first amendment claim against the jaywalking ordinance as applied?[125] If he does, what is that claim, and how will it work out, i.e. will his conviction nonetheless be sustained?[126]

Is the case suitable to analyze under "reasonable time, place, and manner" *speech*-regulating rules?[127] Perhaps, but one needs to do some explaining, if one thinks that it is. The ordinance does not regulate speech as such at all.[128] Compare, for contrast, the *Pacifica Foundation* case.[129] There, an FCC regulation forbidding the use of "vulgar" language over ordinary commercial radio frequencies, during certain daylight hours, was indubitably a regulation of speech. To be sure, it went "merely" to the use of certain words (i.e. vulgar, offensive words) rather than to the content of the broadcaster's message, but even so it was plainly a regulation of speech. This jaywalking ordinance seems quite far removed from regulations of that

---

125. Y, of course, would have no first amendment standing to object to the jaywalking ordinance as applied to him since (by stipulation) Y was not expressing any message at all (rather, Y was merely taking a short cut to cross the street, nothing more).

126. If one concludes that X's conviction cannot be sustained (perhaps by application of the *O'Brien* test?), how does one reconcile that result with the different fate of Y? Why should Y be subject to a fine or a day or two in jail, when he did no more than X did, in jaywalking, and in one sense Y even did less (i.e. Y was neither willfully defying the law as such nor showing some degree of contempt of the law, as X; *why should Y be subject to punishment if X is not likewise to be punished)*? (Why should X get off, *at all* ?)

127. See cases and discussion *infra* at pp. 387-426.

128. Similarly, consider a municipal ordinance of an ordinary sort making it a misdemeanor "to burn anything on the public streets of the town," an ordinance enacted as a simple public safety measure. Would it not be incorrect to review the malicious mischief ordinance under the case law pertinent to "time, place, and manner *speech* regulations"? (The ordinance is not a regulation of "speech," rather, it is a regulation of fires; it regulates when and where fires may (or, rather, may not) take place.) (Cf. Texas v. Johnson, 491 U.S. 397 (1989), and see the notes and discussion following that case, *infra*.)

129. FCC v. Pacifica Foundation, 438 U.S. 726 (1978).

sort.[130] It was solely the illegality of X's walking (rather than talking) that—just as in Y's case— brings him afoul of this law. So cases such as *Pacifica Foundation* are prima facie inapplicable to the kind of case we have put.

I

Beginning with the observation just offered, it would appear that a strong case can be made that X secures *no* first amendment purchase against the jaywalking charge. That is, "jaywalking" is simply not "speech," and *it is solely for jaywalking that X has been charged.* That he committed the offense to dramatize some grievance ought not, perhaps, be held against him vis-à-vis the treatment Y receives in the courts, but even that is far from clear under some not unreasonable views.[131]

Moreover, the case is different not merely from cases such as the *Pacifica Foundation* case, but arguably distinguishable also from cases such as *Tinker v. Des Moines School District*, as well. There, it was said, the wearing of an armband is "akin to pure speech," and, objectively, that may well be true of armbands in general, including (but not limited to) the sort of armband involved in the particular case.[132] Thus a regulation of when and where one may or may not wear an *armband* may be regarded as a regulation of speech, bringing the first amendment directly to bear.

The case may also be different from *Street v. New York*[133] and from *Spence v. State of Washington*,[134] two cases involving flag regulation laws. Flags, especially the standard national flag, are typically communicative—they say something and usually are meant to communicate something. When, therefore, the regulation is one of "flag use," it may be quite right to regard the regulation as, in some measure, a regulation of speech. But, again, we seem to have nothing similar here.

The case is different also from *Stromberg v. California*,[135] where the act (displaying a red flag) was forbidden as a means of expression (of opposition to established government)—it is the same point made by several other examples given in several of the cases noted and distinguished in *O'Brien* itself. To make the jay

130. Similarly, compare City Council v. Taxpayers for Vincent, 466 U.S. 789 (1984) (city ordinance forbidding any posting of notices from utility poles or utility lines in the city, defended as a neutral measure to improve city's appearance, attacked as applied to election posters, as an unreasonable restriction on candidate's committee to hang posters city conceded provided no hazard to traffic or to public safety).

131. See discussion, p. 265 note 126 *supra* (suggesting the appropriateness of a higher fine justified by the deterrence of willful violators).

132. As noted earlier in these materials, a merely generous construction of the words of the first amendment might well include politically expressive insignia (such as armbands) as "speech." To do the same for "jaywalking," in contrast, might well seem to empty the amendment of any coherence at all.

133. 394 U.S. 576 (1969).

134. 417 U.S. 790 (1974).

135. 283 U.S. 359 (1931). See also Barnes v. Glen Theatre, 501 U.S. 560 (1991); Vincent A. Blasi, Six Conservatives in Search of the First Amendment: The Revealing Case of Nude Dancing, 33 Wm. & Mary L. Rev. 611 (1992).

walking case similar to *Stromberg* or to *Street*, would require one to redo the ordinance—to make jaywalking a crime when engaged in as a means of social protest, but not otherwise, thus discriminating between X and Y, which the ordinance does not do.

Neither is our jaywalking case one in which, though the ordinance is neutral on its face (i.e. in its nonspeech concern and apparent ordinariness), there is nonetheless very strong evidence that in fact it was adopted as a means of suppressing a feared message or expression, and would not otherwise have been laid into place. Whatever the proper treatment of any law so conceived and adopted (e.g., in both *Tinker* and in *O'Brien* itself), we have made no similar suggestion here.[136] In each (indeed, perhaps in all) of the above-mentioned distinguishing circumstances, the first amendment might well be deemed to apply. To be sure, that conclusion—that the first amendment applies—would not automatically mean that each involved litigant necessarily prevails, but it clearly will require some first amendment discussion to show why not. Here, in contrast, the cases may have an entirely different feel.[137]

II

Nonetheless, note that *O'Brien* and *Clark* actually both suggest otherwise, i.e. they suggest that the first amendment *can* be invoked by X (although clearly not by Y). Just because O'Brien was trying to make a strong political point by publicly burning his draft card (and just because, likewise, the Community for Creative Non-Violence was trying to make a similar point of its own by maintaining its lived-in tents in Lafayette Park), they evidently did gain a degree of first amendment benefit that the ordinary draft card mutilator, or the ordinary camper, could not claim. Significantly, the majority of the Supreme Court in each case seems to be satisfied this is so, even if in each case the majority also concluded that the regulation was valid as applied.

In this respect (if in no other), it is well worth one's time to note how the cases are something of a first amendment-*favoring* surprise. They treat sleeping out as "speech," and burning a piece of pasteboard as "speech." A priori, there was no reason to suppose that such a concession would necessarily be made, even under a presumption of generous construction of the first amendment.

So far as that concession has been made by the Supreme Court, moreover, presumably it is available in our jaywalking case as well. Looking at that case again, with the hindsight of these remarks, there seems to be no ground to exclude X's case

---

136. In short, the hypothetical case is not one appropriate for analysis pursuant to the "cellophane wrapper" doctrine—where the evidence is clear and convincing that the legislature was *trying to do one thing* (suppress dissent) *under the guise of doing another thing* (regulating traffic). Here, by hypothesis, the ordinance was bona fide in its valid police power concern.

137. Again, if one is inclined to think otherwise, pause for a moment to compare the treatment of Y—why should X get *any* advantage over Y under the circumstances, in being acquitted of the jaywalking offense? (Similarly, in the malicious mischief "burning" cases, compared in an earlier footnote *supra*.)

from the advantage of this development (though it will not apply to Y). In some measure, then, it appears that X's case *will* be treated differently from Y's. And, according to the test now shown to be applicable to X's case (i.e. the test laid out in the *O'Brien* case by Chief Justice Warren), presumably X cannot be validly convicted unless, in addition to proving the usual elements of the jaywalking offense as committed by X, the government can prove the following things as well:

> a) That not only was the jaywalking law well within the constitutional power of government (a standard requirement the government must satisfy in any case whether or not it involves the first amendment), but that the law in question "furthers an important or substantial governmental interest," and not merely one that might suffice if no first amendment interests were involved;
>
> b) That the "important or substantial governmental" interest, moreover, is one that is itself "unrelated to the suppression of free expression"; and
>
> c) That the restriction on free speech (incidental to the restriction as applied) "is (also) no greater than is essential to the furtherance of that (important or substantial) interest."

All of this would clearly imply that the X case might come out differently from the Y case because, by stipulation, the government must meet some burdens (and will fail if it cannot carry those burdens) which burdens it need not meet in the prosecution of Y.[138]

III

Yet, before becoming unduly involved in this matter with high optimism, note the likelihood that in fact rarely will one expect the government to fail to meet the requirements of the *O'Brien* test as it appears to have been applied. Both *O'Brien* and *Clark* tend to show how that is so. Applied to our hypothetical jaywalking case, it is altogether likely that X will also fail.[139]

To be sure, if one applies the last part of the *O'Brien* test by concentrating on X's particular arrest and prosecution, it might well appear that X should tend to

---

138. To consider only the first step, for example, presumably in some instances the government will not be able to show any "substantial" or "important" (as distinct from merely permissible) interest served by the regulation in question, even if, in our particular case, it may be able to do so—as it probably can. And so, too, with the requirement set forth in *O'Brien*, with respect to the third step.

139. The governmental interest will surely be said to be important or substantial, i.e. it will be identified to public safety itself. As to the second step of the test, moreover, we have already passed it (in that we have already stipulated that the jaywalking ordinance is admittedly unrelated to the suppression of free expression as such). And while one might dispute how essential the prohibition of jaywalking is to the furtherance of the substantial and important governmental interest (of safe street use), it is likely to be thought "essential" enough for the ordinance to be sustained as applied. Test it by your own review and comparison of *O'Brien* and *Clark*, and see whether you agree.

prevail.[140] But judging the matter from *O'Brien* and *Clark* cases themselves, the Supreme Court seems wholly disinclined to test these types of cases in any such (limited) case-specific, way. The issue is tested more from a generalized perspective, rather than from an ex post case-specific perspective, i.e. it is tested by viewing the *potential* class of first amendment violators overall as a class, though there is as yet no such real aggregation of violations at hand.[141]

In brief, under *O'Brien* and *Clark*, the question is not whether X created such a traffic danger (or might have created such a danger) in such circumstances as applied to him, sustaining the ordinance was essential to secure traffic safety *at the time*; rather, it is whether, were all persons "like X" to be deemed exempt, the hazard to traffic safety might become substantial. If the reasonable answer to that question is "yes," then X's conviction will, in turn, be sustained. Where treating like future cases, as one says one must treat this case, may lead to the substantial frustration of important public interests (even if this case by itself does not do so), the issue will be treated by the expectation of what would lie ahead, rather than by that which has happened. By this standard, few *O'Brien*-type cases will come out favorably to the first amendment claim.[142]

IV

Even so, note, finally, that the rather undemanding criteria (de facto) of the *O'Brien* approach may control only within its own quite narrowly stated field of regulation, i.e. those regulations which, on their face, do not limit anything one ordinarily would regard as either speech or (even) as "akin" to speech. So, just as a parting counter example, as an example of an ordinance not subject to the *O'Brien* test (but subject, rather, to more stringent first amendment review?),[143] any ordinance

---

140. This would seem to be so, consistent with the last part of the *O'Brien* standard as set out by the Court, because being able to apply the ordinance to X in the particular circumstances seems quite inessential to the furtherance of the common substantial interest in public traffic safety. (Little, if any, actual traffic problem was caused by X.) And, accordingly, by offering this very observation, one might think that, therefore, X should prevail, given the standards said to be applicable to his case.

141. As a mnemonic aid, rock fans may recall a memorable line from a lyric by the Grateful Dead. ("Trouble ahead, trouble behind, and you know this notion just crossed my mind.") So, the Court concludes that were it to sustain the camping "right" of the Creative Non-Violence group on first amendment grounds, it would be bound to treat others equally so to sustain a similar camping right in them in any similar case, i.e. where camping was also part of a political demonstration designed to capture public attention in the same way. Yet, if each group wishing to make its point in this way could do so in the same manner and to the same extent as Creative Non-Violence, under claim of an equal first amendment right, then indeed the park's use as a park would be substantially (perhaps wholly) subverted, i.e. effectively destroyed for ordinary park use.

142. For a generalization and review of this approach to first amendment questions, see Easterbrook, The Supreme Court 1983 Term Forward: The Court and The Economic System, 98 Harv.L.Rev. 4 (1984).

143. Compare and determine whether the different "test" as framed by the Supreme Court in respect to "time, place, and manner" speech regulations (*infra*) are in fact more protective than the *O'Brien* test just reviewed.

in any way presuming to restrict one's use of the streets as places of "public demonstration," or "protest," would presumably remain subject to more stringent first amendment review. Thus qualified, the *O'Brien* test may be limited, and useful, within its narrow area of fit.[144]

SCHACHT v. UNITED STATES

398 U.S. 58 (1970)

MR. JUSTICE BLACK delivered the opinion of the Court.

The petitioner, Daniel Jay Schacht, was indicted in a United States District Court for violating 18 U.S.C. § 702, which makes it a crime for any person "without authority [to wear] the uniform or a distinctive part thereof of any of the armed forces of the United States. ***" He was tried and convicted by a jury, and on February 29, 1968, he was sentenced to pay a fine of $250 and to serve a six-month prison term ***. There is no doubt that Schacht did wear distinctive parts of the uniform of the United States Army[2] and that he was not a member of the Armed Forces. He has defended his conduct since the beginning, however, on the ground that he was authorized to wear the uniform by an Act of Congress, 10 U.S.C. § 772(f), which provides as follows:

"When wearing by persons not on active duty authorized.

***

"(f) While portraying a member of the Army, Navy, Air Force, or Marine Corps, an actor in a theatrical or motion-picture production may wear the uniform of that armed force *if the portrayal does not tend to discredit that armed force*." (Emphasis added.)

Schacht argued in the trial court and in this Court that he wore the army uniform as an "actor" in a "theatrical production" performed several times between 6:30 and 8:30 a.m. on December 4, 1967, in front of the Armed Forces Induction Center at Houston, Texas. The street skit in which Schacht wore the army uniform as a costume was designed, in his view, to expose the evil of the American presence in Vietnam and was part of a larger, peaceful antiwar demonstration at the induction center that morning. ***

---

144. The more serious difficulty with respect to *O'Brien* has been, rather, that some Justices have treated it as a general first amendment test. See, e.g., Barnes v. Glen Theatre, 501 U.S. 560 (1991) (infra at p. 793). See Vincent A. Blasi, Six Conservatives in Search of the First Amendment: The Revealing Case of Nude Dancing, 33 Wm. & Mary L. Rev. 611 (1992).

2. Schacht wore a blouse of the type currently authorized for Army enlisted men with a shoulder patch designating service in Europe. The buttons on his blouse were of the official Army design. On his head Schacht wore an outmoded military hat. Affixed to the hat in an inverted position was the eagle insignia currently worn on the hats of Army officers.

> "The skit was composed of three people. There was Schacht who was dressed in a uniform and cap. A second person was wearing 'military colored' coveralls. The third person was outfitted in typical Viet Cong apparel. The first two men carried water pistols. One of them would yell, 'Be an able American,' and then they would shoot the Viet Cong with their pistols. The pistols expelled a red liquid which, when it struck the victim, created the impression that he was bleeding. Once the victim fell down the other two would walk up to him and exclaim, 'My God, this is a pregnant woman.' Without noticeable variation this skit was reenacted several times during the morning of the demonstration."

Our previous cases would seem to make it clear that 18 U.S.C. § 702, making it an offense to wear our military uniforms without authority is, standing alone, a valid statute on its face. See, e.g., United States v. O'Brien, 391 U.S. 367 (1968). But the general prohibition of 18 U.S.C. § 702 cannot always stand alone in view of 10 U.S.C. § 772, which authorizes the wearing of military uniforms under certain conditions and circumstances including the circumstance of an actor portraying a member of the armed services in a "theatrical production." 10 U.S.C. § 772 (f). The Government's argument in this case seems to imply that somehow what these amateur actors did in Houston should not be treated as a "theatrical production" within the meaning of § 772(f). We are unable to follow such a suggestion. *** We need only find, as we emphatically do, that the street skit in which Schacht participated was a "theatrical production" within the meaning of that section.

This brings us to petitioner's complaint that giving force and effect to the last clause of § 772(f) would impose an unconstitutional restraint on his right of free speech. We agree. This clause on its face simply restricts § 772(f)'s authorization to those dramatic portrayals that do not "tend to discredit" the military, but, when this restriction is read together with 18 U.S.C. § 702, it becomes clear that Congress has in effect made it a crime for an actor wearing a military uniform to say things during his performance critical of the conduct or policies of the Armed Forces. An actor, like everyone else in our country, enjoys a constitutional right to freedom of speech, including the right openly to criticize the Government during a dramatic performance. The last clause of § 772(f) denies this constitutional right to an actor who is wearing a military uniform by making it a crime for him to say things that tend to bring the military into discredit and disrepute. In the present case Schacht was free to participate in any skit at the demonstration that praised the Army, but under the final clause of § 772(f) he could be convicted of a federal offense if his portrayal attacked the Army instead of praising it. In light of our earlier finding that the skit in which Schacht participated was a "theatrical production" within the meaning of § 772(f), it follows that his conviction can be sustained only if he can be punished for speaking out against the role of our Army and our country in Vietnam. Clearly punishment for this reason would be an unconstitutional abridgment of freedom of speech. The final clause of § 772(f), which leaves Americans free to praise the war in Vietnam but can send persons like Schacht to prison for opposing it, cannot survive in a country which has the First Amendment. To preserve the constitutionality of § 772(f) that final clause must be stricken from the section. *** Reversed.

MR. JUSTICE HARLAN, concurring. [Omitted.]

MR. JUSTICE WHITE, with whom THE CHIEF JUSTICE and MR. JUSTICE STEWART join, concurring in the result. [Omitted.]

SPENCE v. STATE OF WASHINGTON
418 U.S. 405 (1974)

PER CURIAM.

Appellant was convicted under a Washington statute forbidding the exhibition of a United States flag to which is attached or superimposed figures, symbols, or other extraneous material. The Supreme Court of Washington affirmed appellant's conviction. *** We reverse on the ground that as applied to appellant's activity the Washington statute impermissibly infringed protected expression.

I

On May 10, 1970, appellant, a college student, hung his United States flag from the window of his apartment on private property in Seattle, Washington. The flag was upside down, and attached to the front and back was a peace symbol (*i. e.*, a circle enclosing a trident) made of removable black tape. The window was above the ground floor. The flag measured approximately three by five feet and was plainly visible to passersby. The peace symbol occupied roughly half of the surface of the flag.

Three Seattle police officers observed the flag and entered the apartment house. Appellant was not charged under Washington's flag-desecration statute. See Wash. Rev. Code § 9.86.030, as amended.[1] Rather, the State relied on the so-called "improper use" statute, Wash.Rev.Code § 9.86.020. This statute provides, in pertinent part:

"No person shall, in any manner, for exhibition or display:

"(1) Place or cause to be placed any word, figure, mark, picture, design, drawing or advertisement of any nature upon any flag, standard, color, ensign or shield of the United States or of this state *** or

---

1. This statute provides in part:

"No person shall knowingly cast contempt upon any flag, standard, color, ensign or shield *** by publicly mutilating, defacing, burning, or trampling upon said flag, standard, color, ensign or shield."

"(2) Expose to public view any such flag, standard, color, ensign or shield upon which shall have been printed, painted or otherwise produced, or to which shall have been attached, appended, affixed or annexed any such word, figure, mark, picture, design, drawing or advertisement ***."[2]

***

The State based its case on the flag itself and the testimony of the three arresting officers, who testified that they had observed the flag displayed from appellant's window and that on the flag was superimposed what they identified as a peace symbol. Appellant took the stand in his own defense. He testified that he put a peace symbol on the flag and displayed it to public view as a protest against the invasion of Cambodia and the killings at Kent State University, events which occurred a few days prior to his arrest. He said that his purpose was to associate the American flag with peace instead of war and violence:

"I felt there had been so much killing and that this was not what America stood for. I felt that the flag stood for America and I wanted people to know that I thought America stood for peace."

Appellant further testified that he chose to fashion the peace symbol from tape so that it could be removed without damaging the flag. The State made no effort to controvert any of appellant's testimony. *** The trial court instructed the jury in essence that the mere act of displaying the flag with the peace symbol attached, if proved beyond a reasonable doubt, was sufficient to convict. There was no requirement of specific intent to do anything more than display the flag in that manner.

II

A number of factors are important in the instant case. First, this was a privately owned flag. In a technical property sense it was not the property of any government. We have no doubt that the State or National Governments constitutionally may forbid anyone from mishandling in any manner a flag that is public property. *** Second, appellant displayed his flag on private property. He engaged in no trespass or disorderly conduct. Nor is this a case that might be analyzed in terms of reasonable time, place, or manner restraints on access to a public area. Third, the record is devoid of proof of any risk of breach of the peace. It was not appellant's purpose to incite violence or even stimulate a public demonstration. There is no evidence that any crowd gathered or that appellant made any effort to attract attention beyond

2. Washington Rev.Code § 9.86.010 defines the flags and other symbols protected by the desecration and improper-use statutes as follows:

"The words flag, standard, color, ensign or shield, as used in this chapter, shall include any flag, standard, color, ensign or shield, or copy, picture or representation thereof, made of any substance or represented or produced thereon, and of any size, evidently purporting to be such flag, standard, color, ensign or shield of the United States of of this state, or a copy, picture or representation thereof."

hanging the flag out of his own window. Indeed, on the facts stipulated by the parties there is no evidence that anyone other than the three police officers observed the flag.

Fourth, the State concedes, as did the Washington Supreme Court, that appellant engaged in a form of communication. *** [T]he nature of appellant's activity, combined with the factual context and environment in which it was undertaken, lead to the conclusion that he engaged in a form of protected expression. *** The Court for decades has recognized the communicative connotations of the use of flags. On this record there can be little doubt that appellant communicated through the use of symbols. The symbolism included not only the flag but also the superimposed peace symbol.

Moreover, the context in which a symbol is used for purposes of expression is important, for the context may give meaning to the symbol. See Tinker v. Des Moines Independent Community School District, 393 U.S. 503 (1969). In *Tinker* the wearing of black armbands in a school environment conveyed an unmistakable message about a contemporaneous issue of intense public concern—the Vietnam hostilities. In this case, appellant's activity was roughly simultaneous with and concededly triggered by the Cambodian incursion and the Kent State tragedy, also issues of great public moment. *** A flag bearing a peace symbol and displayed upside down by a student today might be interpreted as nothing more than bizarre behavior, but it would have been difficult for the great majority of citizens to miss the drift of appellant's point at the time that he made it. ***

We are met at the outset with something of an enigma in the manner in which the case was presented to us. The Washington Supreme Court rejected any reliance on a breach-of-the-peace rationale. *** It based its result primarily on the ground that "the nation and state both have a recognizable interest in preserving the flag as a symbol of the nation."[4] Yet counsel for the State declined to support the highest state court's principal rationale in argument before us. He pursued instead the breach-of-the-peace theory discarded by the state court. Indeed, that was the only basis on which he chose to support the constitutionality of the state statute.

Despite counsel's approach, we think it appropriate to review briefly the range of various state interests that might be thought to support the challenged conviction ***. The first interest at issue is prevention of breach of the peace. In our view, the Washington Supreme Court correctly rejected this notion. It is totally without support in the record.

---

4. A subsidiary ground relied on by the Washington Supreme Court must be rejected summarily. It found the inhibition on appellant's freedom of expression "minuscule and trifling" because there are "thousands of other means available to [him] for the dissemination of his personal view ***." As the Court noted in, *e.g.*, Schneider v. State of New Jersey, 308 U.S. 147 (1939), "one is not to have the exercise of his liberty of expression in appropriate places abridged on the plea that it may be be exercised in some other place."

We are also unable to affirm the judgment below on the ground that the State may have desired to protect the sensibilities of passersby. "It is firmly settled that under our Constitution the public expression of ideas may not be prohibited merely because the ideas are themselves offensive to some of their hearers." *Street v. New York*, [394 U.S.], at 592. Moreover, appellant did not impose his ideas upon a captive audience. Anyone who might have been offended could easily have avoided the display. See Cohen v. California, 403 U.S. 15 (1971). Nor may appellant be punished for failing to show proper respect for our national emblem. *Street v. New York*, *supra*, at 593; *Board of Education v. Barnette*, [319 U.S. 624 (1943)].[6]

We are brought, then, to the state court's thesis that Washington has an interest in preserving the national flag as an unalloyed symbol of our country. The court did not define this interest; it simply asserted it. MR. JUSTICE REHNQUIST's dissenting opinion today adopts essentially the same approach. Presumably, this interest might be seen as an effort to prevent the appropriation of a revered national symbol by an individual, interest group, or enterprise where there was a risk that association of the symbol with a particular product or viewpoint might be taken erroneously as evidence of governmental endorsement.[7] Alternatively, it might be argued that the interest asserted by the state court is based on the uniquely universal character of the national flag as a symbol. For the great majority of us, the flag is a symbol of patriotism, of pride in the history of our country, and of the service, sacrifice, and valor of the millions of Americans who in peace and war have joined together to build and to defend a Nation in which self-government and personal liberty endure. It evidences both the unity and diversity which are America. For others the flag carries in varying degrees a different message. "A person gets from a symbol the meaning he puts into it, and what is one man's comfort and inspiration is another's jest and scorn." *Board of Education v. Barnette*, 319 U.S., at 632-633. It might be said that we all draw something from our national symbol, for it is capable of conveying simultaneously a spectrum of meanings. If it may be destroyed or permanently disfigured, it could be argued that it will lose its capability of mirroring the sentiments of all who view it.

---

6. Counsel for the State conceded that promoting respect for the flag is not a legitimate state interest. ***

7. Undoubtedly such a concern underlies that portion of the improper-use statute forbidding the utilization of representations of the flag in a commercial context. *** There is no occasion in this case to address the application of the challenged statute to commercial behavior. Cf. Halter v. Nebraska, 205 U.S. 34 (1907). MR. JUSTICE REHNQUIST's dissent places major reliance on *Halter*, despite the fact that *Halter* was decided nearly 20 years before the Court concluded that the First Amendment applies to the States by virtue of the Fourteenth Amendment. See Gitlow v. New York, 268 U.S. 652 (1925).

But we need not decide in this case whether the interest advanced by the court below is valid.[8] We assume, *arguendo*, that it is. The statute is nonetheless unconstitutional as applied to appellant's activity.[9] There was no risk that appellant's acts would mislead viewers into assuming that the Government endorsed his viewpoint. To the contrary, he was plainly and peacefully protesting the fact that it did not. Appellant was not charged under the desecration statute, nor did he permanently disfigure the flag or destroy it. He displayed it as a flag of his country in a way closely analogous to the manner in which flags have always been used to convey ideas. Moreover, his message was direct, likely to be understood, and within the contours of the First Amendment. Given the protected character of his expression and in light of the fact that no interest the State may have in preserving the physical integrity of a privately owned flag was significantly impaired on these facts, the conviction must be invalidated. *** The judgment is reversed.

MR. JUSTICE DOUGLAS, concurring. [Omitted]

MR. CHIEF JUSTICE BURGER, dissenting. [Omitted.]

MR. JUSTICE REHNQUIST, with whom THE CHIEF JUSTICE and MR. JUSTICE WHITE join, dissenting.

The Court holds that a Washington statute prohibiting persons from attaching material to the American flag was unconstitutionally applied to appellant. Although I agree with the Court that appellant's activity was a form of communication, I do not agree that the First Amendment prohibits the State from restricting this activity in furtherance of other important interests. And I believe the rationale by which the Court reaches its conclusion is unsound.

---

8. If this interest is valid, we note that it is directly related to expression in the context of activity like that undertaken by appellant. For that reason and because no other governmental interest unrelated to expression has been advanced or can be supported on this record, the four-step analysis of United States v. O'Brien, 391 U. S. 367, 377 (1968), is inapplicable.

9. Because we agree with appellant's as-applied argument, we do not reach the more comprehensive overbreadth contention he also advances. But it is worth noting the nearly limitless sweep of the Washington improper-use flag statute. Read literally, it forbids a veteran's group from attaching, *e.g.*, battalion commendations to a United States flag. It proscribes photographs of war heroes standing in front of the flag. It outlaws newspaper mastheads composed of the national flag with superimposed print. Other examples could easily be listed.

Statutes of such sweep suggest problems of selective enforcement. We are, however, unable to agree with appellant's void-for-vagueness argument. The statute's application is quite mechanical, particularly when implemented with jury instructions like the ones given in this case. The law in Washington, simply put, is that *nothing* may be affixed to or superimposed on a United States flag or a representation thereof. Thus, if selective enforcement has occurred, it has been a result of prosecutorial discretion, not the language of the statute. Accordingly, this case is unlike Smith v. Goguen, 415 U.S. 566 (1974), where the words of the statute at issue ("publicly *** treats contemptuously") were themselves sufficiently indefinite to prompt subjective treatment by prosecutorial authorities.

The Court has recognized that even protected speech may be subject to reasonable limitation when important countervailing interests are involved. Citizens are not completely free to commit perjury, to libel other citizens, to infringe copyrights, to incite riots, or to interfere unduly with passage through a public thoroughfare. The right of free speech, though precious, remains subject to reasonable accommodation to other valued interests.

Since a State concededly may impose some limitations on speech directly, it would seem to follow *a fortiori* that a State may legislate to protect important state interests even though an incidental limitation on free speech results. Virtually any law enacted by a State, when viewed with sufficient ingenuity, could be thought to interfere with some citizen's preferred means of expression. But no one would argue, I presume, that a State could not prevent the painting of public buildings simply because a particular class of protesters believed their message would best be conveyed through that medium. Had appellant here chosen to tape his peace symbol to a federal courthouse, I have little doubt that he could be prosecuted under a statute properly drawn to protect public property. ***

The statute under which appellant was convicted is no stranger to this Court, a virtually identical statute having been before the Court in Halter v. Nebraska, 205 U.S. 34 (1907). In that case the Court held that the State of Nebraska could enforce its statute to prevent use of a flag representation on beer bottles, stating flatly that "a State will be wanting in care for the well-being of its people if it ignores the fact that they regard the flag as a symbol of their country's power and prestige ***." The Court then continued: "Such an use tends to degrade and cheapen the flag in the estimation of the people, as well as to defeat the object of maintaining it as an emblem of national power and national honor."

The Court today finds *Halter* irrelevant to the present case, pointing out that it was decided almost 20 years before the First Amendment was applied to the States and further noting that it involved "commercial behavior," a form of expression the Court presumably will consider another day. Insofar as *Halter* assesses the State's interest, of course, the Court's argument is simply beside the point. But even as the argument relates to appellant's interest, I find it somewhat difficult to grasp. The Court may possibly be suggesting that political expression deserves greater protection than other forms of expression, but that suggestion would seem quite inconsistent with the position taken in *Lehman v. Shaker Heights*,[2] by nearly all Members

---

2. The plurality opinion of MR. JUSTICE BLACKMUN took the position that a ban against political advertising on publicly owned buses was not unconstitutional since "[n]o First Amendment forum is here to be found." MR. JUSTICE DOUGLAS, concurring in the judgment, stated that petitioner in that case had no "constitutional right to spread his message before this captive audience," but specifically noted:

"I do not view the content of the message as relevant either to petitioner's right to express it or to the commuters' right to be free from it. Commercial advertisements may be as offensive and intrusive to captive audiences as any political message." MR. JUSTICE BRENNAN, with whom MR. JUSTICE STEWART, MR. JUSTICE MARSHALL, and MR. JUSTICE POWELL joined, dissenting, stated: "There is some doubt concerning whether the 'commercial speech' distinction announced in Valentine v.

of the majority in the instant case. Yet if the Court is suggesting that*Halter* would now be decided differently, and that the State's interest in the flag falls before any speech which is "direct, likely to be understood, and within the contours of the First Amendment," that view would mean the flag could be auctioned as a background to anyone willing and able to buy or copy one. I find it hard to believe the Court intends to presage that result.

Turning to the question of the State's interest in the flag, it seems to me that the Court's treatment lacks all substance. The suggestion that the State's interest somehow diminishes when the flag is decorated with*removable* tape trivializes something which is not trivial. The State of Washington is hardly seeking to protect the flag's resale value, and yet the Court's emphasis on the lack of actual damage to the flag suggests that this is a significant aspect of the State's interest. Surely the Court does not mean to imply that appellant*could* be prosecuted if he subsequently tore the flag in the process of trying to take the tape off. Unlike flag-desecration statutes, which the Court correctly notes are not at issue in this case, the Washington statute challenged here seeks to prevent personal *use* of the flag, not simply particular forms of *abuse*. The State of Washington has chosen to set the flag apart for a special purpose, and has directed that it not be turned into a common background for an endless variety of superimposed messages. The physical condition of the flag itself is irrelevant to that purpose.

The true nature of the State's interest in this case is not only one of preserving "the physical integrity of the flag," but also one of preserving the flag as "an important symbol of nationhood and unity." Although the Court treats this important interest with a studied inattention, it is hardly one of recent invention and has previously been accorded considerable respect by this Court. In *Halter*, for example, the Court stated:

> "As the statute in question evidently had its origin in a purpose to cultivate a feeling of patriotism among the people of Nebraska, we are unwilling to adjudge that in legislation for that purpose the State erred in duty or has infringed the constitutional right of anyone. On the contrary, it may reasonably be affirmed that a duty rests upon each State in every legal way to encourage its people to love the Union with which the State is indissolubly connected."

There was no question in *Halter* of physical impairment of a flag since no actual flag was even involved. And it certainly would have made no difference to the Court's discussion of the State's interest if the plaintiff in error in that case had chosen to advertise his product by decorating the flag with beer bottles fashioned from some

---

Chrestensen, 316 U.S. 52 (1942), retains continuing validity." referring to Mr. Justice Douglas' concurring opinion in Camarano v. United States, 358 U.S. 498 (1959). The dissent further stated: "Once a public forum for communication has been established, both free speech and equal protection principles prohibit discrimination based *solely* upon subject matter or content." (Emphasis in original.)

removable substance.[5] It is the character, not the cloth, of the flag which the State seeks to protect.

The value of this interest has been emphasized in recent as well as distant times. MR. JUSTICE FORTAS, for example, noted in Street v. New York, 394 U.S. 576, 616 (1969), that "the flag is a special kind of personalty," a form of property "burdened with peculiar obligations and restrictions." *Id.*, at 617 (dissenting opinion).[6] MR. JUSTICE WHITE, has observed that "[t]he flag is a national property, and the Nation may regulate those who would make, imitate, sell, possess, or use it." *Smith v. Goguen*, 415 U.S., at 587 (concurring in judgment). I agree. What appellant here seeks is simply license to use the flag however he pleases, so long as the activity can be tied to a concept of speech, regardless of any state interest in having the flag used only for more limited purposes. I find no reasoning in the Court's opinion which convinces me that the Constitution requires such license to be given.

The fact that the State has a valid interest in preserving the character of the flag does not mean, of course, that it can employ all conceivable means to enforce it. It certainly could not require all citizens to own the flag or compel citizens to salute one. Board of Education v. Barnette, 319 U.S. 624 (1943). It presumably cannot punish criticism of the flag, or the principles for which it stands, any more than it could punish criticism of this country's policies or ideas. But the statute in this case demands no such allegiance. Its operation does not depend upon whether the flag is used for communicative or noncommunicative purposes; upon whether a particular message is deemed commercial or political; upon whether the use of the flag is respectful or contemptuous; or upon whether any particular segment of the State's citizenry might applaud or oppose the intended message. It simply withdraws a unique national symbol from the roster of materials that may be used as a background for communications. Since I do not believe the Constitution prohibits Washington from making that decision, I dissent.

TEXAS v. JOHNSON

491 U.S. 397 (1989)

JUSTICE BRENNAN delivered the opinion of the Court.

After publicly burning an American flag as a means of political protest, Gregory Lee Johnson was convicted of desecrating a flag in violation of Texas law. This case

---

5. It should be noted that *Halter* makes no mention of the argument that allowing use of the flag for a personal or commercial purpose might suggest endorsement of that purpose by the government. While this might be an *additional* state interest in appropriate cases, it is by no means an indispensable element of the State's concern about the integrity of the flag.

6. The majority of the Court in *Street* stated: "We add that disrespect for our flag is to be deplored no less in these vexed times than in calmer periods of our history," 394 U.S., at 594, citing *Halter*.

presents the question whether his conviction is consistent with the First Amendment. We hold that it is not.

I

While the Republican National Convention was taking place in Dallas in 1984, respondent Johnson participated in a political demonstration dubbed the "Repubican War Chest Tour." As explained in literature distributed by the demonstrators and in speeches made by them, the purpose of this event was to protest the policies of the Reagan administration and of certain Dallas-based corporations. The demonstrators marched through the Dallas streets, chanting political slogans and stopping at several corporate locations to stage "die-ins" intended to dramatize the consequences of nuclear war. On several occasions they spray-painted the walls of buildings and overturned potted plants, but Johnson himself took no part in such activities. He did, however, accept an American flag handed to him by a fellow protestor who had taken it from a flag pole outside one of the targeted buildings.

The demonstration ended in front of Dallas City Hall, where Johnson unfurled the American flag, doused it with kerosene, and set it on fire. While the flag burned, the protestors chanted, "America, the red, white, and blue, we spit on you." After the demonstrators dispersed, a witness to the flag-burning collected the flag's remains and buried them in his backyard. No one was physically injured or threatened with injury, though several witnesses testified that they had been seriously offended by the flag-burning.

Of the approximately 100 demonstrators, Johnson alone was charged with a crime. The only criminal offense with which he was charged was the desecration of a venerated object in violation of Tex. Penal Code Ann. § 42.09(a)(3)(1989).[1] After a trial, he was convicted, sentenced to one year in prison, and fined $2,000. The Court of Appeals for the Fifth District of Texas at Dallas affirmed Johnson's conviction, but the Texas Court of Criminal Appeals reversed, holding that the State could not, consistent with the First Amendment, punish Johnson for burning the flag in these circumstances. ***

Because it reversed Johnson's conviction on the ground that § 42.09 was unconstitutional as applied to him, the state court did not address Johnson's argument that

---

1. Tex. Penal Code Ann. § 42.09 (1989) provides in full:

"§ 42.09. Desecration of Venerated Object

"(a) A person commits an offense if he intentionally or knowingly desecrates:

"(1) a public monument;

"(2) a place of worship or burial; or

"(3) a state or national flag.

"(b) For purposes of this section, 'desecrate' means deface, damage, or otherwise physically mistreat in a way that the actor knows will seriously offend one or more persons likely to observe or discover his action.

"(c) An offense under this section is a Class A misdemeanor."

the statute was, on its face, unconstitutionally vague and overbroad. We granted certiorari, and now affirm.

II

Johnson was convicted of flag desecration for burning the flag rather than for uttering insulting words. This fact somewhat complicates our consideration of his conviction under the First Amendment. We must first determine whether Johnson's burning of the flag constituted expressive conduct, permitting him to invoke the First Amendment in challenging his conviction. See, e.g., Spence v. Washington, 418 U.S. 405, 409-411 (1974). If his conduct was expressive, we next decide whether the State's regulation is related to the suppression of free expression. See, e.g., United States v. O'Brien, 391 U.S. 367, 377 (1968); If the State's regulation is not related to expression, then the less stringent standard we announced in *United States v. O'Brien* for regulations of noncommunicative conduct controls. If it is, then we are outside of *O'Brien*'s test, and we must ask whether this interest justifies Johnson's conviction under a more demanding standard.[3]

The First Amendment literally forbids the abridgement only of "speech," but we have long recognized that its protection does not end at the spoken or written word. While we have rejected "the view that an apparently limitless variety of conduct can be labeled 'speech' whenever the person engaging in the conduct intends thereby to express an idea," *United States v. O'Brien*, at 376, we have acknowledged that conduct may be "sufficiently imbued with elements of communication to fall within the scope of the First and Fourteenth Amendments." *Spence*, at 409. ***

Especially pertinent to this case are our decisions recognizing the communicative nature of conduct relating to flags. Attaching a peace sign to the flag, *Spence, supra*, at 409-410; saluting the flag; *Barnette*, 319 U.S., at 632; and displaying a red flag, Stromberg v. California, 283 U.S. 359, 368-369 (1931), we have held, all may find shelter under the First Amendment.

---

3. Although Johnson has raised a facial challenge to Texas' flag-desecration statute, we choose to resolve this case on the basis of his claim that the statute as applied to him violates the First Amendment. Section 42.09 regulates only physical conduct with respect to the flag, not the written or spoken word, and although one violates the statute only if one "knows" that one's physical treatment of the flag "will seriously offend one or more persons likely to observe or discover his action," this fact does not necessarily mean that the statute applies only to *expressive* conduct protected by the First Amendment. *Cf.* Smith v. Goguen, 415 U.S. 566, 588 (1974) (WHITE, J., concurring in judgment) (statute prohibiting "contemptuous" treatment of flag encompasses only expressive conduct). A tired person might, for example, drag a flag through the mud, knowing that this conduct is likely to offend others, and yet have no thought of expressing any idea; neither the language nor the Texas courts' interpretations of the statute precludes the possibility that such a person would be prosecuted for flag desecration. Because the prosecution of a person who had not engaged in expressive conduct would pose a different case and because we are capable of disposing of this case on narrower grounds, we address only Johnson's claim that § 42.09 as applied to political expression like his violates the First Amendment.

We have not automatically concluded, however, that any action taken with respect to our flag is expressive. Instead, in characterizing such action for First Amendment purposes, we have considered the context in which it occurred. In *Spence,* for example, we emphasized that Spence's taping of a peace sign to his flag was "roughly simultaneous with and concededly triggered by the Cambodian incursion and the Kent State tragedy."

The State of Texas conceded for purposes of its oral argument in this case that Johnson's conduct was expressive conduct, and this concession seems to us as prudent as was Washington's in *Spence.* Johnson burned an American flag as part—indeed, as the culmination—of a political demonstration that coincided with the convening of the Republican Party and its renomination of Ronald Reagan for President. The expressive, overtly political nature of this conduct was both intentional and overwhelmingly apparent.

III

The Government generally has a freer hand in restricting expressive conduct than it has in restricting the written or spoken word. See *O'Brien*, 391 U.S., at 376-377; Clark v. Community for Creative Non-Violence, 468 U.S. 299-293 (1984). It may not, however, proscribe particular conduct *because* it has expressive elements. *** A law *directed at* the communicative nature of conduct must, like a law directed at speech itself, be justified by the substantial showing of need that the First Amendment requires." Community for Creative Non-Violence v. Watt, 703 F.2d 586, 622-623 (D.C.Cir. 1983) (Scalia, J., dissenting). ***

Thus, although we have recognized that where "'speech' and 'nonspeech' elements are combined in the same course of conduct, a sufficiently important governmental interest in regulating the nonspeech element can justify incidental limitations on First Amendment freedoms," *O'Brien*, at 376, we have limited the applicability of *O'Brien*'s relatively lenient standard to those cases in which "the governmental interest is unrelated to the suppression of free expression." ***

In order to decide whether *O'Brien*'s test applies here, therefore, we must decide whether Texas has asserted an interest in support of Johnson's conviction that is unrelated to the suppression of expression. If we find that an interest asserted by the State is simply not implicated on the facts before us, we need not ask whether *O'Brien*'s test applies. See *Spence*, at 414, n.8. The State offers two separate interests to justify this conviction: preventing breaches of the peace, and preserving the flag as a symbol of nationhood and national unity. We hold that the first interest is not implicated on this record and that the second is related to the suppression of expression.

Texas claims that its interest in preventing breaches of the peace justifies Johnson's conviction for flag desecration.[4] However, no disturbance of the peace actually occurred or threatened to occur because of Johnson's burning of the flag. Although the State stresses the disruptive behavior of the protestors during their march toward City Hall, it admits that "no actual breach of the peace occurred at the time of the flagburning or in response to the flagburning." The State's emphasis on the protestors' disorderly actions prior to arriving at City Hall is not only somewhat surprising given that no charges were brought on the basis of this conduct, but it also fails to show that a disturbance of the peace was a likely reaction to Johnson's conduct. The only evidence offered by the State at trial to show the reaction to Johnson's actions was the testimony of several persons who had been seriously offended by the flag-burning.

The State's position, therefore, amounts to a claim that an audience that takes serious offense at particular expression is necessarily likely to disturb the peace and that the expression may be prohibited on this basis. Our precedents do not countenance such a presumption. On the contrary, they recognize that a principal "function of free speech under our system of government is to invite dispute. It may indeed best serve its high purpose when it induces a condition of unrest, creates dissatisfaction with conditions as they are, or even stirs people to anger." Terminiello v. Chicago, 337 U.S. 1, 4 (1949). See also *** Hustler Magazine, Inc. v. Falwell, 485 U.S. 46, 55-56 (1988). ***

Nor does Johnson's expressive conduct fall within that small class of "fighting words" that are "likely to provoke the average person to retaliation, and thereby cause a breach of peace." Chaplinsky v. New Hampshire, 315 U.S. 568, 574 (1942). No reasonable onlooker would have regarded Johnson's generalized expression of dissatisfaction with the policies of the Federal Government as a direct personal insult or an invitation to exchange fisticuffs. ***

We thus conclude that the State's interest in maintaining order is not implicated on these facts. The State need not worry that our holding will disable it from preserving the peace. We do not suggest that the First Amendment forbids a State to prevent "imminent lawless action." And, in fact, Texas already has a statute specifically prohibiting breaches of the peace, Tex. Penal Code Ann. § 42.01 (1989),

---

4. Relying on our decision in Boos v. Barry, 485 U.S. 312 (1988), Johnson argues that this state interest is related to the suppression of free expression within the meaning of United States v. O'Brien, 391 U.S. 367 (1968). He reasons that the violent reaction to flag-burnings feared by Texas would be the result of the message conveyed by them, and that this fact connects the State's interest to the suppression of expression. This view has found some favor in the lower courts. See Monroe v. State Court of Fulton County, 739 F.2d 568, 574-575 (CA11 1984). Johnson's theory may overread *Boos* insofar as it suggests that a desire to prevent a violent audience reaction is "related to expression" in the same way that a desire to prevent an audience from being offended is "related to expression." Because we find that the State's interest in preventing breaches of the peace is not implicated on these facts, however, we need not venture further into this area.

which tends to confirm that Texas need not punish this flag desecration in order to keep the peace. ***

The State also asserts an interest in preserving the flag as a symbol of nationhood and national unity. In *Spence,* we acknowledged that the Government's interest in preserving the flag's special symbolic value "is directly related to expression in the context of activity" such as affixing a peace symbol to a flag. We are equally persuaded that this interest is related to expression in the case of Johnson's burning of the flag. The State, apparently, is concerned that such conduct will lead people to believe either that the flag does not stand for nationhood and national unity, but instead reflects other, less positive concepts, or that the concepts reflected in the flag do not in fact exist, that is, we do not enjoy unity as a Nation. These concerns blossom only when a person's treatment of the flag communicates some message, and thus are related "to the suppression of free expression" within the meaning of *O'Brien*'s test altogether.

IV

It remains to consider whether the State's interest in preserving the flag as a symbol of nationhood and national unity justifies Johnson's conviction.

As in *Spence,* "[w]e are confronted with a case of prosecution for the expression of an idea through activity," and "[a]ccordingly, we must examine with particular care the interests advanced by [petitioner] to support its prosecution." Johnson was not, we add, prosecuted for the expression of just any idea; he was prosecuted for his expression of dissatisfaction with the policies of this country, expression situated at the core of our First Amendment values. ***

Moreover, Johnson was prosecuted because he knew that his politically charged expression would cause "serious offense." If he had burned the flag as a means of disposing of it because it was dirty or torn, he would not have been convicted of flag desecration under this Texas law: federal law designates burning as the preferred means of disposing of a flag "when it is in such condition that it is no longer a fitting emblem for display," 36 U.S.C. § 176(k), and Texas has no quarrel with this means of disposal. The Texas law is thus not aimed at protecting the physical integrity of the flag in all circumstances, but is designated instead to protect it only against impairments that would cause serious offense to others.[6] Texas concedes as much: "Section 42.09(b) reaches only those severe acts of physical abuse of the flag carried out in a way likely to be offensive. The statute mandates intentional or knowing abuse, that is, the kind of mistreatment that is not innocent, but rather is intentionally designed to seriously offend other individuals." *** Johnson's political expression was restricted because of the content of the message he conveyed. We must there-

---

6. *Cf.* Smith v. Goguen, 415 U.S., at 590-591 (BLACKMUN. J., dissenting) (emphasizing that lower court appeared to have construed state statute so as to protect physical integrity of the flag in all circumstances); *id.*, at 597-598 (REHNQUIST, J., dissenting) (same).

fore subject the State's asserted interest in preserving the special symbolic character of the flag to "the most exacting scrutiny."[8]

Texas argues that its interest in preserving the flag as a symbol of nationhood and national unity survives this close analysis. Quoting extensively from the writings of this Court chronicling the flag's historic and symbolic role in our society, the State emphasizes the "'special place'" reserved for the flag in our Nation. Brief for Petitioner 22, quoting *Smith v. Goguen*, 415 U.S., at 601 (REHNQUIST, J., dissenting). The State's argument is not that it has an interest simply in maintaining the flag as a symbol of *something*, no matter what it symbolizes; indeed, if that were the State's position, it would be difficult to see how that interest is endangered by highly symbolic conduct such as Johnson's. Rather, the State's claim is that it has an interest in preserving the flag as a symbol of *nationhood* and *national unity*, a symbol with a determinate range of meanings. According to Texas, if one physically treats the flag in a way that would tend to cast doubt on either the idea that nationhood and national unity are the flag's referents or that national unity actually exists, the message conveyed thereby is a harmful one and therefore may be prohibited.[9]

If there is a bedrock principle underlying the First Amendment, it is that the Government may not prohibit the expression of an idea simply because society finds the idea itself offensive or disagreeable. *** In short, nothing in our precedents suggests that a State may foster its own view of the flag by prohibiting expressive conduct relating to it.[10] To bring its argument outside our precedents, Texas attempts

8. Our inquiry is, of course, bounded by the particular facts of this case and by the statute under which Johnson was convicted. There was no evidence that Johnson himself stole the flag he burned, nor did the prosecution or the arguments urged in support of it depend on the theory that the flag was stolen. Thus, our analysis does not rely on the way in which the flag was acquired, and nothing in our opinion should be taken to suggest that one is free to steal a flag so long as one later uses it to communicate an idea. We also emphasize that Johnson was prosecuted *only* for flag desecration—not for trespass, disorderly conduct, or arson.

9. Texas claims that "Texas is not endorsing protecting, avowing or prohibiting any particular philosophy." If Texas means to suggest that its asserted interest does not prefer Democrats over Socialists, or Republicans over Democrats, for example, then it is beside the point, for Johnson does not rely on such an argument. He argues instead that the State's desire to maintain the flag as a symbol of nationhood and national unity assumes that there is only one proper view of the flag. Thus, if Texas means to argue that its interest does not prefer *any* viewpoint over another, it is mistaken; surely one's attitude towards the flag and its referents is a viewpoint.

10. Our decision in Halter v. Nebraska, 205 U.S. 34 (1907), addressing the validity of a state law prohibiting certain commercial uses of the flag, is not to the contrary. That case was decided "nearly 20 years before the Court concluded that the First Amendment applies to the States by virtue of the Fourteenth Amendment." Spence v. Washington, 418 U.S. 405, 413, n. 7 (1974). More important, as we continually emphasized in *Halter* itself, that case involved purely commercial rather than political speech.

Nor does San Francisco Arts & Athletics v. Olympic Committee, 483 U.S. 522, 527 (1987), addressing the validity of Congress' decision to "authoriz[e] the United States Olympic Committee to prohibit certain commercial and promotional uses of the word 'Olympic,'" relied upon by the dissent, *** even begin to tell us whether the Government may criminally punish physical conduct towards the

to convince us that even if its interest in preserving the flag's symbolic role does not allow it to prohibit words or some expressive conduct critical of the flag, it does permit it to forbid the outright destruction of the flag. The State's argument cannot depend here on the distinction between written or spoken words and nonverbal conduct. That distinction, we have shown, is of no moment where the nonverbal conduct is expressive, as it is here, and where the regulation of that conduct is related to expression, as it is here. ***

We never before have held that the Government may ensure that a symbol be used to express only one view of that symbol or its referents. Indeed, in *Schacht v. United States*, we invalidated a federal statute permitting an actor portraying a member of one of our armed forces to "'wear the uniform of that Armed Force if the portrayal does not tend to discredit that armed force.'" This proviso, we held, "which leaves Americans free to praise the war in Vietnam but can send persons like Schacht to prison for opposing it, cannot survive in a country which has the First Amendment."

We perceive no basis on which to hold that the principle underlying our decision in *Schacht* does not apply to this case. To conclude that the Government may permit designated symbols to be used to communicate only a limited set of messages would be to enter territory having no discernible or defensible boundaries. Could the Government, on this theory, prohibit the burning of state flags? Of copies of the Presidential seal? Of the Constitution? In evaluating these choices under the First Amendment, how would we decide which symbols were sufficiently special to warrant this unique status? To do so, we would be forced to consult our own political preferences, and impose them on the citizenry, in the very way that the First Amendment forbids us to do.

There is, moreover, no indication—either in the text of the Constitution or in our cases interpreting it—that a separate juridical category exists for the American flag alone. *** The First Amendment does not guarantee that other concepts virtually sacred to our Nation as a whole—such as the principle that discrimination on the basis of race is odious and destructive—will go unquestioned in the marketplace of ideas. See Brandenburg v. Ohio, 395 U.S. 444 (1969). We decline, therefore, to create for the flag an exception to the joust of principles protected by the First Amendment.

It is not the State's ends, but its means, to which we object. It cannot be gainsaid that there is a special place reserved for the flag in this Nation, and thus we do not doubt that the Government has a legitimate interest in making efforts to "preserv[e] the national flag as an unalloyed symbol of our country." *Spence*, 418 U.S., at 412. We reject the suggestion, urged at oral argument by counsel for Johnson, that the Government lacks "any state interest whatsoever" in regulating the manner in which the flag may be displayed. Congress has, for example, enacted precatory regulations

---

flag engaged in as a means of political protest.

describing the proper treatment of the flag, see 36 U.S.C. §§ 173-177, and we cast no doubt on the legitimacy of its interest in making such recommendations. To say that the Government has an interest in encouraging proper treatment of the flag, however, is not to say that it may criminally punish a person for burning a flag as a means of political protest. ***

The way to preserve the flag's special role is not to punish those who feel differently about these matters. It is to persuade them that they are wrong. ***

V

Johnson was convicted for engaging in expressive conduct. The State's interest in preventing breaches of the peace does not support his conviction because Johnson's conduct did not threaten to disturb the peace. Nor does the State's interest in preserving the flag as a symbol of nationhood and national unity justify his criminal conviction for engaging in political expression. The judgment of the Texas Court of Criminal Appeals is therefore *** affirmed.

JUSTICE KENNEDY, concurring.

***

Our colleagues in dissent advance powerful arguments why respondent may be convicted for his expression, reminding us that among those who will be dismayed by our holding will be some who have had the singular honor of carrying the flag in battle. And I agree that the flag holds a lonely place of honor in an age when absolutes are distrusted and simple truths are burdened by unneeded apologetics.

With all respect to those views, I do not believe the Constitution gives us the right to rule as the dissenting Members of the Court urge, however painful this judgment is to announce. Though symbols often are what we ourselves make of them, the flag is constant in expressing beliefs Americans share, beliefs in law and peace and that freedom which sustains the human spirit. The case here today forces recognition of the costs to which those beliefs commit us. It is poignant but fundamental that the flag protects those who hold it in contempt.

For all the record shows, this respondent was not a philosopher and perhaps did not even possess the ability to comprehend how repellent his statements must be to the Republic itself. But whether or not he could appreciate the enormity of the offense he gave, the fact remains that his acts were speech, in both the technical and the fundamental meaning of the Constitution. So I agree with the Court that he must go free.

CHIEF JUSTICE REHNQUIST, with whom JUSTICE WHITE and JUSTICE O'CONNOR join, dissenting.

*** For more than 200 years, the American flag has occupied a unique position as the symbol of our Nation, a uniqueness that justifies a governmental prohibition against flag burning in the way respondent Johnson did here.

At the time of the American Revolution, the flag served to unify the Thirteen Colonies at home, while obtaining recognition of national sovereignty abroad. By June 14, 1777, after we declared our independence from England, the Continental Congress resolved:

> "That the flag of the thirteen United States be thirteen stripes, alternate red and white: that the union be thirteen stars, white in a blue field, representing a new constellation." 8 Journal of the Continental Congress 1774-1789, p. 464 (Ford Ed. 1907).

One immediate result of the flag's adoption was that American vessels harassing British shipping sailed under an authorized national flag. Without such a flag, the British could treat captured seamen as pirates and hang them summarily; with a national flag, such seamen were treated as prisoners of war.

***

The flag symbolizes the Nation in peace as well as in war. It signifies our national presence on battleships, airplanes, military installations, and public buildings from the United States Capitol to the thousands of county courthouses and city halls throughout the country. ***

*** With the exception of Alaska and Wyoming, all of the States now have statutes prohibiting the burning of the flag. Most of the state statutes are patterned after the Uniform Flag Act of 1917, which in § 3 provides: "No person shall publicly mutilate, deface, defile, defy, trample upon, or by word or act cast contempt upon any such flag, standard, color, ensign or shield." ***

The American flag, then, throughout more than 200 years of our history, has come to be the visible symbol embodying our Nation. It does not represent the views of any particular political party, and it does not represent any particular political philosophy. The flag is not simply another "idea" or "point of view" competing for recognition in the marketplace of ideas. Millions and millions of Americans regard it with an almost mystical reverence regardless of what sort of social, political, or philosophical beliefs they may have. I cannot agree that the First Amendment invalidates the Act of Congress, and the laws of 48 of 50 States, which make criminal the public burning of the flag.

Only two Terms ago, in San Francisco Arts & Athletics, Inc. v. United States Olympic Committee, 483 U.S. 522 (1987), the Court held that Congress could grant exclusive use of the word "Olympic" to the United States Olympic Committee. The Court thought that this "restrictio[n] on expressive speech properly [was] characterized as incidental to the primary congressional purpose of encouraging and rewarding the USOC's activities." ***

Our prior cases dealing with flag desecration statutes have left open the question that the Court resolves today. In Street v. New York, 394 U.S. 576, 579 (1969), the defendant burned a flag in the street, shouting "We don't need no damned flag" and, "[i]f they let that happen to Meredith we don't need an American flag." The Court ruled that since the defendant might have been convicted solely on the basis of his words, the conviction could not stand, but it expressly reserved the question of whether a defendant could constitutionally be convicted for burning the flag.

Chief Justice Warren, in dissent, stated: "I believe that the States and Federal Government do have the power to protect the flag from acts of desecration and disgrace. *** [I]t is difficult for me to imagine that, had the Court faced this issue, it would have concluded otherwise." Justices Black and Fortas also expressed their personal view that a prohibition on flag burning did not violate the Constitution. See *id.*, at 610 (Black, J., dissenting) ("It passes my belief that anything in the Federal Constitution bars a State from making the deliberate burning of the American Flag an offense"); *id.*, at 615-617 (Fortas, J., dissenting) ("[T]he States and the Federal Government have the power to protect the flag from acts of desecration committed in public. *** [T]he flag is a special kind of personality. Its use is traditionally and universally subject to special rules and regulation. *** A person may 'own' a flag, but ownership is subject to special burdens and responsibilities. A flag may be property, in a sense; but it is property burdened with peculiar obligations and restrictions. Certainly *** these special conditions are not *per se* arbitrary or beyond governmental power under our Constitution"). ***

But the Court today will have none of this. The uniquely deep awe and respect for our flag felt by virtually all of us are bundled off under the rubric of "designated symbols," that the First Amendment prohibits the government from "establishing." But the government has not "established" this feeling; 200 years of history have done that. The government is simply recognizing as a fact the profound regard for the American flag created by that history when it enacts statutes prohibiting the disrespectful public burning of the flag. ***

*** The Court decides that the American flag is just another symbol, about which not only must opinions pro and con be tolerated, but for which the most minimal public respect may not be enjoined. The government may conscript men into the Armed Forces where they must fight and perhaps die for the flag, but the government may not prohibit the public burning of the banner under which they fight. I would uphold the Texas statute as applied in this case.

JUSTICE STEVENS, dissenting. [Omitted.]

NOTES ON PROTECTING THE FLAG OF THE UNITED STATES

1. Is there a distinction to be made in cases such as *Texas v. Johnson* between political uses of an intact flag, which uses may be highly offensive to passersby, and acts of burning, tearing, or spitting on the same flag, as in *Texas v. Johnson* itself? Consider the following:

a) A group self-styled as American Nazis, with swastika armbands, brown shirts, and black boots, conducts a parade, at the front of which an American flag is carried. Many whom they pass by on the parade route are affronted by what they regard as an obscene misappropriation of the flag by the (Nazi) marchers, even as the marchers had reason to expect that they would be (and may in fact have wanted them to be);

b) The same group, far from carrying the flag out front, march with a crushed flag held in the fist of the lead marcher. At the parade's end, the leader gives a short speech decrying "mongrelization" of races in the United States. To lend emphasis to his (and the marchers') contempt for what they regard the United States as "representing," the leader sets fire to the crushed flag.

Does the first amendment apply to both instances alike? (May carrying the flag, intact, upright, on a standard, be more protected—because more closely akin to "pure speech"—while burning the flag doesn't make it across the first amendment at all? May the latter be generally, or even specially, prohibited, even assuming the former cannot?)

2. Adopted by Congress in 1968, 18 U.S.C.A. § 700 (captioned "*Desecration* of the flag of the United States")[145] provided as follows:

> (a) Whoever *knowingly casts contempt upon any flag of the United States by publicly* mutilating, defacing, defiling, burning, or trampling upon it shall be fined not more than $1,000 or imprisoned for not more than one year, or both.
>
> (b) The term "flag of the United States" as used in this section shall include any flag, standard colors, ensign, or any picture or representation of either, or of any part of parts of either made of any substance or represented on any substance, of any size evidently purporting to be either of said flag, standard, color, or ensign of the United States of America, or a picture or representation of either, upon which shall be shown the colors, the stars and the stripes, in any number of either thereof, or of any part of parts of either, by which the average person seeing the same without deliberation may believe the same to represent the flag, standards, colors, or ensign of the United States of America.

It was widely assumed that any prosecution brought against Johnson under this statute would fail, given the Supreme Court's decision in *Texas v. Johnson*. Do you agree?

3. On October 12, 1989, three months after the decision in *Texas v. Johnson*, by vote of 371 to 343, the House of Representatives approved the following substitution for (a) of this statute and the Senate speedily concurred (103 Stat. 777, 18 U.S.C.A. § 700):

---

145. Pub. L. 90-381, § 1, July 5, 1968, 82 Stat. 291. (Emphasis added.)

> Whoever knowingly mutilates, defaces, physically defiles, burns, maintains on the floor or ground, or tramples upon any flag of the United States shall be fined under this title or imprisoned for not more than one year or both.

Suppose a case identical to *Texas v. Johnson* were to be prosecuted under the federal statute in its revised form. Upon defense motion to dismiss the charge, on first amendment grounds, what result and why?[146]

4. The same day the House adopted the revised version of the federal statute already noted *supra*, Marlin Fitzwater, White House spokesman, expressed reservations about the sufficiency of the legislative change, in keeping with President Bush's support for a proposed amendment which would provide:

> [Proposed as the 28th Amendment to the Constitution]
> The Congress and the States Shall have Power to Prohibit the Physical Desecration of the Flag of the United States.

Suppose the proposed 28th Amendment were adopted. What would be its effect?

> a) E.g., would the display of a flag, upside down in one's street- facing front apartment window, but intact and unsullied, be subject to legislation based on the power enumerated in the proposed amendment?[147]
>
> b) If it were deemed subject to prohibition based on the provision of the proposed amendment, would its display therefore not be subject to first amendment protection?[148]

5. During the spring of 1989, at the Chicago Art Institute, a controversial exhibit created a very strong protest calling for prosecution of the person who prepared it (and the exhibit was removed by the Institute). The exhibit, in a public gallery, was accompanied by a placard captioned as follows: "What is the proper way to display the flag?" On the wall, photographs were displayed in which the flag was featured in brutal scenes of American involvement in Vietnam and elsewhere. On the floor, a large American flag was stretched out, flat. In front of the flag was a projected shelf with a book laid open for persons to sign on a line of its open blank pages, if they chose to do so. To sign the book, one was likely to step on the laid-out flag.

---

146. See United States v. Eichman, 496 U.S. 310 (1990).

147. Would a Racquel Welch bikini, fashioned from a stars and stripes motif, be subject to any law based on this proposed amendment? (Would it matter that the bikini was not made from a flag, but was made, rather, from bolts of cloth and lycra or spandex that were never parts of a flag?)

148. I.e. note that the proposed amendment does not provide that "the first amendment shall not be construed to extend to any legislation adopted pursuant to this amendment." (Neither does it provide that "legislation adopted pursuant to this amendment shall be immune from first amendment review.")

Consider:

a) Prosecution of the artist under (1) the 1968 version, or (2) the 1989 version, of the federal statute,[149] *supra*;

b) Prosecution instead, or additionally, of any visitor who walked on the flag or stood on one part of it, while signing the book;

c) A civil suit, brought by the artist, to enjoin the removal of the exhibit, i.e. a suit seeking to have the exhibit restored, brought against the Art Institute, a public body of the City of Chicago.[150]

---

149. Under the new form of the Act of Congress, incidentally, note that the exhibit would evidently be subject to the act whether or not anyone actually walked on the flag (i.e. even if a rope barrier were placed around the floor arrangement, and the shelf and sign-in book were removed or placed off to one side). Does this raise any separate or additional problem?

150. One may postpone additional consideration of this case for review *infra*, with cases and materials on "forum" analysis, and/or time, place, and manner regulations of speech.

Chapter 3

THE FIRST AMENDMENT IN SPECIFIC ENVIRONMENTS

A. The Government as employer, contractor, purchaser of services, and provider of benefits, and the extent to which the first amendment may limit its power to set conditions. Herein of the "right-privilege doctrine" and the "unconstitutional conditions" doctrine. The *Pickering-Connick* (balancing) test. Political affiliation and eligibility for public service. First amendment constraints on political litmus tests (*Elrod-Branti*).

The cases and materials we have thus far examined have concerned general laws of general application. These laws typically forbade conduct or utterances of a certain sort,[1] and they provided criminal or civil sanctions for such violations as might occur. Alternatively, they provided mechanisms for restraining or disallowing certain categories of utterances, i.e. they operated as a form of prior restraint.[2]

In contrast, the kinds of laws and regulations now to be considered do not limit what may be published or advocated by citizens or by people in general. Rather, they apply only to persons engaged in certain activities, usually under the control of the government, and they presume merely to regulate the terms of that activity and the freedom of speech of those engaged in that activity, and nothing more. In short, they are not general restrictions on freedom of speech at all. Often, moreover, the restrictions imposed as an incident of the regulated activity do not carry any threat of fine or imprisonment; in fact, even provision for any kind of civil liability is rare. Rather, they typically provide merely for the severance of the offending party from the relationship he or she has had, in the event of breach of the conditions.[3]

---

1. E.g., obstructing the draft, advocating violation of the law, urging the overthrow of the government, inciting to riot, advocating immoral behavior, portraying others as unworthy, advocating discrimination, etc.

2. E.g., permit requirements, licensing requirements, injunctions, restraining orders, arrest prior to speech or publication, etc.

3. This is not always true; a criminal or civil sanction may sometimes also apply. See, e.g., Scopes v. State, 289 S.W. 363 (Tenn. 1927); Snepp v. United States, 444 U.S. 507 (1980), discussed *infra* p. 306, n.25 (In *Scopes*, the offending teacher was not merely dismissed but was also criminally prosecuted; in *Snepp*, the offending ex-employee had a constructive trust imposed on his entire book royalties). Nonetheless, in each case the enforcement technique was otherwise consistent with the rationale of merely keeping the affected party to the terms of the arrangement he was under no duress to have made, so both cases are entirely appropriate to review here.

In all of these cases, the regulated party was a free agent at the beginning, and typically became equally a free agent at the end. Not only is the field marked by an absence of duress in the usual sense (the threatened use of a fine or imprisonment for what one may say or write), but also there is no duress in the sense of the government *compelling* one to enter into the relationship. While the affected party must of course take "the bitter with the sweet"[4] insofar as the terms offered for acceptance may be—and characteristically will be—nonnegotiable (e.g., fixed by statute), there is no duress applied by the government to compel one to enter the relationship in the first place.[5] In a practical view of the matter, one's continuing conformity to the limitations identified by government, and made applicable to the particular activity administered by government, is treated simply as a continuing condition precedent to one's eligibility, and usually nothing more.

The restrictions, in short, are *twice* distinguishable from the general laws we have previously examined. (1) They apply only to those who, with full and reasonable notice of them, accept the relationship to which they are made applicable (usually, a relationship of special advantage, e.g., a government job, contract, grant, or some kind of largesse). (2) Continuing compliance itself is merely a continuing condition of sustaining that relationship, and typically nothing more. So, much as in any ordinary private commercial contract, at most one thus needs to adhere to "the bitter," only so long as one wants to continue to enjoy "the sweet."[6]

---

4. The phrase is lifted from a notable dissent by Justice Rehnquist, in Arnett v. Kennedy, 416 U.S. 134 (1974). The majority held that a nonprobationary federal civil service employee was entitled to some kind of due process hearing before being terminated for cause, despite not having been promised any such hearing. In Justice Rehnquist's view, in dissent, the employee was entitled to as much due process as he was promised and nothing more: "[W]here the grant of a substantive right is inextricably intertwined with the limitations on the procedures which are to be employed in determining that right, a litigant [must] take the bitter with the sweet. [Here] the property interest which appellee had in his employment was itself conditioned by procedural limitations which had accompanied the grant of that interest." The employee got all the due process to which he was entitled; he was entitled to nothing more. Cf. Cleveland City Board of Educ. v. Loudermill, 470 U.S. 572 (1985) (also rejecting Justice Rehnquist's view).

5. Of course, one's personal circumstances may affect one's freedom of choice as a practical matter, but no more so here than in many other areas. Cf., e.g., Harris v. McRae, 448 U.S. 297 (1980) (reimbursement of health care providers by government for women on restricted incomes who elect full term pregnancy and child birth, no reimbursement to health care provider if, instead, the same woman seeks an abortion). See generally, Charles A. Reich, Individual Rights and Social Welfare, 74 Yale L.J. 1245 (1966); Charles A. Reich, The New Property, 73 Yale L.J. 733 (1964).

6. Recall and compare the tenth amendment argument in Massachusetts v. Mellon, 262 U.S. 447 (1923). Congress enacted a measure (the Maternity Act) setting aside certain funds for which states could apply subject to making such reports and meeting such conditions as might be prescribed by a federal agency, the funds to be withheld insofar as it might be determined that they were not being expended in the manner the federal agency prescribed. Massachusetts filed suit in the Supreme Court against Mellon, the Secretary of the Treasury, seeking a declaratory judgment that the "act is invalid because it assumes powers not granted to Congress and usurps the local police power" of the states, due to the strings attached to the grants. The Supreme Court dismissed for lack of jurisdiction, not because

How, if at all, or in what measure, and by what standards, does the first amendment apply in these circumstances? These are the questions we shall next address. The cases and materials chosen for the purpose are illustrative, rather than exhaustive. They should, however, provide a useful guide.

There have been roughly three different perspectives that the courts have brought to bear on the overall problem. Each of the first two of these perspectives is characterized by a particular deductive logic, and each, *within* the limits of its perspective, seems to be compelling and inexorably correct. (As we shall notice, however, they are also 180 degrees apart.) The third manner of addressing the general question considered in this section may be considerably less clear, but the cases which follow in this collection of materials may show how it works out in practice. Here are the three, broadly suggested, approaches variously reflected in the general case law:

a. In cases that fit the general description provided *supra*, we treat the government and the individual equally as free agents, mutually competent to determine their own best interests and we measure the terms of the arrangement according to general principles of the common law of contracts, modified to such extent as statutory law may provide.[7]
b. To the contrary, in cases that fit the general description provided *supra*, the common law of contracts is essentially irrelevant and cannot be invoked. Rather, the first amendment disallows government from imposing restrictions on free speech, as much so by contract as by any other device. The first amendment does not permit the "buying up" of free speech, whether from willing sellers or from unwilling, but necessitous, sellers. All such

---

the case was not within the Court's original jurisdiction (it was), but because, the Court said, the proceeding was itself "not of a justiciable character." Why not? Partly, perhaps, because the issue had not been sufficiently joined between the parties; Massachusetts had not even applied for any funds. But the Court also said: "Probably, it would be sufficient to point out that the powers of the State are not invaded, since the statute imposes no obligation *but simply extends an option which the State is free to accept or reject.* *** In the last analysis, the complaint of the plaintiff State is brought to the naked contention that Congress has usurped the reserved powers of the several States by the mere enactment of the statute, though nothing has been done and *nothing is to be done without their consent*; and it is plain that that question, as it is thus presented, is political and not judicial in character, and therefore is not a matter which admits of the exercise of the judicial power." 262 U.S. at 480-83 (emphasis added). See also South Dakota v. Dole, 483 U.S. 203 (1987); Chas. C. Steward Machine Co. v. Davis, 301 U.S. 548 (1937). But see United States v. Butler, 297 U.S. 1 (1936); McCoy & Friedman, Conditional Spending: Federalism's Trojan Horse, 1988 Supreme Ct.Rev. 85.

7. See, e.g., the discussion in note 6 *supra*, addressing the tenth amendment in a somewhat similar fashion. Cf. also cases condoning the waiver of constitutional rights from criminal procedure (e.g., "waivers" of constitutional rights in guilty plea bargains, or of one's right to counsel following a *Miranda* warning, or of one's right to counsel at trial).

terms, conditions, regulations, or restrictions, insofar as they come from *government*, are constitutionally void.

c. In cases that fit the general description provided *supra*, the first amendment does apply, and it applies unexceptionally,[8] to be sure. Still, one must then struggle to sort out just what that *means* in each case. We have, for instance, already seen that a certain kind of restriction may be valid at certain times though not at other times, or in certain places and circumstances though it might not otherwise be sustainable. Unsurprisingly, much the same will be just as true, here.

It is easier to state the position in *c, supra*, than it is to grasp its actual workings in the Supreme Court. The principal cases immediately ahead of us, however, should be helpful in working it out. Like some comparable cases already behind us (e.g., the post-*New York Times v. Sullivan* libel cases refining first amendment libel law distinctions), moreover, some of these decisions have developed a number of line-drawing distinctions of their own, i.e. somewhat formal distinctions, peculiar to this field.[9] We shall see shortly how well they work here.

These cases all arise from a history in which the first two positions were each separately put forward, however, so it will pay us to understand their respective perspectives a little bit more.[10]

B. A Return to the Early Holmes and the Right-Privilege Distinction of *McAuliffe v. Mayor of New Bedford*

In a famous Massachusetts case, in 1892, dismissing the appeal of a New Bedford policeman who had been fired following some public remarks critical of how

---

8. I.e. compare either the Learned Hand or the Holmes-Brandeis test, and apply either with due care, here.

9. The tendency toward formal complexity in subsets of first amendment law is a recurring tendency, just as it is in criminal procedure or other areas of constitutional review. In some measure, it arises from the inevitability of cases crowding the margin of constitutional uncertainty and the felt need of the Supreme Court to provide clearer guidance to all with a need to know what "the rules" are, whether plaintiffs or defendants, prosecutors or those in danger of prosecution, administrative agencies, lower courts, or legislatures. The complexity of "the rules" thus laid down tends inevitably to engender its own uncertainties. (The distinctions become so esoteric and tenuous and/or so debatable that eventually the whole system may crash under its own weight.) There is, moreover, a serious first amendment hazard at risk in these complex approaches. The risk is, that in trying too hard to figure out which is the "right" rule for the immediate case one may lose sight of some organizing philosophy common to all first amendment cases, and thereby be misled into foregoing access to a far more powerful set of more general observations that might well be important to set matters right.

10. Moreover, each of these prior perspectives continues to be used at the margins of first amendment disputes in the Supreme Court by different Justices: e.g., Chief Justice Rehnquist not infrequently invoked the "right-privilege" distinction, while Justices Brennan, Marshall, and Blackmun invoked the "unconstitutional conditions" doctrine instead.

the police department was run, Justice Holmes dispatched the police officer's first amendment objection with the following epigrammatic response:[11]

> The petitioner may have a constitutional right to talk politics, but he has no constitutional right to be a policeman. There are few employments for hire in which the servant does not agree to *suspend his constitutional right of free speech*, as well as of idleness, by the implied terms of his contract. The servant cannot complain, *as he takes the employment on the terms which are offered him.*

This view of Holmes (a view of the relationship as sounding in contract, with each party competent to determine the acceptability of the terms) was widely quoted and relied upon by other courts, including the Supreme Court, between 1892 and 1954.[12]

In 1927, for example, in the *Scopes* ("Monkey Trial") case,[13] the Tennessee Supreme Court followed this approach. Scopes had been criminally prosecuted for violating a Tennessee law applicable to public school teachers, forbidding the teaching of "any theory that denies the story of the divine creation of man as taught in the Bible," such as Darwin's view respecting the "Origin of the Species."[14] Despite Clarence Darrow's defense efforts on his behalf, Scopes was convicted at trial by the jury. On his appeal on first and fourteenth amendment grounds to the state supreme court, the court responded:

> [Scopes] was under contract with the State to work in an institution of the State. He had no right or privilege to serve the State except upon such terms as the State prescribed. The Statute before us is not an exercise of the police power of the State undertaking to regulate the conduct of individuals.[15] [I]t is an Act of the State as a corporation, a proprietor, an employer. It is a declaration of a master as to the character of work the master's servant will, or rather shall not, perform. *In dealing with its own employees engaged upon its own*

11. McAuliffe v. Mayor of New Bedford, 29 N.E. 517, 518 (Mass. 1892) (emphasis added).

12. For a general review, see William Van Alstyne, The Demise of the Right-Privilege Distinction in Constitutional Law, 83 Harv.L.Rev. 1429 (1968). For a more critical, modern, comprehensive review, see Kathleen M. Sullivan, Unconstitutional Conditions, 102 Harv.L.Rev. 1415 (1989).

13. Scopes v. State, 289 S.W. 363 (Tenn. 1927).

14. H.L. Mencken covered the trial proceedings. William Jennings Bryan, thrice Democratic nominee for the Presidency, appeared as an expert witness for the state.

15. [That is, the statute did *not* regulate persons generally, and did *not* regulate teachers in *private* schools—schools not supported or administered by the state; it is in just this sense, the state supreme court says, that the "police power" of the state is not in any way involved in this case. Cf. Meyer v. Nebraska, 262 U.S. 390 (1923) (state statute forbidding any instruction in any language other than English prior to the eighth grade, held unconstitutional under the fourteenth amendment, as applied to teacher in private, Lutheran school, neither supported nor assisted in any way by the state).]

> *work, the State is not hampered by the limitations of the Fourteenth Amendment* to the Constitution of the United States.[16]

Note, then, the dispositive proposition relied upon by the state supreme court in *Scopes v. State*, i.e. not that the speech restriction was all right under the fourteenth amendment, but, rather, that in dealing with its own employees employed upon its own work, the State is "not hampered" by the limitations of the fourteenth amendment. The same thought is inferable from Holmes' premises in the *McAuliffe* decision: the legal frame of reference is ordinary contract law (and even then as modified by the state statute fixing the terms) and not constitutional law.[17] One's agreement to suspend one's "constitutional right of free speech" is treated in just the same way as one's agreement to suspend one's constitutional right to loaf, i.e. as something for one to decide to do or not to do, neither more nor less, but binding insofar as one does. When the state acts pursuant to its general police power to restrict what its citizens choose to say—whether about the police department, or about the Book of Genesis vs. Darwin, or anything else, it must answer to the first amendment. However, when the state acts differently, as an employer, it need answer merely as any employer need do: Were the terms clear? Were they attached to the position with respect to which they were enforced? Did the employee expressly, or impliedly, agree?

The analogy to the Supreme Court's spending power, tenth amendment "states' rights" position in *Massachusetts v. Mellon* is quite striking.[18] There, in dicta, the state was described also as a free agent to decide for itself whether the changes in its laws that it might not otherwise choose to make were worthwhile making, and it was under no duty to make any changes it deemed inappropriate. Moreover, having made those changes (in order to become eligible for federal assistance), it could at any time change its mind, change its laws back again, and give up the relationship into which it had previously entered.[19] So, too, with the public employee, in *McAuliffe*, and the public school teacher, in *State v. Scopes*. All were free agents, but not more.

C. The Unconstitutional Conditions Doctrine

The preceding approach to public sector free speech restrictions generally fell under the rubric of the "right-privilege" doctrine. As already indicated, it had a very

---

16. 289 S.W. at 364-65 (emphasis added).

17. ("The servant cannot complain, as he takes the employment *on the terms which are offered him.*")

18. See discussion and review in note 6 *supra*.

19. But see William Van Alstyne, "Thirty Pieces of Silver" for the Rights of Your People: Irresistible Offers Reconsidered as a Matter of State Constitutional Law, 16 Harv.J.L. & Pub.Pol. 303 (1993).

substantial career in the courts. Yet, even as it continued to be applied,[20] it faced headwinds within the Supreme Court, headwinds blown by a counter doctrine as old as itself.

The most familiar statement of this "counter doctrine" is forcefully presented in a well known opinion by Justice Sutherland, writing for a majority of the Supreme Court in *Frost & Frost Trucking Co. v. Railroad Commission*, a commercial case (rather than a first amendment case) decided in 1926.[21] Sutherland emphasized that the government is *not* treated like a private party for constitutional purposes, i.e. it is bound by uniform constitutional constraints. *It is government the first and fourteenth amendments are meant to constrain (and do constrain), regardless of the guise or capacity in which government acts.*[22] That government seeks to limit one's speech by the terms of some leasehold, or by the terms of some contract, or by the terms of some permit (e.g., as a condition of using its streets), rather than by direct mandate, should gain it no special ground. In Sutherland's oft quoted words:

> It would be a palpable incongruity to strike down an act of state legislation which, by words of express divestment, seeks to strip the citizen of rights guaranteed by the federal Constitution, but to uphold an act by which the same result is accomplished under the guise of a surrender of a right in exchange for a valuable privilege the state threatens otherwise to withhold. It is inconceivable that guarantees embedded in the Constitution of the United States may be thus manipulated out of existence.[23]

The obvious basis for this view is the observation that government remains government *regardless* of the capacity in which it presumes to act. And *what government cannot do to anyone directly* (because barred by the first amendment), *neither can it do indirectly*, by offering a trade, i.e. the "surrender of a right in exchange for a valuable privilege," such as a public job, a public contract, a rent-controlled apartment, or something else. If, then, the restriction would fail when proposed as a direct restriction on one's speech without reference to the carrot held

---

20. Among the last cases to apply the distinction were Bailey v. Richardson, 182 F.2d 46 (D.C. Cir. 1950), aff'd by an equally divided Court, 341 U.S. 918 (1951), and Adler v. Board of Educ. of City of New York, 341 U.S. 485 (1952). Cf. Keyishian v. Board of Regents, 385 U.S. 589, 607-606 (1967).

21. Interestingly, note that Sutherland also wrote the Court's opinion in *Massachusetts v. Mellon*, in which the dicta are more of a piece with the right-privilege doctrine.

22. Whether the amendment(s) should have stopped with limiting government power alone may be arguable, i.e. perhaps they should also have restricted corporate power as well, but we need not pause to argue it here. For without arguing, much less presuming to settle, that proposition—about corporate power or other varieties of privately-held power—there is no doubt that at least the first amendment controls Congress, and the fourteenth amendment controls the states.

23. 271 U.S. at 593-94. For earlier expressions to the same effect, see, e.g., Doyle v. Continental Ins. Co., 94 U.S. 535, 543 (1876) ("Though a State may have the power *** of prohibiting all foreign corporations from transacting business within its jurisdiction, it has no power to impose *unconstitutional conditions* upon their doing so.") (emphasis added).

out, it should fare no better as a term proposed in a contract, or as a term proposed in a lease, or as a term proposed in a permit. The first amendment makes an offending term substantively void. Accordingly, the result would seem to be the one proposed in *B*, *supra*.[24]

The following cases provide the most recent example of disagreement within the Supreme Court in mapping out the field to which the doctrine of unconstitutional conditions applies.

RUST v. SULLIVAN

500 U.S. 173 (1991)

Chief Justice REHNQUIST delivered the opinion of the Court.

These cases concern a facial challenge to Department of Health and Human Services (HHS) regulations which limit the ability of Title X fund recipients to engage in abortion-related activities. *** In 1970, Congress enacted Title X of the Public Health Service Act. Section 1008 of the Act provides that "[n]one of the funds appropriated under this subchapter shall be used in programs where abortion is a method of family planning." ***

Petitioners are Title X grantees and doctors who supervise Title X funds suing on behalf of themselves and their patients. Respondent is the Secretary of the Department of Health and Human Services. Petitioners challenged the regulations on the grounds that they violate the First and Fifth Amendment rights of Title X clients and the First Amendment rights of Title X health providers. ***

III

Petitioners contend that the regulations violate the First Amendment by impermissibly discriminating based on viewpoint because they prohibit "all discussion about abortion as a lawful option—including counseling, referral, and the provision of neutral and accurate information about ending a pregnancy—while compelling the

---

24. Actually, there are at least two distinct versions of this doctrine of unconstitutional conditions, a stronger and weaker (but still potent) form. In its stronger form, the doctrine may imply that unless the state could forbid the class of activity or speech to citizens in general, it cannot forbid that class of activity or speech by contract or by regulation of others whom it seeks to control by making abstention from such activity or speech a condition of their eligibility for a public contract or public sector "privilege." In its lesser (but still potent) form, it means only that, unless the state could forbid such activity or speech to equivalently situated persons in the *private* sector, it cannot forbid such activity or speech as a condition of eligibility in the *public* sector—the Constitution requires no less. For a discussion of this latter version see Hans Linde, Justice Douglas on Freedom in the Welfare State: Constitutional Rights in the Public Sector, 39 Wash.L.Rev. 4 (1964), 40 Wash.L.Rev. 10 (1965). But see William Van Alstyne, A Comment on the Inappropriate Uses of an Old Analogy, 16 U.C.L.A.L.Rev. 751 (1969).

clinic or counselor to provide information that promotes continuing a pregnancy to term." They assert that the regulations violate the "free speech rights of private health care organizations that receive Title X funds, of their staff, and of their patients" by impermissibly imposing "viewpoint-discriminatory conditions on government subsidies" and thus penaliz[e] speech funded with non-Title X monies." ***

There is no question but that the statutory prohibition contained in § 1008 is constitutional. In *Maher v. Roe*, [432 U.S. 464], we upheld a state welfare regulation under which Medicaid recipients received payments for services related to childbirth, but not for nontherapeutic abortions. The Court rejected the claim that this unequal subsidization worked a violation of the Constitution. We held that the government may "make a value judgment favoring childbirth over abortion, and implement that judgment by the allocation of public funds." Here the Government is exercising the authority it possesses under *Maher* and *McRae* to subsidize family planning services which will lead to conception and childbirth, and declining to "promote or encourage abortion." The Government can, without violating the Constitution, selectively fund a program to encourage certain activities it believes to be in the public interest, without at the same time funding an alternate program which seeks to deal with the problem in another way. In so doing, the Government has not discriminated on the basis of viewpoint; it has merely chosen to fund one activity to the exclusion of the other. *** The challenged regulations implement the statutory prohibition by prohibiting counseling, referral, and the provision of information regarding abortion as a method of family planning. They are designed to ensure that the limits of the federal program are observed.

*** Petitioners' assertions ultimately boil down to the position that if the government chooses to subsidize one protected right, it must subsidize analogous counterpart rights. But the Court has soundly rejected that proposition. Within far broader limits than petitioners are willing to concede, when the government appropriates public funds to establish a program it is entitled to define the limits of that program.

The Secretary's regulations do not force the Title X grantee to give up abortion-related speech; they merely require that the grantee keep such activities separate and distinct from Title X activities. Title X expressly distinguishes between a Title X grantee and a Title X project. The Title X grantee can continue to perform abortions, provide abortion- related services, and engage in abortion advocacy; it simply is required to conduct those activities through programs that are separate and independent from the project that receives Title X funds.

The same principles apply to petitioners' claim that the regulations abridge the free speech rights of the grantee's staff. Individuals who are voluntarily employed for a Title X project must perform their duties in accordance with the regulation's restrictions on abortion counseling and referral. The employees remain free, however, to pursue abortion-related activities when they are not acting under the auspices of the Title X project. The regulations, which govern solely the scope of the Title X project's activities, do not in any way restrict the activities of those persons acting as private individuals. The employees' freedom of expression is limited during the time that they actually work for the project; but this limitation is a consequence of their decision to accept employment in a project, the scope of which is permissibly restricted by the funding authority.[5]

This is not to suggest that funding by the Government, even when coupled with the freedom of the fund recipients to speak outside the scope of the Government-funded project, is invariably sufficient to justify government control over the content of expression. For example, this Court has recognized that the existence of a Government "subsidy," in the form of Government-owned property, does not justify the restriction of speech in areas that have "been traditionally open to the public for expressive activity," United States v. Kokinda, 497 U.S. 720 (1990); Hague v. CIO, 307 U.S. 496, 515 (1939) (opinion of Roberts, J.).

Similarly, we have recognized that the university is a traditional sphere of free expression so fundamental to the functioning of our society that the Government's ability to control speech within that sphere by means of conditions attached to the expenditure of Government funds is restricted by the vagueness and overbreadth doctrines of the First Amendment, Keyishian v. Board of Regents, 385 U.S. 589, 603, 605-606 (1967). It could be argued by analogy that traditional relationships such as that between doctor and patient should enjoy protection under the First Amendment from government regulation, even when subsidized by the Government. We need not resolve that question here, however, because the Title X program regulations do not significantly impinge upon the doctor-patient relationship. Nothing in them requires a doctor to represent as his own any opinion that he does not in fact hold.

---

5. Petitioners also contend that the regulations violate the First Amendment by penalizing speech funded with non-Title X monies. They argue that since Title X requires that grant recipients contribute to the financing of Title X projects through the use of matching funds and grant-related income, the regulation's restrictions on abortion counseling and advocacy penalize privately funded speech.

We find this argument flawed for several reasons. First, Title X subsidies are just that, subsidies. The recipient is in no way compelled to operate a Title X project; to avoid the force of the regulations, it can simply decline the subsidy. *** By accepting Title X funds, a recipient voluntarily consents to any restrictions placed on any matching funds or grant-related income. Potential grant recipients can choose between accepting Title X funds—subject to the Government's conditions that they provide matching funds and forgo abortion counseling and referral in the Title X project—or declining the subsidy and financing their own unsubsidized program. We have never held that the Government violates the First Amendment simply by offering that choice. Second, the Secretary's regulations apply only to Title X programs. A recipient is therefore able to "limi[t] the use of its federal funds to [Title X] activities." FCC v. League of Women Voters of Cal., 468 U.S. 364, at 400 (1984). It is in no way "barred from using even wholly private funds to finance" its pro-abortion activities outside the Title X program. The regulations are limited to Title X funds; the recipient remains free to use private, non-Title X funds to finance abortion-related activities.

Nor is the doctor-patient relationship established by the Title X program sufficiently all-encompassing so as to justify an expectation on the part of the patient of comprehensive medical advice. The program does not provide post-conception medical care, and therefore a doctor's silence with regard to abortion cannot reasonably be thought to mislead a client into thinking that the doctor does not consider abortion an appropriate option for her. The doctor is always free to make clear that advice regarding abortion is simply beyond the scope of the program. In these circumstances, the general rule that the Government may choose not to subsidize speech applies with full force.

IV

That the regulations do not impermissibly burden a woman's Fifth Amendment rights is evident from the line of cases beginning with *Maher* and *McRae* and culminating in our most recent decision in *Webster*. Just as Congress' refusal to fund abortions in *McRae* left "an indigent woman with at least the same range of choice in deciding whether to obtain a medically necessary abortion as she would have had if Congress had chosen to subsidize no health care costs at all," 448 U.S., at 317, and "Missouri's refusal to allow public employees to perform abortions in public hospitals leaves a pregnant woman with the same choices as if the State had chosen not to operate any public hospitals," Webster, 492 U.S., at 509, Congress' refusal to fund abortion counseling and advocacy leaves a pregnant woman with the same choices as if the government had chosen not to fund family-planning services at all. The difficulty that a woman encounters when a Title X project does not provide abortion counseling or referral leaves her in no different position than she would have been if the government had not enacted Title X. ***

[T]he judgment of the Court of Appeals is Affirmed.

Justice BLACKMUN, with whom Justice MARSHALL [and] Justice STEVENS joins dissenting. ***

Until today, the Court never has upheld viewpoint-based suppression of speech simply because that suppression was a condition upon the acceptance of public funds. Whatever may be the Government's power to condition the receipt of its largesse upon the relinquishment of constitutional rights, it surely does not extend to a condition that suppresses the recipient's cherished freedom of speech based solely upon the content or viewpoint of that speech.

It cannot seriously be disputed that the counseling and referral provisions at issue in the present cases constitute content-based regulation of speech. Title X grantees may provide counseling and referral regarding any of a wide range of family planning and other topics, save abortion.

The Regulations are also clearly viewpoint-based. While suppressing speech favorable to abortion with one hand, the Secretary compels antiabortion speech with the other. For example, the Department of Health and Human Services' own description of the regulations makes plain that "Title X projects are *required* to facilitate access to prenatal care and social services, including adoption services, that might be needed by the pregnant client to promote her well-being and that of her child, while making it abundantly clear that the project is not permitted to promote abortion by facilitating access to abortion through the referral process." ***

Moreover, the regulations command that a project refer for prenatal care each woman diagnosed as pregnant, irrespective of the woman's expressed desire to continue or terminate her pregnancy. If a client asks directly about abortion, a Title X physician or counselor is required to say, in essence, that the project does not consider abortion to be an appropriate method of family planning. § 59.8(b)(4). Both requirements are antithetical to the First Amendment. ***

The regulations pertaining to "advocacy" are even more explicitly viewpoint based. These provide: "A Title X project may not *encourage, promote or advocate* abortion as a method of family planning." § 59.10 (emphasis added). They explain: "This requirement prohibits actions to *assist* women to obtain abortions or *increase* the availability or accessibility of abortion for family planning purposes." § 59.10(a) (emphasis added). The regulations do not, however, proscribe or even regulate anti-abortion advocacy. These are clearly restrictions aimed at the suppression of "dangerous ideas."

Remarkably, the majority concludes that "the Government has not discriminated on the basis of viewpoint; it has merely chosen to fund one activity to the exclusion of another." But the majority's claim that the regulations merely limit a Title X project's speech to preventive or preconceptional services rings hollow in light of the broad range of non-preventive services that the regulations authorize Title X projects to provide.[2] By refusing to fund those family-planning projects that advocate abortion *because* they advocate abortion, the Government plainly has targeted a particular viewpoint. *** The majority's reliance on the fact that the regulations pertain solely to funding decisions simply begs the question. Clearly, there are some bases upon which government may not rest its decision to fund or not to fund. For example, the Members of the majority surely would agree that government may not base its decision to support an activity upon considerations of race. [O]ur cases make clear that ideological viewpoint is a similarly repugnant ground upon which to base funding decisions. ***

B

The Court concludes that the challenged regulations do not violate the First Amendment rights of Title X staff members because any limitation of the employees' freedom of expression is simply a consequence of their decision to accept employment at a federally funded project. But it has never been sufficient to justify

---

2. In addition to requiring referral for prenatal care and adoption services, the regulations permit general health services such as physical examinations, screening for breast cancer, treatment of gynecological problems, and treatment for sexually transmitted diseases. None of the latter are strictly preventive, preconceptional services.

an otherwise unconstitutional condition upon public employment that the employee may escape the condition by relinquishing his or her job. It is beyond question "that a government may not require an individual to relinquish rights guaranteed him by the First Amendment as a condition of public employment."

In the cases at bar, the speaker's interest in the communication is both clear and vital. In addressing the family-planning needs of their clients, the physicians and counselors who staff Title X projects seek to provide them with the full range of information and options regarding their health and reproductive freedom. Indeed, the legitimate expectations of the patient and the ethical responsibilities of the medical profession demand no less.

The Government's articulated interest in distorting the doctor/patient dialogue—ensuring that federal funds are not spent for a purpose outside the scope of the program—falls far short of that necessary to justify the suppression of truthful information and professional medical opinion regarding constitutionally protected conduct. ***

[T]he majority's conclusion that "[t]he difficulty that a woman encounters when a Title X project does not provide abortion counseling or referral leaves her in no different position than she would have been if the government had not enacted Title X" is insensitive and contrary to common human experience. Both the purpose and result of the challenged Regulations is to deny women the ability voluntarily to decide their procreative destiny. For these women, the Government will have obliterated the freedom to choose as surely as if it had banned abortions outright. The denial of this freedom is not a consequence of poverty but of the Government's ill-intentioned distortion of information it has chosen to provide.[5]

The majority professes to leave undisturbed the free speech protections upon which our society has come to rely, but one must wonder what force the First Amendment retains if it is read to countenance the deliberate manipulation by the Government of the dialogue between a woman and her physician. While technically leaving intact the fundamental right protected by *Roe v. Wade*, the Court, "through a relentlessly formalistic catechism," *McRae*, 448 U.S., at 341 (Marshall, J., dissenting), once again has rendered the right's substance nugatory.

---

5. In the context of common-law tort liability, commentators have recognized: "If there is no duty to go to the assistance of a person in difficulty or peril, there is at least a duty to avoid any affirmative acts which make his situation worse. *** The same is true, of course, of a physician who accepts a charity patient. Such a defendant will then be liable for a failure to use reasonable care for the protection of the plaintiff's interests." W. Keeton, D. Dobbs, R. Keeton, & D. Owen, Prosser and Keeton on Law of Torts § 56, 378 (5th ed. 1984) (footnotes omitted). This observation seems equally appropriate to the cases at bar.

NOTE

1. *What* "constitutional right" was anyone working in a Title IX project required to give up or to forsake as a condition of organizing, administering, or being a counselor in a Title X project?

2. Suppose it is lawful for parents to spank their children (as generally it is as long as it does not involve criminal abuse of any sort). Suppose, too, that the sparing use of spanking is not disapproved by a number of child psychologists (i.e. that it is instead "regarded as a constructive means of good parenting because, used intelligently, it reassures the child that the parents truly care"). Would a restriction on federally funded family counseling projects be unconstitutional if it forbade "*any* counseling of spanking"? Why would one think so? Would Justice Blackmun? What, if anything, distinguishes this case from *Rust*?[25]

3. What first amendment complaint, if any, would a public school teacher have if the local school board provided by clear rule that such instruction as may be provided even in courses on early American history "shall not include any mention at all of slave ownership by any of the founding fathers (e.g., George Washington, Thomas Jefferson)"? Does the Rehnquist position in *Rust* equally apply to this kind of case as well? Would it apply if the same clear rule also forbade the same thing (i.e. any mention at all of slave ownership by any of the founding fathers) even in

---

25. See William W. Van Alstyne, Second Thoughts on Rust v. Sullivan and the First Amendment, 9 Const. Commentary 5 (1992). Compare Ronald J. Krotoszynski, Jr., *Brind & Rust v. Sullivan*: Free Speech and the Limits of a Written Constitution, 22 Fla.St.U.L.Rev. 1 (1994). For an additional example in which a restriction relating to government employment was sustained, see Snepp v. United States, 444 U.S. 507 (1980) (As an express condition of his employment with the CIA in 1968, plaintiff was required to execute an agreement promising that he would not publish any information relating to the CIA either during or after his employment without first submitting any manuscript for prepublication clearance, a commitment a former employee failed to keep before publishing a book deeply critical of the CIA. Nothing in the book as actually published was alleged by the government to have *in fact* disclosed any classified information, but the government brought suit for breach of contract for Snepp's violation of his promise to secure preclearance review before presuming to submit his manuscript for such publication, frustrating its ability to check the manuscript in advance. *Held*, the agreement was valid and enforceable, three justices dissenting against the Court's approval of a remedy that imposed a constructive trust on all of the book royalties the Court ordered to be paid to the government to avoid "unjust enrichment" of the former employee. The dissenting judges (but not the majority) thought it significant that Congress had made no provision for such a remedy. They also expressed concern that the "covenant [was] a prior restraint on speech" such that "even if such a wide-ranging prior restraint would be good national security policy, [we] would have great difficulty reconciling it with the demands of the First Amendment." (The case may be useful to compare with New York Times Company v. United States, 403 U.S. 713 (1971) (the "Pentagon Papers" case) *supra* at p. 105.)).

such courses in American history as may be taught in the state-funded *university*? Would this be an "unconstitutional condition" or would it not?[26]

LEGAL SERVICES CORPORATION v. VALASQUEZ

121 S.Ct. 1043 (2001)

Justice KENNEDY delivered the opinion of the Court.

In 1974, Congress enacted the Legal Services Corporation Act, 42 U.S.C. § 2996 *et seq*. The Act establishes the Legal Services Corporation (LSC) as a District of Columbia nonprofit corporation. LSC's mission is to distribute funds appropriated by Congress to eligible local grantee organizations "for the purpose of providing financial support for legal assistance in noncriminal proceedings or matters to persons financially unable to afford legal assistance." This suit requires us to decide whether one of the conditions imposed by Congress on the use of LSC funds violates the First Amendment rights of LSC grantees and their clients.

Lawyers employed by New York City LSC grantees, together with private LSC contributors and LSC indigent clients, brought suit to declare the restriction, invalid. *** We agree that the restriction violates the First Amendment, and we affirm the judgment of the Court of Appeals.

I

From the inception of the LSC, Congress has placed restrictions on its use of funds. For instance, the LSC Act prohibits recipients from making available LSC funds, program personnel, or equipment to any political party, to any political campaign, or for use in "advocating or opposing any ballot measures." The Act further proscribes use of funds in most criminal proceedings and in litigation involving nontherapeutic abortions, secondary school desegregation, military desertion, or violations of the Selective Service statute. The restrictions at issue prohibits funding of any organization

> "that initiates legal representation or participates in any other way, in litigation, lobbying, or rulemaking, involving an effort to reform a Federal or State welfare system, except that this paragraph shall not be construed to preclude a recipient from representing an individual eligible client who is seeking specific relief from a welfare agency if such relief does not involve an effort to amend or otherwise challenge existing law in effect on the date of the initiation of the representation."

---

26. Materials, *infra* 314-373, may be helpful to think these questions through. (They are raised here principally to stimulate one's thinking in light of the recent decision in *Rust*.) See also David D. Cole, Beyond Unconstitutional Conditions: Chartering Spheres of Neutrality in Government-Funded Speech, 67 N.Y.U.L.Rev. 675 (1992). Robert C. Post, *Subsidized Speech*, 106 Yale L.J. 151 (1996).

The prohibitions apply to all of the activities of an LSC grantee, including those paid for by non-LSC funds. We are concerned with the statutory provision which excludes LSC representation in cases which "involve an effort to amend or otherwise challenge existing law in effect on the date of the initiation of the representation."

II

The United States and LSC rely on *Rust* v. *Sullivan* as support for the LSC program restrictions. In *Rust*, Congress established program clinics to provide subsidies for doctors to advise patients on a variety of family planning topics. Congress did not consider abortion to be within its family planning objectives, however, and it forbade doctors employed by the program from discussing abortion with their patients.***

We upheld the law, reasoning that Congress had not discriminated against viewpoints on abortion, but had "merely chosen to fund one activity to the exclusion of the other." Title X did not single out a particular idea for suppression because it was dangerous or disfavored; rather, Congress prohibited Title X doctors from counseling that was outside the scope of the project.

The Court in *Rust* did not place explicit reliance on the rationale that the counseling activities of the doctors under Title X amounted to governmental speech; when interpreting the holding in later cases, however, we have explained *Rust* on this understanding. We have said that viewpoint-based funding decisions can be sustained in instances in which the government is itself the speaker, or instances, like *Rust*, in which the government "used private speakers to transmit information pertaining to its own program." *Rosenberger* v. *Rector & Visitors of Univ. of Va.*, 515 U.S. 819, 833 (1995). As we said in *Rosenberger*, "when the government disburses public funds to private entities to convey a governmental message, it may take legitimate and appropriate steps to ensure that its message is neither garbled nor distorted by the grantee."

Neither the latitude for government speech nor its rationale applies to subsidies for private speech in every instance, however. In the specific context of § 504(a)(16) suits for benefits, an LSC-funded attorney speaks on the behalf of the client in a claim against the government for welfare benefits. The lawyer is not the government's speaker. The attorney defending the decision to deny benefits will deliver the government's message in the litigation. The LSC lawyer, however, speaks on the behalf of his or her private, indigent client. ***

The Government has designed this program to use the legal profession and the established Judiciary of the States and the Federal Government to accomplish its end of assisting welfare claimants in determination or receipt of their benefits. The advice from the attorney to the client and the advocacy by the attorney to the courts cannot be classified as governmental speech even under a generous understanding of the concept. In this vital respect this suit is distinguishable from *Rust*.

The private nature of the speech involved here, and the extent of LSC's regulation of private expression, are indicated further by the circumstance that the Government seeks to use an existing medium of expression and to control it, in a class of cases, in ways which distort its usual functioning. At oral argument and in its briefs the LSC advised us that lawyers funded in the Government program may not undertake representation in suits for benefits if they must advise clients respecting the questionable validity of a statute which defines benefit eligibility and the payment structure. The limitation forecloses advice or legal assistance to question the validity of statutes under the Constitution of the United States. It extends further, it must be noted, so that state statutes inconsistent with federal law under the Supremacy Clause may be neither challenged nor questioned.

By providing subsidies to LSC, the Government seeks to facilitate suits for benefits by using the State and Federal courts and the independent bar on which those courts depend for the proper performance of their duties and responsibilities. Restricting LSC attorneys in advising their clients and in presenting arguments and analyses to the courts distorts the legal system by altering the traditional role of the attorneys.

LSC has advised us, furthermore, that upon determining a question of statutory validity is present in any anticipated or pending case or controversy, the LSC-funded attorney must cease the representation at once. This is true whether the validity issue becomes apparent during initial attorney-client consultations or in the midst of litigation proceedings. A disturbing example of the restriction was discussed during oral argument before the Court. It is well understood that when there are two reasonable constructions for a statute, yet one raises a constitutional question, the Court should prefer the interpretation which avoids the constitutional issue. Yet, as the LSC advised the Court, if, during litigation, a judge were to ask an LSC attorney whether there was a constitutional concern, the LSC attorney simply could not answer.

Interpretation of the law and the Constitution is the primary mission of the judiciary when it acts within the sphere of its authority to resolve a case or controversy. *Marbury* v. *Madison*, 5 U.S. 137, 1 Cranch 137, 177, (1803) ("It is emphatically the province and the duty of the judicial department to say what the law is"). An informed, independent judiciary presumes an informed, independent bar. Under § 504(a)(16), however, cases would be presented by LSC attorneys who could not advise the courts of serious questions of statutory validity. The disability is inconsistent with the proposition that attorneys should present all the reasonable and well-grounded arguments necessary for proper resolution of the case. By seeking to prohibit the analysis of certain legal issues and to truncate presentation to the courts, the enactment under review prohibits speech and expression upon which courts must depend for the proper exercise of the judicial power.

The restriction imposed by the statute here threatens severe impairment of the judicial function. Section 504(a)(16) sifts out cases presenting constitutional challenges in order to insulate the Government's laws from judicial inquiry. If the restriction on speech and legal advice were to stand, the result would be two tiers of cases. In cases where LSC counsel were attorneys of record, there would be lingering doubt whether the truncated representation had resulted in complete analysis of the case, full advice to the client, and proper presentation to the court. The courts and the public would come to question the adequacy and fairness of professional representations when the attorney, either consciously to comply with this statute or unconsciously to continue the representation despite the statute, avoided all reference to questions of statutory validity and constitutional authority. A scheme so inconsistent with accepted separation-of-powers principles is an insufficient basis to sustain or uphold the restriction on speech.

It is no answer to say the restriction on speech is harmless because, under LSC's interpretation of the Act, its attorneys can withdraw. This misses the point. The statute is an attempt to draw lines around the LSC program to exclude from litigation those arguments and theories Congress finds unacceptable but which by their nature are within the province of the courts to consider.

The restriction on speech is even more problematic because in cases where the attorney withdraws from a representation, the client is unlikely to find other counsel. The explicit premise for providing LSC attorneys is the necessity to make available representation "to persons financially unable to afford legal assistance." There often will be no alternative source for the client to receive vital information respecting constitutional and statutory rights bearing upon claimed benefits. Thus, with respect to the litigation services Congress has funded, there is no alternative channel for expression of the advocacy Congress seeks to restrict. This is in stark contrast to *Rust*. There, a patient could receive the approved Title X family planning counseling funded by the Government and later could consult an affiliate or independent organization to receive abortion counseling. Unlike indigent clients who seek LSC representation, the patient in *Rust* was not required to forfeit the Government-funded advice when she also received abortion counseling through alternative channels.

Finally, LSC and the Government maintain that § 504(a)(16) is necessary to define the scope and contours of the federal program, a condition that ensures funds can be spent for those cases most immediate to congressional concern. In support of this contention, they suggest the challenged limitation takes into account the nature of the grantees' activities and provides limited congressional funds for the provision of simple suits for benefits. In petitioners' view, the restriction operates neither to maintain the current welfare system nor insulate it from attack; rather, it helps the current welfare system function in a more efficient and fair manner by removing from the program complex challenges to existing welfare laws.

The effect of the restriction, however, is to prohibit advice or argumentation that existing welfare laws are unconstitutional or unlawful. Congress cannot recast a condition on funding as a mere definition of its program in every case, lest the First Amendment be reduced to a simple semantic exercise. Here, notwithstanding

Congress' purpose to confine and limit its program, the restriction operates to insulate current welfare laws from constitutional scrutiny and certain other legal challenges, a condition implicating central First Amendment concerns. *** The attempted restriction is designed to insulate the Government's interpretation of the Constitution from judicial challenge. The Constitution does not permit the Government to confine litigants and their attorneys in this manner. We must be vigilant when Congress imposes rules and conditions which in effect insulate its own laws from legitimate judicial challenge. Where private speech is involved, even Congress' antecedent funding decision cannot be aimed at the suppression of ideas thought inimical to the Government's own interest.

The judgment of the Court of Appeals is [a]ffirmed.

JUSTICE SCALIA, with whom THE CHIEF JUSTICE, JUSTICE O'CONNOR, and JUSTICE THOMAS join, dissenting.

***

I

The Legal Services Corporation Act of 1974 (LSC Act), is a federal subsidy program, the stated purpose of which is to "provide financial support for legal assistance in noncriminal proceedings or matters to persons financially unable to afford legal assistance." Congress, has from the program's inception tightly regulated the use of its funds. No Legal Services Corporation (LSC) funds may be used, for example, for "encouraging . . . labor or antilabor activities," for "litigation relating to the desegregation of any elementary or secondary school or school system," or for "litigation which seeks to procure a nontherapeutic abortion," Congress discovered through experience, however, that these restrictions did not exhaust the politically controversial uses to which LSC funds could be put.

Accordingly, in 1996 Congress added new restrictions to the LSC Act and strengthened existing restrictions. Among the new restrictions is the one at issue here. Section 504(a)(16) withholds LSC funds from every entity that "participates in any way in litigation, lobbying, or rulemaking . . . involving an effort to reform a Federal or State welfare system."

The restrictions relating to rulemaking and lobbying are superfluous; they duplicate general prohibitions on the use of LSC funds for those activities found elsewhere in the Appropriations Act. The restriction on litigation, however, is unique, and it contains a proviso specifying what the restriction does not cover. Funding recipients may "represent an individual eligible client who is seeking specific relief from a welfare agency if such relief does not involve an effort to amend or otherwise challenge existing law in effect on the date of the initiation of the representation." The LSC declares in its brief, and respondents do not deny, that under these provisions the LSC can sponsor neither challenges to *nor* defenses of existing welfare reform law. The litigation ban is symmetrical: Litigants challenging the covered statutes or regulations do not receive LSC funding, and neither do litigants defending those laws against challenge.

If a suit for benefits raises a claim outside the scope of the LSC program, the LSC-funded lawyer may not participate in the suit. As the Court explains, if LSC-funded lawyers anticipate that a forbidden claim will arise in a prospective client's suit, they "may not undertake [the] representation." Likewise, if a forbidden claim arises unexpectedly at trial, "LSC-funded attorneys must cease the representation at once." The lawyers may, however, and indeed *must* explain to the client why they cannot represent him. See 164 F.3d 757, 765 (CA2 1999). They are also free to express their views of the legality of the welfare law to the client, and they may refer the client to another attorney who can accept the representation, ibid.

II

The LSC Act is a federal subsidy program, not a federal regulatory program, and "there is a basic difference between [the two]." *Maher* v. *Roe,* 432 U.S. 464, 475, (1977). Regulations directly restrict speech; subsidies do not. Subsidies, it is true, may *indirectly* abridge speech, but only if the funding scheme is "'manipulated' to have a 'coercive effect'" on those who do not hold the subsidized position. ***

In *Rust* v. *Sullivan, supra,* the Court applied these principles to a statutory scheme that is in all relevant respects indistinguishable from § 504(a)(16). Valid regulations implementing the statute required funding recipients to refer pregnant clients "for appropriate prenatal . . . services by furnishing a list of available providers that promote the welfare of mother and unborn child," but forbade them to refer a pregnant woman specifically to an abortion provider, even upon request. We rejected a First Amendment free-speech challenge to the funding scheme, explaining that "the Government can, without violating the Constitution, selectively fund a program to encourage certain activities it believes to be in the public interest, without at the same time funding an alternative program which seeks to deal with the problem another way." This was not, we said, the type of "discrimination on the basis of viewpoint" that triggers strict scrutiny, because the "'decision not to subsidize the exercise of a fundamental right does not infringe the right,'" *ibid.*

The same is true here. The LSC Act, like the scheme in *Rust*, does not create a public forum. Far from encouraging a diversity of views, it has always, as the Court accurately states, "placed restrictions on its use of funds." Nor does § 504(a)(16) discriminate on the basis of viewpoint, since it funds neither challenges to nor defenses of existing welfare law. The provision simply declines to subsidize a certain class of litigation, and under *Rust* that decision "does not infringe the right" to bring such litigation. *Rust* thus controls these cases and compels the conclusion that § 504(a)(16) is constitutional.

The Court contends that *Rust* is different because the program at issue subsidized government speech, while the LSC funds private speech. This is so unpersuasive it hardly needs response. If the private doctors' confidential advice to their patients at issue in *Rust* constituted "government speech," it is hard to imagine what subsidized speech would *not* be government speech. Moreover, the majority's contention that the subsidized speech in these cases is not government speech because the lawyers have a professional obligation to represent the interests of their clients founders on the reality that the doctors in *Rust* had a professional obligation to serve the interests of their patients.

The Court further asserts that these cases are different from *Rust* because the welfare funding restriction "seeks to use an existing medium of expression and to control it . . . in ways which distort its usual functioning," This is wrong on both the facts and the law. It may well be that the bar of § 504(a)(16) will cause LSC-funded attorneys to decline or to withdraw from cases that involve statutory validity. But that means at most that fewer statutory challenges to welfare laws will be presented to the courts because of the unavailability of free legal services for that purpose. So what? The same result would ensue from excluding LSC-funded lawyers from welfare litigation entirely. It is not the mandated, nondistortable function of the courts to inquire into all "serious questions of statutory validity" in all cases. Courts must consider only those questions of statutory validity *that are presented by litigants*, and if the Government chooses not to subsidize the presentation of some such questions, that in no way "distorts" the courts' role.

Finally, the Court is troubled "because in cases where the attorney withdraws from a representation, the client is unlikely to find other counsel." That is surely irrelevant, since it leaves the welfare recipient in no *worse* condition than he would have been in had the LSC program never been enacted. Respondents properly concede that even if welfare claimants cannot obtain a lawyer anywhere else, the Government is not required to provide one. It is hard to see how providing free legal services to some welfare claimants (those whose claims do not challenge the applicable statutes) while not providing it to others is beyond the range of legitimate legislative choice. *Rust* rejected a similar argument:

> "Petitioners contend, however, that most Title X clients are effectively precluded by indigency and poverty from seeing a health-care provider who will provide abortion-related services. But once again, even these Title X clients are in no worse position than if Congress had never enacted Title X. The financial constraints that restrict an indigent woman's ability to enjoy the full range of constitutionally protected freedom of choice are the product not of governmental restrictions on access to abortion, but rather of her indigency." 500 U.S. at 203 (internal quotation marks omitted).

The only conceivable argument that can be made for distinguishing *Rust* is that there even patients who wished to receive abortion counseling could receive the nonabortion services that the Government-funded clinic offered, whereas here some potential LSC clients who wish to receive representation on a benefits claim that does not challenge the statutes will be unable to do so because their cases raise a reform claim that an LSC lawyer may not present. This difference, of course, is required by the same ethical canons that the Court elsewhere does not wish to distort. Rather than sponsor "truncated representation," Congress chose to subsidize only those cases in which the attorneys it subsidized could work freely.. And it is impossible to see how this difference from *Rust* has any bearing upon the First Amendment question, which, to repeat, is whether the funding scheme is "'manipulated' to have a 'coercive effect'" on those who do not hold the subsidized position. It could be claimed to have such an effect if the client in a case ineligible for LSC representation could eliminate the ineligibility by waiving the claim that the statute is invalid; but he cannot. No *conceivable* coercive effect exists.

This has been a very long discussion to make a point that is embarrassingly simple: The LSC subsidy neither prevents anyone from speaking nor coerces anyone to change speech, and is indistinguishable in all relevant respects from the subsidy upheld in *Rust* v. *Sullivan, supra.* There is no legitimate basis for declaring § 504(a)(16) facially unconstitutional.

III

***

Today's decision is quite simply inexplicable on the basis of our prior law. The only difference between *Rust* and the present case is that the former involved "distortion" of (that is to say, refusal to subsidize) the normal work of doctors, and the latter involves "distortion" of (that is to say, refusal to subsidize) the normal work of lawyers. The Court's decision displays not only an improper special solicitude for our own profession; it also displays, I think, the very fondness for "reform through the courts" -- the making of innumerable social judgments through judge-pronounced constitutional imperatives -- that prompted Congress to restrict publicly funded litigation of this sort. The Court says today, through an unprecedented (and indeed previously rejected) interpretation of the First Amendment, that we will not allow this restriction -- and then, to add insult to injury, permits to stand a judgment that awards the general litigation funding that the statute does not contain. I respectfully dissent.

PICKERING v. BOARD OF EDUCATION OF WILL COUNTY, ILLINOIS

391 U.S. 563 (1968)

MR. JUSTICE MARSHALL delivered the opinion of the Court.

***

I

In February of 1961 the appellee Board of Education asked the voters of the school district to approve a bond issue to raise $4,875,000 to erect two new schools. The proposal was defeated. *** [A] second proposal passed and the schools were built with the money raised by the bond sales. In May of 1964 a proposed increase in the tax rate to be used for educational purposes was submitted to the voters by the

Board and was defeated. Finally, on September 19, 1964, a second proposal to increase the tax rate was submitted by the Board and was likewise defeated. It was in connection with this last proposal of the School Board that appellant wrote the letter to the editor *** that resulted in his dismissal.

Prior to the vote on the second tax increase proposal a variety of articles attributed to the District 205 Teachers' Organization appeared in the local paper. These articles urged passage of the tax increase and stated that failure to pass the increase would result in a decline in the quality of education afforded children in the district's schools. A letter from the superintendent of schools making the same point was published in the paper two days before the election and submitted to the voters in mimeographed form the following day. It was in response to the foregoing material, together with the failure of the tax increase to pass, that appellant submitted the letter in question to the editor of the local paper.

The letter constituted, basically, an attack on the School Board's handling of the 1961 bond issue proposals and its subsequent allocation of financial resources between the schools' educational and athletic programs. It also charged the superintendent of schools with attempting to prevent teachers in the district from opposing or criticizing the proposed bond issue.

The Board dismissed Pickering for writing and publishing the letter. Pursuant to Illinois law, the Board was then required to hold a hearing on the dismissal. At the hearing the Board charged that numerous statements in the letter were false and that the publication of the statements unjustifiably impugned the "motives, honesty, integrity, truthfulness, responsibility and competence" of both the Board and the school administration. The Board also charged that the false statements damaged the professional reputations of its members and of the school administrators, would be disruptive of faculty discipline, and would tend to foment "controversy, conflict and dissension" among teachers, administrators, the Board of Education, and the residents of the district. Testimony was introduced from a variety of witnesses on the truth or falsity of the particular statements in the letter with which the Board took issue. The Board found the statements to be false as charged. No evidence was introduced at any point in the proceedings as to the effect of the publication of the letter on the community as a whole or on the administration of the school system in particular, and no specific findings along these lines were made.

The Illinois courts reviewed the proceeding solely to determine whether the Board's findings were supported by substantial evidence and whether, on the facts as found, the Board could reasonably conclude that appellant's publication of the letter was "detrimental to the best interests of the schools." Pickering's claim that his letter was protected by the First Amendment was rejected on the ground that his acceptance of a teaching position in the public schools obliged him to refrain from making statements about the operation of the schools "which in the absence of such position he would have an undoubted right to engage in." It is not altogether clear whether the Illinois Supreme Court held that the First Amendment had no applicability to appellant's dismissal for writing the letter in question or whether it determined that the particular statements made in the letter were not entitled to First Amendment protection. In any event, it clearly rejected Pickering's claim that, on the facts of this case, he could not constitutionally be dismissed from his teaching position.

II

To the extent that the Illinois Supreme Court's opinion may be read to suggest that teachers may constitutionally be compelled to relinquish the First Amendment rights they would otherwise enjoy as citizens to comment on matters of public interest in connection with the operation of the public schools in which they work, it proceeds on a premise that has been unequivocally rejected in numerous prior decisions of this Court. "[T]he theory that public employment which may be denied altogether may be subjected to any conditions, regardless of how unreasonable, has been uniformly rejected." Keyishian v. Board of Regents, 385 U.S. at 605-606. At the same time it cannot be gainsaid that the State has interests as an employer in regulating the speech of its employees that differ significantly from those it possesses in connection with regulation of the speech of the citizenry in general. The problem in any case is to arrive at a balance between the interests of the teacher, as a citizen, in commenting upon matters of public concern and the interest of the State, as an employer, in promoting the efficiency of the public services it performs through its employees.

III

The Board contends that "the teacher by virtue of his public employment has a duty of loyalty to support his superiors in attaining the generally accepted goals of education and that, if he must speak out publicly, he should do so factually and accurately, commensurate with his education and experience." Appellant, on the other hand, argues that the test applicable to defamatory statements directed against public officials by persons having no occupational relationship with them, namely, that statements to be legally actionable must be made "with knowledge that [they were] false or with reckless disregard of whether [they were] false or not," New York Times Co. v. Sullivan, 376 U.S. 254, 280 (1964), should also be applied to public statements made by teachers. Because of the enormous variety of fact situations in which critical statements by teachers and other public employees may be thought by their superiors, against whom the statements are directed to furnish grounds for dismissal, we do not deem it either appropriate or feasible to attempt to lay down a general standard against which all such statements may be judged. However, in the course of evaluating the conflicts of First Amendment protection and the need for orderly school administration in the context of this case, we shall indicate some of the general lines along which an analysis of the controlling interests should run.

An examination of the statements in appellant's letter objected to by the Board reveals that they, like the letter as a whole, consist essentially of criticism of the Board's allocation of school funds between educational and athletic programs, and of both the Board's and the superintendent's methods of informing, or preventing the informing of, the district's taxpayers of the real reasons why additional tax revenues were being sought for the schools. The statements are in no way directed towards any person with whom appellant would normally be in contact in the course of his daily work as a teacher. Thus no question of maintaining either discipline by immediate superiors or harmony among coworkers is presented here. Appellant's employment relationships with the Board and, to a somewhat lesser extent, with the superintendent are not the kind of close working relationships for which it can persuasively be claimed that personal loyalty and confidence are necessary to their proper functioning. Accordingly, to the extent that the Board's position here can be taken to suggest that even comments on matters of public concern that are substantially correct may furnish grounds for dismissal if they are sufficiently critical in tone, we unequivocally reject it.[3]

We next consider the statements in appellant's letter which we agree to be false. The Board's original charges included allegations that the publication of the letter damaged the professional reputations of the Board and the superintendent and would foment controversy and conflict among the Board, teachers, administrators, and the residents of the district. However, no evidence to support these allegations was introduced at the hearing. So far as the record reveals, Pickering's letter was greeted by everyone but its main target, the Board, with massive apathy and total disbelief. The Board must, therefore, have decided, perhaps by analogy with the law of libel, that the statements were *per se* harmful to the operation of the schools.

However, the only way in which the Board could conclude, absent any evidence of the actual effect of the letter, that the statements contained therein were*per se* detrimental to the interest of the schools was to equate the Board members' own interests with that of the schools. Certainly an accusation that too much money is being spent on athletics by the administrators of the school system (which is precisely the import of that portion of appellant's letter containing the statements that we have found to be false) cannot reasonably be regarded as per se detrimental to the district's schools. Such an accusation reflects rather a difference of opinion between Pickering and the Board as to the preferable manner of operating the school system, a difference of opinion that clearly concerns an issue of general public interest.

---

3. It is possible to conceive of some positions in public employment in which the need for confidentiality is so great that even completely correct public statements might furnish a permissible ground for dismissal. Likewise, positions in public employment in which the relationship between superior and subordinate is of such a personal and intimate nature that certain forms of public criticism of the superior by the subordinate would seriously undermine the effectiveness of the working relationship between them can also be imagined. We intimate no views as to how we would resolve any specific instances of such situations, but merely note that significantly different considerations would be involved in such cases.

In addition, the fact that particular illustrations of the Board's claimed undesirable emphasis on athletic programs are false would not normally have any necessary impact on the actual operation of the schools, beyond its tendency to anger the Board. For example, Pickering's letter was written after the defeat at the polls of the second proposed tax increase. It could, therefore, have had no effect on the ability of the school district to raise necessary revenue, since there was no showing that there was any proposal to increase taxes pending when the letter was written.

More importantly, the question whether a school system requires additional funds is a matter of legitimate public concern on which the judgment of the school administration, including the School Board, cannot, in a society that leaves such questions to popular vote, be taken as conclusive. On such a question free and open debate is vital to informed decision-making by the electorate. Teachers are, as a class, the members of a community most likely to have informed and definite opinions as to how funds allotted to the operation of the schools should be spent. Accordingly, it is essential that they be able to speak out freely on such questions without fear of retaliatory dismissal.

In addition, the amounts expended on athletics which Pickering reported erroneously were matters of public record on which his position as a teacher in the district did not qualify him to speak with any greater authority than any other taxpayer. The Board could easily have rebutted appellant's errors by publishing the accurate figures itself, either via a letter to the same newspaper or otherwise. We are thus not presented with a situation in which a teacher has carelessly made false statements about matters so closely related to the day-to-day operations of the schools that any harmful impact on the public would be difficult to counter because of the teacher's presumed greater access to the real facts. Accordingly, we have no occasion to consider at this time whether under such circumstances a school board could reasonably require that a teacher make substantial efforts to verify the accuracy of his charges before publishing them.[4]

What we do have before us is a case in which a teacher has made erroneous public statements upon issues then currently the subject of public attention, which are critical of his ultimate employer but which are neither shown nor can be presumed to have in any way either impeded the teacher's proper performance of his daily duties in the classroom[5] or to have interfered with the regular operation of the schools

---

4. There is likewise no occasion furnished by this case for consideration of the extent to which teachers can be required by narrowly drawn grievance procedures to submit complaints about the operation of the schools to their superiors for action thereon prior to bringing the complaints before the public.

5. We also note that this case does not present a situation in which a teacher's public statements are so without foundation as to call into question his fitness to perform his duties in the classroom. In such a case, of course, the statements would merely be evidence of the teacher's general competence, or lack thereof, and not an independent basis for dismissal.

generally. In these circumstances we conclude that the interest of the school administration in limiting teachers' opportunities to contribute to public debate is not significantly greater than its interest in limiting a similar contribution by any member of the general public.

IV

The public interest in having free and unhindered debate on matters of public importance—the core value of the Free Speech Clause of the First Amendment—is so great that it has been held that a State cannot authorize the recovery of damages by a public official for defamatory statements directed at him except when such statements are shown to have been made either with knowledge of their falsity or with reckless disregard for their truth or falsity. The same test has been applied to suits for invasion of privacy based on false statements where a "matter of public interest" is involved. Time, Inc. v. Hill, 385 U.S. 374 (1967). It is therefore perfectly clear that, were appellant a member of the general public, the State's power to afford the appellee Board of Education or its members any legal right to sue him for writing the letter at issue here would be limited by the requirement that the letter be judged by the standard laid down in *New York Times*.

While criminal sanctions and damage awards have a somewhat different impact on the exercise of the right to freedom of speech from dismissal from employment, it is apparent that the threat of dismissal from public employment is nonetheless a potent means of inhibiting speech. We have already noted our disinclination to make an across-the-board equation of dismissal from public employment for remarks critical of superiors with awarding damages in a libel suit by a public official for similar criticism. However, in a case such as the present one, in which the fact of employment is only tangentially and insubstantially involved in the subject matter of the public communication made by a teacher, we conclude that it is necessary to regard the teacher as the member of the general public he seeks to be.

In sum, we hold that, in a case such as this, absent proof of false statements knowingly or recklessly made by him,[6] a teacher's exercise of his right to speak on issues of public importance may not furnish the basis for his dismissal from public employment. Since no such showing has been made in this case regarding appellant's letter, his dismissal for writing it cannot be upheld and the judgment of the Illinois Supreme Court must, accordingly, be reversed and the case remanded for further proceedings not inconsistent with this opinion. It is so ordered. ***

MR. JUSTICE WHITE, concurring in part and dissenting in part. [Omitted.]

---

6. Because we conclude that appellant's statements were not knowingly or recklessly false, we have no occasion to pass upon the additional question whether a statement that was knowingly or recklessly false would, if it were neither shown nor could reasonably be presumed to have had any harmful effects, still be protected by the First Amendment. See also n. 5, *supra*.

UNITED STATES CIVIL SERVICE v. NATIONAL ASSOCIATION OF LETTER CARRIERS

413 U.S. 548 (1973)

MR. JUSTICE WHITE delivered the opinion of the Court.

On December 11, 1972, we noted probable jurisdiction of this appeal, 409 U.S. 1058, based on a jurisdictional statement presenting the single question whether the prohibition in § 9(a) of the Hatch Act, now codified in 5 U.S.C. § 7324(a)(2), against federal employees taking "an active part in political management or in political campaigns," is unconstitutional on its face. Section 7324(a) (2) provides:

> An employee in an Executive agency or an individual employed by the government of the District of Columbia may not— 2) take an active part in political campaigns. For the purpose of this subsection, the phrase 'an active part in political management or in political campaigns' means those acts of political management or political campaigning which were prohibited on the part of employees in the competitive service before July 19, 1940, by determinations of the Civil Service Commission under the rules prescribed by the President.

A divided three-judge court sitting in the District of Columbia had held the section unconstitutional. We reverse the judgment of the District Court.

I

The case began when the National Association of Letter Carriers, six individual federal employees and certain local Democratic and Republican political committees filed a complaint, asserting on behalf of themselves and all federal employees that 5 U.S.C. § 7324(a)(2) was unconstitutional on its face and seeking an injunction against its enforcement.

Each of the plaintiffs alleged that the Civil Service Commission was enforcing, or threatening to enforce, the Hatch Act's prohibition against active participation in political management or political campaigns with respect to certain defined activity in which that plaintiff desired to engage.[3] The Union, for example, stated among other things that its members desired to campaign for candidates for public office. The Democratic and Republican Committees complained of not being able to get federal employees to run for state and local offices. Plaintiff Hummel stated that he was aware of the provision of the Hatch Act and that the activities he desired to

---

3. The Union alleged that its members were desirous of

"a. Running in local elections for such offices as school board member, city council member or mayor.

"b. Writing letters on political subjects to newspapers.

"c. Participating as a delegate in a political convention and running for office in a political party.

"d. Campaigning for candidates for political office." ***

II

As the District Court recognized, the constitutionality of the Hatch Act's ban on taking an active part in political management or political campaigns has been here before. This very prohibition was attacked in the *Mitchell* case [1947] by a labor union and various federal employees as being violative of the First, Ninth, and Tenth Amendments and as contrary to the Fifth Amendment by being vague and indefinite, arbitrarily discriminatory, and a deprivation of liberty. The Court there first determined that with respect to all but one of the plaintiffs there was no case or controversy present within the meaning of Art. III As to the plaintiff Poole, however, the Court noted that "[h]e was a ward executive committeeman of a political party and was politically active on election day as a worker at the polls and a paymaster for the services of other party workers." ***

We hesitatingly reaffirm the *Mitchell* holding that Congress had, and has, the power to prevent Mr. Poole and others like him from holding a party office, working at the polls, and acting as party paymaster for other party workers. An Act of Congress going no farther would in our view unquestionably be valid. So would it be if, in plain and understandable language, the statute forbade activities such as organizing a political party or club; actively participating in fund-raising activities for a partisan candidate or political party; becoming a partisan candidate for, or campaigning for, an elective public office; actively managing the campaign of a partisan candidate for public office; initiating or circulating a partisan nominating petition or soliciting votes for a partisan candidate for public office; or serving as a delegate, alternative or proxy to a political party convention. Our judgment is that neither the First Amendment nor any other provision of the Constitution invalidates a law barring this kind of partisan political conduct by federal employees. ***

[A]s the Court held in Pickering v. Board of Education, 391 U.S. 563, 568 (1968), the government has an interest in regulating the conduct and "the speech of its employees that differ[s] significantly from those it possesses in connection with regulation of speech of the citizenry in general. *** Although Congress is free to strike a different balance than it has, if it so chooses, we think the balance it has so far struck is sustainable by the obviously important interests sought to be served by the limitations on partisan political activities now contained in the Hatch Act. ***

III

But however constitutional the proscription of identifiable partisan conduct in understandable language may be, the District Court's judgment was that § 7324(a)(2) was both unconstitutionally vague and fatally overbroad. ***

We take quite a different view of the statute. As we see it, our task is not to destroy the Act if we can, but to construe it, if consistent with the will of Congress, so as to comport with constitutional limitations. ***

Whatever might be the difficulty with a provision against taking "active part in political management or in political campaigns," the Act specifically provides that the employee retains the right to vote as he chooses and to express his opinion on political subjects and candidates. The Act exempts research and educational activities supported by the District of Columbia or by religious, philanthropic, or cultural organizations, 5 U.S.C. § 7324(c); and § 7326 exempts nonpartisan political activity: questions, that is, that are not identified with national or state political parties are not covered by the Act, including issues with respect to constitutional amendments, referendums, approval of municipal ordinances, and the like. Moreover, the plain import of the 1940 amendment to the Hatch Act is that the proscription against taking an active part in the proscribed activities is not open-ended but is limited to those rules and proscriptions that had been developed under Civil Service Rule I up to the date of the passage of the 1940 Act. Those rules, as refined by further adjudications within the outer limits of the 1940 rules, were restated by the Commission in 1970 in the form of regulations specifying the conduct that would be prohibited or permitted by § 7324 and its companion sections. ***

It is also important in this respect that the Commission has established a procedure by which an employee in doubt about the validity of a proposed course of conduct may seek and obtain advice from the Commission and thereby remove any doubt there may be as to the meaning of the law, at least insofar as the Commission itself is concerned. ***

Even if the provisions forbidding partisan campaign endorsements and speechmaking were to be considered in some respects unconstitutionally overbroad, we would not invalidate the entire statute as the District Court did. The remainder of the statute, as we have said, covers a whole range of easily identifiable and constitutionally proscribable partisan conduct on the part of federal employees, and the extent to which pure expression is impermissibly threatened, if at all, by §§ 733.122 (a)(10) and (12), does not in our view make the statute substantially overbroad and so invalid on its face. Broadrick v. Oklahoma, 413 U.S. 601.

For the foregoing reasons, the judgment of the District Court is reversed. ***

MR. JUSTICE DOUGLAS, with whom MR. JUSTICE BRENNAN and MR. JUSTICE MARSHALL concur, dissenting.

The Hatch Act by § 9(a) prohibits federal employees from taking "an active part in political management or in political campaigns." Some of the employees, whose union is speaking for them, want

> to run in state and local elections for the school board, for city council, for mayor;
> to write letters on political subjects to newspapers;
> to be a delegate in a political convention;
> to run for an office and hold office in a political party or political club;
> to campaign for candidates for political office;
> to work at polling places in behalf of a political party.

There is no definition of what "an active part *** in political campaigns" means. The Act incorporates over 3,000 rulings of the Civil Service Commission between 1886 and 1940 and many hundreds of rulings since 1940. But even with that gloss on the Act, the critical phrases lack precision. The chilling effect of these vague and generalized prohibitions is so obvious as not to need elaboration. ***

A nursing assistant at a veterans' hospital put an ad in a news paper reading:

> To All My Many Friends of Poplar Bluff and Butler County I want to take this opportunity to ask your vote and support in the election, TUESDAY, AUGUST 7th. A very special person is seeking the Democratic nomination for Sheriff. I do not have to tell you of his qualifications, his past records stand.
> This person is my dad, Lester (Less) Massingham.
> THANK YOU
> WALLACE (WALLY) MASSINGHAM

He was held to have violated the Act. Massingham, 1 Political Activity Reporter 792, 793 (1959). Is a letter a permissible "expression" of views or a prohibited "solicitation?" The Solicitor General says it is a "permissible" expression; but the Commission ruled otherwise. For an employee who does not have the Solicitor General as counsel great consequences flow from an innocent decision. He may lose his job. Therefore the most prudent thing is to do nothing. Thus is self-imposed censorship imposed on many nervous people who live on narrow economic margins.

I would strike this provision of the law down as unconstitutional so that a new start may be made on this old problem that confuses and restricts nearly five million federal, state, and local public employees today that live under the present Act.

NOTE

Note that in *Letter Carriers*, the federal statute was upheld even though it restricted the affected public employees—not merely (as in *Rust*) while on the job (e.g., as would be the case had the rules merely forbidden soliciting postal patrons or other employees while at work in the post office or while in the course of delivering the mail)—but also while away from work, and entirely on "their own" time as well.[27]

1. How does this differ in any significant way from *McAuliffe v. New Bedford* (the original policeman case from 1892)? In light of *Letter Carriers*, might the *McAuliffe* case still come out the same way today, even without relying on the original rationale?[28]

2. If not (and perhaps *Pickering* suggests why not), may it at least suggest that the doctrine of unconstitutional conditions is nonetheless also less clear cut than one might have thought?[29] In the years immediately following the Court's decision in *Pickering*, litigation involving public employees challenging their dismissal, nonrenewal, suspension (or other adverse treatment), for reinstatement (and for damages) as improperly retaliatory for protected speech, mushroomed in the federal district courts. The next several principal cases present the Court's effort to provide a more systematic overview of the field, refining *Pickering*, but also quite strictly confining it as well.[30] They may best be considered as a group.

---

27. Notwithstanding the decision in *Letter Carriers*, however, in 1995, the Supreme Court struck down a subsequent Act of Congress forbidding any federal employee to accept compensation for making speeches or for writing books or articles on any subject whether or not connected to their work, while employed by the government. See United States v. National Treasury Employees Union, 115 S.Ct. 1003 (1995) (6-3). The act was adopted to forestall possible conflicts of interest, to eliminate possibilities for corrupt influence, and to prevent the appearance of such influence. As applied to those under civil service grade GS-16, the act was held to be an overly broad restriction. The majority relied extensively on *Pickering*, however, though the ban here was merely one on compensation for outside speaking or writing and not a ban on such speech or writing *per se*. The dissent relied on the *Letter Carriers* case. (In dicta, the majority suggested that a more narrowly-drawn restriction, forbidding compensation for outside writing or outside speaking on matters related to one's government position or responsibilities, might be sustained. The majority also declined to pass on the validity of the "no compensation" rule for upper echelon and personnel.)

28. Would a more limited restriction (e.g., one forbidding "such conduct as may affect the efficiency of the police department," as applied to dismiss a police officer who, fully aware of the rule, presumes to become a member of and pay dues to (a) a local Ku Klux Klan chapter; (b) The Man-Boy Love Association; (c) Louis Farrakhan's Nation of Islam; or (d) Operation Rescue come out the same way?

29. Namely, that if the speech or political activity restriction would be invalid when tested without reference to one's public employment (i.e. if it would be invalid as applied to one directly as a private citizen, exercising one's First Amendment rights merely "as a private citizen"), it is likewise invalid when sought to be enforced as a condition of public employment when it presumes to reach conduct separated from such work and pursued on one's own time. (*Letter Carriers* rejects this view, does it not?)

30. See also Perry v. Sindermann, 408 U.S. 593, 598 (1972) (state college professor sued for reinstatement and for damages, alleging he was nonrenewed by state board of regents because of critical testimony he presented in state legislative hearings and because he publicly supported elevation of the college to four-year status—a change opposed by the regents, *held*, "present[s] a bona fide constitutional claim" insofar as he may be able to establish the nonrenewal of his appointment was "in retaliation for his exercise of the constitutional right of free speech," (citing *Pickering*, and declaring, id. at 597: "For at least a quarter-century, this Court has made clear that even though a person has no 'right' to a

MT. HEALTHY CITY SCHOOL DISTRICT BOARD OF EDUCATION v. DOYLE

429 U.S. 274 (1977)

MR. JUSTICE REHNQUIST delivered the opinion of the Court.

Respondent Doyle sued petitioner Mt. Healthy Board of Education in the United States District Court for the Southern District of Ohio. Doyle claimed that the Board's refusal to renew his contract in 1971 violated his rights under the First and Fourteenth Amendments to the United States Constitution. After a bench trial the District Court held that Doyle was entitled to reinstatement with back pay. The Court of Appeals for the Sixth Circuit affirmed the judgment, and we granted the Board's petition for certiorari. ***

Doyle was first employed by the Board in 1966. He worked under one-year contracts for the first three years, and under a two-year contract from 1969 to 1971. In 1969 he was elected president of the Teachers' Association, in which position he worked to expand the subjects of direct negotiation between the Association and the Board of Education. During Doyle's one-year term as president of the Association, and during the succeeding year when he served on its executive committee, there was apparently some tension in relations between the Board and the Association.

Beginning early in 1970, Doyle was involved in several incidents not directly connected with his role in the Teachers' Association. In one instance, he engaged in an argument with another teacher which culminated in the other teacher's slapping him. Doyle subsequently refused to accept an apology and insisted upon some punishment for the other teacher. His persistence in the matter resulted in the suspension of both teachers for one day, which was followed by a walkout by a number of other teachers, which in turn resulted in the lifting of the suspensions.

On other occasions, Doyle got into an argument with employees of the school cafeteria over the amount of spaghetti which had been served him; referred to students, in connection with a disciplinary complaint, as "sons of bitches"; and made an obscene gesture to two girls in connection with their failure to obey commands made in his capacity as cafeteria supervisor. Chronologically the last in the series of incidents which respondent was involved in during his employment by the Board was a telephone call by him to a local radio station. It was the Board's consideration of this incident which the court below found to be a violation of the First and Fourteenth Amendments.

In February 1971, the principal circulated to various teachers a memorandum relating to teacher dress and appearance, which was apparently prompted by the view

---

valuable government benefit and even though the government may deny him the benefit for many reasons, there are some reasons upon which the government may not rely. It may not deny a benefit to a person on a basis that infringes his constitutionally protected interests—especially, his interest in freedom of speech.")).

of some in the administration that there was a relationship between teacher appearance and public support for bond issues. Doyle's response to the receipt of the memorandum — on a subject which he apparently understood was to be settled by joint teacher-administration action—was to convey the substance of the memorandum to a disc jockey at WSAI, a Cincinnati radio station, who promptly announced the adoption of the dress code as a news item. Doyle subsequently apologized to the principal, conceding that he should have made some prior communication of his criticism to the school administration.

Approximately one month later the superintendent made his customary annual recommendations to the Board as to the rehiring of nontenured teachers. He recommended that Doyle not be rehired. The same recommendation was made with respect to nine other teachers in the district, and in all instances, including Doyle's, the recommendation was adopted by the Board. Shortly after being notified of this decision, respondent requested a statement of reasons for the Board's actions. He received a statement citing "a notable lack of tact in handling professional matters which leaves much doubt as to your sincerity in establishing good school relationships." That general statement was followed by references to the radio station incident and to the obscene gesture incident.

The District Court found that all of these incidents had in fact occurred. It concluded that respondent Doyle's telephone call to the radio station was "clearly protected by the First Amendment," and that because it had played a "substantial part" in the decision of the Board not to renew Doyle's employment, he was entitled to reinstatement with back pay. The District Court did not expressly state what test it was applying in determining that the incident in question involved conduct protected by the First Amendment, but simply held that the communication to the radio station was such conduct. The Court of Appeals affirmed in a brief *per curiam* opinion. ***

*** There is no suggestion by the Board that Doyle violated any established policy, or that its reaction to his communication to the radio station was anything more than an ad hoc response to Doyle's action in making the memorandum public. We therefore accept the District Court's finding that the communication was protected by the First and Fourteenth Amendments. We are not, however, entirely in agreement with that court's manner of reasoning from this finding to the conclusion that Doyle is entitled to reinstatement with back pay.

The District Court made the following "conclusions" on this aspect of the case:

> 1) If a non-permissible reason, e.g., exercise of First Amendment rights, played a substantial part in the decision not to renew—even in the face of other permissible grounds—the decision may not stand.
> 2) A non-permissible reason did play a substantial part. That is clear from the letter of the Superintendent immediately following the Board's decision, which stated two reasons—the one, the conversation with the radio station clearly protected by the First Amendment. ***

The difficulty with the rule enunciated by the District Court is that it would require reinstatement in cases where a dramatic and perhaps abrasive incident is inevitably on the minds of those responsible for the decision to rehire, and does indeed play a part in that decision—even if the same decision would have been reached had the incident not occurred. The constitutional principle at stake is sufficiently vindicated if such an employee is placed in no worse a position than if he had not engaged in the conduct. A borderline or marginal candidate should not have the employment question resolved against him because of constitutionally protected conduct. But that same candidate ought not to be able, by engaging in such conduct, to prevent his employer from assessing his performance record and reaching a decision not to rehire on the basis of that record, simply because the protected conduct makes the employer more certain of the correctness of its decision.

Initially, in this case, the burden was properly placed upon respondent to show that his conduct was constitutionally protected, and that this conduct was a "substantial factor"—or, to put in it other words, that it was a "motivating factor" in the Board's decision not to rehire him. Respondent having carried that burden, however, the District Court should have gone on to determine whether the Board had shown by a preponderance of the evidence that it would have reached the same decision as to respondent's reemployment even in the absence of the protected conduct.

We cannot tell from the District Court opinion and conclusions, nor from the opinion of the Court of Appeals affirming the judgment of the District Court, what conclusion those courts would have reached had they applied this test. The judgment of the Court of Appeals is therefore vacated, and the case remanded for further proceedings consistent with this opinion.

GIVHAN v. WESTERN LINE CONSOLIDATED SCHOOL DISTRICT
439 U.S. 410 (1979)

MR. JUSTICE REHNQUIST delivered the opinion of the Court.

Petitioner Bessie Givhan was dismissed from her employment as a junior high English teacher at the end of the 1970-71 school year.[1] At the time of petitioner's termination, respondent Western Line Consolidated School District was the subject of a desegregation order entered by the United States District Court for the Northern

---

1. In a letter to petitioner, dated July 28, 1971, District Superintendent C. L. Morris gave the following reasons for the decision not to renew her contract:

"(1) [A] flat refusal to administer standardized national tests to the pupils in your charge; (2) an announced intention not to co-operate with the administration of the Glen Allan Attendance Center; (3) and an antagonistic and hostile attitude to the administration of the Glen Allan Attendance Center demonstrated throughout the school year."

District of Mississippi. Petitioner filed a complaint *** seeking reinstatement on the dual grounds that nonrenewal of her contract *** infringed her right of free speech secured by the First and Fourteenth Amendments of the United States Constitution. In an effort to show that its decision was justified, respondent School District introduced evidence of, among other things, a series of private encounters between petitioner and the school principal in which petitioner allegedly made "petty and unreasonable demands" in a manner variously described by the principal as "insulting," "hostile," "loud," and "arrogant." After a two-day bench trial, the District Court held that petitioner's termination had violated the First Amendment. Finding that petitioner had made "demands" on but two occasions and that those demands "were neither 'petty' nor 'unreasonable,' insomuch as all the complaints in question involved employment policies and practices at [the] school which [petitioner] conceived to be racially discriminatory in purpose or effect," the District Court concluded that "the primary reason for the school district's failure to renew [petitioner's] contract was her criticism of the policies and the practices of the school district, especially the school to which she was assigned to teach." *** Accordingly, the District Court held that the dismissal violated petitioner's First Amendment rights, as enunciated in Perry v. Sindermann, 408 U.S. 593 (1972), and Pickering v. Board of Education, 391 U.S. 563 (1968), and ordered her reinstatement.

The Court of Appeals for the Fifth Circuit reversed. Although it found the District Court's findings not clearly erroneous, the Court of Appeals concluded that because petitioner had privately expressed her complaints and opinions to the principal, her expression was not protected under the First Amendment. We are unable to agree that private expression of one's views is beyond constitutional protection, and therefore reverse the Court of Appeals' judgment and remand the case so that it may consider the contentions of the parties freed from this erroneous view of the First Amendment.

This Court's decisions in *Pickering, Perry,* and *Mt. Healthy* do not support the conclusion that a public employee forfeits his protection against governmental abridgment of freedom of speech if he decides to express his views privately rather than publicly. While those cases each arose in the context of a public employee's public expression, the rule to be derived from them is not dependent on that largely coincidental fact. Neither the Amendment itself nor our decisions indicate that this freedom is lost to the public employee who arranges to communicate privately with his employer rather than to spread his views before the public. We decline to adopt such a view of the First Amendment.

Since this case was tried before *Mt. Healthy* was decided, it is not surprising that respondents did not attempt to prove in the District Court that the decision not to rehire petitioner would have been made even absent consideration of her "demands." *** Accordingly, the judgment of the Court of Appeals is vacated insofar as it relates to petitioner, and the case is remanded for further proceedings consistent with this opinion.

MR. JUSTICE STEVENS, concurring. [Omitted]

CONNICK v. MYERS
461 U.S. 138 (1983)

JUSTICE WHITE delivered the opinion of the Court.

I

The respondent, Sheila Myers, was employed as an assistant District Attorney in New Orleans for five and a half years. She served at the pleasure of petitioner Harry Connick, the District Attorney for Orleans Parish. During this period Myers competently performed her responsibilities of trying criminal cases.

In the early part of October 1980, Myers was informed that she would be transferred to prosecute cases in a different section of the criminal court. Myers was strongly opposed to the proposed transfer[1] and expressed her view to several of her supervisors, including Connick. Despite her objections, on October 6 Myers was notified that she was being transferred. Myers again spoke with Dennis Waldron, one of the First Assistant District Attorneys, expressing her reluctance to accept the transfer. A number of other office matters were discussed and Myers later testified that, in response to Waldron's suggestion that her concerns were not shared by others in the office, she informed him that she would do some research on the matter.

That night Myers prepared a questionnaire soliciting the views of her fellow staff members concerning office transfer policy, office morale, the need for a grievance committee, the level of confidence in supervisors, and whether employees felt pressured to work in political campaigns. Early the following morning, Myers typed and copied the questionnaire. She also met with Connick who urged her to accept the transfer. She said she would "consider" it. Connick then left the office. Myers then distributed the questionnaire to 15 Assistant District Attorneys. Shortly after noon, Dennis Waldron learned that Myers was distributing the survey. He immediately phoned Connick and informed him that Myers was creating a "mini-insurrection" within the office. Connick returned to the office and told Myers that she was being terminated because of her refusal to accept the transfer. She was also told that her distribution of the questionnaire was considered an act of insubordination. Connick particularly objected to the question which inquired whether employees "had confidence in and would rely on the word" of various superiors in the office, and to a question concerning pressure to work in political campaigns which he felt would be damaging if discovered by the press.

---

1. Myers' opposition was at least partially attributable to her concern that a conflict of interest would have been created by the transfer because of her participation in a counseling program for convicted defendants released on probation in the section of the criminal court to which she was to be assigned.

Myers filed suit under 42 U.S.C. § 1983, contending that her employment was wrongfully terminated because she had exercised her constitutionally protected right of free speech. The District Court agreed, ordered Myers reinstated, and awarded back pay, damages, and attorney's fees. The District Court found that although Connick informed Myers that she was being fired because of her refusal to accept a transfer, the facts showed that the questionnaire was the real reason for her termination. The court then proceeded to hold that Myers' questionnaire involved matters of public concern and that the State had not "clearly demonstrated" that the survey "substantially interfered" with the operations of the District Attorney's office.

Connick appealed to the United States Court of Appeals for the Fifth Circuit, which affirmed on the basis of the District Court's opinion. ***

II

***

A

Connick contends at the outset that no balancing of interests is required in this case because Myers' questionnaire concerned only internal office matters and that such speech is not upon a matter of "public concern," as the term was used in *Pickering*. Although we do not agree that Myers' communication in this case was wholly without First Amendment protection, there is much force to Connick's submission. The repeated emphasis in *Pickering* on the right of a public employee "as a citizen, in commenting upon matters of public concern," was not accidental. This language reiterated in all of *Pickering*'s progeny, reflects both the historical evolvement of the rights of public employees, and the common-sense realization that government offices could not function if every employment decision became a constitutional matter. ***

Pickering, its antecedents, and its progeny lead us to conclude that if Myers' questionnaire cannot be fairly characterized as constituting speech on a matter of public concern, it is unnecessary for us to scrutinize the reasons for her discharge. When employee expression cannot be fairly considered as relating to any matter of political, social, or other concern to the community, government officials should enjoy wide latitude in managing their offices, without intrusive oversight by the judiciary in the name of the First Amendment. Perhaps the government employer's dismissal of the worker may not be fair, but ordinary dismissals from government service which violate no fixed tenure or applicable statute or regulation are not subject to judicial review even if the reasons for the dismissal are alleged to be mistaken or unreasonable. ***

We do not suggest, however, that Myers' speech, even if not touching upon a matter of public concern, is totally beyond the protection of the First Amendment. *** For example, an employee's false criticism of his employer on grounds not of public concern may be cause for his discharge but would be entitled to the same protection in a libel action accorded an identical statement made by a man on the street. We hold only that when a public employee speaks not as a citizen upon matters of public concern, but instead as an employee upon matters only of personal interest, absent the most unusual circumstances, a federal court is not the appropriate forum in which to review the wisdom of a personnel decision taken by a public agency allegedly in reaction to the employee's behavior. *** Our responsibility is to ensure that citizens are not deprived of fundamental rights by virtue of working for the government; this does not require a grant of immunity for employee grievances not afforded by the First Amendment to those who do not work for the State.

Whether an employee's speech addresses a matter of public concern must be determined by the content, form, and context of a given statement, as revealed by the whole record.[7] In this case, with but one exception, the questions posed by Myers to her co-workers do not fall under the rubric matters of "public concern." We view the questions pertaining to the confidence and trust that Myers' co-workers possess in various supervisors, the level of office morale, and the need for a grievance committee as mere extensions of Myers' dispute over her transfer to another section of the criminal court. Unlike the dissent, we do not believe these questions are of public import in evaluating the performance of the District Attorney as an elected official. Myers did not seek to inform the public that the District Attorney's Office was not discharging its governmental responsibilities in the investigation and prosecution of criminal cases. Nor did Myers seek to bring to light actual or potential wrongdoing or breach of public trust on the part of Connick and others. Indeed, the questionnaire, if released to the public, would convey no information at all other than the fact that a single employee is upset with the status quo. While discipline and morale in the workplace are related to an agency's efficient performance of its duties, the focus of Myers' questions is not to evaluate the performance of the office but rather to gather ammunition for another round of controversy with her superiors. These questions reflect one employee's dissatisfaction with a transfer and an attempt to turn that displeasure into a cause célèbre.[8] ***

One question in Myers' questionnaire, however, does touch upon a matter of public concern. Question 11 inquires if assistant district attorneys "ever feel pressured to work in political campaigns on behalf of office supported candidates."***

---

7. The inquiry into the protected status of speech is one of law, not fact. ***

8. This is not a case like *Givhan*, where an employee speaks out as a citizen on a matter of general concern, not tied to a personal employment dispute, but arranges to do so privately. Mrs. Givhan's right to protest racial discrimination—a matter inherently of public concern—is not forfeited by her choice of a private forum. Here, however, a questionnaire not otherwise of public concern does not attain that status because its subject matter could, in different circumstances, have been the topic of communication to the public that might be of general interest. The dissent's analysis of whether discussions of office morale and discipline could be matters of public concern is beside the point—it does not answer whether *this* questionnaire is such speech.

B-C

Because one of the questions in Myers' survey touched upon a matter of public concern and contributed to her discharge, we must determine whether Connick was justified in discharging Myers. Here the District Court erred in imposing an unduly onerous burden on the State to justify Myers' discharge. ***

We agree with the District Court that there is no demonstration here that the questionnaire impeded Myers' ability to perform her responsibilities. The District Court was also correct to recognize that "it is important to the efficient and successful operation of the District Attorney's office for Assistants to maintain close working relationships with their superiors." Connick's judgment, and apparently also that of his first assistant Dennis Waldron, who characterized Myers' actions as causing a "mini-insurrection," was that Myers' questionnaire was an act of insubordination which interfered with working relationships.[11] When close working relationships are essential to fulfilling public responsibilities, a wide degree of deference to the employer's judgment is appropriate. Furthermore, we do not see the necessity for an employer to allow events to unfold to the extent that the disruption of the office and the destruction of working relationships is manifest before taking action. We caution that a stronger showing may be necessary if the employee's speech more substantially involved matters of public concern. ***

Also relevant is the manner, time, and place in which the questionnaire was distributed. Although *** Myers did not violate announced office policy,[14] the fact that Myers, unlike Pickering, exercised her rights to speech at the office supports Connick's fears that the functioning of his office was endangered.

Finally, the context in which the dispute arose is also significant. This is not a case where an employee, out of purely academic interest, circulated a questionnaire so as to obtain useful research. Myers acknowledges that it is no coincidence that the questionnaire followed upon the heels of the transfer notice. When employee speech concerning office policy arises from an employment dispute concerning the very application of that policy to the speaker, additional weight must be given to the supervisor's view that the employee has threatened the authority of the employer to run the office. ***

---

11. Waldron testified that from what he had learned of the events on October 7, Myers "was trying to stir up other people not to accept the changes [transfers] that had been made on the memorandum and that were to be implemented." In his view, the questionnaire was a "final act of defiance" and that, as a result of Myers' action, "there were going to be some severe problems about the changes." Connick testified that he reached a similar conclusion after conducting his own investigation. "After I satisfied myself that not only wasn't she accepting the transfer, but that she was affirmatively opposing it and disrupting the routine of the office by this questionnaire. I called her in *** [and dismissed her]."

14. The violation of such a rule would strengthen Connick's position. See Mt. Healthy City Board of Ed. v. Doyle, 429 U.S., at 284.

III

Myers' questionnaire touched upon matters of public concern in only a most limited sense; her survey, in our view, is most accurately characterized as an employee grievance concerning internal office policy. The limited First Amendment interest involved here does not require that Connick tolerate action which he reasonably believed would disrupt the office, undermine his authority, and destroy close working relationships. Myers' discharge therefore did not offend the First Amendment. We reiterate, however, the caveat we expressed in *Pickering*, 391 U.S., at 569: "Because of the enormous variety of fact situations in which critical statements by public employees may be thought by their superiors *** to furnish grounds for dismissal, we do not deem it either appropriate or feasible to attempt to lay down a standard against which all such statements may be judged."

The judgment of the Court of Appeals is Reversed.

JUSTICE BRENNAN, with whom JUSTICE MARSHALL, JUSTICE BLACKMUN, and JUSTICE STEVENS join, dissenting.

Shelia Myers was discharged for circulating a questionnaire to her fellow Assistant District Attorneys seeking information about the effect of petitioner's personnel policies on employee morale and the overall work performance of the District Attorney's Office. *** Because the questionnaire addressed such matters and its distribution did not adversely affect the operations of the District Attorney's Office or interfere with Myers' working relationship with her fellow employees, I dissent. ***

I would hold that Myers' questionnaire addressed matters of public concern because it discussed subjects that could reasonably be expected to be of interest to persons seeking to develop informed opinions about the manner in which the Orleans Parish District Attorney, an elected official charged with managing a vital governmental agency, discharges his responsibilities. The questionnaire sought primarily to obtain information about the impact of the recent transfers on morale in the District Attorney's Office. *** Because I believe the First Amendment protects the right of public employees to discuss such matters so that the public may be better informed about how their elected officials fulfill their responsibilities, I would affirm the District Court's conclusion that the questionnaire related to matters of public importance and concern.

*** The proper means to ensure that the courts are not swamped with routine employee grievances mischaracterized as First Amendment cases is not to restrict artificially the concept of "public concern," but to require that adequate weight be given to the public's important interests in the efficient performance of governmental functions and in preserving employee discipline and harmony sufficient to achieve that end. ***

III

Although the Court finds most of Myers' questionnaire unrelated to matters of public interest, it does hold that one question—asking whether Assistants felt pressured to work in political campaigns on behalf of office-supported candidates—addressed a matter of public importance and concern. The court also recognizes that this determination of public interest must weigh heavily in the balancing of competing interests required by *Pickering*. Having gone that far, however, the Court misapplies the *Pickering* test and holds—against our previous authorities—that a public employer's mere apprehension that speech will be disruptive justifies suppression of that speech when all the objective evidence suggests that those fears are essentially unfounded. ***

The District Court weighed all of the relevant factors identified by our cases. It found that petitioner failed to establish that Myers violated either a duty of confidentiality or an office policy. Noting that most of the copies of the questionnaire were distributed during lunch, it rejected the contention that the distribution of the questionnaire impeded Myers' performance of her duties, and it concluded that "Connick has not shown *any* evidence to indicate that the plaintiff's work performance was adversely affected by her expression." *** The Court suggests the District Court failed to give sufficient weight to the disruptive potential of Question 10, which asked whether the Assistants had confidence in the word of five named supervisors. The District Court, however, explicitly recognized that this was petitioner's "most forceful argument"; but after hearing the testimony of four of the five supervisors named in the question, it found that the question had no adverse effect on Myers' relationship with her superiors. ***

In this regard, our decision in Tinker v. Des Moines Independent Community School District, 393 U.S. 503 (1969), is controlling. *** At issue was whether public high school students could constitutionally be prohibited from wearing black armbands in school to express their opposition to the Vietnam conflict. The District Court had ruled that such a ban "was reasonable because it was based upon [school officials'] fear of a disturbance from the wearing of armbands." We found that justification inadequate, because "in our system, undifferentiated fear or apprehension of disturbance is not enough to overcome the right to freedom of expression." We concluded:

> "In order for the State *** to justify prohibition of a particular expression of opinion, it must be able to show that its action was caused by something more than a mere desire to avoid the discomfort and unpleasantness that always accompany an unpopular viewpoint. *Certainly where there is no finding and no showing that engaging in the forbidden conduct would 'materially and substantially interfere with the requirements of appropriate discipline in the operation of the school,' the prohibition cannot be sustained.*" ([E]mphasis supplied).

Because the speech at issue addressed matters of public importance, a similar standard should be applied here. ***

IV

The Court's decision today inevitably will deter public employees from making critical statements about the manner in which government agencies are operated for fear that doing so will provoke their dismissal. As a result, the public will be deprived of valuable information with which to evaluate the performance of elected officials. Because protecting the dissemination of such information is an essential function of the First Amendment, I dissent.

NOTE

In light of the Court's decision in *Connick*, evidently the speech of a public employee must be speech about some issue of appropriate public concern (as distinct from some matter of personal job-related grievance) to qualify for First Amendment protection.[31] But suppose that it was speech of that kind, even as in *Pickering*: a signed letter published in the local newspaper critically commenting on public school bond ballot issues. Suppose next, however, that the school superintendent responsible for annual review of local teacher contracts had not seen the letter. Instead, the superintendent merely relied on a *mistaken* report about the letter, a report giving her the impression the letter reflected the teacher's mere irascibility over matters of alleged personal mistreatment in regard to unwelcome job-related duties—matters unprotected according to *Connick*. The superintendent subsequently sends the teacher a form notice of nonrenewal at the end of the school year. The teacher is disappointed by the notice, and telephones the superintendent. He thus learns of the superintendent's basis for sending the notice of nonrenewal (namely, her *impression* of what his letter was about). Anxiously, he tries to explain that her impression was mistaken, and asks her to reconsider. But the superintendent, already somewhat vexed by the call, declines to get further engaged. "It is," she says, "really too late" to discuss the matter further. And so she hangs up.[32] What, if anything,

---

31. For further refinement of this distinction, see the next principal case, *Rankin v. McPherson*.

32. The risk of such misjudgments is a common hazard for a large number of public employees (i.e. in any given year, large numbers of annual contract or "at will" employees may be let go or "nonrenewed" in the course of personnel decisions that may be the result of good faith but *mistaken* impressions of incompetence, or of good faith but *mistaken* impressions of work-related conduct). *Neither the Fifth nor the Fourteenth Amendment has been held to provide such persons any procedural due process safeguards as such* (e.g., notice, a statement of alleged shortcomings, an opportunity to be heard). See, e.g., Board of Regents v. Roth, 408 U.S. 564 (1972).

may the teacher now do?[33] Consider the following possibilities.

If, according to *Pickering*, it is plaintiff's burden *"to show that his conduct was constitutionally protected, and that this conduct was a 'substantial factor'—or, to put it in other words, that it was a 'motivating factor'"* in his adverse treatment, in order to establish a prima facie case in court under *Pickering*,[34] may it be the case here that the employee-plaintiff would lose on a motion for summary judgment once the superintendent submits an uncontested affidavit of how she came to her decision?[35] Or would this outcome seem to be inconsistent with the whole purpose of the *Pickering* doctrine?[36] The Supreme Court recently confronted this question. How do you think this case ought to come out?[37]

RANKIN v. MCPHERSON

483 U.S. 378 (1987)

JUSTICE MARSHALL delivered the opinion of the Court.

The issue in this case is whether a clerical employee in a county Constable's office was properly discharged for remarking, after hearing of an attempt on the life of the President, "If they go for him again, I hope they get him."

---

33. Note that on these facts, the notice of nonrenewal was clearly not motivated by any hostile reaction to any *protected* speech. The superintendent, not even knowing of the teacher's position on the school bond matter, assuredly was not acting from any hostility or animus or defensiveness for what the teacher said or did not say on that matter of public concern. (Indeed, the teacher's actual conduct played no role at all in the superintendent's decision.)

34. The quoted phrase (with the underlined emphasis added), describing the plaintiff's *Pickering* burden, is quoted from the Supreme Court's opinion in *Mt. Healthy*.

35. I.e. that it had nothing whatever to do with any actual public stance the teacher may or may not have taken on any prior school bond expenditures (for indeed the superintendent was wholly unaware the teacher had even taken any position on that matter).

36. What would one say that purpose is?

37. See Waters v. Churchill, 511 U.S. 661 (1994). The Supreme Court divided three ways: (a) three justices (Scalia, Kennedy, and Thomas) concluded that *Pickering* was inapplicable (in their view, once it becomes clear the decision was not retaliatory for any public position the employee may or may not have taken, the first amendment inquiry is at an end); (b) two justices (Stevens and Blackmun) concluded that *Pickering* was fully applicable (i.e. for them, once it becomes clear that but for the employee's exercise of his protected first amendment expression he would have suffered no adverse employment action, he is entitled to be held harmless from any adverse employment action derived from that conduct unless the employer can show that, without reference to that conduct, the adverse action would have been taken anyway); (c) four justices (O'Connor, Rehnquist, Souter, and Ginsburg) concluded that *Pickering* is inapplicable, *but only if* the decision-maker acted in good faith and "reasonably"—but whether the decision-maker acted "reasonably" is not merely a question of good faith. Rather, to assure the adequate protection of the employee's first amendment right of public expression on all subjects of appropriate public concern, *the decision-maker must have made reasonable inquiry before acting*—failure so to do will result in liability in keeping with *Pickering* itself.

I

On January 12, 1981, respondent Ardith McPherson was appointed a deputy in the office of the Constable of Harris County, Texas. The Constable is an elected official who functions as a law enforcement officer. At the time of her appointment, McPherson, a black woman, was 19 years old and had attended college for a year, studying secretarial science. Her appointment was conditional for a 90-day probationary period.

Although McPherson's title was "deputy constable," this was the case only because all employees of the Constable's office, regardless of job function, were deputy constables. *** She was not a commissioned peace officer, did not wear a uniform, and was not authorized to make arrests or permitted to carry a gun.[2] McPherson's duties were purely clerical. Her work station was a desk at which there was no telephone, in a room to which the public did not have ready access. Her job was to type data from court papers into a computer that maintained an automated record of the status of civil process in the county. Her training consisted of two days of instruction in the operation of her computer terminal.

On March 30, 1981, McPherson and some fellow employees heard on an office radio that there had been an attempt to assassinate the President of the United States. Upon hearing that report, McPherson engaged a co-worker, Lawrence Jackson, who was apparently her boyfriend, in a brief conversation, which according to McPherson's uncontroverted testimony went as follows:

> "Q: What did you say?
>
> "A: I said I felt that that would happen sooner or later.
>
> "Q: Okay. And what did Lawrence say?
>
> "A: Lawrence said, yeah, agreeing with me.
>
> "Q: Okay. Now when you—after Lawrence spoke, then what was your next comment?
>
> "A: Well, we were talking—it's a wonder why they did that. I felt like it would be a black person that did that, because I feel like most of my kind is on welfare and CETA, and they use medicaid, and at the time, I was thinking that's what it was.
>
> "*** But then after I said that, and then Lawrence said, yeah, he's cutting back medicaid and food stamps. And I said, yeah, welfare and CETA. I said, shoot, if they go for him again, I hope they get him."

---

2. In order to serve as a commissioned peace officer, as the Court of Appeals noted, a deputy would have to undergo a background check, a psychological examination, and over 300 hours of training in law enforcement. Constable Rankin testified that while his office had on occasion been asked to guard various dignitaries visiting Houston, a deputy who was not a commissioned peace officer would never be assigned to such duty. Nor would such a deputy even be assigned to serve process.

McPherson's last remark was overheard by another deputy constable, who, unbeknownst to McPherson was in the room at the time. The remark was reported to Constable Rankin, who summoned McPherson. McPherson readily admitted that she had made the statement, but testified that she told Rankin, upon being asked if she made the statement, "Yes, but I didn't mean anything by it." After their discussion, Rankin fired McPherson.

II

It is clearly established that a State may not discharge an employee on a basis that infringes that employee's constitutionally protected interest in freedom of speech. *** The determination whether a public employer has properly discharged an employee for engaging in speech requires "a balance between the interests of the [employee], as a citizen, in commenting upon matters of public concern and the interest of the State, as an employer, in promoting the efficiency of the public services it performs through its employees." Pickering v. Board of Education, 391 U.S. 563, 568 (1968); Connick v. Myers, 461 U.S. 138, 140 (1983). This balancing is necessary in order to accommodate the dual role of the public employer as a provider of public services and as a government entity operating under the constraints of the First Amendment. On the one hand, public employers are *employers*, concerned with the efficient function of their operations; review of every personnel decision made by a public employer could in the long run, hamper the performance of public functions. On the other hand, "the threat of dismissal from public employment is *** a potent means of inhibiting speech." *Pickering*, 391 U.S., at 574. Vigilance is necessary to ensure that public employers do not use authority over employees to silence discourse, not because it hampers public functions but simply because superiors disagree with the content of employees' speech.

The threshold question in applying this balancing test is whether McPherson's speech may be "fairly characterized as constituting speech on a matter of public concern." *Connick*, 461 U.S., at 146.[7] ***

Considering the statement in context, as *Connick* requires, discloses that it plainly dealt with a matter of public concern. The statement was made in the course of a conversation addressing the policies of the President's administration.[10] It came

---

7. Even where a public employee's speech does not touch upon a matter of public concern, that speech is not "totally beyond the protection of the First Amendment," *Connick v. Myers*, 461 U.S., at 147, but "absent the most unusual circumstances a federal court is not the appropriate forum in which to review the wisdom of a personnel decision taken by a public agency allegedly in reaction to the employee's behavior." *Ibid.*

10. McPherson actually made the statement at issue not once, but twice, and only in the first instance did she make the statement in the context of a discussion of the President's policies. McPherson repeated the statement to Constable Rankin at his request. We do not consider the second statement independently of the first, however. Having been required by the Constable to repeat her statement, McPherson might well have been deemed insubordinate had she refused. A public employer may not divorce a statement made by an employee from its context by requiring the employee to repeat

on the heels of a news bulletin regarding what is certainly a matter of heightened public attention: an attempt on the life of the President.[11] ***

Because McPherson's statement addressed a matter of public concern, *Pickering* next requires that we balance McPherson's interest in making her statement against "the interest of the State, as an employer, in promoting the efficiency of the public services it performs through its employees." 391 U.S., at 568.[13] The State bears a burden of justifying the discharge on legitimate grounds. *Connick*, 461 U.S., at 150.

We have previously recognized as pertinent considerations whether the statement impairs discipline by superiors or harmony among co-workers, has a detrimental impact on close working relationships for which personal loyalty and confidence are necessary, or impedes the performance of the speaker's duties or interferes with the regular operation of the enterprise. *Pickering*, 391 U.S., at 570-573.

The Constable was evidently not afraid that McPherson had disturbed or interrupted other employees—he did not inquire to whom respondent had made the remark and testified that he "was not concerned who she had made it to," ***. In fact, Constable Rankin testified that the possibility of interference with the functions of the Constable's office had *not* been a consideration in his discharge of respondent and that he did not even inquire whether the remark had disrupted the work of the office.[14]

Nor was there any danger that McPherson had discredited the office by making her statement public. There is no suggestion that any member of the general public was present or heard McPherson's statement. Nor is there any evidence that employees other than Jackson who worked in the room even heard the remark. ***

While the facts underlying Rankin's discharge of McPherson are, despite extensive proceedings in the District Court, still somewhat unclear, it is undisputed that he fired McPherson based on the *content* of her speech. Evidently because McPherson had made the statement, and because the Constable believed that she

---

the statement, and use that statement standing alone as the basis for discharge. Such a tactic could in some cases merely give the employee the choice of being fired for failing to follow orders or for making a statement which, out of context may not warrant the same level of First Amendment protection it merited when originally made.

11. The private nature of the statement does not, contrary to the suggestion of the United States, Brief for United States as *Amicus Curiae* 18, vitiate the status of the statement as addressing a matter of public concern. See Givhan v. Western Line Consolidated School Dist., 439 U.S. 410, 414-416 (1979).

13. We agree with Justice Powell that a purely private statement on a matter of public concern will rarely, if ever, justify discharge of a public employee. *** To the extent petitioner's claim that McPherson's speech rendered her an unsuitable employee for a law enforcement agency implicates a serious state interest and necessitates the application of the balancing element of the *Pickering* analysis, we proceed to that task.

14. He testified: "I did not base my action on whether the work was interrupted or not. I based my action on a statement that was made to me direct."

"meant it," he decided that she was not a suitable employee to have in a law enforcement agency. But in weighing the State's interest in discharging an employee based on any claim that the content of a statement made by the employee somehow undermines the mission of the public employer, some attention must be paid to the responsibilities of the employee within the agency. The burden of caution employees bear with respect to the words they speak will vary with the extent of authority and public accountability the employee's role entails. Where, as here, an employee serves no confidential, policymaking, or public contact role, the danger to the agency's successful functioning from that employee's private speech is minimal. We cannot believe that every employee in Constable Rankin's office, whether computer operator, electrician, or file clerk, is equally required, on pain of discharge, to avoid any statement susceptible of being interpreted by the Constable as an indication that the employee may be unworthy of employment in his law enforcement agency. At some point, such concerns are so removed from the effective functioning of the public employer that they cannot prevail over the free speech rights of the public employee.[18]

This is such a case. McPherson's employment-related interaction with the Constable was apparently negligible. Her duties were purely clerical and were limited solely to the civil process function of the Constable's office. There is no indication that she would ever be in a position to further—or indeed to have any involvement with —the minimal law enforcement activity engaged in by the Constable's office. Given the function of the agency, McPherson's position in the office, and the nature of her statement, we are not persuaded that Rankin's interest in discharging her outweighed her rights under the First Amendment.

Because we agree with the Court of Appeals that McPherson's discharge was improper, the judgment of the Court of Appeals is

Affirmed.

JUSTICE POWELL, concurring.

***

There is no dispute that McPherson's comment was made during a private conversation with a co-worker who happened also to be her boyfriend. She had no intention or expectation that it would be overheard or acted on by others. Given this, I think it is unnecessary to engage in the extensive analysis normally required by Connick v. Myers, 461 U.S. 138 (1983), and Pickering v. Board of Education, 391 U.S. 563 (1968). If a statement is on a matter of public concern, as it was here, it will

18. This is not to say that clerical employees are insulated from discharge where their speech, taking the acknowledged factors into account, truly injures the public interest in the effective functioning of the public employer. Compare McMullen v. Carson, 754 F.2d 936 (CA11 1985) (clerical employee in sheriff's office properly discharged for stating on television news that he was an employee for the sheriff's office and a recruiter for the Ku Klux Klan).

be an unusual case where the employer's legitimate interests will be so great as to justify punishing an employee for this type of private speech that routinely takes place at all levels in the workplace. The risk that a single, offhand comment directed to only one other worker will lower morale, disrupt the work force, or otherwise undermine the mission of the office borders on the fanciful. To the extent that the full constitutional analysis of the competing interests is required, I generally agree with the Court's opinion. ***

JUSTICE SCALIA, with whom THE CHIEF JUSTICE, JUSTICE WHITE, and JUSTICE O'CONNOR join, dissenting.

I agree with the proposition, felicitously put by Constable Rankin's counsel, that no law enforcement agency is required by the First Amendment to permit one of its employees to "ride with the cops and cheer for the robbers." The issue in this case is whether Constable Rankin, a law enforcement official, is prohibited by the First Amendment from preventing his employees from saying of the attempted assassination of President Reagan—on the job and within hearing of other employees—"If they go for him again, I hope they get him." The Court, applying the two-prong analysis of Connick v. Myers, 461 U.S. 138 (1983), holds that McPherson's statement was protected by the First Amendment because (1) it "addressed a matter of public concern," and (2) McPherson's interest in making the statement outweighs Rankin's interest in suppressing it. In so doing, the Court significantly and irrationally expands the definition of "public concern"; it also carves out a new and very large class of employees —i.e., those in "nonpolicymaking" positions—who, if today's decision is to be believed, can never be disciplined for statements that fall within the Court's expanded definition. Because I believe the Court's conclusions rest upon a distortion of both the record and the Court's prior decisions, I dissent.

I

That McPherson's statement does not constitute speech on a matter of "public concern" is demonstrated by comparing it with statements that have been found to fit that description in prior decisions involving public employees. McPherson's statement is a far cry from the question by the assistant district attorney in *Connick* whether her co-workers "ever [felt] pressured to work in political campaigns"; from the letter written by the public school teacher in *Pickering* criticizing the board of education's proposals for financing school construction; from the legislative testimony of a state college teacher in Perry v. Sindermann, 408 U.S. 593, 595 (1972), advocating that a particular college be elevated to 4-year status; from the memorandum given by a teacher to a radio station in Mt. Healthy City Board of Ed. v. Doyle, 429 U.S. 274, 282 (1977), dealing with teacher dress and appearance; and from the complaints about school board policies and practices at issue in Givhan v. Western Line Consolidated School Dist., 439 U.S. 410, 413 (1979). ***

II

Even if I agreed that McPherson's statement was speech on a matter of "public concern," I would still find it unprotected. It is important to be clear on what the issue is in this part of the case. It is not, as the Court suggests, whether "Rankin's interest *in discharging* [McPherson] outweighed her rights under the First Amendment." *** (emphasis added). Rather, it is whether his interest *in preventing the expression of such statements in his agency* outweighed her First Amendment interest in making the statement. We are not deliberating, in other words, (or at least should not be) about whether the sanction of dismissal was, as the concurrence puts it, "an *** intemperat[e] employment decision." It may well have been—and personally I think it was. But we are not sitting as a panel to develop sound principles of proportionality for adverse actions in the state civil service. We are asked to determine whether, given the interests of this law enforcement office, McPherson had a *right* to say what she did—so that she could not only not be fired for it, but could not be formally reprimanded for it, or even prevented from repeating it endlessly into the future. It boggles the mind to think that she has such a right. ***

Because the statement at issue here did not address a matter of public concern, and because, even if it did, a law enforcement agency has adequate reason not to permit such expression, I would reverse the judgment of the court below.

D. A Reprise on the Problem: Applying the "Pickering-Connick" Test

It is surely clear from *Pickering, et al.* that the first amendment does apply even though it is "merely" one's government-linked status that is put at risk by offending a rule or agreement disallowing one to speak. At the same time, it is also clear from the same cases that the analysis will not run according to a simple model of "unconstitutional condition," insofar as it appears to be the case that some restrictions may be sustained though the state could take no action at all if the same things had all been said by someone else, i.e. someone not linked with the government in the manner as the person against whom some adverse action has been taken or proposed. Evidently, some sort of context-specific analysis not wholly dissimilar from Hand's sliding scale, "gravity-of-the evil" formulation is being applied here, adjusted and fine-tuned by elements taken from *New York Times v. Sullivan*, as well. The exact manner in which that calculus has currently worked out is by no means self-evident, however, even as the *Connick* and *Rankin* decisions attest. (Note also all the disclaiming dicta, even in *Pickering* itself.[38])

---

38. E.g., that had Pickering been employed *by the board itself*, or had there been evidence that his published letter actually affected any bond issue adversely (*and* had the margin of falsehood been more substantial than it was), *or* had any of the falsehoods been known by Pickering to be false, *or* were there some evidence that his letter produced friction within the school were he worked, *or* had there been a limited school rule requiring submission of any letter bearing on the operation of the school to

The sheer frequency with which public employment "free speech" claims arise with respect to whether what an employee said about one thing or another is or is not protected by the first amendment in some manner, exerts unusual pressure on the Supreme Court to announce a stylized (i.e. somewhat mechanical) way of going about these questions, principally for the guidance of lower courts. One good way of seeing whether one thinks one has grasped these rather stylized guidelines may be to see whether one can apply them with a certain firm sense of confidence, say, in the following sort of case. So, let's see how you think it ought to proceed.

> An untenured assistant professor of psychiatry at University of North Carolina Medical School made an appointment with the dean. At that time, in the dean's office, he complained to the dean that a senior professor commonly used his assigned parking place in the faculty lot, and he requested the dean to intervene without mentioning how the matter came to the dean's attention. He also complained to the dean that the same senior professor was, in his view, overprescribing barbiturates for his clinical patients at the UNC Medical Center and was having sex in his clinic office with two or three of the patients. The dean assured him he would look into both matters promptly. In the meantime, for the best interests of all concerned, he directed the assistant professor not to speak to anyone else.
>
> Three weeks later, the senior departmental faculty met to review junior faculty members for tenure. On a closely divided vote, tenure was not recommended for the assistant professor to whom we have just referred. The dean voted with the majority; so did the senior professor to whom the dean had spoken about the parking matter (in the course of which he identified the assistant professor who brought the matter to his attention). The dean had said less to the senior professor on the handling of clinical patients because, in his view, the assistant professor had simply not been in a suitable position to know and, in the dean's view, was almost surely mistaken in his perception of the other professor's professional practices. He did, however, ask whether the other man's clinical practice was free of any problems; he assumed that his question was pointed enough such that were there something improper going on, doubtless the other man would get the point—that the dean had evidently

---

be processed internally for the limited purpose of bringing possible factual error to Pickering's attention before he went public (*and* had he failed to go through that process), *then* his dismissal might have been sustained, despite all the Court says about *Sullivan*, etc. And does not *Connick* appear clearly to imply that if one makes complaint to a superior as a public employee (and does not go to the newspapers with the complaint), still [s]he may be fired though the complaint is well taken and quite courteously expressed, if it is "merely" a workplace grievance not deemed by the Court to raise any issue of general public policy? Note also the scope of the political activity ban sustained in the *Letter Carriers* case. On balance, how strongly in fact does the first amendment seem to operate in these several cases? See Steven H. Shiffrin, The First Amendment, Democracy, and Romance 72-80, 106-109 (1990).

heard something—and would quickly desist from anything he may have been doing wrong. As to the parking matter, incidentally, the assistant professor was mistaken; his parking place had been frequently usurped by another staff member, but it was someone other than the senior professor whom he had identified to the dean.

The adverse tenure recommendation was to be forwarded to the Board of Trustees for final action. Under the university's rules, it was not final until the trustees voted, although rarely had the Board reached an outcome at odds with the recommendation they received. In the meantime, the assistant professor, frustrated that the dean had not contacted him again to say what steps had been taken on the matters he had brought to the dean's attention, and discouraged by the adverse vote on his tenure (which, if it were not overturned by the trustees, would mean that he would not be continued in his position beyond the end of the year), felt he could wait no longer— and spoke to a friend on the staff of the *Daily Tarheel* about the likelihood of overprescription of barbiturates at the clinic and possible sexual misconduct with clinic patients as well.

The day following publication of the story in the *Daily Tarheel*, the trustees met in regular session and, among other things, voted unanimously to deny the assistant professor tenure. The same day, the dean so advised the assistant professor and also asked him directly whether he was the source of the *Tarheel* story. When the assistant professor replied that, yes, he was the source, the dean suspended him for the balance of the term altogether. (Coupled with the denial of tenure, this meant that the assistant professor was finished, at once.)

Supposing the assistant professor were at once to bring suit on grounds that he had been punished for his good faith efforts to speak without fear of retribution, consistent with the first amendment, what likely result and why? More particularly, according to the *Pickering-Givhan-Mt. Healthy-Connick* and *Rankin* profile of standards and burdens of proof and procedures applicable to the case, how will it proceed, step by step, and what relief, if any, is the plaintiff entitled to receive?

After you have run through the preceding problem, consider the following reprise as well. A principal case, featured in the introductory materials, was the famous *Scopes* case. It differed from the preceding problem in that Scopes wished to teach materials other than those the state itself specifically prescribed solely for use in its own schools and its own classrooms—but the state law did not restrict what Scopes might say elsewhere (the original doctrine of "unconstitutional conditions" itself thus does not appear to be involved at all). That is, it did not restrict Scopes from writing critical letters publicly complaining of the curricular restriction, criticizing the law, etc., as stridently as much as he might feel inclined. It did not forbid him to go public with anything he might find wrong with the schools or the manner in which they were operated. On what basis, on the strength of the materials you have thus far covered, could a modern Scopes presume to invoke the free speech clause to depart from the school board's (or state law) prescribed materials he is solely to use in class, and defend against being dismissed for insubordination?[39] (Is there any foundation for what is elsewhere sometimes called "academic freedom,"[40] or would it make any difference whether the claim arises at the state university level rather than the state public school level? If you think so, why, and on what grounds?)[41]

---

39. The difficulty and distinction is evident in considering the original logic of the doctrine of unconstitutional conditions itself. Justice Sutherland's quotation *supra* from the *Frost* case spoke of the government requiring "a surrender of a right in exchange for a valuable privilege the state threatens otherwise to withhold." So, the doctrine begins with the observation that one has a right of some sort (e.g., to write letters to the editor of the local newspaper, criticizing the local school board, as in *Pickering*, or the local police department, as in *McAuliffe*) which right one must put aside if, and as long as, one accepts the valuable privilege the state threatens otherwise to withhold. In cases such as *Scopes*, however, the logic does not work, does it? Scopes never had a first amendment "right" to commandeer a public school classroom—access to the classroom is itself part of the "valuable privilege" *he gets*, rather than being a part of some pre-existing right he is made to give up. Moreover, in "exchange" for conducting himself in the classroom as the state-employer dictates, neither is Scopes asked or required to abstain from any pre-existing right he holds (except in the sense Holmes mentioned in passing in *McAuliffe*, i.e. while performing his duties at the appointed time in the classroom, to that extent he does lay aside such "constitutional right" as he might otherwise have used just to loaf). In the *Letter Carriers* case, the postal employees are made to forego off-the-job political activities they were otherwise constitutionally entitled to engage in, so it is logical to talk about the Civil Service restrictions as challengeable under the doctrine of unconstitutional conditions. But what if the restrictions were (merely) that, as lettermen, delivering mail, the postal employee is not to seize the advantage of using that role to ring the doorbell and engage the homeowner in his solicitation of some candidate or political cause he holds dear? Is there any problem with a local rule forbidding one employed as a jailer inside the city jail to solicit for political causes among the inmates—when others are not permitted (i.e. "have a right") to enter the cellblocks and solicit for their causes?

40. See, e.g., Keyishian v. Board of Regents, 385 U.S. 589, 603 (1967) ("[A]cademic freedom *** is *** a special concern of the First Amendment, which does not tolerate laws that cast a pall of orthodoxy over the classroom. *** The classroom is peculiarly the marketplace of ideas. The Nation's future depends upon leaders trained through wide exposure to that robust exchange of ideas which discovers truth out of a multitude of tongues, [rather] than through any kind of authoritative selection."); Sweezy v. New Hampshire, 354 U.S. 234, 262, 263 (1957) (Frankfurter, J., concurring, quoting) ("A university ceases to be true to its own nature if it becomes the tool of Church or State or any sectional interest. A university is characterized by the spirit of free inquiry, its ideal being the ideal of Socrates—to follow the argument where it leads ***."). Compare Rust v. Sullivan, p. 300, *supra*.

41. As a matter of historical fact, the Tennessee statute involved in *Scopes* applied equally to *all* state supported *universities* and colleges as well. For a recent review of academic freedom in the Supreme Court, see William Van Alstyne, The First Amendment and the Usages of Academic Freedom in the Supreme Court of the United States: An Unhurried Historical Review, 53 Law & Contemp.Probs. 78 (1990). See also David Rabban, A Functional Analysis of "Individual" and "Institutional" Academic Freedom Under the First Amendment, in Freedom and Tenure in the Academy 227 (Van Alstyne ed., 1993); Robert O'Neil, Free Speech in the College Community (1997); Louis Menand (ed.)., The Future of Academic Freedom (1966).

Consider the following news item from the *New York Times*.

Book Ban in California School Strikes Down Familiar Target[42]

BORON, Calif., Aug. 30— If a group of local parents had let her speak to them before "The Catcher in the Rye" was banned from her high school, Shelley Keller-Gage says she would have told them she believes it is a highly moral book that deals with the kinds of difficulties their own children are facing.

But Mrs. Keller-Gage, an English teacher, was asked not to speak, and a small group of people led by a woman who says she has not read —and never would read—such a book, persuaded the school board to ban it this month from the Boron High School supplementary reading list.

The school board's 4-to-1 vote has aroused this small sunbaked town of 4,000 at the edge of the Mojave Desert. *** Ed Roberts, a school board member who works for a transportation company, carries a copy in the front seat of his pickup truck. He has shown one passage to people so often that the book frequently falls open to that section, whose profanity he finds objectionable.

Jim Sommers, the head of the school board, who operates Jim's Mobil Service, says he is halfway through the book, though he is having a hard time keeping up his interest. ***

Vickie Swindler, the parent who raised the first objections when her 14-year-old daughter, Brook, showed her the book, has been calling her friends, reading passages from it, mostly the one on page 32 with three goddamns in it.

When she found out about the language in it, Mrs. Swindler said, "I called the school, and I said, 'How the hell did this teacher get this book?'"

"Yes, there's harshness and profanity in society," said F.O. Roe, a school board member who runs a furniture and flower shop, responding to the argument that the book's contents are no longer as shocking as they once were. "But we don't have to accept them, just the same as we don't have to accept the narcotics that are in the streets and the murders that are happening all over the country. We live in harmony in this little town."

---

42. N.Y. Times, Sept. 4, 1989, § 1, p. 1, col. 5. In addition to the following principal case, see Parducci v. Rutland, 316 F. Supp. 352 (M.D.Ala. 1970) (high school English teacher reinstated on first amendment grounds by federal court following dismissal for refusal of principal's demand to discontinue reading assignment to Kurt Vonnegut's Slaughterhouse Five); Hazelwood School Dist. v. Kuhlmeier, 484 U.S. 260 (1988) (6-3, high school principal's censorship of school financed student newspaper sustained); Bethel School Dist. No. 403 v. Fraser, 478 U.S. 675 (1986) (suspension of student using sexual reference in student assembly address supporting another student for elective office, sustained). *Cf.* Papish v. Board of Curators of Univ. of Missouri, 410 U.S. 667 (1973) (graduate student reinstated on first amendment grounds following expulsion for on campus distribution of student newspaper not financially subsidized by the state university, containing sexually explicit political cartoon and "M*** F***" word).

Mrs. Keller-Gage said the Salinger book might carry a particular message for people like these.

"These people are being just like Holden, the ones who are trying to censor the book," she said. "They are trying to be catchers in the rye." The book derives its title from a passage in which Holden Caulfield describes his vision of himself as a protector of innocence. ***

As the school year began this week, Mrs. Keller-Gage's three dozen copies of "The Catcher in the Rye" were on a top shelf of her classroom closet, inside a tightly taped cardboard box.

In their place, she said, she would be assigning "Farenheit 451," by Ray Bradbury, a novel about book burning.

If Ms. Keller-Gage untaped the cardboard box, returned "The Catcher in the Rye," to her high school English class supplementary list, and then promptly was dismissed (for insubordination) for having done so, under the circumstances, what result in court if the dismissal were challenged on first amendment ground? In the following case, what difference would there be, if any, had the school board forbidden acquisition (rather than directed removal) of the named books?

BOARD OF EDUCATION v. PICO

457 U.S. 853 (1982)

JUSTICE BRENNAN announced the judgment of the Court and delivered an opinion, in which JUSTICE MARSHALL and JUSTICE STEVENS joined, and in which JUSTICE BLACKMUN joined except for Part II-A-(1).

The principal question presented is whether the First Amendment imposes limitations upon the exercise by a local school board of its discretion to remove library books from high school and junior high school libraries.

I

Petitioners are the Board of Education of the Island Trees Union Free School District No. 26, in New York, and Richard Ahrens, Frank Martin, Christina Fasulo, Patrick Hughes, Richard Melchers, Richard Michaels, and Louis Nessim. When this suit was brought, Ahrens was the President of the Board, Martin was the Vice President, and the remaining petitioners were Board members. *** Respondents are Steven Pico, Jacqueline Gold, Glenn Yarris, Russell Rieger, and Paul Sochinski. *** Pico, Gold, Yarris, and Rieger were students at the High School, and Sochinski was a student at the Junior High School.

In September 1975, petitioners Ahrens, Martin, and Hughes attended a conference sponsored by Parents of New York United (PONYU), a politically conservative organization of parents concerned about education legislation in the State of

New York. At the conference these petitioners obtained lists of books described by Ahrens as "objectionable," *** and by Martin as "improper fare for school students," ***. It was later determined that the High School library contained nine of the listed books, and that another listed book was in the Junior High School library.[3] In February 1976, at a meeting with the Superintendent of Schools and the Principals of the High School and Junior High School, the Board gave an "unofficial direction" that the listed books be removed from the library shelves and delivered to the Board's offices, so that Board members could read them. When this directive was carried out, it became publicized, and the Board issued a press release justifying its action. It characterized the removed books as "anti-American, anti-Christian, anti-Sem[i]tic, and just plain filthy," and concluded that "[i]t is our duty, our moral obligation, to protect the children in our schools from this moral danger as surely as from physical and medical dangers." ***

A short time later, the Board appointed a "Book Review Committee," consisting of four Island Trees parents and four members of the Island Trees schools staff, to read the listed books and to recommend to the Board whether the books should be retained, taking into account the books' "educational suitability," "good taste," "relevance," and "appropriateness to age and grade level." In July, the Committee made its final report to the Board, recommending that five of the listed books be retained and that two others be removed from the school libraries. As for the remaining four books, the Committee could not agree on two, took no position on one, and recommended that the last book be made available to students only with parental approval. The Board substantially rejected the Committee's report later that month, deciding that only one book should be returned to the High School library without restriction[10] that another should be made available subject to parental approval,[11] but that the remaining nine books should "be removed from elementary and secondary libraries and [from] use in the curriculum." ***[12] The Board gave no reasons for rejecting the recommendations of the Committee that it had appointed.

---

3. The nine books in the High School library were: Slaughter House Five, by Kurt Vonnegut, Jr.; The Naked Ape, by Desmond Morris; Down These Mean Streets, by Piri Thomas; Best Short Stories of Negro Writers, edited by Langston Hughes; Go Ask Alice, of anonymous authorship; Laughing Boy, by Oliver LaFarge; Black Boy, by Richard Wright; A Hero Ain't Nothin' But A Sandwich, by Alice Childress; and Soul On Ice, by Eldridge Cleaver. The book in the Junior High School library was A Reader for Writers, edited by Jerome Archer. Still another listed book, The Fixer, by Bernard Malamud, was found to be included in the curriculum of a 12th grade literature course. ***

10. Laughing Boy. 474 F.Supp., at 391, n.12.

11. Black Boy. 474 F.Supp., at 391, n.13.

12. As a result, the nine removed books could not be assigned or suggested to students in connection with school work. However, teachers were not instructed to refrain from discussing the removed books or the ideas and positions expressed in them.

Respondents reacted to the Board's decision by bringing the present action under 42 U.S.C. § 1983 in the United States District Court for the Eastern District of New York. They alleged that petitioners had

> "ordered the removal of the books from school libraries and proscribed their use in the curriculum because particular passages in the books offended their social, political and moral tastes and not because the books, taken as a whole, were lacking in educational value."

Respondents claimed that the Board's actions denied them their rights under the First Amendment. They asked the court for a declaration that the Board's actions were unconstitutional, and for preliminary and permanent injunctive relief ordering the Board to return the nine books to the school libraries and to refrain from interfering with the use of those books in the schools' curricula.

The District Court granted summary judgment in favor of petitioners. In the court's view, "the parties substantially agree[d] about the motivation behind the board's actions,"—namely, that

> "the board acted not on religious principles but on its conservative educational philosophy, and on its belief that the nine books removed from the school library and curriculum were irrelevant, vulgar, immoral, and in bad taste, making them educationally unsuitable for the district's junior and senior high school students."

With this factual premise as its background, the court rejected respondents' contention that their First Amendment rights had been infringed by the Board's actions. *** A three-judge panel of the United States Court of Appeals for the Second Circuit reversed the judgment of the District Court, and remanded the action for a trial on respondents' allegations. ***

II A (1)

***

Of course, courts should not "intervene in the resolution of conflicts which arise in the daily operation of school systems" unless "basic constitutional values" are "directly and sharply implicate[d]" in those conflicts. Epperson v. Arkansas, 393 U.S., at 104. But we think that the First Amendment rights of students may be directly and sharply implicated by the removal of books from the shelves of a school library. *** [W]e have recognized that "the State may not, consistently with the spirit of the First Amendment, contract the spectrum of available knowledge." Griswold v. Connecticut, 381 U.S. 479, 482 (1965). In keeping with this principle, we have held that in a variety of contexts "the Constitution protects the right to receive information and ideas." Stanley v. Georgia, 394 U.S. 557, 564 (1969); see Kleindienst v. Mandel, 408 U.S. 753, 762-763 (1972) (citing cases). This right is an inherent corollary of the rights of free speech and press that are explicitly guaranteed by the Constitution, in two senses. First, the right to receive ideas follows ineluctably from the *sender*'s First Amendment right to send them: "The right of freedom of speech and press *** embraces the right to distribute literature, and necessarily protects the right to receive it." Martin v. Struthers, 319 U.S. 141, 143 (1943) (citation omitted). ***

More importantly, the right to receive ideas is a necessary predicate to the*recipient*'s meaningful exercise of his own rights of speech, press, and political freedom. Madison admonished us:

> "A popular Government, without popular information, or the means of acquiring it, is but a Prologue to a Farce or a Tragedy; or, perhaps both. Knowledge will forever govern ignorance: And a people who mean to be their own Governors, must arm themselves with the power which knowledge gives." 9 Writings of James Madison 103 (G. Hunt ed. 1910).

*** Petitioners emphasize the inculcative function of secondary education, and argue that they must be allowed *unfettered* discretion to "transmit community values" through the Island Trees schools. But that sweeping claim overlooks the unique role of the school library. It appears from the record that use of the Island Trees school libraries is completely voluntary on the part of students. Their selection of books from these libraries is entirely a matter of free choice; the libraries afford them an opportunity at self-education and individual enrichment that is wholly optional. Petitioner might well defend their claim of absolute discretion in matters of *curriculum* by reliance upon their duty to inculcate community values. But we think that petitioners' reliance upon that duty is misplaced where, as here, they attempt to extend their claim of absolute discretion beyond the compulsory environment of the classroom, into the school library and the regime of voluntary inquiry that there holds sway.

(2)

In rejecting petitioners' claim of absolute discretion to remove books from their school libraries, we do not deny that local school boards have a substantial legitimate role to play in the determination of school library content. We thus must turn to the question of the extent to which the First Amendment places limitations upon the discretion of petitioners to remove books from their libraries. In this inquiry we enjoy the guidance of several precedents. *West Virginia Board of Education v. Barnette* stated:

> "If there is any fixed star in our constitutional constellation, it is that no official, high or petty, can prescribe what shall be orthodox in politics, nationalism, religion, or other matters of opinion ***. If there are any circumstances which permit an exception, they do not now occur to us."

This doctrine has been reaffirmed in later cases involving education. For example, *Keyishian v. Board of Regents*, at 603, noted that "the First Amendment *** does not tolerate laws that cast a pall of orthodoxy over the classroom;" see also Epperson v.

Arkansas, 393 U.S., at 104-105. And Mt. Healthy City Board of Ed. v. Doyle, 429 U.S. 274 (1977), recognized First Amendment limitations upon the discretion of a local school board to refuse to rehire a nontenured teacher. ***

With respect to the present case, the message of these precedents is clear. Petitioners rightly possess significant discretion to determine the content of their school libraries. But that discretion may not be exercised in a narrowly partisan or political manner. If a Democratic school board, motivated by party affiliation, ordered the removal of all books written by or in favor of Republicans, few would doubt that the order violated the constitutional rights of the students denied access to those books. The same conclusion would surely apply if an all-white school board, motivated by racial animus, decided to remove all books authored by blacks or advocating racial equality and integration. Our Constitution does not permit the official suppression of *ideas*. Thus whether petitioners' removal of books from their school libraries denied respondents their First Amendment rights depends upon the motivation behind petitioners actions. If petitioners *intended* by their removal decision to deny respondents access to ideas with which petitioners disagreed, and if this intent was the decisive factor in petitioners' decision,[22] then petitioners have exercised their discretion in violation of the Constitution. To permit such intentions to control official actions would be to encourage the precise sort of officially prescribed orthodoxy unequivocally condemned in *Barnette*. On the other hand, respondents implicitly concede that an unconstitutional motivation would *not* be demonstrated if it were shown that petitioners had decided to remove the books at issue because those books were pervasively vulgar. *** And again, respondents concede that if it were demonstrated that the removal decision was based solely upon the "educational suitability" of the books in question, then their removal would be "perfectly permissible." *** In other words, in respondents' view such motivations, if decisive of petitioners' actions, would not carry the danger of an official suppression of ideas, and thus would not violate respondents' First Amendment rights.

As noted earlier, nothing in our decision today affects in any way the discretion of a local school board to choose books to *add* to the libraries of their schools. Because we are concerned in this case with the suppression of ideas, our holding today affects only the discretion to *remove* books. In brief, we hold that local school boards may not remove books from school library shelves simply because they dislike the ideas contained in those books and seek by their removal to "prescribe what shall be orthodox in politics, nationalism, religion, or other matters of opinion." West Virginia Board of Education v. Barnette, 319 U.S., at 642. Such purposes stand inescapably condemned by our precedents.

---

22. By "decisive factor" we mean a "substantial factor" in the absence of which the opposite decision would have been reached. See Mt. Healthy City Board of Ed. v. Doyle, 429 U.S. 274, 287 (1977).

B

We now turn to the remaining question presented by this case: Do the evidentiary materials that were before the District Court, when construed most favorably to respondents, raise a genuine issue of material fact whether petitioners exceeded constitutional limitations in exercising their discretion to remove the books from the school libraries? We conclude that the materials do raise such a question, which forecloses summary judgment in favor of petitioners. ***

Construing these claims, affidavit statements, and other evidentiary materials in a manner favorable to respondents, we cannot conclude that petitioners were "entitled to a judgment as a matter of law." The evidence plainly does not foreclose the possibility that petitioners' decision to remove the books rested decisively upon disagreement with constitutionally protected ideas in those books, or upon a desire on petitioners' part to impose upon the students of the Island Trees High School and Junior High School a political orthodoxy to which petitioners and their constituents adhered. Of course, some of the evidence before the District Court might lead a finder of fact to accept petitioners' claim that their removal decision was based upon constitutionally valid concerns. But that evidence at most creates a genuine issue of material fact on the critical question of the credibility of petitioners' justifications for their decision: On that issue, it simply cannot be said that there is no genuine issue as to any material fact. ***

Affirmed.

JUSTICE BLACKMUN, concurring in part and concurring in the judgment.

While I agree with much in today's plurality opinion, and while I accept the standard laid down by the plurality to guide proceedings on remand, I write separately because I have a somewhat different perspective on the nature of the First Amendment right involved. ***

In my view, then, the principle involved here is both narrower and more basic than the "right to receive information" identified by the plurality. I do not suggest that the State has any affirmative obligation to provide students with information or ideas, something that may well be associated with a "right to receive." *** And I do not believe, as the plurality suggests, that the right at issue here is somehow associated with the peculiar nature of the school library; if schools may be used to inculcate ideas, surely libraries may play a role in that process. Instead, I suggest that certain forms of state discrimination *between* ideas are improper. In particular, our precedents command the conclusion that the State may not act to deny access to an idea simply because state officials disapprove of that idea for partisan or political reasons.[2] *** In my view, we strike a proper balance here by holding that school

2. In effect, my view presents the obverse of the plurality's analysis: while the plurality focuses on the failure to provide information, I find crucial the State's decision to single out an idea for disapproval and then deny access to it.

officials may not remove books for the *purpose* of restricting access to the political ideas or social perspectives discussed in them, when that action is motivated simply by the officials' disapproval of the ideas involved.

[I] believe that tying the First Amendment right to the *purposeful* suppression of ideas makes the concept more manageable than Justice Rehnquist acknowledges. Most people would recognize that refusing to allow discussion of current events in Latin class is a policy designed to "inculcate" Latin, not to suppress ideas. Similarly, removing a learned treatise criticizing American foreign policy from an elementary school library because the students would not understand it is an action unrelated to the *purpose* of suppressing ideas. In my view, however, removing the same treatise because it is "anti-American" raises a far more difficult issue. ***

Arguing that the majority in the community rejects the ideas involved, (BURGER, C. J., dissenting), does not refute this principle: "The very purpose of a Bill of Rights was to withdraw certain subjects from the vicissitudes of political controversy, to place them beyond the reach of majorities and officials ***."

Because I believe that the plurality has derived a standard similar to the one compelled by my analysis, I join all but Part II-A(1) of the plurality opinion.

JUSTICE WHITE, concurring in the judgment.

The District Court found that the books were removed from the school library because the school board believed them "to be, in essence, vulgar." Both Court of Appeals judges in the majority concluded, however, that there was a material issue of fact that precluded summary judgment sought by petitioners. The unresolved factual issue, as I understand it, is the reason or reasons underlying the school board's removal of the books. I am not inclined to disagree with the Court of Appeals on such a fact-bound issue and hence concur in the judgment of affirmance. Presumably this will result in a trial and the making of a full record and findings on the critical issues. ***

CHIEF JUSTICE BURGER, with whom JUSTICE POWELL, JUSTICE REHNQUIST, and JUSTICE O'CONNOR join, dissenting. [Omitted.]

JUSTICE POWELL, dissenting.

The plurality opinion today rejects a basic concept of public school education in our country: that the States and locally elected school boards should have the responsibility for determining the educational policy of the public schools. After today's decision any junior high school student, by instituting a suit against a school board or teacher, may invite a judge to overrule an educational decision by the official body designated by the people to operate the schools. ***

As JUSTICE REHNQUIST tellingly observes, how does one limit—on a principled basis—today's new constitutional right? If a 14-year-old child may challenge a school board's decision to remove a book from the library, upon what theory is a court to prevent a like challenge to a school board's decision not to purchase that identical book? And at the even more "sensitive" level of "receiving ideas," does today's decision entitle student oversight of which courses may be added or removed from the curriculum, or even of what a particular teacher elects to teach or not teach in the classroom? Is not the "right to receive ideas" as much—or indeed even more—implicated in these educational questions?[2]

***

APPENDIX TO OPINION OF POWELL, J., DISSENTING

"The excerpts which led the Board to look into the educational suitability of the books in question are set out (with minor corrections after comparison with the text of the books themselves) below. The pagination and the underlinings are retained from the original report used by the board. In new editions of some of the books, the quotes appear at different pages.

"1) *SOUL ON ICE* by Eldridge Cleaver

PAGE QUOTE

157-158 '*** There are white men who will pay you to fuck their wives. They approach you and say, "How would you like to fuck a white woman?" "What is this?" you ask. "On the up-and-up," he assures you. "It's all right. She's my wife. She needs black rod, is all. It's like a medicine or drug to her. She has to have it. I'll pay you. It's all on the level, no trick involved. Interested?"' ***

***

"4) *GO ASK ALICE* by Anonymous

PAGE QUOTE

31 'I wonder if sex without acid could be so exciting, so wonderful, so indescribable. I always thought it just took a minute, or that it would be like dogs mating.'

47 'Chris and I walked into Richie and Ted's apartment to find the bastards stoned and making love to each other *** low class queer.'

81 'shitty, goddamned, pissing, ass, goddamned beJesus, screwing life's, ass, shit. Doris was ten and had *humped* with who knows how many men in between *** her current stepfather started having sex with her but good *** *sonofabitch balling her*'

***

2. The plurality suggests that the books in a school library derive special protection under the Constitution because the school library is a place in which students exercise unlimited choice. *** This suggestion is without support in law or fact. It is contradicted by this very case. The school board in this case does not view the school library as a place in which students pick from an unlimited range of books—some of which may be inappropriate for young people. Rather, the school library is analogous to an assigned reading list within which students may exercise a degree of choice.

"7) *BLACK BOY* by Richard Wright
PAGE QUOTE
70-71 'We black children—seven or eight or nine years of age—used to run to the Jew's store and shout:
*** Bloody Christ Killers
Never trust a Jew
Bloody Christ Killers
What won't a Jew do ***
Red, white and blue
Your pa was a Jew
Your ma a dirty dago
What the hell is you?'
265 'Crush that nigger's nuts, nigger!' 'Hit that nigger!' 'Aw, fight, you goddam niggers!' 'Sock 'im, in his f-k-g-piece!' 'Make 'im bleed!'

***

JUSTICE REHNQUIST, with whom THE CHIEF JUSTICE and JUSTICE POWELL join, dissenting.

*** Though for reasons stated in Part II of this opinion I entirely disagree with JUSTICE BRENNAN's treatment of the constitutional issue, I also disagree with his opinion for the entirely separate reason that it is not remotely tailored to the facts presented by this case.

In the course of his discussion, JUSTICE BRENNAN states:

> "Petitioners rightly possess significant discretion to determine the content of their school libraries. But that discretion may not be exercised in a narrowly partisan or political manner. If a Democratic school board, motivated by party affiliation, ordered the removal of all books written by or in favor of Republicans, few would doubt that the order violated the constitutional rights of the students. *** The same conclusion would surely apply if an all-white school board, motivated by racial animus, decided to remove all books authored by blacks or advocating racial equality and integration. Our Constitution does not permit the official suppression of *ideas*." *** (emphasis in original).

I can cheerfully concede all of this, but as in so many other cases the extreme examples are seldom the ones that arise in the real world of constitutional litigation. In *this case* the facts taken most favorably to respondents suggest that nothing of this sort happened. The nine books removed undoubtedly can contain "ideas," but in the light of the excerpts from them found in the dissenting opinion of Judge Mansfield in the Court of Appeals, it is apparent that eight of them contained demonstrable amounts of vulgarity and profanity, and the ninth contained nothing that could be considered partisan or political. As already demonstrated, respondents admitted as much. Petitioners did not, for the reasons stated hereafter, run afoul of the First and Fourteenth Amendments by removing these particular books from the library in the manner in which they did. I would save for another day—feeling quite confident that that day will not arrive—the extreme examples posed in JUSTICE BRENNAN's opinion.

B

Considerable light is shed on the correct resolution of the constitutional question in this case by examining the role played by petitioners. Had petitioners been the members of a town council, I suppose all would agree that, absent a good deal more than is present in this record, they could not have prohibited the sale of these books by private booksellers within the municipality. But we have also recognized that the government may act in other capacities than as sovereign, and when it does the First Amendment may speak with a different voice:

> "[I]t cannot be gainsaid that the State has interests as an employer in regulating the speech of its employees that differ significantly from those it possesses in connection with regulation of the speech of the citizenry in general. The problem in any case is to arrive at a balance between the interests of the teacher, as a citizen, in commenting upon matters of concern and the interest of the State, as an employer, in promoting the efficiency of the public services it performs through its employees." Pickering v. Board of Education, 391 U.S. 563, 568 (1968).

With these differential roles of government in mind, it is helpful to assess the role of government as educator, as compared with the role of government as sovereign. When it acts as an educator, at least at the elementary and secondary school level, the government is engaged in inculcating social values and knowledge in relatively impressionable young people. Obviously there are innumerable decisions to be made as to what courses should be taught, what books should be purchased, or what teachers should be employed. In every one of these areas the members of a school board will act on the basis of their own personal or moral values, will attempt to mirror those of the community, or will abdicate the making of such decisions to so-called "experts."[5] In this connection I find myself entirely in agreement with the observation of the Court of Appeals for the Seventh Circuit in Zykan v. Warsaw Community School Corp., 631 F.2d 1300, 1305 (1980), that it is "permissible and appropriate for local boards to make educational decisions based upon their personal social, political and moral views." ***

5. There are intimations in JUSTICE BRENNAN's opinion that if petitioners had only consulted literary experts, librarians, and teachers their decision might better withstand First Amendment attack. *** These observations seem to me wholly fatuous; surely ideas are no more accessible or no less suppressed if the school board merely ratifies the opinion of some group rather than following its own opinion.

II

Justice Brennan would hold that the First Amendment gives high school and junior high school students a "right to receive ideas" in the school. This right is a curious entitlement. It exists only in the library of the school, and only if the idea previously has been acquired by the school in book form. It provides no protection against a school board's decision not to acquire a particular book, even though that decision denies access to ideas as fully as removal of the book from the library, and it prohibits removal of previously acquired books only if the remover "dislike[s] the ideas contained in those books," even though removal for any other reason also denies the students access to the books.

But it is not the limitations which Justice Brennan places on the right with which I disagree; they simply demonstrate his discomfort with the new doctrine which he fashions out of whole cloth. It is the very existence of a right to receive information, in the junior high school and high school setting, which I find wholly unsupported by our past decisions and inconsistent with the necessarily selective process of elementary and secondary education. ***

As already mentioned, elementary and secondary schools are inculcative in nature. The libraries of such schools serve as supplements to this inculcative role. Unlike university or public libraries, elementary and secondary school libraries are not designed for freewheeling inquiry; they are tailored, as the public school curriculum is tailored, to the teaching of basic skills and ideas. Thus, Justice Brennan cannot rely upon the nature of school libraries to escape the fact that the First Amendment right to receive information simply has no application to the one public institution which, by its very nature, is a place for the selective conveyance of ideas.

After all else is said, however, the most obvious reason that petitioners' removal of the books did not violate respondents' right to receive information is the ready availability of the books elsewhere. Students are not denied books by their removal from a school library. The books may be borrowed from a public library, read at a university library, purchased at a bookstore, or loaned by a friend. The government as educator does not seek to reach beyond the confines of the school. Indeed, following the removal from the school library of the books at issue in this case, the local public library put all nine books on display for public inspection. Their contents were fully accessible to any inquisitive student. ***

Intertwined as a basis for JUSTICE BRENNAN's opinion, along with the "right to receive information," is the statement that "[o]ur Constitution does not permit the official suppression of *ideas*." *** (emphasis in original). There would be few champions, I suppose, of the idea that our Constitution *does* permit the official suppression of ideas; my difficulty is not with the admittedly appealing catchiness of the phrase, but with my doubt that it is really a useful analytical tool in solving difficult First Amendment problems.

In the case before us the petitioners may in one sense be said to have "suppressed" the "ideas" of vulgarity and profanity, but that is hardly an apt description of what was done. They ordered the removal of books containing vulgarity and profanity, but they did not attempt to preclude discussion about the themes of the books or the books themselves. Such a decision, on respondents' version of the facts in this case, is sufficiently related to "educational suitability" to pass muster under the First Amendment. ***

I think the Court will far better serve the cause of First Amendment jurisprudence by candidly recognizing that the role of government as sovereign is subject to more stringent limitations than is the role of government as employer, property owner, or educator. It must also be recognized that the government as educator is subject to fewer strictures when operating an elementary and secondary school system than when operating an institution of higher learning. Cf. Tilton v. Richardson, 403 U.S. 672, 685-686 (1971) (opinion of JUSTICE BURGER, C. J.). ***

JUSTICE O'CONNOR, dissenting.

If the school board can set the curriculum, select teachers, and determine initially what books to purchase for the school library, it surely can decide which books to discontinue or remove from the school library so long as it does not also interfere with the right of students to read the material and to discuss it. As JUSTICE REHNQUIST persuasively argues, the plurality's analysis overlooks the fact that in this case the government is acting in its special role as educator.

I do not personally agree with the Board's action with respect to some of the books in question here, but it is not the function of the courts to make the decisions that have been properly relegated to the elected members of school boards. It is the school board that must determine educational suitability, and it has done so in this case. I therefore join The Chief Justice's dissent.

ELROD v. BURNS
427 U.S. 347 (1976)

MR. JUSTICE BRENNAN announced the judgment of the Court and delivered an opinion in which MR. JUSTICE WHITE and MR. JUSTICE MARSHALL joined.

This case presents the question whether public employees who allege that they were discharged or threatened with discharge solely because of their partisan political affiliation or nonaffiliation state a claim for deprivation of constitutional rights secured by the First and Fourteenth Amendments. ***

II

In December 1970, the Sheriff of Cook County, a Republican, was replaced by Richard Elrod, a Democrat. At that time, respondents, all Republicans, were employees of the Cook County Sheriff's Office. They were non-civil-service employees and, therefore, not covered by any statute, ordinance, or regulation protecting them from arbitrary discharge. One respondent, John Burns, was Chief Deputy of the Process Division and supervised all departments of the Sheriff's Office working on the seventh floor of the building housing that office. Frank Vargas was a bailiff and security guard at the Juvenile Court of Cook County. Fred L. Buckley was employed as a process server in the office. Joseph Dennard was an employee in the office.

It has been the practice of the Sheriff of Cook County, when he assumes office from a Sheriff of a different political party, to replace non-civil-service employees of the Sheriff's Office with members of his own party when the existing employees lack or fail to obtain requisite support from, or fail to affiliate with, that party. Consequently, subsequent to Sheriff Elrod's assumption of office, respondents, with the exception of Buckley, were discharged from their employment solely because they did not support and were not members of the Democratic Party and had failed to obtain the sponsorship of one of its leaders. Buckley is in imminent danger of being discharged solely for the same reasons. ***

IV

The Cook County Sheriff's practice of dismissing employees on a partisan basis is but one form of the general practice of political patronage. The practice also includes placing loyal supporters in government jobs that may or may not have been made available by political discharges. Nonofficeholders may be the beneficiaries of lucrative government contracts for highway construction, buildings, and supplies.[*] Favored wards may receive improved public services. Members of the judiciary may even engage in the practice through the appointment of receiverships, trusteeships, and refereeships. Although political patronage comprises a broad range of activities, we are here concerned only with the constitutionality of dismissing public employees for partisan reasons.

Patronage practice is not new to American politics. It has existed at the federal level at least since the Presidency of Thomas Jefferson, although its popularization and legitimation primarily occurred later, in the Presidency of Andrew Jackson. The practice is not unique to American politics. It has been used in many European countries, and in darker times, it played a significant role in the Nazi rise to power in Germany and other totalitarian states. ***

V

The cost of the practice of patronage is the restraint it places on freedoms of belief and association. In order to maintain their jobs, respondents were required to pledge their political allegiance to the Democratic Party, work for the election of other candidates of the Democratic Party, contribute a portion of their wages to the Party, or obtain the sponsorship of a member of the Party, usually at the price of one

---

*. **[Ed. Note**. See note on p. 374, *infra*, about political patronage and independent contractors.]

of the first three alternatives. Regardless of the incumbent party's identity, Democratic or otherwise, the consequences for association and belief are the same. An individual who is a member of the out-party maintains affiliation with his own party at the risk of losing his job. He works for the election of his party's candidates and espouses its policies at the same risk. The financial and campaign assistance that he is induced to provide to another party furthers the advancement of that party's policies to the detriment of his party's views and ultimately his own beliefs, and any assessment of his salary is tantamount to coerced belief. Even a pledge of allegiance to another party, however ostensible, only serves to compromise the individual's true beliefs. Since the average public employee is hardly in the financial position to support his party and another, or to lend his time to two parties, the individual's ability to act according to his beliefs and to associate with others of his political persuasion is constrained, and support for his party is diminished. ***

Our concern with the impact of patronage on political belief and association does not occur in the abstract, for political belief and association constitute the core of those activities protected by the First Amendment.

*** Patronage, therefore, to the extent it compels or restrains belief and association, is inimical to the process which undergirds our system of government and is "at war with the deeper traditions of democracy embodied in the First Amendment." Illinois State Employees Union v. Lewis, 473 F.2d, at 576. As such, the practice unavoidably confronts decisions by this Court either invalidating or recognizing as invalid government action that inhibits belief and association through the conditioning of public employment on political faith.

Particularly pertinent to the constitutionality of the practice of patronage dismissals are Keyishian v. Board of Regents, 385 U.S. 589 (1967), and Perry v. Sindermann, 408 U.S. 593 (1972). In *Keyishian*, the Court invalidated New York statutes barring employment merely on the basis of membership in "subversive" organizations. *Keyishian* squarely held that political association alone could not, consistently with the First Amendment, constitute an adequate ground for denying public employment.[11] In *Perry*, the Court broadly rejected the validity of limitations on First Amendment rights as a condition to the receipt of a governmental benefit, standing that the government "may not deny a benefit to a person on a basis that infringes his constitutionally protected interests—especially, his interest in freedom of speech." ***

Patronage practice falls squarely within the prohibitions of*Keyishian* and *Perry*. Under that practice, public employees hold their jobs on the condition that they provide, in some acceptable manner, support for the favored political party. ***

---

11. Thereafter, United States v. Robel, 389 U.S. 258 (1967), similarly held that mere membership in the Communist Party could not bar a person from employment in private defense establishments important to national security.

VI

Although the practice of patronage dismissals clearly infringes First Amendment interests, our inquiry is not at an end, for the prohibition on encroachment of First Amendment protections is not an absolute. Restraints are permitted for appropriate reasons. Before examining those justifications, however, it is necessary to have in mind the standards according to which their sufficiency is to be measured. It is firmly established that a significant impairment of First Amendment rights must survive exacting scrutiny. The interest advanced must be paramount, one of vital importance, and the burden is on the government to show the existence of such an interest. [I]f conditioning the retention of public employment on the employee's support of the in- party is to survive constitutional challenge, it must further some vital government end by a means that is least restrictive of freedom of belief and association in achieving that end, and the benefit gained must outweigh the loss of constitutionally protected rights.[17]

One interest which has been offered in justification of patronage is the need to insure effective government and the efficiency of public employees. It is argued that employees of political persuasions not the same as that of the party in control of public office will not have the incentive to work effectively and may even be motivated to subvert the incumbent administration's efforts to govern effectively. We are not persuaded. The inefficiency resulting from the wholesale replacement of large numbers of public employees every time political office changes hands belies this justification. And the prospect of dismissal after an election in which the incumbent party has lost is only a disincentive to good work.[18] Further, it is not clear that dismissal in order to make room for a patronage appointment will result in replacement by a person more qualified to do the job since appointment often occurs in exchange for the delivery of votes, or other party service, not job capability. ***

Even if the first argument that patronage serves effectiveness and efficiency be rejected, it still may be argued that patronage serves those interests by giving the employees of an incumbent party the incentive to perform well in order to insure their

---

17. The Court's decision in United States v. O'Brien, 391 U.S. 367 (1968), does not support petitioners. *O'Brien* dealt with the constitutionality of laws regulating the "nonspeech" elements of expressive conduct. No such regulation is involved here, for it is association and belief *per se*, not any particular form of conduct, which patronage seeks to control. ***

18. It does not appear that efficiency and effective government were the concerns of elected officials in this case. Employees originally dismissed were reinstated after obtaining sponsorship letters, a practice hardly promotive of efficiency if the employee's work had been less than par or if the employee had previously behaved in an insubordinate manner. Complaints by one supervisor that too many people were being discharged too fast, without adequately trained replacements, were met with the response that the number of dismissals was to be maintained because the job openings were needed for partisan appointments. One Republican employee of the Sheriff's Office was told that his dismissal had nothing to do with the quality of his work, but that his position was needed for a Democratic replacement.

party's incumbency and thereby their jobs. Patronage, according to the argument, thus makes employees highly accountable to the public. But the ability of officials more directly accountable to the electorate to discharge employees for cause and the availability of merit systems, growth in the use of which has been quite significant, convince us that means less intrusive than patronage still exist for achieving accountability in the public work force and, thereby, effective and efficient government. The greater effectiveness of patronage over these less drastic means, if any, is at best marginal, a gain outweighed by the absence of intrusion on protected interests under the alternatives.

The lack of any justification for patronage dismissals as a means of furthering government effectiveness and efficiency distinguishes this case from CSC v. Letter Carriers, 413 U.S. 548 (1973), and United Public Workers v. Mitchell, 330 U.S. 75 (1949). In both of those cases, legislative restraints on political management and campaigning, by public employees were upheld despite their encroachment on First Amendment rights because, *inter alia*, they did serve in a necessary manner to foster and protect efficient and effective government.[20] Interestingly, the activities that were restrained by the legislation involved in those cases are characteristic of patronage practices. ***

A second interest advanced in support of patronage is the need for political loyalty of employees, not to the end that effectiveness and efficiency be insured, but to the end that representative government not be undercut by tactics obstructing the implementation of policies of the new administration, policies presumably sanctioned by the electorate. The justification is not without force, but is nevertheless inadequate to validate patronage wholesale. Limiting patronage dismissals to policymaking positions is sufficient to achieve this governmental end. Nonpolicy making individuals usually have only limited responsibility and are therefore not in a position to thwart the goals of the in-party.

No clear line can be drawn between policymaking and nonpolicymaking positions. While nonpolicymaking individuals usually have limited responsibility, that is not to say that one with a number of responsibilities is necessarily in a policymaking position. *** Since, as we have noted, it is the government's burden to demonstrate an overriding interest in order to validate an encroachment on protected interests, the burden of establishing this justification as to any particular respondent will rest on the petitioners on remand, cases of doubt being resolved in favor of the particular respondent.

It is argued that a third interest supporting patronage dismissals is the preservation of the democratic process. According to petitioners, "'we have contrived no system for the support of party that does not place considerable reliance on

20. Legislative restraints on political management and campaigning were also upheld in *Letter Carriers* and *Mitchell* because they served to protect individual belief and association and, thereby, the political process.

patronage. The party organization makes a democratic government work and charges a price for its services.'"[21] ***

But however important preservation of the two party system or any system involving a fixed number of parties may or may not be,[22] we are not persuaded that the elimination of patronage practice or, as is specifically involved here, the interdiction of patronage dismissals, will bring about the demise of party politics. Political parties existed in the absence of active patronage practice prior to the administration of Andrew Jackson, and they have survived substantial reduction in their patronage power through the establishment of merit systems.

Patronage dismissals thus are not the least restrictive alternative to achieving the contribution they may make to the democratic process. The process functions as well without the practice, perhaps even better, for patronage dismissals clearly also retard that process. Patronage can result in the entrenchment of one or a few parties to the exclusion of others. And most indisputably, as we recognized at the outset, patronage is a very effective impediment to the associational and speech freedoms which are essential to a meaningful system of democratic government. Thus, if patronage contributes at all to the elective process, that contribution is diminished by the practice's impairment of the same. ***

More fundamentally, however, any contribution of patronage dismissals to the democratic process does not suffice to override their severe encroachment on First Amendment freedoms. We hold, therefore, that the practice of patronage dismissals is unconstitutional under the First and Fourteenth Amendments, and that respondents thus stated a valid claim for relief.

VII

There remains the question whether the issuance of a preliminary injunction was properly directed by the Court of Appeals. The District Court predicated its denial of respondents' motion for a preliminary injunction on its finding that the allegations in their complaints and affidavits did not constitute a sufficient showing of irreparable injury and that respondents had an adequate remedy at law. The Court of Appeals held, however: "Inasmuch as this case involves First Amendment rights of association which must be carefully guarded against infringement by public office

---

21. Brief for Petitioners 43, quoting V. Key, Politics, Parties and Pressure Groups 369 (5th ed. 1964).

22. Partisan politics bears the imprimatur only of tradition, not the Constitution.

> "It may be correct that the patronage system has been followed for 'almost two hundred years' and therefore was in existence when the Constitution was adopted. However, the notoriety of the practice in the administration of Andrew Jackson in 1828 implies that it was not prevalent theretofore; we are not aware of any discussion of the practice during the drafting of the Constitution or the First Amendment. In any event, if the age of a pernicious practice were a sufficient reason for its continued acceptance, the constitutional attack on racial discrimination would, of course, have been doomed to failure."

Illinois State Employees Union v. Lewis, 473 F.2d 561, 568 n. 14 (CA7 1972).

holders, we judge that injunctive relief is clearly appropriate in these cases." We agree. *** The judgment of the Court of Appeals is affirmed.

MR. JUSTICE STEVENS did not participate in the consideration of this case.

MR. JUSTICE STEWART, with whom MR. JUSTICE BLACKMUN joins, concurring in the judgment. [Omitted]

MR. CHIEF JUSTICE BURGER, dissenting. [Omitted.]

MR. JUSTICE POWELL, with whom THE CHIEF JUSTICE and MR. JUSTICE REHNQUIST join, dissenting.

***

The question is whether it is consistent with the First and Fourteenth Amendments for a State to offer some employment conditioned, explicitly or implicitly, on partisan political affiliation and on the political fortunes of the incumbent officeholder. This is to be determined, as the plurality opinion agrees, by whether patronage hiring practices sufficiently advance important state interests to justify the consequent burdening of First Amendment interests. ***

[P]atronage hiring practices have contributed to American democracy by stimulating political activity and by strengthening parties, thereby helping to make government accountable.[6] It cannot be questioned seriously that these contributions promote important state interests. ***

The complaining parties are or were employees of the Sheriff. In many communities, the sheriff's duties are as routine as process serving, and his election attracts little or no general public interest. In the States, and especially in the thousands of local communities, there are large numbers of elective offices, and many are as relatively obscure as that of the local sheriff or constable. Despite the importance of elective offices to the ongoing work of local governments, election campaigns for lesser offices in particular usually attract little attention from the media, with consequent disinterest and absence of intelligent participation on the part of the public. Unless the candidates for these offices are able to dispense the traditional patronage that has accrued to the offices, they also are unlikely to attract donations of time or money from voluntary groups. *** The candidates for these offices derive their support at the precinct level, and their modest funding for publicity, from cadres of friends and political associates who hope to benefit if their "man" is elected. The activities of the latter are often the principal source of political information for the

6. Some commentators have believed that patronage hiring practices promote other social interests as well: "Patronage is peculiarly important for minority groups, involving much more than the mere spoils of office. Each first appointment given a member of any underdog element is a boost in that element's struggle for social acceptance. It means that another barrier to their advance has been lifted, another shut door has swung open." S. Lubell, The Future of American Politics 76-77 (1952).

voting public. The "robust" political discourse that the plurality opinion properly emphasizes is furthered—not restricted—by the time-honored system. ***

It is naive to think that these types of political activities are motivated at these levels by some academic interest in "democracy" or other public service impulse. For the most part, as every politician knows, the hope of some reward generates a major portion of the local political activity supporting parties. It is difficult to overestimate the contributions to our system by the major political parties, fortunately limited in number compared to the fractionalization that has made the continued existence of democratic government doubtful in some other countries. Parties generally are stable, high-profile, and permanent institutions. Voters can and do hold parties to long-term accountability, and it is not too much to say that, in their absence, responsive and responsible performance in low-profile offices, particularly, is difficult to maintain.

I thus conclude that patronage hiring practices sufficiently serve important state interests, including some interest sought to be advanced by the First Amendment, to justify a tolerable intrusion on the First Amendment interests of employees or potential employees. *** This intrusion, while not insignificant, must be measured in light of the limited role of patronage hiring in most government employment. The pressure to abandon one's beliefs and associations to obtain government employment—especially employment of such uncertain duration—does not seem to me to assume impermissible proportions in light of the interests to be served.

BRANTI v. FINKEL

445 U.S. 507 (1980)

MR. JUSTICE STEVENS delivered the opinion of the Court.

The question presented is whether the First and Fourteenth Amendments to the Constitution protect an assistant public defender who is satisfactorily performing his job from discharge solely because of his political beliefs.

The two respondents have served as assistants since their respective appointments in March 1971 and September 1975; they are both Republicans.[4]

Petitioner Branti's predecessor, a Republican, was appointed in 1972 by a Republican-dominated County Legislature. By 1977, control of the legislature had shifted to the Democrats and petitioner, also a Democrat, was appointed to replace the incumbent when his term expired. As soon as petitioner was formally appointed

---

4. The District Court noted that Finkel had changed his party registration from Republican to Democrat in 1977 in the apparent hope that such action would enhance his chances of being reappointed as an assistant when a new, Democratic public defender was appointed. The court concluded that, despite Finkel's formal change of party registration, the parties had regarded him as a Republican at all relevant times.

on January 3, 1978, he began executing termination notices for six of the nine assistants then in office. Respondents were among those who were to be terminated. With one possible exception, the nine who were to be appointed or retained were all Democrats and were all selected by Democratic legislators or Democratic town chairmen on a basis that had been determined by the Democratic caucus.

The District Court found that Finkel and Tabakman had been selected for termination solely because they were Republicans and thus did not have the necessary Democratic sponsors:

> "The sole grounds for the attempted removal of plaintiffs were the facts that plaintiffs' political beliefs differed from those of the ruling Democratic majority in the County Legislature and that the Democratic majority had determined that Assistant Public Defender appointments were to be made on political bases." ***

The court rejected petitioner's belated attempt to justify the dismissals on nonpolitical grounds. Noting that both Branti and his predecessor had described respondents as "competent attorneys," the District Court expressly found that both had been "satisfactorily performing their duties as Assistant Public Defenders." ***

Having concluded that respondents had been discharged solely because of their political beliefs, the District Court held that those discharges would be permissible under this Court's decision in Elrod v. Burns, 427 U.S. 347, only if assistant public defenders are the type of policymaking, confidential employees who may be discharged solely on the basis of their political affiliations. The court concluded that respondents clearly did not fall within that category. Although recognizing that they had broad responsibilities with respect to particular cases that were assigned to them, the court found that respondents had "very limited, if any, responsibility" with respect to the overall operation of the public defender's office. They did not "act as advisors or formulate plans for the implementation of the broad goals of the office" and, although they made decisions in the context of specific cases, "they do not make decisions about the orientation and operation of the office in which they work."

The District Court also rejected the argument that the confidential character of respondents' work justified conditioning their employment on political grounds. The court found that they did not occupy any confidential relationship to the policymaking process, and did not have access to confidential documents that influenced policymaking deliberations. Rather, the only confidential information to which they had access was the product of their attorney-client relationship with the office's clients; to the extent that such information was shared with the public defender, it did not relate to the formulation of office policy.

In light of these factual findings, the District Court concluded that petitioner could not terminate respondents' employment as assistant public defenders consistent with the First and Fourteenth Amendments. On appeal, a panel of the Second Circuit affirmed, specifically holding that the District Court's findings of fact were adequately supported by the record. That court also expressed "no doubt" that the District Court "was correct in concluding that an assistant public defender was neither a policymaker nor a confidential employee." We granted certiorari *** and now affirm.

Petitioner advances two principal arguments for reversal: First, that the holding in *Elrod v. Burns* is limited to situations in which government employees are coerced into pledging allegiance to a political party that they would not voluntarily support and does not apply to a simple requirement that an employee be sponsored by the party in power; and, second, that, even if party sponsorship is an unconstitutional condition of continued public employment for clerks, deputies, and janitors, it is an acceptable requirement for an assistant public defender.

I

***

Petitioner argues that *Elrod v. Burns* should be read to prohibit only dismissals resulting from an employee's failure to capitulate to political coercion. Thus, he argues that, so long as an employee is not asked to change his political affiliation or to contribute to or work for the party's candidates, he may be dismissed with impunity— even though he would not have been dismissed if he had had the proper political sponsorship and even though the sole reason for dismissing him was to replace him with a person who did have such sponsorship. Such an interpretation would surely emasculate the principles set forth in *Elrod.* While it would perhaps eliminate the more blatant forms of coercion described in *Elrod,* it would not eliminate the coercion of belief that necessarily flows from the knowledge that one must have a sponsor in the dominant party in order to retain one's job.[11] More importantly, petitioner's interpretation would require the Court to repudiate entirely the conclusion of both Mr. Justice BRENNAN and Mr. Justice STEWART that the First Amendment prohibits the dismissal of a public employee solely because of his private political beliefs.

In sum, there is no requirement that dismissed employees prove that they, or other employees, have been coerced into changing, either actually or ostensibly, their political allegiance. To prevail in this type of an action, it was sufficient as *Elrod* holds, for respondents to prove that they were discharged "solely for the reason that they were not affiliated with or sponsored by the Democratic Party." 427 U.S., at 350.

---

11. As Mr. Justice BRENNAN pointed out in *Elrod,* political sponsorship is often purchased at the price of political contributions or campaign work in addition to a simple declaration of allegiance to the party. Thus, an employee's realization that he must obtain a sponsor in order to retain his job is very likely to lead to the same type of coercion as that described by the plurality in *Elrod.* While there was apparently no overt political pressure exerted on respondents in this case, the potentially coercive effect of requiring sponsorship was demonstrated by Mr. Finkel's change of party registration in a futile attempt to retain his position.

II

Both opinions in *Elrod* recognize that party affiliation may be an acceptable requirement for some types of government employment. Thus, if an employee's private political beliefs would interfere with the discharge of his public duties, his First Amendment rights may be required to yield to the State's vital interest in maintaining governmental effectiveness and efficiency. In *Elrod*, it was clear that the duties of the employees—the chief deputy of the process division of the sheriff's office, a process server and another employee in that office, and a bailiff and security guard at the Juvenile Court of Cook County—were not of that character, for they were, as Mr. Justice Stewart stated, "nonpolicymaking, nonconfidential" employees. *Id.*, at 375.[12]

As Mr. Justice BRENNAN noted in *Elrod*, it is not always easy to determine whether a position is one in which political affiliation is a legitimate factor to be considered. Under some circumstances, a position may be appropriately considered political even though it is neither confidential nor policymaking in character. As one obvious example, if a State's election laws require that precincts be supervised by two election judges of different parties, a Republican judge could be legitimately discharged solely for changing his party registration. That conclusion would not depend on any finding that the job involved participation in policy decisions or access to confidential information. Rather, it would simply rest on the fact that party membership was essential to the discharge of the employee's governmental responsibilities.

It is equally clear that party affiliation is not necessarily relevant to every policymaking or confidential position. The coach of a state university's football team formulates policy, but no one could seriously claim that Republicans make better coaches than Democrats, or vice versa, no matter which party is in control of the state government. On the other hand, it is equally clear that the Governor of a State may appropriately believe that the official duties of various assistants who help him write speeches, explain his views to the press, or communicate with the legislature cannot be performed effectively unless those persons share his political beliefs and party

---

12. The plurality emphasized that patronage dismissals could be justified only if they advanced a governmental, rather than a partisan, interest. 427 U.S., at 362. That standard clearly was not met to the extent that employees were expected to perform extracurricular activities for the party, or were being rewarded for past services to the party. Government funds, which are collected from taxpayers of all parties on a nonpolitical basis, cannot be expended for the benefit of one political party simply because that party has control of the government. The compensation of government employees, like the distribution of other public benefits, must be justified by a governmental purpose.

The Sheriff argued that his employees' political beliefs did have a bearing on the official duties they were required to perform because political loyalty was necessary to the continued efficiency of the office. But after noting the tenuous link between political loyalty and efficiency where process servers and clerks were concerned, the plurality held that any small gain in efficiency did not outweigh the employees' First Amendment rights. *Id.*, at 366.

commitments. In sum, the ultimate inquiry is not whether the label "policymaker" or "confidential" fits a particular position; rather, the question is whether the hiring authority can demonstrate that party affiliation is an appropriate requirement for the effective performance of the public office involved.

Having thus framed the issue, it is manifest that the continued employment of an assistant public defender cannot properly be conditioned upon his allegiance to the political party in control of the county government. The primary, if not the only, responsibility of an assistant public defender is to represent individual citizens in controversy with the State.[13] As we recently observed in commenting on the duties of counsel appointed to represent indigent defendants in federal criminal proceedings:

> "[T]he primary office performed by appointed counsel parallels the office of privately retained counsel. Although it is true that appointed counsel serves pursuant to statutory authorization and in furtherance of the federal interest in insuring effective representation of criminal defendants, his duty is not to the public at large, except in that general way. His principal responsibility is to serve the undivided interests of his client. Indeed, an indispensable element of the effective performance of his responsibilities is the ability to act independently of the government and to oppose it in adversary litigation." Ferri v. Ackerman, 444 U.S. 193, 204.

Thus, whatever policymaking occurs in the public defender's office must relate to the needs of individual clients and not to any partisan political interests. Similarly, although an assistant is bound to obtain access to confidential information arising out of various attorney-client relationships, that information has no bearing whatsoever on partisan political concerns. Under these circumstances, it would undermine, rather than promote, the effective performance of an assistant public defender's office to make his tenure dependent on his allegiance to the dominant political party.

Accordingly, the entry of an injunction against termination of respondents' employment on purely political grounds was appropriate and the judgment of the Court of Appeals is affirmed.

MR. JUSTICE STEWART, dissenting.

I joined the judgment of the Court in Elrod v. Burns, because it is my view that, under the First and Fourteenth Amendments, "a nonpolicymaking, nonconfidential government employee can[not] be discharged *** from a job that he is satisfactorily performing upon the sole ground of his political beliefs." That judgment in my

---

13. This is in contrast to the broader public responsibilities of an official such as a prosecutor. We express no opinion as to whether the deputy of such an official could be dismissed on grounds of political party affiliation or loyalty. Cf. Newcomb v. Brennan, 558 F.2d 825 (CA7 1977), cert. denied, 434 U.S. 968 (dismissal of deputy city attorney).

opinion does not control the present case for the simple reason that the respondents here clearly are not "nonconfidential" employees.

The respondents in the present case are lawyers, and the employment positions involved are those of assistants in the office of the Rockland County Public Defender. *** I believe that the petitioner, upon his appointment as Public Defender, was not constitutionally compelled to enter such a close professional and necessarily confidential association with the respondents if he did not wish to do so.

MR. JUSTICE POWELL, with whom MR. JUSTICE REHNQUIST joins, and with whom MR. JUSTICE STEWART joins as to Part I, dissenting.

I

The Court contends that its holding is compelled by the First Amendment. In reaching this conclusion, the Court largely ignores the substantial governmental interests served by patronage. Patronage is a long-accepted practice[1] that never has been eliminated totally by civil service laws and regulations. The flaw in the Court's opinion lies not only in its application of First Amendment principles, see Parts II-IV, *infra*, but also in its promulgation of a new, and substantially expanded, standard for determining which governmental employees may be retained or dismissed on the basis of political affiliation.[2] ***

The standard articulated by the Court is framed in vague and sweeping language certain to create vast uncertainty. Elected and appointed officials at all levels who now receive guidance from civil service laws, no longer will know when political affiliation is an appropriate consideration in filling a position. *** Prudent individuals requested to accept a public appointment must consider whether their predecessors will threaten to oust them through legal action.

One example at the national level illustrates the nature and magnitude of the problem created by today's holding. The President customarily has considered political affiliation in removing and appointing United States attorneys. Given the critical role that these key law enforcement officials play in the administration of the Depart-

---

1. When Thomas Jefferson became the first Chief Executive to succeed a President of the opposing party, he made substantial use of appointment and removal powers. Andrew Jackson, the next President to follow an antagonistic administration, used patronage extensively when he took office. The use of patronage in the early days of our Republic played an important role in democratizing American politics. Elrod v. Burns, 427 U.S., at 378-379 (POWELL, J., dissenting). President Lincoln's patronage practices and his reliance upon the newly formed Republican Party enabled him to build support for his national policies during the Civil War. See E. McKitrick, Party Politics and the Union and Confederate War Efforts, in The American Party System 117, 131-133 (W. Chambers & W. Burnham eds. 1967).

2. The Court purports to limit the issue in this case to the dismissal of public employees. Yet the Court also states that "it is difficult to formulate any justification of tying either the selection or retention of an assistant public defender to his party affiliation." *** If this latter statement is not a holding of the Court, it at least suggests that the Court perceives no constitutional distinction between selection and dismissal of public employees. **[Ed. Note**. See Rutan v. Republican Party of Illinois, 497 U.S. 62 (1990).]

ment of Justice, both Democratic and Republican Attorneys General have concluded, not surprisingly, that they must have the confidence and support of the United States attorneys. And political affiliation has been used as one indicator of loyalty.

Yet, it would be difficult to say, under the Court's standard, that "partisan" concerns properly are relevant to the performance of the duties of a United States attorney. ***

III

*** The Court's opinion appears to recognize that the implementation of policy is a legitimate goal of the patronage system and that some, but not all, policymaking employees may be placed on the basis of their political affiliation. But the Court does not recognize that the implementation of policy often depends upon the cooperation of public employees who do not hold policymaking posts. As one commentator has written: "What the Court forgets is that, if government is to work, policy implementation is just as important as policymaking. No matter how wise the chief, he has to have the right Indians to transform his ideas into action, to get the job done."[13] The growth of the civil service system already has limited the ability of elected politicians to effect political change. Public employees immune to public pressure "can resist changes in policy without suffering either the loss of their jobs or a cut in their salary." Such effects are proper when they follow from legislative or executive decisions to withhold some jobs from the patronage system. But the Court tips the balance between patronage and nonpatronage positions, and, in my view, imposes unnecessary constraints upon the ability of responsible officials to govern effectively and to carry out new policies. ***

IV-V

The facts of this case also demonstrate that the Court's decision well may impair the right of local voters to structure their government. Consideration of the form of local government in Rockland County, N. Y., demonstrates the antidemocratic effect of the Court's decision.

The voters of the county elect a legislative body. Among the responsibilities that the voters give to the legislature is the selection of a county public defender. In 1972, when the county voters elected a Republican majority in the legislature a Republican was selected as public defender. The public defender retained one respondent and appointed the other as assistant public defenders. Not surprisingly, both respondents are Republican. In 1976, the voters elected a majority of Democrats to the legislature. The Democratic majority, in turn, selected a Democratic Public Defender who replaced both respondents with Assistant Public Defenders approved by the Democratic legislators. ***

The voters of Rockland County are free to elect their public defender and assistant public defenders instead of delegating their selection to elected and appointed

13. Peters, A Kind Word for the Spoils System, The Washington Monthly, Sept. 1976, p. 30.

officials. Certainly the Court's holding today would not preclude the voters, the ultimate "hiring authority," from choosing both public defenders and their assistants by party membership. The voters' choice of public officials on the basis of political affiliation is not yet viewed as an inhibition of speech; it is democracy. Nor may any incumbent contend seriously that the voters' decision not to re-elect him because of his political views is an impermissible infringement upon his right of free speech or affiliation. In other words, the operation of democratic government depends upon the selection of elected officials on precisely the basis rejected by the Court today.

Although the voters of Rockland County could have elected both the public defender and his assistants, they have given their legislators a representative proxy to appoint the public defender. And they have delegated to the public defender the power to choose his assistants. Presumably the voters have adopted this course in order to facilitate more effective representative government. Of course, the voters could have instituted a civil service system that would preclude the selection of either the public defender or his assistants on the basis of political affiliation. But the continuation of the present system reflects the electorate's decision to select certain public employees on the basis of political affiliation. *** In my view, the First Amendment does not incorporate a national civil service system. I would reverse the judgment of the Court of Appeals.

NOTE

1990 the Court applied *Elrod* to hirings, promotions, and transfers of government employees.[43] *Pickering, Elrod, Branti*, and *Rutan* accordingly provide government *employees* with substantial protection for their political affiliations, their speech critical of the government, and their decisions to support—or not support—particular candidates for office. Several courts of appeal, however, refused to apply the same protections to independent contractors. Is there any reason why those who independently contract with the government should not be similarly insulated from the spoils system?[44] In 1996,the Supreme Court ended the controversy. By vote of seven-to-two (Scalia and Thomas, J.I., dissenting), the Court

---

43. Rutan v. Republican Party of Illinois, 497 U.S. 62 (1990).

44. See, e.g., O'Hare Truck Serv., Inc. v. City of Northlake, 47 F.3d 883 (7th Cir. 1995) (sustaining police department removal of independent towing company from rotation list for vehicle tows after owner of company publicly supported opponent of incumbent mayor for election); Downtown Auto Parks, Inc. v. City of Milwaukee, 938 F.2d 705 (7th Cir. 1991) (holding that city may refuse to renew a parking lot lease with an independent contractor based upon that contractor's political affiliation); Horn v. Kean, 796 F.2d 668 (3d Cir. 1986) (holding that independent contractors whose contracts were terminated following a change in administration were not protected by the First Amendment). But see Umbehr v. McClure, 44 F.3d 876, 883 (10th Cir. 1995) (explicitly rejecting the reasoning of the Seventh and Third Circuits, concluding that "an independent contractor is protected under the First Amendment from retaliatory government action, just as an employee would be," and applying the *Pickering* test).

extended the doctrines of *Pickering* and of *Elrod* to apply to independent contractors. See Board of County Commissioners v. Umbehr, 518 U.S. 668 (1996), and O'Hare Truck Service, Inc. v. City of Northlake, 518 U.S. 712 (1996).

E. The Government's Management of Public Property: First Amendment Rights of Access and Use.

The movement of doctrine from *Davis v. Commonwealth* to *Hague v. CIO*, and subsequent general distinctions of "time, place, and manner," affecting first amendment rights of free speech. The emergence of "forum" analysis in lieu of time, place, and manner review.

To what extent may government restrict access and use of property under its own ownership or control? In the course of his dissent in *Board of Education v. Pico*,[45] Justice Rehnquist said the following:[46]

> Had petitioners been the members of a town council, I suppose all would agree that, absent a good deal more than is present in this record, they could not have prohibited the sale of these books by private booksellers within the municipality. But we have also recognized that the government may act in other capacities than as sovereign, and when it does the First Amendment may speak with a different voice:
>
> [I]t cannot be gainsaid that the State has interests as an employer in regulating the speech of its employees that differ significantly from those it possesses in connection with regulation of the speech of the citizenry in general. ***[47]
>
> By the same token, expressive conduct which may not be prohibited by the State as sovereign may be proscribed by the State *as property owner*: "*The State, <u>no less</u> than a private party has power to preserve the property under its control for the use to which it is lawfully dedicated.*"[48]

---

45. 457 U.S. 853 (1982) (school board removal of certain objectionable books from public school library) (the case is reproduced *supra* at p. 347).

46. 457 U.S. at 908.

47. (Quoting from *Pickering*).

48. (Quoting from the majority opinion in Adderley v. Florida, 385 U.S. 39, 47 (1966) (emphasis added) (five-to-four decision sustaining criminal trespass conviction of demonstrators within curtilage of a local jail, following request to leave the outside yard where the protestors had gathered to protest the arrest and confinement of others held in the jail, opinion by Justice Black concluding that a total bar of persons from the immediate external premises was all right under the first amendment, despite focused nature of the demonstration and lack of requirement that there be any actual threat to jail security by the particular demonstration).) See also Greer v. Spock, 424 U.S. 828 (1976) (divided decision, total ban on handbill distribution even at open intersection of vast military base, sustained). Cf. Brown v. Louisiana, 383 U.S. 131 (1966) (breach of peace conviction for standing inside public library anteroom

"*No* less than *** a *private* party?" But a private party could close his property entirely, or admit to its use only those whom it pleased himself so to do, pretty much at will. To what extent may government restrict access and use of property under public ownership, consistent with the first amendment?[49] *May* it do so as much as a private party may do with such property as such private party otherwise lawfully possesses?

Presumably a municipality may be under no original constitutional obligation to acquire land for a park or to commit such land as it may already hold to any particular local use—such as to provide some sort of public park. For that matter, neither a city nor a state may be under any constitutional duty to acquire private property by eminent domain to provide for sidewalks or streets. May a city, a state (or, for that matter, the federal government itself), upon undertaking to provide for parks, thoroughfares, public buildings, schools, military bases, etc., enact enforceable regulations carefully restricting the lawful uses of each solely to the lawfully dedicated, exactly specified, function of each? May it do so "*no less than a private party* has power" equivalently to do, in respect to such property as such private party might likewise own?[50]

For instance, may a municipality decide to bear the ownership and maintenance responsibilities to provide a public park exclusively as a *haven* within the community— for residents to stroll the pathways, to view the garden, to picnic in quiet places, to read poetry, to reflect, and to relax: a sheltered place away from the

---

as form of mute protest reversed). See also Tinker v. Des Moines Indep. Community School Dist., 393 U.S. 503 (1969) (armbands worn on public school premises held to be protected by first amendment).

49. May the question be affected somewhat by the equal protection clause, apart from the first amendment? That is, although the state need not provide public schools or public parks, and though admission to either may, in that original sense, be a "privilege" rather than a "right," still, once embarked on the venture, the state is then controlled by the equal protection clause in determining standards of admission and standards of treatment of those admitted. Will an equal protection analysis respond to all questions in this area? (E.g., if those who are Republicans or Democrats are permitted speech uses on public property, does equal protection require equal terms of use to those who are Nazis, Klan members, Communists, pedophiles, militant Shiite Muslims, etc.?) If the issue is approached solely through the equal protection clause, uninformed by the first amendment, which standard of substantive judicial review will be applied ("strict scrutiny" or "mere rationality" review)? Suppose, moreover, the public property at issue is not authorized for speech uses by anyone else (i.e. there is no favored group, person, or point of view extended speaking privileges but, rather, no political speech uses are allowed at all), on what basis will one attempt to mount an equal protection claim in such a case? (Equal protection jurisprudence usually requires the leverage of comparing one's less favored treatment with the more favored treatment of others, shifting the burden to the government to justify the disparity of treatment. *But if no one is favored, what then*?)

50. E.g., Busch Gardens outside Williamsburg, Virginia, or Sarah Duke Gardens, inside Duke University, Durham, North Carolina, each being private property neither owned nor managed under government auspices.

hurly-burly of business, of noise, of electioneering, of the cacophony of vendors, leafleteers, petition- circulators, itinerant ministers, political demonstrators, and the like? May it not do so, and, if not, *why* not?

Might the city council make provision solely for such speech presentations as might be conducted in moderate tones, on constructive subjects as in its view may be conducive to the general welfare of the local community (while declining to authorize any other speech presentations within the park)?[51] What constitutional clause or principle can plausibly be interposed against such decisions? Such is the general question we shall be reviewing, through the general case law, here.

Likewise in the case of a proposed street, the felt local need for a street (furnished or maintained at public expense) may be solely "to facilitate the more efficient movement of pedestrian and vehicular traffic from point A to point B," i.e. the facilitation of traffic and movement with more efficiency and with less congestion, inconvenience, and lost time occasioned by having to circumnavigate the area through which the proposed street is newly to be provided. No other uses are allowed.

May stationary assembly therefore be prohibited? May lingering also be prohibited, at least when not strictly incidental to getting from one end of the street to the other, or not incidental solely to the completion of such errands as one may have with such businesses, public offices, or homes, as may happen to grow up on this street? In short, may all uses other than those incidental to the use of the sidewalk and street as a passageway, whether through the area, or to-and-from public and private premises lawfully located along its way, be forbidden? Does the first amendment have anything to say about this?[52]

---

51. Recall that in Maher v. Roe, 432 U.S. 464 (1977), the Supreme Court sustained a state law providing Medicaid funds to reimburse low-income eligible women for the costs of childbirth, but not for the costs of low-income women electing nontherapeutic first trimester abortions. See also Harris v. McRae, 448 U.S. 297 (1980) (similar case sustaining a similar, more strict federal limitation on federal funds available for state Medicaid reimbursement). The rationale was that the act placed "no affirmative obstacle" in the path "of a woman's exercise of her freedom of choice," in leaving the woman electing an abortion to such private resources as she might (or might not) possess to exercise that choice. Will a similar rationale apply here? I.e. may tax funds or public property be made available to assist those whose speech is deemed constructive and a positive good (like subsidizing low income persons who choose childbirth vis-à-vis abortion) and not otherwise? Cf. Board of Educ. v. Pico, 457 U.S. 853 (1982) (the very function of public schools is, in part, to "inculcate" "community" values.)

52. May news vendors thus be forbidden to utilize the sidewalks and streets for hawking such newspapers as they seek to sell? May the sidewalks be kept clean by forbidding persons who neither have relevant errands nor an interest simply to pass through, to distribute political handbills or anything else, there? May fixed-in-place machines be forbidden from being installed (e.g., news vending machines)? (Cf. City of Lakewood v. Plain Dealer Pub. Co., 486 U.S. 750, 770-781 (1988) (dissenting opinion) ("The right to leaflet does not create a right to build a booth on city streets from which leafletting can be conducted.").) If, on the other hand, to defray the expenses of putting in and maintaining the streets, the city decides to auction street corner machine-installation space, may it do so? May it seek a higher price than it otherwise might hope to secure, by offering an exclusive license to the highest bidder (as a private business might do in leasing equivalent space inside a shopping mall),

Another property the municipality may own might be a civic center auditorium. Alternatively, it may merely be a line of utility poles edging residential or city streets. In rationing the possible uses of each of these, is public authority also entitled to "no less" than the full power a private party may exercise in respect to his equivalent private property (e.g., a privately-owned auditorium, a private company's own utility poles),[53] so far as the first amendment is concerned? Recall, too, from the *Tornillo* case, that what a private newspaper owner decides as appropriate editorial policy is virtually conclusive of what goes into that newspaper, i.e. that neither the first amendment requires—nor can any state generally require—such a newspaper to carry material it does not see fit to print. Is the same true of government when it operates not as regulator of private property uses (as Florida attempted to do in respect to the Miami Herald), but merely as owner of property itself?[54]

As one can see simply from these few casual examples, the questions raised here are far from obviously self-answering. Perhaps that ought not be a surprise. For aside from such early examples as the Post Office, the assumption of ownership and management responsibility by the public sector for other kinds of property (housing, for instance) is a relatively recent phenomenon. To what extent does the first amendment create—or not create—claims against government when it manages public property? Or, to frame the same question somewhat differently, to what extent may each kind of government managed property be some kind of "public forum" in fact? The answer, such as it is, tends to track a great deal of our earlier work.[55]

---

if it so elects? See Gerald Goldberger, A Reconsideration of Cox v. New Hampshire: Can Demonstrators Be Required to Pay the Costs of Using America's Public Forums?, 62 Tex.L.Rev. 403 (1983).

53. Consider, too, a common variation of a case of this sort where the utility poles along a public right of way are owned by a private utility company, but the company is also a state or local regulated service monopoly, subject to having its rates and business practices closely controlled by government agencies. To what extent: (a) may the private company be forbidden by government directive from using its own "property" (e.g., its utility poles) to post *its own* speech messages; (b) may the private company be required by government to permit third-party speech use of its utility poles; and (c) may the private company be required to yield such third-party access rights—to post speech notices on its poles—by force of the first amendment itself, even if not so required by government directive? (When does private property become a first amendment public forum of some sort?)

54. May it lawfully dedicate certain public property solely to the end of communicating its own views, for instance, excluding all replies, rebuttals, and other communications? Why not? Suppose a city decides to acquire its own cablevision company. Having once acquired the company, may the city put on exactly what it sees fit (as presumably the Miami Herald may do with its own newspaper pages)? For a general (useful but inconclusive) review, see Mark G. Yudof, When Government Speaks (1993); cf. Robert D. Kamenshine, The First Amendment's Implied Political Establishment Clause, 67 Cal. L.Rev. 1104 (1979). See also Steven H. Shiffrin, Government Speech, 27 UCLA L.Rev. 565 (1980).

55. For comprehensive critical review of the general subject, see Keith Werhan, The Supreme Court's Public Forum Doctrine and the Return of Formalism, 7 Cardozo L.Rev. 335 (1986). See also Ronald A. Cass, First Amendment Access to Government Facilities, 65 Va.L.Rev. 1287 (1979); Daniel A. Farber & John E. Nowak, The Misleading Nature of Public Forum Analysis: Content and Context in First Amendment Adjudication, 70 Va.L.Rev. 1219 (1984); R. Allan Hornung, The First Amendment Right to A Public Forum, 1969 Duke L.J. 931; Harry Kalven, The Concept of the Public Forum: Cox

I

The dictum by Justice Rehnquist (quoting from an earlier opinion by Justice Black) with which this section began, harkens back to the perspective of the very first case to be reviewed in the Supreme Court on this subject, in 1897. That case was *Davis v. Commonwealth.*[56] The *Davis* case was altogether contemporary with *Patterson v. Colorado*[57] and *McAuliffe v. Mayor of New Bedford,*[58] the two turn- of-the-century decisions authored by Justice Holmes, and prior to the opinions and dissents Holmes and Brandeis authored in the twenties, opinions and dissents that marked the first great movement in this country in the protection of freedom of speech. The *Davis* case treated restrictions on the speech-use of government-held property very much in the manner the Rehnquist dictum would even now suggest.

Davis, an itinerant minister, had been convicted of speaking in Boston Common without a permit as required by city ordinance.[59] Relying heavily on Justice Holmes's opinion in the Supreme Judicial Court of Massachusetts affirming Davis's conviction, a unanimous Supreme Court gave Davis's appeal very short shrift. In the Supreme Judicial Court of Massachusetts, this had been Holmes's dispositive view:[60]

> For the Legislature absolutely or conditionally to forbid public speaking in a highway or public park is no more an infringement of the rights of a member of the public *than for the owner of a private house* to forbid it in his house. When no proprietary right interferes, the Legislature may end the right of the public to enter upon the public place by putting an end to the dedication to public uses. *So it may take the lesser step of limiting the public use to certain purposes.*

Doing little more than to quote this portion of Justice Holmes's opinion (the whole report of the case in the Supreme Court is barely three pages), the Supreme Court unanimously affirmed.[61]

---

v. Louisiana, 1965 Sup.Ct.Rev. 1; Geoffrey R. Stone, Fora Americana: Speech in Public Places, 1974 Sup.Ct.Rev. 233; Shelia M. Cahill, Note, The Public Forum: Minimum Access, Equal Access, and the First Amendment, 28 Stan.L.Rev. 117 (1975).

56. 167 U.S. 43 (1897).

57. 205 U.S. 454 (1907). See *supra* p. 8.

58. 29 N.E. 517 (Mass. 1892). See *supra* p. 296.

59. The ordinance (see 39 N.E. at 113) provided: "No person shall, in or upon any of the public grounds, make any public address *** except in accordance with a permit from the mayor."

60. Commonwealth v. Davis, 39 N.E. 113 (1895) (emphasis added).

61. The Court made no more of Davis's separate objection that, assuming public addresses might be altogether forbidden in Boston Common, the ordinance did not do so but, rather, held out the possibility of such a use pursuant to a permit that the mayor was authorized to grant or deny seemingly at will. (167 U.S. at 48) ("The plaintiff in error cannot avail himself of the right granted by the state and yet obtain exemption from the lawful regulations to which this right on his part was subjected by law."). Subsequent cases have abandoned this branch of the *Davis* case; permit systems, to be constitutional (as a form of prior restraint), must minimally have: (a) clear substantive standards limiting the administrator's discretion to (b) tightly confined, valid grounds for disallowing the permit under specified cir-

In 1920 (shortly following the *Schenck* and *Abrams* Espionage Act cases from World War I), in contrast with *Davis*, Justice Holmes and Justice Brandeis dissented in a case involving the Postmaster General's revocation of second-class mailing privileges for a newspaper editorially promoting pro-German views, *The Milwaukee Leader*. The second-class rates denied the publisher—because of the content of his newspaper—were far lower than the third-class rates the *Leader* would have to pay were the revocation sustained. In fact, they were estimated to represent but one-sixth of the Post Office's estimated *actual* cost of carrying the kind of mail thus favored by this rate, i.e. the rates provided a heavily tax-subsidized advantage to newspapers delivered by mail. A majority of the Supreme Court sustained the Postmaster General's decision. Brandeis and Holmes dissented, albeit, technically, on statutory grounds.[62] Even so, Justice Brandeis expressed doubts about the constitutionality of

---

cumstances; (c) a virtually costless opportunity for a party denied a permit to secure immediate review of any adverse administrative decision, in (d) a regular adversary proceeding before a neutral party (e.g., a regular judge, rather than an administrator), in which proceeding (e) the burden rests with the state to sustain the denial of the permit (rather than the burden resting with the private party to show why it should not be sustained).

A permit system not complying with these standards need not be complied with and may, when a prosecution is brought for one's failure to have applied as required by the law, be attacked as void on its face. See also Lovell v. Griffin, 303 U.S. 444, 452-53 (1938) ("[A]s the ordinance is void on its face, it was not necessary for appellant to seek a permit under it. She was entitled to contest its validity in answer to the charge against her."); City of Lakewood v. Plain Dealer Pub. Co., 486 U.S. 750 (1988); Southeastern Promotions, Ltd. v. Conrad, 420 U.S. 546 (1975); Shuttlesworth v. Birmingham, 394 U.S. 147 (1969); Carroll v. President & Comm'rs, 393 U.S. 175 (1968); Staub v. Baxley, 355 U.S. 313 (1958); Kunz v. New York, 340 U.S. 290 (1951); Niemotko v. Maryland, 340 U.S. 268 (1951); Saia v. New York, 334 U.S. 558 (1948); Thomas v. Collins, 323 U.S. 516 (1945).

The exceptional first amendment requirements for (prior restraint) administrative permit systems, where permission turns on administrative discretion by officials who are likely to err on the side of avoiding blame for a demonstration or an address that might be disruptive or offensive, was anticipated even in Blackstone's Commentaries (vol. iv, p. 150 (1769)) on press licensing, as we noted earlier. ("To subject the press to the restrictive power of a licenser, as was formerly done, *** is to subject all freedom of sentiment to the prejudices of one man, and make him the arbitrary and infallible judge of all controverted points in learning, religion and government ***.") See also Bantam Books v. Sullivan, 372 U.S. 58 (1963) ("Any system of prior restraints of expression comes to this Court bearing a heavy presumption against its constitutional validity."); Freedman v. Maryland, 380 U.S. 51 (1965). But see other cases and discussion in Vincent A. Blasi, Prior Restraints on Demonstrations, 68 Mich.L.Rev. 1482 (1970). See also Vincent A. Blasi, Toward a Theory of Prior Restraint, 66 Minn.L.Rev. 11 (1981); Thomas L. Emerson, The Doctrine of Prior Restraint, 20 Law & Contemp.Probs. 648 (1955); Henry P. Monaghan, First Amendment "Due Process," 83 Harv. L.Rev. 518 (1970); Martin H. Redish, The Proper Role of the Prior Restraint Doctrine in First Amendment Theory, 70 Va.L.Rev. 53 (1984).

62. Recall that technically, in *Abrams v. United States*, the 1919 Espionage Act case in which Holmes wrote his principal dissent defending a robust standard of free speech protection under the first amendment, the dissent similarly first held that the acts for which Abrams was prosecuted were not, in its view, reached by the Espionage Act. The general rule of statutory interpretation where constitutional issues of a substantial nature would be raised if one view of the statute were taken but are fairly avoided under a different view of the statute itself, has frequently been pressed into service in first amendment cases, sometimes even when it has seemed to strain the words of the act in question at the time. See,

the Postmaster's actions along the following lines. Note the strong similarity of some of this passage to the development of the doctrine of unconstitutional conditions in the public status (employment) cases:[63]

> Congress may not through its postal police power put limitations upon the freedom of the press which if directly attempted would be unconstitutional. *** Government might, of course, decline altogether to distribute newspapers; or it might decline to carry any at less than the cost of the service; and it would not thereby abridge the freedom of the press, since to all papers other means of transportation would be left open. But to carry newspapers generally at a sixth of the cost of the service and to deny that service to one paper of the same general character, because to the Postmaster General views therein expressed in the past seem illegal, would prove an effective censorship and abridge seriously freedom of expression.

The dissent in *Burleson* is of a piece with the simultaneous emergence in the twenties of the stronger perspectives Brandeis and Holmes contributed to first amendment jurisprudence generally. It seems quite far from the view reflected in 1897 in *Davis v. Commonwealth.* Moreover, a dictum Holmes added in his concurrence to the Brandeis dissent in *Burleson* went a step further. "The United States," Holmes suggested, "may give up the Post Office when it sees fit, *but while it carries it on the use of the mails is almost as much a part of free speech as the right to use our tongues* ***."[64]

---

e.g., Yates v. United States, 354 U.S. 298 (1957) (follow-up case to *Dennis v. United States*, narrowly construing Smith Act to reach only active incitement of violence to overthrow government, despite statutory language making the teaching of the desirability of such action a felony). On the other hand, once the Court appears to have confronted and settled the first amendment controlling standard in what it may deem to be a clear and substantial fashion, there is sometimes less disposition to "save" a statute by interpreting it to hold that it does not, as sparingly interpreted, violate that standard. An excellent example is United States v. Robel, 389 U.S. 258 (1967). For an excellent general discussion of the point, see Gerald Gunther, Reflections on Robel: It's Not What the Court Did But the Way It Did It, 20 Stan.L.Rev. 1140 (1968).

63. U.S. ex rel. Milwaukee Publishing Co. v. Burleson, 255 U.S. 407, 430-431 (1920). See also Hannegan v. Esquire, Inc., 327 U.S. 146 (1946) (finding no statutory discretion for the Postmaster General to revoke second class mailing privileges of Esquire Magazine). In *Hannegan*, the Postmaster General had acted pursuant to his view that the statute's second class mailing advantage (a stipulated $500,000 advantage or annual indirect subsidy) was limited to such magazines as might "contribute to the public good and the public welfare." In his view, Esquire ("The Magazine for Men") was *not* such a magazine, given Esquire's "dominant tone" ("smoking-room type of humor, featuring, in the main, sex," which some witnesses regarded as "highly objectionable, calling [it] salacious and indecent"). The Court construed the statute narrowly, because "grave constitutional questions are immediately raised once it is said that the uses of the mails is a privilege which may be extended or withheld on any grounds whatsoever." 327 U.S. at 156, citing to Brandeis and Holmes in *Burleson.*

64. 255 U.S. at 437 (Holmes, J., dissenting) (emphasis added).

But if use of the mails actually *were* regarded as "almost as much a part of free speech as the right to *use our tongues*," as Holmes suggests, note the difference it would at once make in the relevant legal standard in measuring the terms of access and use of the mails. Presumably, restrictions on using the mails would have to satisfy first amendment standards not significantly different from those that apply to the right to use "our tongues."[65] In 1939, as the following case shows, this idea began to take hold in a more general way.[66]

HAGUE v. COMMITTEE FOR INDUSTRIAL ORGANIZATION
307 U.S. 496 (1939)

MR. JUSTICE ROBERTS delivered an opinion in which MR. JUSTICE BLACK concurred.

***

The bill alleges that respondents have repeatedly applied for permits to hold public meetings in the city for the stated purpose, as required by ordinance,[1] the petitioners have consistently refused to issue any permits for meetings to be held by, or sponsored by, respondents, and have thus prevented the holding of such meetings; that the respondents did not, and do not, propose to advocate the destruction or overthrow of the Government of the United States, or that of New Jersey, but that their sole purpose is to explain to workingmen the purposes of the National Labor Relations Act, the benefits to be derived from it, and the aid which the Committee for Industrial Organization would furnish workingmen to that end.

---

65. See Lamont v. Postmaster Gen., 381 U.S. 301 (1965) (relying on Holmes dictum and holding unconstitutional statute requiring post office to detain and destroy unsealed mail, from foreign countries, determined to be communist propaganda unless addressee affirmatively indicated desire to receive such mail). Cf. Rowan v. Post Office Dept., 397 U.S. 728 (1970) (federal statute forbidding mailings to homeowners filing notice with Post Office of desire not to receive certain mail they, not the Post Office, deem undesirable, sustained).

66. For a comprehensive review, see John H. Gibbons, Hague v. CIO: A Retrospective, 52 N.Y.U.L.Rev. 731 (1977).

1. "The Board of Commissioners of Jersey City Do Ordain:

"1. From and after the passage of this ordinance, no public parades or public assembly in or upon the public streets, highways, public parks or public buildings of Jersey City shall take place or be conducted until a permit shall be obtained from the Director of Public Safety. ***

"3. The Director of Public Safety is hereby authorized to refuse to issue said permit when, after investigation of all of the facts and circumstances pertinent to said application, he believes it to be proper to refuse the issuance thereof; provided, however, that said permit shall only be refused for the purpose of preventing riots, disturbances or disorderly assemblage.

"4. Any person or persons violating any of the provisions of this ordinance shall upon conviction before a police magistrate of the City of Jersey City be punished by a fine not exceeding two hundred dollars or imprisonment in the Hudson County jail for a period not exceeding ninety days or both."

The bill charges that the ordinances are unconstitutional and void, or are being enforced against respondents in an unconstitutional and discriminatory way; and that the petitioners, as officials of the city, purporting to act under the ordinances, have deprived respondents of the privileges of free speech and peaceable assembly secured to them, as citizens of the United States, by the Fourteenth Amendment. It prays an injunction against continuance of petitioners' conduct. ***

The findings are that the petitioners, as officials, have adopted and enforced a deliberate policy of forbidding the respondents and their associates from communicating their views respecting the National Labor Relations Act to the citizens of Jersey City by holding meetings or assemblies in the open air and at public places; that there is no competent proof that the proposed speakers have ever spoken at an assembly where a breach of the peace occurred or at which any utterances were made which violated the canons of proper discussion or gave occasion for disorder consequent upon what was said; that there is no competent proof that the parks of Jersey City are dedicated to any general purpose other than the recreation of the public and that there is competent proof that the municipal authorities have granted permits to various persons other than the respondents to speak at meetings in the streets of the city.***

The question now presented is whether freedom to disseminate information concerning the provisions of the National Labor Relations Act, to assemble peaceably for discussion of the Act, and of the opportunities and advantages offered by it, is a privilege or immunity of a citizen of the United States secured against State abridgment by § 1 of the Fourteenth Amendment; and whether R.S. 1979 and § 24 (14) of the Judicial Code afford redress in a federal court for such abridgment. This is the narrow question presented by the record, and we confine our decision to it, without consideration of broader issues which the parties urge.***

Although it has been held that the Fourteenth Amendment created no rights in citizens of the United States, but merely secured existing rights against state abridgment, it is clear that the right peaceably to assemble and to discuss these topics, and to communicate respecting them, whether orally or in writing, is a privilege inherent in citizenship of the United States which the Amendment protects. *** Natural persons, and they alone, are entitled to the privileges and immunities which § 1 of the Fourteenth Amendment secures for "citizens of the United States." Only the individual respondents may, therefore, maintain this suit.

*** What has been said demonstrates that, in the light of the facts found, privileges and immunities of the individual respondents as citizens of the United States, were infringed by the petitioners, by virtue of their official positions, under color of ordinances of Jersey City, unless, as petitioners contend, the city's ownership of streets and parks is as absolute as one's ownership of his home, with consequent power altogether to exclude citizens from the use thereof, or unless, though the city holds the streets in trust for public use, the absolute denial of their use to the respondents is a valid exercise of the police power. In support of the former the petitioners rely upon *Davis v. Massachusetts*, 167 U. S. 43.

The decision seems to be grounded on the holding of the State court that the Common "was absolutely under the control of the legislature," and that it was thus "conclusively determined there was no right in the plaintiff in error to use the common except in such mode and subject to such regulations as the legislature, in its wisdom, may have deemed proper to prescribe."

We have no occasion to determine whether, on the facts disclosed, the *Davis* case was rightly decided, but we cannot agree that it rules the instant case. Wherever the title of streets and parks may rest, they have immemorially been held in trust for the use of the public and, time out of mind, have been used for purposes of assembly, communicating thoughts between citizens, and discussing public questions. Such use of the streets and public places has, from ancient times, been a part of the privileges, immunities, rights, and liberties of citizens. The privilege of a citizen of the United States to use the streets and parks for communication of views on national questions may be regulated in the interest of all; it is not absolute, but relative, and must be exercised in subordination to the general comfort and convenience, and in consonance with peace and good order; but it must not, in the guise of regulation, be abridged or denied.

We think the court below was right in holding the ordinance quoted in Note 1 void upon its face. It does not make comfort or convenience in the use of streets or parks the standard of official action. It enables the Director of Safety to refuse a permit on his mere opinion that such refusal will prevent "riots, disturbances or disorderly assemblage." It can thus, as the record discloses, be made the instrument of arbitrary suppression of free expression of views on national affairs for the prohibition of all speaking will undoubtedly "prevent" such eventualities. But uncontrolled official suppression of the privilege cannot be made a substitute for the duty to maintain order in connection with the exercise of the right.

Although the court below held the ordinance void, the decree enjoins the petitioners as to the manner in which they shall administer it. We think this is wrong. As the ordinance is void, the respondents are entitled to a decree so declaring and an injunction against its enforcement by the petitioners. They are free to hold meetings without a permit and without regard to the terms of the void ordinance. The courts cannot rewrite the ordinance, as the decree, in effect, does.

MR. JUSTICE STONE:

I do not doubt that the decree below, modified as has been proposed, is rightly affirmed, but I am unable to follow the path by which some of my brethren have attained that end, and I think the matter is of sufficient importance to merit discussion in some detail.

It has been explicitly and repeatedly affirmed by this Court, without a dissenting voice, that freedom of speech and of assembly for any lawful purpose are rights of personal liberty secured to all persons, without regard to citizenship, by the due process clause of the Fourteenth Amendment. ***

No more grave and important issue can be brought to this Court than that of freedom of speech and assembly, which the due process clause guarantees to all persons regardless of their citizenship, but which the privileges and immunities clause secures only to citizens, and then only to the limited extent that their relationship to the national government is affected. I am unable to rest decision here on the assertion, which I think the record fails to support, that respondents must depend upon their limited privileges as citizens of the United States in order to sustain their cause, or upon so palpable an avoidance of the real issue in the case, which respondents have raised by their pleadings and sustained by their proof. *** I think respondents' right to maintain it does not depend on their citizenship and cannot rightly be made to turn on the existence or non-existence of a purpose to disseminate information about the National Labor Relations Act. It is enough that petitioners have prevented respondents from holding meetings and disseminating information whether for the organization of labor unions or for any other lawful purpose. ***

SCHNEIDER v. STATE
308 U.S. 147 (1939)

MR. JUSTICE ROBERTS delivered the opinion of the Court.

Four cases are here, each of which presents the question whether regulations embodied in a municipal ordinance abridge the freedom of speech and of the press secured against state invasion by the Fourteenth Amendment of the Constitution.

No. 13

The Municipal Code of the City of Los Angeles, 1936, provides:

> "Sec. 28.00. 'Hand-Bill' shall mean any hand-bill, dodger, commercial advertising circular, folder, booklet, letter, card, pamphlet, sheet, poster, sticker, banner, notice or other written, printed or painted matter calculated to attract attention of the public."
>
> "Sec. 28.01. No person shall distribute any hand-bill to or among pedestrians along or upon any street, sidewalk or park, or to passengers on any street car, or throw, place or attach any hand-bill in, to, or upon any automobile or other vehicle."

The appellant was charged in the Municipal Court with a violation of § 28.01. Upon his trial it was proved that he distributed handbills to pedestrians on a public sidewalk and had more than three hundred in his possession for that purpose. Judgment of conviction was entered and sentence imposed. The Superior Court of Los Angeles County affirmed the judgment. The hand-bill which the appellant was distributing bore a notice of a meeting to be held under the auspices of "Friends of Lincoln Brigade" at which speakers would discuss the war in Spain.

The court below sustained the validity of the ordinance on the ground that experience shows littering of the streets results from the indiscriminate distribution of handbills.[3] It held that the right of free expression is not absolute but subject to reasonable regulation and that the ordinance does not transgress the bounds of reasonableness. ***

No. 18

An ordinance of the City of Milwaukee, Wisconsin, provides: "It is hereby made unlawful for any person ***to *** throw *** paper *** or to circulate or distribute any circular, handbills, cards, posters, dodgers, or other printed or advertising matter *** in or upon any sidewalk, street, alley, wharf, boat landing, dock or other public place, park or ground within the City of Milwaukee ***."

The petitioner, who was acting as a picket, stood in the street in front of a meat market and distributed to passing pedestrians handbills which pertained to a labor dispute with the meat market, set forth the position of organized labor with respect to the market, and asked citizens to refrain from patronizing it. Some of the bills were thrown in the street by the persons to whom they were given and it resulted that many of the papers lay in the gutter and in the street. The police officers who arrested the petitioner and charged him with a violation of the ordinance did not arrest any of those who received the bills and threw them away. The testimony was that the action of the officers accorded with a policy of the police department in enforcement of the ordinance to the effect that, when such distribution resulted in littering of the streets the one who was the cause of the littering, that is, he who passed out the bills, was arrested rather than those who received them and afterwards threw them away. The Milwaukee County court found the petitioner guilty and fined him. On appeal the judgment was affirmed by the Supreme Court.

The court held that the purpose of the ordinance was to prevent an unsightly, untidy, and offensive condition of the sidewalks. ***

---

3. On the hand-bill were the words "Admission 25¢ and 50¢." The Superior Court adverted to these and said: "Whatever traffic in ideas the Friends Lincoln Brigade may have planned for the meeting, the cards themselves seem to fall within the classification of commercial advertising rather than the expression of one's views. But if this be so, our conclusion is not thereby changed."

No. 29

An ordinance of the City of Worcester, Massachusetts, provides: "No person shall distribute in, or place upon any street or way, any placard, handbill, flyer, poster, advertisement or paper of any description.***"

The appellants distributed in a street leaflets announcing a protest meeting in connection with the administration of state unemployment insurance. They did not throw any of the leaflets on the sidewalk or scatter them. Some of those to whom the leaflets were handed threw them on the sidewalk and the street, with the result that some thirty were lying about.

The appellants were arrested and charged with a violation of the ordinance. The Superior Court of Worcester County rendered a judgment of conviction and imposed sentence. *** Referring to the ordinance the court said: "It interferes in no way with the publication of anything in the city of Worcester, except only that it excludes the public streets and ways from the places available for free distribution. It leaves open such distribution all other places in the city, public and private." ***

This court has characterized the freedom of speech and that of the press as fundamental personal rights and liberties. The phrase is not an empty one and was not lightly used. It reflects the belief of the framers of the Constitution that exercise of the rights lies at the foundation of free government by free men. It stresses, as do many opinions of this court, the importance of preventing the restriction of enjoyment of these liberties.

In every case, therefore, where legislative abridgment of the rights is asserted, the courts should be astute to examine the effect of the challenged legislation. Mere legislative preferences or beliefs respecting matters of public convenience may well support regulation directed at other personal activities, but be insufficient to justify such as diminishes the exercise of rights so vital to the maintenance of democratic institutions. And so, cases arise, the delicate and difficult task falls upon the courts to weigh the circumstances and to appraise the substantiality of the reasons advanced in support of the regulation of the free enjoyment of the rights. ***

The motive of the legislation under attack in Numbers 13, 18, and 29 is held by the courts below to be the prevention of littering of the streets and, although the alleged offenders were not charged with themselves scattering paper in the streets, their convictions were sustained upon the theory that distribution by them encouraged or resulted in such littering. We are of opinion that the purpose to keep the streets clean and of good appearance is insufficient to justify an ordinance which prohibits a person rightfully on a public street from handing literature to one willing to receive it. Any burden imposed upon the city authorities in cleaning and caring for the streets as an indirect consequence of such distribution results from the constitutional protection of the freedom of speech and press. This constitutional protection does not deprive a city of all power to prevent street littering. There are obvious methods of preventing littering. Amongst these is the punishment of those who actually throw papers on the street.

It is argued that the circumstance that in the actual enforcement of the Milwaukee ordinance the distributor is arrested only if those who receive the literature throw it in the streets, renders it valid. But, even as thus construed, the ordinance cannot be enforced without unconstitutionally abridging the liberty of free speech. As we have pointed out, the public convenience in respect of cleanliness of the streets does not justify an exertion of the police power which invades the free communication of information and opinion secured by the Constitution.

It is suggested that the Los Angeles and Worcester ordinances are valid because their operation is limited to streets and alleys and leaves persons free to distribute printed matter in other public places. But, as we have said, the streets are natural and proper places for the dissemination of information and opinion; and one is not to have the exercise of his liberty of expression in appropriate places abridged on the plea that it may be exercised in some other place. ***

The judgment in each case is reversed and the causes are remanded for further proceedings not inconsistent with this opinion.

Reversed.

MR. JUSTICE MCREYNOLDS is of opinion that the judgment in each case should be affirmed.

NOTE

Hague, *Schneider*, and similar cases suggest that to some extent the first amendment creates a tentative free speech easement of access and use in certain kinds of publicly-owned property, at least for politically-related speech, and perhaps for some other kinds (e.g., religiously-impelled speech) as well. These cases appear also to reject exclusionary rationales based on public interest claims that the avoidance of certain costs, disruptions, and other minor harms is a sufficient ground to disallow certain kinds of proposed uses of publicly-held property. (E.g., the Court in *Schneider* concedes that punishing only those who throw leaflets into the streets might not keep the sidewalks and streets free of litter as efficiently as would forbidding the distribution of leaflets in the first place.)

How far do these new kinds of first amendment protections extend? And if they extend in some measure to other sorts of publicly-held property, do they extend there with the same, rather full measure of protection as in streets, parks, and sidewalks, or are they subject to greater restriction the less "traditional" the nature of the "public forum" may chance to be? Note, incidentally, that these kinds of forums, such as they are, are sometimes all that some groups and individuals (for example, those lacking extensive private property holdings) may have. Is it arguable, moreover, that *whenever* and *wherever* it is *public* property, the burden does not rest with the free speech user to show some legal entitlement other than the first amendment itself to use that property to communicate his or her message? That the burden, rather, is on government at all times to justify the kind of restriction it has presumed to impose, or else to step aside—a burden, moreover, (again as illustrated in the *Schneider* decision) with a bite?

As to what kind of restriction(s) may or may not be sustainable, the following several cases, decided together in the Supreme Court, may furnish some further clues.[68]

---

2. Time, Place, and Manner Regulation

KUNZ v. NEW YORK

340 U.S. 290 (1951)

MR. CHIEF JUSTICE VINSON delivered the opinion of the Court.

New York City has adopted an ordinance which makes it unlawful to hold public worship meetings on the streets without first obtaining a permit from the city police commissioner. Appellant, Carl Jacob Kunz, was convicted and fined $10 for violating this ordinance by holding a religious meeting without a permit. The conviction was affirmed by the Appellate Part of the Court of Special Sessions, and by the New York Court of Appeals, three judges dissenting. The case is here on appeal, it having been urged that the ordinance is invalid under the Fourteenth Amendment.

Appellant is an ordained Baptist minister who speaks under the auspices of the "Outdoor Gospel Work," of which he is the director. He has been preaching for about six years, and states that it is his conviction and duty to "go out on the highways and byways and preach the word of God." In 1946, he applied for and received a permit under the ordinance in question, there being no question that appellant comes within the classes of persons entitled to receive permits under the ordinance.[2] This permit, like all others, was good only for the calendar year in which issued. In November, 1946, his permit was revoked after a hearing by the police commissioner. The revocation was based on evidence that he had ridiculed and denounced other religious beliefs in his meetings. ***

Although the penalties of the ordinance apply to anyone who "ridicules and denounces other religious beliefs," the ordinance does not specify this as a ground

---

68. See also Cohen v. California, 403 U.S. 15 (1971); Tinker v. Des Moines Indep. School Dist., 393 U.S. 503 (1969), each of which in several respects previewed the first amendment considerations once again at work here as well, and each of which postdates the following cases from the Supreme Court.

2. The New York Court of Appeals has construed the ordinance to require that all initial requests for permits by eligible applicants must be granted.

for permit revocation. Indeed, there is no mention in the ordinance of any power of revocation. However, appellant did not seek judicial or administrative review of the revocation proceedings, and any question as to the propriety of the revocation is not before us in this case. In any event, the revocation affected appellant's rights to speak in 1946 only. Appellant applied for another permit in 1947, and again in 1948, but was notified each time that his application was "disapproved," with no reason for the disapproval being given. On September 11, 1948, appellant was arrested for speaking at Columbus Circle in New York City without a permit. It is from the conviction which resulted that this appeal has been taken.

Appellant's conviction was thus based upon his failure to possess a permit for 1948. We are here concerned only with the propriety of the action of the police commissioner in refusing to issue that permit. Disapproval of the 1948 permit application by the police commissioner was justified by the New York courts on the ground that a permit had previously been revoked "for good reasons."[3] It is noteworthy that there is no mention in the ordinance of reasons for which such a permit application can be refused. This interpretation allows the police commissioner, an administrative official, to exercise discretion in denying subsequent permit applications on the basis of his interpretation, at that time, of what is deemed to be conduct condemned by the ordinance. We have here, then, an ordinance which gives an administrative official discretionary power to control in advance the right of citizens to speak on religious matters on the streets of New York. As such, the ordinance is clearly invalid as a prior restraint on the exercise of First Amendment rights. ***

*** We do not express any opinion on the propriety of punitive remedies which the New York authorities may utilize. We are here concerned with suppression—not punishment. It is sufficient to say that New York cannot vest restraining control over the right to speak on religious subjects in an administrative official where there are no appropriate standards to guide his action.*

Reversed.

MR. JUSTICE BLACK concurs in the result. ***

MR. JUSTICE JACKSON, dissenting. ***

I

To know what we are doing, we must first locate the point at which rights asserted by Kunz conflict with powers asserted by the organized community. New York City has placed no limitation upon any speech Kunz may choose to make on private property, but it does require a permit to hold religious meetings in its streets.

3. The New York Court of Appeals said: "The commissioner had no reason to assume, and no promise was made, that defendant wanted a new permit for any uses different from the disorderly ones he had been guilty of before." 90 N.E. 2d at 457.

*. [**Ed. Note**. See also Lakewood v. Plain Dealer Publishing Co., 486 U.S. 750 (1988) (confirming that permit requirements lacking narrowly tailored criteria are void on their face, when a general prohibition would be sustained).]

The ordinance, neither by its terms nor as it has been applied, prohibited Kunz, even in street meetings, from preaching his own religion or making any temperate criticism or refutation of other religions; indeed, for the year 1946, he was given a general permit to do so. His meetings, however, brought "a flood of complaints" to city authorities that he was engaging in scurrilous attacks on Catholics and Jews. On notice, he was given a hearing at which eighteen complainants appeared. The Commissioner revoked his permit and applications for 1947 and 1948 were refused. For a time he went on holding meetings without a permit in Columbus Circle, where in September, 1948, he was arrested for violation of the ordinance. He was convicted and fined ten dollars.

At these meetings, Kunz preached, among many other things of like tenor, that "The Catholic Church makes merchandise out of souls," that Catholicism is "a religion of the devil," and that the Pope is "the anti-Christ." The Jews he denounced as "Christ-killers," and he said of them, "All the garbage that didn't believe in Christ should have been burnt in the incinerators. It's a shame they all weren't."

II-III

This Court today initiates the doctrine that language such as this, in the environment of the street meeting, is immune from prior municipal control. We would have a very different question if New York had presumed to say that Kunz could not speak his piece in his own pulpit or hall. But it has undertaken to restrain him only if he chooses to speak at street meetings. There is a world of difference. The street preacher takes advantage of people's presence on the streets to impose his message upon what, in a sense, is a captive audience. A meeting on private property is made up of an audience that has volunteered to listen. The question, therefore, is not whether New York could, if it tried, silence Kunz, but whether it must place its streets at his service to hurl insults at the passer-by. ***

These terse epithets come down to our generation weighted with hatreds accumulated through centuries of bloodshed. They are recognized words of art in the profession of defamation. They are not the kind of insult that men bandy and laugh off when the spirits are high and the flagons are low. They are not in that class of epithets whose literal sting will be drawn if the speaker smiles when he uses them. They are always, and in every context, insults which do not spring from reason and can be answered by none. Their historical associations with violence are well understood, both by those who hurl and those who are struck by these missiles. Jews, many of whose families perished in extermination furnaces of Dachau and Auschwitz, are more than tolerant if they pass off lightly the suggestion that unbelievers in Christ should all have been burned. Of course, people might pass this speaker by as a mental case, and so they might file out of a theatre in good order at the cry of "fire." But in both cases there is genuine likelihood that someone will get hurt. ***

The Court of Appeals did not treat the ordinance as existing in a vacuum but considered all the facts of the controversy. While it construed the ordinance "as *re-*

quiring the commissioner to give an annual permit for street preaching, *to anyone* who, like defendant, is a minister of religion," 90 N.E. 2d 455, 456 (emphasis supplied), it held on the facts that when, as here, the applicant "claims a constitutional right to incite riots, and a constitutional right to the services of policemen to quell those riots," then a permit need not be issued. Id. at 457. ***

IV

***

Of course, as to the press, there are the best of reasons against any licensing or prior restraint. Decisions such as *Near v. Minnesota* hold any licensing or prior restraint of the press unconstitutional, and I heartily agree. But precedents from that field cannot reasonably be transposed to the street-meeting field. The impact of publishing on public order has no similarity with that of a street meeting. Publishing does not make private use of public property. It reaches only those who choose to read, and, in that way, is analogous to a meeting held in a hall where those who come do so by choice. Written words are less apt to incite or provoke to mass action than spoken words, speech being the primitive and direct communication with the emotions. Few are the riots caused by publication alone, few are the mobs that have not had their immediate origin in harangue. The vulnerability of various forms of communication to community control must be proportioned to their impact upon other community interests.

It is suggested that a permit for a street meeting could be required if the ordinance would prescribe precise standards for its grant or denial.***

Of course, standards for administrative action are always desirable, and the more exact the better. But I do not see how this Court can condemn municipal ordinances for not setting forth comprehensive First Amendment standards. This Court never has announced what those standards must be, it does not now say what they are, and it is not clear that any majority could agree on them. *** It seems hypercritical to strike down local laws on their faces for want of standards when we have no standards. And I do not find it required by existing authority. I think that where speech is outside of constitutional immunity the local community or the State is left a large measure of discretion as to the means for dealing with it. ***

FEINER v. NEW YORK

340 U.S. 315 (1951)

MR. CHIEF JUSTICE VINSON delivered the opinion of the Court.

Petitioner was convicted of the offense of disorderly conduct, a misdemeanor under the New York penal laws, in the Court of Special Sessions of the City of Syracuse and was sentenced to thirty days in the county penitentiary. The conviction was affirmed by the Onondaga County Court and the New York Court of Appeals. The case is here on certiorari, petitioner having claimed that the conviction is in violation of his right of free speech under the Fourteenth Amendment. ***

On the evening of March 8, 1949, petitioner Irving Feiner was addressing an open-air meeting at the corner of South McBride and Harrison Streets in the City of Syracuse. At approximately 6:30 p.m., the police received a telephone complaint concerning the meeting, and two officers were detailed to investigate. One of these officers went to the scene immediately, the other arriving some twelve minutes later. They found a crowd of about seventy-five or eighty people, both Negro and white, filling the sidewalk and spreading out into the street. Petitioner, standing on a large wooden box on the sidewalk, was addressing the crowd through a loud-speaker system attached to an automobile. Although the purpose of his speech was to urge his listeners to attend a meeting to be held that night in the Syracuse Hotel, in its course he was making derogatory remarks concerning President Truman, the American Legion, the Mayor of Syracuse, and other local political officials.

The police officers made no effort to interfere with petitioner's speech, but were first concerned with the effect of the crowd on both pedestrian and vehicular traffic. They observed the situation from the opposite side of the street, noting that some pedestrians were forced to walk in the street to avoid the crowd. Since traffic was passing at the time, the officers attempted to get the people listening to petitioner back on the sidewalk. The crowd was restless and there was some pushing, shoving and milling around. One of the officers telephoned the police station from a nearby store, and then both policemen crossed the street and mingled with the crowd without any intention of arresting the speaker.

At this time, petitioner was speaking in a "loud, high-pitched voice." He gave the impression that he was endeavoring to arouse the Negro people against the whites, urging that they rise up in arms and fight for equal rights. The statements before such a mixed audience "stirred up a little excitement." Some of the onlookers made remarks to the police about their inability to handle the crowd and at least one threatened violence if the police did not act. There were others who appeared to be favoring petitioner's arguments. Because of the feeling that existed in the crowd both for and against the speaker, the officers finally "stepped in to prevent it from resulting in a fight." One of the officers approached the petitioner, not for the purpose of arresting him, but to get him to break up the crowd. He asked petitioner to get down off the box, but the latter refused to accede to his request and continued talking. The officer waited for a minute and then demanded that he cease talking. Although the officer had thus twice requested petitioner to stop over the course of several minutes, petitioner not only ignored him but continued talking. During all this time, the crowd was pressing closer around petitioner and the officer. Finally, the officer told petitioner he was under arrest and ordered him to get down from the box, reaching up to grab him. Petitioner stepped down, announcing over the microphone that "the law has arrived, and I suppose they will take over now." In all, the officer had asked petitioner to get down off the box three times over a space of four or five minutes. Petitioner had been speaking for over a half hour.

On these facts, petitioner was specifically charged with violation of § 722 of the Penal Law of New York ***. The bill of particulars, demanded by petitioner and furnished by the State, gave in detail the facts upon which the prosecution relied to support the charge of disorderly conduct. Paragraph C is particularly pertinent here: "By ignoring and refusing to heed and obey reasonable police orders issued at the time and place mentioned in the Information to regulate and control said crowd and to prevent a breach or breaches of the peace and to prevent injury to pedestrians attempting to use said walk, and being forced into the highway adjacent to the place in question, and prevent injury to the public generally."

We are not faced here with blind condonation by a state court of arbitrary police action. Petitioner was accorded a full, fair trial. The trial judge heard testimony supporting and contradicting the judgment of the police officers that a clear danger of disorder was threatened. After weighing this contradictory evidence, the trial judge reached the conclusion that the police officers were justified in taking action to prevent a breach of the peace. The exercise of the police officers' proper discretionary power to prevent a breach of the peace was thus approved by the trial court and later by two courts on review.[2] The courts below recognized petitioner's right to hold a street meeting at this locality, to make use of loud-speaking equipment in giving his speech, and to make derogatory remarks concerning public officials and the American Legion. They found that the officers in making the arrest were motivated solely by a proper concern for the preservation of order and protection of the general welfare, and that there was no evidence which could lend color to a claim that the acts of the police were a cover for suppression of petitioner's views and opinions. Petitioner was thus neither arrested nor convicted for the making or the content of his speech. Rather, it was the reaction which it actually engendered.

*** The findings of the New York courts as to the condition of the crowd and the refusal of petitioner to obey the police requests, supported as they are by the record of this case, are persuasive that the conviction of petitioner for violation of public peace, order and authority does not exceed the bounds of proper state police action. This Court respects, as it must, the interest of the community in maintaining peace and order on its streets. We cannot say that the preservation of that interest here encroaches on the constitutional rights of this petitioner.

---

2. The New York Court of Appeals said: "An imminent danger of a breach of the peace, of a disturbance of public order, perhaps even of riot, was threatened. *** The defendant, as indicated above, disrupted pedestrian and vehicular traffic on the sidewalk and street, and, with intent to provoke a breach of the peace and with knowledge of the consequences, so inflamed and agitated a mixed audience of sympathizers and opponents that, in the judgment of the police officers present, a clear danger of disorder and violence was threatened. Defendant then deliberately refused to accede to the reasonable request of the officer, made within the lawful scope of his authority, that the defendant desist in the interest of public welfare and safety."

We are well aware that the ordinary murmurings and objections of a hostile audience cannot be allowed to silence a speaker, and are also mindful of the possible danger of giving overzealous police officials complete discretion to break up otherwise lawful public meetings. "A State may not unduly suppress free communication of views, religious or other, under the guise of conserving desirable conditions." But we are not faced here with such a situation. It is one thing to say that the police cannot be used as an instrument for the suppression of unpopular views, and another to say that, when as here the speaker passes the bounds of argument or persuasion and undertakes incitement to riot, they are powerless to prevent a breach of the peace. Nor in this case can we condemn the considered judgment of three New York courts approving the means which the police, faced with a crisis, used in the exercise of their power and duty to preserve peace and order. The findings of the state courts as to the existing situation and the imminence of greater disorder coupled with petitioner's deliberate defiance of the police officers convince us that we should not reverse this conviction in the name of free speech.

Affirmed.

MR. JUSTICE BLACK, dissenting.

The record before us convinces me that petitioner, a young college student, has been sentenced to the penitentiary for the unpopular views he expressed on matters of public interest while lawfully making a street-corner speech in Syracuse, New York.[2] Today's decision, however, indicates that we must blind ourselves to this fact because the trial judge fully accepted the testimony of the prosecution witnesses on all important points.***

The Court's opinion apparently rests on this reasoning: The policeman, under the circumstances detailed, could reasonably conclude that serious fighting or even riot was imminent; therefore he could stop petitioner's speech to prevent a breach of peace; accordingly, it was "disorderly conduct" for petitioner to continue speaking in disobedience of the officer's request. As to the existence of a dangerous situation on the street corner, it seems far-fetched to suggest that the "facts" show any imminent threat of riot or uncontrollable disorder. It is neither unusual nor unexpected that some people at public street meetings mutter, mill about, push, shove, or disagree, even violently, with the speaker. Indeed, it is rare where controversial topics

---

2. There was no charge that any city or state law prohibited such a meeting at the place or time it was held. Evidence showed that it was customary to hold public gatherings on that same corner every Friday night, and the trial judge who convicted petitioner admitted that he understood the meeting was a lawful one. Nor did the judge treat the lawful meeting as unlawful because a crowd congregated on the sidewalk. Consequently, any discussion of disrupted pedestrian and vehicular traffic, while suggestive coloration, is immaterial under the charge and conviction here. It is implied in a concurring opinion that the use of sound amplifiers in some way caused the meeting to become less lawful. This fact, however, had nothing to do with the conviction of petitioner. In sentencing him the trial court said: "You had a perfect right to appear there and to use that implement, the loud speaker. You had a right to have it in the street." ***

are discussed that an outdoor crowd does not do some or all of these things. Nor does one isolated threat to assault the speaker forebode disorder. Especially should the danger be discounted where, as here, the person threatening was a man whose wife and two small children accompanied him and who, so far as the record shows, was never close enough to petitioner to carry out the threat.

Moreover, assuming that the "facts" did indicate a critical situation, I reject the implication of the Court's opinion that the police had no obligation to protect petitioner's constitutional right to talk. The police of course have power to prevent breaches of the peace. But if, in the name of preserving order, they ever can interfere with a lawful public speaker, they first must make all reasonable efforts to protect him.[8] Here the policemen did not even pretend to try to protect petitioner. *** Their duty was to protect petitioner's right to talk, even to the extent of arresting the man who threatened to interfere.[9] Instead, they shirked that duty and acted only to suppress the right to speak. ***

In this case I would reverse the conviction, thereby adhering to the great principles of the First and Fourteenth Amendments as announced for this Court in 1940 by Mr. Justice Roberts:

> "In the realm of religious faith, and in that of political belief, sharp differences arise. In both fields the tenets of one man may seem the rankest error to his neighbor. To persuade others to his own point of view, the pleader, as we know, at times, resorts to exaggeration, to vilification of men who have been, or are, prominent in church or state, and even to false statement. But the people of this nation have ordained in the light of history, that, in spite of the probability of excesses and abuses, these liberties are, in the long view, essential to enlightened opinion and right conduct on the part of the citizens of a democracy." Cantwell v. Connecticut, 310 U.S. 296, 310.

I regret my inability to persuade the Court not to retreat from this principle.

MR. JUSTICE DOUGLAS, with whom MR. JUSTICE MINTON concurs, dissenting. [Omitted.]

---

8. Cf. Hague v. C.I.O., 307 U.S. 496; Terminiello v. Chicago, 337 U.S. 1; Sellers v. Johnson, 163 F.2d 877; see also summary of Brief for Committee on the Bill of Rights of the American Bar Association as *amicus curiae, Hague v. C.I.O.*, reprinted at 307 U.S. 678-682.

9. In Schneider v. State, 308 U.S. 147, we held that a purpose to prevent littering of the streets was insufficient to justify an ordinance which prohibited a person lawfully on the street from handing literature to one willing to receive it. We said at page 162, "There are obvious methods of preventing littering. Amongst these is the punishment of those who actually throw papers on the streets." In the present case as well, the threat of one person to assault a speaker does not justify suppression of the speech. There are obvious available alternative methods of preserving public order. One of these is to arrest the person who threatens an assault. ***

NOTE

The preceding cases illustrate and apply a general doctrine of "reasonable time, place, and manner" regulation of speech-related activities. Is this doctrine confined to regulations applicable only to public places (i.e. premises owned or managed under government auspices), or is it, rather, a more general doctrine (e.g., applicable just as well to noise-level controls regarding speech-activities on *private* property—like the common law of nuisance, permitting a homeowner to seek injunctive relief from excessive noise broadcast from the neighboring house)? In either case, what are the elements of this test? For example, to satisfy the first amendment, (a) must the regulation be drawn as the "least restrictive" means consistent with accomplishing its objectives, and (b) may it have to give way, even so, for the acceptance of at least some minor inconveniences, so to allow adequate breathing space for such speech uses as those who are otherwise lawfully present may wish to pursue? Consider these more recent cases.

CITY COUNCIL v. TAXPAYERS FOR VINCENT
466 U.S. 789 (1984)

JUSTICE STEVENS delivered the opinion of the Court.

Section 28.04 of the Los Angeles Municipal Code prohibits the posting of signs on public property.[10] The question presented is whether that prohibition abridges appellees' freedom of speech within the meaning of the First Amendment.

In March 1979, Roland Vincent was a candidate for election to the Los Angeles City Council. A group of his supporters known as Taxpayers for Vincent (Taxpayers) entered into a contract with a political sign service company known as Candidates' Outdoor Graphics Service (COGS) to fabricate and post signs with Vincent's name on them. COGS produced 15- by 44-inch cardboard signs and attached them to utility poles at various locations by draping them over crosswires which support the poles and stapling the cardboard together at the bottom. The signs' message was: "Roland Vincent—City Council."

Acting under the authority of § 28.04 of the Municipal Code, employees of the city's Bureau of Street Maintenance routinely removed all posters attached to utility poles and similar objects covered by the ordinance, including the COGS signs. The

---

10. The ordinance reads as follows:

"Sec. 28.04. Hand-bills, signs-public places and objects:

"(a) No person shall paint, mark or write on, or post or otherwise affix, any hand-bill or sign to or upon any sidewalk, crosswalk, curb, curbstone, street lamp post, hydrant, tree, shrub, tree stake or guard, railroad trestle, electric light or power or telephone or telegraph or trolley wire pole, or wire appurtenance thereof or upon any fixture of the fire alarm or police telegraph system or upon any lighting system, public bridge, drinking fountain, life buoy, life preserve, life boat or other life saving equipment, street sign or traffic sign. ***"

weekly sign removal report covering the period March 1-March 7, 1979, indicated that among the 1,207 signs removed from public property during that week, 48 were identified as "Roland Vincent" signs. Most of the other signs identified in that report were apparently commercial in character. ***

In its conclusions of law the District Court characterized the esthetic and economic interests in improving the beauty of the City "by eliminating clutter and visual blight" as "legitimate and compelling." Those interests, together with the interest in protecting the safety of workmen who must scale utility poles and the interest in eliminating traffic hazards, adequately supported the sign prohibition as a reasonable regulation affecting the time, place, and manner of expression.

The Court of Appeals did not question any of the District Court's findings of fact, but it rejected some of its conclusions of law. The Court of Appeals reasoned that the ordinance was presumptively unconstitutional because significant First Amendment interests were involved. *** The Court of Appeals held that the City had failed to make a sufficient showing that its asserted interests in esthetics and preventing visual clutter were substantial because it had not offered to demonstrate that the City was engaged in a comprehensive effort to remove other contributions to an unattractive environment in commercial and industrial areas. The City's interest in minimizing traffic hazards was rejected because it was readily apparent that no substantial traffic problems would result from permitting the posting of certain kinds of signs on many of the publicly owned objects covered by the ordinance. Finally, while acknowledging that a flat prohibition against signs on certain objects such as fire hydrants and traffic signals would be a permissible method of preventing interference with the intended use of public property, and that regulation of the size, design, and construction of posters, or of the method of removing them, might be reasonable, the Court of Appeals concluded that the City had not justified its total ban. ***

II-III

The ordinance prohibits appellees from communicating with the public in a certain manner, and presumably diminishes the total quantity of their communication in the City. The application of the ordinance to appellees' expressive activities surely raises the question whether the ordinance abridges their "freedom of speech" within the meaning of the First Amendment, and the appellees certainly have standing to challenge the application of the ordinance to their own expressive activities. "But to say the ordinance presents a First Amendment *issue* is not necessarily to say that it constitutes a First Amendment *violation*." Metromedia, Inc. v. San Diego, 453 U.S., at 561 (BURGER, C. J., dissenting). It has been clear since this Court's earliest decisions concerning the freedom of speech that the state may sometimes curtail speech when necessary to advance a significant and legitimate state interest. Schenck v. United States, 249 U.S. 47, 52 (1919). ***

In United States v. O'Brien, 391 U.S. 367 (1968), the Court set forth the appropriate framework for reviewing a viewpoint-neutral regulation of this kind:

> "[A] government regulation is sufficiently justified if it is within the constitutional power of the Government; if it furthers an important or substantial governmental interest; if the governmental interest is unrelated to the suppression of free expression; and if the incidental restriction on alleged First Amendment freedoms is no greater than is essential to the furtherance of that interest."

It is well settled that the state may legitimately exercise its police powers to advance esthetic values. *** *Metromedia, Inc. v. San Diego,* dealt with San Diego's prohibition of certain forms of outdoor billboards. There the Court considered the city's interest in avoiding visual clutter, and seven Justices explicitly concluded that this interest was sufficient to justify a prohibition of billboards, see [453 U.S.], at 507-508 (opinion of WHITE, J., joined by STEWART, MARSHALL, and POWELL, JJ.); *id.*, at 552 (STEVENS, J. dissenting in part); *id.*, at 559-561 (BURGER, C.J., dissenting); *id.*, at 570 (REHNQUIST, J., dissenting).

We reaffirm the conclusion of the majority in *Metromedia.* The problem addressed by this ordinance—the visual assault on the citizens of Los Angeles presented by an accumulation of signs posted on public property—constitutes a significant substantive evil within the City's power to prohibit.

IV

We turn to the question whether the scope of the restriction on appellees' expressive activity is substantially broader than necessary to protect the City's interest in eliminating visual clutter. The incidental restriction on expression which results from the City's attempt to accomplish such a purpose is considered justified as a reasonable regulation of the time, place, or manner of expression if it is narrowly tailored to serve that interest. *** The District Court found that the signs prohibited by the ordinance do constitute visual clutter and blight. By banning these signs, the City did no more than eliminate the exact source of the evil it sought to remedy. ***

It is true that the esthetic interest in preventing the kind of litter that may result from the distribution of leaflets on the public streets and sidewalks cannot support a prophylactic prohibition against the citizen's exercise of that method of expressing his views. In Schneider v. State, 308 U.S. 147 (1939), the Court held that ordinances that absolutely prohibited handbilling on the streets were invalid. The Court explained that cities could adequately protect the esthetic interest in avoiding litter without abridging protected expression merely by penalizing those who actually litter. ***

The rationale of *Schneider* is inapposite in the context of the instant case. *** In *Schneider*, an antilittering statute could have addressed the substantive evil without prohibiting expressive activity, whereas application of the prophylactic rule actually employed gratuitously infringed upon the right of an individual to communicate directly with a willing listener. Here, the substantive evil—visual blight—is not merely a possible byproduct of the activity, but is created by the medium of expression itself. In contrast to *Schneider*, therefore, the application of the ordinance in this case responds precisely to the substantive problem which legitimately concerns the City. The ordinance curtails no more speech than is necessary to accomplish its purpose.

V

The Court of Appeals accepted the argument that a prohibition against the use of unattractive signs cannot be justified on esthetic grounds if it fails to apply to all equally unattractive signs wherever they might be located. A comparable argument was categorically rejected in *Metromedia.* In that case it was argued that the city could not simultaneously permit billboards to be used for onsite advertising and also justify the prohibition against offsite advertising on esthetic grounds, since both types of advertising were equally unattractive. The Court held, however, that the city could reasonably conclude that the esthetic interest was outweighed by the countervailing interest in one kind of advertising even thought it was not outweighed by the other. So here, the validity of the esthetic interest in the elimination of signs on public property is not compromised by failing to extend the ban to private property. The private citizen's interest in controlling the use of his own property justifies the disparate treatment. ***

VI

While the First Amendment does not guarantee the right to employ every conceivable method of communication at all times and in all places, a restriction on expressive activity may be invalid if the remaining modes of communication are inadequate. *** The Los Angeles ordinance does not affect any individual's freedom to exercise the right to speak and to distribute literature in the same place where the posting of signs on public property is prohibited. To the extent that the posting of signs on public property has advantages over these forms of expression, there is no reason to believe that these same advantages cannot be obtained through other means. To the contrary, the findings of the District Court indicate that there are ample alternative modes of communication in Los Angeles. ***

VIII

Finally, Taxpayers and COGS argue that Los Angeles could have written an ordinance that would have had a less severe effect on expressive activity such as theirs, by permitting the posting of any kind of sign at any time on some types of public property, or by making a variety of other more specific exceptions to the ordinance: for signs carrying certain types of messages (such as political campaign signs), for signs posted during specific time periods (perhaps during political campaigns), for particular locations (perhaps for areas already cluttered by an excessive number of signs on adjacent private property), or for signs meeting design specifications (such as size or color). Plausible public policy arguments might well be made in support of any such exception, but it by no means follows that it is therefore constitutionally mandated, nor is it clear that some of the suggested exceptions would even be constitutionally permissible. For example, even though political speech is entitled to the fullest possible measure of constitutional protection, there are a host of other communications that command the same respect. An assertion that "Jesus Saves," that "Abortion is Murder," that every woman has the "Right to Choose," or that "Alcohol Kills," may have a claim to a constitutional exemption from the ordinance that is just as strong as "Roland Vincent—City Council." ***

The judgment of the Court of Appeals is reversed, and the case is remanded to that Court.

JUSTICE BRENNAN, with whom JUSTICE MARSHALL and JUSTICE BLACKMUN join, dissenting.

***

The Court finds that the City's "interest [in eliminating visual clutter] is sufficiently substantial to justify the effect of the ordinance on appellees' expression" and that the effect of the ordinance on speech is "no greater than necessary to accomplish the City's purpose." *** These are the right questions to consider when analyzing the constitutionality of the challenged ordinance, but the answers that the Court provides reflect a startling insensitivity to the principles embodied in the First Amendment. ***

I

***

In deciding this First Amendment question, the critical importance of the posting of signs as a means of communication must not be overlooked. Use of this medium of communication is particularly valuable in part because it entails a relatively small expense in reaching a wide audience, allows flexibility in accommodating various formats, typographies, and graphics, and conveys its message in a manner that is easily read and understood by its reader or viewer. ***

Nevertheless, the City of Los Angeles asserts that ample alternative avenues of communication are available. The City notes that, although the posting of signs on public property is prohibited, the posting of signs on private property and the distribution of handbills are not. But *** there is no proof that a sufficient number of private parties would allow the posting of signs on their property. Indeed, common sense suggests the contrary at least in some instances. A speaker with a message that is generally unpopular or simply unpopular among property owners is hardly likely to get his message across if forced to rely on this medium. It is difficult to believe, for example, that a group advocating an increase in the rate of a property tax would succeed in persuading private property owners to accept its signs.

Similarly, the adequacy of distributing handbills is dubious, despite certain advantages of handbills over signs. Particularly when the message to be carried is best expressed by a few words or a graphic image, a message on a sign will typically reach far more people than one on a handbill. The message on a posted sign remains to be seen by passersby as long as it is posted, while a handbill is typically read by a single reader and discarded. Thus, not only must handbills be printed in large quantity, but many hours must be spent distributing them. The average cost of communicating by handbill is therefore likely to be far higher than the average cost of communicating by poster. For that reason, signs posted on public property are doubtless "essential to the poorly financed causes of little people," and their prohibition constitutes a total ban on an important medium of communication. ***

III

***

Initially, a reviewing court faces substantial difficulties determining whether the actual objective is related to the suppression of speech. The asserted interest in aesthetics may be only a facade of content-based suppression. *** For example, in evaluating the ordinance before us in this case, the City might be pursuing either of two objectives, motivated by two very different judgments. One objective might be the elimination of "visual clutter," attributable in whole or in part to signs posted on public property. The aesthetic judgment underlying this objective would be that the clutter created by these signs offends the community's desire for an orderly, visually pleasing environment. A second objective might simply be the elimination of the messages typically carried by the signs. In that case, the aesthetic judgment would be that the signs' messages are themselves displeasing. The first objective is lawful, of course, but the second is not. Yet the City might easily mask the second objective by asserting the first and declaring that signs constitute visual clutter. In short, we must avoid the unquestioned acceptance of the City's bare declaration of an aesthetic objective lest we fail in our duty to prevent unlawful trespasses upon First Amendment protections.

In my view, such statements of aesthetic objectives should be accepted as substantial and unrelated to the suppression of speech only if the government demonstrates that it is pursuing an identified objective seriously and comprehensively and in ways that are unrelated to the restriction of speech. *Metromedia*, 453 U.S., at 531 (BRENNAN, J., concurring in judgment). Without such a demonstration, I would invalidate the restriction as violative of the First Amendment.

This does not mean that a government must address all aesthetic problems at one time or that a government should hesitate to pursue aesthetic objectives. What it does mean, however, is that when such an objective is pursued, it may not be pursued solely at the expense of First Amendment freedoms, nor may it be pursued by arbitrarily discriminating against a form of speech that has the same aesthetic characteristics as other forms of speech that are also present in the community.

*** In this case, as the Court of Appeals found, there is no indication that the City has addressed its visual clutter problem in any way other than by prohibiting the posting of signs—throughout the City and without regard to the density of their presence. Therefore, I would hold that the prohibition violates appellees' First Amendment rights. ***

In the absence of such a showing in this case, I believe that Los Angeles' total ban sweeps so broadly and trenches so completely on the appellees' use of an important medium of political expression that it must be struck down as violative of the First Amendment.[7]

I therefore dissent.

CITY OF LADUE v. GILLEO

512 U.S. 43 (1994)

JUSTICE STEVENS delivered the opinion of the Court.

I

[Margaret P. Gilleo] placed on her front lawn a 24- by 36-inch sign printed with the words "Say No to War in the Persian Gulf, Call Congress Now." After that sign disappeared, Gilleo put up another but it was knocked to the ground. When Gilleo reported these incidents to the police, they advised her that such signs were prohibited in Ladue.

The District Court issued a preliminary injunction against enforcement of the ordinance. The Ladue City Council responded to the injunction by repealing its ordinance and enacting a replacement. The ordinance prohibits all signs except those that fall within one of ten exemptions.[6] *** Unlike its predecessor, the new ordinance contains a lengthy "Declaration of Findings, Policies, Interests, and Purposes," part of which recites that the

> "proliferation of an unlimited number of signs in private, residential, commercial, industrial, and public areas of the City of Ladue would create ugliness, visual blight and clutter, tarnish the natural beauty of the landscape as well as the residential and commercial architecture, impair property values, substantially impinge upon the privacy and special ambience of the community, and may cause safety and traffic hazards to motorists, pedestrians, and children[.]"

---

7. Although the Court does not reach the question, appellants argue that the City's interest in traffic safety provides an independent and significant justification for its ban on signs. As the Court of Appeals concluded, however, "[t]he City has not offered to prove facts that raise any genuine issue regarding traffic safety hazards with respect to the posting of signs on many of the objects covered by the ordinance."

6. The full catalog of exceptions, each subject to special size limitations, is as follows: "municipal signs"; "[s]ubdivision and residence identification" signs; "[r]oad signs and driveway signs for danger, direction, or identification"; "[h]ealth inspection signs"; "[s]igns for churches, religious institutions, and schools" (subject to regulations set forth in § 35-5); "identification signs" for other not-for-profit organizations; signs "identifying the location of public transportation stops"; "[g]round signs advertising the sale or rental of real property," subject to the conditions, set forth in § 35-10, that such signs may "not be attached to any tree, fence or utility pole" and may contain only the fact of proposed sale or rental and the seller or agent's name and address or telephone number; "[c]ommercial signs in commercially zoned or industrial zoned districts," subject to restrictions set out elsewhere in the ordinance; and signs that "identif[y] safety hazards."

Gilleo amended her complaint to challenge the new ordinance. *** Relying on the plurality opinion in Metromedia, Inc. v. San Diego, 453 U.S. 490 (1981), the Court of Appeals held the ordinance invalid as a "content based" regulation because the City treated commercial speech more favorably than noncommercial speech and favored some kinds of noncommercial speech over others. ***

Under the Court of Appeals' content discrimination rationale, the City might theoretically remove the defects in its ordinance by simply repealing all of the exemptions. If, however, the ordinance is also vulnerable because it prohibits too much speech, that solution would not save it. Moreover, if the prohibitions in Ladue's ordinance are impermissible, resting our decision on its exemptions would afford scant relief for respondent Gilleo. She is primarily concerned not with the scope of the exemptions available in other locations, such as commercial areas and on church property. She asserts a constitutional right to display an antiwar sign at her own home. Therefore, we first ask whether Ladue may properly *prohibit* Gilleo from displaying her sign, and then, only if necessary, consider the separate question whether it was improper for the City simultaneously to *permit* certain other signs. ***

IV

*** Ladue contends that its ordinance is a mere regulation of the "time, place, or manner" of speech because residents remain free to convey their desired messages by other means, such as *hand-held* signs, "letters, handbills, flyers, telephone calls, newspaper advertisements, bumper stickers, speeches, and neighborhood or community meetings." However, even regulations that do not foreclose an entire medium of expression, but merely shift the time, place, or manner of its use, must "leave open ample alternative channels for communication." In this case, we are not persuaded that adequate substitutes exist for the important medium of speech that Ladue has closed off.

Displaying a sign from one's own residence often carries a message quite distinct from placing the same sign someplace else, or conveying the same text or picture by other means. ***

Residential signs are an unusually cheap and convenient form of communication. Especially for persons of modest means or limited mobility, a yard or window sign may have no practical substitute. Even for the affluent, the added costs in money or time of taking out a newspaper advertisement, handing out leaflets on the street, or standing in front of one's house with a hand-held sign may make the difference between participating and not participating in some public debate. ***

A special respect for individual liberty in the home has long been part of our culture and our law; that principle has special resonance when the government seeks to constrain a person's ability to *speak* there. See Spence v. Washington, 418 U.S. 405, 406, 409, 411 (1974) (*per curiam*). *** Whereas the government's need to mediate among various competing uses, including expressive ones, for public streets and facilities is constant and unavoidable, its need to regulate temperate speech from the home is surely much less pressing.

Our decision that Ladue's ban on almost all residential signs violates the First Amendment by no means leaves the City powerless to address the ills that may be associated with residential signs.[17] *** We are confident that more temperate measures could in large part satisfy Ladue's stated regulatory needs without harm to the First Amendment rights of its citizens. As currently framed, however, the ordinance abridges those rights.

Accordingly, the judgment of the Court of Appeals is Affirmed.

JUSTICE O'CONNOR, concurring. [Omitted.]

WARD v. ROCK AGAINST RACISM

491 U.S. 781 (1989)

JUSTICE KENNEDY delivered the opinion of the Court.

In the southeast portion of New York City's Central Park, about 10 blocks upward from the park's beginning point at 59th Street, there is an amphitheater and stage structure known as the Naumberg Acoustic Bandshell. The bandshell faces west across the remaining width of the park. In close proximity to the bandshell, and lying within the directional path of its sound, is a grassy open area called the Sheep Meadow. The city has designated the Sheep Meadow as a quiet area for passive recreations like reclining, walking, and reading. Just beyond the park, and also within the potential sound range of the bandshell, are the apartments and residences of Central Park West.

This case arises from the city's attempt to regulate the volume of amplified music at the bandshell so the performances are satisfactory to the audience without intruding upon those who use the Sheep Meadow or live on Central Park West and in its vicinity.

The city's regulation requires bandshell performers to use sound-amplification equipment and a sound technician provided by the city. The challenge to this volume control technique comes from the sponsor of a rock concert. The trial court sustained the noise control measures, but the Court of Appeals for the Second Circuit reversed. We granted certiorari to resolve the important First Amendment issues presented by the case.

---

17. Nor do we hold that every kind of sign must be permitted in residential areas. Different considerations might well apply, for example, in the case of signs (whether political or otherwise) displayed by residents for a fee, or in the case of off-site commercial advertisements on residential property. We also are not confronted here with mere regulations short of a ban.

I

Rock Against Racism, respondent in this case, is an unincorporated association which, in its own words, is "dedicated to the espousal and promotion of antiracist views." Each year from 1979 through 1986, RAR has sponsored a program of speeches and rock music at the Bandshell. RAR has furnished the sound equipment and sound technician used by the various performing groups at these annual events.

Over the years, the city received numerous complaints about excessive sound amplification at respondent's concerts from park users and residents of areas adjacent to the park. On some occasions RAR was less than cooperative when city officials asked that the volume be reduced; at one concert, police felt compelled to cut off the power to the sound system, an action that caused the audience to become unruly and hostile.

The city considered various solutions to the sound amplification problem. The idea of a fixed decibel limit for all performers using the bandshell was rejected because the impact on listeners of a single decibel level is not constant, but varies in response to changes in air temperature, foliage, audience size, and like factors. The city also rejected the possibility of employing a sound technician to operate the equipment provided by the various sponsors of bandshell events, because the city's technician might have had difficulty satisfying the needs of sponsors while operating unfamiliar, and perhaps inadequate, sound equipment. *** Instead, the city concluded that the most effective way to achieve adequate but not excessive sound amplification would be for the city to furnish high quality sound equipment and retain an independent, experienced sound technician for all performances at the bandshell. After an extensive search the city hired a private sound company capable of meeting the needs of all the varied users of the bandshell.

The Use Guidelines were promulgated on March 21, 1986. After learning that it would be expected to comply with the guidelines at its upcoming annual concert in May 1986, respondent returned to the District Court and filed a motion for an injunction against the enforcement of certain aspects of the guidelines. The District Court preliminarily enjoined enforcement of the sound-amplification rule on May 1, 1986. ***

After the concert, respondent amended its complaint to seek damages and a declaratory judgment striking down the guidelines as facially invalid. After hearing five days of testimony about various aspects of the guidelines, the District Court issued its decision upholding the sound-amplification guideline.

The Court of Appeals reversed. After recognizing that "[c]ontent neutral time, place and manner regulations are permissible so long as they are narrowly tailored to serve a substantial government interest and do not unreasonably limit alternative avenues of expression," the court added the proviso that "the method and extent of such regulation must be reasonable, that is, it must be the least intrusive upon the freedom of expression as is reasonably necessary to achieve a legitimate purpose of regulation."

*** Because the Court of Appeals erred in requiring the city to prove that its regulation was the least intrusive means of furthering its legitimate governmental interests, and because the ordinance is valid on its face, we now reverse.

II

Music is one of the oldest forms of human expression. From Plato's discourse in the Republic to the totalitarian state in our own times, rulers have known its capacity to appeal to the intellect and to the emotions, and have censored musical compositions to serve the needs of the state. See 2 Dialogues of Plato, Republic, bk. III, pp. 231, 245-248 (B. Jowett trans., 4th ed. 1953) ("Our poets must sing in another and a nobler strain"); Musical Freedom and Why Dictators Fear It, N.Y. Times, Aug. 23, 1981, section 2, p. 1, col. 5; Soviet Schizophrenia toward Stravinsky, N.Y. Times, June 26, 1982, section 1, p. 25, col. 2; Symphonic Voice from China Is Heard Again, N.Y. Times, Oct. 11, 1987, section 2, p. 27, col. 1. The Constitution prohibits any like attempts in our own legal order. Music, as a form of expression and communication, is protected under the First Amendment. ***

*** Our cases make clear, however, that even in a public forum the government may impose reasonable restrictions on the time, place, or manner of protected speech, provided the restrictions "are justified without reference to the content of the regulated speech, that they are narrowly tailored to serve a significant governmental interest, and that they leave open ample alternative channels for communication of information." ***

A

***

The principal justification for the sound-amplification guideline is the city's desire to control noise levels at Bandshell events, in order to retain the character of the Sheep Meadow and its more sedate activities, and to avoid undue intrusion into residential areas and other areas of the park. This justification for the guideline "ha[s] nothing to do with content," and it satisfies the requirement that time, place, or manner regulations be content-neutral.

The only other justification offered below was the city's interest in "ensur[ing] the quality of sound at Bandshell events." Respondent urges that this justification is not content-neutral because it is based upon the quality, and thus the content, of the speech being regulated. In respondent's view, the city is seeking to assert artistic control over performers at the bandshell by enforcing a bureaucratically determined, value-laden conception of good sound. ***

While respondent's arguments that the government may not interfere with artistic judgment may have much force in other contexts, they are inapplicable to the facts of this case. The city has disclaimed in express terms any interest in imposing its own view of appropriate sound mix on performers. To the contrary, as the District Court found, the city requires its sound technician to defer to the wishes of event sponsors concerning sound mix. On this record, the city's concern with sound quality extends only to the clearly content-neutral goals of ensuring adequate sound amplification and avoiding the volume problems associated with inadequate sound mix. Any governmental attempt to serve purely aesthetic goals by imposing subjective standards of acceptable sound mix on performers would raise serious First Amendment concerns, but this case provides us with no opportunity to address those questions. As related above, the District Court found that the city's equipment and its sound technician could meet all of the standards requested by the performers, including RAR. ***

B

The city's regulation is also "narrowly tailored to serve a significant governmental interest." Community for Creative Non-Violence, 468 U.S., at 293. Despite respondent's protestations to the contrary, it can no longer be doubted that government "ha[s] a substantial interest in protecting its citizens from unwelcome noise." ***

We think it also apparent that the city's interest in ensuring the sufficiency of sound amplification at Bandshell events is a substantial one. The record indicates that inadequate sound amplification has had an adverse affect on the ability of some audiences to hear and enjoy performances at the Bandshell. The city enjoys a substantial interest in ensuring the ability of its citizens to enjoy whatever benefits the city parks have to offer, from amplified music to silent meditation.

The Court of Appeals recognized the city's substantial interest in limiting the sound emanating from the bandshell. The court concluded, however, that the city's sound-amplification guideline was not narrowly tailored to further this interest, because "it has not [been] shown *** that the requirement of the use of the city's sound system and technical was the *least intrusive means* of regulating the volume." In the court's judgment, there were several alternative methods of achieving the desired end that would have been less restrictive of respondent's First Amendment rights.

The Court of Appeals erred in sifting through all the available or imagined alternative means of regulating sound volume in order to determine whether the city's solution was "the least intrusive means" of achieving the desired end. This "less- restrictive-alternative analysis has never been a part of the inquiry into the validity of a time, place, and manner regulation." *** Lest any confusion on the point remain, we reaffirm today that a regulation of time, place, or manner of protected speech must be narrowly tailored to serve the government's legitimate content-neutral interests but that it need not be the least- restrictive or least-intrusive means of doing so. Rather, the requirement of narrow tailoring is satisfied "so long as the *** regulation promotes a substantial government interest that would be achieved less effectively absent the regulation." *** To be sure, this standard does not mean that a time, place, or manner regulation may burden substantially more speech than is necessary to further the government's legitimate interests. Government may not regulate expression in such a manner that a substantial portion of the burden on speech does not serve to advance its goals.[7] ***

It is undeniable that the city's substantial interest in limiting sound volume is served in a direct and effective way by the requirement that the city's sound technician control the mixing board during performances. Absent this requirement, the city's interest would have been served less well, as is evidenced by the complaints about excessive volume generated by respondent's past concerts. ***

The city's second content-neutral justification for the guideline, that of ensuring "that the sound amplification [is] sufficient to reach all listeners within the defined concertground," also supports the city's choice of regulatory methods. By providing competent sound technicians and adequate amplification equipment, the city eliminated the problems of inexperienced technicians and insufficient sound volume that had plagued some bandshell performers in the past. ***

Respondent nonetheless argues that the sound-amplification guideline is not narrowly tailored because, by placing control of sound mix in the hands of the city's technician, the guideline sweeps far more broadly than is necessary to further the city's legitimate concern with sound volume. According to respondent, the guideline "targets *** more than the exact source of the 'evil' it seeks to remedy." ***

If the city's regulatory scheme had a substantial deleterious effect on the ability of bandshell performers to achieve the quality of sound they desired, respondent's concerns would have considerable force. The District Court found, however, that pursuant to city policy, the city's sound technician "give[s] the sponsor autonomy with respect to the sound mix [and] does all that he can to accommodate the sponsor's desires in those regards." The court squarely rejected respondent's claim that the city's "technician is not able properly to implement a sponsor's instructions as to sound quality or mix," finding that "[n]o evidence to that effect was offered at trial; as noted, the evidence is to the contrary."

C

The final requirement, that the guideline leave open ample alternative channels of communication, is easily met. Indeed, in this respect the guideline is far less restrictive than regulations we have upheld in other cases, for it does not attempt to ban any particular manner or type of expression at a given place or time. *** Rather, the

---

7. The dissent's attempt to analogize the sound-amplification guideline to a total ban on distribution of handbills is imaginative but misguided. *** The guideline does not ban all concerts, or even all rock concerts, but instead focuses on the source of the evils the city seeks to eliminate—excessive and inadequate sound amplification—and eliminates them without at the same time banning or significantly restricting a substantial quantity of speech that does not create the same evils. This is the essence of narrow tailoring. A ban on handbilling, of course, would suppress a great quantity of speech that does not cause the evils that it seeks to eliminate, whether they be fraud, crime, litter, traffic congestion, or noise. See Martin v. Struthers, 319 U. S. 141, 145-146 (1943). For that reason a complete ban on handbilling would be substantially broader than necessary to achieve the interests justifying it.

guideline continues to permit expressive activity in the bandshell, and has no effect on the quantity or content of that expression beyond regulating the extent of amplification. That the city's limitations on volume may reduce to some degree the potential audience for respondent's speech is of no consequence, for there has been no showing that the remaining avenues of communication are inadequate. ***

*** The judgment of the Court of Appeals is Reversed.

JUSTICE BLACKMUN concurs in the result.

JUSTICE MARSHALL, with whom JUSTICE BRENNAN and JUSTICE STEVENS join, dissenting.

The majority sets forth the appropriate standard for assessing the constitutionality of the Guidelines. A time, place, and manner regulation of expression must be content neutral, serve a significant government interest, be narrowly tailored to serve that interest, and leave open ample alternative channels of communication. ***

My complaint is with the majority's serious distortion of the narrow tailoring requirement. Our cases have not, as the majority asserts, "clearly" rejected a less-restrictive-alternative test. *** In *Schneider*, for example, the Court invalidated a ban on handbill distribution on public streets, notwithstanding that it was the most effective means of serving government's legitimate interest in minimizing litter, noise, and traffic congestion, and in preventing fraud. The Court concluded that punishing those who actually litter or perpetrate frauds was a much less intrusive, albeit not quite as effective, means to serve those significant interests. *** Indeed, after today's decision, a city could claim that bans on handbill distribution or on door-to-door solicitation are the most effective means of avoiding littering and fraud, or that a ban on loudspeakers and radios in a public park is the most effective means of avoiding loud noise. Logically extended, the majority's analysis would permit such far-reaching restrictions on speech. ***

Had the majority not abandoned the narrow tailoring requirement, the Guidelines could not possibly survive constitutional scrutiny. Government's interest in avoiding loud sounds cannot justify giving government total control over sound equipment, any more than its interest in avoiding litter could justify a ban on handbill distribution. In both cases, government's legitimate goals can be effectively and less intrusively served by directly punishing the evil—the persons responsible for excessive sounds and the persons who litter. Indeed, the city concedes that it has an ordinance generally limiting noise but has chosen not to enforce it.[6] ***

---

6. Because I conclude that the Guidelines are not narrowly tailored, there is no need to consider whether there are ample alternative channels for communication. I note only that the availability of alternative channels of communication outside a public park does not magically validate a government restriction on protected speech within it. See *Southeastern Promotions, Ltd. v. Conrad*, 420 U. S. 546, 556 (1975) ("'[O]ne is not to have the exercise of his liberty of expression in appropriate places abridged on the plea that it may be exercised in some other place,'" quoting *Schneider v. State*, 308 U.

III

Today's decision has significance far beyond the world of rock music. Government no longer need balance the effectiveness of regulation with the burdens on free speech. After today, government need only assert that it is most effective to control speech in advance of its expression. Because such a result eviscerates the First Amendment, I dissent.

MADSEN v. WOMEN'S HEALTH CENTER

512 U.S. 753 (1994)

CHIEF JUSTICE REHNQUIST delivered the opinion of the Court.

***

Respondents operate abortion clinics throughout central Florida. Petitioners and other groups and individuals are engaged in activities near the site of one such clinic in Melbourne, Florida. They picketed and demonstrated where the public street gives access to the clinic. In September 1992, a Florida state court permanently enjoined petitioners from blocking or interfering with public access to the clinic, and from physically abusing persons entering or leaving the clinic. Six months later, respondents sought to broaden the injunction, complaining that access to the clinic was still impeded by petitioners' activities and that such activities had also discouraged some potential patients from entering the clinic, and had deleterious physical effects on others. The trial court thereupon issued a broader injunction, which is challenged here. ***

If this were a content-neutral, generally applicable statute, instead of an injunctive order, its constitutionality would be assessed under the standard set forth in *Ward v. Rock Against Racism.* Given that the forum around the clinic is a traditional public forum, we would determine whether the time, place, and manner regulations were "narrowly tailored to serve a significant governmental interest."

There are obvious differences, however, between an injunction and a generally applicable ordinance. *** We believe that these differences require a somewhat more stringent application of general First Amendment principles in this context. In past cases evaluating injunctions restricting speech, we have relied upon such general principles while also seeking to ensure that the injunction was no broader than necessary to achieve its desired goals. Our close attention to the fit between the objectives of an injunction and the restrictions it imposes on speech is consistent with the general rule, quite apart from First Amendment considerations, "that injunctive relief should be no more burdensome to the defendants than necessary to provide complete relief to the plaintiffs." *** [W]e think that our standard time, place, and manner analysis is not sufficiently rigorous. We must ask instead whether the chal-

---

S. 147, 163 (1939).)

lenged provisions of the injunction burden no more speech than necessary to serve a significant government interest. ***

A

We begin with the 36-foot buffer zone. The state court prohibited petitioners from "congregating, picketing, patrolling, demonstrating or entering" any portion of the public right-of-way or private property within 36 feet of the property line of the clinic as a way of ensuring access to the clinic. This speech-free buffer zone requires that petitioners move to the other side of Dixie Way and away from the driveway of the clinic, where the state court found that they repeatedly had interfered with the free access of patients and staff. ***

The 36-foot buffer zone protecting the entrances to the clinic and the parking lot is a means of protecting unfettered ingress to and egress from the clinic, and ensuring that petitioners do not block traffic on Dixie Way. *** The state court was convinced that allowing the petitioners to remain on the clinic's sidewalk and driveway was not a viable option in view of the failure of the first injunction to protect access. And allowing the petitioners to stand in the middle of Dixie Way would obviously block vehicular traffic.

The need for a complete buffer zone near the clinic entrances and driveway may be debatable, but some deference must be given to the state court's familiarity with the facts and the background of the dispute between the parties even under our heightened review. *** We also bear in mind the fact that the state court originally issued a much narrower injunction, providing no buffer zone, and that this order did not succeed in protecting access to the clinic. *** On balance, we hold that the 36-foot buffer zone around the clinic entrances and driveway burdens no more speech than necessary to accomplish the governmental interest at stake.

The inclusion of private property on the back and side of the clinic in the 36-foot buffer zone raises different concerns. The accepted purpose of the buffer zone is to protect access to the clinic and to facilitate the orderly flow of traffic on Dixie Way. Patients and staff wishing to reach the clinic do not have to cross the private property abutting the clinic property on the north and west, and nothing in the record indicates that petitioners' activities on the private property have obstructed access to the clinic. *** We hold that on the record before us the 36-foot buffer zone as applied to the private property to the north and west of the clinic burdens more speech than necessary to protect access to the clinic.

B

In response to high noise levels outside the clinic, the state court restrained the petitioners from "singing, chanting, whistling, shouting, yelling, use of bullhorns, auto horns, sound amplification equipment or other sounds or images observable to or within earshot of the patients inside the [c]linic" during the hours of 7:30 a.m. through noon on Mondays through Saturdays. We must, of course, take account of the place to which the regulations apply in determining whether these restrictions burden more speech than necessary. *** Noise control is particularly important around hospitals and medical facilities during surgery and recovery periods.***

We hold that the limited noise restrictions imposed by the state court order burden no more speech than necessary to ensure the health and well-being of the patients at the clinic. The First Amendment does not demand that patients at a medical facility undertake Herculean efforts to escape the cacophony of political protests. ***

C

The same, however, cannot be said for the "images observable" provision of the state court's order. Clearly, threats to patients or their families, however communicated, are proscribable under the First Amendment. But rather than prohibiting the display of signs that could be interpreted as threats or veiled threats, the state court issued a blanket ban on all "images observable." This broad prohibition on all "images observable" burdens more speech than necessary to achieve the purpose of limiting threats to clinic patients or their families. Similarly, if the blanket ban on "images observable" was intended to reduce the level of anxiety and hypertension suffered by the patients inside the clinic, it would still fail. The only plausible reason a patient would be bothered by "images observable" inside the clinic would be if the patient found the expression contained in such images disagreeable. But it is much easier for the clinic to pull its curtains than for a patient to stop up her ears, and no more is required to avoid seeing placards through the windows of the clinic. This provision of the injunction violates the First Amendment.

D

The state court ordered that petitioners refrain from physically approaching any person seeking services of the clinic "unless such person indicates a desire to communicate" in an area within 300 feet of the clinic. The state court was attempting to prevent clinic patients and staff from being "stalked" or "shadowed" by the petitioners as they approached the clinic. ***

But it is difficult, indeed, to justify a prohibition on *all* uninvited approaches of persons seeking the services of the clinic, regardless of how peaceful the contact may be, without burdening more speech than necessary to prevent intimidation and to ensure access to the clinic. Absent evidence that the protesters' speech is independently proscribable (*i.e.*, "fighting words" or threats), or is so infused with violence as to be indistinguishable from a threat of physical harm, this provision cannot stand. "As a general matter, we have indicated that in public debate our own citizens must tolerate insulting, and even outrageous, speech in order to provide adequate breathing space to the freedoms protected by the First Amendment." Boos v. Barry, 485 U.S., at 322 (internal quotation marks omitted). The "consent" requirement alone invalidates this provision; it burdens more speech than is necessary to prevent intimidation and to ensure access to the clinic.

E

The final substantive regulation challenged by petitioners relates to a prohibition against picketing, demonstrating, or using sound amplification equipment within 300 feet of the residences of clinic staff. The prohibition also covers impeding access to streets that provide the sole access to streets on which those residences are located. The same analysis applies to the use of sound amplification equipment here as that discussed above: the government may simply demand that petitioners turn down the volume if the protests overwhelm the neighborhood.

As for the picketing, our prior decision upholding a law banning targeted residential picketing remarked on the unique nature of the home, as "'the last citadel of the tired, the weary, and the sick.'" *Frisby*, 487 U.S., at 484. ***

But the 300-foot zone around the residences in this case is much larger than the zone provided for in the ordinance which we approved in *Frisby*. The ordinance at issue there made it "unlawful for any person to engage in picketing before or about the residence or dwelling of any individual." The prohibition was limited to "focused picketing taking place solely in front of a particular residence." By contrast, the 300-foot zone would ban "[g]eneral marching through residential neighborhoods, or even walking a route in front of an entire block of houses." The record before us does not contain sufficient justification for this broad a ban on picketing; it appears that a limitation on the time, duration of picketing, and number of pickets outside a smaller zone could have accomplished the desired result.

IV

Petitioners also challenge the state court's order as being vague and overbroad. They object to the portion of the injunction making it applicable to those acting "in concert" with the named parties. But petitioners themselves are named parties in the order, and they therefore lack standing to challenge a portion of the order applying to persons who are not parties. Nor is that phrase subject, at the behest of petitioners, to a challenge for "overbreadth"; the phrase itself does not prohibit any conduct, but is simply directed at unnamed parties who might later be found to be acting "in concert" with the named parties. ***

Affirmed in part, and reversed in part.

JUSTICE SOUTER, concurring. [Omitted.]

JUSTICE STEVENS, concurring in part and dissenting in part.

*** [A] statute prohibiting demonstrations within 36 feet of an abortion clinic would probably violate the First Amendment, but an injunction directed at a limited group of persons who have engaged in unlawful conduct in a similar zone might well be constitutional. ***

In this case, the trial judge heard three days of testimony and found that petitioners not only had engaged in tortious conduct, but also had repeatedly violated an earlier injunction. The injunction is thus twice removed from a legislative proscription applicable to the general public and should be judged by a standard that gives appropriate deference to the judge's unique familiarity with the facts.

JUSTICE SCALIA, with whom JUSTICE KENNEDY and JUSTICE THOMAS join, concurring in the judgment in part and dissenting in part.

The judgment in today's case has an appearance of moderation and Solomonic wisdom, upholding as it does some portions of the injunction while disallowing others. That appearance is deceptive. The entire injunction in this case departs so far from the established course of our jurisprudence that in any other context it would have been regarded as a candidate for summary reversal. ***

Under this Court's jurisprudence, there is no question that this public sidewalk area is a "public forum," where citizens generally have a First Amendment right to speak. United States v. Grace, 461 U.S. 171, 177 (1983). The parties to this case invited the Court to employ one or the other of the two well established standards applied to restrictions upon this First Amendment right. Petitioners claimed the benefit of so-called "strict scrutiny," the standard applied to content-based restrictions: the restriction must be "necessary to serve a compelling state interest and *** narrowly drawn to achieve that end." Respondents, on the other hand, contended for what has come to be known as "intermediate scrutiny" (midway between the "strict scrutiny" demanded for content-based regulation of speech, and the "rational basis" standard that is applied-under the Equal Protection Clause-to government regulation of non-speech activities). ***

*** [A] restriction upon speech imposed by injunction (whether nominally content based or nominally content neutral) is *at least* as deserving of strict scrutiny as a statutory, content-based restriction.

That is so for several reasons: The danger of content-based statutory restrictions upon speech is that they may be designed and used precisely to suppress the ideas in question rather than to achieve any other proper governmental aim. But that same danger exists with injunctions. Although a speech-restricting injunction may not attack content *as content* (in the present case, as I shall discuss, even that is not true), it lends itself just as readily to the targeted suppression of particular ideas. When a judge, on the motion of an employer, enjoins picketing at the site of a labor dispute, he enjoins (and he *knows* he is enjoining) the expression of pro-union views. Such targeting of one or the other side of an ideological dispute cannot readily be achieved in speech-restricting general legislation except by making content the basis of the restriction; it is achieved in speech-restricting injunctions almost invariably. ***

The second reason speech-restricting injunctions are at least as deserving of strict scrutiny is obvious enough: they are the product of individual judges rather than of legislatures-and often of judges who have been chagrined by prior disobedience of their orders. The right to free speech should not lightly be placed within the control of a single man or woman. And the third reason is that the injunction is a much more powerful weapon than a statute, and so should be subjected to greater safeguards. Normally, when injunctions are enforced through contempt proceedings, only the defense of factual innocence is available. The collateral bar rule of Walker v. Birmingham, 388 U.S. 307 (1967), eliminates the defense that the injunction itself was unconstitutional. Thus, persons subject to a speech-restricting injunction who have not the money or not the time to lodge an immediate appeal face a Hobson's choice: they must remain silent, since if they speak their First Amendment rights are no defense in subsequent contempt proceedings. This is good reason to require the strictest standard for issuance of such orders. ***

I turn now to the Court's performance in the present case. I am content to evaluate it under the lax *** standard that the Court has adopted, because even by that distorted light it is inadequate. ***

Assuming then that the "significant interests" the Court mentioned must in fact be significant enough to be protected by state law (a concept that includes a prior court order), which law has been, or is about to be, violated, the question arises: what state law is involved here? The only one even mentioned is the original September 30, 1992, injunction, which had been issued (quite rightly, in my judgment) in response to threats by the originally named parties (including petitioners here) that they would "'[p]hysically close down abortion mills,'" "bloc[k] access to clinics," "ignore the law of the State," and "shut down a clinic." That original injunction prohibited petitioners from:

> "1) trespassing on, sitting in, blocking, impeding or obstructing ingress into or egress from any facility at which abortions are performed in Brevard and Seminole County Florida;
>
> "2) physically abusing persons entering, leaving, working, or using any services of any facility at which abortions are performed in Brevard and Seminole County, Florida; and
>
> "3) attempting or directing others to take any of the actions described in Paragraphs 1 and 2 above." ***

If the original injunction is read as it must be, there is nothing in the trial court's findings to suggest that it was violated. The Court today speaks of "the failure of the first injunction to protect access." *** There was no sitting down, no linking of arms, no packing en masse in the driveway; the most that can be alleged (and the trial court did not even make this a finding) is that on one occasion protestors "took their time to get out of the way." If that is enough to support this one-man proscription of free speech, the First Amendment is in grave peril.

I almost forgot to address the facts showing prior violation of law (including judicial order) with respect to the other portion of the injunction the Court upholds: the no-noise-within-earshot-of-patients provision. That is perhaps because, amazingly, neither the Florida courts *nor this Court* makes the slightest attempt to link that provision to prior violations of law.*** The pro-abortion demonstrators who were often making (if respondents' videotape is accurate) *more* noise than the petitioners, can continue to shout their chants at their opponents exiled across the street to their hearts' content. ***

Perhaps there is a local ordinance in Melbourne, Florida, prohibiting loud noise in the vicinity of hospitals and abortion clinics. Or perhaps even a Florida common-law prohibition applies, rendering such noise-making tortious. But the record in this case shows (and, alas, the Court's opinion today demands) neither indication of the existence of any such law nor a finding that it had been violated. The fact that such a law would be reasonable is enough, according to the Court, to justify a single judge in imposing it upon these protesters alone. The First Amendment reels in disbelief.

*** [I] turn to the Court's application of the second part of its test: whether the provisions of the injunction "burden no more speech than necessary" to serve the significant interest protected.

This test seems to me amply and obviously satisfied with regard to the noise restriction that the Court approves: it is only such noise as would reach the patients in the abortion clinic that is forbidden—and not even at all times, but only during certain fixed hours and "during surgical procedures and recovery periods." *** With regard to the 36-foot speech-free zone, however, it seems to me just as obvious that the test which the Court sets for itself has not been met.

Assuming a "significant state interest" of the sort cognizable for injunction purposes (*i.e.*, one protected by a law that has been or is threatened to be violated) in both (1) keeping pedestrians off the paved portion of Dixie Way, and (2) enabling cars to cross the public sidewalk at the clinic's driveways without having to slow down or come to even a "momentary" stop, there are surely a number of ways to protect those interests short of banishing the entire protest demonstration from the 36-foot zone. *** In application, in other words, the "burden no more speech than is necessary" test has become an "arguably burden no more speech than is necessary" test. This renders the Court's intermediate-intermediate scrutiny not only no *more* stringent than plain old intermediate scrutiny, but considerably *less* stringent. ***

NOTES

1. See also *Schenck v. Pro-Choice Network of Western New York,* 519 U.S. 357 (1997) (*sustaining* injunction (a) forbidding acts of physical obstruction and (b) providing a "buffer zone" forbidding further demonstrations within 15 feet of abortion clinic doorway and driveway entries [following hearings and findings of record by trial court of failure of more limited injunction effectively to restrain protestors]; but *reversing* injunction (c) securing "floating buffer zones" requiring any demonstrator or leafletter to move 15 feet from any person approaching or departing from an affected facility indicating her wish not to be confronted more closely). (Part (c) held to be overly broad restriction on first amendment right

peacefully to remonstrate or persuade.) (opinion for the Court by Rehnquist, C.J.; dissent by Kennedy, Scalia, and Thomas, JJ., insofar as the Court sustained (b)).[68]
2. Note that plantiffs in *Madsen* and in *Schenck* labored under the burden of having to initiate a civil action at their own expense, and having also to prove specific acts on defendants' part–acts both unprotected by the First Amendment and substantially interfering with their rights–before being entitled to any relief. Such will usually be the case, of course, at least where there is no legislation in place, pursuant to which plaintiffs might instead merely call the police and have the demonstrator(s) arrested, and held for trial under "an appropriate" law.

But now suppose that plaintiffs and those strongly in sympathy with them seek help from the legislature, to provide just such a law. Perhaps in the form of the following criminal statute:

> No person shall knowingly approach another person within eight feet of such person, unless such person consents, for the purpose of passing a leaflet or handbill to, displaying a sign to, or engaging in oral protest, education, or counseling, with such person in the public way or sidewalk area within a radius of one hundred feet from any entrance door to a health care facility. Any person who violates this [ordinance] commits a class 3 misdeamor.

Were this ordinance to be applied, say, to a leafletter who approached an employee as (s)he was about to enter the doorway of a health clinic offering abortion services, to try to press into her reluctant hand a leaflet with a picture (a picture of a "dismembered fetus") while displaying a small sign (a sign declaring "please don't

68. *Schenck* is a clarifying close sequel to *Madsen*, re first amendment requirements of injunctions restricting persons or groups engaged in acts of remonstrance outside health care clinics providing abortion services. As in *Madsen*, the Court in *Schenck* held that injunctions issued to restrain public, on-site politically expressive anti-abortion activity (e.g., leafletting, sign carrying, remonstrating) are subject to "heightened scrutiny" under the first amendment. While declining to regard such injunctions as a form of prior restraint deemed presumptively forbidden by the first amendment, the Court in *Schenck* again holds they are nonetheless subject to rigorous requirements of specific fact-finding and of narrow tailoring. A close fit between the specific terms of the injunction, the specific activities it enjoins, and adequate findings of record to justify such restrictions, must be achieved to withstand heightened scrutiny appellate review. These requirements are imposed on first amendment grounds partly because of the effect of the "collateral bar" rule (briefly noted in *Madsen*). (The "collateral bar" rule may disallow one cited for contempt for violating an injunction to defend against the citation for contempt by asserting that the acts were constitutionally protected and ought not to have been enjoined. See, e.g., *Walker v. City of Birmingham*, 388 U.S. 308 (1967); *United States v. United Mine Workers of America*, 330 U.S. 258, 293 (1947).) As noted (text *supra*), the Court in *Schenck* agreed the first part of the injunction restraining physical obstruction met the appropriate standard; it divided on the part forbidding approach by protestors within 15 feet of entryways and driveways (the majority sustaining it on the strength of findings by the district court that more narrowly tailored restrictions had proven ineffective); and reversed on part (c) as overly broad.

work at this terrible place"), what would you say? Is the ordinance unconstitutional on its face?[1]

---

3. Defraying the Costs of Public Forum Use—Who Pays?

In *Ward v. Rock Against Racism*, the issue before the Court was whether the city could require groups wishing to use a public park bandshell to use the sound equipment and technician provided by the city, rather than their own equipment and their own technicians, as a means of regulating overall sound level of the performance. Insofar as the city's requirement was upheld (despite plaintiff's objections), *Ward* was significant for its de-emphasis (or abandonment?) of the "least restrictive means" branch of strict scrutiny time, place, and manner review.[2]

Not dealt with in *Ward* would be the separate question of who is expected to pay the expenses of maintaining the park bandshell, the sound equipment the city provides, and the city-supplied technician in charge of the equipment. But in many circumstances, just this kind of question does arise, especially in the new age of shifting from the use of general tax funds to "user fees" in operating public amenities. This separate issue can be crucial for reasons that should be obvious.

Those most likely to demonstrate in the streets or parks, for example, may also be the most likely to generate municipal expenses in policing the demonstration itself. Yet they may also be among those least likely to have money to contribute to those costs. Does it matter whether they can afford to pay "their own way"? And what does it mean to require them to pay the city for expenses the city incurs? *What* expenses may or may not be constitutionally assigned to them?

Such an expense might include a standard minimum fifty dollar fee simply as a fixed charge to process issuance of a municipal parade permit for a street assembly, parade, or demonstration. It might likewise extend to the deposit of an amount sufficient to reimburse the city for estimated overtime police duty occasioned by the parade— special traffic detail or crowd control personnel. Might it extend likewise to clean-up costs from the extra clutter left over from the parade, demonstration, or the march? To extraordinary measures the city takes in order to protect the marchers or onlookers from possible harm that may well be expected in light of the character of the demonstration and the inflammatory or unwanted message it presents? Are there any limits and, if there are, what are they?

---

1. *See Hill v. Colorado*, 530 U.S. 703 (2000) (Ordinance sustained against void-on-its-face "overbreadth" challenge, six-to-three, Scalia, J., Thomas, J., and Kennedy, J. dissenting.

2. See also Board of Trustees v. Fox, 491 U.S. 469 (1989) (least restrictive means of regulation *not* required to be met to sustain a public university ban on sales persons seeking access to campus dormitories, whether or not invited there by resident students).

In the Court's first address to this kind of question, *Cox v. New Hampshire*,[3] it sustained an advance payment requirement imposed by a city. The law provided that a specific charge up to (but not greater than) three hundred dollars could be assessed, the specific amount to be based on an objectively reasonable estimate of expenses likely to be incurred as an incident of city park use—in this case, an assembly by Jehovah's Witnesses in a city park. But this feature of the *Cox* case was not the issue principally reviewed at the time. Nor is it clear that the holding—that the provision was not void on its face—survived subsequent developments expanding first amendment public forum doctrine during the civil rights era of the 1960s and 1970s.[4] In 1992, the Supreme Court again addressed this kind of question to resolve a disagreement among federal courts of appeals as to whether the first amendment would prohibit anything greater than "nominal" (i.e. minimal) fees or charges from being imposed as a condition of free speech uses of traditional public forums. How definitively does it do so? What *is* the extent to which, and the reasons for which, charges may be imposed as a condition of parading, marching, leafletting, or demonstrating?

FORSYTH COUNTY v. NATIONALIST MOVEMENT

505 U.S. 123 (1992)

JUSTICE BLACKMUN delivered the opinion of the Court.

In this case *** we must decide whether the free speech guarantees of the First and Fourteenth Amendments are violated by an assembly and parade ordinance that permits a government administrator to vary the fee for assembling or parading to reflect the estimated cost of maintaining public order.

I

Petitioner Forsyth County is a primarily rural Georgia county approximately 30 miles northeast of Atlanta. *** [T]he Forsyth County Board of Commissioners enacted Ordinance 34 on January 27, 1987. *** The ordinance recites that it is "to provide for the issuance of permits for parades, assemblies, demonstrations, road closings, and other uses of public property and roads by private organizations and groups of private persons for private purposes." [It] was amended on June 8, 1987,

---

3. 312 U.S. 569 (1941).

4. For two of many critical reviews of *Cox* and the relevant cases and general issues raised in this area prior to *Forsyth County*, see Eric Neisser, Charging for Free Speech: User Fees and Insurance Requirements in the Marketplace of Ideas, 174 Geo.L.J. 257 (1985), and David Goldberger, [C]an Demonstrators be Required to Pay the Costs of Using America's Public Forums?, 62 Tex.L.Rev. 403 (1983). And see generally Vincent A. Blasi, Prior Restraints on Demonstrations, 68 Mich.L.Rev. 1481 (1970). (For recent elaborate reviews subsequent to Forsyth County, see Pinette v. Capitol Square Review & Advisory Bd., 874 F.Supp. 791 (S.D. Ohio 1994); Long Beach Lesbian & Gay Pride, Inc. v. City of Long Beach, 17 Cal.Rptr.2d 861 (1993).)

to provide that every permit applicant "shall pay in advance for such permit, for the use of the County, a sum not more than $1000.00 for each day such parade, procession, or open air public meeting shall take place." *** In addition, the county administrator was empowered to "adjust the amount to be paid in order to meet the expense incident to the administration of the Ordinance and to the maintenance of public order in the matter licensed." ***

In January 1989, respondent The Nationalist Movement proposed to demonstrate in opposition to the federal holiday commemorating the birthday of Martin Luther King, Jr. In Forsyth County, the Movement sought to "conduct a rally and speeches for one and a half to two hours" on the courthouse steps on a Saturday afternoon. *** The county imposed a $100 fee. The fee did not include any calculation for expenses incurred by law enforcement authorities, but was based on 10 hours of the county administrator's time in issuing the permit. The county administrator testified that the cost of his time was deliberately undervalued and that he did not charge for the clerical support involved in processing the application. ***

The Movement did not pay the fee and did not hold the rally. Instead, it instituted this action, requesting a temporary restraining order and permanent injunction prohibiting Forsyth County from interfering with the Movement's plans.

The District Court denied the temporary restraining order and injunction. *** The United States Court of Appeals for the Eleventh Circuit reversed this aspect of the District Court's judgment. [T]he Court of Appeals held: "An ordinance which charges more than a nominal fee for using public forums for public issue speech, violates the First Amendment." *** The court determined that a permit fee of up to $1000 a day exceeded this constitutional threshold. ***

We granted certiorari to resolve a conflict among the Courts of Appeals concerning the constitutionality of charging a fee for a speaker in a public forum. ***

II

Respondent mounts a facial challenge to the Forsyth County ordinance. It is well established that in the area of freedom of expression an overbroad regulation may be subject to facial review and invalidation, even though its application in the case under consideration may be constitutionally unobjectionable. *** This exception from general standing rules is based on an appreciation that the very existence of some broadly written laws has the potential to chill the expressive activity of others not before the court. ***

The Forsyth County ordinance requiring a permit and a fee before authorizing public speaking, parades, or assemblies in "the archetype of a traditional public forum," Frisby v. Schultz, 487 U.S. 474, 480 (1988), is a prior restraint on speech. Although there is a "heavy presumption" against the validity of a prior restraint, Bantam Books, Inc. v. Sullivan, 372 U.S. 58, 70 (1963), the Court has recognized that government, in order to regulate competing uses of public forums, may impose a permit requirement on those wishing to hold a march, parade, or rally. *** Such a scheme, however, must meet certain constitutional requirements. It may not delegate overly broad licensing discretion to a government official. Further, any permit scheme controlling the time, place, and manner of speech must not be based on the content of the message, must be narrowly tailored to serve a significant governmental interest, and must leave open ample alternatives for communication. See United States v. Grace, 461 U.S. 171, 177 (1983).

A

***

In evaluating petitioner's facial challenge, we must consider the county's authoritative constructions of the ordinance, including its own implementation and interpretation of it. *** In the present litigation, the county has made clear how it interprets and implements the ordinance. The ordinance can apply to any activity on public property—from parades, to street corner speeches, to bike races—and the fee assessed may reflect the county's police and administrative costs. Whether or not, in any given instance, the fee would include any or all of the county's administrative and security expenses is decided by the county administrator.[9]

In this case, according to testimony at the District Court hearing, the administrator based the fee on his own judgment of what would be reasonable. Although the county paid for clerical support and staff as an "expense incident to the administration" of the permit, the administrator testified that he chose in this instance not to include that expense in the fee. The administrator also attested that he had deliberately kept the fee low by undervaluing the cost of the time he spent processing the application. Even if he had spent more time on the project, he claimed, he would not have charged more. He further testified that, in this instance, he chose not to include any charge for expected security expense. *** The administrator also once charged bike-race organizers $25 to hold a race on county roads, but he did not explain why processing a bike-race permit demanded less administrative time than processing a parade permit or why he had chosen to assess $25 in that instance. ***

Based on the county's implementation and construction of the ordinance, it simply cannot be said that there are any "narrowly drawn, reasonable and definite standards," *Niemotko*, 340 U.S., at 271, guiding the hand of the Forsyth County administrator. The decision how much to charge for police protection or administrative time—or even whether to charge at all— is left to the whim of the administrator. There are no articulated standards either in the ordinance or in the county's established practice. The administrator is not required to rely on any objective factors.

---

9. In pertinent part, the ordinance, as amended, states that the administrator "*shall* adjust the amount to be paid in order to meet the expense incident to the administration of the Ordinance and to the maintenance of public order." § 3(6) (emphasis added). This could suggest that the administrator has no authority to reduce or waive these expenses. It has not been so understood, however, by the county. See 934 F.2d, at 1488, n. 12 (opinion concurring in part and dissenting in part). ***

He need not provide any explanation for his decision, and that decision is unreviewable. Nothing in the law or its application prevents the official from encouraging some views and discouraging others through the arbitrary application of fees.[10] The First Amendment prohibits the vesting of such unbridled discretion in a government official.[11]

B

The Forsyth County ordinance contains more than the possibility of censorship through uncontrolled discretion. As construed by the county, the ordinance often requires that the fee be based on the content of the speech.

The county envisions that the administrator, in appropriate instances, will assess a fee to cover "the cost of necessary and reasonable protection of persons participating in or observing said *** activit[y]." *** In order to assess accurately the cost of security for parade participants, the administrator "'must necessarily examine the content of the message that is conveyed,'" *** estimate the response of others to that content, and judge the number of police necessary to meet that response. The fee assessed will depend on the administrator's measure of the amount of hostility likely to be created by the speech based on its content. Those wishing to express views unpopular with bottle-throwers, for example, may have to pay more for their permit.

Although petitioner agrees that the cost of policing relates to content, *** it contends that the ordinance is content-neutral because it is aimed only at a secondary effect—the cost of maintaining public order. ***

The costs to which petitioner refers are those associated with the public's reaction to the speech. Listeners' reaction to speech is not a content-neutral basis for regulation. *** [C]f. Schneider v. State, 308 U.S. 147, 162 (1939) (fact that city is financially burdened when listeners throw leaflets on the street does not justify restriction on distribution of leaflets). Speech cannot be financially burdened, any more than it can be punished or banned, simply because it might offend a hostile

10. The District Court's finding that in this instance the Forsyth County administrator applied legitimate, content-neutral criteria, even if correct, is irrelevant to this facial challenge. Facial attacks on the discretion granted a decisionmaker are not dependent on the facts surrounding any particular permit decision. See Lakewood v. Plain Dealer Publishing Co., 486 U.S. 750, 770 (1988). ***

11. Petitioner also claims that Cox v. New Hampshire, 312 U.S. 569 (1941), excuses the administrator's discretion in setting the fee. Reliance on *Cox* is misplaced. Although the discretion granted to the administrator under the language in this ordinance is the same as in the statute at issue in *Cox*, the interpretation and application of that language are different. Unlike this case, there was in *Cox* no testimony or evidence that the statute granted unfettered discretion to the licensing authority. ***

mob.[12] See Gooding v. Wilson, 405 U.S. 518 (1972); Terminiello v. Chicago, 337 U.S. 1 (1949).

This Court has held time and again: "Regulations which permit the Government to discriminate on the basis of the content of the message cannot be tolerated under the First Amendment." Regan v. Time, Inc., 468 U.S. 641, 648-649 (1984) ***. The county offers only one justification for this ordinance: raising revenue for police services. While this undoubtedly is an important government responsibility, it does not justify a content-based permit fee. ***

Petitioner insists that its ordinance cannot be unconstitutionally content-based because it contains much of the same language as did the state statute upheld in Cox v. New Hampshire, 312 U.S. 569 (1941). Although the Supreme Court of New Hampshire had interpreted the statute at issue in *Cox* to authorize the municipality to charge a permit fee for the "maintenance of public order," no fee was actually assessed. *** Nothing in this Court's opinion suggests that the statute, as interpreted by the New Hampshire Supreme Court, called for charging a premium in the case of a controversial political message delivered before a hostile audience. In light of the Court's subsequent First Amendment jurisprudence, we do not read *Cox* to permit such a premium.

C

Petitioner, as well as the Court of Appeals and the District Court, all rely on the maximum allowable fee as the touchstone of constitutionality. Petitioner contends that the $1,000 cap on the fee ensures that the ordinance will not result in content-based discrimination. The ordinance was found unconstitutional by the Court of Appeals because the $1,000 cap was not sufficiently low to be "nominal." Neither the $1,000 cap on the fee charged, nor even some lower nominal cap, could save the ordinance because in this context, the level of the fee is irrelevant. A tax based on the content of speech does not become more constitutional because it is a small tax.

The lower courts derived their requirement that the permit fee be "nominal" from a sentence in the opinion in Murdock v. Pennsylvania, 319 U.S. 105 (1943). In *Murdock*, the Court invalidated a flat license fee levied on distributors of religious literature. In distinguishing the case from *Cox*, where the Court upheld a permit fee, the Court stated: "And the fee is not a nominal one, imposed as a regulatory measure

12. The dissent prefers a remand because there are no lower court findings on the question whether the county plans to base parade fees on hostile crowds. *** We disagree. A remand is unnecessary because there is no question that petitioner intends the ordinance to recoup costs that are related to listeners' reaction to the speech. Petitioner readily admits it did not charge for police protection for the 4th of July parades, although they were substantial parades, which required the closing of streets and drew large crowds. Petitioner imposed a fee only when it became necessary to provide security for parade participants from angry crowds opposing their message. *** The ordinance itself makes plain that the costs at issue are those needed for "necessary and reasonable protection of persons participating in or observing" the speech. *** We find no disputed interpretation of the ordinance necessitating a remand.

and calculated to defray the expense of protecting those on the streets and at home against the abuses of solicitors." 319 U.S., at 116. This sentence does not mean that an invalid fee can be saved if it is nominal, or that only nominal charges are constitutionally permissible. It reflects merely one distinction between the facts in*Murdock* and those in *Cox*.

The tax at issue in *Murdock* was invalid because it was unrelated to any legitimate state interest, not because it was of a particular size. Similarly, the provision of the Forsyth County ordinance relating to fees is invalid because it unconstitutionally ties the amount of the fee to the content of the speech and lacks adequate procedural safeguards; no limit on such a fee can remedy these constitutional violations.

The judgment of the Court of Appeals is affirmed.

CHIEF JUSTICE REHNQUIST, with whom JUSTICE WHITE, JUSTICE SCALIA, and JUSTICE THOMAS join, dissenting.

We granted certiorari in this case to consider the following question:

> "Whether the provisions of the First Amendment to the United States Constitution limit the amount of a license fee assessed pursuant to the provisions of a county parade ordinance to a nominal sum or whether the amount of the license fee may take into account the actual expense incident to the administration of the ordinance and the maintenance of public order in the matter licensed, up to the sum of $1,000.00 per day of the activity." ***

The Court's discussion of this question is limited to an ambiguous and noncommittal paragraph toward the very end of the opinion. *** The rest of the opinion takes up and decides other perceived unconstitutional defects in the Forsyth County ordinance. None of these claims were passed upon by the Court of Appeals; that court decided only that the First Amendment forbade the charging of more than a nominal fee for a permit to parade on public streets. Since that was the question decided by the Court of Appeals below, the question which divides the courts of appeals, and the question presented in the petition for certiorari, one would have thought that the Court would at least authoritatively decide, if not limit itself to, that question.

I

The answer to this question seems to me quite simple, because it was authoritatively decided by this Court more than half a century ago in Cox v. New Hampshire, 312 U.S. 569 (1941). There we confronted a State statute which required payment of a license fee of up to $300 to local governments for the right to parade in the public streets. The Supreme Court of New Hampshire had construed the provision as requiring that the amount of the fee be adjusted based on the size of the parade, as the fee "for a circus parade or a celebration procession of length, each drawing crowds of observers, would take into account the greater public expense of policing the spectacle, compared with the slight expense of a less expansive and attractive parade or procession." *** Under the state court's construction, the fee provision was "not a revenue tax, but one to meet the expense incident to the administration of the Act and to the maintenance of public order in the matter licensed." *** This Court, in a unanimous opinion by Chief Justice Hughes, upheld the statute, saying:

> "There is nothing contrary to the Constitution in the charge of a fee limited to the purpose stated. The suggestion that a flat fee should have been charged fails to take account of the difficulty of framing a fair schedule to meet all circumstances, and we perceive no constitutional ground for denying to local governments that flexibility of adjustment of fees which in the light of varying conditions would tend to conserve rather than impair the liberty sought.
>
> "There is no evidence that the statute has been administered otherwise than in the fair and nondiscriminatory manner which the state court has construed it to require." ***

*** I believe that the decision in *Cox* squarely controls the disposition of the question presented in this case, and I therefore would explicitly hold that the Constitution does not limit a parade license fee to a nominal amount.

II

Instead of deciding the particular question on which we granted certiorari, the Court concludes that the county ordinance is facially unconstitutional because it places too much discretion in the hands of the county administrator and forces parade participants to pay for the cost of controlling those who might oppose their speech. *** But, because the lower courts did not pass on these issues, the Court is forced to rely on its own interpretation of the ordinance in making these rulings. The Court unnecessarily reaches out to interpret the ordinance on its own at this stage, even though there are no lower court factual findings on the scope or administration of the ordinance. Because there are no such factual findings, I would not decide at this point whether the ordinance fails for lack of adequate standards to guide discretion or for incorporation of a "heckler's veto," but would instead remand the case to the lower courts to initially consider these issues.

*** The Court's analysis on this issue rests on an assumption that the county will interpret the phrase "maintenance of public order" to support the imposition of fees based on opposition crowds. There is nothing in the record to support this assumption, however, and I would remand for a hearing on this question.

For the foregoing reasons, I dissent.

NOTE

The decision in *Forsyth* is doubtless helpful in clarifying two points: (a) that whatever charges for public permits are to be imposed in advance, they must be settled by readily ascertainable, objective standards minimizing subjectivity and personal discretion in the administering public agency;[73] and (b) that they may not take into account even objectively determinable costs likely to be incurred (or even actually incurred) as a consequence of attendance or activity by "anti-demonstrators" or others offended by or hostile to the proposed public forum use.[74] Each is doubtless a significant point. But what of the following questions?

1. What of the *original* question posed by *Forsyth* (the question that had divided the courts of appeal)? Consistent with the limitations just noted, may "the amount of [a] license fee *** take into account [all] reasonable expense incident to the administration of the ordinance and to the maintenance of public order in the matter licensed?" May it do so, that is, though the required amount (objectively computed) is far from being merely "nominal"—though it is, in fact, well beyond the means of the permit seeker? Does it matter if the permit seeker is "unable" to pay, as opposed to "unwilling" to pay, or likely to suffer "hardship" in paying?

2. If it does matter, doesn't this mean that, in a real sense, the poor would have *more* rights that those less poor—and that others (namely taxpayers) would pay for the expenses the poor generate by their activity, while others will not be permitted to parade unless they *themselves* pay? If it doesn't make a difference, however, wouldn't unpopular and financially unsupported causes have less access than popular well-supported causes? Wouldn't it mean that unpopular causes would be deprived of access to even the traditional public forum, such places now to be "cost-reserved" for those with the means to pay?[75]

3. Is it likewise clear, with respect to both of the preceding questions, that no distinctions can be made to depend upon the pedigree of the group (e.g., the same rule for the NAACP as for the Ku Klux Klan), or the nature of the cause for which a group seeks to ventilate its felt grievance? So, for example, if the direct costs incidental to a Selma-to-Montgomery march—to protect the alleged denial of equal protection of the law to racial minorities in Alabama—were the same as, say, the direct costs incidental to a "St. Patrick's Day" celebratory parade on Fifth Avenue

73. This point is merely a reiteration of standard doctrine regarding regimes of prior restraint. See, e.g., Kunz v. New York, 340 U.S. 290 (1951); Lakewood v. Plain Dealer Publishing Co., 486 U.S. 750 (1988).

74. This point is an amplification and application of standard "heckler's veto" doctrine.

75. The Court has struck down, on equal protection grounds, several "mere cost" schemes, when inability to pay foreclosed a plaintiff from access to an essential service or from exercise of a fundamental right. See, e.g., Harper v. Virginia Bd. of Elections, 383 U.S. 663 (1966) (poll tax); Griffin v. Illinois, 351 U.S. 12 (1956) (costs of producing record, including transcript, from criminal trial for purposes of appeal); Boddie v. Connecticut, 401 U.S. 371 (1971) (court fees and costs incident to divorce proceedings); Memorial Hosp. v. Maricopa County, 415 U.S. 250 (1974) (one year residency requirement for indigents to receive nonemergency medical care at county's expense).

in New York (each objectively determined to entail direct public expense)—a "neutral" denial of the required permit would be required, insofar as the sponsoring group (whether unable or not) failed to deposit that sum in advance?[76]

---

4. Forum Analysis

INTRODUCTORY NOTE

The preceding materials, culminating in *Ward v. Rock Against Racism* (and the stylized "three-part *Ward* test"), have elaborately illustrated the Supreme Court's review of time, place, and manner restrictions on speech in public places. The cases cover a half century of litigation in a wide variety of settings (e.g., leafletting, picketing, posting, parading, demonstrating, marching, even singing), all since the seminal 1939 decision, *Hague v. Committee for Industrial Organization*.[77] The nature of the governmentally-controlled place in which one's communicative conduct took place obviously mattered in many of these cases,[78] but it was virtually never conclusive. Rather, it was but one salient factor, among many, to be taken into account. Consistent with the general framework of "time, place, and manner" review developed steadily in the decades following *Hague*, even though the place of one's expression or expressive conduct was not the "traditional" forum of the public streets or parks (as in *Hague*), the first amendment nevertheless often disallowed the restriction at issue.[79]

In the past two decades, however, a refinement has been added. Called "forum analysis," this refinement identifies a special (sometimes conclusive) significance to the *place* to which a given restriction of access, and of forum use, may be tied. It permits significantly greater discretion of public regulation of what may (and also of what may *not*) be expressed in some places than in others, and a significantly greater

---

76. For one approach to this question, see Ronald J. Krotoszynski, Jr., Celebrating Selma: The Importance of Context in Public Forum Analysis, 104 Yale L.J. 1411 (1995).

77. 307 U.S. 496 (1939). For two more matched examples of divided cases in the Supreme Court, compare Brown v. Louisiana, 383 U.S. 131 (1966) (reversing breach of peace conviction for silent sit-in protesters in a public library who had refused to leave when requested) with Adderley v. Florida, 385 U.S. 39 (1966) (sustaining trespass conviction of protesters who refused to leave outside jail grounds), and compare Flower v. United States, 407 U.S. 197 (1972) (finding protected the distribution of peace leaflets on streets open to the public within a large military base) with Greer v. Spock, 424 U.S. 828 (1976) (finding a similar distribution not protected against base commander's evenhanded administration of rule requiring prior approval—which the leafletters had not sought and would not have received).

78. As did the *time* at which one chose to engage in that conduct, and the *manner* in which one did so.

79. See, e.g., Tinker v. Des Moines Indep. Sch. Dist., 393 U.S. 503 (1969) (public school students and political protest armbands worn during school hours on school premises); Cohen v. California, 403 U.S. 15 (1971) ("Fuck the Draft" jacket exhibited in corridor of county courthouse during business hours); Rankin v. McPherson, 483 U.S. 378 (1987) (political views expressed inside sheriff's office by one worker to a co-worker).

public discretion of who may (and also of who may *not*) be permitted to share access and first amendment use of particular governmentally-managed facilities.

We track this development in this section, to take the full measure of this new "forum analysis." It makes one of its first appearances in the dissenting opinion of Justice Rehnquist in the case immediately following this Note, *Southeastern Promotions, Ltd. v. Conrad.* On grounds he found pertinent to the distinctive nature of this kind of taxpayer-supported facility, Justice Rehnquist suggested that public authority may disallow third parties to rent and to use a publicly-held civic auditorium for performances of a kind it could, admittedly, not keep from being presented in a privately owned theater.[81] One might usefully come back to this case after completing the balance of the section, to determine whether a restriction of the kind Justice Rehnquist thought sustainable would, in fact, now be upheld.

SOUTHEASTERN PROMOTIONS, LTD. v. CONRAD
420 U.S. 546 (1975)

MR. JUSTICE BLACKMUN delivered the opinion of the Court.

The issue in this case is whether First Amendment rights were abridged when respondents denied petitioner the use of a municipal facility in Chattanooga, Tenn., for the showing of the controversial rock musical "Hair." ***

I

Petitioner, Southeastern Promotions, Ltd., is a New York corporation engaged in the business of promoting and presenting theatrical productions for profit. On October 29, 1971, it applied for the use of the Tivoli, a privately owned Chattanooga theater under long-term lease to the city, to present "Hair" there for six days beginning November 23. This was to be a road company showing of the musical that had played for three years on Broadway, and had appeared in over 140 cities in the United States.[1]

Respondents are the directors of the Chattanooga Memorial Auditorium, a municipal theater. Shortly after receiving Southeastern's application, the directors met, and, after a brief discussion, voted to reject it. None of them had seen the play or read the script, but they understood from outside reports that the musical, as produced elsewhere, involved nudity and obscenity on stage. Although no conflicting engagement was scheduled for the Tivoli, respondents determined that the production

---

81. The majority found no occasion to consider his point.

1. Twice previously, petitioner informally had asked permission to use the Tivoli, and had been refused. In other cities, it had encountered similar resistance and had successfully sought injunctions ordering local officials to permit use of municipal facilities.***

would not be "in the best interest of the community." Southeastern was so notified but no written statement of reasons was provided.

On November 1 petitioner, alleging that respondents' action abridged its First Amendment rights, sought a preliminary injunction from the United States District Court for the Eastern District of Tennessee. *** The District Court took evidence as to the play's content, and respondent Conrad gave the following account of the board's decision:

> "We use the general terminology in turning down the request for its use that we felt it was not in the best interest of the community and I can't speak beyond that. That was the board's determination.
>
> "Now, I would have to speak for myself, the policy to which I would refer, as I mentioned, basically indicates that we will, as a board, allow those productions which are clean and healthful and culturally uplifting, or words to that effect. They are quoted in the original dedication booklet of the Memorial Auditorium."[4]

The court denied preliminary relief, concluding that petitioner had failed to show that it would be irreparably harmed pending a final judgment since scheduling was "purely a matter of financial loss or gain" and was compensable.

Southeastern some weeks later pressed for a permanent injunction permitting it to use the larger auditorium, rather than the Tivoli, on Sunday, April 9, 1972. The District Court held three days of hearings beginning April 3. On the issue of obscenity *vel non*, presented to an advisory jury, it took evidence consisting of the full script and libretto, with production notes and stage instructions, a recording of the musical numbers, a souvenir program, and the testimony of seven witnesses who had seen the production elsewhere. The jury returned a verdict that "Hair" was obscene. The District Court agreed. It concluded that conduct in the production—group nudity and simulated sex—would violate city ordinances and state statutes making public nudity and obscene acts criminal offenses. This criminal conduct, the court reasoned, was neither speech nor symbolic speech, and was to be viewed separately from the musical's speech elements. Being pure conduct, comparable to rape or murder, it

---

4. The Memorial Auditorium, completed in 1924, was dedicated to the memory of Chattanooga citizens who had "offered their lives" in World War I. The booklet referred to is entitled Souvenir of Dedication of Soldiers & Sailors Auditorium Chattanooga, Tenn. It contains the following:

"It will be [the board's] endeavor to make [the auditorium] the community center of Chattanooga; where civic, educational, religious, patriotic and charitable organizations and associations may have a common meeting place to discuss and further the upbuilding and general welfare of the city and surrounding territory.

"It will not be operated for profit, and no effort to obtain financial returns above the actual operating expenses will be permitted. Instead its purpose will be devoted for cultural advancement, and for clean, healthful, entertainment which will make for the upbuilding of a better citizenship."

was not entitled to First Amendment protection. Accordingly, the court denied the injunction.

On appeal, the United States Court of Appeals for the Sixth Circuit, by a divided vote, affirmed. The majority relied primarily on the lower court's reasoning. Neither the judges of the Court of Appeals nor the District Court saw the musical performed. Because of the First Amendment overtones, we granted certiorari.

Petitioner urges reversal on the grounds that (1) respondents' action constituted an unlawful prior restraint, (2) the courts below applied an incorrect standard for the determination of the issue of obscenity *vel non*, and (3) the record does not support a finding that "Hair" is obscene. We do not reach the latter two contentions, for we agree with the first. We hold that respondents' rejection of petitioner's application to use this public forum accomplished a prior restraint under a system lacking in constitutionally required minimal procedural safeguards. Accordingly, on this narrow ground, we reverse.

II

***

Respondents' action was no less a prior restraint because the public facilities under their control happened to be municipal theaters. The Memorial Auditorium and the Tivoli were public forums designed for and dedicated to expressive activities. There was no question as to the usefulness of either facility for petitioner's production. There was no contention by the board that these facilities could not accommodate a production of this size. ***

Whether petitioner might have used some other, privately owned, theater in the city for the production is of no consequence. There is reason to doubt on this record whether any other facility would have served as well as these, since none apparently had the seating capacity, acoustical features, stage equipment, and electrical service that the show required. Even if a privately owned forum had been available, that fact alone would not justify an otherwise impermissible prior restraint. "[O]ne is not to have the exercise of his liberty of expression in appropriate places abridged on the plea that it may be exercised in some other place." Schneider v. State, 308 U.S., at 163.

Thus, it does not matter for purposes of this case that the board's decision might not have had the effect of total suppression of the musical in the community. Denying use of the municipal facility under the circumstances present here constituted the prior restraint. That restraint was final.***

III

***

*** In *Freedman* [v. Maryland, 380 U.S. 51 (1965)] the Court struck down a state scheme for the licensing of motion pictures, holding "that, because only a judicial determination in an adversary proceeding ensures the necessary sensitivity to freedom of expression, only a procedure requiring a judicial determination suffices to impose a valid final restraint." 380 U.S., at 58. We held in *Freedman*, and we reaffirm here, that a system of prior restraint runs afoul of the First Amendment if it lacks certain safeguards: *First*, the burden of instituting judicial proceedings, and of proving that the material is unprotected, must rest on the censor. *Second*, any restraint prior to judicial review can be imposed only for a specified brief period and only for the purpose of preserving the status quo. *Third*, a prompt final judicial determination must be assured.

Although most of our cases have pertained to motion picture licensing or censorship, this Court has applied *Freedman* to the system by which federal customs agents seize imported materials, *United States v. Thirty-seven Photographs*, [402 U.S. 363 (1971)] and to that by which postal officials restrict use of the mails,*Blount v. Rizzi*, [400 U.S. 410 (1971)]. In *Blount* we held unconstitutional provisions of the postal laws designed to control use of the mails for commerce in obscene materials. The provisions enabled the Postmaster General to halt delivery of mail to an individual and prevent payment of money orders to him. The administrative order became effective without judicial approval, and the burden of obtaining judicial review was placed upon the user.

If a scheme that restricts access to the mails must furnish the procedural safeguards set forth in *Freedman*, no less must be expected of a system that regulates use of a public forum. Respondents here had the same powers of licensing and censorship exercised by postal officials in *Blount*, and by boards and officials in other cases.

Procedural safeguards were lacking here in several respects. The board's system did not provide a procedure for prompt judicial review. Although the District Court commendably held a hearing on petitioner's motion for a preliminary injunction within a few days of the board's decision, it did not review the merits of the decision at that time. The question at the hearing was whether petitioner should receive *preliminary* relief, i.e., whether here was likelihood of success on the merits and whether petitioner would suffer irreparable injury pending full review. Effective review on the merits was not obtained until more than five months later. Throughout, it was petitioner, not the board, that bore the burden of obtaining judicial review. It was petitioner that had the burden of persuasion at the preliminary hearing if not at the later stages of the litigation. Respondents did not file a formal answer to the complaint for five months after petitioner sought review. During the time prior to judicial determination, the restraint altered the status quo. Petitioner was forced to forgo the initial dates planned for the engagement and to seek to schedule the performance at a later date. The delay and uncertainty inevitably discouraged use of the forum.

The procedural shortcomings that form the basis for our decision are unrelated to the standard that the board applied. Whatever the reasons may have been for the board's exclusion of the musical, it could not escape the obligation to afford appropriate procedural safeguards. We need not decide whether the standard of obscenity applied by respondents or the courts below was sufficiently precise or substantively correct, or whether the production is in fact obscene. *** The standard, whatever it may be, must be implemented under a system that assures prompt judicial review with a minimal restriction of First Amendment rights necessary under the circumstances.

Reversed.

MR. JUSTICE DOUGLAS, dissenting in part and concurring in the result in part.

***

A municipal theater is no less a forum for the expression of ideas than is a public park, or a sidewalk; the forms of expression adopted in such a forum may be more expensive and more structured than those typically seen in our parks and streets, but they are surely no less entitled to the shelter of the First Amendment. As soon as municipal officials are permitted to pick and choose, as they are in all existing socialist regimes, between those productions which are "clean and healthful and culturally uplifting" in content and those which are not, the path is cleared for a regime of censorship under which full voice can be given only to those views which meet with the approval of the powers that be.

There was much testimony in the District Court concerning the pungent social and political commentary which the musical "Hair" levels against various sacred cows of our society: The Vietnam war, the draft, and the puritanical conventions of the Establishment. This commentary is undoubtedly offensive to some, but its contribution to social consciousness and intellectual ferment is a positive one. In this respect, the musical's often ribald humor and trenchant social satire may someday merit comparison to the most highly regarded works of Aristophanes, a fellow debunker of established tastes and received wisdom, yet one whose offerings would doubtless meet with a similarly cold reception at the hands of Establishment censors. No matter how many procedural safeguards may be imposed, any system which permits governmental officials to inhibit or control the flow of disturbing and unwelcome ideas to the public threatens serious diminution of the breadth and richness of our cultural offerings.

MR. JUSTICE WHITE, with whom THE CHIEF JUSTICE joins, dissenting. [Omitted.]

MR. JUSTICE REHNQUIST, dissenting.

The Court treats this case as if it were on all fours with Freedman v. Maryland, 380 U.S. 51 (1965), which it is not. *Freedman* dealt with the efforts of the State of Maryland to prohibit the petitioner in that case from showing a film "at his Baltimore theater." Petitioner here did not seek to show the musical production "Hair" at *its* Chattanooga theater, but rather at a Chattanooga theater owned by the city of Chattanooga.

The Court glosses over this distinction by treating a community-owned theater as if it were the same as a city park or city street, which it is not. The Court's decisions have recognized that city streets and parks are traditionally open to the public, and that permits or licenses to use them are not ordinarily required. "[O]ne who is rightfully on a street which the state has left open to the public carries with him there as elsewhere the constitutional right to express his views in an orderly fashion. This right extends to the communication of ideas by handbills and literature as well as by the spoken word." Jamison v. Texas, 318 U.S. 413, 416 (1943). The Court has therefore held that where municipal authorities seek to exact a license or permit for those who wish to use parks or streets for the purpose of exercising their right of free speech, the standards governing the licensing authority must be objective, definite, and nondiscriminatory. Shuttlesworth v. City of Birmingham, 394 U.S. 147 (1969). But until this case the Court has not equated a public auditorium, which must of necessity schedule performances by a process of inclusion and exclusion, with public streets and parks. ***

[T]he auditoriums in question here have historically been devoted to "clean, healthful entertainment"; they have accepted only productions not inappropriate for viewing by children so that the facilities might serve as a place for entertaining the whole family. Viewed apart from any constitutional limitations, such a policy would undoubtedly rule out much worthwhile adult entertainment. But if it is the desire of the citizens of Chattanooga, who presumably have paid for and own the facilities, that the attractions to be shown there should not be of the kind which would offend any substantial number of potential theatergoers, I do not think the policy can be described as arbitrary or unreasonable.[2] Whether or not the production of the version of "Hair" here under consideration is obscene, the findings of fact made by the District Court and affirmed on appeal do indicate that it is not entertainment designed for the whole family. ***

A municipal theater may not be run by municipal authorities as if it were a private theater, free to judge on a content basis alone which plays it wishes to have performed and which it does not. But, just as surely, that element of it which is "theater" ought to be accorded some constitutional recognition along with that element of it which is "municipal." I do not believe fidelity to the First Amendment requires the exaggerated and rigid procedural safeguards which the Court insists upon in this case. I think that the findings of the District Court and the Court of Appeals support the conclusion that petitioner was denied a lease for constitutionally adequate and nondiscriminatory reasons. I would therefore affirm the judgment of the Court of Appeals.

---

2. Limitations on the use of municipal auditoriums by government must be sufficiently reasonable to satisfy the Due Process Clause and cannot unfairly discriminate in violation of the Equal Protection Clause. A municipal auditorium which opened itself to Republicans while closing itself to Democrats would run afoul of the Fourteenth Amendment. There is no allegation in the instant case that the auditoriums accepted equally graphic productions while unfairly discriminating against "Hair" because of its expressions of political and social belief.

PERRY EDUCATION ASSOCIATION v. PERRY LOCAL EDUCATORS' ASSOCIATION

460 U.S. 37 (1983)

JUSTICE WHITE delivered the opinion of the Court.

Perry Education Association is the duly elected exclusive bargaining representative for the teachers of the Metropolitan School District of Perry Township, Ind. A collective-bargaining agreement with the Board of Education provided that Perry Education Association, but no other union, would have access to the interschool mail system and teacher mailboxes in the Perry Township schools. The issue in this case is whether the denial of similar access to the Perry Local Educators' Association, a rival teacher group, violates the First and Fourteenth Amendments.

I

***

Prior to 1977, both the Perry Education Association (PEA) and the Perry Local Educators' Association (PLEA) represented teachers in the School District and apparently had equal access to the interschool mail system. In 1977, PLEA challenged PEA's status as *de facto* bargaining representative for the Perry Township teachers by filing an election petition with the Indiana Education Employment Relations Board (Board). PEA won the election and was certified as the exclusive representative, as provided by Indiana law. ***

The Board permits a school district to provide access to communication facilities to the union selected for the discharge of the exclusive representative duties of representing the bargaining unit and its individual members without having to provide equal access to rival unions. Following the election, PEA and the School District negotiated a labor contract in which the School Board gave PEA "access to teachers' mailboxes in which to insert material" and the right to use the interschool mail delivery system to the extent that the School District incurred no extra expense by such use. The labor agreement noted that these access rights were being accorded to PEA "acting as the representative of the teachers" and went on to stipulate that these access rights shall not be granted to any other "school employee organization" —a term of art defined by Indiana law to mean "any organization which has school employees as members and one of whose primary purposes is representing school employees in dealing with their school employer." The PEA contract with these provisions was renewed in 1980 and is presently in force.

The exclusive-access policy applies only to use of the mailboxes and school mail system. PLEA is not prevented from using other school facilities to communicate with teachers. PLEA may post notices on school bulletin boards; may hold meetings on school property after school hours; and may, with approval of the building principals, make announcements on the public address system. Of course, PLEA also may communicate with teachers by word of mouth, telephone, or the United States mail. Moreover, under Indiana law, the preferential access of the bargaining agent may continue only while its status as exclusive representative is insulated from challenge. *** While a representation contest is in progress, unions must be afforded equal access to such communication facilities.

PLEA and two of its members filed this action under 42 U.S.C. § 1983 against PEA and individual members of the Perry Township School Board. Plaintiffs contended that PEA's preferential access to the internal mail system violates the First Amendment and the Equal Protection Clause of the Fourteenth Amendment. They sought injunctive and declaratory relief and damages. Upon cross-motions for summary judgment, the District Court entered judgment for the defendants. *** The Court of Appeals for the Seventh Circuit reversed. PEA now seeks review of this judgment by way of appeal. ***

III

The primary question presented is whether the First Amendment, applicable to the States by virtue of the Fourteenth Amendment, is violated when a union that has been elected by public school teachers as their exclusive bargaining representative is granted access to certain means of communication, while such access is denied to a rival union. There is no question that constitutional interests are implicated by denying PLEA use of the interschool mail system. "It can hardly be argued that either students or teachers shed their constitutional rights to freedom of speech or expression at the schoolhouse gate." Tinker v. Des Moines School District, 393 U.S. 503, 506 (1969); Healy v. James, 408 U.S. 169 (1972). The First Amendment's guarantee of free speech applies to teachers' mailboxes as surely as it does elsewhere within the school, *Tinker v. Des Moines School District,* and on sidewalks outside. But this is not to say that the First Amendment requires equivalent access to all parts of a school building in which some form of communicative activity occurs. *** The existence of a right of access to public property and the standard by which limitations upon such a right must be evaluated differ depending on the character of the property at issue.

A

In places which by long tradition or by government fiat have been devoted to assembly and debate, the rights of the State to limit expressive activity are sharply circumscribed. At one end of the spectrum are streets and parks which "have immemorially been held in trust for the use of the public and, time out of mind, have been used for purposes of assembly, communicating thoughts between citizens, and discussing public questions." Hague v. CIO, 307 U.S. 496, 515 (1939). In these quintessential public forums, the government may not prohibit all communicative activity. For the State to enforce a content-based exclusion it must show that its regulation is necessary to serve a compelling state interest and that it is narrowly drawn to achieve that end. *** The State may also enforce regulations of the time, place, and manner of expression which are content-neutral, are narrowly tailored to serve a significant government interest, and leave open ample alternative channels of communication. ***

A second category consists of public property which the State has opened for use by the public as a place for expressive activity. The Constitution forbids a State to enforce certain exclusions from a forum generally open to the public even if it was not required to create the forum in the first place. Widmar v. Vincent, 454 U.S. 263 (1982) (university meeting facilities); City of Madison Joint School District v. Wisconsin Employment Relations Comm'n, 429 U.S. 167 (1976) (school board meeting); Southeastern Promotions, Ltd. v. Conrad, 420 U.S. 546 (1975) (municipal theater).[7] Although a State is not required to indefinitely retain the open character of the facility, as long as it does so it is bound by the same standards as apply in a traditional public forum. Reasonable time, place, and manner regulations are permissible, and a content-based prohibition must be narrowly drawn to effectuate a compelling state interest.

Public property which is not by tradition or designation a forum for public communication is governed by different standards. We have recognized that the "First Amendment does not guarantee access to property simply because it is owned or controlled by the government." *United States Postal Service v. Council of Greenburgh Civic Assns.*, [453 U.S.], at 129. In addition to time, place, and manner regulations, the State may reserve the forum for its intended purposes, communicative or otherwise, as long as the regulation on speech is reasonable and not an effort to suppress expression merely because public officials oppose the speaker's view.

The school mail facilities at issue here fall within this third category. The Court of Appeals recognized that Perry School District's interschool mail system is not a traditional public forum: "We do not hold that a school's internal mail system is a public forum in the sense that a school board may not close it to all but official business if it chooses." On this point the parties agree. Nor do the parties dispute that, as the District Court observed, the "normal and intended function [of the school mail facilities] is to facilitate internal communication of school-related matters to the teachers." The internal mail system, at least by policy, is not held open to the general public. It is instead PLEA's position that the school mail facilities have become a "limited public forum" from which it may not be excluded because of the periodic use of the system by private non-school-connected groups, and PLEA's own unrestricted access to the system prior to PEA's certification as exclusive representative.

Neither of these arguments is persuasive. The use of the internal school mail by groups not affiliated with the schools is no doubt a relevant consideration. If by policy or by practice the Perry School District has opened its mail system for indiscriminate use by the general public, then PLEA could justifiably argue a public forum has been created. This, however, is not the case. As the case comes before us, there is no indication in the record that the school mailboxes and interschool delivery

7. A public forum may be created for a limited purpose such as use by certain groups, e.g., *Widmar v. Vincent* (student groups), or for the discussion of certain subjects, e.g., *City of Madison, Joint School District v. Wisconsin Public Employment Relations Comm'n* (school board business).

system are open for use by the general public. Permission to use the system to communicate with teachers must be secured from the individual building principal. There is no court finding or evidence in the record which demonstrates that this permission has been granted as a matter of course to all who seek to distribute material. We can only conclude that the schools do allow some outside organizations such as the YMCA, Cub Scouts, and other civic and church organizations to use the facilities. This type of selective access does not transform government property into a public forum. ***

Moreover, even if we assume that by granting access to the Cub Scouts, YMCA's, and parochial schools, the School District has created a "limited" public forum, the constitutional right of access would in any event extend only to other entities of similar character. While the school mail facilities thus might be a forum generally open for use by the Girl Scouts, the local boys' club, and other organizations that engage in activities of interest and educational relevance to students, they would not as a consequence be open to an organization such as PLEA, which is concerned with the terms and conditions of teacher employment.

PLEA also points to its ability to use school mailboxes and delivery system on an equal footing with PEA prior to the collective-bargaining agreement signed in 1978. Its argument appears to be that the access policy in effect at that time converted the school mail facilities into a limited public forum generally open for use by employee organizations, and that once this occurred, exclusions of employee organizations thereafter must be judged by the constitutional standard applicable to public forums. The fallacy in the argument is that it is not the forum, but PLEA itself, which has changed. Prior to 1977, there was no exclusive representative for the Perry School District teachers. PEA and PLEA each represented its own members. Therefore the School District's policy of allowing both organizations to use the school mail facilities simply reflected the fact that both unions represented the teachers and had legitimate reasons for use of the system. PLEA's previous access was consistent with the School District's preservation of the facilities for school-related business, and did not constitute creation of a public forum in any broader sense.

*** In the Court of Appeals' view, however, the access policy adopted by the Perry schools favors a particular viewpoint, that of PEA, on labor relations, and consequently must be strictly scrutinized regardless of whether a public forum is involved. There is, however, no indication that the School Board intended to discourage one viewpoint and advance another. We believe it is more accurate to characterize the access policy as based on the *status* of the respective unions rather than their views. Implicit in the concept of the nonpublic forum is the right to make distinctions in access on the basis of subject matter and speaker identity. These distinctions may be impermissible in a public forum but are inherent and inescapable in the process of limiting a nonpublic forum to activities compatible with the intended purpose of the property. The touchstone for evaluating these distinctions is whether they are reasonable in light of the purpose which the forum at issue serves.

B

*** Use of school mail facilities enables PEA to perform effectively its obligations as exclusive representative of *all* Perry Township teachers. Conversely, PLEA does not have any official responsibility in connection with the School District and need not be entitled to the same rights of access to school mailboxes. We observe that providing exclusive access to recognized bargaining representatives is a permissible labor practice in the public sector.

The Court of Appeals accorded little or no weight to PEA's special responsibilities. In its view these responsibilities, while justifying PEA's access, did not justify denying equal access to PLEA. The Court of Appeals would have been correct if a public forum were involved here. But the internal mail system is not a public forum. As we have already stressed, when government property is not dedicated to open communication the government may—without further justification—restrict use to those who participate in the forum's official business.[13]

Finally, the reasonableness of the limitations of PLEA's access to the school mail system is also supported by the substantial alternative channels that remain open for union-teacher communication to take place. These means range from bulletin boards to meeting facilities to the United States mail. During election periods, PLEA is assured of equal access to all modes of communication. There is no showing here that PLEA's ability to communicate with teachers is seriously impinged by the restricted access to the internal mail system. ***

IV

The Court of Appeals also held that the differential access provided the rival unions constituted impermissible content discrimination in violation of the Equal Protection Clause of the Fourteenth Amendment. We have rejected this contention when cast as a First Amendment argument, and it fares no better in equal protection garb. As we have explained above, PLEA did not have a First Amendment or other right

---

13. The Court of Appeals was also mistaken in finding that the exclusive-access policy was not closely tailored to the official responsibilities of PEA. The Court of Appeals thought the policy over-inclusive—because the collective-bargaining agreement does not limit PEA's use of the mail system to messages related to its special legal duties. The record, however, does not establish that PEA enjoyed or claimed unlimited access by usage or otherwise; indeed, the collective-bargaining agreement indicates that the right of access was accorded to PEA "acting as the representative of the teachers." In these circumstances, we do not find it necessary to decide the reasonableness of a grant of access for unlimited purposes.

The Court of Appeals also indicated that the access policy was underinclusive because the School District permits outside organizations with no special duties to teachers to use the system. As we have already noted in text, *** there was no District policy of open access for private groups and, in any event, the provision of access to these private groups does not undermine the reasons for not allowing similar access by a rival labor union. ***

of access to the interschool mail system. The grant of such access to PEA, therefore, does not burden a fundamental right of PLEA. Thus, the decision to grant such privileges to PEA need not be tested by the strict scrutiny applied when government action impinges upon a fundamental right protected by the Constitution. See San Antonio Independent School District v. Rodriguez, 411 U.S. 1, 17 (1973). The School District's policy need only rationally further a legitimate state purpose. That purpose is clearly found in the special responsibilities of an exclusive bargaining representative.

The Seventh Circuit and PLEA rely on Police Department of Chicago v. Mosley, 408 U.S. 92 (1972), and Carey v. Brown, 447 U.S. 455 (1980). In *Mosley* and *Carey*, we struck down prohibitions on peaceful picketing in a public forum. In *Mosley*, the city of Chicago permitted peaceful picketing on the subject of a school's labor-management dispute, but prohibited other picketing in the immediate vicinity of the school. In *Carey*, the challenged state statute barred all picketing of residences and dwellings except the peaceful picketing of a place of employment involved in a labor dispute. In both cases, we found the distinction between classes of speech violative of the Equal Protection Clause. The key to those decisions, however, was the presence of a public forum. In a public forum, by definition, all parties have a constitutional right of access and the State must demonstrate compelling reasons for restriction of access to a single class of speakers, a single viewpoint, or a single subject.

When speakers and subjects are similarly situated, the State may not pick and choose. Conversely on government property that has not been made a public forum, not all speech is equally situated, and the State may draw distinctions which relate to the special purpose for which the property is used. As we have explained above, for a school mail facility, the difference in status between the exclusive bargaining representative and its rival is such a distinction. *** The judgment of the Court of Appeals is reversed.

JUSTICE BRENNAN, with whom JUSTICE MARSHALL, JUSTICE POWELL, and JUSTICE STEVENS join, dissenting.

I

***

The Court fundamentally misperceives the essence of the respondents' claims and misunderstands the thrust of the Court of Appeals' well-reasoned opinion. This case does not involve an "absolute access" claim. It involves an "equal access" claim. As such it does not turn on whether the internal school mail system is a "public forum." In focusing on the public forum issue, the Court disregards the First Amendment's central proscription against censorship, in the form of viewpoint discrimination, in any forum, public or nonpublic.

The First Amendment's prohibition against government discrimination among viewpoints on particular issues falling within the realm of protected speech has been noted extensively in the opinions of this Court. In Niemotko v. Maryland, 340 U.S.

268 (1951), two Jehovah's Witnesses were denied access to a public park to give Bible talks. Members of other religious groups had been granted access to the park for purposes related to religion. The Court found that the denial of access was based on public officials' disagreement with the Jehovah's Witnesses views, and held it invalid. During the course of its opinion, the Court stated: "The right to equal protection of the laws, in the exercise of those freedoms of speech and religion protected by the First and Fourteenth Amendments, has a firmer foundation than the whims or personal opinions of a local governing body." In an opinion concurring in the result, Justice Frankfurter stated that "[t]o allow expression of religious views by some and deny the same privilege to others merely because they or their views are unpopular, even deeply so, is a denial of equal protection of the law forbidden by the Fourteenth Amendment." ***

Once the government permits discussion of certain subject matter, it may not impose restrictions that discriminate among viewpoints on those subjects whether a nonpublic forum is involved or not. *** We have never held that government may allow discussion of a subject and then discriminate among viewpoints on that particular topic, even if the government for certain reasons may entirely exclude discussion of the subject from the forum. In this context, the greater power does not include the lesser because for First Amendment purposes exercise of the lesser power is more threatening to core values. Viewpoint discrimination is censorship in its purest form and government regulation that discriminates among viewpoints threatens the continued vitality of "free speech." ***

Addressing the question of viewpoint discrimination directly, free of the Court's irrelevant public forum analysis, it is clear that the exclusive-access policy discriminates on the basis of viewpoint. The Court of Appeals found that "[t]he access policy adopted by the Perry schools, in form a speaker restriction, favors a particular viewpoint on labor relations in the Perry schools *** : the teachers inevitably will receive from [the petitioner] self-laudatory descriptions of its activities on their behalf and will be denied the critical perspective offered by [the respondents]." ***

*** The Court of Appeals also suggested that even if the Board had attempted to tailor the policy more carefully by denying outside groups access to the system and by expressly limiting the petitioner's use of the system to messages relating to its official duties, "the fit would still be questionable, for it might be difficult—both in practice and in principle—effectively to separate 'necessary' communications from propaganda." The Court of Appeals was justly concerned with this problem, because the scope of the petitioner's "legal duties" might be difficult, if not impossible, to define with precision.

The petitioner also argues, that the exclusive-access policy is justified by the State's interest in preserving labor peace. *** Although the State's interest in preserving labor peace in the schools in order to prevent disruption is unquestionably substantial, merely articulating the interest in not enough to sustain the exclusive-access policy in this case. There must be some showing that the asserted interest is advanced by the policy. In the absence of such a showing, the exclusive-access policy must fail.[13] ***

CORNELIUS v. NAACP LEGAL DEFENSE & EDUCATIONAL FUND
473 U.S. 788 (1985)

JUSTICE O'CONNOR delivered the opinion of the Court.

I

The CFC [Combined Federal Campaign] is an annual charitable fundraising drive conducted in the federal workplace during working hours largely through the voluntary efforts of federal employees. [P]articipating organizations confine their fundraising activities to a 30-word statement submitted by them for inclusion in the Campaign literature. Volunteer federal employees distribute to their coworkers literature describing the Campaign and the participants along with pledge cards. Contributions may take the form of either a payroll deduction or a lump-sum payment made to a designated agency or to the general Campaign fund. Undesignated contributions are distributed on the local level by a private umbrella organization to certain participating organizations. Designated funds are paid directly to the specified recipient. Through the CFC, the Government employees contribute in excess of $ 100 million to charitable organizations each year. ***

The CFC is a relatively recent development. Prior to 1957, charitable solicitation in the federal workplace occurred on an ad hoc basis. *** Eventually, the increasing number of entities seeking access to federal buildings and the multiplicity of appeals disrupted the work environment and confused employees who were unfamiliar with the groups seeking contributions. *** From 1963 until 1982, the CFC was implemented by guidelines set forth in the Civil Service Commission's Manual on Fund-Raising. Only tax-exempt, nonprofit charitable organizations that were supported by contributions from the public and that provided direct health and welfare services to individuals were eligible to participate in the CFC. ***

Respondents in this case are the NAACP Legal Defense and Educational Fund, Inc., the Sierra Club Legal Defense Fund, the Puerto Rican Legal Defense and Education Fund, the Federally Employed Women Legal Defense and Education Fund,

---

13. The Court also cites the availability of alternative channels of communication in support of the "reasonableness" of the exclusive-access policy. *** In a detailed discussion, the Court of Appeals properly concluded that the other channels of communication available to the respondents were "not nearly as effective as the internal mail system." Perry Local Educators' Assn. v. Hohlt, 652 F.2d, at 1299. See also *id.*, at 1299-1300. In addition, the Court apparently disregards the principle that "one is not to have the exercise of his liberty of expression in appropriate places abridged on the plea that it may be exercised in some other place." Schneider v. State, 308 U.S. 147, 163 (1939). In this case, the existence of inferior alternative channels of communication does not affect the conclusion that the petitioner has failed to justify the viewpoint-discriminatory exclusive-access policy.

the Indian Law Resource Center, the Lawyers' Committee for Civil Rights under Law, and the Natural Resources Defense Council. Each of the respondents attempts to influence public policy through one or more of the following means: political activity, advocacy, lobbying, or litigation on behalf of others. ***

In the first action the Legal Defense Funds challenged the "direct services" requirement on the grounds that it violated the First Amendment and the equal protection component of the Fifth Amendment. The District Court did not reach the equal protection challenge, because it found that the "direct services" requirement as formulated in the Manual on Fund-Raising was too vague to satisfy the strict standards of specificity required by the First Amendment. ***

In response to the District Court's decision, President Reagan took several steps to restore the CFC to what he determined to be its original purpose. In 1982, the President issued [an] Executive Order which limited participation to "voluntary, charitable, health and welfare agencies that provide or support direct health and welfare services to individuals or their families," and specifically excluded those "[a]gencies that seek to influence the outcomes of elections or the determination of public policy through political activity or advocacy, lobbying, or litigation on behalf of parties other than themselves." *** Respondents brought this action challenging their threatened exclusion under the new Executive Order. ***

II

The issue presented is whether respondents have a First Amendment right to solicit contributions that was violated by their exclusion from the CFC. To resolve this issue we must first decide whether solicitation in the context of the CFC is speech protected by the First Amendment, for, if it is not, we need go no further. Assuming that such solicitation is protected speech, we must identify the nature of the forum, because the extent to which the Government may limit access depends on whether the forum is public or nonpublic. *** Applying this analysis, we find that respondents' solicitation is protected speech occurring in the context of a nonpublic forum and that the Government's reasons for excluding respondents from the CFC appear, at least facially, to satisfy the reasonableness standard. We express no opinion on the question whether petitioner's explanation is merely a pretext for viewpoint discrimination. Accordingly, we reverse and remand for further proceedings consistent with this opinion.

A

Charitable solicitation of funds has been recognized by this Court as a form of protected speech. *** Notwithstanding the significant distinctions between in-person solicitation and solicitation in the abbreviated context of the CFC, we find that the latter deserves First Amendment protection. The brief statements in the CFC literature directly advance the speaker's interest in informing readers about its existence and its goals. Moreover, an employee's contribution in response to a request for funds functions as a general expression of support for the recipient and its views.

B

The conclusion that the solicitation which occurs in the CFC is protected speech merely begins our inquiry. Even protected speech is not equally permissible in all places and at all times. Nothing in the Constitution requires the Government freely to grant access to all who wish to exercise their right to free speech on every type of Government property without regard to the nature of the property or to the disruption that might be caused by the speaker's activities. *** [T]he Court has adopted a forum analysis as a means of determining when the Government's interest in limiting the use of its property to its intended purpose outweighs the interest of those wishing to use the property for other purposes. Accordingly, the extent to which the Government can control access depends on the nature of the relevant forum. Because a principal purpose of traditional public fora is the free exchange of ideas, speakers can be excluded from a public forum only when the exclusion is necessary to serve a compelling state interest and the exclusion is narrowly drawn to achieve that interest. Similarly, when the Government has intentionally designated a place or means of communication as a public forum speakers cannot be excluded without a compelling governmental interest. Access to a nonpublic forum, however, can be restricted as long as the restrictions are "reasonable and [are] not an effort to suppress expression merely because public officials oppose the speaker's view." ***

We agree with respondents that the relevant forum for our purposes is the CFC. Although petitioner is correct that as an initial matter a speaker must seek access to public property or to private property dedicated to public use to evoke First Amendment concerns, forum analysis is not completed merely by identifying the government property at issue. *** Here, as in *Perry Education Assn.*, respondents seek access to a particular means of communication. Consistent with the approach taken in prior cases, we find that the CFC, rather than the federal workplace, is the forum. This conclusion does not mean, however, that the Court will ignore the special nature and function of the federal workplace in evaluating the limits that may be imposed on an organization's right to participate in the CFC. ***

Having identified the forum as the CFC, we must decide whether it is nonpublic or public in nature. Most relevant in this regard, of course, is *Perry Education Assn.* There the Court identified three types of fora: the traditional public forum, the public forum created by government designation, and the nonpublic forum. Traditional public fora are those places which "by long tradition or by government fiat have been devoted to assembly and debate." Public streets and parks fall into this category. See Hague v. CIO, 307 U.S. 496, 515 (1939). In addition to traditional public fora, a public forum may be created by government designation of a place or channel of communication for use by the public at large for assembly and speech, for use by certain speakers, or for the discussion of certain subjects. Of course, the government "is not required to indefinitely retain the open character of the facility."

The government does not create a public forum by inaction or by permitting limited discourse, but only by intentionally opening a nontraditional forum for public discourse. Accordingly, the Court has looked to the policy and practice of the government to ascertain whether it intended to designate a place not traditionally open to assembly and debate as a public forum. The Court has also examined the nature of the property and its compatibility with expressive activity to discern the government's intent. For example, in Widmar v. Vincent, 454 U.S. 263 (1981), we found that a state university that had an express policy of making its meeting facilities available to registered student groups had created a public forum for their use. *** Additionally, we noted that a university campus, at least as to its students, possesses many of the characteristics of a traditional public forum. And in Madison Joint School District v. Wisconsin Employment Relations Comm'n, 429 U.S. 167 (1976), the Court held that a forum for citizen involvement was created by a state statute providing for open school board meetings. Similarly, the Court found a public forum where a municipal auditorium and a city-leased theater were designed for and dedicated to expressive activities. Southeastern Promotions, Ltd. v. Conrad, 420 U.S. 546, 555 (1975). ***

Here the parties agree that neither the CFC nor the federal workplace is a traditional public forum. Respondents argue, however, that the Government created a limited public forum for use by all charitable organizations to solicit funds from federal employees. Petitioner contends, and we agree, that neither its practice nor its policy is consistent with an intent to designate the CFC as a public forum open to all tax-exempt organizations. In 1980, an estimated 850,000 organizations qualified for tax-exempt status. ***

Nor does the history of the CFC support a finding that the Government was motivated by an affirmative desire to provide an open forum for charitable solicitation in the federal workplace when it began the Campaign. The historical background indicates that the Campaign was designed to minimize the disruption to the workplace that had resulted from unlimited ad hoc solicitation activities by *lessening* the amount of expressive activity occurring on federal property. ***

An examination of the nature of the Government property involved strengthens the conclusion that the CFC is a nonpublic forum. The federal workplace, like any place of employment, exists to accomplish the business of the employer. In light of the Government policy in creating the CFC and its practice in limiting access, we conclude that the CFC is a nonpublic forum.

C

Control over access to a nonpublic forum can be based on subject matter and speaker identity so long as the distinctions drawn are reasonable in light of the purpose served by the forum and are viewpoint neutral. *Perry Education Assn.*, at 49. Although a speaker may be excluded from a nonpublic forum if he wishes to address a topic not encompassed within the purpose of the forum, see Lehman v. City of Shaker Heights, 418 U.S. 298 (1974), or if he is not a member of the class of speakers for whose especial benefit the forum was created, see *Perry Education Assn.*, the government violates the First Amendment when it denies access to a speaker solely to suppress the point of view he espouses on an otherwise includible subject. The Court of Appeals found it unnecessary to resolve whether the government's denial of access to respondents was viewpoint based, because it determined that respondents' exclusion was unreasonable in light of the purpose served by the CFC.

Petitioner maintains that the purpose of the CFC is to provide a means for traditional health and welfare charities to solicit contributions in the federal workplace, while at the same time maximizing private support of social programs that would otherwise have to be supported by Government funds and minimizing costs to the Federal Government by controlling the time that federal employees expend on the Campaign. Petitioner posits that excluding agencies that attempt to influence the outcome of political elections or the determination of public policy is reasonable in light of this purpose. First, petitioner contends that there is likely to be a general consensus among employees that traditional health and welfare charities are worthwhile, as compared with the more diverse views concerning the goals of organizations like respondents. Limiting participation to widely accepted groups is likely to contribute significantly to employees' acceptance of the Campaign and consequently to its ultimate success. In addition, because the CFC is conducted largely through the efforts of federal employees during their working hours, any controversy surrounding the CFC would produce unwelcome disruption. Finally, the President determined that agencies seeking to affect the outcome of elections or the determination of public policy should be denied access to the CFC in order to avoid the reality and the appearance of Government favoritism or entanglement with particular viewpoints. In such circumstances, petitioner contends that the decision to deny access to such groups was reasonable.

In respondents' view, the reasonableness standard is satisfied only when there is some basic incompatibility between the communication at issue and the principal activity occurring on the Government property. Respondents contend that the purpose of the CFC is to permit solicitation by groups that provide health and welfare services. By permitting such solicitation to take place in the federal workplace, respondents maintain, the Government has concluded that such activity is consistent with the activities usually conducted here. Because respondents are seeking to solicit such contributions and their activities result in direct, tangible benefits to the groups they represent, the Government's attempt to exclude them is unreasonable. Respondents reject petitioner's justifications on the ground that they are unsupported by the record.

The Court of Appeals accepted the position advanced by respondents. When the excluded and included speakers share a similar "status," the court asserted that a heightened reasonableness inquiry is appropriate. Here the status of respondents, in the court's view, is analogous to that of traditional health and welfare organizations, because both provide direct health and welfare services and are tax exempt under 26 U.S.C. § 501(c)(3). ***

Based on the present record, we disagree and conclude that respondents may be excluded from the CFC. The Court of Appeals' conclusion to the contrary fails to reflect the nature of a nonpublic forum. The Government's decision to restrict access to a nonpublic forum need only be *reasonable*; it need not be the most reasonable or the only reasonable limitation. In contrast to a public forum, a finding of strict incompatibility between the nature of the speech or the identity of the speaker and the functioning of the nonpublic forum is not mandated. *** Even if some incompatibility with general expressive activity were required, the CFC would meet the requirement because it would be administratively unmanageable if access could not be curtailed in a reasonable manner. Nor is there a requirement that the restriction be narrowly tailored or that the Government's interest be compelling. The First Amendment does not demand unrestricted access to a nonpublic forum merely because use of that forum may be the most efficient means of delivering the speaker's message. ***

The reasonableness of the Government's restriction of access to a nonpublic forum must be assessed in the light of the purpose of the forum and all the surrounding circumstances. Here the President could reasonably conclude that a dollar directly spent on providing food or shelter to the needy is more beneficial than a dollar spent on litigation that might or might not result in aid to the needy. Moreover, avoiding the appearance of political favoritism is a valid justification for limiting speech in a nonpublic forum. In furthering this interest, the Government is not bound by decisions of other executive agencies made in other contexts. Thus, respondents' tax status, while perhaps relevant, does not determine the reasonableness of the Government's conclusion that participation by such agencies in the CFC will create the appearance of favoritism. ***

Finally, the record amply supports an inference that respondents' participation in the CFC jeopardized the success of the Campaign. OPM submitted a number of letters from federal employees and managers, as well as from Chairmen of local Federal Coordinating Committees and Members of Congress expressing concern about the inclusion of groups termed "political" or "nontraditional" in the CFC. *** [T]he record adequately supported petitioner's position that respondents' continued participation in the Campaign would be detrimental to the Campaign and disruptive of the federal workplace. Although the avoidance of controversy is not a valid ground for restricting speech in a public forum, a nonpublic forum by definition is not dedicated to general debate or the free exchange of ideas. The First Amendment does not forbid a viewpoint-neutral exclusion of speakers who would disrupt a nonpublic forum and hinder its effectiveness for its intended purpose.

D

*** We decline to decide in the first instance whether the exclusion of respondents was impermissibly motivated by a desire to suppress a particular point of view. Respondents are free to pursue this contention on remand.

III

We conclude that the Government does not violate the First Amendment when it limits participation in the CFC in order to minimize disruption to the federal workplace, to ensure the success of the fundraising effort, or to avoid the appearance of political favoritism without regard to the viewpoint of the excluded groups. Accordingly, we reverse the judgment of the Court of Appeals that the exclusion of respondents was unreasonable, and we remand this case for further proceedings consistent with this opinion.

JUSTICE MARSHALL took no part in the consideration or decision of this case. JUSTICE POWELL took no part in the decision of this case.

JUSTICE BLACKMUN, with whom JUSTICE BRENNAN joins, dissenting.

I agree with the Court that the Combined Federal Campaign (CFC) is not a traditional public forum. I also agree with the Court that our precedents indicate that the Government may create a "forum by designation" (or, to use the term our cases have adopted, a "limited public forum") by allowing public property that traditionally has not been available for assembly and debate to be used as a place for expressive activity by certain speakers or about certain subjects. I cannot accept, however, the Court's circular reasoning that the CFC is not a limited public forum because the Government intended to limit the forum to a particular class of speakers. Nor can I agree with the Court's conclusion that distinctions the Government makes between speakers in defining the limits of a forum need not be narrowly tailored and necessary to achieve a compelling governmental interest. Finally, I would hold that the exclusion of the several respondents from the CFC was, on its face, viewpoint-based discrimination. Accordingly, I dissent.

I

***

Access to government property can be crucially important to those who wish to exercise their First Amendment rights. Government property often provides the only space suitable for large gatherings, and it often attracts audiences that are otherwise difficult to reach. Access to government property permits the use of the less costly means of communication so "essential to the poorly financed causes of little people," Martin v. Struthers, 319 U.S. 141, 146 (1943), and "allow[s] challenge to governmental action at its locus." Cass, First Amendment Access to Government Facilities, 65 Va. L. Rev. 1287, 1288 (1979). ***

[T]he public forum, limited-public-forum, and nonpublic forum categories are but analytical shorthand for the principles that have guided the Court's decisions regarding claims to access to public property for expressive activity. The interests served by the expressive activity must be balanced against the interests served by the uses for which the property was intended and the interests of all citizens to enjoy the property. *** The Court's analysis, it seems to me, turns these principles on end. *** Rather than taking the nature of the property into account in balancing the First Amendment interests of the speaker and society's interests in freedom of speech against the interests served by reserving the property to its normal use, the Court simply labels the property and dispenses with the balancing.

*** The Court offers no explanation why attaching the label "nonpublic forum" to particular property frees the Government of the more stringent constraints imposed by the First Amendment in other contexts. The Government's interests in being able to use the property for the purposes for which it was intended obviously are important; that is why a compatibility requirement is imposed. ***

Nor should tradition or governmental "designation" be completely determinative of the rights of a citizen to speak on public property. Many places that are natural sites for expressive activity have no long tradition of use for expressive activity. Airports, for example, are a relatively recent phenomenon, as are government- sponsored shopping centers. Other public places may have no history of expressive activity because only recently have they become associated with the issue that citizens wish to use the property to discuss. It is likely that the library in*Brown v. Louisiana,* historically had not been used for demonstrations for the obvious reason that its association with the subject of segregation became a topic of public protest only during the civil rights movement.[2] Another reason a particular parcel of property may have little history of expressive use is that the Government has excluded expressive activity from the property unjustifiably. Cf. *United States v. Grace*, 461 U.S., at 180.

The guarantees of the First Amendment should not turn entirely on either an accident of history or the grace of the Government. Thus, the fact that the Government "owns" the property to which a citizen seeks access for expressive activity does not dispose of the First Amendment claim; it requires that we balance the First Amendment interests of those who seek access for expressive activity against the interests of the other users of the property and the interests served by reserving the property for its intended uses. The Court's analysis forsakes that balancing, and abandons the compatibility test that always has served as a threshold indicator of the proper balance. ***

III

***

The Court would point to three "justifications" for the exclusion of respondents. First, the Court states that "the President could reasonably conclude that a dollar

---

2. See generally Note, A Unitary Approach to Claims of First Amendment Access to Publicly Owned Property, 35 Stan. L. Rev. 121, 137 (1982).

directly spent on providing food or shelter to the needy is more beneficial than a dollar spent on litigation that might or might not result in aid to the needy." *** I fail to see how the President's view of the relative benefits obtained by various charitable activities translates into a compelling governmental interest. The Government may have a compelling interest in increasing charitable contributions because charities provide services that the Government otherwise would have to provide. But that interest does not justify the exclusion of respondents, for respondents work to enforce the rights of minorities, women, and others through litigation, a task that various Government agencies otherwise might be called upon to undertake.

The Court next states that "avoiding the appearance of political favoritism is a valid justification for limiting speech in a nonpublic forum." *** The Court, however, flatly has rejected that justification in the context of limited public forums. *Widmar v. Vincent,* 454 U.S., at 274. In addition, petitioner's proffered justification again fails to explain why respondents are excluded when other groups, such as the National Right to Life Educational Trust Fund and Planned Parenthood, at least one of which the Government presumably would wish to avoid the appearance of supporting, are allowed to participate. And petitioner offers no explanation why a simple disclaimer in the brochure would not suffice to achieve the Government's interest in avoiding the appearance of support.

Nor is the Government's "interest in avoiding controversy" a compelling state interest that would justify the exclusion of respondents. The managers of the theater in *Southeastern Promotions* no doubt thought the exclusion of the rock musical "Hair" was necessary to avoid controversy, see 420 U.S., at 563-564 (Douglas, J., dissenting in part and concurring in result in part); and the school officials in *Tinker* thought their exclusion of students protesting the activities of the United States in Vietnam was necessary to avoid controversy, see 393 U.S., at 509-510. Yet in those cases, both of which involved limited public forums, the Court did not accept the mere avoidance of controversy as a compelling governmental interest. *** Further, even if the avoidance of controversy in the forum itself could ever serve as a legitimate governmental purpose, the record here does not support a finding that the inclusion of respondents in the CFC threatened a material and substantial disruption. In fact, the evidence shows that contributions to the CFC increased during each of the years respondents participated in the Campaign. The "hundreds" of phone calls and letters expressing a preference that groups other than "traditional" charities be excluded from the CFC reflect nothing more than the discomfort that can be expected whenever a change is made, and whenever any opinion is expressed on a topic of concern to the huge force in 1983 of some 2.7 million civilian federal employees. The letters objecting to the inclusion of respondents in the Campaign must be considered against the fact that many federal employees obviously supported their inclusion in the CFC, as is evidenced by the substantial contributions respondents received through the Campaign.

It is true that unions organized boycotts of the CFC in some areas because of their opposition to the participation in the CFC of the National Right to Work Legal Defense and Education Fund, and that, in those areas, contributions sometimes declined. But the evidence also showed that after some initial confusion regarding whether the organization the unions found objectionable was receiving undesignated contributions, the major unions urged their members simply to designate their contributions so that none went to that group. ***

I would affirm the judgment of the Court of Appeals.

JUSTICE STEVENS, dissenting. [Omitted.]

HAZELWOOD SCHOOL DISTRICT v. KUHLMEIER

484 U.S. 260 (1988)

JUSTICE WHITE delivered the opinion of the Court.

This case concerns the extent to which educators may exercise editorial control over the contents of a high school newspaper produced as part of the school's journalism curriculum.

I

Petitioners are the Hazelwood School District in St. Louis County, Missouri; various school officials; Robert Eugene Reynolds, the principal of Hazelwood East High School; and Howard Emerson, a teacher in the school district. Respondents are three former Hazelwood East students who were staff members of Spectrum, the school newspaper. They contend that school officials violated their First Amendment rights by deleting two pages of articles from the May 13, 1983, issue of Spectrum.

Spectrum was written and edited by the Journalism II class at Hazelwood East. The newspaper was published every three weeks or so during the 1982-1983 school year. More than 4,500 copies of the newspaper were distributed during that year to students, school personnel, and members of the community.

The Board of Education allocated funds from its annual budget for the printing of Spectrum. These funds were supplemented by proceeds from sales of the newspaper. The printing expenses during the 1982-1983 school year totaled $4,668.50; revenue from sales was $1,166.84. The other costs associated with the newspaper—such as supplies, textbooks, and a portion of the journalism teacher's salary—were borne entirely by the Board.

The Journalism II course was taught by Robert Stergos for most of the 1982-1983 academic year. Stergos left Hazelwood East to take a job in private industry on April 29, 1983, when the May 13 edition of Spectrum was nearing completion, and petitioner Emerson took his place as newspaper adviser for the remaining weeks of the term.

The practice at Hazelwood East during the spring 1983 semester was for the journalism teacher to submit page proofs of each Spectrum issue to Principal Reynolds for his review prior to publication. On May 10, Emerson delivered the proofs of the May 13 edition to Reynolds, who objected to two of the articles scheduled to appear in that edition. One of the stories described three Hazelwood East students' experiences with pregnancy; the other discussed the impact of divorce on students at the school.

Reynolds was concerned that, although the pregnancy story used false names "to keep the identity of these girls a secret," the pregnant students still might be identifiable from the text. He also believed that the article's references to sexual activity and birth control were inappropriate for some of the younger students at the school. In addition, Reynolds was concerned that a student identified by name in the divorce story had complained that her father "wasn't spending enough time with my mom, my sister and I" prior to the divorce, "was always out of town on business or out late playing cards with the guys," and "always argued about everything" with her mother. Reynolds believed that the student's parents should have been given an opportunity to respond to these remarks or to consent to their publication. He was unaware that Emerson had deleted the student's name from the final version of the article.

Reynolds believed that there was no time to make the necessary changes in the stories before the scheduled press run and that the newspaper would not appear before the end of the school year if printing were delayed to any significant extent. He concluded that his only options under the circumstances were to publish a four-page newspaper instead of the planned six-page newspaper, eliminating the two pages on which the offending stories appeared, or to publish no newspaper at all. Accordingly, he directed Emerson to withhold from publication the two pages containing the stories on pregnancy and divorce.[1] He informed his superiors of the decision, and they concurred.

Respondents subsequently commenced this action in the United States District Court for the Eastern District of Missouri seeking a declaration that their First Amendment rights had been violated, injunctive relief, and monetary damages. After a bench trial, the District Court denied an injunction, holding that no First Amendment violation had occurred. *** The Court of Appeals for the Eighth Circuit reversed. The court held at outset that Spectrum was not only "a part of the school adopted curriculum," but also a public forum, because the newspaper was "intended to be and operated as a conduit for student viewpoint." *** We granted certiorari, and we now reverse.

1. The two pages deleted from the newspaper also contained articles on teenage marriage, runaways, and juvenile delinquents, as well as a general article on teenage pregnancy. Reynolds testified that he had no objection to these articles and that they were deleted only because they appeared on the same pages as the two objectionable articles.

II

We deal first with the question whether Spectrum may appropriately be characterized as a forum for public expression. The public schools do not possess all of the attributes of streets, parks, and other traditional public forums that "time out of mind, have been used for purposes of assembly, communicating thoughts between citizens, and discussing public questions." Hague v. CIO, 307 U.S. 496, 515 (1939). Hence, school facilities may be deemed to be public forums only if school authorities have "by policy or by practice" opened those facilities "for indiscriminate use by the general public," Perry Education Assn. v. Perry Local Educators' Assn., 460 U.S. 37, 47 (1983), or by some segment of the public, such as student organizations. *** If the facilities have instead been reserved for other intended purposes, "communicative or otherwise," then no public forum has been created, and school officials may impose reasonable restrictions on the speech of students, teachers, and other members of the school community. ***

The evidence relied upon by the Court of Appeals in finding Spectrum to be a public forum, is equivocal at best. For example, Board Policy 348.51, which stated in part that "[s]chool sponsored student publications will not restrict free expression or diverse viewpoints within the rules of responsible journalism," also stated that such publications were "developed within the adopted curriculum and its educational implications." One might reasonably infer from the full text of Policy 348.51 that school officials retained ultimate control over what constituted "responsible journalism" in a school-sponsored newspaper. Although the Statement of Policy published in the September 14, 1982, issue of Spectrum declared that "*Spectrum*, as a student-press publication, accepts all rights implied by the First Amendment," this statement, understood in the context of the paper's role in the school's curriculum, suggests at most that the administration will not interfere with the students' exercise of those First Amendment rights that attend the publication of a school-sponsored newspaper. It does not reflect an intent to expand those rights by converting a curricular newspaper into a public forum. Finally, that students were permitted to exercise some authority over the contents of Spectrum was fully consistent with the Curriculum Guide objective of teaching the Journalism II students "leadership responsibilities as issue and page editors." A decision to teach leadership skills in the context of a classroom activity hardly implies a decision to relinquish school control over that activity. *** Accordingly, school officials were entitled to regulate the contents of Spectrum in any reasonable manner. *** It is this standard, rather than our decision in *Tinker*, that governs this case.

The question whether the First Amendment requires a school to tolerate particular student speech—the question that we addressed in *Tinker*—is different from the question whether the First Amendment requires a school affirmatively to promote particular student speech. The former question addresses educators' ability to silence a student's personal expression that happens to occur on the school premises. The latter question concerns educators' authority over school-sponsored publications, theatrical productions, and other expressive activities that students, parents, and members of the public might reasonably perceive to bear the imprimatur of the school. These activities may fairly be characterized as part of the school curriculum, whether or not they occur in a traditional classroom setting, so long as they are supervised by faculty members and designed to impart particular knowledge or skills to student participants and audiences.[3]

Educators are entitled to exercise greater control over this second form of student expression to assure that participants learn whatever lessons the activity is designed to teach, that readers or listeners are not exposed to material that may be inappropriate for their level of maturity, and that the views of the individual speaker are not erroneously attributed to the school. *** A school must also retain the authority to refuse to sponsor student speech that might reasonably be perceived to advocate drug or alcohol use, irresponsible sex, or conduct otherwise inconsistent with "the shared values of a civilized social order," *Fraser*, [478 U.S.] at 683, or to associate the school with any position other than neutrality on matters of political controversy.[*]

Accordingly, we conclude that the standard articulated in *Tinker* for determining when a school may punish student expression need not also be the standard for determining when a school may refuse to lend its name and resources to the dissemination of student expression. Instead, we hold that educators do not offend the First Amendment by exercising editorial control over the style and content of student speech in school-sponsored expressive activities so long as their actions are reasonably related to legitimate pedagogical concerns.

This standard is consistent with our oft-expressed view that the education of the Nation's youth is primarily the responsibility of parents, teachers, and state and local school officials and not of federal judges. *** It is only when the decision to censor

3. The distinction that we draw between speech that is sponsored by the school and speech that is not is fully consistent with Papish v. Board of Curators, 410 U.S. 667 (1973) (*per curiam*), which involved an off-campus "underground" newspaper that school officials merely had allowed to be sold on a state university campus.

*. [**Ed. Note.** Bethel School Dist. v. Fraser, 478 U.S. 675 (1986), reversed a court of appeals decision based on *Tinker* in favor of a high school student who had been suspended by a school principal for sexually suggestive remarks worked into a nominating speech he had offered in support of another student for class president during a school assembly. He had described his candidate as "a man who is firm *** who takes his point and pounds it in *** who will go to the very end—even the climax, for each and everyone of you." A school rule prohibited "[c]onduct which materially and substantially interferes with the educational process *** including the use of obscene, profane language or gestures." Finding insufficient evidence of material disruption (as required by *Tinker*), the court of appeals affirmed the district court decision in favor of the student (the district court did not reach the merits—it held that the rule was void on first amendment grounds of vagueness and overbreadth). Reversing (7-2, Marshall and Stevens, JJ., dissenting), the Court distinguished *Tinker* as not involving a school-sponsored event (the scheduled assembly). Dicta in *Fraser* went beyond that distinction, however, declaring that "the process of educating our youth for citizenship in public schools is not confined to *** the curriculum," and as in incident of the public school "inculcative" function, a range of vulgar speech, whether or not obscene may be prohibited.]

a school-sponsored publication, theatrical production, or other vehicle of student expression has no valid educational purpose that the First Amendment is so "directly and sharply implicate[d]," as to require judicial intervention to protect students' constitutional rights.[7]

We also conclude that Principal Reynolds acted reasonably in requiring the deletion from the May 13 issue of Spectrum of the pregnancy article, the divorce article, and the remaining articles that were to appear on the same pages of the newspaper.

The initial paragraph of the pregnancy article declared that "[a]ll names have been changed to keep the identity of these girls a secret." The principal concluded that the students' anonymity was not adequately protected, however, given the other identifying information in the article and the small number of pregnant students at the school. Indeed, a teacher at the school credibly testified that she could positively identify at least one of the girls and possibly all three. It is likely that many students at Hazelwood East would have been at least as successful in identifying the girls. Reynolds therefore could reasonably have feared that the article violated whatever pledge of anonymity had been given to the pregnant students. In addition, he could reasonably have been concerned that the article was not sufficiently sensitive to the privacy interests of the students' boyfriends and parents, who were discussed in the article but who were given no opportunity to consent to its publication or to offer a response. The article did not contain graphic accounts of sexual activity. The girls did comment in the article, however, concerning their sexual histories and their use or nonuse of birth control. It was not unreasonable for the principal to have concluded that such frank talk was inappropriate in a school-sponsored publication distributed to 14-year-old freshmen and presumably taken home to be read by students' even younger brothers and sisters.

The student who was quoted by name in the version of the divorce article seen by Principal Reynolds made comments sharply critical of her father. The principal could reasonably have concluded that an individual publicly identified as an inattentive parent—indeed, as one who chose "playing cards with the guys" over home and family —was entitled to an opportunity to defend himself as a matter of journalistic fairness. These concerns were shared by both of Spectrum's faculty advisers for the 1982-1983 school year, who testified that they would not have allowed the article to be printed without deletion of the student's named.[8] ***

---

7. *** We need not now decide whether the same degree of deference is appropriate with respect to school-sponsored expressive activities at the college and university level.

8. The reasonableness of Principal Reynolds' concerns about the two articles was further substantiated by the trial testimony of Martin Duggan, a former editorial page editor of the St. Louis Globe Democrat and a former college journalism instructor and newspaper adviser. Duggan testified that the divorce story did not meet journalistic standards of fairness and balance because the father was not given an opportunity to respond, and that the pregnancy story was not appropriate for publication in a high school newspaper because it was unduly intrusive into the privacy of the girls, their parents, and

Finally, we conclude that the principal's decision to delete two pages of Spectrum, rather than to delete only the offending articles or to require that they be modified, was reasonable under the circumstances as he understood them. Accordingly, no violation of First Amendment rights occurred.[9]

JUSTICE BRENNAN, with whom JUSTICE MARSHALL and JUSTICE BLACKMUN join, dissenting.

***

Public education serves vital national interests in preparing the Nation's youth for life in our increasingly complex society and for the duties of citizenship in our democratic Republic. See Brown v. Board of Education, 347 U.S. 483, 493 (1954). The public school conveys to our young the information and tools required not merely to survive in, but to contribute to, civilized society. It also inculcates in tomorrow's leaders the "fundamental values necessary to the maintenance of a democratic political system ***." Ambach v. Norwick, 441 U.S. 68, 77 (1979). All the while, the public educator nurtures students' social and moral development by transmitting to them an official dogma of "'community values.'" Board of Education v. Pico, 457 U.S. 853, 864 (1982) (plurality opinion) (citation omitted). ***

Free student expression undoubtedly sometimes interferes with the effectiveness of the school's pedagogical functions. Some brands of student expression do so by directly preventing the school from pursuing its pedagogical mission: The young polemic who stands on a soapbox during calculus class to deliver an eloquent political diatribe interferes with the legitimate teaching of calculus.*** Other student speech, however, frustrates the school's legitimate pedagogical purposes merely by expressing a message that conflicts with the school's, without directly interfering with the school's expression of its message: A student who responds to a political science teacher's question with the retort, "socialism is good," subverts the school's inculcation of the message that capitalism is better. Even the maverick who sits in class passively sporting a symbol of protest against a government policy, cf. Tinker v. Des Moines Independent Community School Dist., 393 U.S. 503 (1969), or the gossip who sits in the student commons swapping stories of sexual escapade could readily muddle a clear official message condoning the government policy or condemning teenage sex. Likewise, the student newspaper that, like Spectrum, conveys

---

their boyfriends. The District Court found Duggan to be "an objective and independent witness" whose testimony was entitled to significant weight.

9. It is likely that the approach urged by the dissent would as a practical matter have far more deleterious consequences for the student press than does the approach that we adopt today. The dissent correctly acknowledges "[t]he State's prerogative to dissolve the student newspaper entirely." *** It is likely that many public schools would do just that rather than open their newspapers to all student expression that does not threaten "materia[l] disrup[tion of] classwork" or violation of "rights that are protected by law," *** regardless of how sexually explicit, racially intemperate, or personally insulting that expression otherwise might be.

a moral position at odds with the school's official stance might subvert the administration's legitimate inculcation of its own perception of community values.

If mere incompatibility with the school's pedagogical message were a constitutionally sufficient justification for the suppression of student speech, school officials could censor each of the students or student organizations in the foregoing hypotheticals, converting our public schools into "enclaves of totalitarianism," *id.*, at 511, that "strangle the free mind at its source," *West Virginia State Board of Education v. Barnette*, at 637. The First Amendment permits no such blanket censorship authority. *** [P]ublic educators must accommodate some student expression even if it offends them or offers views or values that contradict those the school wishes to inculcate.

*** The Court today casts no doubt on *Tinker*'s vitality. Instead it erects a taxonomy of school censorship, concluding that *Tinker* applies to one category and not another. On the one hand is censorship "to silence a student's personal expression that happens to occur on the school premises." On the other hand is censorship of expression that arises in the context of "school-sponsored expressive activities that students, parents, and members of the public might reasonably perceive to bear the imprimatur of the school." ***

The Court does not, for it cannot, purport to discern from our precedents the distinction it creates. Nor has this Court ever intimated a distinction between personal and school- sponsored speech in any other context. Particularly telling is this Court's heavy reliance on *Tinker* in two cases of First Amendment infringement on state college campuses. See Papish v. University of Missouri Board of Curators, 410 U.S. 667, 671, n. 6 (1973) (*per curiam*); Healy v. James, 408 U.S. 169, 180, 189, and n.18, 191 (1972). One involved the expulsion of a student for lewd expression in a newspaper that she sold on campus pursuant to university authorization, and the other involved the denial of university recognition and concomitant benefits to a political student organization. Tracking *Tinker*'s analysis, the Court found each act of suppression unconstitutional. In neither case did this Court suggest the distinction, which the Court today finds dispositive, between school-sponsored and incidental student expression.

II

Even if we were writing on a clean slate, I would reject the Court's rationale for abandoning *Tinker* in this case. The Court offers no more than an obscure tangle of three excuses to afford educators "greater control" over school-sponsored speech than the *Tinker* test would permit: the public educator's prerogative to control curriculum; the pedagogical interest in shielding the high school audience from objectionable viewpoints and sensitive topics; and the school's need to dissociate itself from student expression. *** None of the excuses, once disentangled, supports the distinction that the Court draws. *Tinker* fully addresses the first concern; the second is illegitimate; and the third is readily achievable through less oppressive means. ***

B

The Court's *** excuse for deviating from precedent is the school's interest in shielding an impressionable high school audience from material whose substance is "unsuitable for immature audiences." *** Specifically, the majority decrees that we must afford educators authority to shield high school students from exposure to "potentially sensitive topics" (like "the particulars of teenage sexual activity") or unacceptable social viewpoints (like the advocacy of "irresponsible se[x] or conduct otherwise inconsistent with 'the shared values of a civilized social order'") through school-sponsored student activities. ***

The mere fact of school sponsorship does not, as the Court suggests, license such thought control in the high school, whether through school suppression of disfavored viewpoints or through official assessment of topic sensitivity. The former would constitute unabashed and unconstitutional viewpoint discrimination, see *Board of Education v. Pico*, 457 U.S., at 878-879 (BLACKMUN, J., concurring in part and concurring in judgment), as well as an impermissible infringement of the students' "'right to receive information and ideas,'" *id.*, at 867. The State's prerogative to dissolve the student newspaper entirely (or to limit its subject matter) no more entitles it to dictate which viewpoints students may express on its pages, than the State's prerogative to close down the schoolhouse entitles it to prohibit the nondisruptive expression of antiwar sentiment within its gates. ***

C

The sole concomitant of school sponsorship that might conceivably justify the distinction that the Court draws between sponsored and nonsponsored student expression is the risk "that the views of the individual speaker [might be] erroneously attributed to the school." *** Dissociative means short of censorship are available to the school. It could, for example, require the student activity to publish a disclaimer, such as the "Statement of Policy" that Spectrum published each school year announcing that "[a]ll *** editorials appearing in this newspaper reflect the opinions of the Spectrum staff, which are not necessarily shared by the administrators or faculty of Hazelwood East".

III

*** Nor did the censorship fall within the category that *Tinker* described as necessary to prevent student expression from "inva[ding] the rights of others". If that term is to have any content, it must be limited to rights that are protected by law. And, as the Court of Appeals correctly reasoned, whatever journalistic impropriety these articles may have contained, they could not conceivably be tortious, much less criminal. ***

Finally, even if the majority were correct that the principal could constitutionally have censored the objectionable material, I would emphatically object to the brutal manner in which he did so. Where "[t]he separation of legitimate from illegitimate speech calls for more sensitive tools" Speiser v. Randall, 357 U.S. 513, 525 (1958) the principal used a paper shredder. He objected to some material in two articles, but excised six entire articles. He did not so much as inquire into obvious alternatives, such as precise deletions or additions (one of which had already been made), rearranging the layout, or delaying publication. Such unthinking contempt for individual rights is intolerable from any state official. It is particularly insidious from one to whom the public entrusts the task of inculcating in its youth an appreciation for the cherished democratic liberties that our Constitution guarantees.

The young men and women of Hazelwood East expected a civics lesson, but not the one the Court teaches them today.

ROSENBERGER v. RECTOR AND VISITORS OF THE UNIVERSITY OF VIRGINIA

515 U.S. 819 (1995)

Justice KENNEDY delivered the opinion of the Court.**

The University of Virginia authorizes the payment of outside contractors for the printing costs of a variety of student publications. It withheld any authorization for payments on behalf of petitioners for the sole reason that their student paper "primarily promotes or manifests a particular belie[f] in or about a deity or an ultimate reality." The challenge is to the University's regulation and its denial of authorization, the case raising issues under the Speech and Establishment Clauses of the First Amendment.

I

*** Before a student group is eligible to submit bills from its outside contractors for payment by the fund described below, it must become a "Contracted Independent Organization" (CIO). CIO status is available to any group the majority of whose

---

. [Ed. Note**: *Rosenberger* was decided by a closely divided five-to-four vote. The dissent (Souter, Ginsburg, Stevens, and Breyer, JJ.) did not except to Justice Kennedy's general observations on forum analysis (i.e. his review of "forums," "content," and "viewpoint" discrimination re public universities and funding of various student organizations). Rather, it disagreed mainly with the Court's characterization of the facts of the case, and disagreed with its treatment of the Establishment Clause issue — an issue also present in this case. Relevant portions of the Opinions revisiting these matters and bearing on the Establishment Clause are omitted here, but included *infra*, at pp. 109-114.

Also not considered here is any discussion of a different kind of First Amendment claim — one left over for possible consideration in light of the manner in which this case was decided. That issue is identified in one part of the concurring Opinion by Justice O'Connor, 515 U.S.at 850, where she observes: "[A]lthough the question is not presented here, I note the possibility that the student fee is susceptible to a Free Speech Clause challenge by an objecting student that she should not be compelled to pay for speech with which she disagrees." Her Opinion cites pertinent case law elaborating the bases for this kind of claim. (Those cases are considered in the casebook (*see* pp. 561-567) where this different kind of challenge is analyzed and reviewed, and with respect to which it may well be appropriate to consider the "possibility" Justice O'Connor notes.) (*See* also *Board of Regents v. Southworth*, this supplement at pp. 568-572)]

members are students, whose managing officers are full-time students, and that complies with certain procedural requirements. A CIO must file its constitution with the University; must pledge not to discriminate in its membership; and must include in dealings with third parties and in all written materials a disclaimer, stating that the CIO is independent of the University and that the University is not responsible for the CIO. CIO's enjoy access to University facilities, including meeting rooms and computer terminals. A standard agreement signed between each CIO and the University provides that the benefits and opportunities afforded to CIO's "should not be misinterpreted as meaning that those organizations are part of or controlled by the University, that the University is responsible for the organizations' contracts or other acts or omissions, or that the University approves of the organizations' goals or activities."

All CIO's may exist and operate at the University, but some are also entitled to apply for funds from the Student Activities Fund (SAF). The SAF receives its money from a mandatory fee of $14 per semester assessed to each full-time student. Some, but not all, CIO's may submit disbursement requests to the SAF. The Guidelines recognize 11 categories of student groups that may seek payment to third-party contractors because they "are related to the educational purpose of the University of Virginia." One of these is "student news, information, opinion, entertainment, or academic communications media groups." The Guidelines also specify, however, that the costs of certain activities of CIO's that are otherwise eligible for funding will not be reimbursed by the SAF. The student activities that are excluded from SAF support are religious activities, philanthropic contributions and activities, political activities, activities that would jeopardize the University's tax-exempt status, those which involve payment of honoraria or similar fees, or social entertainment or related expenses. The prohibition on "political activities" is defined so that it is limited to electioneering and lobbying. The Guidelines provide that "[t]hese restrictions on funding political activities are not intended to preclude funding of any otherwise eligible student organization which ... espouses particular positions or ideological viewpoints, including those that may be unpopular or are not generally accepted." A "religious activity," by contrast, is defined as any activity that "primarily promotes or manifests a particular belie[f] in or about a deity or an ultimate reality." ***

Petitioners' organization, Wide Awake Productions (WAP), qualified as a CIO. *** WAP was established "[t]o publish a magazine of philosophical and religious expression," "[t]o facilitate discussion which fosters an atmosphere of sensitivity to and tolerance of Christian viewpoints," and "[t]o provide a unifying focus for Christians of multicultural backgrounds." WAP publishes Wide Awake: A Christian Perspective at the University of Virginia. *** The editors committed the paper to a two-fold mission: "to challenge Christians to live, in word and deed, according to the faith they proclaim and to encourage students to consider what a personal relationship with Jesus Christ means." Each page of Wide Awake, and the end of each article or review, is marked by a cross. By June 1992, WAP had distributed about 5,000 copies of Wide Awake to University students, free of charge.

WAP had acquired CIO status soon after it was organized. This is an important consideration in this case, for had it been a "religious organization," WAP would not have been accorded CIO status. As defined by the Guidelines, a "[r]eligious [o]rganization" is "an organization whose purpose is to practice a devotion to an acknowledged ultimate reality or deity." At no stage in this controversy has the University contended that WAP is such an organization.

A few months after being given CIO status, WAP requested the SAF to pay its printer $5,862 for the costs of printing its newspaper. The Appropriations Committee of the Student Council denied WAP's request on the ground that Wide Awake was a "religious activity" within the meaning of the Guidelines, i.e., that the newspaper "promote[d] or manifest[ed] a particular belie[f] in or about a deity or an ultimate reality." It made its determination after examining the first issue. *** WAP, Wide Awake, and three of its editors and members filed suit in the United States District Court for the Western District of Virginia, challenging the SAF's action as violative of 42 U.S.C. § 1983. ***

II

It is axiomatic that the government may not regulate speech based on its substantive content or the message it conveys. *** [T]he government offends the First Amendment when it imposes financial burdens on certain speakers based on the content of their expression. When the government targets not subject matter, but particular views taken by speakers on a subject, the violation of the First Amendment is all the more blatant. See *R.A.V. v. St. Paul*, 505 U.S. 377, 391 (1992). Viewpoint discrimination is thus an egregious form of content discrimination. The government must abstain from regulating speech when the specific motivating ideology or the opinion or perspective of the speaker is the rationale for the restriction.

These principles provide the framework forbidding the State to exercise viewpoint discrimination, even when the limited public forum is one of its own creation. The necessities of confining a forum to the limited and legitimate purposes for which it was created may justify the State in reserving it for certain groups or for the discussion of certain topics. See, e.g., *Cornelius v. NAACP Legal Defense & Ed. Fund, Inc.*, 473 U.S. 788, 806 (1985); *Perry Ed. Assn.*, at 49. Once it has opened a limited forum, however, the State must respect the lawful boundaries it has itself set. *** Thus, in determining whether the State is acting to preserve the limits of the forum it has created so that the exclusion of a class of speech is legitimate, we have observed a distinction between, on the one hand, content discrimination, which may be permissible if it preserves the purposes of that limited forum, and, on the other hand, viewpoint discrimination, which is presumed impermissible when directed against speech otherwise within the forum's limitations.

The SAF is a forum more in a metaphysical than in a spatial or geographic sense, but the same principles are applicable. *See, e.g., Perry Ed. Assn.*, at 46-47 (forum analysis of a school mail system); *Cornelius*, at 801 (forum analysis of charitable contribution program). The most recent and most apposite case is our decision in *Lamb's Chapel v. Center Moriches School Dist.*, 508U.S.384(1993). There, a school district had opened school facilities for use after school hours by community groups for a wide variety of social, civic, and recreational purposes. The district, however, had enacted a formal policy against opening facilities to groups for religious purposes. Invoking its policy, the district rejected a request from a group desiring to show a film series addressing various child-rearing questions from a "Christian perspective." There was no indication in the record in Lamb's Chapel that the request to use the school facilities was "denied, for any reason other than the fact that the presentation would have been from a religious perspective." Our conclusion was unanimous: "[I]t discriminates on the basis of viewpoint to permit school property to be used for the presentation of all views about family issues and childrearing except those dealing with the subject matter from a religious standpoint." *

The University does acknowledge (as it must in light of our precedents) that "ideologically driven attempts to suppress a particular point of view are presumptively unconstitutional in funding, as in other contexts," but insists that this case does not present that issue because the Guidelines draw lines based on content, not viewpoint. As we have noted, discrimination against one set ofviews or ideas is but a subset or particular instance of the more general phenomenon of content discrimination. And, it must be acknowledged, the distinction is not a precise one. It is, in a sense, something of an understatement to speak of religious thought and discussion as just a viewpoint, as distinct from a comprehensive body of thought. The nature of our origins and destiny and their dependence upon the existence of a

---

*. **[Ed. Note.** *See also* Good News Club v. Milford Central School, 121 S.Ct. 2093 (2001) (applying and extending *Lamb's Chapel*). (In *Good News*, the local school board also provided that community groups could use public school rooms after school hours, either "for instruction in any branch of education, learning or the arts," or for "social, civic and recreational meetings and entertainment events." The Court treated the policy as one establishing a "limited public forum" and then held (five-to-four) that a local Christian Club ("Good News") could not be refused equal access and use for regularly scheduling rooms immediately following the regular school day, engaging elementary school children in Christian songs, Bible reading, prayer, and Christian teachings.) --The majority in an Opinion by Thomas, J., (with whom Rehnquist, C.J., O'Connor, Scalia, and Kennedy, JJ., joined), regarded the refusal to allow the requested access and use as a form of "viewpoint" discrimination, as in *Lamb's Chapel*. The dissent (Stevens, Breyer, Ginsburg, and Souter, JJ.) distinguished *Lamb's Chapel* as "viewpoint" discrimination (insofar as the denied use forbade a group access and use to show films addressing the alleged wrongfulness of abortion from a "Christian" perspective), from a more general "use" restriction-a restriction according to the *kind* of use (namely "proselytizing," defined as "use by organized groups whether religious, political or otherwise, to hold meetings, *the principal purpose of which is not to discuss current-event topics from their unique point of view but rather to recruit others to join their respective groups*") (emphasis added); in their view, a general and neutral restriction of that kind, in regulating outside group-use of elementary grade classrooms, with school youngsters still at the school, was a permissible line to draw in providing a "limited public forum" in respect to the local public schools.

divine being have been subjects of philosophic inquiry throughout human history. We conclude, nonetheless, that here, as in *Lamb's Chapel*, viewpoint discrimination is the proper way to interpret the University's objections to Wide Awake. By the very terms of the SAF prohibition, the University does not exclude religion as a subject matter but selects for disfavored treatment those student journalistic efforts with religious editorial viewpoints. Religion may be a vast area of inquiry, but it also provides, as it did here, a specific premise, a perspective, a standpoint from which a variety of subjects may be discussed and considered. The prohibited perspective, not the general subject matter, resulted in the refusal to make third-party payments, for the subjects discussed were otherwise within the approved category of publications. ***

The University tries to escape the consequences of our holding in *Lamb's Chapel* by urging that this case involves the provision of funds rather than access to facilities. The University begins with the unremarkable proposition that the State must have substantial discretion in determining how to allocate scarce resources to accomplish its educational mission. Citing our decisions in *Rust v. Sullivan, 500 U.S. 173 (1991)* and *Widmar v. Vincent*, 454 U.S. 263 (1981), the University argues that content-based funding decisions are both inevitable and lawful. Were the reasoning of *Lamb's Chapel* to apply to funding decisions as well as to those involving access to facilities, it is urged, its holding "would become a judicial juggernaut, constitutionalizing the ubiquitous content-based decisions that schools, colleges, and other government entities routinely make in the allocation of public funds."

*** When the University determines the content of the education it provides, it is the University speaking, and we have permitted the government to regulate the content of what is or is not expressed when it is the speaker or when it enlists private entities to convey its own message. In the same vein, in *Rust v. Sullivan*, we upheld the government's prohibition on abortion-related advice applicable to recipients of federal funds for family planning counseling. There, the government did not create a program to encourage private speech but instead used private speakers to transmit specific information pertaining to its own program. We recognized that when the government appropriates public funds to promote a particular policy of its own it is entitled to say what it wishes. When the government disburses public funds to private entities to convey a governmental message, it may take legitimate and appropriate steps to ensure that its message is neither garbled nor distorted by the grantee.

It does not follow, however, that viewpoint-based restrictions are proper when the University does not itself speak or subsidize transmittal of a message it favors but instead expends funds to encourage a diversity of views from private speakers. A holding that the University may not discriminate based on the viewpoint of private persons whose speech it facilitates does not restrict the University's own speech, which is controlled by different principles. ***

The distinction between the University's own favored message and the private speech of students is evident in the case before us. The University itself has taken steps to ensure the distinction in the agreement each CIO must sign. The University declares that the student groups eligible for SAF support are not the University's agents, are not subject to its control, and are not its responsibility. Having offered to pay the third-party contractors on behalf of private speakers who convey their own messages, the University may not silence the expression of selected viewpoints.

The University urges that, from a constitutional standpoint, funding of speech differs from provision of access to facilities because money is scarce and physical facilities are not. *** The government cannot justify viewpoint discrimination among private speakers on the economic fact of scarcity. ***

Vital First Amendment speech principles are at stake here. The first danger to liberty lies in granting the State the power to examine publications to determine whether or not they are based on some ultimate idea and, if so, for the State to classify them. The second, and corollary, danger is to speech from the chilling of individual thought and expression. That danger is especially real in the University setting, where the State acts against a background and tradition of thought and experiment that is at the center of our intellectual and philosophic tradition. ***

The prohibition on funding on behalf of publications that "primarily promot[e] or manifes[t] a particular belie[f] in or about a deity or an ultimate reality," in its ordinary and commonsense meaning, has a vast potential reach. *** Were the prohibition applied with much vigor at all, it would bar funding of essays by hypothetical student contributors named Plato, Spinoza, and Descartes. And if the regulation covers, as the University says it does, those student journalistic efforts that primarily manifest or promote a belief that there is no deity and no ultimate reality, then under-graduates named Karl Marx, Bertrand Russell, and Jean-Paul Sartre would likewise have some of their major essays excluded from student publications. *** Based on the principles we have discussed, we hold that the regulation invoked to deny SAF support, both in its terms and in its application to these petitioners, is a denial of their right of free speech guaranteed by the First Amendment. ***

---

5. A "Forum" Discussion and Review

The Court's recent decisions appear to trifurcate first amendment review of restrictions on publicly-held property according to "forum analysis." Additionally, these cases suggest that one must take a step *preceding* the application of time, place, and manner, regulation review. For if the public property in question is not judicially regarded as some kind of public forum,[81] even the moderately protective *(Ward)* standards of "time, place, and manner" first amendment review appear not to apply,

---

81. Whether "traditional" or "dedicated," or whether "limited" (rather than unlimited).

i.e. they need *not* be met by the state.[82] In 1987, moreover, a majority of the Supreme Court reiterated the position that this three-forum threshold approach is correct:

> In balancing the government's interest in limiting the use of its property against the interests of those who wish to use the property for expressive activity, the Court has identified three types of fora: the traditional public forum, the public forum created by government designation, and the nonpublic forum. *The proper First Amendment analysis differs depending on whether the area in question falls in one category rather than another.*[83]

Some public agencies responded quite aggressively to this development of forum categorization. Immediately following the Supreme Court's decision in *Perry Education Association*, for instance, on July 13, 1983, the Board of Airport Commissioners for the Los Angeles International Airport adopted a broad resolution applicable to the entire Los Angeles International Airport Terminal. The new regulation provided that "the Central Terminal Area of Los Angeles International Airport is not open for First Amendment activities by any individual and/or entity." Its object was to make the entire interior of that vast terminal a "nonpublic forum," a place restricted to the services incidental to travel, thus putting an end to various kinds of solicitations, petitions, leafletting activities, and the like, by *banishing them all.* Plainly the new rule sought to avoid the perplexities of more finely-tuned "time, place, and manner" restrictions, and the unwelcome task of drawing fine lines.

In the actual case as it came to the Supreme Court, the Airport Authority's particular attempt to clear out the airport of speech-users was held to fail. Tested in the Court "on its face," rather than "as applied," the regulation was held to be void on overbreadth grounds (the idea that *all* "first amendment activities" were forbidden was readily found to be quite absurd.[84]) But the decision was otherwise inconclusive on the main point for which it was originally meant to be reviewed (namely, the

---

82. In other words, where the government-held property is a "nonpublic forum," the interest deemed sufficient to exclude a wide range of speech uses need not be "compelling" but merely "not prohibited," and the regulation need not be "narrowly tailored," but merely "rationally related." There is also no question regarding ample alternative means for communicating elsewhere. And likewise, the regulation need not be "content neutral", or "speaker neutral." (It is enough that the regulation is (a) "viewpoint neutral", (b) rationally related to preserving the facility for its (lawful) use, and (c) not enacted from a mere desire to suppress expression or speech as such.)

83. Airport Commissioners v. Jews For Jesus, Inc., 482 U.S. 569, 482-83 (1987) (citing *Perry*) (emphasis added).

84. The Court unanimously held the regulation void on its face for overbreadth because, on its face, the regulation was addressed to literally *all* "first amendment activity" and thus appeared to cover "even talking (politics) and reading (newspapers), or the wearing of campaign buttons or symbolic clothing" while in the terminal. 482 U.S. at 575. Even treating the whole of the terminal as a "nonpublic forum"— the Court expressly declined to say whether it was—the Court held that "no conceivable governmental interest would justify an absolute prohibition of speech" within the terminal of the sort just illustrated, i.e. the regulation lacked even a rational nexus with a proper purpose, viewed this way, and so was invalid *per se*.

extent to which a government-owned terminal might or might not be sheltered as a "nonpublic forum" subject only to the Court's least demanding kind of forum test).

On the other hand, the case may also cause one to pause over the usefulness of the "three-kinds-of-forum"[86] approach the Court appears to have adopted, as either a very exacting or as a wholly reliable new tool. For instance, note that in this case, *Jews for Jesus,* while the Court expressly declined to decide whether the entirety of a major airport terminal could be cordoned off as a nonpublic forum, the Court nonetheless added that, assuming it could be, even then, in some measure some confrontational forms of unwanted political speech might still be protected from regulations prohibiting some forms of such speech.[87] But if that is so, might there be less actual clarity and certainty gained from the overall "forum" categories the Court has proposed than one might first have supposed, after all?[88] Yet, surely, these advantages (i.e. greater categorical clarity and greater regulatory certainty) were among the principal objects meant to be secured by this new approach.

Taking the new approach seriously, consider the following case.

---

86. Or is it, rather, a four-forum approach: (a) traditional public forum, (b) dedicated public forum, (c) "limited" public forum, (d) "nonpublic" forum? Are (a) and (b) treated identically under the first amendment? If not, what is the distinction, if any, between the two? (Is the distinction between (a) and (b) the distinction that the first kind is not subject to more than time, place, and manner regulations, but that the second kind, while subject only to the same kinds of regulations while it *remains* "dedicated" as a public forum, can be withdrawn as such when government so elects an option not applicable to the first kind)? Similarly, what difference in first amendment review standards distinguishes (c) from (d)? And is there any first amendment limitation forbidding government from *changing* a (b) forum to a (c) forum, and/or a (c) forum to (d)?

87. Specifically, for example, Justice O'Connor wrote: "Much nondisruptive speech—such as the wearing of a T-shirt or button that contains a political message—may not be 'airport related,' *but is still protected speech even in a nonpublic forum.*" 482 U.S. at 576, citing Cohen v. California, 403 U.S. 15 (1971) (the "Fuck the draft" t-shirt case) (emphasis added).

88. For a post hoc refinement, consider again the *Taxpayers for Vincent* case, *supra*, decided at the time under a "time, place, and manner" rationale (sustaining the *complete* ban even of election posters on public utility poles or lines, solely on aesthetic grounds, though the lines were along the public streets, and the posters were conventional political posters, and the city disclaimed safety concerns, a less restrictive regulation requiring removal within so many hours or days following the relevant election was not deemed required on first amendment grounds, nor was a more narrowly drawn restriction deemed required). Under an application of the *Perry* and *Cornelius* cases, would it have been plausible to argue that the "forum" to which Taxpayers for Vincent sought "access" was *not* the "traditional forum" of the public streets and sidewalks, but, rather, the lesser part thereof consisting of the utility lines and poles— and, as to these, they were neither "traditional" public fora, "dedicated" public fora, nor limited public fora, but *nonpublic fora* such that the flat ban, being viewpoint neutral, and rationally related to a legitimate police power interest in aesthetics, as imposed on a nonpublic forum, was valid, whether or not related to a "substantial" or "compelling" government objective, whether or not "narrowly" tailored?

INTERNATIONAL SOCIETY FOR KRISHNA CONSCIOUSNESS v. LEE
505 U.S. 672 (1992)*

CHIEF JUSTICE REHNQUIST delivered the opinion of the Court [in 91-155].

In this case we consider whether an airport terminal operated by a public authority is a public forum and whether a regulation prohibiting solicitation in the interior of an airport terminal violates the First Amendment.

The relevant facts in this case are not in dispute. Petitioner International Society for Krishna Consciousness, Inc. (ISKCON) is a not-for-profit religious corporation whose members perform a ritual known as *sankirtan*. The ritual consists of "going into public places, disseminating religious literature and soliciting funds to support the religion."

Respondent Walter Lee, now deceased, was the police superintendent of the Port Authority of New York and New Jersey and was charged with enforcing the regulation at issue. The Port Authority owns and operates three major airports in the greater New York City area: John F. Kennedy International Airport (Kennedy), La Guardia Airport (La Guardia), and Newark International Airport (Newark). The three airports collectively form one of the world's busiest metropolitan airport complexes. They serve approximately 8% of this country's domestic airline market and more than 50% of the trans-Atlantic market. By decade's end they are expected to serve at least 110 million passengers annually.

*** The terminals are generally accessible to the general public and contain various commercial establishments such as restaurants, snack stands, bars, newsstands, and stores of various types. Virtually all who visit the terminals do so for purposes related to air travel. These visitors principally include passengers, those meeting or seeing off passengers, flight crews, and terminal employees.

The Port Authority has adopted a regulation forbidding within the terminals the repetitive solicitation of money or distribution of literature. The regulation states:

> 1. The following conduct is prohibited within the interior areas of buildings or structures at an air terminal if conducted by a person to or with passers-by in a continuous or repetitive manner:
> (a) The sale or distribution of any merchandise, including but not limited to jewelry, food stuffs, candles, flowers, badges and clothing.

---

*. **[Ed. Note.** The Court of Appeals for the Second Circuit upheld a ban on solicitation of funds within the airport terminals operated by the Port Authority of New York and New Jersey, and the International Society for Krishna Consciousness petitioned for certiorari (No. 91-155). In the same opinion, however, the Second Circuit also struck down a ban on the distribution of printed or written materials, and the Port Authority petitioned for certiorari (No. 91-339). The majority opinion (authored by Rehnquist) for 91-155 is printed at 505 U.S. 672 , and the *per curiam* opinion for 91-339 appears at 505 U.S. 830 Concurrences and dissents mostly appear in the "opinion" at 505 U.S. 672. The opinions of the justices have been rearranged here for clarity.]

(b) The sale or distribution of flyers, brochures, pamphlets, books or any other printed or written material.
(c) Solicitation and receipt of funds. ***

The regulation governs only the terminals; the Port Authority permits solicitation and distribution on the sidewalks outside the terminal buildings. The regulation effectively prohibits petitioner from performing *sankirtan* in the terminals.

It is uncontested that the solicitation at issue in this case is a form of speech protected under the First Amendment. Heffron v. International Society for Krishna Consciousness, Inc., 452 U.S. 640 (1981). But it is also well settled that the government need not permit all forms of speech on property that it owns and controls. United States Postal Service v. Council of Greenburgh Civic Assns., 453 U.S. 114, 129 (1981); Greer v. Spock, 424 U.S. 828 (1976).

These cases reflect a "forum-based" approach for assessing restrictions that the government seeks to place on the use of its property. Cornelius v. NAACP Legal Defense and Educational Fund, Inc., 473 U.S. 788, 800 (1985). Under this approach, regulation of speech on government property that has traditionally been available for public expression is subject to the highest scrutiny. Such regulations survive only if they are narrowly drawn to achieve a compelling state interest. *Perry* [Education Ass'n v. Perry Local Educators' Ass'n, 460 U.S.] at 45. The second category of public property is the designated public forum, whether of a limited or unlimited character—property that the state has opened for expressive activity by part or all of the public. Regulation of such property is subject to the same limitations as that governing a traditional public forum. Finally, there is all remaining public property. Limitations on expressive activity conducted on this last category of property must survive only a much more limited review. The challenged regulation need only be reasonable, as long as the regulation is not an effort to suppress the speaker's activity due to disagreement with the speaker's view.

Our recent cases provide additional guidance on the characteristics of a public forum. In *Cornelius* we noted that a traditional public forum is property that has as "a principal purpose ... the free exchange of ideas." 473 U.S., at 800. Moreover, consistent with the notion that the government—like other property owners—"has power to preserve the property under its control for the use to which it is lawfully dedicated," *Greer*, at 836, the government does not create a public forum by inaction. Nor is a public forum created "whenever members of the public are permitted freely to visit a place owned or operated by the Government." *Ibid.* The decision to create a public forum must instead be made "by intentionally opening a nontraditional forum for public discourse." *Cornelius*, at 802. Finally, we have recognized that the location of property also has bearing because separation from acknowledged public areas may serve to indicate that the separated property is a special enclave, subject to greater restriction. *United States v. Grace*, 461 U.S. 171, 179-180 (1983).

[G]iven the lateness with which the modern air terminal has made its appearance, it hardly qualifies for the description of having "immemorially time out of mind" been held in the public trust and used for purposes of expressive activity. Moreover, even within the rather short history of air transport, it is only "[i]n recent years [that] it has become a common practice for various religious and non- profit organizations to use commercial airports as a forum for the distribution of literature, the solicitation of funds, the proselytizing of new members, and other similar activities." 45 Fed. Reg. 35314 (1980). Thus, the tradition of airport activity does not demonstrate that airports have historically been made available for speech activity. Nor can we say that these particular terminals, or airport terminals generally have been intentionally opened by their operators to such activity; the frequent and continuing litigation evidencing the operators' objections belies any such claim. In short, there can be no argument that society's time-tested judgment, expressed through acquiescence in a continuing practice, has resolved the issue in petitioner's favor.

Petitioner attempts to circumvent the history and practice governing airport activity by pointing our attention to the variety of speech activity that it claims historically occurred at various "transportation nodes" such as rail stations, bus stations, wharves, and Ellis Island. Even if we were inclined to accept petitioner's historical account describing speech activity at these locations, an account respondent contests, we think that such evidence is of little import for two reasons. First, much of the evidence is irrelevant to *public* fora analysis, because sites such as bus and rail terminals traditionally have had *private* ownership. The development of privately owned parks that ban speech activity would not change the public fora status of publicly held parks. But the reverse is also true. The practices of privately held transportation centers do not bear on the government's regulatory authority over a publicly owned airport.

Second, the relevant unit for our inquiry is an airport, not "transportation nodes" generally. When new methods of transportation develop, new methods for accommodating that transportation are also likely to be needed. And with each new step, it therefore will be a new inquiry whether the transportation necessities are compatible with various kinds of expressive activity. To make a category of "transportation nodes," therefore, would unjustifiably elide what may prove to be critical differences of which we should rightfully take account. To blithely equate airports with other transportation centers, therefore, would be a mistake.

The differences among such facilities are unsurprising since, as the Court of Appeals noted, airports are commercial establishments funded by users fees and designed to make a regulated profit, and where nearly all who visit do so for some travel related purpose. As commercial enterprises, airports must provide services attractive to the marketplace. In light of this, it cannot fairly be said that an airport terminal has as a principal purpose "promoting the free exchange of ideas." To the contrary, the record demonstrates that Port Authority management considers the purpose of the terminals to be the facilitation of passenger air travel, not the promotion of expression. Even if we look beyond the intent of the Port Authority to the manner in which the terminals have been operated, the terminals have never been dedicated (except under the threat of court order) to expression in the form sought to be exercised here: *i.e.*, the solicitation of contributions and the distribution of literature.

*** Thus, we think that neither by tradition nor purpose can the terminals be described as satisfying the standards we have previously set out for identifying a public forum.

The restrictions here challenged, therefore, need only satisfy a requirement of reasonableness. We reiterate what we stated in *Kokinda*, the restriction "'need only be *reasonable*; it need not be the most reasonable or the only reasonable limitation.'" We have no doubt that under this standard the prohibition on solicitation passes muster.

We have on many prior occasions noted the disruptive effect that solicitation may have on business. "Solicitation requires action by those who would respond: The individual solicited must decide whether or not to contribute (which itself might involve reading the solicitor's literature or hearing his pitch), and then, having decided to do so, reach for a wallet, search it for money, write a check, or produce a credit card." Delays may be particularly costly in this setting, as a flight missed by only a few minutes can result in hours worth of subsequent inconvenience.

In addition, face-to-face solicitation presents risks of duress that are an appropriate target of regulation. [T]he targets of such activity frequently are on tight schedules. This in turn makes such visitors unlikely to stop and formally complain to airport authorities. As a result, the airport faces considerable difficulty in achieving its legitimate interest in monitoring solicitation activity to assure that travelers are not interfered with unduly.

The Port Authority has concluded that its interest in monitoring the activities can best be accomplished by limiting solicitation and distribution to the sidewalk areas outside the terminals. This sidewalk area is frequented by an overwhelming percentage of airport users. Thus the resulting access of those who would solicit the general public is quite complete. In turn we think it would be odd to conclude that the Port Authority's terminal regulation is unreasonable despite the Port Authority having otherwise assured access to an area universally traveled.

The inconveniences to passengers and the burdens on Port Authority officials flowing from solicitation activity may seem small, but viewed against the fact that "pedestrian congestion is one of the greatest problems facing the three terminals," 925 F.2d, at 582, the Port Authority could reasonably worry that even such incremental effects would prove quite disruptive. Moreover, the justification for the Rule should not be measured by the disorder that would result from granting an exemption solely to ISKCON. For if petitioner is given access, so too must other groups. As a result, we conclude that the solicitation ban is reasonable.

For the foregoing reasons, the judgment of the Court of Appeals sustaining the ban on solicitation in Port Authority terminals is affirmed.

JUSTICE KENNEDY, with whom JUSTICE BLACKMUN, JUSTICE STEVENS, and JUSTICE SOUTER join as to Part I, concurring in the judgment [in 91-155].

***

I

*** The Court today holds that traditional public forums are limited to public property which have as "'a principal purpose ... the free exchange of ideas'" and that this purpose must be evidenced by a long-standing historical practice of permitting speech. The Court also holds that designated forums consist of property which the government intends to open for public discourse. All other types of property are, in the Court's view, nonpublic forums (in other words, not public forums), and government-imposed restrictions of speech in these places will be upheld so long as reasonable and viewpoint-neutral.

This analysis is flawed at its very beginning. It leaves the government with almost unlimited authority to restrict speech on its property by doing nothing more than articulating a non-speech-related purpose for the area, and it leaves almost no scope for the development of new public forums absent the rare approval of the government. In my view, the inquiry must be an objective one, based on the actual, physical characteristics and uses of the property.

The First Amendment is a limitation on government, not a grant of power. Its design is to prevent the government from controlling speech. Yet under the Court's view the authority of the government to control speech on its property is paramount, for in almost all cases the critical step in the Court's analysis is a classification of the property that turns on the government's own definition or decision, unconstrained by an independent duty to respect the speech its citizens can voice there. The Court acknowledges as much, by reintroducing today into our First Amendment law a strict doctrinal line between the proprietary and regulatory functions of government which I thought had been abandoned long ago.*** [C]ompare Davis v. Massachusetts, 167 U.S. 43 (1897); with Hague v. Committee for Industrial Organization, [307 U.S.] at 515; Schneider v. State, 308 U.S. 147 (1939).***

The Court's approach is contrary to the underlying purposes of the public forum doctrine. The liberties protected by our doctrine derive from the Assembly, as well as the Speech and Press Clauses of the First Amendment, and are essential to a functioning democracy. Public places are of necessity the locus for discussion of public issues, as well as protest against arbitrary government action. At the heart of our jurisprudence lies the principle that in a free nation citizens must have the right to gather and speak with other persons in public places. The recognition that certain government-owned property is a public forum provides open notice to citizens that their freedoms may be exercised there without fear of a censorial government, adding tangible reinforcement to the idea that we are a free people.

A fundamental tenet of our Constitution is that the government is subject to constraints which private persons are not. The public forum doctrine vindicates that principle by recognizing limits on the government's control over speech activities on property suitable for free expression. The doctrine focuses on the physical characteristics of the property because government ownership is the source of its purported authority to regulate speech. The right of speech protected by the doctrine, however, comes not from a Supreme Court dictum but from the constitutional recognition that the government cannot impose silence on a free people.

The effect of the Court's narrow view of the first category of public forums is compounded by its description of the second purported category, the so-called "designated" forum. The requirements for such a designation are so stringent that I cannot be certain whether the category has any content left at all. In any event, it seems evident that under the Court's analysis today few if any types of property other than those already recognized as public forums will be accorded that status.

One of the places left in our mobile society that is suitable for discourse is a metropolitan airport. It is of particular importance to recognize that such spaces are public forums because in these days an airport is one of the few government-owned spaces where many persons have extensive contact with other members of the public. Given that private spaces of similar character are not subject to the dictates of the First Amendment, it is critical that we preserve these areas for protected speech. In my view, our public forum doctrine must recognize this reality, and allow the creation of public forums which do not fit within the narrow tradition of streets, sidewalks, and parks. We have allowed flexibility in our doctrine to meet changing technologies in other areas of constitutional interpretation, see, e.g., Katz v. United States, 389 U.S. 347 (1967), and I believe we must do the same with the First Amendment.

*** Under this analysis, it is evident that the public spaces of the Port Authority's airports are public forums. First, the District Court made detailed findings regarding the physical similarities between the Port Authority's airports and public streets. These findings show that the public spaces in the airports are broad, public thoroughfares full of people and lined with stores and other commercial activities. An airport corridor is of course not a street, but that is not the proper inquiry. The question is one of physical similarities, sufficient to suggest that the airport corridor should be a public forum for the same reasons that streets and sidewalks have been treated as public forums by the people who use them.

*** [M]ost important, it is apparent from the record, and from the recent history of airports, that when adequate time, place, and manner regulations are in place, expressive activity is quite compatible with the uses of major airports. The Port Authority's primary argument to the contrary is that the problem of congestion in its airports' corridors makes expressive activity inconsistent with the airports' primary purpose, which is to facilitate air travel. The First Amendment is often inconvenient. But that is besides the point. Inconvenience does not absolve the government of its obligation to tolerate speech. The Authority makes no showing that any real impediments to the smooth functioning of the airports cannot be cured with reasonable time, place, and manner regulations. In fact, the history of the Authority's own airports, as well as other major airports in this country, leaves little doubt that such a solution is quite feasible. ***

The danger of allowing the government to suppress speech is shown in the case now before us. A grant of plenary power allows the government to tilt the dialogue heard by the public, to exclude many, more marginal voices. The Port Authority's rule, which prohibits almost all such activity, is among the most restrictive possible of those liberties. The regulation is in fact so broad and restrictive of speech, JUSTICE O'CONNOR finds it void even under the standards applicable to government regulations in nonpublic forums. I have no difficulty deciding the regulation cannot survive the far more stringent rules applicable to regulations in public forums. The regulation is not drawn in narrow terms and it does not leave open ample alternative channels for communication. See Ward v. Rock Against Racism, 491 U.S. 781, 791 (1989). The Port Authority's concerns with the problem of congestion can be addressed through narrow restrictions on the time and place of expressive activity (see opinion of O'CONNOR, J.). I would strike down the regulation as an unconstitutional restriction of speech.

II

It is my view, however, that the Port Authority's ban on the "solicitation and receipt of funds" within its airport terminals should be upheld under the standards applicable to speech regulations in public forums. The regulation may be upheld as either a reasonable time, place, and manner restriction, or as a regulation directed at the nonspeech element of expressive conduct. The two standards have considerable overlap in a case like this one. *** The confluence of the two tests is well demonstrated by a case like this, where the government regulation at issue can be described with equal accuracy as a regulation of the manner of expression, or as a regulation of conduct with an expressive component.

I am in full agreement with the statement of the Court that solicitation is a form of protected speech. If the Port Authority's solicitation regulation prohibited all speech which requested the contribution of funds, I would conclude that it was a direct, content-based restriction of speech in clear violation of the First Amendment. The Authority's regulation does not prohibit all solicitation, however; it prohibits the "solicitation and receipt of funds." I do not understand this regulation to prohibit all speech that solicits funds. It reaches only personal solicitations for immediate payment of money. ***

So viewed, I believe the Port Authority's rule survives our test for speech restrictions in the public forum. In-person solicitation of funds, when combined with immediate receipt of that money, creates a risk of fraud and duress which is well recognized, and which is different in kind from other forms of expression or conduct. Travelers who are unfamiliar with the airport, perhaps even unfamiliar with this country, its customs and its language, are an easy prey for the money solicitor.***

I have little difficulty in deciding that the Port Authority has left open ample alternative channels for the communication of the message which is an aspect of solicitation. As already discussed, the Authority's rule does not prohibit all solicitation of funds: It restricts only the manner of the solicitation, or the conduct associated with solicitation, to prohibit immediate receipt of the solicited money. Requests for money continue to be permitted, and in the course of requesting money solicitors may explain their cause, or the purposes of their organization, without violating the regulation. It is only if the solicitor accepts immediate payment that a violation occurs. Thus the solicitor can continue to disseminate his message, for example by distributing preaddressed envelopes in which potential contributors may mail their donations.

Much of what I have said about the solicitation of funds may seem to apply to the sale of literature, but the differences between the two activities are of sufficient significance to require they be distinguished for constitutional purposes. The Port Authority's flat ban on the distribution or sale of printed material must, in my view, fall in its entirety. The application of our time, place, and manner test to the ban on sales leads to a result quite different from the solicitation ban. *** Attempting to collect money at another time or place is a far less plausible option in the context of a sale than when soliciting donations, because the literature sought to be sold will under normal circumstances be distributed within the forum. These distinctions have been recognized by the National Park Service, which permits the sale or distribution of literature, while prohibiting solicitation. [T]he Port Authority's regulation allows no practical means for advocates and organizations to sell literature within the public forums which are its airports.

"It should be remembered that the pamphlets of Thomas Paine were not distributed free of charge." The effect of a rule of law distinguishing between sales and distribution would be to close the marketplace of ideas to less affluent organizations and speakers, leaving speech as the preserve of those who are able to fund themselves. One of the primary purposes of the public forum is to provide persons who lack access to more sophisticated media the opportunity to speak. A prohibition on sales forecloses that opportunity for the very persons who need it most. And while the same arguments might be made regarding solicitation of funds, the answer is that the Port Authority has not prohibited all solicitation, but only a narrow class of conduct associated with a particular manner of solicitation.

For these reasons I agree that the Court of Appeals should be affirmed in full in finding the Port Authority's ban on the distribution or sale of literature unconstitutional, but upholding the prohibition on solicitation and immediate receipt of funds.

JUSTICE O'CONNOR, concurring in 91-155 and concurring in the judgment in 91-339.

In the decision below, the Court of Appeals upheld a ban on solicitation of funds within the airport terminals operated by the Port Authority of New York and New Jersey, but struck down a ban on the repetitive distribution of printed or written material within the terminals. I would affirm both parts of that judgment.

I concur in the Court's opinion in No. 91-155, and agree that publicly owned airports are not public fora. Unlike public streets and parks, both of which our First Amendment jurisprudence has identified as "traditional public fora," airports do not count among their purposes the "free exchange of ideas." *** I also agree with the Court that the Port Authority has not expressly opened its airports to the types of expression at issue here and therefore has not created a "limited" or "designated" public forum relevant to this case. For these reasons, the Port Authority's restrictions on solicitation and leafletting within the airport terminals do not qualify for the strict scrutiny that applies to restriction of speech in public fora. ***

"The reasonableness of the Government's restriction [on speech in a nonpublic forum] must be assessed in light of the purpose of the forum and all the surrounding circumstances." *** In this case, the "special attributes" and "surrounding circumstances" of the airports operated by the Port Authority are determinative. Not only has the Port Authority chosen *not* to limit access to the airports under its control, it has created a huge complex open to travelers and nontravelers alike. The airports house restaurants, cafeterias, snack bars, coffee shops, cocktail lounges, post offices, banks, telegraph offices, clothing shops, drug stores, food stores, nurseries, barber shops, currency exchanges, art exhibits, commercial advertising displays, bookstores, newsstands, dental offices and private clubs. The International Arrivals Building at JFK Airport even has two branches of Bloomingdale's.

In my view, the Port Authority is operating a shopping mall as well as an airport. The reasonableness inquiry, therefore, is not whether the restrictions on speech are "consistent with preserving the property" for air travel, but whether they are reasonably related to maintaining the multipurpose environment that the Port Authority has deliberately created.

Applying that standard, I agree with the Court in No. 91-155 that the ban on solicitation is reasonable. Face-to-face solicitation is incompatible with the airport's functioning in a way that the other, permitted activities are not. We have previously observed that "[s]olicitation impedes the normal flow of traffic [because it] requires action by those who would respond: The individual solicited must decide whether or not to contribute (which itself might involve reading the solicitor's literature or hearing his pitch), and then, having decided to do so, reach for a wallet, search it for money, write a check, or produce a credit card. *** As residents of metropolitan areas know from daily experience, confrontation by a person asking for money disrupts passage and is more intrusive and intimidating than an encounter with a person giving out information."

In my view, however, the regulation banning leafletting-or, in the Port Authority's words, the "continuous or repetitive distribution of printed or written material" cannot be upheld as reasonable on this record. I therefore concur in the judgment in No. 91-339 striking down that prohibition. ***

*** Because I cannot see how peaceful pamphleteering is incompatible with the multipurpose environment of the Port Authority airports, I cannot accept that a total ban on that activity is reasonable without an explanation as to why such a restriction "preserv[es] the property" for the several uses to which it has been put.

I would affirm the judgment of the Court of Appeals in both No. 91-155 and No. 91-339.

JUSTICE SOUTER, with whom JUSTICE BLACKMUN and JUSTICE STEVENS join, concurring in the judgment in No. 91-339 and dissenting in No. 91-155.

I

I join in Part I of JUSTICE KENNEDY's opinion and the judgment of affirmance in No. 91-339. I agree with JUSTICE KENNEDY's view of the rule that should determine what is a public forum and with his conclusion that the public areas of the airports at issue here qualify as such. The designation of a given piece of public property as a traditional public forum must not merely state a conclusion that the property falls within a static category including streets, parks, sidewalks and perhaps not much more, but must represent a conclusion that the property is no different in principle from such examples, which we have previously described as "archetypes" of property from which the government was and is powerless to exclude speech.*** To treat the class of such forums as closed by their description as "traditional," taking that word merely as a charter for examining the history of the particular public property claimed as a forum, has no warrant in a Constitution whose values are not to be left behind in the city streets that are no longer the only focus of our community life. If that were the line of our direction, we might as well abandon the public forum doctrine altogether.

*** I also agree with JUSTICE KENNEDY's statement of the public forum principle: we should classify as a public forum any piece of public property that is "suitable for discourse" in its physical character, where expressive activity is "compatible" with the use to which it has actually been put. *** Applying this test, I have no difficulty concluding that the unleased public areas at airports like the metropolitan New York airports at issue in this case are public forums.

II

From the Court's conclusion in No. 91-155, however, sustaining the total ban on solicitation of money for immediate payment, I respectfully dissent.

As JUSTICE KENNEDY's opinion indicates, the respondent comes closest to justifying the restriction as one furthering the government's interest in preventing coercion and fraud.[1] The claim to be preventing coercion is weak to start with. While a solicitor can be insistent, a pedestrian on the street or airport concourse can simply walk away or walk on. Since there is here no evidence of any type of coercive

1. Respondent also attempts to justify its regulation on the alternative basis of "interference with air travelers," referring in particular to problems of "annoyance," and "congestion." The First Amendment inevitably requires people to put up with annoyance and uninvited persuasion. Indeed, in such cases we need to scrutinize restrictions on speech with special care. ***

conduct, over and above the merely importunate character of the open and public solicitation, that might justify a ban, the regulation cannot be sustained to avoid coercion.

As for fraud, our cases do not provide government with plenary authority to ban solicitation just because it could be fraudulent. The evidence of fraudulent conduct here is virtually nonexistent. *** Petitioners claim, and respondent does not dispute, that by the Port Authority's own calculation, there has not been a single claim of fraud or misrepresentation since 1981. As against these facts, respondent's brief is ominous in adding that "[t]he Port Authority is also aware that members of [International Society for Krishna Consciousness] have engaged in misconduct elsewhere." This is precisely the type of vague and unsubstantiated allegation that could never support a restriction on speech.

Finally, I do not think the Port Authority's solicitation ban leaves open the "ample" channels of communication required of a valid content-neutral time, place and manner restriction. A distribution of preaddressed envelopes is unlikely to be much of an alternative. The practical reality of the regulation, which this Court can never ignore, is that it shuts off a uniquely powerful avenue of communication for organizations like the International Society for Krishna Consciousness, and may, in effect, completely prohibit unpopular and poorly funded groups from receiving funds in response to protected solicitation.

Accordingly, I would reverse the judgment of the Court of Appeals in No. 91-155, and strike down the ban on solicitation.

PER CURIAM [in 91-339].

For the reasons expressed in the opinions of JUSTICE O'CONNOR, JUSTICE KENNEDY, and JUSTICE SOUTER in *International Society for Krishna Consciousness, Inc. v. Lee*, the judgment of the Court of Appeals holding that the ban on distribution of literature in the Port Authority airport terminals is invalid under the First Amendment is affirmed.

CHIEF JUSTICE REHNQUIST, with whom JUSTICE WHITE, JUSTICE SCALIA and JUSTICE THOMAS join, dissenting [in 91-339].

Leafletting presents risks of congestion similar to those posed by solicitation. It presents, in addition, some risks unique to leafletting. And of course, as with solicitation, these risks must be evaluated against a backdrop of the substantial congestion problem facing the Port Authority and with an eye to the cumulative impact that will result if all groups are permitted terminal access. Viewed in this light, I conclude that the distribution ban, no less than the solicitation ban, is reasonable. I therefore dissent from the Court's holding striking the distribution ban. ***

---

6. Who Owns the Airwaves?

The Judicial Response to First Amendment Issues Arising from Government Management of Airwave Access and Use through licensing subject to conditions licensed broadcasters may be required to accept, or forfeit their license and step aside for others who will adhere to the conditions thus prescribed.

RED LION BROADCASTING COMPANY v. FCC
395 U.S. 367 (1969)

Mr. Justice White delivered the opinion of the Court.

***

The Red Lion Broadcasting Company is licensed to operate a Pennsylvania radio station, WGCB. On November 27, 1964, WGCB carried a 15-minute broadcast by the Reverend Billy James Hargis as part of a "Christian Crusade" series. A book by Fred J. Cook entitled "Goldwater—Extremist on the Right" was discussed by Hargis, who said that Cook had been fired by a newspaper for making false charges against city officials; that Cook had then worked for a Communist-affiliated publication; that he had defended Alger Hiss and attacked J. Edgar Hoover and the Central Intelligence Agency; and that he had now written a "book to smear and destroy Barry Goldwater." When Cook heard of the broadcast he concluded that he had been personally attacked and demanded free reply time, which the station refused. After an exchange of letters among Cook, Red Lion, and the FCC, the FCC declared that the Hargis broadcast constituted a personal attack on Cook; that Red Lion had failed to meet its obligation under the fairness doctrine as expressed in Times-Mirror Broadcasting Co., 24 P & F Radio Reg. 404 (1962), to send a tape, transcript, or summary of the broadcast to Cook and offer him reply time; and that the station must provide reply time whether or not Cook would pay for it. ***

As they now stand amended, the regulations read as follows:

> "Personal attacks; political editorials.
>
> "(a) When, during the presentation of views on a controversial issue of public importance, an attack is made upon the honesty, character, integrity or like personal qualities of an identified person or group, the licensee shall, within a reasonable time and in no event later than 1 week after the attack, transmit to the person or group attacked (1) notification of the date, time and identification of the broadcast; (2) a script or tape (or an accurate summary if a script or tape is not available) of the attack and (3) an offer of a reasonable opportunity to respond over the licensee's facilities.

***

The broadcasters challenge the fairness doctrine and its specific manifestations in the personal attack and political editorial rules on conventional First Amendment grounds, alleging that the rules abridge their freedom of speech and press. Their contention is that the First Amendment protects their desire to use their allotted frequencies continuously to broadcast whatever they choose, and to exclude whomever they choose from ever using that frequency. No man may be prevented from saying or publishing what he thinks, or from refusing in his speech or other utterances to give equal weight to the views of his opponents. This right, they say, applies equally to broadcasters.

A

Although broadcasting is clearly a medium affected by a First Amendment interest, United States v. Paramount Pictures, Inc., 334 U.S. 131, 166 (1948), differences in the characteristics of new media justify differences in the First Amendment standards applied to them. *** The lack of know-how and equipment may keep many from the air, but only a tiny fraction of those with resources and intelligence can hope to communicate by radio at the same time if intelligible communication is to be had, even if the entire radio spectrum is utilized in the present state of technology. ***

Where there are substantially more individuals who want to broadcast than there are frequencies to allocate, it is idle to posit an unabridgeable First Amendment right to broadcast comparable to the right of every individual to speak, write, or publish. If 100 persons want broadcast licenses but there are only 10 frequencies to allocate, all of them may have the same "right" to a license; but if there is to be any effective communication by radio, only a few can be licensed and the rest must be barred from the airwaves. It would be strange if the First Amendment, aimed at protecting and furthering communications, prevented the Government from making radio communication possible by requiring licenses to broadcast and by limiting the number of licenses so as not to overcrowd the spectrum. ***

By the same token, as far as the First Amendment is concerned those who are licensed stand no better than those to whom licenses are refused. A license permits broadcasting, but the licensee has no constitutional right to be the one who holds the license or to monopolize a radio frequency to the exclusion of his fellow citizens. There is nothing in the First Amendment which prevents Government from requiring a licensee to share his frequency with others and to conduct himself as a proxy or fiduciary with obligations to present those views and voices which are representative of his community and which would otherwise, by necessity, be barred from the airwaves. ***

B

Rather than confer frequency monopolies on a relatively small number of licensees, in a Nation of 200,000,000, the Government could surely have decreed that each frequency should be shared among all of some of those who wish to use it, each being assigned a portion of the broadcast day or the broadcast week. The ruling and regulations at issue here do not go quite so far. They assert that under specified circumstances, a licensee must offer to make available a reasonable amount of broadcast time to those who have a view different from that which has already been expressed on his station. The expression of a political endorsement, or of a personal attack while dealing with a controversial public issue, simply triggers this time sharing. As we have said, the First Amendment confers no right on licensees to prevent others from broadcasting on "their" frequencies and no right to an unconditional monopoly of a scarce resource which the Government has denied others the right to use.

Nor can we say that it is inconsistent with the First Amendment goal of producing an informed public capable of conducting its own affairs to require a broadcaster to permit answers to personal attacks occurring in the course of discussing controversial issues, or to require that the political opponents of those endorsed by the station be given a chance to communicate with the public.[18] Otherwise, station owners and a few networks would have unfettered power to make time available only to the highest bidders, to communicate only their own views on public issues, people and candidates, and to permit on the air only those with whom they agreed. There is no sanctuary in the First Amendment for unlimited private censorship operating in a medium not open to all. "Freedom of the press from governmental interference under the First Amendment does not sanction repression of that freedom by private interests." Associated Press v. United States, 326 U.S. 1, 20 (1945).

C

It is strenuously argued, however, that if political editorials or personal attacks will trigger an obligation in broadcasters to afford the opportunity for expression to speakers who need not pay for time and whose views are unpalatable to the licensees, then broadcasters will be irresistibly forced to self-censorship and their coverage of controversial public issues will be eliminated or at least rendered wholly ineffective. Such a result would indeed be a serious matter, for should licensees actually eliminate their coverage of controversial issues, the purposes of the doctrine would be stifled.

At this point, however, as the Federal Communications Commission has indicated, that possibility is at best speculative. The communications industry, and in particular the networks, have taken pains to present controversial issues in the past, and even now they do not assert that they intend to abandon their efforts in this regard. It would be better if the FCC's encouragement were never necessary to induce the broadcasters to meet their responsibility. And if experience with the administration of these doctrines indicates that they have the net effect of reducing rather than enhancing the volume and quality of coverage, there will be time enough to

18. The expression of views opposing those which broadcasters permit to be aired in the first place need not be confined solely to the broadcasters themselves as proxies. "Nor is it enough that he should hear the arguments of adversaries from his own teachers, presented as they state them, and accompanied by what they offer as refutations. That is not the way to do justice to the arguments, or bring them into real contact with his own mind. He must be able to hear them from persons who actually believe them; who defend them in earnest, and do their very utmost for them." J. Mill, On Liberty 32. (R. McCallum ed. 1947).

reconsider the constitutional implications. The fairness doctrine in the past has had no such overall effect.

That this will occur now seems unlikely, however, since if present licensees should suddenly prove timorous, the Commission is not powerless to insist that they give adequate and fair attention to public issues. It does not violate the First Amendment to treat licensees given the privilege of using scarce radio frequencies as proxies for the entire community, obligated to give suitable time and attention to matters of great public concern. To condition the granting or renewal of licenses on a willingness to present representative community views on controversial issues is consistent with the ends and purposes of those constitutional provisions forbidding the abridgment of freedom of speech and freedom of the press. Congress need not stand idly by and permit those with licenses to ignore the problems which beset the people or to exclude from the airways anything but their own views of fundamental questions. The statute, long administrative practice, and cases are to this effect. ***

We need not and do not now ratify every past and future decision by the FCC with regard to programming. There is no question here of the Commission's refusal to permit the broadcaster to carry a particular program or to publish his own views; of a discriminatory refusal to require the licensee to broadcast certain views which have been denied access to the airwaves; of government censorship of a particular program contrary to § 326; or of the official government view dominating public broadcasting. Such questions would raise more serious First Amendment issues. But we do hold that the Congress and the Commission do not violate the First Amendment when they require a radio or television station to give reply time to answer personal attacks and political editorials. ***

E

It is argued that even if at one time the lack of available frequencies for all who wished to use them justified the Government's choice of those who would best serve the public interest by acting as proxy for those who would present differing views, or by giving the latter access directly to broadcast facilities, this condition no longer prevails so that continuing control is not justified. To this there are several answers.

Scarcity is not entirely a thing of the past. Advances in technology, such as microwave transmission, have led to more efficient utilization of the frequency spectrum but uses for that spectrum have also grown apace. ***

In a view of the scarcity of broadcast frequencies, the Government's role in allocating those frequencies, and the legitimate claims of those unable without governmental assistance to gain access to those frequencies for expression of their views, we hold the regulations and ruling at issue here are both authorized by statute and constitutional. The judgment of the Court of Appeals in *Red Lion* is affirmed and that in *RTNDA* reversed and the causes remanded for proceedings consistent with this opinion.

Not having heard oral argument in these cases, MR. JUSTICE DOUGLAS took no part in the Court's decision.

7. Notes on *Red Lion* and "Public Forum" Use

Red Lion, should immediately bring to mind (for comparison and contrast)*Miami Herald Publishing Co. v. Tornillo*.[92] There, as one may recall, a unanimous Supreme Court held that the first amendment forbids a state-created right-of-reply entitlement, even for a candidate for public office whose character has been assailed in the columns of a newspaper, just prior to a pending election, and under circumstances where the impugned person may have no practical equivalent forum to rebut the disparagements or mischaracterizations the newspaper editorial contained. Moreover, whatever the self-censoring effect the Court felt was implicit in the Florida right-of-reply statute, surely it is at least as great in a*Red Lion* kind of case. How are the cases best explained? To be sure, *Tornillo* did involve a newspaper rather than a radio or television station, and perhaps the case is thought to be influenced by the express separate mention in the first amendment of "the freedom of the press."

Yet, by itself, that distinction seems extremely weak. It is obvious that CBS, NBC, ABC, and CNN provide news coverage and other features of a like sort. In many other first amendment settings (e.g., first amendment limitations on the application of libel laws), moreover, we have seen that media defendants are treated without distinction under *New York Times v. Sullivan*: radio and television news and commentary are equally protected under the first amendment as news and commentary that appears in print. It would be odd at this late date to suppose a constitutional distinction would turn upon an adventitious distinction that radio and television were unknown in 1791 (the date of the first amendment's ratification), but that newspapers were already a well established fact of life. Moreover, in other areas of constitutional adjudication (e.g., fourth amendment privacy protection), the Bill of Rights has not been arrested by the state of the existing technology of the era.[93] Neither has the first amendment otherwise been limited to some time-bound notion of the communicative state of the art.[94] For that matter, neither did the Court in *Red Lion* deny the full relevance of the first amendment to communication by airwave. So this suggested distinction would not appear to explain the difference between the two cases.

Rather, *Red Lion* is expressly distinguished from *Miami Herald* on two other grounds, noted in the opinion by Justice White. Both grounds of distinction apparently are closely tied to the subject we have been considering here, namely, government-owned or government-managed *public* property, and the rules that may govern *that* property as such.

---

92. 418 U.S. 241 (1974). See p. 200 *supra*.

93. See, e.g., Katz v. United States, 389 U.S. 347 (1967) (fourth amendment is applicable to telephone wiretaps though telephones did not exist when the fourth amendment was framed, and though the wiretap may not involve any act of trespass upon the premises of the property of the person whose messages are intercepted and recorded), overruling Olmstead v. United States, 277 U.S. 438 (1928).

94. See, e.g., the public figure libel cases and the similar treatment of television reports and newspaper reports on public figures.

First, the Court noted that, strictly speaking, no private property is permitted to exist in the airwaves, by fiat of federal law. In that strict sense, the airwaves are more appropriately thought of as "socialized" property, i.e. they belong to us all, as a common resource, held in public trust. They are thus also akin to a public park, held in public trust, subject to rationing by permit, issued by the FCC. Second, in awarding an exclusive three-year license to the Red Lion Broadcasting Company, respecting the use of a given FM signal of a given transmitting strength, the government has thereby locked out all other would-be users of the same broadcast frequency, thus withdrawing *any* use of that same "forum" (i.e. that FM frequency), during the whole time of the licensee's grant. From then on, during the time of the license, the public forum is severely restricted by government fiat, and restricted by mere "speaker identity" alone. The government has appointed a speaker to put in charge of a public forum and granted him virtual *carte blanche* power to admit or deny anyone else the privilege to speak in that "forum". In generally forbidding others to broadcast over the same frequency without the licensee's permission, the government creates a monopoly which is mitigated only somewhat by the "fairness doctrine." After satisfying every tittle and jot of the fairness doctrine, the licensee is still a vastly more privileged party, vis-à-vis others: the licensee retains a monopoly on the use of the public forum (the FM broadcast frequency).

In contrast, no similar thing can be said in respect to the *Miami Herald* case. There, there was no public property committed to the newspaper's exclusive use, and no public forum with respect to which the Miami Herald was granted any privileged use. Any cost barriers to starting up a newspaper, and any other problems faced by Pat Tornillo as he conveyed his own message (by means of a newspaper, pamphlet, or even handbill), to subscribers of the Miami Herald, would have been faced equally by anyone else. They did not result from state action allocating public property (or a public forum) and vesting exclusive speaking rights in that forum, in a single company for a three year, renewable period.[95]

Additionally, though the matter was not particularly emphasized by the Court in *Red Lion*, note that the grant of the public property speech monopoly-privilege (i.e. exclusive broadcast rights to a given broadcast frequency for three years renewable), was also made by the FCC to the Red Lion Broadcasting Company *rent free*.[96] May

---

95. Nor did the state or the city favor the Miami Herald by granting it an advantage with respect to any "public forum" *means* for delivering its publication—for example by granting the Miami Herald an exclusive license to distribute through the network of public streets. (Any public property to which the Miami Herald had access for distribution of its newspaper was equally available for the same purpose to anyone else.)

96. If full market price value had been charged, would the outcome then be different? Suppose the Miami Herald happens to rent the property on which it constructs its editorial offices and/or publishing plant from the City of Miami. Would the additional datum of the city's relationship to the Miami Herald as "landlord" have been at all persuasive to the Supreme Court in determining whether the state right-of-reply statute was valid as applied?

not this also make some difference in the case? First, Red Lion Broadcasting Company received a privileged use of a natural public forum. And for this exclusionary advantage vis-à-vis others who might want to broadcast from time to time over the same frequency, whether to reply to some message Red Lion broadcast or simply to present some original programs of their own, Red Lion had paid absolutely nothing at all.[97]

In the *Miami Herald* case, there is no equivalent public forum argument to be made. The government does not lock out anyone from the use of any public property or "public forum," and, obviously, neither is there any foregone rent so to favor a given publisher in the (rent free) exclusive use of a scarce public good.[98] In essence, then, from this perspective, *Red Lion* is both a distinguishable, and a very modest, Supreme Court case. The government has taken a natural forum (the public property of an airwave broadcast frequency), which formerly anyone might have used, and made it into a very limited public forum. Indeed, *rent free* it is made available to a *single* user, except to the extent of providing an assurance of access when one otherwise denied access to it is specifically mentioned in a disparaging way: albeit at a later time than the original broadcast, he or she may appear briefly to make some reply. Viewed *this* way, the case may seem both easy and right.[99]

---

97. Whether the actual rental value of the particular FCC license involved in the *Red Lion* case was large or small, the case does not enable us to say. Obviously the rental value of *particular* broadcast frequencies may differ greatly, from an estimated several million dollars in certain top ten VHF television markets, down to virtually nothing for certain rural AM radio frequencies, even as sometimes evidenced insofar as some available frequencies may even go unclaimed for lack of a suitable applicant convinced that there is any money to be made by setting up a suitable broadcast facility and incurring the costs necessary to operate the station, though the license is free. The surer way of determining the real value of an FCC license would be to modify the current system and allocate licenses according to open market, competitive, sealed bids. A good proxy, absent the institution of a real bid auction system, is nonetheless available simply by determining what whole sum a transferee of an FCC license (the transfer of which the FCC approves prior to the closing of the deal) pays the transferor for the broadcast facilities the transferee purchases from the transferor, and by subtracting such amount as one can fairly determine to represent the fair market value merely of the facilities as such; the difference reflects the value of the license. (Consider buying a used taxicab in New York City, on the one hand, and an identical used taxicab-with-medallion-included, on the other hand. The latter purchase is likely to cost about $100,000 more.)

98. In contrast, arguably, were the state to charge full market price in allocating the airwaves (as in a bid auction system), it may be argued that the price paid by the successful bidder would make the "property" private property for first amendment purposes. (In paying full market price, for the property rental, the buyer is made to internalize the costs of his own freedom of speech preferences in respect to that property, just as The Miami Herald, The National Review, The Durham Morning Herald, Ms. Magazine, or any other private publisher does, with theirs.) See also discussion *infra*, note 104.

99. Note, however, in contrast, that this kind of public forum analysis will not work to rationalize certain other kinds of FCC rules such as those that forbid profanity, indecency, or vulgarity by broadcasters. Such rules obviously do not enlarge the opportunities for free speech. Neither do they compensate those lacking licenses, by providing some opportunity for them to address issues they might wish to present, in the manner they think best to do. Rather, the rules substantively restrict what may

Indeed, viewed this way, perhaps several other questions might be raised.

1. For instance, is it even arguable that were the fairness doctrine dropped by the FCC (as it might be),[100] the first amendment would itself mandate third party rights of access to a broadcast frequency in circumstances like those in *Red Lion*—on the basis that the frequency is public property and a natural public forum, with respect to which the government cannot, constitutionally, discriminate by "speaker identity" in a totally exclusionary (i.e. licensee-favoring) way?[101]

2. To what extent, moreover, might the favored "forum status" of an FCC licensee support the statutory imposition of even *greater* (if different) restrictions on the licensee, such as common carrier obligations, i.e. rules obliging the licensee to carry third party programs without discrimination because of their content whether the licensee finds them absolutely contrary to the licensee's own program prefer-

---

be said, regardless of by whom, and regardless of listener or viewer interest (which may in fact be very substantial). Nothing in the reasoning of *Red Lion* explains any such case at all. Cf. FCC v. Pacifica Foundation, 438 U.S. 726 (1978).

100. In August 1987, the FCC unanimously moved to repeal the fairness doctrine. The FCC pointed to evidence that the fairness doctrine chilled broadcasters from presenting controversial subjects, and to evidence of greater diversity in the available means of communication (for example, cable channels had vastly expanded carrying capacity). It then concluded, on first amendment grounds, that different standards for newspapers and broadcast media were unwarranted.

The "fairness doctrine" abandoned by the FCC in 1987, however, spoke generally to the "obligations" of broadcasters to "afford reasonable opportunity for the discussion of conflicting views on issues of public importance." See 47 C.F.R. 73.1910 (Fairness Doctrine); 2 F.C.C.R. 5043 (1987) (decision to end enforcement of Fairness Doctrine). Although the FCC abandoned this doctrine in 1987, it continues to apply to broadcasters two other related rules, one of which reads largely like the regulations at issue in *Red Lion Broadcasting Co v. FCC.*

According to the first of these, the "political editorial rule," if a station broadcasts an editorial endorsing or opposing a candidate, it must notify the candidate's opponents (or the candidate that the editorial opposed) of the date and time of the editorial; it must provide a script or tape of the broadcast; and it must offer the affected candidate a reasonable opportunity to respond using the station's or system's facilities. 47 C.F.R. 73.1930.

According to the second, the "personal attack rule," if an attack on the "honesty, character, integrity, or like personal qualities" of a specific person or group is made during the presentation of views on a controversial issue of public importance, the station airing the attack must notify the attacked person or group of the date and time of the attack and the program in which it took place; provide a script, tape, or accurate summary of the attack; and offer the attacked person or group a reasonable opportunity to respond to the attack using the station's or system's facilities. 47 C.F.R. 73.1920. In 1995, the FCC dismissed a personal attack complaint on the merits (because the petitioners had failed to show that the personal attack took place during the presentation of a controversial issue of public importance) but reaffirmed that broadcasters remain subject to the rule.

101. Cf. CBS v. Democratic Nat'l Committee, 412 U.S. 94 (1973) (in light of fairness doctrine, first amendment does not require broadcast licensee otherwise to yield air time to third party requests). See Note, Constitutional Ramifications of a Repeal of the Fairness Doctrine, 64 Geo.L.J. 1293 (1976).

ences, economic interests, or point of view, and although clearly no such obligations could be imposed upon the ordinary private press?[102]

3. On the other hand, to what extent may the fairness doctrine nonetheless in fact tend to induce self-censorship[103] and thus merely add to general tendencies of industry risk-averseness in broadcasting, providing *less* diversity than one might reasonably otherwise expect were the doctrine either dropped or (as in the *Miami Herald* case) deemed unconstitutional *per se*?

4. In the domain of the (private) print media, note that the paradigm of "freedom of the press" is that each publisher marches solely to his or her own tune, leaving other publishers—large or small, mainstream or idiosyncratic—to march solely to theirs. The success or failure of the publisher is, in turn, principally contingent on finding subscribers or at least willing readers (without whom they will ordinarily lack advertisers and thus will go broke). And, accordingly, Ms. Magazine is not expected to look like, or read like, The National Review. Those who prefer either Ms. Magazine or The National Review, moreover, may not be the same ones who prefer Playboy, or those who prefer Commentary, or those who prefer Elijah Speaks, though one may, if one wants, seek to subscribe to all five (why not?).

Neither the selection of the subjects covered in any of these journals, nor the slant, the presentation, or the "fairness" of the publisher matters in resisting any effort by government to make them more alike, or more moderate, or more uplifting, or more in "the public interest" (whatever that is). Indeed, as to each, the point of the first amendment is that, as to all such matters, the government is to keep out of the way.

The paradigm of private speech property is freedom to publish whatever one thinks best (or can find a market to satisfy)—and the reciprocal freedom of each to read what one wants, however narrow, one-sided, and satisfying to oneself it may be, culled from a blizzard of alternative publishers, unleavened by what some agency of

---

102. See, e.g., Henry Geller & Donna Lampert, Cable, Content Regulation and the First Amendment, 32 Cath.U.L.Rev. 603 (1983).

103. **Note** that unless an identifiable person is mentioned in a disparaging fashion in the course of the broadcast of a controversial social or political issue, there of course arises no duty to furnish free air time for a reply. The access right is thus triggered only by the broadcaster's own broadcast; to avoid having to subsidize the reply (a shadow cost to be added to the cost of the original broadcast), the broadcaster need merely be prudent and keep still. **Note** also that setting aside equal air time for a reply may also be far more expensive, in terms of opportunity cost to a licensee broadcaster, than furnishing "reply space" in a newspaper. The medium is strictly limited (i.e. a fixed number of broadcast minutes), unlike the flexibility of pages, print size, width of margins, and columns in print. The resulting shadow cost may therefore be proportionately higher and the disincentive of controversy comparatively great. See David L. Lange, The Role of the Access Doctrine in the Regulation of the Mass Media: A Critical Review and Assessment, 52 N.C.L.Rev. 1 (1973).

government deems consistent with the public interest.[104] It is ultimately from the competition of this ideological marketplace, each publication having its own pronounced attitude, format, features, and editorial preferences, that "truth," popularity and success are in some sense sorted out. Consumers subscribe to, read, reject, boycott, or pick what they want, whether of the right, the center, or the left, whether the good, the bad, or the profane. This unchecked diversity, itself subject principally to the sole check of marketplace failure—failure against the appeal for subscribers and advertisers by rivals—seems to be the general first amendment rule.

Compare this model with the "social" model of the FCC, given the proliferation of cable, of UHF, VHF, AM, FM, FAX, the Internet, etc. (and given, too, their substantial overlapping communications markets with the print media as well). Is there any principled distinction for treating the airwaves in the manner the*Red Lion* case presumes to do?[105]

---

104. For a provocative recent book suggesting a more active role by government in this regard, however, *See* Cass Sunstein, Republic.com (2001)

105. Cf. the following view by Justice Douglas, writing separately in CBS v. Democratic Nat'l Committee, 412 U.S. at 148-161 (1973): "I did not participate in [*Red Lion*] and, with all respect, would not support it. *** The struggle for liberty has been a struggle against Government *** [I]t is anathema to the First Amendment to allow Government any role of censorship over newspapers, magazines, books, art, music, TV, radio, or any other aspect of the press." (Justice Douglas would have confined the FCC principally to (a) application of antitrust responsibilities and (b) facilitation of new broadcast technologies; he would have taken the FCC out of program content controls virtually altogether.) (See also discussion at n. 103 p. 484 *supra.*)

Insofar as a licensee derives any advantage from having a license "rent free," consider the proposal to offset any such advantage by extracting a fair, market price rent, putting the ensuing risks entirely on the license holder—just as they are with Ms. Magazine, Time, or anyone else who must internalize the costs of what they publish, according to whatever position or positions they choose to take. See, e.g., Bruce M. Owen, Economics and Freedom of Expression: Media Structure and The First Amendment (1975); R. H. Coase, Evaluation of Public Policy Relating to Radio and Television Broadcasting: Social and Economic Issues, 41 Land Econ. 161 (1965); R. H. Coase, The Federal Communications Commission, 2 J.L. & Econ. 1 (1959); Fowler & Brenner, A Marketplace Approach to Broadcast Regulation, 60 Tex.L.Rev. 207 (1982); Abbott B. Lipsky, Jr., Note, Reconciling Red Lion and Tornillo: A Consistent Theory of Media Regulation, 28 Stan.L.Rev. 563 (1976). Nor (to anticipate the obvious objection) does this approach neglect "diversity," for what one will aim at in markets already saturated with tuned-in, mere ordinary audience appeal fare will be to provide a specialized niche—by capturing an element previously not as well served by others on the airwaves, one maximizes the highest possible use of the channel or frequency on which one seeks to bid. (In a word, the invisible hand works.)

For example, it may be that in Durham, North Carolina, the highest bid for an FM radio frequency, given what is already on the air, would in fact be submitted by a small company intending to devote the entirety of its programming to the African-American community; that proposed format may give it a product edge, so to speak, i.e. bring with it an array of advertisers, given the listening audience those advertisers find they now reach more effectively per dollar charged than on any other medium through which they might try to promote sales. (In what way is the African-American-oriented radio station different from an African-American-oriented magazine, in this regard?) Note, too, that in this circumstance, it has received no subsidy (for it is paying full rent for the airwave). And why should its legal duty to afford access, reply, balance, etc., be any different from a particular foreign language

5. Consider also the following idea. "Newsprint" is what newspapers are printed on (it is "inexpensive paper made from wood pulp, used chiefly for printing newspapers")[106] but it is also, like the airwaves, not a free good. To the extent one cannot afford to buy newsprint, to the same extent one may not be able to have the same practical influence as someone who can, for one will lack the same stock of material to use to print one's message in bulk to sell or give away, whether on a simple handbill or on the full equivalent of the New York Times.

Suppose, on this account, that newsprint were effectively *socialized* in the United States[107](as the airwaves were socialized in the 1920s by Act of Congress, and have remained so in contemplation of basic property ownership theory ever since). What then? The rationale for doing so, incidentally, might be that, as with airwaves, newsprint is a scarce good: that at any point in time, it is finite and its finitude matters, i.e. the relatively greater amounts demanded by those wanting it and the relatively lesser amounts then physically available, the relatively higher price the market price becomes for any stated quantity, and, correspondingly, the less equal each person's ability to have as much as someone else has on any given day or month or year. The fundamental reason for socializing newsprint is to recognize that all who might want it cannot simultaneously be supplied at the zero (or near zero) price level necessary to put it within the reach of all on equal terms, and the accompanying social resolve that access to newsprint ought *not* rest on inequalities of ability to pay.

The "real" value of newsprint, one may say, is its value in the printing of newspapers, just as the "real" value of airwaves is their value in facilitating broadcast speech. By first making some (or most, or all newsprint a form of*public* property (as the airwaves are public property, or a public park is public property), we can better allocate free press rights more equitably than a price system allegedly does, where the queue of applicants for newsprint is simply sorted out by letting the price rise in light of demand until at the marginal price, the effective demand (i.e. ability-plus- willingness-to-buy) establishes an equilibrium between price and supply.

We do not allocate the airwaves by a price system though we obviously could.[108] So why should we allocate newsprint by a price system, either? Rather, why not collectively acquire (a) some, (b) most, or (c) all of the existing supply of newsprint, even while providing incentives for additional sources of newsprint to be developed, as well. And, having publicly reserved or acquired (a) some, (b) most, or (c) all of the existing supply of newsprint, might one also establish an NNLC (*National Newsprint Licensing Commission*), patterned on the existing FCC?

---

magazine subscribed to by those who think it just fine as it is?

106. The American Heritage Dictionary 885 (1971 ed.).

107. It might be done by government purchase of all forests in which trees useful as newsprint can be grown, constitutionally pursued by the eminent domain clause in the fifth amendment. Alternatively, it might be done by establishing the government as a monopsonist (monopoly buyer) of all newsprint produced in the United States or permitted to be imported with its approval and consent.

108. See discussion and references in note 104 p. 484 *supra*.

Following the FCC model, the NNLC could similarly provide for the issuance of licenses, each good for a three-year, renewable term, pursuant to which the licensees might pay merely in keeping with their ability to do so, for such stock as may be issued for their newsprint use. To the extent that the existing newsprint stock were too limited to meet all demand on this basis (as seems likely) then, in keeping with the FCC example, newsprint stock could be issued to licensees pursuant to comparative license application hearings under standards not unlike those now used by the FCC, including the feature upheld in *Red Lion*.[109]

Among the several questions one might want to raise about such a proposal, consider these:

a. If the proposed NNLC somehow strikes one as too closely resembling a system of government licensed presses (i.e. licensing with strings attached) to withstand first amendment scrutiny even under the conservative (i.e. Blackstone) understanding of that amendment, how is it distinguishable from the airwaves and the FCC?

b. If the treatment of the airwaves we currently have is constitutional (as certainly the Court in *Red Lion* assumes), however, why would it be any less constitutional to proceed with the proposal just described, in respect to such newsprint stock as the government may either acquire or control?[110]

NOTE AND INTRODUCTION TO *TURNER BROADCASTING*

Cable television companies carry programs and communication services to cable service subscribers through the co-axial cable systems they own and maintain at their own expense. Cable companies of course may take a great deal of their material from the airwaves. Still, they do not themselves use or "occupy" the airwaves in the sense involved in the *Red Lion* case. Nothing a cable company does reduces electromagnetic spectrum availability to others. None is given any "exclusive" (licensed) use over any frequency and their business does not depend upon having any frequency or frequencies assigned to them by the FCC.

---

109. E.g., a rule that such newsprint as one receives pursuant to application to the NNLC, will be impressed with a duty to notify in advance any person whom the recipient intends to identify and criticize, and provide free space for reply, in a column of equal length and prominence as the critical column in which they are disparaged.

110. For new (and contrasting) views of the problems raised by *Red Lion* and regulation of other technologies and further comparisons with "the press," see Cass Sunstein, Republic.com (2001); Lee C. Bollinger, Images of a Free Press (1991); Jonathan Emord, Freedom, Technology, and the First Amendment (1991); Rodney A. Smolla, Free Speech in an Open Society 321-342 (1992). See also L. A. Scot Powe, Jr., American Broadcasting and the First Amendment (1987); William W. Van Alstyne, Interpretations of the First Amendment 68-90 (1984).

May government nonetheless presume to dictate to cable companies what they must carry whether they (or, for that matter, their subscribers) might prefer a different selection of channels and of programs? Or would the reasoning of the *Miami Herald* case so clearly apply that *any* such "must-carry" rules should be struck down under the first amendment (as an interference with the editorial autonomy of the cable company)?

If government may impose certain must-carry rules on cable companies notwithstanding the first amendment, on what possible grounds, on what reasoning, and *to what extent*? *Red Lion* assuredly doesn't provide a satisfactory basis for answering that question, does it? Does *Miami Herald*? In 1994, in *Turner Broadcasting*, the Supreme Court addressed this question, in the following (five-to-four) decision. Who in your view was more nearly correct?

TURNER BROADCASTING SYSTEM v. FEDERAL COMMUNICATIONS COMMISSION

512 U.S. 622 (1994)

JUSTICE KENNEDY announced the judgment of the Court and delivered the opinion of the Court, except as to Part III-B. ***

On October 5, 1992, Congress overrode a Presidential veto to enact the Cable Television Consumer Protection and Competition Act of 1992. At issue in this case is the constitutionality of the so-called must-carry provisions, contained in §§ 4 and 5 of the Act.

Section 4 requires carriage of "local commercial television stations," defined to include all full power television broadcasters, other than those qualifying as "noncommercial educational" stations under § 5, that operate within the same television market as the cable system. Cable systems with more than 12 active channels, and more than 300 subscribers, are required to set aside up to one-third of their channels for commercial broadcast stations that request carriage. Cable systems with more than 300 subscribers, but only 12 or fewer active channels, must carry the signals of three commercial broadcast stations.

The broadcast signals carried under this provision must be transmitted on a continuous, uninterrupted basis, and must be placed in the same numerical channel position as when broadcast over the air. Further, subject to a few exceptions, a cable operator may not charge a fee for carrying broadcast signals in fulfillment of its must-carry obligations.

Section 5 of the Act imposes similar requirements regarding the carriage of local public broadcast television stations, referred to in the Act as local "noncommercial educational television stations." A cable system with 12 or fewer channels must carry one of these stations; a system of between 13 and 36 channels must carry between one and three; and a system with more than 36 channels must carry each local public broadcast station requesting carriage. As with commercial broadcast stations, § 5 requires cable system operators to carry the program schedule of the public broadcast station in its entirety and at its same over-the-air channel position.

Congress enacted the 1992 Cable Act after conducting three years of hearings on the structure and operation of the cable television industry. In brief, Congress found that the physical characteristics of cable transmission, compounded by the increasing concentration of economic power in the cable industry, are endangering the ability of over-the-air broadcast television stations to compete for a viewing audience and thus for necessary operating revenues.

In particular, Congress found that over 60 percent of the households with television sets subscribe to cable, and for these households cable has replaced over-the-air broadcast television as the primary provider of video programming. This is so, Congress found, because "[m]ost subscribers to cable television systems do not or cannot maintain antennas to receive broadcast television services, do not have input selector switches to convert from a cable to antenna reception system, or cannot otherwise receive broadcast television services." In addition, Congress concluded that due to "local franchising requirements and the extraordinary expense of constructing more than one cable television system to serve a particular geographic area," the overwhelming majority of cable operators exercise a monopoly over cable service.

According to Congress, this market position gives cable operators the power and the incentive to harm broadcast competitors. The power derives from the cable operator's ability, as owner of the transmission facility, to "terminate the retransmission of the broadcast signal, refuse to carry new signals, or reposition a broadcast signal to a disadvantageous channel position." The incentive derives from the economic reality that "[c]able television systems and broadcast television stations increasingly compete for television advertising revenues." By refusing carriage of broadcasters' signals, cable operators, as a practical matter, can reduce the number of households that have access to the broadcasters' programming, and thereby capture advertising dollars that would otherwise go to broadcast stations.

In light of these technological and economic conditions, Congress concluded that unless cable operators are required to carry local broadcast stations, "[t]here is a substantial likelihood that additional local broadcast signals will be deleted, repositioned, or not carried," the "marked shift in market share" from broadcast to cable will continue to erode the advertising revenue base which sustains free local broadcast television. and that, as a consequence, "the economic viability of free local broadcast television and its ability to originate quality local programming will be seriously jeopardized."

[T]he District Court, in a divided opinion, granted summary judgment in favor of the Government and the other intervenor-defendants, ruling that the must- carry provisions are consistent with the First Amendment. This direct appeal followed.

II (A)

We address first the Government's contention that regulation of cable television should be analyzed under the same First Amendment standard that applies to regulation of broadcast television. It is true that our cases have permitted more intrusive regulation of broadcast speakers than of speakers in other media. Compare Red Lion Broadcasting Co. v. FCC, 395 U.S. 367 (1969) (television) with Miami Herald Publishing Co. v. Tornillo, 418 U.S. 241 (1974) (print). But the broadcast cases are inapposite in the present context because cable television does not suffer from the inherent limitations that characterize the broadcast medium. Indeed, given the rapid advances in fiber optics and digital compression technology, soon there may be no practical limitation on the number of speakers who may use the cable medium. Nor is there any danger of physical interference between two cable speakers attempting to share the same channel.* In light of these fundamental technological differences between broadcast and cable transmission, application of the more relaxed standard of scrutiny adopted in *Red Lion* and the other broadcast cases is inapt when determining the First Amendment validity of cable regulation.

Although the Government acknowledges the substantial technological differences between broadcast and cable, it advances a second argument for application of the *Red Lion* framework to cable regulation. It asserts that the foundation of our broadcast jurisprudence is not the physical limitations of the electromagnetic spectrum, but rather the "market dysfunction" that characterizes the broadcast market. *** While we agree that the cable market suffers certain structural impediments, the Government's argument is flawed in two respects. First, as discussed above, the special physical characteristics of broadcast transmission, not the economic characteristics of the broadcast market, are what underlies our broadcast jurisprudence. Second, the mere assertion of dysfunction or failure in a speech market, without more, is not sufficient to shield a speech regulation from the First Amendment standards applicable to nonbroadcast media. See, e.g., Miami Herald Publishing Co. v. Tornillo, 418 U.S., at 248-258.

By a related course of reasoning, the Government and some appellees maintain that the must-carry provisions are nothing more than industry-specific antitrust legislation, and thus warrant rational basis scrutiny under this Court's "precedents governing legislative efforts to correct market failure in a market whose commodity is speech," such as Associated Press v. United States, 326 U.S. 1 (1945), and Lorain Journal Co. v. United States, 342 U.S. 143 (1951). This contention is unavailing. *Associated Press* and *Lorain Journal* both involved actions against members of the press brought under the Sherman Antitrust Act, a law of general application. But

---

*. **[Ed. Note.** In City of Los Angeles v. Preferred Communications, Inc., 476 U.S. 488 (1986), the Supreme Court held that cities and other units of state and local government may not constitutionally confer a cable monopoly.]

while the enforcement of a generally applicable law may or may not be subject to heightened scrutiny under the First Amendment, laws that single out the press, or certain elements thereof, are always subject to at least some degree of heightened First Amendment scrutiny. Because the must-carry provisions impose special obligations upon cable operators and special burdens upon cable programmers, some measure of heightened First Amendment scrutiny is demanded.

B

At the heart of the First Amendment lies the principle that each person should decide for him or herself the ideas and beliefs deserving of expression, consideration, and adherence. Our political system and cultural life rest upon this ideal. Government action that stifles speech on account of its message, or that requires the utterance of a particular message favored by the Government, contravenes this essential right. Laws of this sort pose the inherent risk that the Government seeks not to advance a legitimate regulatory goal, but to suppress unpopular ideas or information or manipulate the public debate through coercion rather than persuasion.

For these reasons, the First Amendment, subject only to narrow and well-understood exceptions, does not countenance governmental control over the content of messages expressed by private individuals. In contrast, regulations that are unrelated to the content of speech are subject to an intermediate level of scrutiny, see Clark v. Community for Creative Non-Violence, 468 U.S. 288, 293 (1984), because in most cases they pose a less substantial risk of excising certain ideas or viewpoints from the public dialogue.

Insofar as they pertain to the carriage of full power broadcasters, the must-carry rules, on their face, impose burdens and confer benefits without reference to the content of speech. Although the provisions interfere with cable operators' editorial discretion by compelling them to offer carriage to a certain minimum number of broadcast stations, the extent of the interference does not depend upon the content of the cable operators' programming. Cf. Miami Herald Publishing Co. v. Tornillo, 418 U.S., at 256-257 (newspaper may avoid access obligations by refraining from speech critical of political candidates). The must-carry provisions also burden cable programmers by reducing the number of channels for which they can compete. But, again, this burden is unrelated to content, for it extends to all cable programmers irrespective of the programming they choose to offer viewers.

It is true that the must-carry provisions distinguish between speakers in the television programming market. But they do so based only upon the manner in which speakers transmit their messages to viewers, and not upon the messages they carry: Broadcasters, which transmit over the airwaves, are favored, while cable programmers, which do not, are disfavored.

Appellants contend, in this regard, that the must-carry regulations are content-based because Congress' purpose in enacting them was to promote speech of a favored content. We do not agree. Our review of the Act and its various findings persuades us that Congress' overriding objective in enacting must-carry was not to favor programming of a particular subject matter, viewpoint, or format, but rather to preserve access to free television programming for the 40 percent of Americans without cable. ***

By preventing cable operators from refusing carriage to broadcast television stations, the must-carry rules ensure that broadcast television stations will retain a large enough potential audience to earn necessary advertising revenue—or, in the case of noncommercial broadcasters, sufficient viewer contributions—to maintain their continued operation. In so doing, the provisions are designed to guarantee the survival of a medium that has become a vital part of the Nation's communication system, and to ensure that every individual with a television set can obtain access to free television programming. ***

In short, Congress' acknowledgment that broadcast television stations make a valuable contribution to the Nation's communications system does not render the must-carry scheme content-based. The scope and operation of the challenged provisions make clear, in our view, that Congress designed the must-carry provisions not to promote speech of a particular content, but to prevent cable operators from exploiting their economic power to the detriment of broadcasters, and thereby to ensure that all Americans, especially those unable to subscribe to cable, have access to free television programming—whatever its content.

We likewise reject the suggestion, advanced by appellants and by Judge Williams in dissent, that the must-carry rules are content-based because the preference for broadcast stations "*automatically* entails content requirements." It is true that broadcast programming, unlike cable programming, is subject to certain limited content restraints imposed by statute and FCC regulation. But it does not follow that Congress mandated cable carriage of broadcast television stations as a means of ensuring that particular programs will be shown, or not shown, on cable systems.

In a regime where Congress or the FCC exercised more intrusive control over the content of broadcast programming, an argument similar to appellants' might carry greater weight. But in the present regulatory system, those concerns are without foundation. ***

D

Appellants advance three additional arguments to support their view that the must-carry provisions warrant strict scrutiny. In brief, appellants contend that the provisions (1) compel speech by cable operators, (2) favor broadcast programmers over cable programmers, and (3) single out certain members of the press for disfavored treatment. None of these arguments suffices to require strict scrutiny in the present case. ***

First, unlike the access rules struck down in [*Tornillo*], the must-carry rules are content-neutral in application. They are not activated by any particular message spoken by cable operators and thus exact no content-based penalty. ***

Second, appellants do not suggest, nor do we think it the case, that must-carry will force cable operators to alter their own messages to respond to the broadcast programming they are required to carry. See Brenner, Cable Television and the Freedom of Expression, 1988 Duke L. J., at 379 ("Other than adding new ideas—offensive, insightful or tedious—the [speaker granted access to cable] does not influence an operator's agenda"). Given cable's long history of serving as a conduit for broadcast signals, there appears little risk that cable viewers would assume that the broadcast stations carried on a cable system convey ideas or messages endorsed by the cable operator.

Finally, the asserted analogy to *Tornillo* ignores an important technological difference between newspapers and cable television. Although a daily newspaper and a cable operator both may enjoy monopoly status in a given locale, the cable operator exercises far greater control over access to the relevant medium. A daily newspaper, no matter how secure its local monopoly, does not possess the power to obstruct readers' access to other competing publications—whether they be weekly local newspapers, or daily newspapers published in other cities.

The same is not true of cable. When an individual subscribes to cable, the physical connection between the television set and the cable network gives the cable operator bottleneck, or gatekeeper, control over most (if not all) of the television programming that is channeled into the subscriber's home. Hence, simply by virtue of its ownership of the essential pathway for cable speech, a cable operator can prevent its subscribers from obtaining access to programming it chooses to exclude. A cable operator, unlike speakers in other media, can thus silence the voice of competing speakers with a mere flick of the switch.[8]

The potential for abuse of this private power over a central avenue of communication cannot be overlooked. *** We thus reject appellants' contention that *Tornillo* and *Pacific Gas & Electric* require strict scrutiny of the access rules in question here. *** The must-carry provisions, as we have explained above, are justified by special characteristics of the cable medium: the bottleneck monopoly power exercised by cable operators and the dangers this power poses to the viability of broadcast television. ***

III (A)

[W]e agree with the District Court that the appropriate standard by which to evaluate the constitutionality of must-carry is the intermediate level of scrutiny applicable to content-neutral restrictions that impose an incidental burden on speech. See Ward v. Rock Against Racism, 491 U.S. 781 (1989); United States v. O'Brien, 391 U.S. 367 (1968).

---

8. As one commentator has observed: "The central dilemma of cable is that it has unlimited capacity to accommodate as much diversity and as many publishers as print, yet all of the producers and publishers use the same physical plant. *** If the cable system is itself a publisher, it may restrict the circumstances under which it allows others also to use its system." I. de Sola Pool, Technologies of Freedom 168 (1983).

Under *O'Brien*, a content-neutral regulation will be sustained if "it furthers an important or substantial governmental interest; if the governmental interest is unrelated to the suppression of free expression; and if the incidental restriction on alleged First Amendment freedoms is no greater than is essential to the furtherance of that interest."

To satisfy this standard, a regulation need not be the least speech-restrictive means of advancing the Government's interests. "Rather, the requirement of narrow tailoring is satisfied 'so long as the regulation promotes a substantial government interest that would be achieved less effectively absent the regulation.'" *Ward, supra*, at 799 (quoting United States v. Albertini, 472 U.S. 675, 689 (1985)). Narrow tailoring in this context requires, in other words, that the means chosen do not "burden substantially more speech than is necessary to further the government's legitimate interests."

Congress declared that the must-carry provisions serve three interrelated interests: (1) preserving the benefits of free, over-the-air local broadcast television, (2) promoting the widespread dissemination of information from a multiplicity of sources, and (3) promoting fair competition in the market for television programming. And viewed in the abstract, we have no difficulty concluding that each of them is an important governmental interest. ***

B

That the Government's asserted interests are important in the abstract does not mean, however, that the must-carry rules will in fact advance those interests. When the Government defends a regulation on speech as a means to redress past harms or prevent anticipated harms, it must do more than simply "posit the existence of the disease sought to be cured." Quincy Cable TV, Inc. v. FCC, 768 F. 2d 1434, 1455 (CADC 1985). ***

Thus, in applying *O'Brien* scrutiny we must ask first whether the Government has adequately shown that the economic health of local broadcasting is in genuine jeopardy and in need of the protections afforded by must-carry. Assuming an affirmative answer to the foregoing question, the Government still bears the burden of showing that the remedy it has adopted does not "burden substantially more speech than is necessary to further the government's legitimate interests." *Ward*, 491 U.S., at 799. On the state of the record developed thus far, and in the absence of findings of fact from the District Court, we are unable to conclude that the Government has satisfied either inquiry.

***

The paucity of evidence indicating that broadcast television is in jeopardy is not the only deficiency in this record. Also lacking are any findings concerning the actual effects of must-carry on the speech of cable operators and cable programmers—*i.e.*, the extent to which cable operators will, in fact, be forced to make changes in their current or anticipated programming selections; the degree to which cable programmers will be dropped from cable systems to make room for local broadcasters; and the extent to which cable operators can satisfy their must-carry obligations by devoting previously unused channel capacity to the carriage of local broadcasters. Finally, the record fails to provide any judicial findings concerning the availability and efficacy of "constitutionally acceptable less restrictive means" of achieving the Government's asserted interests. See Sable Communications, 492 U.S., at 129.

In sum, because there are genuine issues of material fact still to be resolved on this record, we hold that the District Court erred in granting summary judgment in favor of the Government. The judgment below is vacated, and the case is remanded for further proceedings consistent with this opinion.

JUSTICE BLACKMUN, concurring. [Omitted.]

JUSTICE STEVENS, concurring in part and concurring in the judgment. [Omitted]

JUSTICE O'CONNOR, with whom JUSTICE SCALIA and JUSTICE GINSBURG join, and with whom JUSTICE THOMAS joins as to Parts I and III, concurring in part and dissenting in part.

***

I

The 1992 Cable Act implicates the First Amendment rights of two classes of speakers. First, it tells cable operators which programmers they must carry, and keeps cable operators from carrying others that they might prefer. Though cable operators do not actually originate most of the programming they show, the Court correctly holds that they are, for First Amendment purposes, speakers. Selecting which speech to retransmit is, as we know from the example of publishing houses, movie theaters, bookstores, and Reader's Digest, no less communication than is creating the speech in the first place.

Second, the Act deprives a certain class of video programmers—those who operate cable channels rather than broadcast stations—of access to over one-third of an entire medium. Cable programmers may compete only for those channels that are not set aside by the must-carry provisions. A cable programmer that might otherwise have been carried may well be denied access in favor of a broadcaster that is less appealing to the viewers but is favored by the must-carry rules. It is as if the government ordered all movie theaters to reserve at least one-third of their screening for films made by American production companies, or required all bookstores to devote one- third of their shelf space to nonprofit publishers.

Under the First Amendment, it is normally not within the government's power to decide who may speak and who may not, at least on private property or in traditional public fora. ***

The controversial judgment at the heart of the statute is not that broadcast television has some value—obviously it does—but that broadcasters should be preferred over cable programmers. The best explanation for the findings, it seems to me, is that they represent Congress' reasons for adopting this preference; and, according to the findings, these reasons rest in part on the content of broadcasters' speech. To say in the face of the findings that the must-carry rules "impose burdens and confer benefits without reference to the content of speech," cannot be correct, especially in light of the care with which we must normally approach speaker-based restrictions.

The interest in localism, either in the dissemination of opinions held by the listeners' neighbors or in the reporting of events that have to do with the local community, cannot be described as "compelling" for the purposes of the compelling state interest test. It is a legitimate interest, perhaps even an important one—certainly the government can foster it by, for instance, providing subsidies from the public fisc —but it does not rise to the level necessary to justify content-based speech restrictions. It is for private speakers and listeners, not for the government, to decide what fraction of their news and entertainment ought to be of a local character and what fraction ought to be of a national (or international) one. And the same is true of the interest in diversity of viewpoints: While the government may subsidize speakers that it thinks provide novel points of view, it may not restrict other speakers on the theory that what they say is more conventional.

The interests in public affairs programming and educational programming seem somewhat weightier, though it is a difficult question whether they are compelling enough to justify restricting other sorts of speech. We have never held that the Government could impose educational content requirements on, say, newsstands, bookstores, or movie theaters; and it is not clear that such requirements would in any event appreciably further the goals of public education.

But even assuming arguendo that the Government could set some channels aside for educational or news programming, the Act is insufficiently tailored to this goal. To benefit the educational broadcasters, the Act burdens more than just the cable entertainment programmers. It equally burdens CNN, C-SPAN, the Discovery Channel, the New Inspirational Network, and other channels with as much claim as PBS to being educational or related to public affairs.

Finally, my conclusion that the must-carry rules are content based leads me to conclude that they are an impermissible restraint on the cable operators' editorial discretion as well as on the cable programmers' speech. For reasons related to the content of speech, the rules restrict the ability of cable operators to put on the programming they prefer, and require them to include programming they would rather avoid. This, it seems to me, puts this case squarely within the rule of Pacific Gas & Electric Co., 475 U.S., at 14-15 (plurality); see also Miami Herald Publishing Co. v. Tornillo, 418 U.S. 241, 257-258 (1974).

II

Even if I am mistaken about the must-carry provisions being content based, however, in my view they fail content-neutral scrutiny as well. Assuming arguendo that the provisions are justified with reference to the content-neutral interests in fair competition and preservation of free television, they nonetheless restrict too much speech that does not implicate these interests.

Sometimes, a cable system's choice to carry a cable programmer rather than a broadcaster may be motivated by anticompetitive impulses, or might lead to the broadcaster going out of business. That some speech within a broad category causes harm, however, does not justify restricting the whole category. If Congress wants to protect those stations that are in danger of going out of business, or bar cable operators from preferring programmers in which the operators have an ownership stake, it may do that. But it may not, in the course of advancing these interests, restrict cable operators and programmers in circumstances where neither of these interests is threatened. ***

III

Having said all this, it is important to acknowledge one basic fact: The question is not whether there will be control over who gets to speak over cable—the question is who will have this control. Under the FCC's view, the answer is Congress, acting within relatively broad limits. Under my view, the answer is the cable operator. Most of the time, the cable operator's decision will be largely dictated by the preferences of the viewers; but because many cable operators are indeed monopolists, the viewers' preferences will not always prevail. Our recognition that cable operators are speakers is bottomed in large part on the very fact that the cable operator has editorial discretion.

I have no doubt that there is danger in having a single cable operator decide what millions of subscribers can or cannot watch. And I have no doubt that Congress can act to relieve this danger. In other provisions of the Act, Congress has already taken steps to foster competition among cable systems. § 3(a), 47 U.S.C. § 543(a)(2) (1988 ed., Supp. IV). Congress can encourage the creation of new media, such as inexpensive satellite broadcasting, or fiber-optic networks with virtually unlimited channels, or even simple devices that would let people easily switch from cable to over-the-air broadcasting. And of course Congress can subsidize broadcasters that it thinks provide especially valuable programming.

Congress might also conceivably obligate cable operators to act as common carriers for some of their channels, with those channels being open to all through some sort of lottery system or timesharing arrangement. Setting aside any possible Takings Clause issues, it stands to reason that if Congress may demand that telephone companies operate as common carriers, it can ask the same of cable companies; such an approach would not suffer from the defect of preferring one speaker to another.

But the First Amendment as we understand it today rests on the premise that it is government power, rather than private power, that is the main threat to free expression; and as a consequence, the Amendment imposes substantial limitations on the Government even when it is trying to serve concededly praiseworthy goals. Perhaps Congress can to some extent restrict, even in a content-based manner, the speech of cable operators and cable programmers. But it must do so in compliance with the constitutional requirements, requirements that were not complied with here. Accordingly, I would reverse the judgment below.

JUSTICE GINSBURG, concurring in part and dissenting in part.

Substantially for the reasons stated by Circuit Judge Williams in his opinion dissenting from the three-judge District Court's judgment, 819 F.Supp. 32, 57 (DC 1993), I conclude that Congress' "must-carry" regime, which requires cable operators to set aside just over one-third of their channels for local broadcast stations, reflects an unwarranted content-based preference and hypothesizes a risk to local stations that remains imaginary. I therefore concur in Parts I, II-A, and II-B of the Court's opinion, and join JUSTICE O'CONNOR's opinion concurring in part and dissenting in part.

The "must-carry" rules Congress has ordered do not differentiate on the basis of "viewpoint," and therefore do not fall in the category of speech regulation that Government must avoid most assiduously. *** The rules, however, do reflect a content preference, and on that account demand close scrutiny.

***

As Circuit Judge Williams stated: "Congress rested its decision to promote [local broadcast] stations in part, but quite explicitly, on a finding about their content —that they were 'an important source of local news and public affairs programming and other local broadcast services critical to an informed electorate.'" 819 F. Supp., at 58, quoting 1992 Cable Act, § 2(a)(11). Moreover, as Judge Williams persuasively explained, "[the] facts do not support an inference that over-the-air TV is at risk," 819 F. Supp., at 63, see *id.*, at 62-65; "[w]hatever risk there may be in the abstract has completely failed to materialize." *Id.*, at 63. "The paucity of evidence indicating that broadcast television is in jeopardy," if it persists on remand, should impel an ultimate judgment for the petitioners.

NOTES AND QUESTIONS ON *TURNER*

1. Note that the Court rejected the comparison with *Miami Herald*, even while agreeing that the rationale of *Red Lion* could not be used to justify the (local over-the-air, and local "nonprofit" broadcaster) mandated must-carry requirements imposed by the Act on cable companies. Why did the comparison with the *Miami Herald* fail to persuade the Court?

2. The majority describes the first amendment "test" it applies as one of "intermediate scrutiny." More exactly, what are the elements of that standard of review? Note the majority says it is the standard provided by the *O'Brien* case. Then, again, note the majority also quotes from the "time, place, and manner" test of *Ward*, suggesting that this, too, is a proper statement of the "intermediate scrutiny" standard of

First Amendment review as well.[110] Finally, if the majority of the Court regards the *Ward* standard essentially the same as the *O'Brien* standard (despite their different articulated parts), with both now being merged into some sort of more general purpose "intermediate scrutiny" first amendment standard of judicial review, how will one know when this standard (rather than some more stringent standard) is to be applied? What are its essential components, and how protective or unprotective do they seem to be?

3. One (of the two) significant legitimate interests served by the must-carry rules imposed by Congress the Court accepted as sufficient to warrant the requirement of a minimum number of channels set aside for certain broadcasters,[111] was the expressed concern by Congress for the maintenance of "free" television reception. But if the manufacturers of television sets were required (as they might readily be required by Congress) to include as part of each set a simple switch readily enabling set owners to switch off cable (and thereby at once resume whatever over-the-air reception they had the capacity to receive before subscribing to cable), so there would be no "prejudice" to over-the-air broadcasters merely because many or most set owners subscribed to cable, wouldn't that have been a vastly less restrictive means of proceeding under the circumstances?[112] If, notwithstanding such switches, cable subscribers simply no longer find it useful or interesting to "switch out" to over-the-air stations (perhaps because they don't find the content of the programs as interesting), how is that any different than when the same thing happens in other areas of technology, competition, and free speech?[113]

---

110. But was *O'Brien* not concerned exclusively with statutes on their face having nothing to do with speech as such? Here, in contrast, the government directive is directed expressly to speech as such (i.e. what—or whose—speech must be carried whether the defendant wants to present it or not). Does the Court's use of the *O'Brien* test in *Turner* indicate that the test (one of the weaker tests we have seen) is not now confined to the narrower category of cases of the special sort in which it first appeared? And the actual wording of the "time, place, and manner" standard from *Ward* is not the same as actual wording of the *O'Brien* test, is it? Moreover, was it not an express limitation of the *Ward* standard (itself not a very demanding standard) that it applies only to general restrictions of "time, place, or manner" and not to content? And is not content (namely, that x amount of local broadcast fare and y amount of nonprofit broadcast fare must be carried) the direct object of the Act? How did the majority reconcile this difficulty?

111. The other being of an antitrust or unfair competitive practice rationale. (Is this one sufficient to warrant the kind of directive written by Congress?)

112. Note that earlier in the development of new markets for previously unused (UHF) television frequencies, this is essentially the approach that was used: to require television set manufacturers to build in a capacity for UHF reception (to provide an incentive for broadcast companies to seek UHF, and not merely VHF, frequency licenses).

113. E.G., when the new availability of the New York Times on a same-day basis in Durham, North Carolina, as in New York itself comes to be so commonplace such that enough Durham subscribers drop the Durham Sun to put it into bankruptcy, not because they dislike the Sun but simply because they are better satisfied with the Times and no longer care to pay the same degree of attention as they once did to the Sun, no doubt many may believe that Durham has lost an "important" voice (the

---

SUBSEQUENT REVIEW OF *TURNER BROADCASTING*

In Turner Broadcasting System, Inc. v. Federal Communications Comm'n, 520 U.S. 180 (1997), in a virtual replay of Turner Broadcasting v. FCC, 512 U.S. 622 (1994), the Cable Act's "must-carry" rules were sustained. Essentially, there was no change within the Court in *Turner II*, following the proceedings on remand; Justice Breyer provides the fifth vote for the vote previously provided by Justice Blackmun, for the same majority in *Turner I*. And in *Turner II*, Justice Kennedy again wrote the majority Opinion, and Justice O'Connor wrote the dissent. Nor did the substantive position on either side significantly change.

Just as in *Turner I*, Turner Broadcasting complained that its first amendment's rights of editorial control, content selection, and selection of program array, were unconstitutionally abridged by the must-carry provisions of the Cable Act. Once again, however, the majority rejected the comparison of a cable television company with a newspaper, and reviewed the case under the far less exacting "*O'Brien* intermediate scrutiny test" (set out in *United States v. O'Brien*, 391 U.S. 367 (1968)). Once again the majority concluded that the must-carry rules were "content neutral"; that they were reasonably regarded by Congress as necessary to "advance important government interests unrelated to the suppression of free speech" (specifically, protection of free, over-the-air local broadcasting, of assuring a multiplicity of program sources, and promoting fair competition for television programming); and that they did "not burden substantially more speech than necessary" to serve these valid government interests.

And, as in *Turner I*, the dissent disagreed at virtually every step. It rejected the application of the *O'Brien* test as inappropriate.[114] Moreover, the dissent could find no sufficient justification for requiring free, enhanced cable carriage of local over-the-air broadcasters in lieu of displaced remote sources, whether as an anti-trust measure, or otherwise, especially given the availability of less editorially-intrusive measures available to Congress (e.g., subsidies), to preserve such local, over-the-air broadcasters it might deem sufficiently important so to assist.

Such clarification as *Turner II* provides over the major doctrinal differences as previously ventilated in *Turner I*, lies principally in the majority's new statement that "[t]he question is not whether Congress, as an objective matter, was correct to determine must-carry is necessary to prevent a substantial number of broadcast stations from losing cable carriage and suffering financial hardship, [but merely] whether the legislative conclusion was reasonable and supported by substantial evidence in the record before Congress." In brief, considerable deference to Congress's views, re-

---

Sun). Could Congress on that account restrict the New York Times in some way (to save the Sun)? In what way?

114. Rather, the dissent insisted that the must-carry rules were not "content neutral" and accordingly were subject to more rigorous review).

specting the need for legislation of this sort, appears in *Turner II.* Likewise, in sustaining the act imposing the must-carry rules, the majority reiterated that it was not necessary for the government to establish that no less restrictive provisions applicable to cable television companies would suffice. Again, however, as in *Turner I*, the dissent substantially disagreed and also concluded that there was no sufficient evidence in the record establishing the must-carry obligations (including free carriage) as demonstrably "narrowly tailored" to meeting any real problems allegedly meant to be addressed by the rules. Overall, however, the disagreement is pretty much the same as in *Turner I.* The principal effect of the case is largely just to lift the uncertainty as to whether the original decision would hold, despite the serious shortcomings it was thought to contain.

In the meantime, while *Turner* was on remand to the district court, a related set of questions was examined in the Supreme Court in respect to cable companies and editorial control over program content. The issue involved in these newer cases was not whether cablevision companies had been unconstitutionally restricted by the requirement that they carry certain other parties' programs against their will and carry them wholly unedited. Instead, it was whether in changing its mind, in *permitting* cable companies to *refuse* to carry certain material (even on the must-carry channels), Congress acted to abridge freedom of speech—*not* that of the cable company, rather, the freedom of speech of those the cable company was previously required to carry unedited.

So, here, suddenly, was seemingly a virtual reverse twist to the cablevision must-carry debate. When Congress merely "gives back" to cable companies *some* portion of such control as they would have had more completely if Congress had simply left them alone in the first place (i.e. had it never subjected them to any must-carry rules), and a cable company merely acts within the limits of the granted-back authority, wherein can one find grounds to frame a suitable first amendment complaint?

To be sure, anyone whose program the cable company is now permitted to turn away (and *does* turn away) may feel badly treated by the cable company. But so much as this would be true were there no must-carry rules at all.[115] Even assuming the must-carry rules are not themselves an unconstitutional interference by Congress with the first amendment rights of cable companies as "publishers," to what extent would mere forbearance by Congress from requiring cable companies to carry certain

---

115. Note that in respect to all of its programming except that which is subject to the must-carry rules, cable companies have all along been free generally to decide what to carry or not. (Generally, a cable company is no more obliged to permit programs it disdains to carry any more than the Miami Herald need publish stories it disdains to publish, however "unfair" someone considers its policy to be.)

types of programs (e.g., "indecent" programs)[116] present a first amendment basis for complaint? Consider the following case.

DENVER AREA EDUCATIONAL TELECOMMUNICATIONS CONSORTIUM V. FEDERAL COMMUNICATIONS COMMISSION

518 U.S. 727 (1996)

JUSTICE BREYER announced the judgment of the Court and delivered the opinion of the Court.

These cases present First Amendment challenges to three statutory provisions that seek to regulate the broadcasting of "patently offensive" sex-related material on cable television. ***

I

Certain special channels here at issue, called "leased channels" and "public, educational, or governmental channels," carry programs provided by those to whom the law gives special cable system access rights.

A "leased channel" is a channel that federal law requires a cable system operator to reserve for commercial lease by unaffiliated third parties. About 10 to 15 percent of a cable system's channels would typically fall into this category. "[P]ublic, educational, or governmental channels" (which we shall call "public access" channels) are channels that, over the years, local governments have required cable system operators to set aside for public, educational, or governmental purposes as part of the consideration an operator gives in return for permission to install cables under city streets and to use public rights-of-way. Between 1984 and 1992 federal law prohibited cable system operators from exercising any editorial control over the content of any program broadcast over either leased or public access channels.

In 1992, in an effort to control sexually explicit programming conveyed over access channels, Congress enacted the three provisions before us. The federal law before us (the statute as implemented through regulations) now permits cable operators either to allow or to forbid the transmission of "patently offensive" sex-related materials over both leased and public access channels, and requires those operators, at a minimum, to segregate and to block transmission of that same material on leased channels.

Petitioners, claiming that the three statutory provisions, as implemented by the Commission regulations, violate the First Amendment, sought judicial review. ***

---

116. What if the *only* programs Congress permitted cable companies to refuse to carry (over its must-carry channels) were programs "denigrative of others," or programs "the cable company deems morally objectionable"? (May there be a problem when the "giving back" of the cable company's "editorial discretion" is limited or partial, rather than in whole?)

II

We turn initially to the provision that permits cable system operators to prohibit "patently offensive" (or "indecent") programming transmitted over leased access channels. *** [T]he problem Congress addressed here is remarkably similar to the problem addressed by the FCC in *Pacifica* [438 U.S. 726], and the balance Congress struck is commensurate with the balance we approved there. In *Pacifica* this Court considered a governmental ban of a radio broadcast of "indecent" materials, defined in part, like the provisions before us, to include

> language that describes, in terms patently offensive as measured by contemporary community standards for the broadcast medium, sexual or excretory activities and organs, at times of the day when there is a reasonable risk that children may be in the audience.'"

The Court found this ban constitutionally permissible primarily because "broadcasting is uniquely accessible to children" and children were likely listeners to the program there at issue—an afternoon radio broadcast. Cable television broadcasting, including access channel broadcasting, is as "accessible to children" as over- the-air broadcasting, if not more so. Cable television systems, including access channels, "have established a uniquely pervasive presence in the lives of all Americans." *Pacifica*, [438 U.S.] at 748. ***

[T]he permissive nature of § 10(a) means that it likely restricts speech less than, not more than, the ban at issue in *Pacifica*. The provision removes a restriction as to some speakers—namely, cable operators. Moreover, although the provision does create a risk that a program will not appear, that risk is not the same as the certainty that accompanies a governmental ban. In fact, a glance at the programming that cable operators allow on their own (nonaccess) channels suggests that this distinction is not theoretical, but real. Finally, the provision's permissive nature brings with it a flexibility that allows cable operators, for example, not to ban broadcasts, but, say, to rearrange broadcast times, better to fit the desires of adult audiences while lessening the risks of harm to children.

The existence of this complex balance of interests persuades us that the permissive nature of the provision, coupled with its viewpoint-neutral application, is a constitutionally permissible way to protect children from the type of sexual material that concerned Congress, while accommodating both the First Amendment interests served by the access requirements and those served in restoring to cable operators a degree of the editorial control that Congress removed in 1984.

III

The statute's second provision significantly differs from the first. [T]his provision and its implementing regulations require cable system operators to place "patently offensive" leased channel programming on a separate channel; to block that channel; to unblock the channel within 30 days of a subscriber's written request for access; and to reblock the channel within 30 days of a subscriber's request for re-blocking. Also, leased channel programmers must notify cable operators of an intended "patently offensive" broadcast up to 30 days before its scheduled broadcast date.

These restrictions will prevent programmers from broadcasting to viewers who select programs day by day (or, through "surfing," minute by minute); to viewers who would like occasionally to watch a few, but not many, of the programs on the "patently offensive" channel; and to viewers who simply tend to judge a program's value through channel reputation, i.e., by the company it keeps. Moreover, the "written notice" requirement will further restrict viewing by subscribers who fear for their reputations should the operator, advertently or inadvertently, disclose the list of those who wish to watch the "patently offensive" channel. Cf. Lamont v. Postmaster General, 381 U.S. 301, 307 (1965) (finding unconstitutional a requirement that recipients of Communist literature notify the Post Office that they wish to receive it). Further, the added costs and burdens that these requirements impose upon a cable system operator may encourage that operator to ban programming that the operator would otherwise permit to run, even if only late at night.

We agree with the Government that protection of children is a "compelling interest." But we do not agree that the "segregate and block" requirements properly accommodate the speech restrictions they impose and the legitimate objective they seek to attain.

Several circumstances lead us to this conclusion. For one thing, the law, as recently amended, uses other means to protect children from similar "patently offensive" material broadcast on unleased cable channels, i.e., broadcast over any of a system's numerous ordinary, or public access, channels. The law, as recently amended, requires cable operators to "scramble or block" such programming on any (unleased) channel "primarily dedicated to sexually-oriented programming." In addition, cable operators must honor a subscriber's request to block any, or all, programs on any channel to which he or she does not wish to subscribe. And manufacturers, in the future, will have to make television sets with a so-called "V-chip"—a device that will be able automatically to identify and block sexually explicit or violent programs.

Although we cannot, and do not, decide whether the new provisions are themselves lawful (a matter not before us), we note that they are significantly less restrictive than the provision here at issue. They do not force the viewer to receive (for days or weeks at a time) all "patently offensive" programming or none; they will not lead the viewer automatically to judge the few by the reputation of the many; and they will not automatically place the occasional viewer's name on a special list. They therefore inevitably lead us to ask why, if they adequately protect children from "patently offensive" material broadcast on ordinary channels, they would not offer adequate protection from similar leased channel broadcasts as well?

The record does not answer these questions. It does not explain why a simple subscriber blocking request system, perhaps a phone-call based system, would adequately protect children from "patently offensive" material broadcast on ordinary non-sex-dedicated channels (i.e., almost all channels) but a far more restrictive segregate/block/written-access system is needed to protect children from similar broadcasts on what (in the absence of the segregation requirement) would be non-sex-dedicated channels that are leased.

The record's description and discussion of a different alternative—the "lockbox"—leads, through a different route, to a similar conclusion. The Cable Communications Policy Act of 1984 required cable operators to provide "upon the request of a subscriber, a device by which the subscriber can prohibit viewing of a particular cable service during periods selected by the subscriber." 47 U.S.C. § 544(d)(2). This device—the "lockbox"—would help protect children by permitting their parents to "lock out" those programs or channels that they did not want their children to see. ***

Consequently, we cannot find that the "segregate and block" restrictions on speech are a narrowly, or reasonably, tailored effort to protect children. Rather, they are overly restrictive, "sacrific[ing]" important First Amendment interests for too "speculative a gain."***

IV

The statute's third provision, as implemented by FCC regulation, is similar to its first provision, in that it too *permits* a cable operator to prevent transmission of "patently offensive" programming, in this case on public access channels. But there are important differences.

The first is the historical background. As JUSTICE KENNEDY points out, cable operators have traditionally agreed to reserve channel capacity for public, governmental, and educational channels as part of the consideration they give municipalities that award them cable franchises. Significantly, these are channels over which cable operators have not historically exercised editorial control. Unlike § 10(a) therefore, § 10(c) does not restore to cable operators editorial rights that they once had, and the countervailing First Amendment interest is nonexistent, or at least much diminished.

The second difference is the institutional background that has developed as a result of the historical difference. Public access channels are normally subject to complex supervisory systems of various sorts, often with both public and private elements. This system of public, private, and mixed nonprofit elements, through its supervising boards and nonprofit or governmental access managers, can set programming policy and approve or disapprove particular programming services. *** Whether these locally accountable bodies prescreen programming, promulgate rules for the use of public access channels, or are merely available to respond when problems arise, the upshot is the same: there is a locally accountable body capable of addressing the problem, should it arise, of patently offensive programming broadcast to children, making it unlikely that many children will in fact be exposed to programming considered patently offensive in that community. [W]e conclude that the Government cannot sustain its burden of showing that § 10(c) is necessary to protect children or that it is appropriately tailored to secure that end. Consequently, we find that this third provision violates the First Amendment. ***

[Concurring opinions by STEVENS and SOUTER, JJ., Omitted.]

JUSTICE O'CONNOR, concurring in part and dissenting in part. ***

The distinctions upon which the Court relies in deciding that § 10(c) must fall while § 10(a) survives are not, in my view, constitutionally significant. *** The interest in protecting children remains the same, whether on a leased access channel or a public access channel, and allowing the cable operator the option of prohibiting the transmission of indecent speech seems a constitutionally permissible means of addressing that interest. Nor is the fact that public access programming may be subject to supervisory systems in addition to the cable operator, sufficient in my mind to render § 10(c) so ill-tailored to its goal as to be unconstitutional.

JUSTICE KENNEDY, with whom JUSTICE GINSBURG joins, concurring in part, concurring in the judgment in part, and dissenting in part. ***

Sections 10(a) and (c) are unusual. They do not require direct action against speech, but do authorize a cable operator to deny the use of its property to certain forms of speech. As a general matter, a private person may exclude certain speakers from his or her property without violating the First Amendment, Hudgens v. NLRB, 424 U.S. 507 (1976), and if §§ 10(a) and (c) were no more than affirmations of this principle they might be unremarkable. Access channels, however, are property of the cable operator dedicated or otherwise reserved for programming of other speakers or the government. A public access channel is a public forum, and laws requiring leased access channels create common carrier obligations. When the government identifies certain speech on the basis of its content as vulnerable to exclusion from a common carrier or public forum, strict scrutiny applies. These laws cannot survive this exacting review. However compelling Congress' interest in shielding children from indecent programming, the provisions in this case are not drawn with enough care to withstand scrutiny under our precedents. *** The straightforward issue here is whether the Government can deprive certain speakers, on the basis of the content of their speech, of protections afforded all others. There is no reason to discard our existing First Amendment jurisprudence in answering this question.

Laws removing common-carriage protection from a single form of speech based on its content should be reviewed under the same standard as content-based restrictions on speech in a public forum. Making a cable operator a common carrier does not create a public forum in the sense of taking property from private control and dedicating it to public use; rather, regulations of a common carrier dictate the manner in which private control is exercised. A common-carriage mandate, nonetheless, serves the same function as a public forum. It ensures open, nondiscriminatory access to the means of communication.

The provisions here are content-based discriminations in the strong sense of suppressing a certain form of expression that the Government dislikes, or otherwise wishes to exclude on account of its effects, and there is no justification for anything but strict scrutiny here. ***

[The] concerns [for children] are weighty and will be relevant to whether the law passes strict scrutiny. They do not justify, however, a blanket rule of lesser protection for indecent speech. [T]o the extent cable operators prohibit indecent programming on access channels, not only children but adults will be deprived of it. The Government may not "reduce the adult population to [viewing] only what is fit for children." When applying strict scrutiny, we will not assume plausible alternatives will fail to protect compelling interests; there must be some basis in the record, in legislative findings or otherwise, establishing the law enacted as the least restrictive means. *** I dissent from the judgment of the Court insofar as it upholds the constitutionality of § 10(a).

JUSTICE THOMAS, joined by the CHIEF JUSTICE and JUSTICE SCALIA, concurring in the judgment in part and dissenting in part.

I agree with the plurality's conclusion that § 10(a) is constitutionally permissible, but I disagree with its conclusion that §§ 10(b) and (c) violate the First Amendment.

The text of the First Amendment makes no distinction between print, broadcast, and cable media, but we have done so. In Red Lion Broadcasting Co. v. FCC, 395 U.S. 367 (1969), we held that, in light of the scarcity of broadcasting frequencies, the Government may require a broadcast licensee "to share his frequency with others and to conduct himself as a proxy or fiduciary with obligations to present those views and voices which are representative of his community and which would otherwise, by necessity, be barred from the airwaves." ***

In contrast, we have not permitted that level of government interference in the context of the print media. In Miami Herald Publishing Co. v. Tornillo, 418 U.S. 241 (1974), for instance, we invalidated a Florida statute that required newspapers to allow, free of charge, a right of reply to political candidates whose personal or professional character the paper assailed. ***

Our First Amendment distinctions between media, dubious from their infancy, placed cable in a doctrinal wasteland in which regulators and cable operators alike could not be sure whether cable was entitled to the substantial First Amendment protections afforded the print media or was subject to the more onerous obligations shouldered by the broadcast media. Over time, however, we have drawn closer to recognizing that cable operators should enjoy the same First Amendment rights as the nonbroadcast media.

We implicitly recognized in *Turner* that the programmer's right to compete for channel space is derivative of, and subordinate to, the operator's editorial discretion. Like a free-lance writer seeking a paper in which to publish newspaper editorials, a programmer is protected in searching for an outlet for cable programming, but has no free-standing First Amendment right to have that programming transmitted. Likewise, the rights of would-be viewers are derivative of the speech rights of operators and programmers. *** By recognizing the general primacy of the cable operator's editorial rights over the rights of programmers and viewers, *Turner* raises serious questions about the merits of petitioners' claims. None of the petitioners in these cases are cable operators; they are all cable viewers or access programmers or their representative organizations. ***

Because the access provisions are part of a scheme that restricts the free speech rights of cable operators, and expands the speaking opportunities of access programmers, who have no underlying constitutional right to speak through the cable medium, I do not believe that access programmers can challenge the scheme, or a particular part of it, as an abridgment of their "freedom of speech."

The permissive nature of §§ 10(a) and (c) is important in this regard. If Congress had forbidden cable operators to carry indecent programming on leased and public access channels, that law would have burdened the programmer's right, recognized in *Turner*, to compete for space on an operator's system. The Court would undoubtedly strictly scrutinize such a law. But §§ 10(a) and (c) do not burden a programmer's right to seek access for its indecent programming on an operator's system. Rather, they merely restore part of the editorial discretion an operator would have absent government regulation without burdening the programmer's underlying speech rights. ***

Unlike §§ 10(a) and (c), § 10(b) clearly implicates petitioners' free speech rights. Though § 10(b) by no means bans indecent speech, it clearly places content-based restrictions on the transmission of private speech by requiring cable operators to block and segregate indecent programming that the operator has agreed to carry. Consequently, § 10(b) must be subjected to strict scrutiny and can be upheld only if it furthers a compelling governmental interest by the least restrictive means available. ***

The Court strikes down § 10(b) by pointing to alternatives, such as reverse-blocking and lockboxes, that it says are less restrictive than segregation and blocking. Though these methods attempt to place in parents' hands the ability to permit their children to watch as little, or as much, indecent programming as the parents think proper, they do not effectively support parents' authority to direct the moral upbringing of their children. *** Rather than being able to simply block out certain channels at certain times, a subscriber armed with only a lockbox must carefully monitor all leased-access programming and constantly reprogram the lockbox to keep out undesired programming. Thus, even assuming that cable subscribers generally have the technical proficiency to properly operate a lockbox, by no means a given, this distinguishing characteristic of leased access channels makes lockboxes and reverse-blocking largely ineffective.

The FCC regulation requires only that the cable operator receive written consent. Other statutory provisions make clear that the cable operator may not share that, or any other, information with any other person, including the Government. *** The United States has carried its burden of demonstrating that § 10(b) and its implementing regulations are narrowly tailored to satisfy a compelling governmental interest. Accordingly, I would affirm the judgment of the Court of Appeals in its entirety. ***

QUESTIONS AND PROBLEMS

1. Note how sharply five members of the Court divided in defining the threshold first amendment issues—i.e. how to characterize the case for purposes of determining *which* first amendment test to apply. Two justices (Kennedy and Ginsburg) contended that all three sections of the 1992 Act were subject to "strict scrutiny," and that all three sections failed that test. What made "strict scrutiny" appropriate in their view? Did they have the matter right?)[117] By way of contrast, three others (Thomas, Scalia, and Rehnquist) voted to sustain all three sections, but only after concluding that the first amendment *barely* applied to sections 10(a) and 10(c). (On what basis did they so thoroughly disagree as to the proper way to view the case?)[118]

In contrast, none of the remaining justices agreed with *either* of the sharply differing models offered by their colleagues. But neither did they offer an alternative description, one providing a better fit (in their view). Indeed, the plurality opinion authored by Justice Breyer expressly disavowed any intent (on the part of the plurality) to be bound by *any* particular analogy—e.g., the broadcast model from *Red Lion*, the private publisher model from *Miami Herald*, the public forum or limited

---

117. With respect to § 10(a) of the Act, which applied to "leased access channels," and with respect to the "common carrier" model—suppose an Act of Congress designated certain kinds of major interstate freight haulers (railroads) as common carriers, then forbade them to reject any safely packaged and lawful goods, but permitted them to refuse to carry materials "unsuitable for minors." Why might this be unconstitutional? (Note that seven of the justices voted to sustain § 10(a) of the Act involved in *Denver Area*. Is there any reason to think some of them might not sustain this variation?)

118. The dissent relied heavily on the "editorial discretion" of the cable operator. The New York Times, of course, may decline to publish what it does not regard as "fit to print." Can a cable television company appropriately be compared with the New York Times? Why or why not?

The concurring/dissenting opinion by Kennedy and Ginsburg distinguished leased access channels and public access channels from conventional privately owned property, even while otherwise agreeing that, "[a]s a general matter, a private person *may* exclude certain speakers from his or her property without violating the first amendment," citing Hudgens v. NLRB, 424 U.S. 507 (1976) (emphasis added). Further consideration of the extent to which "private property" may be subject (or not subject) to third party first amendment claims of access and speech-use is provided *infra*, ch. III, § 9, pp. 528-548 ("The Blurred Boundary Between Private and Public Property"). The *Hudgens* case is included as a principal case (casebook at pp. 533-537).

public forum model, or the common carrier model.[119] Granted that they may have had good reason to be wary of appropriating pre-existing "models," still—how would you describe the method of first amendment review as explained and applied by them?[120]

2. To move beyond cable television, suppose restrictions were imposed by Congress on users of the Internet, and on owners of certain Internet service providers, to forbid the knowing transmission of sexually-explicit, indecent, patently offensive material (as defined by the statute in *Denver Area* or as defined in the FCC regulation in *Pacifica*)[121] over networks readily accessed by minors.[122]

---

8. The First Amendment as a "Freedom of Information Act"

Introductory Note

In 1964, a few months after its newsworthy decision in *New York Times Co. v. Sullivan*,[1] the Supreme Court decided a different case that drew far less notice in the press. This less noticed case, *Aptheker v. United States*,[2] reviewed the government's revocation of passports of two members of the Communist Party, Herbert Aptheker and Elizabeth Gurley Flynn. Elizabeth Flynn was quite well known as National Chairman of the Communist Party of the United States. Herbert Aptheker was a well known Marxist, also a "top-ranking leader" of the Communist Party, as well as editor of *Political Affairs*, the "theoretical organ" of the Party. Their passports had been re-

---

119. Rather, Justice Breyer demurred to what he described as a premature undertaking to force descriptions of new technologies into one or another pre-existing model for purposes of first amendment review.

120. Note the observation in the plurality opinion by Justice Breyer that sections 10(a) and (c) are "viewpoint neutral" (even if not "content neutral")—a matter obviously critical for Justice Breyer's vote to sustain even § 10(a) (which six of the other eight also voted to uphold). *Is* it altogether "viewpoint neutral"? No doubt it is, in comparison with the type of ordinance held invalid in the *Hudnut* case (sexually explicit material depicting women in positive ways permitted, sexually explicit material depicting women as "subordinate" or as "objects" forbidden) (see casebook at pp. 222-228) But is it "viewpoint neutral" in a larger sense? May not one's choice of words (four-letter or otherwise) capture and offer "viewpoints" very distinctive from depictions or descriptions composed from an abridged dictionary? If one is equally forbidden to use four-letter expletives whether to praise the draft or to condemn the draft, is "viewpoint neutrality" preserved—or, rather, are certain "viewpoints" thereby banished on *both* sides, as it were, by stripping out certain features of expression (and thus also certain competing perspectives) as well? Cf. Cohen v. California, 403 U.S. 15 (1971) (Harlan, J.) (casebook at pp. 134-136).

121. FCC v. Pacifica Found., 438 U.S. 726 (1978) (reviewed in the principal opinion in *Denver Area*, and see also casebook at p. 482, n.99).

122. For a first response to the problem, see Reno v. ACLU, 520 U.S. 1113, (1997), this casebook at p. 46 *infra*.

1. 376 U.S. 254 (1964). See *supra* p. 190.

2. 378 U.S. 500 (1964).

voked pursuant to § 6 of the Subversive Activities Control Act of 1950.[3] This section of the Act expressly prohibited the issuance of passports to persons holding membership in an organization under final order to register with the Subversive Activities Control Board. Neither Aptheker or Flynn contested the registration order outstanding against the Party. The Communist Party had already presented such a challenge, and it had failed.[4] Even so, Aptheker and Flynn did challenge the passport control section of the Act, § 6.

Their basic attack on this section of the Subversive Activities Control Act was not grounded in the first amendment (the free speech and free press clause) but on a fifth amendment, substantive due process liberty, "right to travel," claim. Even if, despite the first amendment, the Communist Party (of which they were ranking members) could be compelled to register as a Communist-action organization, as the Court had held, Aptheker contended that Congress could not also act to deny a passport to a person who belonged to that Party simply from some vague apprehension of how, or to what end, that passport might be used by such a person while abroad. To be sure, denial of a passport did not make it unlawful *per se* for them to leave the country or to return. Nevertheless, because of its obvious importance as a travel document to anyone seeking to go abroad, its deprivation was effectively an infringement of their constitutional right to travel—or so Aptheker alleged.[5]

Without deciding that either Flynn or Aptheker could not be denied a passport individually, the Court effectively held in their favor by holding § 6 of the Subversive Activities Control Act *void on its face*. As the Court observed, the Act would apply even to mere passive members of the Communist Party, none of whom, while outside the country, would necessarily present any real risk of activities likely to compromise any legitimate security or foreign relations interests of the United States. Denying *all* such persons passports, "without regard to their knowledge [or lack thereof] concerning the organization, [their] degree of activity, commitment to its purpose, or likelihood that travel by such a person would be attended by the type of activity which Congress sought to control,"[6] was clearly unwarranted. Without deciding whether a more narrowly drafted statute would be constitutional (i.e. one

3. 64 Stat. 993, 50 U.S.C §782 (since expired and not renewed).

4. Communist Party of the United States v. Subversive Activities Control Board, 367 U.S. 1 (1961) (rejecting argument that the registration and disclosure requirements infringed first amendment rights and denied due process of law).

5. Specifically, Aptheker stated that he wished to travel to Europe and elsewhere, partly "for study [and] to observe social, political and economic conditions abroad, and thereafter to write, publish, teach and lecture in this country about [his] observations." 378 U.S. at 511-12 n.10. Without a passport, however, he was unlikely to be admitted into the countries he wanted to visit. Effectively, then, confiscation of his passport was the same as denying his right to travel abroad, a right the Court had already said was an aspect of personal liberty of any American citizen subject only to reasonable limits as Congress might provide pursuant to its powers in respect to foreign commerce, national security and defense, and foreign relations. See Kent v. Dulles, 357 U.S. 116 (1958).

6. 378 U.S. at 510.

applicable only to persons who, like Flynn and Aptheker, might hold high ranking Party positions),[7] the Court struck the act down as void on its face

Despite how inconclusive the case was in some respects, the *Aptheker* decision was quite significant at the time. For one thing, it did establish a "right to travel" as a right implicitly protected by the (substantive) due process clause of the fifth amendment. For another, the Court also treated that right as "fundamental," and as therefore subject to special standards of judicial review ("strict scrutiny review"). Moreover— and this was a real surprise—it also appeared to say that laws restricting the right to travel more broadly than the government could adequately justify would be subject to attack as void on their face.

This last proposition was a most surprising development because, until now, recourse to "void on its face" attacks on statutes had been allowed almost exclusively only in first amendment cases. Since *Aptheker* was not treated as a first amendment case (rather, as a right to travel case), the manner in which the Court had presumed to decide the case seemed at odds with its usual refusal to consider a statute other than as applied to the facts in each case. The oddity drew a sharp dissent.[8]

In the dissent's view, even as the majority itself had acknowledged, there was no suggestion in this case that either Aptheker or Flynn fell within the margin of mere passive or mere casual Communist Party membership. Since that was so, there was no reason to relieve them of the Act if it could *validly* apply to them, regardless of its fate as applied to others. As the dissent noted, in reference to such others, "[N]o such party is here and no such claim is asserted. It will be soon enough to test this situation when it comes here."[9] They admonished the other justices that this was not a first amendment case. Absent such a case, they noted, the Court's doctrines strictly confined parties to challenging the constitutionality of statutes as applied to themselves, and not to hythothetical third parties.[10]

In fact, however, although *Aptheker* was decided on fifth amendment grounds, the majority had acknowledged that it also did raise first amendment issues.

---

7. From what was said in the case, moreover it appeared quite likely the narrower act would be sustained. For subsequent, related, fifth amendment cases, see Zemel v. Rusk, 381 U.S. 1 (1965), and Regan v. Wald, 468 U.S. 222 (1984) (both sustaining passport area restrictions on travel to Cuba); Haig v. Agee, 453 U.S. 280 (1981) (sustaining passport revocation of former CIA operative disclosing CIA intelligence operations while abroad).

8. The Court divided, six to three, Warren, C.J., and Justices Black, Douglas, Brennan, and Stewart joining the opinion of the Court by Justice Goldberg, Justices Harlan and White joining a dissent by Justice Clark.

9. Id. at 525 (Clark, J.,dissenting).

10. The most often cited case for this view is United States v. Raines, 362 U.S. 17, 21 (1960) (reviewing the Court's jurisdictional doctrines on standing and *ius tertii*–the inability of a litigant to invoke the hypothetical claim of someone not before the court as a basis for objecting to its application to himself–and holding: "[O]ne to whom application of a statute is constitutional will not be heard to attack the statute on the ground that impliedly it might also be taken as applying to other persons or other situations in which its application might be unconstitutional").

Aptheker had declared his interest in visiting several countries in Europe to see for himself whether conditions in those countries matched up with other people's impressions. He had also said that he would use what he learned to inform himself and others when he returned.[11] To the extent that he would be foreclosed from information bearing on the integrity of American foreign or domestic policy, were he not permitted to travel, perhaps his complaint could be seen as raising a serious first amendment issue after all. An overly broad access restriction may result in an imposed ignorance as readily as in an overly broad restriction on speech itself. James Madison, the principal author of the first amendment, had himself suggested the basic point:

> A popular Government, without popular information, or the means of acquiring it, is but a Prologue to a Farce or a Tragedy; or, perhaps both. Knowledge will forever govern ignorance: And a people who mean to be their own Governors, must arm themselves with the power which knowledge gives.[12]

"The means of acquiring" information is a kind of first amendment right in this view. If so, perhaps overly broad restrictions on its acquisition may themselves be subject to first amendment standards of judicial review.[13] *Aptheker*, though not nearly as prominent as *New York Times v. Sullivan* three decades ago, did set in motion the use of the first amendment to secure access to information in places traditionally under government management regulation and control. We now turn briefly to see several principal developments in this expanding, albeit highly unsettled field.

HOUCHINS v. KQED, INC.

438 U.S. 1 (1978)

MR. CHIEF JUSTICE BURGER announced the judgment of the Court and delivered an opinion, in which MR. JUSTICE WHITE and MR. JUSTICE REHNQUIST joined.

The question presented is whether the news media have a constitutional right of access to a county jail, over and above that of other persons, to interview inmates and make sound recordings, films, and photographs for publication and broadcasting by newspapers, radio, and television.

---

11. See note 4 *supra*.

12. 9 Writings of James Madison 103 (G. Hunt ed. 1910).

13. Which is what the majority also implied in *Aptheker*, drawing the connection to the first amendment pretty much as we have drawn it here. See 378 U.S. at 517 ("[S]ince freedom of travel is a constitutional liberty *closely related to rights of free speech and association*, we believe that appellants in this case should not be required to assume the burden of demonstrating that Congress could not have written a statute constitutionally prohibiting their travel.") (emphasis added).

I

Petitioner Houchins, as Sheriff of Alameda County, Cal., controls all access to the Alameda County Jail at Santa Rita. Respondent KQED operates licensed television and radio broadcasting stations which have frequently reported newsworthy events relating to penal institutions in the San Francisco Bay Area. On March 31, 1975, KQED reported the suicide of a prisoner in the Greystone portion of the Santa Rita jail. The report included a statement by a psychiatrist that the conditions at the Greystone facility were responsible for the illnesses of his patient-prisoners there, and a statement from petitioner denying that prison conditions were responsible for the prisoners' illnesses.

KQED requested permission to inspect and take pictures within the Greystone facility. After permission was refused, KQED and the Alameda and Oakland branches of the National Association for the Advancement of Colored People (NAACP) filed suit under 42 U.S.C. § 1983. They alleged that petitioner had violated the First Amendment by refusing to permit media access and failing to provide any effective means by which the public could be informed of conditions prevailing in the Greystone facility or learn of the prisoners' grievances. Public access to such information was essential, they asserted, in order for NAACP members to participate in the public debate on jail conditions in Alameda County. They further asserted that television coverage of the conditions in the cells and facilities was the most effective way of informing the public of prison conditions.

The complaint requested a preliminary and permanent injunction to prevent petitioner from "excluding KQED news personnel from the Greystone cells and Santa Rita facilities and generally preventing full and accurate news coverage of the conditions prevailing therein." On June 17, 1975, when the complaint was filed, there appears to have been no formal policy regarding public access to the Santa Rita jail. However, according to petitioner, he had been in the process of planning a program of regular monthly tours since he took office six months earlier. On July 8, 1975, he announced the program and invited all interested persons to make arrangements for the regular public tours. News media were given notice in advance of the public and presumably could have made early reservations. ***

Each tour was limited to 25 persons and permitted only limited access to the jail. The tours did not include the disciplinary cells or the portions of the jail known as "Little Greystone," the scene of alleged rapes, beatings, and adverse physical conditions. Photographs of some parts of the jail were made available, but no cameras or tape recorders were allowed on the tours. Those on the tours were not permitted to interview inmates, and inmates were generally removed from view. ***

After considering the testimony, affidavits, and documentary evidence presented by the parties, the District Court preliminarily enjoined petitioner from denying KQED news personnel and "responsible representatives" of the news media access to the Santa Rita facilities, including Greystone, "at reasonable times and hours" and "from preventing KQED news personnel and responsible representatives of the news media from utilizing photographic and sound equipment or from utilizing inmate interviews in providing full and accurate coverage of the Santa Rita facilities."

On interlocutory appeal from the District Court's order, *** [t]he Court of Appeals *** concluded, albeit in three separate opinions, that the public and the media had a First and Fourteenth Amendment right of access to prisons and jails, and sustained the District Court's order. ***

III

We can agree with many of the respondents' generalized assertions; conditions in jails and prisons are clearly matters "of great public importance." *** Penal facilities are public institutions which require large amounts of public funds, and their mission is crucial in our criminal justice system. Each person placed in prison becomes, in effect, a ward of the state for whom society assumes broad responsibility. It is equally true that with greater information, the public can more intelligently form opinions about prison conditions. Beyond question, the role of the media is important; acting as the "eyes and ears" of the public, they can be a powerful and constructive force, contributing to remedial action in the conduct of public business. They have served that function since the beginning of the Republic, but like all other components of our society media representatives are subject to limits.

The public importance of conditions in penal facilities and the media's role of providing information afford no basis for reading into the Constitution a right of the public or the media to enter these institutions, with camera equipment, and take moving and still pictures of inmates for broadcast purposes. This Court has never intimated a First Amendment guarantee of a right of access to all sources of information within government control. Nor does the rationale of the decisions upon which respondents rely lead to the implication of such a right.

Grosjean v. American Press Co. and *Mills v. Alabama* emphasized the importance of informed public opinion and the traditional role of a free press as a source of public information. But an analysis of those cases reveals that the Court was concerned with the freedom of the media to communicate information once it is obtained; neither case intimated that the Constitution compels the government to provide the media with information or access to it on demand. *Grosjean* involved a challenge to a state tax on advertising revenues of newspapers, the "plain purpose" of which was to penalize the publishers and curtail the publication of a selected group of newspapers. *** *Mills* involved a statute making it a crime to publish an editorial about election issues on election day. In striking down the statute, the Court noted that "a major purpose of [the First] Amendment was to protect the free discussion of governmental affairs." *** As in *Grosjean*, however, the Court did not remotely imply a constitutional right guaranteeing anyone access to government information beyond that open to the public generally. ***

IV

The respondents' argument is flawed, not only because it lacks precedential support and is contrary to statements in this Court's opinions, but also because it invites the Court to involve itself in what is clearly a legislative task which the Constitution has left to the political processes. *** Unarticulated but implicit in the assertion that media access to the jail is essential for informed public debate on jail conditions is the assumption that media personnel are the best qualified persons for the task of discovering malfeasance in public institutions. But that assumption finds no support in the decisions of this Court or the First Amendment. Editors and newsmen who inspect a jail may decide to publish or not to publish what information they acquire. *** Public bodies and public officers, on the other hand, may be coerced by public opinion to disclose what they might prefer to conceal. No comparable pressures are available to anyone to compel publication by the media of what they might prefer not to make known.

There is no discernible basis for a constitutional duty to disclose, or for standards governing disclosure of or access to information. Because the Constitution affords no guidelines, absent statutory standards, hundreds of judges would, under the Court of Appeals' approach, be at large to fashion ad hoc standards, in individual cases, according to their own ideas of what seems "desirable" or "expedient." We, therefore, reject the Court of Appeals' conclusory assertion that the public and the media have a First Amendment right to government information regarding the conditions of jails and their inmates and presumably all other public facilities such as hospitals and mental institutions.

> "*** The Constitution itself is neither a Freedom of Information Act nor an Official Secrets Act. *** "The Constitution, in other words, establishes the contest, not its resolution. Congress may provide a resolution, at least in some instances, through carefully drawn legislation. For the rest, we must rely, as so often in our system we must, on the tug and pull of the political forces in American society." ***
>
> Stewart, "Or of the Press," 26 Hastings L.J. 631, 636 (1975).

Petitioner cannot prevent respondents from learning about jail conditions in a variety of ways, albeit not as conveniently as they might prefer. Respondents have a First Amendment right to receive letters from inmates criticizing jail officials and reporting on conditions. See Procunier v. Martinez, 416 U.S., at 413-418. Respondents are free to interview those who render the legal assistance to which inmates are entitled. See *id.*, at 419. They are also free to seek out former inmates, visitors to the prison, public officials, and institutional personnel, as they sought out the complaining psychiatrist here.

***

Neither the First Amendment nor the Fourteenth Amendment mandates a right of access to government information or sources of information within the government's control. [And] under our holdings in *Pell v. Procunier* and *Saxbe v. Washington Post Co.*, until the political branches decree otherwise, as they are free to do, the media have no special right of access to the Alameda County Jail different from or greater than that accorded the public generally.

The judgment of the Court of Appeals is reversed, and the case is remanded for further proceedings.

MR. JUSTICE MARSHALL and MR. JUSTICE BLACKMUN took no part in the consideration or decision of this case.

MR. JUSTICE STEWART, concurring in the judgment.

I agree that the preliminary injunction issued against the petitioner was unwarranted, and therefore concur in the judgment. In my view, however, KQED was entitled to injunctive relief of more limited scope.

The First and Fourteenth Amendments do not guarantee the public a right of access to information generated or controlled by government, nor do they guarantee the press any basic right of access superior to that of the public generally. The Constitution does no more than assure the public and the press equal access once government has opened its doors. Accordingly, I agree substantially with what the opinion of THE CHIEF JUSTICE has to say on that score.

We part company, however, in applying these abstractions to the facts of this case. Whereas he appears to view "equal access" as meaning access that is identical in all respects, I believe that the concept of equal access must be accorded more flexibility in order to accommodate the practical distinctions between the press and the general public.

When on assignment, a journalist does not tour a jail simply for his own edification. He is there to gather information to be passed on to others, and his mission is protected by the Constitution for very specific reasons. ***

That the First Amendment speaks separately of freedom of speech and freedom of the press is no constitutional accident, but an acknowledgment of the critical role played by the press in American society. The Constitution requires sensitivity to that role, and to the special needs of the press in performing it effectively. A person touring Santa Rita jail can grasp its reality with his own eyes and ears. But if a television reporter is to convey the jail's sights and sounds to those who cannot personally visit the place, he must use cameras and sound equipment. In short, terms of access that are reasonably imposed on individual members of the public may, if they impede effective reporting without sufficient justification, be unreasonable as applied to journalists who are there to convey to the general public what the visitors see.

Under these principles, KQED was clearly entitled to some form of preliminary injunctive relief. At the time of the District Court's decision, members of the public were permitted to visit most parts of the Santa Rita jail, and the First and Fourteenth Amendments required the Sheriff to give members of the press *effective* access to the same areas. The Sheriff evidently assumed that he could fulfill this obligation simply by allowing reporters to sign up for tours on the same terms as the public. I think he was mistaken in this assumption, as a matter of constitutional law. ***

MR. JUSTICE STEVENS, with whom MR. JUSTICE BRENNAN and MR. JUSTICE POWELL join, dissenting.

***

Respondent KQED, Inc., has televised a number of programs about prison conditions and prison inmates, and its reporters have been granted access to various correctional facilities in the San Francisco Bay area, including San Quentin State Prison, Soledad Prison, and the San Francisco County Jails at San Bruno and San Francisco, to prepare program material. They have taken their cameras and recording equipment inside the walls of those institutions and interviewed inmates. No disturbances or other problems have occurred on those occasions. ***

An evidentiary hearing on the motion for a preliminary injunction was held after the first four guided tours had taken place. The evidence revealed the inadequacy of the tours as a means of obtaining information about the inmates and their conditions of confinement for transmission to the public. The tours failed to enter certain areas of the jail.[9] They afforded no opportunity to photograph conditions within the facility, and the photographs which the county offered for sale to tour visitors omitted certain jail characteristics, such as catwalks above the cells from which guards can observe the inmates.[10] The tours provided no opportunity to question randomly encountered inmates about jail conditions. Indeed, to the extent possible, inmates were kept out of sight during the tour, preventing the tour visitors from obtaining a realistic picture of the conditions of confinement within the jail. ***

For two reasons, which will be discussed separately, the decisions in *Pell* and *Saxbe* do not control the propriety of the District Court's preliminary injunction. First, the unconstitutionality of petitioner's policies which gave rise to this litigation does not rest on the premise that the press has a greater right of access to information regarding prison conditions than do other members of the public. Second, relief tailored to the needs of the press may properly be awarded to a representative of the press which is successful in proving that it has been harmed by a constitutional violation and need not await the grant of relief to members of the general public who may also have been injured by petitioner's unconstitutional access policy but have not yet sought to vindicate their rights. ***

In Pell v. Procunier, 417 U.S., at 834, the Court stated that "newsmen have no constitutional right of access to prisons or their inmates beyond that afforded the general public." But the Court has never intimated that a nondiscriminatory policy

---

9. The tour did not include Little Greystone, which was the subject of reports of beatings, rapes, and poor conditions, or the disciplinary cells.

10. There were also no photos of the women's cells, of the "safety cell," of the "disciplinary cells," or of the interior of Little Greystone. In addition, the photograph of the dayroom omits the television monitor that maintains continuous observation of the inmates and the open urinals.

of excluding entirely both the public and the press from access to information about prison conditions would avoid constitutional scrutiny.[15]

*** What *Pell* does indicate is that the question whether respondents established a probability of prevailing on their constitutional claim is inseparable from the question whether petitioner's policies unduly restricted the opportunities of the general public to learn about the conditions of confinement in Santa Rita jail. As in *Pell*, in assessing its adequacy, the total access of the public and the press must be considered. *** Here, the broad restraints on access to information regarding operation of the jail that prevailed on the date this suit was instituted are plainly disclosed by the record. ***

II

The preservation of a full and free flow of information to the general public has long been recognized as a core objective of the First Amendment to the Constitution. It is for this reason that the First Amendment protects not only the dissemination but also the receipt of information and ideas. *** Without some protection for the acquisition of information about the operation of public institutions such as prisons by the public at large, the process of self-governance contemplated by the Framers would be stripped of its substance.[22]

For that reason information gathering is entitled to some measure of constitutional protection. *** The question is whether petitioner's policies, which cut off the flow of information at its source, abridged the public's right to be informed about those conditions.

The answer to that question does not depend upon the degree of public disclosure which should attend the operation of most governmental activity. Such

---

15. In Zemel v. Rusk, 381 U.S. 1, 17, the Court said:

> "The right to speak and publish does not carry with it the *unrestrained* right to gather information." (Emphasis added.)

And in Branzburg v. Hayes, 408 U.S. 665, 681:

> "We do not question the significance of free speech, press, or assembly to the country's welfare. Nor is it suggested that news gathering does not qualify for First Amendment protection; without some protection for seeking out the news, freedom of the press could be eviscerated."

Both statements imply that there is a right to acquire knowledge that derives protection from the First Amendment. See *id.*, at 728 n. 4 (Stewart, J. dissenting).

22. Admittedly, the right to receive or acquire information is not specifically mentioned in the Constitution. But "the protection of the Bill of Rights goes beyond the specific guarantees to protect from *** abridgement those equally fundamental personal rights necessary to make the express guarantees fully meaningful. *** The dissemination of ideas can accomplish nothing if otherwise willing addressees are not free to receive and consider them. It would be a barren marketplace of ideas that had only sellers and no buyers." Lamont v. Postmaster General, 381 U.S., at 308 (BRENNAN, J., concurring). It would be an even more barren marketplace that had willing buyers and sellers and no meaningful information to exchange.

matters involve questions of policy which generally must be resolved by the political branches of government. Moreover, there are unquestionably occasions when governmental activity may properly be carried on in complete secrecy. For example, the public and the press are commonly excluded from "grand jury proceedings, our own conferences, [and] the meetings of other official bodies gathered in executive session ***." Branzburg v. Hayes, 408 U.S., at 684; Pell v. Procunier, 417 U.S., at 834. In addition, some functions of government—essential to the protection of the public and indeed our country's vital interests—necessarily require a large measure of secrecy, subject to appropriate legislative oversight. In such situations the reasons for withholding information from the public are both apparent and legitimate. ***

In this case, the record demonstrates that both the public and the press had been consistently denied any access to the inner portions of the Santa Rita jail, that there had been excessive censorship of inmate correspondence, and that there was no valid justification for these broad restraints on the flow of information. An affirmative answer to the question whether respondents established a likelihood of prevailing on the merits did not depend, in final analysis, on any right of the press to special treatment beyond that accorded the public at large. Rather, the probable existence of a constitutional violation rested upon the special importance of allowing a democratic community access to knowledge about how its servants were treating some of its members who have been committed to their custody. An official prison policy of concealing such knowledge from the public by arbitrarily cutting off the flow of information at its source abridges the freedom of speech and of the press protected by the First and Fourteenth Amendments to the Constitution. ***

RICHMOND NEWSPAPERS, INC. v. VIRGINIA

448 U.S. 555 (1980)

MR. CHIEF JUSTICE BURGER announced the judgment of the Court and delivered an opinion, in which MR. JUSTICE WHITE and MR. JUSTICE STEVENS joined.

The narrow question presented in this case is whether the right of the public and press to attend criminal trials is guaranteed under the United States Constitution.

I

In March 1976, one Stevenson was indicted for the murder of a hotel manager who had been found stabbed to death on December 2, 1975. Tried promptly in July 1976, Stevenson was convicted of second-degree murder in the Circuit Court of Hanover County, Va. The Virginia Supreme Court reversed the conviction in October 1977, holding that a bloodstained shirt reportedly belonging to Stevenson had been improperly admitted into evidence. Stevenson was retried in the same court. This second trial ended in a mistrial on May 30, 1978, when a juror asked to be excused after trial had begun and no alternate was available.[1]

A third trial, which began in the same court on June 6, 1978, also ended in a mistrial. It appears that the mistrial may have been declared because a prospective juror had read about Stevenson's previous trials in a newspaper and had told other prospective jurors about the case before the retrial began. ***

Stevenson was tried in the same court for a fourth time beginning on September 11, 1978. Present in the courtroom when the case was called were appellants Wheeler and McCarthy, reporters for appellant Richmond Newspapers, Inc. Before the trial began, counsel for the defendant moved that it be closed to the public:

> "[T]here was this woman that was with the family of the deceased when we were here before. She had sat in the Courtroom. I would like to ask that everybody be excluded from the Courtroom because I don't want any information being shuffled back and forth when we have a recess as to what— who testified to what."

The trial judge, who had presided over two of the three previous trials, asked if the prosecution had any objection to clearing the courtroom. The prosecutor stated he had no objection and would leave it to the discretion of the court. Presumably referring to Va. Code § 19.2-266 (Supp. 1980), the trial judge then announced: "[T]he statute gives me that power specifically and the defendant has made the motion." He then ordered "that the Courtroom be kept clear of all parties except the witnesses when they testify." The record does not show that any objections to the closure order were made by anyone present at the time, including appellants Wheeler and McCarthy.

Later that same day, however, appellants sought a hearing on a motion to vacate the closure order. *** At the closed hearing, counsel for appellants observed that no evidentiary findings had been made by the court prior to the entry of its closure order and pointed out that the court had failed to consider any other, less drastic measures within its power to ensure a fair trial. Counsel for appellants argued that constitutional considerations mandated that before ordering closure, the court should first decide that the rights of the defendant could be protected in no other way.

Counsel for defendant Stevenson pointed out that this was the fourth time he was standing trial. He also referred to "difficulty with information between the jurors," and stated that he "didn't want information to leak out," be published by the media, perhaps inaccurately, and then be seen by the jurors. Defense counsel argued that these things, plus the fact that "this is a small community," made this a proper case

---

1. A newspaper account published the next day reported the mistrial and went on to note that "[a] key piece of evidence in Stevenson's original conviction was a bloodstained shirt obtained from Stevenson's wife soon after the killing. The Virginia Supreme Court, however, ruled that the shirt was entered into evidence improperly."

for closure. *** The court denied the motion to vacate and ordered the trial to continue the following morning "with the press and public excluded."

What transpired when the closed trial resumed the next day was disclosed in the following manner by an order of the court entered September 12, 1978:

> "[I]n the absence of the jury, the defendant by counsel made a Motion that a mistrial be declared, which motion was taken under advisement.
> "At the conclusion of the Commonwealth's evidence, the attorney for the defendant moved the Court to strike the Commonwealth's evidence on grounds stated to the record, which Motion was sustained by the Court.
> "And the jury having been excused, the Court doth find the accused NOT GUILTY of Murder, as charged in the Indictment, and he was allowed to depart."[3]

***

II

We begin consideration of this case by noting that the precise issue presented here has not previously been before this Court for decision. In *Gannett Co. v. DePasquale,* the Court was not required to decide whether a right of access to *trials*, as distinguished from hearings on *pre*trial motions, was constitutionally guaranteed. The Court held that the Sixth Amendment's guarantee to the accused of a public trial gave neither the public nor the press an enforceable right of access to a pretrial suppression hearing. *** Moreover, the Court did not decide whether the First and Fourteenth Amendments guarantee a right of the public to attend trials ***.

*** [H]ere for the first time the Court is asked to decide whether a criminal trial itself may be closed to the public upon the unopposed request of a defendant, without any demonstration that closure is required to protect the defendant's superior right to a fair trial, or that some other overriding consideration requires closure. ***

[T]he historical evidence demonstrates conclusively that at the time when our organic laws were adopted, criminal trials both here and in England had long been presumptively open. *** Both Hale in the 17th century and Blackstone in the 18th saw the importance of openness to the proper functioning of a trial; it gave assurance that the proceedings were conducted fairly to all concerned, and it discouraged perjury, the misconduct of participants, and decisions based on secret bias or partiality. *** Looking back, we see that when the ancient "town meeting" form of trial became too cumbersome, 12 members of the community were delegated to act as its surrogates, but the community did not surrender its right to observe the conduct of trials. The people retained a "right of visitation" which enabled them to satisfy themselves that justice was in fact being done.

***

---

3. At oral argument, it was represented to the Court that tapes of the trial were available to the public as soon as the trial terminated.

From this unbroken, uncontradicted history, supported by reasons as valid today as in centuries past, we are bound to conclude that a presumption of openness inheres in the very nature of a criminal trial under our system of justice. ***

Despite the history of criminal trials being presumptively open since long before the Constitution, the State presses its contention that neither the Constitution nor the Bill of Rights contains any provision which by its terms guarantees to the public the right to attend criminal trials. Standing alone, this is correct, but there remains the question whether, absent an explicit provision, the Constitution affords protection against exclusion of the public from criminal trials.

III

***

The Bill of Rights was enacted against the backdrop of the long history of trials being presumptively open. Public access to trials was then regarded as an important aspect of the process itself; the conduct of trials "before as many of the people as chuse to attend" was regarded as one of "the inestimable advantages of a free English constitution of government." 1 Journals 106, 107. In guaranteeing freedoms such as those of speech and press, the First Amendment can be read as protecting the right of everyone to attend trials so as to give meaning to those explicit guarantees. "[T]he First Amendment goes beyond protection of the press and the self-expression of individuals to prohibit government from limiting the stock of information from which members of the public may draw." First National Bank of Boston v. Bellotti, 435 U.S. 765, 783 (1978). ***

It is not crucial whether we describe this right to attend criminal trials to hear, see, and communicate observations concerning them as a "right of access," cf. *Gannett*, 433 U.S. at 397 (POWELL, J., concurring); Saxbe v. Washington Post Co., 417 U.S. 843 (1974); Pell v. Procunier, 417 U.S. 817 (1974),[11] or a "right to gather information," for we have recognized that "without some protection for seeking out the news, freedom of the press could be eviscerated." Branzburg v. Hayes, 408 U.S. 665, 681 (1972). The explicit, guaranteed rights to speak and to publish concerning what takes place at a trial would lose much meaning if access to observe the trial could, as it was here, be foreclosed arbitrarily.[12]

---

11. *Procunier* and *Saxbe* are distinguishable in the sense that they were concerned with penal institutions which, by definition, are not "open" or public places. Penal institutions do not share the long tradition of openness, although traditionally there have been visiting committees of citizens, and there is no doubt that legislative committees could exercise plenary oversight and "visitation rights." ***

12. That the right to attend may be exercised by people less frequently today when information as to trials generally reaches them by way of print and electronic media in no way alters the basic right. Instead of relying on personal observation or reports from neighbors as in the past, most people receive information concerning trials through the media whose representatives "are entitled to the same rights [to attend trials] as the general public." ***

The right of access to places traditionally open to the public, as criminal trials have long been, may be seen as assured by the amalgam of the First Amendment guarantees of speech and press; and their affinity to the right of assembly is not without relevance. *** People assemble in public places not only to speak or to take action, but also to listen, observe, and learn; indeed, they may "assembl[e] for any lawful purpose," Hague v. CIO, 307 U.S. 496, 519 (1939) (opinion of Stone, J.). Subject to the traditional time, place, and manner restrictions, streets, sidewalks, and parks are places traditionally open, where First Amendment rights may be exercised, a trial courtroom also is a public place where the people generally—and representatives of the media—have a right to be present, and where their presence historically has been thought to enhance the integrity and quality of what takes place.[13]

The State argues that the Constitution nowhere spells out a guarantee for the right of the public to attend trials, and that accordingly no such right is protected. The possibility that such a contention could be made did not escape the notice of the Constitution's draftsmen; they were concerned that some important rights might be thought disparaged because not specifically guaranteed. It was even argued that because of this danger no Bill of Rights should be adopted. See, e.g., The Federalist No. 84 (A. Hamilton). In a letter to Thomas Jefferson in October 1788, James Madison explained why he, although "in favor of a bill of rights," had "not viewed it in an important light" up to that time: "I conceive that in a certain degree *** the rights in question are reserved by the manner in which the federal powers are granted." He went on to state that "there is great reason to fear that a positive declaration of some of the most essential rights could not be obtained in the requisite latitude." 5 Writings of James Madison 271 (G. Hunt ed. 1904).[14]

But arguments such as the State makes have not precluded recognition of important rights not enumerated. Notwithstanding the appropriate caution against reading into the Constitution rights not explicitly defined, the Court has acknowl-

---

13. It is of course true that the right of assembly in our Bill of Rights was in large part drafted in reaction to restrictions on such rights in England. See, *e.g.*, 1 Geo. 1, stat. 2, ch. 5 (1714); cf. 36 Geo. 3, ch. 8 (1795). As we have shown, the right of Englishmen to attend trials was not similarly limited; but it would be ironic indeed if the very historic openness of the trial could militate against protection of the right to attend it. The Constitution guarantees more than simply freedom from those abuses which led the Framers to single out particular rights. The very purpose of the First Amendment is to guarantee all facets of each right described; its draftsmen sought both to protect the "rights of Englishmen" and to enlarge their scope. See Bridges v. California, 314 U.S. 252, 263-265 (1941).

14. Madison's comments in Congress also reveal the perceived need for some sort of constitutional "saving clause," which, among other things, would serve to foreclose application to the Bill of Rights of the maxim that the affirmation of particular rights implies a negation of those not expressly defined. See 1 Annals of Cong. 438-440 (1789). See also, e.g., 2 J. Story, Commentaries on the Constitution of the United States 651 (5th ed. 1891). Madison's efforts, culminating in the Ninth Amendment, served to allay the fears of those who were concerned that expressing certain guarantees could be read as excluding others.

edged that certain unarticulated rights are implicit in enumerated guarantees. For example, the rights of association and of privacy, the right to be presumed innocent, and the right to be judged by a standard of proof beyond a reasonable doubt in a criminal trial, as well as the right to travel, appear nowhere in the Constitution or Bill of Rights. Yet these important but unarticulated rights have nonetheless been found to share constitutional protection in common with explicit guarantees. The concerns expressed by Madison and others have thus been resolved; fundamental rights, even though not expressly guaranteed, have been recognized by the Court as indispensable to the enjoyment of rights explicitly defined.

We hold that the right to attend criminal trials[17] is implicit in the guarantees of the First Amendment; without the freedom to attend such trials, which people have exercised for centuries, important aspects of freedom of speech and "of the press could be eviscerated." *Branzburg*, 408 U.S., at 681.

D

Having concluded there was a guaranteed right of the public under the First and Fourteenth Amendments to attend the trial of Stevenson's case, we return to the closure order challenged by appellants. The Court in *Gannett* made clear that although the Sixth Amendment guarantees the accused a right to a public trial, it does not give a right to a private trial. Despite the fact this was the fourth trial of the accused, the trial judge made no findings to support closure; no inquiry was made as to whether alternative solutions would have met the need to ensure fairness; there was no recognition of any right under the Constitution for the public or press to attend the trial. There was no suggestion that any problems with witnesses could not have been dealt with by their exclusion from the courtroom or their sequestration during the trial. Nor is there anything to indicate that sequestration of the jurors would not have guarded against their being subjected to any improper information. All of the alternatives admittedly present difficulties for trial courts, but none of the factors relied on here was beyond the realm of the manageable. Absent an overriding interest articulated in findings, the trial of a criminal case must be open to the public. Accordingly, the judgment under review is [r]eversed.

MR. JUSTICE POWELL took no part in the consideration or decision of this case.

MR. JUSTICE WHITE, concurring.

This case would have been unnecessary had Gannett Co. v. DePasquale, 443 U.S. 368 (1979), construed the Sixth Amendment to forbid excluding the public from criminal proceedings except in narrowly defined circumstances. But the Court there rejected the submission of four of us to this effect, thus requiring that the First

---

17. Whether the public has a right to attend trials of civil cases is a question not raised by the case, but we note that historically both civil and criminal trials have been presumptively open.

Amendment issue involved here be addressed. On this issue, I concur in the opinion of THE CHIEF JUSTICE.

MR. JUSTICE STEVENS, concurring.

This is a watershed case. Until today the Court has accorded virtually absolute protection to the dissemination of information or ideas, but never before has it squarely held that the acquisition of newsworthy matter is entitled to any constitutional protection whatsoever. An additional word of emphasis is therefore appropriate.

Twice before, the Court has implied that any governmental restriction on access to information, no matter how severe and no matter how unjustified, would be constitutionally acceptable so long as it did not single out the press for special disabilities not applicable to the public at large. [I]n Houchins v. KQED, Inc., 438 U.S. 1, 19-40, I explained at length why MR. JUSTICE BRENNAN, MR. JUSTICE POWELL, and I were convinced that "[a]n official prison policy of concealing *** knowledge from the public by arbitrarily cutting off the flow of information at its source abridges the freedom of speech and of the press protected by the First and Fourteenth Amendments to the Constitution." Since MR. JUSTICE MARSHALL and MR. JUSTICE BLACKMUN were unable to participate in that case, a majority of the Court neither accepted nor rejected that conclusion or the contrary conclusion expressed in the prevailing opinions. Today, however, for the first time, the Court unequivocally holds that an arbitrary interference with access to important information is an abridgment of the freedoms of speech and of the press protected by the First Amendment.

It is somewhat ironic that the Court should find more reason to recognize a right of access today than it did in *Houchins*. For *Houchins* involved the plight of a segment of society least able to protect itself, an attack on a long-standing policy of concealment, and an absence of any legitimate justification for abridging public access to information about how government operates. In this case we are protecting the interests of the most powerful voices in the community, we are concerned with an almost unique exception to an established tradition of openness in the conduct of criminal trials, and it is likely that the closure order was motivated by the judge's desire to protect the individual defendant from the burden of a fourth criminal trial.

In any event, for the reasons stated in Part II of my *Houchins* opinion, as well as those stated by THE CHIEF JUSTICE today, I agree that the First Amendment protects the public and the press from abridgment of their rights of access to information about the operation of their government, including the Judicial Branch; given the total absence of any record justification for the closure order entered in this case, that order violated the First Amendment.

MR. JUSTICE BRENNAN, with whom MR. JUSTICE MARSHALL joins, concurring in the judgment. [Omitted.]

MR. JUSTICE STEWART, concurring in the judgment. [Omitted.]

MR. JUSTICE BLACKMUN, concurring in the judgment. [Omitted]

***

MR. JUSTICE REHNQUIST, dissenting.

***

For the reasons stated in my separate concurrence in Gannett Co. v. DePasquale, 443 U.S. 368, 403 (1979), I do not believe that either the First or Sixth Amendment, as made applicable to the States by the Fourteenth, requires that a State's reasons for denying public access to a trial, where both the prosecuting attorney and the defendant have consented to an order of closure approved by the judge, are subject to any additional constitutional review at our hands. And I most certainly do not believe that the Ninth Amendment confers upon us any such power to review orders of state trial judges closing trials in such situations. ***

The issue here is not whether the "right" to freedom of the press conferred by the First Amendment to the Constitution overrides the defendant's "right" to a fair trial conferred by other Amendments to the Constitution; it is instead whether any provision in the Constitution may fairly be read to prohibit what the trial judge in the Virginia state-court system did in this case. Being unable to find any such prohibition in the First, Sixth, Ninth, or any other Amendment to the United States Constitution, or in the Constitution itself, I dissent.

NOTE

1. Why should it make any difference whether there has, or has not, been a long standing tradition of public or press access in determining whether one has a first amendment right of access for informational purposes? Suppose there were no long-standing tradition of public access to certain portions of certain criminal trials (for example, during testimony by minors in sex offense cases). Would a statute that merely hardened this general rule—by requiring that the courtroom be cleared during such proceedings—be valid notwithstanding *Richmond Newspapers*? (A majority of the Court concluded that such a rule was not sustainable after *Richmond Newspapers*. See Globe Newspaper Co. v. Superior Court, 482 U.S. 596 (1982).)[137]

2. *Richmond Newspapers* dealt only with press and public courtroom access at the trial stage of a criminal proceeding. But what of identical claims of access during *pre*trial proceedings (for example, when motions to suppress evidence or motions to dismiss the charges are heard and decided, or when *voir dire* jury selection takes place). See Press-Enterprise Co. v. Superior Court, 464 U.S. 501 (1984) and Press-

---

137. Might government restriction on public access to the identity of victims of sexual offenses also be unconstitutional under *Richmond Newspapers* and *Globe*? See Sarah Henderson Hutt, Note, In Praise of Public Access: Why the Government Should Disclose the Identities of Alleged Crime Victims, 1991 Duke L.J. 368.

Enterprise Co. v. Superior Court, 478 U.S. 1 (1986) (holding that *Richmond Newspapers* also extends to these proceedings).

3. To what extent does press (or public) access to judicial proceedings extend to recording events (as well as being able to attend these events)—to take pictures, or (in the case of the press) to provide live or taped video coverage? (Are cameras permitted in the Supreme Court? See Todd Piccus, Note, Demystifying the Least Understood Branch: Opening the Supreme Court to Broadcast Media, 71 Tex.L Rev. 1053 (1993).)

4. More generally, what other government-conducted business may also be open to direct press or public first amendment "right to know" entitlements, either to attend certain kinds of meetings, or to copy certain records, or both? Would the *Houchins* case come out differently, if relitigated subsequent to *Richmond News*? Why or why not? What of a citizen's challenge to gain access to "closed executive sessions" held by ordinary city councils meeting to consider personnel matters, or to sessions of state university trustees or public school boards? What might courts do with press challenges brought to test restrictions on press access to areas of military action (as military command decisions forbidding press presence other than in designated tours during "Operation Desert Storm," or the prohibition of journalists during the quick strike in Grenada)? For an early reflection, see Anthony Lewis, A Public Right to Know About Public Institutions: The First Amendment as a Sword, 1980 Sup.Ct. Rev. 1. For more recent critical commentary, see Michael J. Hayes, Note, Whatever Happened to "The Right to Know"?: Access to Government Information Since Richmond Newspapers, 73 Va.L.Rev. 1111 (1987).

5. Is the case for press access in any respect stronger than general public access?[138] If so, why? (Assuming that it might be, what would define "the press" for purposes of making such a distinction?)

---

9. The Blurred Boundary Separating Private from Public Property for Purposes of Deciding First Amendment Rights of Access and of Use. (Herein also of the "State Action" Requirement of First and Fourteenth Amendment Review)

MARSH v. ALABAMA

326 U.S. 501 (1946)

MR. JUSTICE BLACK delivered the opinion of the Court.

In this case we are asked to decide whether a State, consistently with the First and Fourteenth Amendments, can impose criminal punishment on a person who undertakes to distribute religious literature on the premises of a company-owned town

138. For further discussion of the notion that the press has a "preferred position" in our constitutional scheme, see William Van Alstyne, Interpretations of the First Amendment 50-67 (1984).

contrary to the wishes of the town's management. The town, a suburb of Mobile, Alabama, known as Chickasaw, is owned by the Gulf Shipbuilding Corporation. Except for that it has all the characteristics of any other American town. The property consists of residential buildings, streets, a system of sewers, a sewage disposal plant and a "business block" on which business places are situated. A deputy of the Mobile County Sheriff, paid by the company, serves as the town's policeman. Merchants and service establishments have rented the stores and business places on the business block and the United States uses one of the places as a post office from which six carriers deliver mail to the people of Chickasaw and the adjacent area. The town and the surrounding neighborhood, which can not be distinguished from the Gulf property by anyone not familiar with the property lines, are thickly settled, and according to all indications the residents use the business block as their regular shopping center. ***

Appellant, a Jehovah's Witness, came onto the sidewalk we have just described, stood near the post office and undertook to distribute religious literature. In the stores the corporation had posted a notice which read as follows: "This Is Private Property, and Without Written Permission, No Street, or House Vendor, Agent or Solicitation of Any Kind Will Be Permitted." Appellant was warned that she could not distribute the literature without a permit and told that no permit would be issued to her. She protested that the company rule could not be constitutionally applied so as to prohibit her from distributing religious writings. When she was asked to leave the sidewalk and Chickasaw she declined. The deputy sheriff arrested her and she was charged in the state court with violating Title 14, § 426 of the 1940 Alabama Code which makes it a crime to enter or remain on the premises of another after having been warned not to do so. ***

Had the title to Chickasaw belonged not to a private but to a municipal corporation and had appellant been arrested for violating a municipal ordinance rather than a ruling by those appointed by the corporation to manage a company town it would have been clear that appellant's conviction must be reversed. Under our decision in Lovell v. Griffin, 303 U.S. 444, and others which have followed that case, neither a State nor a municipality can completely bar the distribution of literature containing religious or political ideas on its streets, sidewalks and public places or make the right to distribute dependent on a flat license tax or permit to be issued by an official who could deny it at will. *** Our question then narrows down to this: Can those people who live in or come to Chickasaw be denied freedom of press and religion simply because a single company has legal title to all the town? For it is the State's contention that the mere fact that all the property interests in the town are held by a single company is enough to give that company power, enforceable by a state statute, to abridge these freedoms.

We do not agree that the corporation's property interests settle the question. The State urges in effect that the corporation's right to control the inhabitants of Chickasaw is coextensive with the right of a homeowner to regulate the conduct of his guests. We cannot accept that contention. Ownership does not always mean absolute dominion. The more an owner, for his advantage, opens up his property for use by the public in general, the more do his rights become circumscribed by the statutory and constitutional rights of those who use it. *** Thus, the owners of privately held bridges, ferries, turnpikes and railroads may not operate them as freely as a farmer does his farm. Since these facilities are built and operated primarily to benefit the public and since their operation is essentially a public function, it is subject to state regulation. *** As we have heretofore stated, the town of Chickasaw does not function differently from any other town. ***

In our view the circumstance that the property rights to the premises where the deprivation of liberty, here involved, took place, were held by others than the public, is not sufficient to justify the State's permitting a corporation to govern a community of citizens so as to restrict their fundamental liberties and the enforcement of such restraint by the application of a state statute. Insofar as the State has attempted to impose criminal punishment on appellant for undertaking to distribute religious literature in a company town, its action cannot stand. The case is reversed and the cause remanded for further proceedings not inconsistent with this opinion.

MR. JUSTICE JACKSON took no part in the consideration or decision of this case.

MR. JUSTICE FRANKFURTER, concurring. [Omitted.]

***

MR. JUSTICE REED, dissenting.

This is the first case to extend by law the privilege of religious exercises beyond public places or to private places without the assent of the owner. ***

As the rule now announced permits this intrusion, without possibility of protection of the property by law, and apparently is equally applicable to the freedom of speech and the press, it seems appropriate to express a dissent to this, to us, novel Constitutional doctrine. Of course, such principle may subsequently be restricted by this Court to the precise facts of this case—that is to private property in a company town where the owner for his own advantage has permitted a restricted public use by his licensees and invitees. Such distinctions are of degree and require new arbitrary lines, judicially drawn, instead of those hitherto established by legislation and precedent. ***

Appellant was distributing religious pamphlets on a privately owned passway or sidewalk thirty feet removed from a public highway of the State of Alabama and remained on these private premises after an authorized order to get off. We do not understand from the record that there was objection to appellant's use of the nearby public highway and under our decisions she could rightfully have continued her activities a few feet from the spot she insisted upon using. An owner of property may very well have been willing for the public to use the private passway for business purposes and yet have been unwilling to furnish space for street trades or a location for the practice of religious exhortations by itinerants. The passway here in question was not put to any different use than other private passways that lead to privately owned areas, amusement places, resort hotels or other businesses. There had been no dedication of the sidewalk to the public use, express or implied. Alabama so decided and we understand that this Court accepts that conclusion. Alabama, also, decided that appellant violated by her activities the above-quoted state statute. ***

Our Constitution guarantees to every man the right to express his views in an orderly fashion. An essential element of "orderly" is that the man shall also have a right to use the place he chooses for his exposition. The rights of the owner, which the Constitution protects as well as the right of free speech, are not outweighed by the interests of the trespasser, even though he trespasses in behalf of religion or free speech. We cannot say that Jehovah's Witnesses can claim the privilege of a license, which has never been granted, to hold their meetings in other private places, merely because the owner has admitted the public to them for other limited purposes. ***

THE CHIEF JUSTICE and MR. JUSTICE BURTON join in this dissent.

NOTE

There are several different points of emphasis in *Marsh v. Alabama*. Which do you find most persuasive?[139] Why?

A. At the beginning and again at the end, the Court emphasizes the state's own reviewable action as follows:

> In this case, we are asked to decide whether a State, consistently with the First and Fourteenth Amendments, can impose criminal sanctions on a person who undertakes to distribute religious literature on the premises of a company-owned town contrary to the wishes of the town's management.

Is it, then, the use of state power to describe the conduct of the defendant as a crime, and *its* actions in imposing criminal sanctions, that violates the first amendment? Why? Compare these cases:

1. A person who enters or remains on the premises of another for the purpose of distributing religious literature after having been warned not to do so, is guilty of criminal trespass and subject to 30 days in jail, $500 fine, or both.

---

139. Cf. Justice Harlan's dissent in Evans v. Newton, 382 U.S. 297, 319 (1966) (describing *Marsh* as "a shaky precedent"), and see also his dissenting opinion in Burton v. Wilmington Parking Auth., 365 U.S. 715, 728 (1961) ("The Court's opinion, by a process of first undiscriminatingly throwing together various factual bits and pieces and then undermining the resulting structure by an equally vague disclaimer, seems to me to leave completely at sea just what it is in this record that satisfies the requirement of 'state action.'")

2. A person who enters or remains on the premises of another after having been warned not to do so, is guilty of criminal trespass and subject to 30 days in jail, $500 fine, or both.[140]

B. If it is the state's use of criminal sanctions, and not the company's policy *per se* that offends the fourteenth amendment, what follows from that? Suppose the next week Marsh returned to Chickasaw, again to distribute Jehovah's Witness pamphlets in the same place as before. On this occasion, too, an authorized agent of the company, after pointing to the same signs as before (still in place) again asks Marsh to leave. Suppose Marsh refuses, following which the company sues Marsh in state court for civil trespass, but not pressing any criminal charge. Would state court recognition of the validity of the plaintiff's privately brought common law civil trespass action violate the first amendment? Why?[141]

C. In *Marsh*, the entirety of the town was under one corporate ownership, with power akin to that of a city council. But what if it were not so clear a case? Suppose the Gulf Shipbuilding Company, requiring capital to stay in the shipbuilding business, sells off half of its property such that an independent company (e.g., RJR Nabisco) becomes the sole owner of all the land, buildings, streets, etc., on one half of the Main Street, Gulf now being owner of merely the remaining half. Gulf retains the same signage as before. It has nothing to say as to how RJR Nabisco admits or does not admit solicitors to its property. Marsh seeks to distribute Jehovah's Witness pamphlets on Gulf property. As before, Gulf says "no." How will *this* case come out?[142]

---

140. In case 1, the state's position seems to be that of disfavoring acts of trespass by criminal sanction only if they involve religious speech (for only one who attempts to distribute religious literature contrary to the owner's wishes is subject to arrest and no one else). Cf. Burton v. Wilmington Parking Auth., 365 U.S. at 728 (Stewart, J., concurring) (a state law generally disallowing restaurants to refuse service to customers of good deportment but nonetheless permitting them to refuse such service on the grounds of race is violative of the fourteenth amendment). In case 2, the state's position is strictly a general position of protecting "private property rights." If it is nonetheless unconstitutional as applied, what makes it so?

141. Alternatively, suppose merely that employees of the company used minimum reasonable self-help to eject Marsh following Marsh's refusal to leave as requested, and Marsh sued the company for civil assault and battery (or sued for an injunction); if the state court acknowledged that the company's nonviolent ejection of Marsh was privileged under its common law (or refused an injunction), would the state court's acceptance of the defense of privilege be deemed to violate the fourteenth amendment? (Does *Marsh v. Alabama* stand for the proposition that unless the state affirmatively sides with Marsh, i.e. to enable Marsh to distribute her pamphlets at the time, in the place, and in the manner she sought to do, the state is guilty of abridging Marsh's freedom of speech?)

142. Will it make a difference that RJR Nabisco may have no equivalent "no trespass" policy, i.e. it may welcome such activity, such that Marsh could have handed out her pamphlets just a few feet away? Suppose RJR Nabisco and Gulf both subsequently sell off half of each of their respective holdings, such that each now does not control either a town or half a town, but a quarter "town." At what point will *Marsh* no longer control? Why?

In many communities, the downtown area has been pretty well deserted such that efforts to engage residents by handing them leaflets, by engaging them in conversation, or by peaceful demonstration or soapbox talks in the town plaza, may go relatively unnoticed. Businesses have moved out to the suburbs and to large shopping malls surrounded by extensive parking aprons, taking the activity of the community to the malls. To what extent may the first amendment extend free speech easements to these locations as well? Consider the following principal cases.[143]

HUDGENS v. NLRB

424 U.S. 507 (1976)

MR. JUSTICE STEWART delivered the opinion of the Court.

I

The petitioner, Scott Hudgens, is the owner of the North DeKalb Shopping Center, located in suburban Atlanta, Ga. The center consists of a single large building with an enclosed mall. Surrounding the building is a parking area which can accommodate 2,640 automobiles. The shopping center houses 60 retail stores leased to various businesses. One of the lessees is the Butler Shoe Co. Most of the stores, including Butler's, can be entered only from the interior mall.

In January 1971, warehouse employees of the Butler Shoe Co. went on strike to protest the company's failure to agree to demands made by their union in contract negotiations. The strikers decided to picket not only Butler's warehouse but its nine retail stores in the Atlanta area as well, including the store in the North DeKalb Shopping Center. [F]our of the striking warehouse employees entered the center's enclosed mall carrying placards which read: "Butler Shoe Warehouse on Strike, AFL-CIO, Local 315." The general manager of the shopping center informed the employees that they could not picket within the mall or on the parking lot and threatened them with arrest if they did not leave. The employees departed but returned a short time later and began picketing in an area of the mall immediately adjacent to the entrances of the Butler store. After the picketing had continued for approximately 30 minutes, the shopping center manager again informed the pickets that if they did not leave they would be arrested for trespassing. The pickets departed.

The union subsequently filed with the Board an unfair labor practice charge against Hudgens, alleging interference with rights protected by § 7 of the Act, 29

---

143. See Herbert Wechsler, Toward Neutral Principles of Constitutional Law, 73 Harv.L.Rev. 1, 31 (1959) ("Many understandably would like to perceive in [cases such as *Marsh*] a principle susceptible of broad extension, applying to the other power aggregates in our society limitations of the kind the Constitution has imposed on government.") (citing Adolf A. Berle, Constitutional Limitations on Corporate Activity—Protection of Personal Rights from Invasion Through Economic Power, 100 U.Pa. L.Rev. 933 (1952)).

U.S.C. § 157. Relying on this Court's decision in Food Employees v. Logan Valley Plaza, 391 U.S. 308, the Board entered a cease-and-desist order against Hudgens, reasoning that because the warehouse employees enjoyed a First Amendment right to picket on the shopping center property, the owner's threat of arrest violated § 8(a)(1) of the Act, 29 U.S.C. § 158(a)(1). ***

II

***

It is, of course, a commonplace that the constitutional guarantee of free speech is a guarantee only against abridgment by government, federal or state. Thus, while statutory or common law may in some situations extend protection or provide redress against a private corporation or person who seeks to abridge the free expression of others, no such protection or redress is provided by the Constitution itself.

This elementary proposition is little more than a truism. But even truisms are not always unexceptionably true, and an exception to this one was recognized almost 30 years ago in Marsh v. Alabama, 326 U.S. 501. In *Marsh,* a Jehovah's Witness who had distributed literature without a license on a sidewalk in Chickasaw, Ala., was convicted of criminal trespass. Chickasaw was a so-called company town, wholly owned by the Gulf Shipbuilding Corp. ***

The Court pointed out that if the "title" to Chickasaw had "belonged not to a private but to a municipal corporation and had appellant been arrested for violating a municipal ordinance rather than a ruling by those appointed by the corporation to manage a company town it would have been clear that appellant's conviction must be reversed." Concluding that Gulf's "property interests" should not be allowed to lead to a different result in Chickasaw, which did "not function differently from any other town," the Court invoked the First and Fourteenth Amendments to reverse the appellant's conviction.

It was the *Marsh* case that in 1968 provided the foundation for the Court's decision in Amalgamated Food Employees Union v. Logan Valley Plaza, 391 U.S. 308. That case involved peaceful picketing within a large shopping center near Altoona, Pa. One of the tenants of the shopping center was a retail store that employed a wholly nonunion staff. Members of a local union picketed the store, carrying signs proclaiming that it was nonunion and that its employees were not receiving union wages or other union benefits. The picketing took place on the shopping center's property in the immediate vicinity of the store. *** This Court held that the doctrine of the *Marsh* case required reversal of that judgment. ***

There were three dissenting opinions in the *Logan Valley* case, one of them by the author of the Court's opinion in *Marsh,* Mr. Justice Black. His disagreement with the Court's reasoning was total:

> ***
>
> "The question is, Under what circumstances can private property be treated as though it were public? The answer that *Marsh* gives is when that property has taken on all the attributes of a town, *i.e.*, 'residential buildings, streets, a system

of sewers, a sewage disposal plant and a "business block" on which business places are situated.' 326 U.S., at 502. I can find nothing in *Marsh* which indicates that if one of these features is present, *e.g.*, a business district, this is sufficient for the Court to confiscate a part of an owner's private property and give its use to people who want to picket on it." ***

Four years later the Court had occasion to reconsider the *Logan Valley* doctrine in Lloyd Corp. v. Tanner, 407 U.S. 551. That case involved a shopping center covering some 50 acres in downtown Portland, Ore. On a November day in 1968 five young people entered the mall of the shopping center and distributed handbills protesting the then ongoing American military operations in Vietnam. Security guards told them to leave, and they did so, "to avoid arrest." They subsequently brought suit in a Federal District Court, seeking declaratory and injunctive relief. The trial court ruled in their favor, holding that the distribution of handbills on the shopping center's property was protected by the First and Fourteenth Amendments. The Court of Appeals for the Ninth Circuit affirmed the judgment, expressly relying on this Court's *Marsh* and *Logan Valley* decisions. This Court reversed the judgment of the Court of Appeals.

The Court in its *Lloyd* opinion did not say that it was overruling the *Logan Valley* decision. Indeed, a substantial portion of the Court's opinion in *Lloyd* was devoted to pointing out the differences between the two cases, noting particularly that, in contrast to the handbilling in *Lloyd*, the picketing in *Logan Valley* had been specifically directed to a store in the shopping center and the pickets had had no other reasonable opportunity to reach their intended audience. *** But the fact is that the reasoning of the Court's opinion in *Lloyd* cannot be squared with the reasoning of the Court's opinion in *Logan Valley*. ***

If a large self-contained shopping center *is* the functional equivalent of a municipality, as *Logan Valley* held, then the First and Fourteenth Amendments would not permit control of speech within such a center to depend upon the speech's content. For while a municipality may constitutionally impose reasonable time, place, and manner regulations on the use of its streets and sidewalks for First Amendment purposes, see Cox v. New Hampshire, 312 U.S. 569; Poulos v. New Hampshire, 345 U.S. 395, and may even forbid altogether such use of some of its facilities, see Adderley v. Florida, 385 U.S. 39; what a municipality may not do under the First and Fourteenth Amendments is to discriminate in the regulation of expression on the basis of the content of that expression, Erznoznik v. City of Jacksonville, 422 U.S. 205. "[A]bove all else, the First Amendment means that government has no power to restrict expression because of its message, its ideas, its subject matter, or its content." Police Dept. of Chicago v. Mosley, 408 U.S. 92, 95. It conversely follows, therefore, that if the respondents in the *Lloyd* case did not have a First Amendment right to enter that shopping center to distribute handbills concerning Vietnam, then the pickets in the present case did not have a First Amendment right to enter this shopping center for the purpose of advertising their strike against the Butler Shoe Co.

We conclude, in short, that under the present state of the law the constitutional guarantee of free expression has no part to play in a case such as this. ***

For the reasons stated in this opinion, the judgment is vacated and the case is remanded to the Court of Appeals with directions to remand to the National Labor Relations Board, so that the case may be there considered under the statutory criteria of the National Labor Relations Act alone.

MR. JUSTICE STEVENS took no part in the consideration or decision of this case.

MR. JUSTICE POWELL, with whom THE CHIEF JUSTICE joins, concurring.

Although I agree with MR. JUSTICE WHITE's view concurring in the result that Lloyd Corp. v. Tanner, 407 U.S. 551 (1972), did not overrule Food Employees v. Logan Valley Plaza, 391 U.S. 308 (1968), and that the present case can be distinguished narrowly from *Logan Valley*, I nevertheless have joined the opinion of the Court today. *** I now agree with Mr. Justice Black that the opinions in these cases cannot be harmonized in a principled way. Upon more mature thought, I have concluded that we would have been wiser in *Lloyd Corp.* to have confronted this disharmony rather than draw distinctions based upon rather attenuated factual differences.

The Court's opinion today clarifies the confusion engendered by these cases by accepting Mr. Justice Black's reading of *Marsh* and by recognizing more sharply the distinction between the First Amendment and labor law issues that may arise in cases of this kind. It seems to me that this clarification of the law is desirable.

MR. JUSTICE WHITE, concurring in the result.

While I concur in the result reached by the Court, I find it unnecessary to inter Food Employees v. Logan Valley Plaza, 391 U.S. 308 (1968), and therefore do not join the Court's opinion. ***

MR. JUSTICE MARSHALL, with whom MR. JUSTICE BRENNAN joins, dissenting.

***

The Court adopts the view that *Marsh* has no bearing on this case because the privately owned property in *Marsh* involved all the characteristics of a typical town. But there is nothing in *Marsh* to suggest that its general approach was limited to the particular facts of that case. The underlying concern in *Marsh* was that traditional public channels of communication remain free, regardless of the incidence of ownership. Given that concern, the crucial fact in *Marsh* was that the company owned the traditional forums essential for effective communication; it was immaterial that the company also owned a sewer system and that its property in other respects resembled a town.

In *Logan Valley* we recognized what the Court today refuses to recognize—that the owner of the modern shopping center complex, by dedicating his property to public use as a business district, to some extent displaces the "State" from control of historical First Amendment forums, and may acquire a virtual monopoly of places suitable for effective communication. The roadways, parking lots, and walkways of the modern shopping center may be as essential for effective speech as the streets and sidewalks in the municipal or company-owned town. I simply cannot reconcile the Court's denial of any role for the First Amendment in the shopping center with *Marsh*'s recognition of a full role for the First Amendment on the streets and sidewalks of the company-owned town. ***

PRUNEYARD SHOPPING CENTER v. ROBINS

447 U.S. 74 (1980)

MR. JUSTICE REHNQUIST delivered the opinion of the Court.

We postponed jurisdiction of this appeal from the Supreme Court of California to decide the important federal constitutional questions it presented. Those are whether state constitutional provisions, which permit individuals to exercise free speech and petition rights on the property of a privately owned shopping center to which the public is invited, violate the shopping center owner's property rights under the Fifth and Fourteenth Amendments or his free speech rights under the First and Fourteenth Amendments.

I

Appellant PruneYard is a privately owned shopping center in the city of Campbell, Cal. It covers approximately 21 acres—5 devoted to parking and 16 occupied by walkways, plazas, sidewalks, and buildings that contain more than 65 specialty shops, 10 restaurants, and a movie theater. The PruneYard is open to the public for the purpose of encouraging the patronizing of its commercial establishments. It has a policy not to permit any visitor or tenant to engage in any publicly expressive activity, including the circulation of petitions, that is not directly related to its commercial purposes. This policy has been strictly enforced in a nondiscriminatory fashion. ***

Appellees are high school students who sought to solicit support for their opposition to a United Nations resolution against "Zionism." On a Saturday afternoon they set up a card table in a corner of PruneYard's central courtyard. They distributed pamphlets and asked passersby to sign petitions, which were to be sent to the President and Members of Congress. Their activity was peaceful and orderly and so far as the record indicates was not objected to by PruneYard's patrons.

Soon after appellees had begun soliciting signatures, a security guard informed them that they would have to leave because their activity violated PruneYard regulations. The guard suggested that they move to the public sidewalk at the PruneYard's perimeter. Appellees immediately left the premises and later filed this lawsuit in the California Superior Court of Santa Clara County. ***

The California Supreme Court [held] that the California Constitution protects "speech and petitioning, reasonably exercised, in shopping centers even when the centers are privately owned." It concluded that appellees were entitled to conduct their activity on PruneYard property. *** Before this Court, appellants contend that their constitutionally established rights under the Fourteenth Amendment to exclude appellees from adverse use of appellants' private property cannot be denied by invocation of a state constitutional provision or by judicial reconstruction of a State's laws of private property. We postponed consideration of the question of jurisdiction until the hearing of the case on the merits. *** We now affirm.

Appellants first contend that Lloyd Corp. v. Tanner, 407 U.S. 551 (1972), prevents the State from requiring a private shopping center owner to provide access to persons exercising their state constitutional rights of free speech and petition when adequate alternative avenues of communication are available. *** Respondents in *Lloyd* argued that because the shopping center was open to the public, the First Amendment prevents the private owner from enforcing the handbilling restriction on shopping center premises. In rejecting this claim we substantially repudiated the rationale of Food Employees v. Logan Valley Plaza, 391 U.S. 308 (1968), which was later overruled in Hudgens v. NLRB, 424 U.S. 507 (1976). We stated that property does not "lose its private character merely because the public is generally invited to use it for designated purposes," and that "[t]he essentially private character of a store and its privately owned abutting property does not change by virtue of being large or clustered with other stores in a modern shopping center." ***

Our reasoning in *Lloyd*, however, does not *ex proprio vigore* limit the authority of the State to exercise its police power or its sovereign right to adopt in its own Constitution individual liberties more expansive than those conferred by the Federal Constitution. *** It is, of course, well established that a State in the exercise of its police power may adopt reasonable restrictions on private property so long as the restrictions do not amount to a taking without just compensation or contravene any other federal constitutional provision. ***

Appellants next contend that a right to exclude others underlies the Fifth Amendment guarantee against the taking of property without just compensation and the Fourteenth Amendment guarantee against the deprivation of property without due process of law.

It is true that one of the essential sticks in the bundle of property rights is the right to exclude others. Kaiser Aetna v. United States, 444 U.S. 164, 179-180 (1979). And here there has literally been a "taking" of that right to the extent that the California Supreme Court has interpreted the State Constitution to entitle its citizens to exercise free expression and petition rights on shopping center property.[6] But it is well established that "not every destruction or injury to property by governmental action has been held to be a 'taking' in the constitutional sense." Armstrong v. United States, 364 U.S. 40, 48 (1960). Rather, the determination whether a state law unlawfully infringes a landowner's property in violation of the Taking Clause requires an examination of whether the restriction on private property "forc[es] some people alone to bear public burdens which, in all fairness and justice, should be borne by the public as a whole." *Id.*, at 49. This examination entails inquiry into such factors as the character of the governmental action, its economic impact, and its interference with reasonable investment-backed expectations. When "regulation goes too far it will be recognized as a taking." Pennsylvania Coal Co. v. Mahon, 260 U.S. 393, 415 (1922).

Here the requirement the appellants permit appellees to exercise state-protected rights of free expression and petition on shopping center property clearly does not amount to an unconstitutional infringement of appellants' property rights under the Taking Clause. There is nothing to suggest that preventing appellants from prohibiting this sort of activity will unreasonably impair the value or use of their property as a shopping center. The PruneYard is a large commercial complex that covers several city blocks, contains numerous separate business establishments, and is open to the public at large. The decision of the California Supreme Court makes it clear that the PruneYard may restrict expressive activity by adopting time, place, and manner regulations that will minimize any interference with its commercial functions. Appellees were orderly, and they limited their activity to the common areas of the shopping center. In these circumstances, the fact that they may have "physically invaded" appellants' property cannot be viewed as determinative. ***

Appellants finally contend that a private property owner has a First Amendment right not to be forced by the State to use his property as a forum for the speech of others. They state that in Wooley v. Maynard, 430 U.S. 705 (1977), this Court concluded that a State may not constitutionally require an individual to participate in the dissemination of an ideological message by displaying it on his private property in a manner and for the express purpose that it be observed and read by the public. This rationale applies here, they argue, because the message of *Wooley* is that the State may not force an individual to display any message at all.

Wooley, however, was a case in which the government itself prescribed the message, required it to be displayed openly on appellee's personal property that was

---

6. The term "property" as used in the Taking Clause includes the entire "group of rights inhering in the citizen's [ownership]." United States v. General Motors Corp., 323 U.S. 373 (1945). It is not used in the "vulgar and untechnical sense of the physical thing with respect to which the citizen exercises rights recognized by law. [Instead, it] denote[s] the group of rights inhering in the citizen's relation to the physical thing, as the right to possess, use and dispose of it ***. The constitutional provision is addressed to every sort of interest the citizen may possess." *Id.*, at 377-378.

used "as part of his daily life," and refused to permit him to take any measures to cover up the motto even though the Court found that the display of the motto served no important state interest. Here, by contrast, there are a number of distinguishing factors. Most important, the shopping center by choice of its owner is not limited to the personal use of appellants. It is instead a business establishment that is open to the public to come and go as they please. The views expressed by members of the public in passing out pamphlets or seeking signatures for a petition thus will not likely be identified with those of the owner. Second, no specific message is dictated by the State to be displayed on appellants' property. There consequently is no danger of governmental discrimination for or against a particular message. Finally, as far as appears here appellants can expressly disavow any connection with the message by simply posting signs in the area where the speakers or handbillers stand. Such signs, for example, could disclaim any sponsorship of the message and could explain that the persons are communicating their own messages by virtue of state law.

Appellants also argue that their First Amendment rights have been infringed in light of *** Miami Herald Publishing Co. v. Tornillo, 418 U.S. 241 (1974). ***

Tornillo struck down a Florida statute requiring a newspaper to publish a political candidate's reply to criticism previously published in that newspaper. It rests on the principle that the State cannot tell a newspaper what it must print. The Florida statute contravened this principle in that it "exact[ed] a penalty on the basis of the content of a newspaper." There also was a danger in *Tornillo* that the statute would "dampe[n] the vigor and limi[t] the variety of public debate" by deterring editors from publishing controversial political statements that might trigger the application of the statute. Thus, the statute was found to be an "intrusion into the function of editors." These concerns obviously are not present here.

We conclude that neither appellants' federally recognized property rights nor their First Amendment rights have been infringed by the California Supreme Court's decision recognizing a right of appellees to exercise state-protected rights of expression and petition on appellants' property. The judgment of the Supreme Court of California is therefore affirmed.

MR. JUSTICE MARSHALL, concurring. [Omitted.]

MR. JUSTICE WHITE, concurring in part and concurring in the judgment.

***

I concur in this judgment, but I agree with MR. JUSTICE POWELL that there are other circumstances that would present a far different First Amendment issue. May a State require the owner of a shopping center to subsidize any and all political, religious, or social-action groups by furnishing a convenient place for them to urge their views on the public and to solicit funds from likely prospects? Surely there are some limits on state authority to impose such requirements; and in this respect, I am not in entire accord with Part V of the Court's opinion.

MR. JUSTICE POWELL, with whom MR. JUSTICE WHITE joins, concurring in part and in the judgment.

***

Restrictions on property use, like other state laws, are invalid if they infringe the freedom of expression and belief protected by the First and Fourteenth Amendments. In Part V of today's opinion, the Court rejects appellants' contention that "a private property owner has a First Amendment right not to be forced by the State to use his property as a forum for the speech of others." *** I agree that the owner of this shopping center has failed to establish a cognizable First Amendment claim in this case. But some of the language in the Court's opinion is unnecessarily and perhaps confusingly broad. In my view, state action that transforms privately owned property into a forum for the expression of the public's views could raise serious First Amendment questions. ***

If a state law mandated public access to the bulletin board of a freestanding store, hotel, office, or small shopping center, customers might well conclude that the messages reflect the view of the proprietor. The same would be true if the public were allowed to solicit or distribute pamphlets in the entrance area of a store or in the lobby of a private building. The property owner or proprietor would be faced with a choice: he either could permit his customers to receive a mistaken impression or he could disavow the messages. Should he take the first course, he effectively has been compelled to affirm someone else's belief. Should he choose the second, he has been forced to speak when he would prefer to remain silent. In short, he has lost control over his freedom to speak or not to speak on certain issues. The mere fact that he is free to dissociate himself from the views expressed on his property, *** cannot restore his "right to refrain from speaking at all." *Wooley v. Maynard*, at 714. ***

To require the owner to specify the particular ideas he finds objectionable enough to compel a response would force him to relinquish his "freedom to maintain his own beliefs without public disclosure." *** Thus, the right to control one's own speech may be burdened impermissibly even when listeners will not assume that the messages expressed on private property are those of the owner. *** I do not interpret our decision today as a blanket approval for state efforts to transform privately owned commercial property into public forums. Any such state action would raise substantial federal constitutional questions not present in this case.

NOTES

Cases like *Marsh* and *Hudgens* trace out an uncertain line in applying the first amendment to private property.[144] Additionally, where a rule has been formulated by a private entity to limit speech activity of those subject to the private entity, but the rule itself was expressly encouraged by an agency of government, courts have sometimes found the rule is subject to direct first amendment review.[145] And the *PruneYard* case provides a good example of the practical wisdom to see whether state constitutional clauses may cover more than either the first or the fourteenth amendment—by way of providing speech access to private enclaves.[146]

More recently still, some agencies of government have begun to "privatize" portions of the public sector (e.g., charter schools, private prisons under contract to the state). So the same "state action-free speech" question may now arise in this new setting as well: at what point may the disassociation of a company from direct operation by government, or at what point may delegation of responsibilities previously fulfilled by some government agency, become sufficiently detached to enable the new, separate entity the same freedom to make business decisions as other private companies —freed from third-party first amendment claims? The Supreme Court recently addressed this question in respect to Pennsylvania Station in New York City, under the control of Amtrak.

---

144. Would *Marsh* enable labor organizers to go onto privately owned farms to contact migratory farm workers temporarily housed there, or would *Hudgens* sustain the validity of a trespass prosecution as brought on behalf of the owner who forbade such entry? See Note, First Amendment and the Problem of Access to Migrant Labor Camps, 60 Cornell L.Rev. 560 (1976).

145. See, e.g., Alliance for Community Media v. FCC, 10 F.3d 812, 818 (D.C. Cir. 1993) and cases cited therein (private cable television operator's ban disallowing certain speech over its facility struck down on first amendment grounds, where the company's policy resulted from "significant encourage[ment of] the private actor to commit the infringement," by the FCC). Universities receiving federal assistance funds are expected to adopt rules forbidding sexually harassing speech, pursuant to Title IX of the Educational Amendments Act of 1972. (*Query*, would a private university rule adopted in order to be in compliance with federal requirements be subject to first amendment review?)

146. See also Gerald E. Weiss, Stepping into the Breach: State Constitutional Protection of Expressive Rights in Private Owned Commercial Establishments, 4 Emerging Issues in St.Const.L. 159 (1991) (noting that New Jersey, Massachusetts, Oregon and Washington have followed *PruneYard*, while Michigan, Connecticut, New York, North Carolina, Pennsylvania, and Wisconsin have not). At least one state supreme court has applied the state constitutional free speech clause to the open parts of a private university campus (Princeton). State v. Schmid, 423 A.2d 615 (N.J. 1980), appeal dismissed sub. nom. Princeton University v. Schmid, 455 U.S. 100 (1982).

LEBRON v. NATIONAL RAILROAD PASSENGER CORPORATION

513 U.S. 374 (1995)

JUSTICE SCALIA delivered the opinion of the Court.

In this case we consider whether actions of the National Railroad Passenger Corporation, commonly known as Amtrak, are subject to the constraints of the Constitution.

I

Petitioner, Michael A. Lebron, creates billboard displays that involve commentary on public issues, and that seemingly propel him into litigation. In August 1991, he contacted Transportation Displays, Incorporated (TDI), which manages the leasing of the billboards in Amtrak's Pennsylvania Station in New York City, seeking to display an advertisement on a billboard of colossal proportions, known to New Yorkers as "the Spectacular." The Spectacular is a curved, illuminated billboard, approximately 103 feet long and 10 feet high, which dominates the main entrance to Penn Station's waiting room and ticket area.

Lebron signed a contract with TDI to display an advertisement on the Spectacular for two months beginning in January 1993. The contract provided that "[a]ll advertising copy is subject to approval of TDI and [Amtrak] as to character, text, illustration, design and operation." Lebron declined to disclose the specific content of his advertisement throughout his negotiations with TDI, although he did explain to TDI that it was generally political. On December 2 he submitted to TDI (and TDI later forwarded to Amtrak) an advertisement described by the District Court as follows: "The work is a photomontage, accompanied by considerable text. Taking off on a widely circulated Coors beer advertisement which proclaims Coors to be the 'Right Beer,' Lebron's piece is captioned 'Is it the Right's Beer Now?' It includes photographic images of convivial drinkers of Coors beer, juxtaposed with a Nicaraguan village scene in which peasants are menaced by a can of Coors that hurtles towards them, leaving behind a trail of fire, as if it were a missile. The accompanying text, appearing on either end of the montage, criticizes the Coors family for its support of right-wing causes, particularly the contras in Nicaragua. Again taking off on Coors' advertising which uses the slogan of 'Silver Bullet' for its beer cans, the text proclaims that Coors is 'The Silver Bullet that aims The Far Right's political agenda at the heart of America.'" Amtrak's vice president disapproved the advertisement, invoking Amtrak's policy, inherited from its predecessor as landlord of Penn Station, the Pennsylvania Railroad Company, "that it will not allow political advertising on the [S]pectacular advertising sign."

Lebron then filed suit against Amtrak and TDI, claiming *** that the refusal to place his advertisement on the Spectacular had violated his First and Fifth Amendment rights. After expedited discovery, the District Court ruled that Amtrak, because of its close ties to the Federal Government, was a Government actor, at least for First Amendment purposes, and that its rejection of Lebron's proposed advertisement as unsuitable for display in Penn Station had violated the First Amendment. The court granted Lebron an injunction and ordered Amtrak and TDI to display Lebron's advertisement on the Spectacular.

The United States Court of Appeals for the Second Circuit reversed. *** We granted certiorari.

II-III

We have held once, Burton v. Wilmington Parking Authority, 365 U.S. 715 (1961), and said many times, that actions of private entities can sometimes be regarded as governmental action for constitutional purposes. *** It may be unnecessary to traverse that difficult terrain in the present case, since Lebron's first argument is that Amtrak is not a private entity but Government itself. Before proceeding to consider Lebron's contention that Amtrak, though nominally a private corporation, must be regarded as a Government entity for First Amendment purposes, we examine the nature and history of Amtrak and of Government-created corporations in general.

Congress established Amtrak in order to avert the threatened extinction of passenger trains in the United States. The statute that created it begins with the congressional finding, redolent of provisions of the Interstate Commerce Act, that "the public convenience and necessity require the continuance and improvement" of railroad passenger service. Rail Passenger Service Act of 1970 (RPSA), § 101, 84 Stat. 1328. In the current version of the RPSA, the congressional findings are followed by a section entitled "Goals," which include items of such detail as the following:

> (3) Improvement of the number of passenger miles generated systemwide per dollar of Federal funding by at least 30 percent within the two- year period beginning on October 1, 1981.
>
> (4) Elimination of the deficit associated with food and beverage services by September 30, 1982. ***
>
> (6) Operation of Amtrak trains, to the maximum extent feasible, to all station stops within 15 minutes of the time established in public timetables for such operation. ***
>
> (8) Implementation of schedules which provide a systemwide average speed of at least 60 miles per hour. ***"

Later sections of the statute authorize Amtrak's incorporation, set forth its structure and powers, and outline procedures under which Amtrak will relieve private railroads of their passenger-service obligations and provide intercity and commuter rail passenger service itself ***.

Amtrak is incorporated under the District of Columbia Business Corporation Act, but is subject to the provisions of that Act only insofar as the RPSA does not provide to the contrary. It does provide to the contrary with respect to many matters of structure and power, including the manner of selecting the company's board of directors. The RPSA provides for a board of nine members, six of whom are appointed directly by the President of the United States. The Secretary of Transportation, or his designee, sits ex officio. The President appoints three more directors with the advice and consent of the Senate, selecting one from a list of individuals recommended by the Railway Labor Executives Association, one "from among the Governors of States with an interest in rail transportation," and one as a "representative of business with an interest in rail transportation." Since the United States presently holds all of Amtrak's preferred stock, which it received (and still receives) in exchange for its subsidization of Amtrak's perennial losses, the Secretary of Transportation selects these two directors. The ninth member of the board is Amtrak's president, who serves as the chairman of the board, is selected by the other eight directors, and serves at their pleasure. Amtrak's four private shareholders have not been entitled to vote in selecting the board of directors since 1981. By § 548 of the RPSA, Amtrak is required to submit three different annual reports to the President and Congress. ***

Amtrak is not a unique, or indeed even a particularly unusual, phenomenon. In considering the question before us, it is useful to place Amtrak within its proper context in the long history of corporations created and participated in by the United States for the achievement of governmental objectives.

***

The first large-scale use of Government-controlled corporations came with the First World War. In 1917 and 1918 Congress created, among others, the United States Grain Corporation, the United States Emergency Fleet Corporation, the United States Spruce Production Corporation, and the War Finance Corporation. *** The growth of federal corporations during the Depression and the World War II era was not limited to the numerous entities specifically approved by Congress. ***

By the end of World War II, Government-created and -controlled corporations had gotten out of hand, in both their number and their lack of accountability. ***

*** [I]n the years immediately following World War II, many Government corporations were dissolved, and to our knowledge only one, the Saint Lawrence Seaway Development Corporation, was created. In the 1960's, however, the allure of the corporate form was felt again, and new entities proliferated. Many of them followed the traditional model, often explicitly designated as Government agencies and located within the existing Government structure. Beginning in 1962, the Government turned to sponsoring corporations which it specifically designated not to be agencies or establishments of the United States Government, and declined to subject to the control mechanisms of the GCCA. The first of these, the Communications Satellite Corporation (Comsat), was incorporated under the District of Columbia Business Corporation Act, with the purpose of entering the private sector, but doing so with Government- conferred advantages. Comsat was capitalized entirely with private funds. *** In contrast to the corporations that had in the past been deemed part of the Government, Comsat's board was to be controlled by its private shareholders; only 3 of its 15 directors were appointed by the President.

The Comsat model, which was seen as allowing the Government to act unhindered by the restraints of bureaucracy and politics, was soon followed in creating other corporations. But some of these new "private" corporations, though said by their charters not to be agencies or instrumentalities of the Government, see, e.g., 47 U.S.C. § 396(b) (Corporation for Public Broadcasting (CPB)); 42 U.S.C. § 2996d(e)(1) (Legal Services Corporation (LSC)), and though not subjected to the restrictions of the GCCA, were (unlike Comsat) managed by boards of directors on which Government appointees had not just a few votes but voting control.

Amtrak is yet another variation upon the Comsat theme. Like Comsat, CPB and LSC, its authorizing statute declares that it "will not be an agency or establishment of the United States Government." Unlike Comsat, but like CPB and LSC, its board of directors is controlled by Government appointees. And unlike all three of those "private" corporations, it has been added to the list of corporations covered by the GCCA, see 31 U.S.C. § 9101 (1988 ed. and Supp. V). As one perceptive observer has concluded with regard to the post-Comsat Government-sponsored "private" enterprises: "There is no valid basis for distinguishing between many government-sponsored enterprises and other types of government activities, except for the fact that they are designed [designated?] by law as 'not an agency and instrumentality of the United States Government.'"

IV

Amtrak claims that, whatever its relationship with the Federal Government, its charter's disclaimer of agency status prevents it from being considered a Government entity in the present case. This reliance on the statute is misplaced. *** [I]t is not for Congress to make the final determination of Amtrak's status as a government entity for purposes of determining the constitutional rights of citizens affected by its actions. If Amtrak is, by its very nature, what the Constitution regards as the Government, congressional pronouncement that it is not such can no more relieve it of its First Amendment restrictions than a similar pronouncement could exempt the Federal Bureau of Investigation from the Fourth Amendment. ***

V

The question before us today is unanswered, therefore, by governing statutory text or by binding precedent of this Court. Facing the question of Amtrak's status for the first time, we conclude that it is an agency or instrumentality of the United States for the purpose of individual rights guaranteed against the Government by the Constitution.

This conclusion seems to us in accord with public and judicial understanding of the nature of Government-created and -controlled corporations over the years. A remarkable feature of the heyday of those corporations, in the 1930's and 1940's, was that, even while they were praised for their status "as agencies separate and distinct, administratively and financially and legally, from the government itself, [which] has facilitated their adoption of commercial methods of accounting and financing, avoidance of political controls, and utilization of regular procedures of business management," it was fully acknowledged that they were a "device" of "government," and constituted "federal corporate agencies" apart from "regular government departments." Pritchett, 40 Am.Pol.Sci.Rev., at 495. ***

That Government-created and -controlled corporations are (for many purposes at least) part of the Government itself has a strong basis, not merely in past practice and understanding, but in reason itself. It surely cannot be that government, state or federal, is able to evade the most solemn obligations imposed in the Constitution by simply resorting to the corporate form. On that thesis, Plessy v. Ferguson, 163 U.S. 537 (1896), can be resurrected by the simple device of having the State of Louisiana operate segregated trains through a state-owned Amtrak. In Pennsylvania v. Board of Directors of City Trusts of Philadelphia, 353 U.S. 230 (1957) (per curiam), we held that Girard College, which had been built and maintained pursuant to a privately erected trust, was nevertheless a governmental actor for constitutional purposes because it was operated and controlled by a board of state appointees, which was itself a state agency. Amtrak seems to us an *a fortiori* case. ***

We hold that where, as here, the Government creates a corporation by special law, for the furtherance of governmental objectives, and retains for itself permanent authority to appoint a majority of the directors of that corporation, the corporation is part of the Government for purposes of the First Amendment. We express no opinion as to whether Amtrak's refusal to display Lebron's advertisement violated that Amendment, but leave it to the Court of Appeals to decide that. The judgment of the Court of Appeals is reversed, and the case is remanded for further proceedings consistent with this opinion.

JUSTICE O'CONNOR, dissenting.

The Court holds that Amtrak is a Government entity and therefore all of its actions are subject to constitutional challenge. Lebron, however, expressly disavowed this argument below, and consideration of this broad and unexpected question is precluded because it was not presented in the petition for certiorari. The question on which we granted certiorari is narrower: Whether the alleged suppression of Lebron's speech by Amtrak, as a concededly private entity, should be imputed to the Government. Because Amtrak's decision to reject Lebron's billboard proposal was a matter of private business judgment and not of Government coercion, I would affirm the judgment below. ***

QUESTION

In *Lebron*, the Court ruled that Amtrak was an instrumentality of the United States for the purposes of Michael Lebron's challenge. But what of the substance of his challenge—did Amtrak's refusal to place Lebron's political advertisement on a colossal billboard in the main entrance to Pennsylvania Station violate Lebron's first amendment rights?[147]

---

147. *See Lebron v. National Railroad Passenger Corp.*, 69 .F3d 650, *rehearing denied* 89 F.3d 39 (2d cir. 1995). Cf. Lehman v. Shaker Heights, 418 U.S. 298 (1974) (sustaining a ban on all political advertisements inside buses of city transit system, though transit system accepted commercial advertising); Lebron v. Washington Metropolitan Area Transit Auth., 749 F.2d 893 (D.C. Cir. 1984) (invalidating WMATA's refusal—on the grounds of "deceptiveness"—to accept political poster critical of Reagan administration, where subway system accepted other political advertisements, but not ruling on whether WMATA could decline political advertisements in general).

See also New York Magazine v. Metropolitan Transportation Authority, 136 F.3d 123 (2nd Cir. 1998), *cert. denied*, 119 S. Ct. 68 (1998). (The New York MTA leases commercial and political advertising space on outsides of public buses in New York City. All contracts contain an indemnity clause to hold MTA harmless in respect to liability arising from any ads placed with MTA. New York Magazine contracted, for $85,000, for ads to be carried on seventy-five city buses, each prominently featuring the magazine logo and the following eye-catching caption: "Possibly the only good thing in New York Rudy hasn't taken credit for." The name reference ("Rudy") was to Rudolph W. Giuliani, Mayor of New York City. Shortly after the first ads appeared on the buses pursuant to the contract, however, MTA removed them. It did so following complaint to MTA from the mayor's office, requesting prompt removal, and calling to MTA's attention § 50 of N.Y. Civil Rights Law. §50 of the N.Y. Civil Rights Law makes it a misdemeanor and an actionable tort for "any person, firm, or corporation [to] use for advertising purposes...the name, portrait, or picture of any living person without having obtained the consent of such person." In response to MTA's action, New York Magazine at once brought suit in federal court to enjoin MTA, asserting first amendment claims for entitlement to requested relief to have the ads displayed.) (Consider the case in relation to *Lebron*; cases on privacy and misappropriation of personal likeness for commercial gain, casebook, p. 187, n. 96; and with *Hustler*, casebook at p. 215.)

Chapter 4

COERCED EXPRESSION AND FREEDOM NOT TO SPEAK:
THE EXTENT TO WHICH PERSONS MAY BE MADE TO EXPRESS VIEWS OR SUPPORT THE EXPRESSION OF VIEWS, THEY DO NOT HOLD.

INTRODUCTION

In several cases already considered in these cases and materials, we have had occasion to examine the extent to which the First Amendment (and not merely the Fifth Amendment) may or may not limit the power of the government to grant third party speech-access rights to privately held property whose owners would not themselves grant any such rights. Among such cases were *Miami Herald Publishing Co. v. Tornillo; Red Lion Broadcasting Co. v. FCC; Turner Broadcasting Co. v. FCC*; and *Pruneyard Shopping Center v. Robins.*[1] In each, by operation of some force of law, the property owner was required to step aside and permit some person or some group to use their facility as a forum for the expression of their own views. In a number of these cases, moreover, the government's requirement was sustained *e.g., Red Lion* (free access to radio broadcasting facility for right of reply), *Turner* (cablevision company's cable system-free carriage of local broadcasters), and *Robins* (shopping center plaza access for leaflet distribution), albeit not in all (*e.g., Miami Herald*).

In none, however, though there certainly were some significant first amendment rights to consider in these cases, was the imposed-upon party *also* required to express any affirmative endorsement of the person or group thus imposed upon them; much less any obligation to endorse or to parrot their views, or (perish the thought) to contribute money to support them or their activity. Rather, generally, "all" that was required was: (a) not to deny access, and (b) not to presume to control the content or point of view presented. Beyond that, the private property owner could generally proceed as he or she thought best (e.g., to make plain their disassociation from the activity by appropriate disclaimers or sign, or say nothing and just let the matter play itself out, or indeed themselves to offer "countervailing" speech).

To be sure, we have considered some cases in which persons not in fact holding the views they express to others, nonetheless do express those views which they may not agree with– and do so, moreover, under government directive so to do, obliged

---

1. Miami Hearld Publishing Co. v. Tornillo 418 US 241 (1974) p. 200; Red Lion Broadcasting Co. v. FCC 395 US 367 (1969) p. 476; Turner Broadcasting Co. v. FCC 512 US 622 (1994) p. 488; and Pruneyard Shopping Center v. Robins 447 US (1980) p. 537.

to keep silent their dissent, and not advert to countervailing, or additional, information–information which in their own view would be necessary to convey the "truth" as they themselves see that truth. Such is (sometimes) obviously the case of being in the government's own employment: to proceed not as an independent speaker, but as government agent, accepting the job description, without liberty to "distort" or detract from (or even correct?) the message or information the government has seen fit to provide through those whom it will employ, or with whom it will contract, to communicate "its own" speech. Up to a point (it is admittedly still an uncertain one[2]) this remains an area where, indeed, one may be obliged to subordinate one's own freedom of expression inconsistent with the undertaking one has accepted though without duress.

The cases now to be considered, however, though thematically certainly connected (sometimes even overlapping) with these other subjects, go more directly to core first amendment limits on government coercing speech and compelling financial support for groups, expressions, and points of view one would not willingly support, indeed, groups and views one may find anathema to one's own beliefs. Here, one is neither a willing contractor nor an employee or other agent of government (i.e., one who may be significantly circumscribed in conducting oneself *within* that position by the terms of engagement). And neither is it the case that one is a property owner who may (in some circumstances) be obliged to provide some degree of third party access, which, while doubtless compromising of one's freedom to control that property as an exclusionary fief, may otherwise leave one's own freedom of expression, and choice of causes to support, or not, unimpaired. We turn now to see how some of these other matters of coerced expression and support may tend to play themselves out.

WEST VIRGINIA BOARD OF EDUCATION v. BARNETTE
319 U.S. 624 (1943)

MR. JUSTICE JACKSON delivered the opinion of the Court.

Following the decision by this Court on June 3, 1940, in Minersville School District v. Gobitis, 310 U.S. 586, the West Virginia *** Board of Education on January 9, 1942, adopted a resolution containing recitals taken largely from the Court's *Gobitis* opinion and ordering that the salute to the flag become "a regular part of the program of activities in the public schools," that all teachers and pupils "shall be required to participate in the salute honoring the Nation represented by the Flag;

---

2. E.g., compare Rust v. Sullivan (cite and cite also to casebook page) with Legal Services case (121 S.Ct. 1043 (2001) casebook p. 307). Compare also Pickering (391 U.S. 563 (1968) casebook p. 314) and Rankin (483 U.S. 378 (1987) casebook p. 336) with Connick (461 U.S. 138 (1983) casebook p. 329).

provided, however, that refusal to salute the Flag be regarded as an act of insubordination, and shall be dealt with accordingly." ***

Appellees, citizens of the United States and of West Virginia, brought suit in the United States District Court for themselves and others similarly situated asking its injunction to restrain enforcement of these laws and regulations against Jehovah's Witnesses. The Witnesses are an unincorporated body teaching that the obligation imposed by law of God is superior to that of laws enacted by temporal government. Their religious beliefs include a literal version of Exodus, Chapter 20, verses 4 and 5, which says: "Thou shalt not make unto thee any graven image, or any likeness of anything that is in heaven above, or that is in the earth beneath, or that is in the water under the earth; thou shalt not bow down thyself to them nor serve them." They consider that the flag is an "image" within this command. For this reason they refuse to salute it. ***

This case calls us to reconsider a precedent decision, as the Court throughout its history often has been required to do. Before turning to the *Gobitis* case, however, it is desirable to notice certain characteristics by which this controversy is distinguished.

The freedom asserted by these appellees does not bring them into collision with rights asserted by any other individual. It is such conflicts which most frequently require intervention of the State to determine where the rights of one end and those of another begin. But the refusal of these persons to participate in the ceremony does not interfere with or deny rights of others to do so. Nor is there any question in this case that their behavior is peaceable and orderly. The sole conflict is between authority and rights of the individual. The State asserts power to condition access to public education on making a prescribed sign and profession and at the same time to coerce attendance by punishing both parent and child. The latter stand on a right of self-determination in matters that touch individual opinion and personal attitude.

As the present CHIEF JUSTICE said in dissent in the *Gobitis* case, the State may "require teaching by instruction and study of all in our history and in the structure and organization of our government, including the guaranties of civil liberty, which tend to inspire patriotism and love of country." 310 U.S. at 604. Here, however, we are dealing with a compulsion of students to declare a belief. They are not merely made acquainted with the flag salute so that they may be informed as to what it is or even what it means. The issue here is whether this slow and easily neglected route to aroused loyalties constitutionally may be short-cut by substituting a compulsory salute and slogan. ***

There is no doubt that, in connection with the pledges, the flag salute is a form of utterance. Symbolism is a primitive but effective way of communicating ideas. The use of an emblem or flag to symbolize some system, idea, institution, or personality, is a short cut from mind to mind. Causes and nations, political parties, lodges and ecclesiastical groups seek to knit the loyalty of their followings to a flag or banner, a color or design. The State announces rank, function, and authority through crowns and maces, uniforms and black robes; the church speaks through the Cross, the Crucifix, the altar and shrine, and clerical raiment. Symbols of State often convey political ideas just as religious symbols come to convey theological ones. Associated with many of these symbols are appropriate gestures of acceptance or respect: a salute, a bowed or bared head, a bended knee. A person gets from a symbol the meaning he puts into it, and what is one man's comfort and inspiration is another's jest and scorn.

Over a decade ago Chief Justice Hughes led this Court in holding that the display of a red flag as a symbol of opposition by peaceful and legal means to organized government was protected by the free speech guaranties of the Constitution. Stromberg v. California, 283 U.S. 359. Here it is the State that employs a flag as a symbol of adherence to government as presently organized. It requires the individual to communicate by word and sign his acceptance of the political ideas it thus bespeaks. Objection to this form of communication when coerced is an old one, well known to the framers of the Bill of Rights.[13]

It is also to be noted that the compulsory flag salute and pledge requires affirmation of a belief and an attitude of mind. It is not clear whether the regulation contemplates that pupils forego any contrary convictions of their own and become unwilling converts to the prescribed ceremony or whether it will be acceptable if they simulate assent by words without belief and by a gesture barren of meaning. It is now a commonplace that censorship or suppression of expression of opinion is tolerated by our Constitution only when the expression presents a clear and present danger of action of a kind the State is empowered to prevent and punish. It would seem that involuntary affirmation could be commanded only on even more immediate and urgent grounds than silence. But here the power of compulsion is invoked without any allegation that remaining passive during a flag salute ritual creates a clear and present danger that would justify an effort even to muffle expression. To sustain the compulsory flag salute we are required to say that a Bill of Rights which guards the individual's right to speak his own mind, left it open to public authorities to compel him to utter what is not in his mind.

Whether the First Amendment to the Constitution will permit officials to order observance of ritual of this nature does not depend upon whether as a voluntary exercise we would think it to be good, bad or merely innocuous. Any credo of nationalism is likely to include what some disapprove or to omit what others think essential,

---

13. Early Christians were frequently persecuted for their refusal to participate in ceremonies before the statue of the emperor or other symbol of imperial authority. The story of William Tell's sentence to shoot an apple off his son's head for refusal to salute a bailiff's hat is an ancient one. 21 Encyclopedia Britannica (14th ed.) 911-912. The Quakers, William Penn included, suffered punishment rather than uncover their heads in deference to any civil authority. Braithwaite, The Beginnings of Quakerism (1912) 200, 229-230, 232-233, 447, 451; Fox, Quakers Courageous (1941) 113.

and to give off different overtones as it takes on different accents or interpretations.[14] If official power exists to coerce acceptance of any patriotic creed, what it shall contain cannot be decided by courts, but must be largely discretionary with the ordaining authority, whose power to prescribe would no doubt include power to amend. Hence validity of the asserted power to force an American citizen publicly to profess any statement of belief or to engage in any ceremony of assent to one, presents questions of power that must be considered independently of any idea we may have as to the utility of the ceremony in question.

Nor does the issue as we see it turn on one's possession of particular religious views or the sincerity with which they are held. While religion supplies appellees' motive for enduring the discomforts of making the issue in this case, many citizens who do not share these religious views hold such a compulsory rite to infringe constitutional liberty of the individual. It is not necessary to inquire whether non-conformist beliefs will exempt from the duty to salute unless we first find power to make the salute a legal duty.

The *Gobitis* decision, however, *assumed*, as did the argument in that case and in this, that power exists in the State to impose the flag salute discipline upon school children in general. The Court only examined and rejected a claim based on religious beliefs of immunity from an unquestioned general rule. The question which underlies the flag salute controversy is whether such a ceremony so touching matters of opinion and political attitude may be imposed upon the individual by official authority under powers committed to any political organization under our Constitution. We examine rather than assume existence of this power and, against this broader definition of issues in this case, reexamine specific grounds assigned for the *Gobitis* decision.

1. It was said that the flag-salute controversy confronted the Court with "the problem which Lincoln cast in memorable dilemma: 'Must a government of necessity be too *strong* for the liberties of its people, or too *weak* to maintain its own existence?'" and that the answer must be in favor of strength. *Minersville School District v. Gobitis*, at 596.

We think these issues may be examined free of pressure or restraint growing out of such considerations.*** If validly applied to this problem, the utterance cited would resolve every issue of power in favor of those in authority and would require us to override every liberty thought to weaken or delay execution of their policies.

Government of limited power need not be anemic government. Assurance that rights are secure tends to diminish fear and jealousy of strong government, and by making us feel safe to live under it makes for its better support. Without promise of

14. For example: Use of "Republic," if rendered to distinguish our government from a "democracy," or the words "one Nation," if intended to distinguish it from a "federation," open up old and bitter controversies in our political history; "liberty and justice for all," if it must be accepted as descriptive of the present order rather than an ideal, might to some seem an overstatement.

a limiting Bill of Rights it is doubtful if our Constitution could have mustered enough strength to enable its ratification. To enforce those rights today is not to choose weak government over strong government. It is only to adhere as a means of strength to individual freedom of mind in preference to officially disciplined uniformity for which history indicates a disappointing and disastrous end.

The subject now before us exemplifies this principle. Free public education, if faithful to the ideal of secular instruction and political neutrality, will not be partisan or enemy of any class, creed, party, or faction. If it is to impose any ideological discipline, however, each party or denomination must seek to control, or failing that, to weaken the influence of the educational system. Observance of the limitations of the Constitution will not weaken government in the field appropriate for its exercise.

2. It was also considered in the *Gobitis* case that functions of educational officers in States, counties and school districts were such that to interfere with their authority "would in effect make us the school board for the country."

The Fourteenth Amendment, as now applied to the States, protects the citizen against the State itself and all of its creatures—Boards of Education not excepted. These have, of course, important, delicate, and highly discretionary functions, but none that they may not perform within the limits of the Bill of Rights. That they are educating the young for citizenship is reason for scrupulous protection of Constitutional freedoms of the individual, if we are not to strangle the free mind at its source and teach youth to discount important principles of our government as mere platitudes. ***

The very purpose of a Bill of Rights was to withdraw certain subjects from the vicissitudes of political controversy, to place them beyond the reach of majorities and officials and to establish them as legal principles to be applied by the courts. One's right to life, liberty, and property, to free speech, a free press, freedom of worship and assembly, and other fundamental rights may not be submitted to vote: they depend on the outcome of no elections.

*** Nor does our duty to apply the Bill of Rights to assertions of official authority depend upon our possession of marked competence in the field where the invasion of rights occurs. *** [W]e act in these matters not by authority of our competence but by force of our commissions. We cannot, because of modest estimates of our competence in such specialities as public education, withhold the judgment that history authenticates as the function of this Court when liberty is infringed.

4. Lastly, and this is the very heart of the *Gobitis* opinion, it reasons that "National unity is the basis of national security," that the authorities have "the right to select appropriate means for its attainment," and hence reaches the conclusion that such compulsory measures toward "national unity" are constitutional. Upon the verity of this assumption depends our answer in this case.

National unity as an end which officials may foster by persuasion and example is not in question. The problem is whether under our Constitution compulsion as here employed is a permissible means for its achievement.

Struggles to coerce uniformity of sentiment in support of some end thought essential to their time and country have been waged by many good as well as by evil men. Nationalism is a relatively recent phenomenon but at other times and places the ends have been racial or territorial security, support of a dynasty or regime, and particular plans for saving souls. As first and moderate methods to attain unity have failed, those bent on its accomplishment must resort to an ever-increasing severity. As governmental pressure toward unity becomes greater, so strife becomes more bitter as to whose unity it shall be. *** Those who begin coercive elimination of dissent soon find themselves exterminating dissenters. Compulsory unification of opinion achieves only the unanimity of the graveyard.

It seems trite but necessary to say that the First Amendment to our Constitution was designed to avoid these ends by avoiding these beginnings. There is no mysticism in the American concept of the State or of the nature or origin of its authority. We set up government by consent of the governed, and the Bill of Rights denies those in power any legal opportunity to coerce that consent. ***

The case is made difficult not because the principles of its decision are obscure but because the flag involved is our own. Nevertheless, we apply the limitations of the Constitution with no fear that freedom to be intellectually and spiritually diverse or even contrary will disintegrate the social organization. To believe that patriotism will not flourish if patriotic ceremonies are voluntary and spontaneous instead of a compulsory routine is to make an unflattering estimate of the appeal of our institutions to free minds. [F]reedom to differ is not limited to things that do not matter much. That would be a mere shadow of freedom. The test of its substance is the right to differ as to things that touch the heart of the existing order.

If there is any fixed star in our constitutional constellation, it is that no official, high or petty, can prescribe what shall be orthodox in politics, nationalism, religion, or other matters of opinion or force citizens to confess by word or act their faith therein. If there are any circumstances which permit an exception, they do not now occur to us.[19]

We think the action of the local authorities in compelling the flag salute and pledge transcends constitutional limitations on their power and invades the sphere of intellect and spirit which it is the purpose of the First Amendment to our Constitution to reserve from all official control.

The decision of this Court in *Minersville School District v. Gobitis* and the holdings of those few *per curiam* decisions which preceded and foreshadowed it are

---

19. The Nation may raise armies and compel citizens to give military service. Selective Draft Law Cases, 245 U.S. 366. It follows, of course, that those subject to military discipline are under many duties and may not claim many freedoms that we hold inviolable as to those in civilian life. [**Ed. Note.** True to this dictum, the Supreme Court has sustained a variety of first amendment restrictions on military personnel nearly certain to fail in a civilian setting. See, e.g., Brown v. Glines, 444 U.S. 348 (1980); Parker v. Levy, 417 U.S. 733 (1974).]

overruled, and the judgment enjoining enforcement of the West Virginia Regulation is Affirmed.

MR. JUSTICE ROBERTS and MR. JUSTICE REED adhere to the views expressed by the Court in Minersville School District v. Gobitis, 310 U.S. 586, and are of the opinion that the judgment below should be reversed.

MR. JUSTICE BLACK and MR. JUSTICE DOUGLAS, concurring. [Omitted.]

MR. JUSTICE MURPHY, concurring. [Omitted.]

MR. JUSTICE FRANKFURTER, dissenting.

One who belongs to the most vilified and persecuted minority in history is not likely to be insensible to the freedoms guaranteed by our Constitution. Were my purely personal attitude relevant I should wholeheartedly associate myself with the general libertarian views in the Court's opinion, representing as they do the thought and action of a lifetime. But as judges we are neither Jew nor Gentile, neither Catholic nor agnostic. We owe equal attachment to the Constitution and are equally bound by our judicial obligations whether we derive our citizenship from the earliest or the latest immigrants to these shores. As a member of this Court I am not justified in writing my private notions of policy into the Constitution, no matter how deeply I may cherish them or how mischievous I may deem their disregard. *** In the light of all the circumstances, including the history of this question in this Court, it would require more daring than I possess to deny that reasonable legislators could have taken the action which is before us for review. ***

The present action is one to enjoin the enforcement of this requirement by those in school attendance. We have not before us any attempt by the State to punish disobedient children or visit penal consequences on their parents. All that is in question is the right of the State to compel participation in this exercise by those who choose to attend the public school. ***

The right of West Virginia to utilize the flag salute as part of its educational process is denied because, so it is argued, it cannot be justified as a means of meeting a "clear and present danger" to national unity. *** To apply such a test is for the Court *** to take a felicitous phrase out of the context of the particular situation where it arose and for which it was adapted. Mr. Justice Holmes *** meant merely to indicate that, in view of the protection given to utterance by the First Amendment, in order that mere utterance may not be proscribed, "the words used are used in such circumstances and are of such a nature as to create a clear and present danger that they will bring about the substantive evils that Congress has a right to prevent." ***

Saluting the flag suppresses no belief nor curbs it. Children and their parents may believe what they please, avow their belief and practice it. It is not even remotely suggested that the requirement for saluting the flag involves the slightest restriction against the fullest opportunity on the part both of the children and of their parents to disavow as publicly as they choose to do so the meaning that others attach to the gesture of salute. All channels of affirmative free expression are open to both children and parents. Had we before us any act of the state putting the slightest curbs upon such free expression, I should not lag behind any member of this Court in striking down such an invasion of the right to freedom of thought and freedom of speech protected by the Constitution.

I am fortified in my view of this case by the history of the flag salute controversy in this Court. Five times has the precise question now before us been adjudicated. Four times the Court unanimously found that the requirement of such a school exercise was not beyond the powers of the states. Indeed in the first three cases to come before the Court the constitutional claim now sustained was deemed so clearly unmeritorious that this Court dismissed the appeals for want of a substantial federal question.

WOOLEY v. MAYNARD

430 U.S. 705 (1977)

MR. CHIEF JUSTICE BURGER delivered the opinion of the Court.

The issue on appeal is whether the State of New Hampshire may constitutionally enforce criminal sanctions against persons who cover the motto "Live Free or Die" on passenger vehicle license plates because that motto is repugnant to their moral and religious beliefs.

Since 1969 New Hampshire has required that noncommercial vehicles bear license plates embossed with the state motto, "Live Free or Die." Another New Hampshire statute makes it a misdemeanor "knowingly [to obscure] the figures or letters on any number plate." The term "letters" in this section has been interpreted by the State's highest court to include the state motto.

Appellees George Maynard and his wife Maxine are followers of the Jehovah's Witnesses faith. The Maynards consider the New Hampshire State motto to be repugnant to their moral, religious, and political beliefs,[2] and therefore assert it objectionable to disseminate this message by displaying it on their automobiles. Pursuant to these beliefs, the Maynards began early in 1974 to cover up the motto on their license plates.

On December 28, 1974, Mr. Maynard was again charged with violating §

---

2. Mr. Maynard described his objection to the state motto:
"[B]y religious training and belief, I believe my 'government'—Jehovah's Kingdom—offers everlasting life. It would be contrary to that belief to give up my life for the state, even if it meant living in bondage. Although I obey all laws of the State not in conflict with my conscience, this slogan is directly at odds with my deep religious convictions.

" *** I also disagree with the motto on political grounds. I believe that life is more precious than freedom." Affidavit of George Maynard, App. 3.

262:27-c. He appeared in court on January 31, 1975, and again chose to represent himself; he was found guilty, fined $50, and sentenced to six months in the Grafton County House of Corrections. *** He has served the full sentence.

On March 4, 1975, appellees brought the present action pursuant to 42 U. S. C. § 1983 in the United States District Court for the District of New Hampshire. They sought injunctive and declaratory relief against enforcement of N. H. Rev. Stat. Ann. § 262:27-c, 263:1, insofar as these required displaying the state motto on their vehicle license plates, and made it a criminal offense to obscure the motto. ***

The District Court held that by covering up the state motto "Live Free or Die" on his automobile license plate, Mr. Maynard was engaging in symbolic speech and that "New Hampshire's interest in the enforcement of its defacement statute is not sufficient to justify the restriction on [appellee's] constitutionally protected expression." We find it unnecessary to pass on the "symbolic speech" issue, since we find more appropriate First Amendment grounds to affirm the judgment of the District Court.[10] We turn instead to what in our view is the essence of appellees' objection to the requirement that they display the motto "Live Free or Die" on their automobile license plates. This is succinctly summarized in the statement made by Mr. Maynard in his affidavit filed with the District Court:

> "I refuse to be coerced by the State into advertising a slogan which I find morally, ethically, religiously and politically abhorrent."

We are thus faced with the question of whether the State may constitutionally require an individual to participate in the dissemination of an ideological message by displaying it on his private property in a manner and for the express purpose that it be observed and read by the public. We hold that the State may not do so.

We begin with the proposition that the right of freedom of thought protected by the First Amendment against state action includes both the right to speak freely and the right to refrain from speaking at all. See Board of Education v. Barnette, 319 U.S. 624, 633-634 (1943). ***

The Court in *Barnette*, was faced with a state statute which required public school students to participate in daily public ceremonies by honoring the flag both with words and traditional salute gestures. Compelling the affirmative act of a flag salute involved a more serious infringement upon personal liberties than the passive act of carrying the state motto on a license plate, but the difference is essentially one of degree. Here, as in *Barnette*, we are faced with a state measure which forces an

---

10. We note that appellees' claim of symbolic expression is substantially undermined by their prayer in the District Court for issuance of special license plates not bearing the state motto. This is hardly consistent with the stated intent to communicate affirmative opposition to the motto. Whether or not we view appellees' present practice of covering the motto with tape as sufficiently communicative to sustain a claim of symbolic expression, display of the "expurgated" plates requested by appellees would surely not satisfy that standard. See Spence v. Washington, 418 U.S. 405, 410-411 (1974); United States v. O'Brien, 391 U.S. 367, 376 (1968). (MR. JUSTICE BRENNAN does not join in this note.)

individual, as part of his daily life—to be an instrument for fostering public adherence to an ideological point of view he finds unacceptable. In doing so, the State "invades the sphere of intellect and spirit which it is the purpose of the First Amendment to our Constitution to reserve from all official control."

New Hampshire's statute in effect requires that appellees use their private property as a "mobile billboard" for the State's ideological message—or suffer a penalty, as Maynard already has. As a condition to driving an automobile—a virtual necessity for most Americans—the Maynards must display "Live Free or Die" to hundreds of people each day.[11] The fact that most individuals agree with the thrust of New Hampshire's motto is not the test; most Americans also find the flag salute acceptable. The First Amendment protects the right of individuals to hold a point of view different from the majority and to refuse to foster, in the way New Hampshire commands, an idea they find morally objectionable.

Identifying the Maynards' interests as implicating First Amendment protections does not end our inquiry however. We must also determine whether the State's countervailing interest is sufficiently compelling to justify requiring appellees to display the state motto on their license plates. See, e.g., United States v. O'Brien, 391 U.S. 367, 376-377 (1968). The two interests advanced by the State are that display of the motto (1) facilitates the identification of passenger vehicles,[12] and (2) promotes appreciation of history, individualism, and state pride.

The State first points out that passenger vehicles, but not commercial, trailer, or other vehicles are required to display the state motto. Thus, the argument proceeds, officers of the law are more easily able to determine whether passenger vehicles are carrying the proper plates. However, the record here reveals that New Hampshire passenger license plates normally consist of a specific configuration of letters and numbers, which makes them readily distinguishable from other types of plates, even without reference to the state motto. Even were we to credit the State's reasons and "even though the governmental purpose be legitimate and substantial, that purpose cannot be pursued by means that broadly stifle fundamental personal liberties when the end can be more narrowly achieved. The breadth of legislative abridgment must be viewed in the light of less drastic means for achieving the same basic purpose." Shelton v. Tucker, 364 U.S. 479, 488 (1960) (footnotes omitted).

The State's second claimed interest is not ideologically neutral. The State is

---

11. Some States require that certain documents bear the seal of the State or some other official stamp for purposes of recordation. Such seals might contain, albeit obscurely, a symbol or motto having political or philosophical implications. The purpose of such seal, however, is not to advertise the message it bears but simply to authenticate the document by showing the authority of its origin.

12. The Chief of Police of Lebanon, N. H., testified that "enforcement of the motor vehicle laws is facilitated by the State Motto appearing on non-commercial license plates, the benefits being the ease of distinguishing New Hampshire license plates from those of similar colors of other states and the ease of discovering misuse of license plates, for instance, the use of a 'trailer' license plate on a non-commercial vehicle."

seeking to communicate to others an official view as to proper appreciation of history, state pride, and individualism. Of course, the State may legitimately pursue such interests in any number of ways. However, where the State's interest is to disseminate an ideology, no matter how acceptable to some, such interest cannot outweigh an individual's First Amendment right to avoid becoming the courier of such message.

We conclude that the State of New Hampshire may not require appellees to display the state motto[15] upon their vehicle license plates; and accordingly, we affirm the judgment of the District Court.

Affirmed.

MR. JUSTICE REHNQUIST, with whom MR. JUSTICE BLACKMUN joins, dissenting.

***

I not only agree with the Court's implicit recognition that there is no protected "symbolic speech" in this case, but I think that that conclusion goes far to undermine the Court's ultimate holding that there is an element of protected expression here. The State has not forced appellees to "say" anything; and it has not forced them to communicate ideas with nonverbal actions reasonably likened to "speech," such as wearing a lapel button promoting a political candidate or waving a flag as a symbolic gesture. The State has simply required that *all* noncommercial automobiles bear license tags with the state motto, "Live Free or Die." Appellees have not been forced to affirm or reject that motto; they are simply required by the State, under its police power, to carry a state auto license tag for identification and registration purposes.

[T]he Court relies almost solely on Board of Education v. Barnette, 319 U.S. 624 (1943). The Court cites *Barnette* for the proposition that there is a constitutional right, in some cases, to "refrain from speaking." What the Court does not demonstrate is that there is any "speech" or "speaking" in the context of this case. The Court also relies upon the "right to decline to foster [religious, political, and ideological] concepts," and treats the state law in this case as if it were forcing appellees to proselytize, or to advocate an ideological point of view. But this begs the question. The issue, confronted by the Court, is whether appellees, in displaying as they are required to do, state license tags, the format of which is known to all as having been prescribed by the State, would be considered to be advocating political of ideological views.

The Court recognizes, as it must, that this case substantially differs from *Barnette*, in which schoolchildren were forced to recite the pledge of allegiance while

---

15. It has been suggested that today's holding be read as sanctioning the obliteration of the national motto, "In God We Trust," from United States coins and currency. That question is not before us today but we note that currency, which is passed from hand to hand, differs in significant respects from an automobile, which is readily associated with its operator. Currency is generally carried in a purse or pocket and need not be displayed to the public. The bearer of currency is thus not required to publicly advertise the national motto.

giving the flag salute. *** But having recognized the rather obvious differences between these two cases, the Court does not explain why the same result should obtain. The Court suggests that the test is whether the individual is forced "to be an instrument for fostering public adherence to an ideological point of view he finds unacceptable." But, once again, these are merely conclusory words, barren of analysis. For example, were New Hampshire to erect a multitude of billboards, each proclaiming "Live Free or Die," and tax all citizens for the cost of erection and maintenance, clearly the message would be "fostered" by the individual citizen-taxpayers and just as clearly those individuals would be "instruments" in that communication. Certainly, however, that case would not fall within the ambit of *Barnette*. In that case, as in this case, there is no *affirmation* of belief. For First Amendment principles to be implicated, the State must place the citizen in the position of either apparently or actually "asserting as true" the message. This was the focus of *Barnette*, and clearly distinguishes this case from that one.

In holding that the New Hampshire statute does not run afoul of our holding in *Barnette*, the New Hampshire Supreme Court in *Hoskin*, at 295 A.2d, at 457, aptly articulated why there is no required affirmation of belief in this case:

> "The defendants' membership in a class of persons required to display plates bearing the State motto carries no implication and is subject to no requirement that they endorse that motto or profess to adopt it as matter of belief."

As found by the New Hampshire Supreme Court in *Hoskin*, there is nothing in state law which precludes appellees from displaying their disagreement with the state motto as long as the methods used do not obscure the license plates. Thus appellees could place on their bumper a conspicuous bumper sticker explaining in no uncertain terms that they do not profess the motto "Live Free or Die" and that they violently disagree with the connotations of that motto. Since any implication that they affirm the motto can be so easily displaced, I cannot agree that the state statutory system for motor vehicle identification and tourist promotion may be invalidated under the fiction that appellees are unconstitutionally forced to affirm, or profess belief in, the state motto.

The logic of the Court's opinion leads to startling, and I believe totally unacceptable, results. For example, the mottoes "In God We Trust" and "E Pluribus Unum" appear on the coin and currency of the United States. I cannot imagine that the statutes, proscribing defacement of United States currency impinge upon the First Amendment rights of an atheist. The fact that an atheist carries and uses United States currency does not, in any meaningful sense, convey any affirmation of belief on his part in the motto "In God We Trust." Similarly, there is no affirmation of belief involved in the display of state license tags upon the private automobiles involved here.

I would reverse the judgment of the District Court.

ABOOD v. DETROIT BOARD OF EDUCATION
431 U.S. 209 (1977)

MR. JUSTICE STEWART delivered the opinion of the Court.

The State of Michigan has enacted legislation authorizing a system for union representation of local governmental employees. A union and a local government employer are specifically permitted to agree to an "agency shop" arrangement, whereby every employee represented by a union—even though not a union member—must pay to the union, as a condition of employment, a service fee equal in amount to union dues. The issue before us is whether this arrangement violates the constitutional rights of government employees who object to public-sector unions as such or to various union activities financed by the compulsory service fees.

I

After a secret ballot election, the Detroit Federation of Teachers (Union) was certified in 1967 pursuant to Michigan law as the exclusive representative of teachers employed by the Detroit Board of Education (Board). The Union and the Board thereafter concluded a collective-bargaining agreement effective from July 1, 1969, to July 1, 1971. Among the agreement's provisions was an "agency shop" clause, requiring every teacher who had not become a Union member within 60 days of hire (or within 60 days of January 26, 1970, the effective date of the clause) to pay the Union a service charge equal to the regular dues required of Union members. A teacher who failed to meet this obligation was subject to discharge. Nothing in the agreement, however, required any teacher to join the Union, espouse the cause of unionism, or participate in any other way in Union affairs.

On November 7, 1969—more than two months before the agency-shop clause was to become effective—Christine Warczak and a number of other named teachers filed a class action in a state court, naming as defendants the Board, the Union, and several Union officials. Their complaint, as amended, alleged that they were unwilling or had refused to pay dues and that they opposed collective bargaining in the public sector. The amended complaint further alleged that the Union "carries on various social activities for the benefit of its members which are not available to non-members as a matter of right," and that the Union is engaged

> "in a number and variety of activities and programs which are economic, political, professional, scientific and religious in nature of which Plaintiffs do not approve, and in which they will have no voice, and which are not and will not be collective bargaining activities, i.e., the negotiation and administration of contracts with Defendant Board, and that a substantial part of the sums required to be paid under Agency Shop Clause are used and will continue to be used for the support of such activities and programs, and not solely for the purpose of defraying the cost of Defendant Federation of its activities as bargaining agent for teachers employed by Defendant Board."

The complaint prayed that the agency-shop clause be declared invalid under state law and also under the United States Constitution as a deprivation of, *inter alia*, the plaintiffs' freedom of association protected by the First and Fourteenth Amendments, and for such further relief as might be deemed appropriate.

Upon the defendants' motion for summary judgment, the trial court dismissed the action for failure to state a claim upon which relief could be granted. ***

II (A)

Consideration of the question whether an agency-shop provision in a collective-bargaining agreement covering governmental employees is, as such, constitutionally valid must begin with two cases in this Court that on their face go far toward resolving the issue. The cases are Railway Employees' Dept. v. Hanson, [351 U.S. 225], and Machinists v. Street, 367 U.S. 740.

In the *Hanson* case a group of railroad employees brought an action in a Nebraska court to enjoin enforcement of a union-shop agreement.[10] *** The record in *Hanson* contained no evidence that union dues were used to force ideological conformity or otherwise to impair the free expression of employees, and the Court noted that "[i]f 'assessments' are in fact imposed for purposes not germane to collective bargaining, a different problem would be presented." But the Court squarely held that "the requirement for financial support of the collective-bargaining agency by all who receive the benefits of its work does not violate the First Amendmen[t]."

The Court faced a similar question several years later in the *Street* case, which also involved a challenge to the constitutionality of a union shop authorized by the Railway Labor Act. In *Street*, however, the record contained findings that the union treasury to which all employees were required to contribute had been used "to finance the campaigns of candidates for federal and state offices whom [the plaintiffs] opposed, and to promote the propagation of political and economic doctrines, concepts and ideologies with which [they] disagreed."

The Court recognized that these findings presented constitutional "questions of the utmost gravity" not decided in *Hanson*, and therefore considered whether the Act

---

10. Under a union-shop agreement, an employee must become a member of the union within a specified period of time after hire, and must as a member pay whatever union dues and fees are uniformly required. Under both the National Labor Relations Act and the Railway Labor Act, "[i]t is permissible to condition employment upon membership, but membership, insofar as it has significance to employment rights, may in turn be conditioned only upon payment of fees and dues." ***

Hanson was concerned simply with the requirement of financial support for the union, and did not focus on the question whether the additional requirement of a union-shop arrangement that each employee formally join the union is constitutionally permissible. *** See *NLRB v. General Motors* ("Such a difference between the union and agency shop may be of great importance in some contexts ***") As the agency shop before us does not impose that additional requirement, we have no occasion to address that question.

could fairly be construed to avoid these constitutional issues.[13] The Court concluded that the Act could be so construed, since only expenditures related to the union's functions in negotiating and administering the collective-bargaining agreement and adjusting grievances and disputes fell within "the reasons accepted by Congress why authority to make union-shop agreements was justified." The Court ruled, therefore, that the use of compulsory union dues for political purposes violated the Act itself. ***

The designation of a union as exclusive representative carries with it great responsibilities. The tasks of negotiating and administering a collective-bargaining agreement and representing the interests of employees in settling disputes and processing grievances are continuing and difficult ones. They often entail expenditure of much time and money. *** Moreover, in carrying out these duties, the union is obliged "fairly and equitably to represent all employees, union and non-union," within the relevant unit. A union-shop arrangement has been thought to distribute fairly the cost of these activities among those who benefit, and it counteracts the incentive that employees might otherwise have to become "free riders"—to refuse to contribute to the union while obtaining benefits of union representation that necessarily accrue to all employees.

To compel employees financially to support their collective-bargaining representative has an impact upon their First Amendment interests. An employee may very well have ideological objections to a wide variety of activities undertaken by the union in its role as exclusive representative. His moral or religious views about the desirability of abortion may not square with the union's policy in negotiating a medical benefits plan. One individual might disagree with a union policy of negotiating limits on the right to strike, believing that to be the road to serfdom for the working class, while another might have economic or political objections to unionism itself. An employee might object to the union's wage policy because it violates guidelines designed to limit inflation, or might object to the union's seeking a clause in the collective-bargaining agreement proscribing racial discrimination. The examples could be multiplied. To be required to help finance the union as a collective-bargaining agent might well be thought, therefore, to interfere in some way with an employee's freedom to associate for the advancement of ideas, or to refrain from doing so, as he sees fit. But the judgment clearly made in *Hanson* and *Street* is that such interference as exists is constitutionally justified by the legislative assessment of the important contribution by the union shop to the system of labor relations established by Congress. "The furtherance of the common cause leaves some leeway for the leadership of the group. As long as they act to promote the cause which

---

13. In suggesting that *Street* "significantly undercut," and constituted a "rethinking" of, *Hanson*, the opinion concurring in the judgment loses sight of the fact that the record in *Street*, unlike that in *Hanson*, potentially presented constitutional questions arising from union expenditures for ideological purposes unrelated to collective bargaining.

justified bringing the group together, the individual cannot withdraw his financial support merely because he disagrees with the group's strategy. If that were allowed, we would be reversing the *Hanson* case, *sub silentio*." Machinists v. Street, 367 U.S., at 778 (Douglas, J., concurring).

B

***

Our province is not to judge the wisdom of Michigan's decision to authorize the agency shop in public employment. Rather, it is to adjudicate the constitutionality of that decision. The same important government interests recognized in the *Hanson* and *Street* cases presumptively support the impingement upon associational freedom created by the agency shop here at issue. Thus, insofar as the service charge is used to finance expenditures by the Union for the purposes of collective bargaining, contract administration, and grievance adjustment, those two decisions of this Court appear to require validation of the agency-shop agreement before us.

While recognizing the apparent precedential weight of the *Hanson* and *Street* cases, the appellants advance two reasons why those decisions should not control decision of the present case. First, the appellants note that it is *government employment* that is involved here, thus directly implicating constitutional guarantees, in contrast to the private employment that was the subject of the *Hanson* and *Street* decisions. Second, the appellants say that in the public sector collective bargaining itself is inherently "political," and that to require them to give financial support to it is to require the "ideological conformity" that the Court expressly found absent in the *Hanson* case. We find neither argument persuasive.

Because it is employment by the State that is here involved, the appellants suggest that this case is governed by a long line of decisions holding that public employment cannot be conditioned upon the surrender of First Amendment rights. But, while the actions of public employers surely constitute "state action," the union shop, as authorized by the Railway Labor Act, also was found to result from governmental action in *Hanson*. The plaintiffs' claims in *Hanson* failed, not because there was no governmental action, but because there was no First Amendment violation. The appellants' reliance on the "unconstitutional conditions" doctrine is therefore misplaced.

*** We conclude that the Michigan Court of Appeals was correct in viewing this Court's decisions in *Hanson* and *Street* as controlling in the present case insofar as the service charges are applied to collective-bargaining, contract administration, and grievance-adjustment purposes.

C

Because the Michigan Court of Appeals ruled that state law "sanctions the use of nonunion members' fees for purposes other than collective bargaining," and because the complaints allege that such expenditures were made, this case presents constitutional issues not decided in *Hanson* and *Street*.

Our decisions establish with unmistakable clarity that the freedom of an individual to associate for the purpose of advancing beliefs and ideas is protected by the

First and Fourteenth Amendments. Equally clear is the proposition that a government may not require an individual to relinquish rights guaranteed him by the First Amendment as a condition of public employment. The appellants argue that they fall within the protection of these cases because they have been prohibited, not from actively associating, but rather from refusing to associate. They specifically argue that they may constitutionally prevent the Union's spending a part of their required service fees to contribute to political candidates and to express political views unrelated to its duties as exclusive bargaining representative. We have concluded that this argument is a meritorious one.

The fact that the appellants are compelled to make, rather than prohibited from making, contributions for political purposes works no less an infringement of their constitutional rights.[31] For at the heart of the First Amendment is the notion that an individual should be free to believe as he will, and that in a free society one's beliefs should be shaped by his mind and his conscience rather than coerced by the State. ***

These principles prohibit the appellees from requiring any of the appellants to contribute to the support of an ideological cause he may oppose as a condition of holding a job as a public school teacher.

We do not hold that a union cannot constitutionally spend funds for the expression of political views, on behalf of political candidates, or toward the advancement of other ideological causes not germane to its duties as collective-bargaining representative. Rather, the Constitution requires only that such expenditures be financed from charges, dues, or assessments paid by employees who do not object to advancing those ideas and who are not coerced into doing so against their will by the threat of loss of governmental employment.

There will, of course, be difficult problems in drawing lines between collective-bargaining activities, for which contributions may be compelled, and ideological activities unrelated to collective bargaining, for which such compulsion is prohibited.[33] *** We have no occasion in this case, however, to try to define such a dividing line. All that we decide is that the general allegations in the complaints, if proved, establish a cause of action under the First and Fourteenth Amendments.

---

31. This view has long been held. James Madison, the First Amendment's author, wrote in defense of religious liberty: "Who does not see *** [t]hat the same authority which can force a citizen to contribute three pence only of his property for the support of any one establishment, may force him to conform to any other establishment in all cases whatsoever?" 2 The Writings of James Madison 186 (Hunt ed. 1901). Thomas Jefferson agreed that "'to compel a man to furnish contributions of money for the propagation of opinions which he disbelieves, is sinful and tyrannical.'" I. Brant, James Madison: The Nationalist 354 (1948).

33. The appellants' complaints also alleged that the Union carries on various "social activities" which are not open to nonmembers. It is unclear to what extent such activities fall outside the Union's duties as exclusive representative or involve constitutionally protected rights of association. Without greater specificity in the description of such activities and the benefit of adversary argument, we leave these questions in the first instance to the Michigan courts.

III

In determining what remedy will be appropriate if the appellants prove their allegations, the objective must be to devise a way of preventing compulsory subsidization of ideological activity by employees who object thereto without restricting the Union's ability to require every employee to contribute to the cost of collective- bargaining activities.[35] ***

The judgment is vacated, and the case is remanded for further proceedings not inconsistent with this opinion.*

***

MR. JUSTICE STEVENS, concurring. [Omitted.]

MR. JUSTICE POWELL, with whom THE CHIEF JUSTICE and MR. JUSTICE BLACKMUN join, concurring in the judgment.

***

Before today it had been well established that when state law intrudes upon protected speech, the State itself must shoulder the burden of proving that its action is justified by overriding state interests. See *Elrod v. Burns,* at 363; Healy v. James, 408 U.S. 169, 184 (1972); Speiser v. Randall, 357 U.S. 513, 525-526 (1958). The Court, for the first time in a First Amendment case, simply reverses this principle. Under today's decision a nonunion employee who would vindicate his First Amendment rights apparently must initiate a proceeding to prove that the union has allocated some portion of its budget to "ideological activities unrelated to collective bargaining." I would adhere to established First Amendment principles and require the State to come forward and demonstrate, as to each union expenditure for which

---

35. It is plainly not an adequate remedy to limit the use of the actual dollars collected from dissenting employees to collective-bargaining purposes:

> "[Such a limitation] is of bookkeeping significance only rather than a matter of real substance. It must be remembered that the service fee is admittedly the exact equal of membership initiation fees and monthly dues *** If the union's total budget is divided between collective bargaining and institutional expenses and if nonmember payments, equal to those of a member, go entirely for collective bargaining costs, the nonmember will pay more of these expenses than his pro rata share. The member will pay less and to that extent a portion of his fees and dues is available to pay institutional expenses. The union's budget is balanced. By paying a larger share of collective bargaining costs the nonmember subsidizes the union's institutional activities." Retail Clerks v. Schermerhorn, 373 U.S. 746, 753-754.

*. [**Ed. Note.** See also Keller v. State Bar of Cal., 496 U.S. 1(1990), which applied *Abood* to a state bar association in which membership dues were required of all attorneys as a condition of practicing law in the state. The Court held that dues may be required in respect to bar expenses incidental to professional regulation, but not for activities of an ideological nature (e.g., dues-funded state bar conference at which delegates endorsed gun control legislation, nuclear weapons freeze, and opposed federal legislation limiting federal-court jurisdiction over abortions, public school prayer, busing), remanded the case for the lower court to work out mechanics of excludable dues fraction under formula suggested in an earlier agency shop, Teachers v. Hudson, 475 U.S. 292 (1986), and remanded also on issue of whether membership itself (as distinct from partial dues contribution) may not be required if the bar association continues to assert ideological partisan positions.]

it would exact support from minority employees, that the compelled contribution is necessary to serve overriding governmental objectives. This placement of the burden of litigation, not the Court's, gives appropriate protection to First Amendment rights without sacrificing ends of government that may be deemed important.

NOTE

1. Following *Abood* (and *Keller*), suppose that a student enrolled at the University of Illinois files suit to enjoin the university from requiring a payment of a $25 student activity fee a portion of which is allocated by the student Government Association to a student Public Interest Research Group (PIRG). The PIRG is an organization on campus, open to all students, that devotes some organizational efforts to lobby in Springfield, Illinois, where the state legislature meets, for causes the PIRG believes to be in the public interest: higher minimum wages for workers, state-financed abortion assistance for low income women, additional laws limiting cigarette smoking, community service by students in lieu of tuition fees at state schools. What should the outcome of this case be?[148]

BOARD OF REGENTS OF THE UNIVERSITY OF WISCONSIN v. SOUTHWORTH

529 U.S. 217 (2000)

JUSTICE KENNEDY delivered the opinion of the Court.

Respondents are a group of students at the University of Wisconsin. They brought a First Amendment challenge to a mandatory student activity fee imposed by petitioner Board of Regents of the University of Wisconsin and used in part by the University to support student organizations engaging in political or ideological speech. Respondents object to the speech and expression of some of the student organizations. Relying upon our precedents which protect members of unions and bar associations from being required to pay fees used for speech the members find objectionable, both the District Court and the Court of Appeals invalidated the University's student fee program.

We reverse. The First Amendment permits a public university to charge its students an activity fee used to fund a program to facilitate extracurricular student speech if the program is viewpoint neutral. We do not sustain, however, the student

---

148. As a variation, suppose the mandatory $25 student activity fee is also allocated through the student government association partly to fund the student campus newspaper—a paper that operates under its own staff, with the editor-in-chief being chosen each year by election within the student staff. The newspaper decides its own editorial policy. Generally, that policy has been "center left." What, if anything, may students who disagree with that policy do?

referendum mechanism of the University's program, which appears to permit the exaction of fees in violation of the viewpoint neutrality principle. As to that aspect of the program, we remand for further proceedings.

I

[S]ince its founding the University has required full-time students enrolled at its Madison campus to pay a nonrefundable activity fee. For the 1995-1996 academic year, when this suit was commenced, the activity fee amounted to $331.50 per year. The allocable portion of the fee supports extracurricular endeavors pursued by the University's registered student organizations or RSO's. To qualify for RSO status students must organize as a not-for-profit group, limit membership primarily to students, and agree to undertake activities related to student life on campus. As one would expect, the expressive activities undertaken by RSO's are diverse in range and content, from displaying posters and circulating newsletters throughout the campus, to hosting campus debates and guest speakers, and to what can best be described as political lobbying.

RSO's obtain funding support on a reimbursement basis by submitting receipts or invoices to the University. Guidelines identify expenses appropriate for reimbursement. Permitted expenditures include, in the main, costs for printing, postage, office supplies, and use of University facilities and equipment. Materials printed with student fees must contain a disclaimer that the views expressed are not those of the [Associated Students of Madison]. In March 1996, respondents, each of whom attended or still attend the University's Madison campus, filed suit in the United States District Court for the Western District of Wisconsin against members of the board of regents.***On cross-motions for summary judgment, the District Court ruled in their favor, declaring the University's segregated fee program invalid under *Abood v. Detroit Bd. of Ed.*, 431 U.S. 209 (1977), and *Keller v. State Bar of Cal.*, 496 U.S. 1 (1990).

II

We must begin by recognizing that the complaining students are being required to pay fees which are subsidies for speech they find objectionable, even offensive.***The proposition that students who attend the University cannot be required to pay subsidies for the speech of other students without some First Amendment protection follows from the *Abood* and *Keller* cases. Students enroll in public universities to seek fulfillment of their personal aspirations and of their own potential. If the University conditions the opportunity to receive a college education, an opportunity comparable in importance to joining a labor union or bar association, on an agreement to support objectionable, extracurricular expression by other students, the rights acknowledged in *Abood* and *Keller* become implicated. It infringes on the speech and beliefs of the individual to be required, by this mandatory student activity fee program, to pay subsidies for the objectionable speech of others without any recognition of the State's corresponding duty to him or her. Yet recognition must be given as well to the important and substantial purposes of the

University, which seeks to facilitate a wide range of speech.

In *Abood* and *Keller* the constitutional rule took the form of limiting the required subsidy to speech germane to the purposes of the union or bar association. The standard of germane speech as applied to student speech at a university is unworkable, however, and gives insufficient protection both to the objecting students and to the University program itself. Even in the context of a labor union, whose functions are, or so we might have thought, well known and understood by the law and the courts after a long history of government regulation and judicial involvement, we have encountered difficulties in deciding what is germane and what is not. The difficulty manifested itself in our decision in *Lehnert v. Ferris Faculty Assn.*, 500 U.S. 507 (1991), where different members of the Court reached varying conclusions regarding what expressive activity was or was not germane to the mission of the association. If it is difficult to define germane speech with ease or precision where a union or bar association is the party, the standard becomes all the more unmanageable in the public university setting, particularly where the State undertakes to stimulate the whole universe of speech and ideas.

Just as the vast extent of permitted expression makes the test of germane speech inappropriate for intervention, so too does it underscore the high potential for intrusion on the First Amendment rights of the objecting students. It is all but inevitable that the fees will result in subsidies to speech which some students find objectionable and offensive to their personal beliefs. If the standard of germane speech is inapplicable, then, it might be argued the remedy is to allow each student to list those causes which he or she will or will not support. If a university decided that its students' First Amendment interests were better protected by some type of optional or refund system it would be free to do so. We decline to impose a system of that sort as a constitutional requirement, however. The restriction could be so disruptive and expensive that the program to support extracurricular speech would be ineffective. The First Amendment does not require the University to put the program at risk.

The University may determine that its mission is well served if students have the means to engage in dynamic discussions of philosophical, religious, scientific, social, and political subjects in their extracurricular campus life outside the lecture hall. If the University reaches this conclusion, it is entitled to impose a mandatory fee to sustain an open dialogue to these ends.

The University must provide some protection to its students' First Amendment interests, however. The proper measure, and the principal standard of protection for objecting students, we conclude, is the requirement of viewpoint neutrality in the allocation of funding support. Viewpoint neutrality was the obligation to which we gave substance in *Rosenberger v. Rector and Visitors of Univ. of Va.*, 515 U.S. 819 (1995).***While *Rosenberger* was concerned with the rights a student has to use an extracurricular speech program already in place, today's case considers the antecedent question, acknowledged but unresolved in *Rosenberger*: whether a public university may require its students to pay a fee which creates the mechanism for the extracurricular speech in the first instance. When a university requires its students to pay fees to support the extracurricular speech of other students, all in the interest of open discussion, it may not prefer some viewpoints to others. There is symmetry then in our holding here and in *Rosenberger*: Viewpoint neutrality is the justification for requiring the student to pay the fee in the first instance and for ensuring the integrity of the program's operation once the funds have been collected. We conclude that the University of Wisconsin may sustain the extracurricular dimensions of its programs by using mandatory student fees with viewpoint neutrality as the operational principle.***If the rule of viewpoint neutrality is respected, our holding affords the University latitude to adjust its extracurricular student speech program to accommodate these advances and opportunities.

Our decision ought not to be taken to imply that in other instances the University, its agents or employees, or--of particular importance--its faculty, are subject to the First Amendment analysis which controls in this case. Where the University speaks, either in its own name through its regents or officers, or in myriad other ways through its diverse faculties, the analysis likely would be altogether different.***In the instant case, the speech is not that of the University or its agents. It is not, furthermore, speech by an instructor or a professor in the academic context, where principles applicable to government speech would have to be considered.

III

It remains to discuss the referendum aspect of the University's program. While the record is not well developed on the point, it appears that by majority vote of the student body a given RSO may be funded or defunded. It is unclear to us what protection, if any, there is for viewpoint neutrality in this part of the process. To the extent the referendum substitutes majority determinations for viewpoint neutrality it would undermine the constitutional protection the program requires. The whole theory of viewpoint neutrality is that minority views are treated with the same respect as are majority views. Access to a public forum, for instance, does not depend upon majoritarian consent. That principle is controlling here. A remand is necessary and appropriate to resolve this point; and the case in all events must be reexamined in light of the principles we have discussed.

It is so ordered.

JUSTICE SOUTER, with whom JUSTICE STEVENS AND JUSTICE BREYER join, concurring in the judgment.

The majority today validates the University's student activity fee after recognizing a new category of First Amendment interests and a new standard of viewpoint neutrality protection. I agree that the University's scheme is permissible, but do not believe that the Court should take the occasion to impose a cast-iron viewpoint neutrality requirement to uphold it.

***Our understanding of academic freedom has included not merely liberty from restraints on thought, expression, and association in the academy, but also the idea that universities and schools should have the freedom to make decisions about how and what to teach. In *Regents of Univ. of Mich. v. Ewing*, 474 U.S. 214 (1985), we recognized these related conceptions: "Academic freedom thrives not only on the independent and uninhibited exchange of ideas among teachers and students, but also, and somewhat inconsistently, on autonomous decisionmaking by the academy itself." Some of the opinions in our books emphasize broad conceptions of academic freedom that if accepted by the Court might seem to clothe the University with an immunity to any challenge to regulations made or obligations imposed in the discharge of its educational mission......

[Even so] our cases on academic freedom thus far have dealt with more limited subjects, and do not compel the conclusion that the objecting university student is without a First Amendment claim here.[4] While we have spoken in terms of a wide protection for the academic freedom and autonomy that bars legislatures (and courts) from imposing conditions on the spectrum of subjects taught and viewpoints expressed in college teaching (as the majority recognizes), we have never held that universities lie entirely beyond the reach of students' First Amendment rights. Thus our prior cases do not go so far as to control the result in this one, and going beyond those cases would be out of order, simply because the University has not litigated on grounds of academic freedom. As to that freedom and university autonomy, then, it is enough to say that protecting a university's discretion to shape its educational mission may prove to be an important consideration in First Amendment analysis of objections to student fees.

NOTES AND QUESTIONS

1. Suppose a state legislature concludes that further labor organization in the state may adversely affect the state's general economy by discouraging capital investment and by driving new companies either to other states or, indeed, to relocate outside the United States. The state currently has a "Right to Work" law, disallowing union shops. The legislature believes this legislation to be sound. Nevertheless, trade union organizational and political activity in the state is at such a level that members of the state legislature feel under pressure to repeal that law, a move that a clear majority of the legislature believes would be extremely unwise.

Convinced that the repeal of the state right to work law would be damaging to the state's economy, and convinced, too, that the public does not understand how

4. Our university cases have dealt with restrictions imposed from outside the academy on individual teachers' speech or associations, and cases dealing with the right of teaching institutions to limit expressive freedom of students have been confined to high schools [citations omitted], whose students and their schools' relation to them are different and at least arguably distinguishable from their counterparts in college education.

capital markets operate and how trade union practices can (in the legislature's view) lead to their own serious abuses (e.g., misappropriation of members' dues by union officials, infiltration by organized crime), the legislature appropriates $50 million to be allocated to the State Department of Development specifically to enter into contracts with private advertising firms that will undertake to prepare newspaper and television advertisements. The aim of the advertisements is to bring to public attention the *negative* aspects of trade unions and the *negative* aspects of repealing the right to work law. The purpose is "to serve the public interest as the legislature sees that interest." Is there a first amendment basis to seek to enjoin the expenditure? Who may bring such an action? Where? On what theory might it be based? What relief, if any, are they entitled to receive?[5]

Does the first amendment permit a faction not merely to take control of the legislative process when it succeeds through fair and open elections, but also to harness the power of government to levy taxes to finance tax-funded, government sponsored propaganda respecting the "proper" attitude toward, response to, and treatment of, social, political, and economic issues?[6]

2. Despite *Abood*, may a public school teacher be required to lead the pledge of allegiance as part of his or her regular school duty each day whether or not the teacher disagreed with the contents; or would the reasoning of *Wooley v. Maynard* and *Abood* require that an unwilling teacher be excused from leading this daily recitation? See Opinion of Justices, 371 Mass. 874 (1977) (state supreme court advisory opinion holding state legislative requirement of daily teacher-conducted pledge of allegiance unconstitutional). But see Sherman v. Community Consolidated School District 21, 980 F.2d 437 (7th Cir. 1992), *cert. denied*, 113 S.Ct. 2439 (1993) (suit on behalf of student to enjoin daily pledge in elementary school rejected, dicta broadly accept claim of state authority to inculcate loyalty and patriotism in public

---

5. Is it, at most, that no objecting taxpayer may be denied such pro rata refund of such state taxes as may be reflected by this appropriation, or is there a stronger first amendment object to be made (e.g., that the first amendment disallows "domestic partisan ideological speech" under official government auspices in the United States?)

6. For a troubling treatment of "government speech," see Meese v. Keane, 481 U.S. 465 (1987) (sustaining Department of Justice's labeling as "political propaganda" films which contained political material and were disseminated by "agents" of foreign "principals," and construing such label as "neutral and evenhanded," and without "pejorative connotation," despite appellee's argument that the label would adversely affect his reputation). See also Paul v. Davis, 424 U.S. 693 (1975) (no Fourteenth Amendment due process claim for state-imposed injury to personal reputation alone). For some attempts to come to terms with this kind of question, see Thomas L. Emerson, The System of Free Expression 697-716 (1970); Mark G. Yudof, When Governments Speak: Politics, Law and Government Expression in America (1983); Robert D. Kamenshine, The First Amendment's Implied Establishment Clause, 67 Cal.L.Rev. 1104 (1979); John E. Nowak, Using the Press Clause to Limit Government Speech, 30 Ariz.L.Rev. 1 (1988); Steven H. Shiffrin, Government Speech, 27 UCLA L. Rev. 656 (1980); Mark G. Yudof, Personal Speech and Government Expression, 30 Ariz.L.Rev. 671 (1988); Edward H. Ziegler, Jr., Government Speech and the Constitution: The Limits of Official Partisanship, 21 B.C.L.Rev. 578 (1980).

school curriculum); Palmer v. Board of Education, 603 F.2d 1271 (7th Cir. 1979) (sustaining such a requirement).

JOHN HURLEY AND SOUTH BOSTON ALLIED WAR VETERANS COUNCIL v. IRISH-AMERICAN GAY, LESBIAN AND BISEXUAL GROUP OF BOSTON

515 U.S. 557 (1995).

JUSTICE SOUTER delivered the opinion of the Court.

The issue in this case is whether Massachusetts may require private citizens who organize a parade to include among the marchers a group imparting a message the organizers do not wish to convey. We hold that such a mandate violates the First Amendment.

I

March 17 is set aside for two celebrations in South Boston. As early as 1737, some people in Boston observed the feast of the apostle to Ireland, and since 1776 the day has marked the evacuation of royal troops and Loyalists from the city, prompted by the guns captured at Ticonderoga and set up on Dorchester Heights under General Washington's command. Although the General Court of Massachusetts did not officially designate March 17 as Evacuation Day until 1938, the City Council of Boston had previously sponsored public celebrations of Evacuation Day, including notable commemorations on the centennial in 1876, and on the 125th anniversary in 1901, with its parade, salute, concert, and fireworks display.

The tradition of formal sponsorship by the city came to an end in 1947, when Mayor James Michael Curley granted authority to organize and conduct the St. Patrick's Day-Evacuation Day Parade to the petitioner South Boston Allied War Veterans Council, an unincorporated association of individuals elected from various South Boston veterans groups. Every year since that time the Council has applied for and received a permit for the parade, which at times has included as many as 20,000 marchers and drawn up to 1 million watchers. No other applicant has ever applied for that permit.

1992 was the year that a number of gay, lesbian, and bisexual descendants of the Irish immigrants joined together with other supporters to form the respondent organization, GLIB, to march in the parade. Although the Council denied GLIB's application to take part in the 1992 parade, GLIB obtained a state-court order to include its contingent, which marched "uneventfully" among that year's 10,000 participants and 750,000 spectators.

In 1993, after the Council had again refused to admit GLIB to the upcoming parade, the organization and some of its members filed this suit against the Council, the individual petitioner John J. "Wacko" Hurley, and the City of Boston, alleging violations of the State and Federal Constitutions and of the state public accommodations law, which prohibits "any distinction, discrimination or restriction on account of *** sexual orientation relative to the admission of any person to, or treatment in any place of public accommodation, resort or amusement." [T]he state trial court ruled that the parade fell within the statutory definition of a public accommodation. While noting that the Council had indeed excluded the Ku Klux Klan and ROAR (an antibusing group), it attributed little significance to these facts, concluding ultimately that "[t]he only common theme among the participants and sponsors is their public involvement in the Parade."

The court rejected the Council's assertion that the exclusion of "groups with sexual themes merely formalized [the fact] that the Parade expresses traditional religious and social values." It concluded that the parade is "not an exercise of [the Council's] constitutionally protected right of expressive association," but instead "an open recreational event that is subject to the public accommodations law." The Supreme Judicial Court of Massachusetts affirmed, seeing nothing clearly erroneous in the trial judge's findings that GLIB was excluded from the parade based on the sexual orientation of its members, that it was impossible to detect an expressive purpose in the parade, that there was no state action, and that the parade was a public accommodation within the meaning of § 272:92A.

We granted certiorari to determine whether the requirement to admit a parade contingent expressing a message not of the private organizers' own choosing violates the First Amendment. We hold that it does and reverse.

II

Given the scope of the issues as originally joined in this case, it is worth noting some that have fallen aside in the course of the litigation, before reaching us. [R]espondents originally argued that the Council's conduct was not purely private, but had the character of state action. [T]hey "do not press that issue here." In this Court, then, their claim for inclusion in the parade rests solely on the Massachusetts public accommodations law. ***

III (A-B)

If there were no reason for a group of people to march from here to there except to reach a destination, they could make the trip without expressing any message beyond the fact of the march itself. Some people might call such a procession a parade, but it would not be much of one. Real "[p]arades are public dramas of social relations, and in them performers define who can be a social actor and what subjects and ideas are available for communication and consideration." S. Davis, Parades and Power: Street Theatre in Nineteenth- Century Philadelphia 6 (1986). Hence, we use the word "parade" to indicate marchers who are making some sort of collective point, not just to each other but to bystanders along the way. Indeed a parade's dependence on watchers is so extreme that nowadays, as with Bishop Berkeley's celebrated tree, "if a parade or demonstration receives no media coverage, it may as well not have happened."

The protected expression that inheres in a parade is not limited to its banners and songs, for the Constitution looks beyond written or spoken words as mediums of expression. Noting that "[s]ymbolism is a primitive but effective way of communicating ideas," West Virginia Bd. of Ed. v. Barnette, 319 U.S. 624, 632 (1943), our cases have recognized that the First Amendment shields such acts as saluting a flag (and refusing to do so), wearing an arm band to protest a war, displaying a red flag, and even "[m]arching, walking or parading" in uniforms displaying the swastika, National Socialist Party of America v. Skokie, 432 U.S. 43 (1977). As some of these examples show, a narrow, succinctly articulable message is not a condition of constitutional protection, which if confined to expressions conveying a "particularized message," cf. Spence v. Washington, 418 U.S. 405, 411 (1974) (per curiam), would never reach the unquestionably shielded painting of Jackson Pollock, music of Arnold Schonberg, or Jabberwocky verse of Lewis Carroll.

Not many marches, then, are beyond the realm of expressive parades, and the South Boston celebration is not one of them. To be sure, we agree with the state courts that in spite of excluding some applicants, the Council is rather lenient in admitting participants. But a private speaker does not forfeit constitutional protection simply by combining multifarious voices, or by failing to edit their themes to isolate an exact message as the exclusive subject matter of the speech. Nor, under our precedent, does First Amendment protection require a speaker to generate, as an original matter, each item featured in the communication. Cable operators, for example, are engaged in protected speech activities even when they only select programming originally produced by others. Turner Broadcasting System, Inc. v. FCC. For that matter, the presentation of an edited compilation of speech generated by other persons is a staple of most newspapers' opinion pages, which, of course, fall squarely within the core of First Amendment security, Miami Herald Publishing Co. v. Tornillo, 418 U.S. 241, 258 (1974), as does even the simple selection of a paid noncommercial advertisement for inclusion in a daily paper, see New York Times, 376 U. S., at 265-266. The selection of contingents to make a parade is entitled to similar protection.

Respondents' participation as a unit in the parade was equally expressive. GLIB was formed for the very purpose of marching in it, as the trial court found, in order to celebrate its members' identity as openly gay, lesbian, and bisexual descendants of the Irish immigrants, to show that there are such individuals in the community, and to support the like men and women who sought to march in the New York parade. GLIB understandably seeks to communicate its ideas as part of the existing parade, rather than staging one of its own.

C

In the case before us, the Massachusetts law has been applied in a peculiar way. Its enforcement does not address any dispute about the participation of openly gay, lesbian, or bisexual individuals in various units admitted to the parade. The petitioners disclaim any intent to exclude homosexuals as such, and no individual member of GLIB claims to have been excluded from parading as a member of any group that the Council has approved to march. Instead, the disagreement goes to the admission of GLIB as its own parade unit carrying its own banner. Although the state courts spoke of the parade as a place of public accommodation, once the expressive character of both the parade and the marching GLIB contingent is understood, it becomes apparent that the state courts' application of the statute had the effect of declaring the sponsors' speech itself to be the public accommodation. Under this approach any contingent of protected individuals with a message would have the right to participate in petitioners' speech, so that the communication produced by the private organizers would be shaped by all those protected by the law who wished to join in with some expressive demonstration of their own. But this use of the State's power violates the fundamental rule of protection under the First Amendment, that a speaker has the autonomy to choose the content of his own message.

Petitioners' claim to the benefit of this principle of autonomy to control one's own speech is as sound as the South Boston parade is expressive. Rather like a composer, the Council selects the expressive units of the parade from potential participants, and though the score may not produce a particularized message, each contingent's expression in the Council's eyes comports with what merits celebration on that day. Even if this view gives the Council credit for a more considered judgment than it actively made, the Council clearly decided to exclude a message it did not like from the communication it chose to make, and that is enough to invoke its right as a private speaker to shape its expression by speaking on one subject while remaining silent on another. The message it disfavored is not difficult to identify.

Respondents argue that any tension between this rule and the Massachusetts law falls short of unconstitutionality, citing the most recent of our cases on the general subject of compelled access for expressive purposes, Turner Broadcasting, 512 U.S. 622, 641. There we reviewed regulations requiring cable operators to set aside channels for designated broadcast signals, and applied only intermediate scrutiny. Respondents contend on this authority that admission of GLIB to the parade would not threaten the core principle of speaker's autonomy because the Council, like a cable operator, is merely "a conduit" for the speech of participants in the parade "rather than itself a speaker." But this metaphor is not apt here, because GLIB's participation would likely be perceived as having resulted from the Council's customary determination about a unit admitted to the parade, that its message was worthy of presentation and quite possibly of support as well. A newspaper, similarly, "is more than a passive receptacle or conduit for news, comment, and advertising," and we have held that "[t]he choice of material and the decisions made as to limitations on the size and content and treatment of public issues —whether fair or unfair—constitute the exercise of editorial control and judgment" upon which the State can not intrude.

In *Turner Broadcasting,* we found this problem absent in the cable context, because "[g]iven cable's long history of serving as a conduit for broadcast signals, there appears little risk that cable viewers would assume that the broadcast stations carried on a cable system convey ideas or messages endorsed by the cable operator."

Parades and demonstrations, in contrast, are not understood to be so neutrally presented or selectively viewed. Without deciding on the precise significance of the likelihood of misattribution, it nonetheless becomes clear that in the context of an expressive parade, as with a protest march, the parade's overall message is distilled from the individual presentations along the way, and each unit's expression is perceived by spectators as part of the whole.

An additional distinction between *Turner Broadcasting* and this case points to the fundamental weakness of any attempt to justify the state court order's limitation on the Council's autonomy as a speaker. A cable is not only a conduit for speech produced by others and selected by cable operators for transmission, but a franchised channel giving monopolistic opportunity to shut out some speakers. This power gives rise to the government's interest in limiting monopolistic autonomy in order to allow for the survival of broadcasters who might otherwise be silenced and consequently destroyed. The government's interest in *Turner Broadcasting* was not the alteration of speech, but the survival of speakers.

In this case, of course, there is no assertion comparable to the *Turner Broadcasting* claim that some speakers will be destroyed in the absence of the challenged law. True, the size and success of petitioners' parade makes it an enviable vehicle for the dissemination of GLIB's views, but that fact, without more, would fall far short of supporting a claim that petitioners enjoy an abiding monopoly of access to spectators.

*** Our tradition of free speech commands that a speaker who takes to the street corner to express his views in this way should be free from interference by the State based on the content of what he says. While the law is free to promote all sorts of conduct in place of harmful behavior, it is not free to interfere with speech for no better reason than promoting an approved message or discouraging a disfavored one, however enlightened either purpose may strike the government.

IV

Our holding today rests not on any particular view about the Council's message but on the Nation's commitment to protect freedom of speech. Disapproval of a private speaker's statement does not legitimize use of the Commonwealth's power to compel the speaker to alter the message by including one more acceptable to others. Accordingly, the judgment of the Supreme Judicial Court is reversed and the case remanded for proceedings not inconsistent with this opinion.

BOY SCOUTS OF AMERICA v. JAMES DALE*
530 U.S. 640 [June 28, 2000]

CHIEF JUSTICE REHNQUIST delivered the opinion of the Court.

The Boy Scouts asserts that homosexual conduct is inconsistent with the values it seeks to instill. Respondent is James Dale, a former Eagle Scout whose adult membership in the Boy Scouts was revoked when the Boy Scouts learned that he is an avowed homosexual and gay rights activist. The New Jersey Supreme Court held that New Jersey's public accommodations law requires that the Boy Scouts admit Dale. This case presents the question whether applying New Jersey's public accommodations law in this way violates the Boy Scouts' First Amendment right of expressive association. We hold that it does.

I

James Dale became a Boy Scout in 1981 and remained a Scout until he turned 18. By all accounts, Dale was an exemplary Scout. In 1988, he achieved the rank of Eagle Scout, one of Scouting' s highest honors. [H]e applied for adult membership in the Boy Scouts in 1989. The Boy Scouts approved his application for the position of assistant scoutmaster of Troop 73. Around the same time, Dale left home to attend Rutgers University. After arriving at Rutgers, Dale first acknowledged to himself and others that he is gay. He quickly became involved with, and eventually became the co-president of, the Rutgers University Lesbian/Gay Alliance. In 1990, Dale attended a seminar addressing the psychological and health needs of lesbian and gay teenagers. A newspaper covering the event interviewed Dale about his advocacy of homosexual teenagers' need for gay role models. [I]t published the interview and Dale' s photograph over a caption identifying him as the co-president of the Lesbian/Gay Alliance.

Later that month, Dale received a letter from Monmouth Council Executive James Kay revoking his adult membership. Dale wrote to Kay requesting the reason for Monmouth Council's decision. Kay responded by letter that the Boy Scouts "specifically forbid membership to homosexuals."

In 1992, Dale filed a complaint against the Boy Scouts in the New Jersey Superior Court. The complaint alleged that the Boy Scouts had violated New Jersey's public accommodations statute and its common law by revoking Dale's membership based solely on his sexual orientation. New Jersey's public accommodations statute prohibits, among other things, discrimination on the basis of sexual orientation in places of public accommodation.

---

*. [**Ed. Note**: See also and compare, *California Democratic Party et al. v. Bill Jones, Secretary of State of California*, 530 U.S. 567 (June 26, 2000). (First amendment right of "expressive association" of political parties to select their candidates to appear on the general election ballot, recognized and applied; state "blanket primary" election law authorizing non-party members–including members of parties with ideology different from or even opposite of that the party espouses –to vote to determine each political party's nominees for election for statewide offices, held unconstitutional.)

The New Jersey Superior Court's Chancery Division granted summary judgment in favor of the Boy Scouts. The New Jersey Superior Court's Appellate Division reversed [and] rejected the Boy Scouts' federal constitutional claims. The New Jersey Supreme Court affirmed the judgment of the Appellate Division. [T]he court held "that Dale's membership does not violate the Boy Scouts' right of expressive association because his inclusion would not affect in any significant way [the Boy Scouts'] existing members' ability to carry out their various purposes. ***We granted the Boy Scouts' petition for certiorari to determine whether the application of New Jersey's public accommodations law violated the First Amendment.

II

In *Roberts* v. *United States Jaycees,* 468 U. S. 609 (1984), we observed that "implicit in the right to engage in activities protected by the First Amendment" is "a corresponding right to associate with others in pursuit of a wide variety of political, social, economic, educational, religious, and cultural ends." This right is crucial in preventing the majority from imposing its views on groups that would rather express other, perhaps unpopular, ideas. See *ibid*. (stating that protection of the right to expressive association is "especially important in preserving political and cultural diversity and in shielding dissident expression from suppression by the majority"). Government actions that may unconstitutionally burden this freedom may take many forms, one of which is "intrusion into the internal structure or affairs of an association" like a "regulation that forces the group to accept members it does not desire." Forcing a group to accept certain members may impair the ability of the group to express those views, and only those views, that it intends to express. Thus, "[f]reedom of association ...plainly presupposes a freedom not to associate."

The forced inclusion of an unwanted person in a group infringes the group's freedom of expressive association if the presence of that person affects in a significant way the group's ability to advocate public or private viewpoints. *New York State Club Assn., Inc.* v. *City of New York,* 487 U. S. 1, 13 (1988). But the freedom of expressive association, like many freedoms, is not absolute. We have held that the freedom could be overridden "by regulations adopted to serve compelling state interests, unrelated to the suppression of ideas, that cannot be achieved through means significantly less restrictive of associational freedoms." *Roberts,* at 623.

To determine whether a group is protected by the First Amendment's expressive associational right, we must determine whether the group engages in "expressive association." The First Amendment's protection of expressive association is not reserved for advocacy groups. But to come within its ambit, a group must engage in some form of expression, whether it be public or private.

Because this is a First Amendment case where the ultimate conclusions of law are virtually inseparable from findings of fact, we are obligated to independently review the factual record to ensure that the state court' s judgment does not unlawfully intrude on free expression. See *Hurley,* at 567–568. The record reveals the following. The Boy Scouts is a private, nonprofit organization. According to its mission statement: "It is the mission of the Boy Scouts of America to serve others by helping to instill values in young people and, in other ways, to prepare them to make ethical choices over their lifetime in achieving their full potential. The values we strive to instill are based on those found in the Scout Oath and Law:

Scout Oath	**Scout Law**
"On my honor I will do my best To do my duty to God and my country and to obey the Scout Law; To help other people at all times; To keep myself physically strong, mentally, awake, and morally straight	A Scout is: Trustworthy, Obedient, Loyal, Cheerful, Helpful, Thrifty, Friendly, Brave, Courteous, Clean, Kind, Reverent."

Thus, the general mission of the Boy Scouts is clear: "[T]o instill values in young people." The Boy Scouts seeks to instill these values by having its adult leaders spend time with the youth members, instructing and engaging them in activities like camping, archery, and fishing. During the time spent with the youth members, the scoutmasters and assistant scoutmasters inculcate them with the Boy Scouts' values—both expressly and by example. It seems indisputable that an association that seeks to transmit such a system of values engages in expressive activity. Given that the Boy Scouts engages in expressive activity, we must determine whether the forced inclusion of Dale as an assistant scoutmaster would significantly affect the Boy Scouts' ability to advocate public or private viewpoints. This inquiry necessarily requires us first to explore, to a limited extent, the nature of the Boy Scouts' view of homosexuality.

The Boy Scouts explains that the Scout Oath and Law provide "a positive moral code for living; they are a list of 'do's' rather than 'don'ts.'" Brief for Petitioners 3. The Boy Scouts asserts that homosexual conduct is inconsistent with the values embodied in the Scout Oath and Law, particularly with the values represented by the terms "morally straight" and "clean."

Obviously, the Scout Oath and Law do not expressly mention sexuality or sexual orientation. And the terms "morally straight" and "clean" are by no means self-defining. Different people would attribute to those terms very different meanings. For example, some people may believe that engaging in homosexual conduct is not at odds with being "morally straight" and "clean." And others may believe that engaging in homosexual conduct is contrary to being "morally straight" and "clean." The Boy Scouts says it falls within the latter category.

The New Jersey Supreme Court analyzed the Boy Scouts' beliefs and found that the "exclusion of members solely on the basis of their sexual orientation is inconsistent with Boy Scouts' commitment to a diverse and 'representative' membership... [and] contradicts Boy Scouts' overarching objective to reach 'all eligible youth.'" The court concluded that the exclusion of members like Dale "appears antithetical to the organization' s goals and philosophy." But our cases reject this sort of inquiry; it is not the role of the courts to reject a group's expressed values because they disagree with those values or find them internally inconsistent. See *Thomas* v. *Review Bd. of Indiana Employment Security Div.*, ("[R]eligious beliefs need not be acceptable, logical, consistent, or comprehensible to others to merit First Amendment protection").

The Boy Scouts asserts that it "teach[es] that homosexual conduct is not morally straight," Brief for Petitioners 39, and that it does "not want to promote homosexual conduct as a legitimate form of behavior," Reply Brief for Petitioners 5. We accept the Boy Scouts' assertion. We need not inquire further to determine the nature of the Boy Scouts' expression with respect to homosexuality. But because the record before us contains written evidence of the Boy Scouts' viewpoint, we look to it as instructive, if only on the question of the sincerity of the professed beliefs.

A 1978 position statement to the Boy Scouts' Executive Committee, signed by Downing B. Jenks, the President of the Boy Scouts, and Harvey L. Price, the Chief Scout Executive, expresses the Boy Scouts' "official position" with regard to "homosexuality and Scouting":

> "Q. May an individual who openly declares himself to be a homosexual be a volunteer Scout leader?
>
> "A. No. The Boy Scouts of America is a private, membership organization and leadership therein is a privilege and not a right. We do not believe that homosexuality and leadership in Scouting are appropriate. We will continue to select only those who in our judgment meet our standards and qualifications for leadership."

Thus, at least as of 1978—the year James Dale entered Scouting—the official position of the Boy Scouts was that avowed homosexuals were not to be Scout leaders. A position statement promulgated by the Boy Scouts in 1991 (after Dale's membership was revoked but before this litigation was filed) also supports its current view:

> "We believe that homosexual conduct is inconsistent with the requirement in the Scout Oath that a Scout be morally straight and in the Scout Law that a Scout be clean in word and deed, and that homosexuals do not provide a desirable role model for Scouts."

This position statement was redrafted numerous times but its core message remained consistent. For example, a 1993 position statement, the most recent in the record, reads, in part:

> "The Boy Scouts of America has always reflected the expectations that Scouting families have had for the organization. We do not believe that homosexuals

provide a role model consistent with these expectations. Accordingly, we do not allow for the registration of avowed homosexuals as members or as leaders of the BSA."

The Boy Scouts publicly expressed its views with respect to homosexual conduct by its assertions in prior litigation. For example, throughout a California case with similar facts filed in the early 1980's, the Boy Scouts consistently asserted the same position with respect to homosexuality that it asserts today. We cannot doubt that the Boy Scouts sincerely holds this view.

We must then determine whether Dale's presence as an assistant scoutmaster would significantly burden the Boy Scouts' desire to not "promote homosexual conduct as a legitimate form of behavior." Reply Brief for Petitioners 5. As we give deference to an association' s assertions regarding the nature of its expression, we must also give deference to an association's view of what would impair its expression. That is not to say that an expressive association can erect a shield against anti-discrimination laws simply by asserting that mere acceptance of a member from a particular group would impair its message. But here Dale, by his own admission, is one of a group of gay Scouts who have "become leaders in their community and are open and honest about their sexual orientation." Dale was the copresident of a gay and lesbian organization at college and remains a gay rights activist. Dale's presence in the Boy Scouts would, at the very least, force the organization to send a message, both to the youth members and the world, that the Boy Scouts accepts homosexual conduct as a legitimate form of behavior.

Hurley is illustrative on this point. There we considered whether the application of Massachusetts' public accommodations law to require the organizers of a private St. Patrick' s Day parade to include among the marchers an Irish-American gay, lesbian, and bisexual group, GLIB, violated the parade organizers' First Amendment rights. We noted that the parade organizers did not wish to exclude the GLIB members because of their sexual orientations, but because they wanted to march behind a GLIB banner.*** As the presence of GLIB in Boston's St. Patrick's Day parade would have interfered with the parade organizers' choice not to propound a particular point of view, the presence of Dale as an assistant scoutmaster would just as surely interfere with the Boy Scout's choice not to propound a point of view contrary to its beliefs.

The New Jersey Supreme Court determined that the Boy Scouts' ability to disseminate its message was not significantly affected by the forced inclusion of Dale as an assistant scoutmaster because of the following findings: "Boy Scout members do not associate for the purpose of disseminating the belief that homosexuality is immoral; Boy Scouts discourages its leaders from disseminating *any* views on sexual issues; and Boy Scouts includes sponsors and members who subscribe to different views in respect of homosexuality." We disagree with the New Jersey Supreme Court's conclusion drawn from these findings.

First, associations do not have to associate for the "purpose" of disseminating a certain message in order to be entitled to the protections of the First Amendment. An association must merely engage in expressive activity that could be impaired in order to be entitled to protection. For example, the purpose of the St. Patrick's Day parade in *Hurley* was not to espouse any views about sexual orientation, but we held that the parade organizers had a right to exclude certain participants nonetheless.

Second, even if the Boy Scouts discourages Scout leaders from disseminating views on sexual issues—a fact that the Boy Scouts disputes with contrary evidence—the First Amendment protects the Boy Scouts' method of expression. If the Boy Scouts wishes Scout leaders to avoid questions of sexuality and teach only by example, this fact does not negate the sincerity of its belief discussed above.

Third, the First Amendment simply does not require that every member of a group agree on every issue in order for the group's policy to be "expressive association." The Boy Scouts takes an official position with respect to homosexual conduct, and that is sufficient for First Amendment purposes. In this same vein, Dale makes much of the claim that the Boy Scouts does not revoke the membership of heterosexual Scout leaders that openly disagree with the Boy Scouts' policy on sexual orientation. But if this is true, it is irrelevant. The presence of an avowed homosexual and gay rights activist in an assistant scoutmaster's uniform sends a distinctly different message from the presence of a heterosexual assistant scoutmaster who is on record as disagreeing with Boy Scouts policy. The Boy Scouts has a First Amendment right to choose to send one message but not the other. The fact that the organization does not trumpet its views from the housetops, or that it tolerates dissent within its ranks, does not mean that its views receive no First Amendment protection.

Having determined that the Boy Scouts is an expressive association and that the forced inclusion of Dale would significantly affect its expression, we inquire whether the application of New Jersey's public accommodations law to require that the Boy Scouts accept Dale as an assistant scoutmaster runs afoul of the Scouts' freedom of expressive association. We conclude that it does.

State public accommodations laws were originally enacted to prevent discrimination in traditional places of public accommodation—like inns and trains. Over time, the public accommodations laws have expanded to cover more places.[1] New Jersey' s statutory definition of "' [a] place of public accommodation'" is extremely broad. In this case, the New Jersey Supreme Court went a step further and applied its public accommodations law to a private entity without even attempting

1. Public accommodations laws have also broadened in scope to cover more groups; they have expanded beyond those groups that have been given heightened equal protection scrutiny under our cases. Some municipal ordinances have even expanded to cover criteria such as prior criminal record, prior psychiatric treatment, military status, personal appearance, source of income, place of residence, and political ideology.

to tie the term "place" to a physical location.[2] As the definition of "public accommodation" has expanded from clearly commercial entities, such as restaurants, bars, and hotels, to membership organizations such as the Boy Scouts, the potential for conflict between state public accommodations laws and the First Amendment rights of organizations has increased.

Dale contends that we should apply the intermediate standard of review enunciated in *United States* v. *O' Brien,* 391 U. S. 367 (1968), to evaluate the competing interests. There the Court enunciated a four-part test for review of a governmental regulation that has only an incidental effect on protected speech–in that case the symbolic burning of a draft card. A law prohibiting the destruction of draft cards only incidentally affects the free speech rights of those who happen to use a violation of that law as a symbol of protest. But New Jersey' s public accommodations law directly and immediately affects associational rights, in this case associational rights that enjoy First Amendment protection. Thus,*O' Brien* is inapplicable.

In *Hurley,* we applied traditional First Amendment analysis to hold that the application of the Massachusetts public accommodations law to a parade violated the First Amendment rights of the parade organizers. Although we did not explicitly deem the parade in *Hurley* an expressive association, the analysis we applied there is similar to the analysis we apply here. We have already concluded that a state requirement that the Boy Scouts retain Dale as an assistant scoutmaster would significantly burden the organization's right to oppose or disfavor homosexual conduct. The state interests embodied in New Jersey's public accommodations law do not justify such a severe intrusion on the Boy Scouts' rights to freedom of expressive association. That being the case, we hold that the First Amendment prohibits the State from imposing such a requirement through the application of its public accommodations law.[3]

We are not, as we must not be, guided by our views of whether the Boy Scouts' teachings with respect to homosexual conduct are right or wrong; public or judicial disapproval of a tenet of an organization's expression does not justify the State's effort to compel the organization to accept members where such acceptance would derogate from the organization's expressive message. "While the law is free to promote all sorts of conduct in place of harmful behavior, it is not free to interfere

---

2. Four State Supreme Courts and one United States Court of Appeals have ruled that the Boy Scouts is not a place of public accommodation. No federal appellate court or state supreme court—except the New Jersey Supreme Court in this case—has reached a contrary result.

3. We anticipated this result in *Hurley* when we illustrated the reasons for our holding in that case by likening the parade to a private membership organization. 515 U. S., at 580. We stated: "Assuming the parade to be large enough and a source of benefits (apart from its expression) that would generally justify a mandated access provision, GLIB could nonetheless be refused admission as an expressive contingent with its own message just as readily as a private club could exclude an applicant whose manifest views were at odds with a position taken by the club's existing members." *Id.,* at 580–581.

with speech for no better reason than promoting an approved message or discouraging a disfavored one, however enlightened either purpose may strike the government." *Hurley,* 515 U. S., at 579.

The judgment of the New Jersey Supreme Court is reversed, and the cause remanded for further proceedings not inconsistent with this opinion.

It is so ordered.

JUSTICE STEVENS, with whom JUSTICE SOUTER, JUSTICE GINSBURG and JUSTICE BREYER join, dissenting.

The majority holds that New Jersey law violates BSA's right to associate and its right to free speech. But that law does not "impos[e] any serious burdens" on BSA's "collective effort on behalf of [its] shared goals," *Roberts* v. *United States Jaycees,* 468 U. S. 609, 622 (1984), nor does it force BSA to communicate any message that it does not wish to endorse. New Jersey's law, therefore, abridges no constitutional right of the Boy Scouts.

I

***

BSA's mission statement reads as follows: "It is the mission of the Boy Scouts of America to serve others by helping to instill values in young people and, in other ways, to prepare them to make ethical choices over their lifetime in achieving their full potential." Its federal charter declares its purpose is "to promote, through organization, and cooperation with other agencies, the ability of boys to do things for themselves and others, to train them in scoutcraft, and to teach them patriotism, courage, self-reliance, and kindred values, using the methods which were in common use by Boy Scouts on June 15, 1916." In particular, the group emphasizes that "[n]either the charter nor the bylaws of the Boy Scouts of America permits the exclusion of any boy...."

To bolster its claim that its shared goals include teaching that homosexuality is wrong, BSA directs our attention to two terms[,] the phrase "morally straight," in the Oath, [and] the word "clean," which appears in a list of 12 characteristics comprising the Scout Law.

The Boy Scout Handbook defines "morally straight," as such:

> [G]uide your life with honesty, purity, and justice. Respect and defend the rights of all people. Your relationships with others should be honest and open. Be clean in your speech and actions, and faithful in your religious beliefs. The values you follow as a Scout will help you become virtuous and self-reliant.

As for the term "clean," the Boy Scout Handbook offers the following:

> A Scout is CLEAN. A Scout keeps his body and mind fit and clean. He chooses the company of those who live by these same ideals. He helps keep his home and community clean. You never need to be ashamed of dirt that will wash off.*** There's another kind of dirt that won't come off by washing. It is the

> kind that shows up in foul language and harmful thoughts. Swear words, profanity, and dirty stories are weapons that ridicule other people and hurt their feelings. A Scout knows there is no kindness or honor in such mean-spirited behavior. He avoids it in his own words and deeds. He defends those who are targets of insults.

It is plain as the light of day that neither one of these principles—"morally straight" and "clean"—says the slightest thing about homosexuality. Indeed, neither term in the Boy Scouts' Law and Oath expresses any position whatsoever on sexual matters.

BSA's published guidance on that topic underscores this point. *** More specifically, BSA has set forth a number of rules for Scoutmasters when these types of issues come up:

> You may have boys asking you for information or advice about sexual matters.... How should you handle such matters?
> Rule number 1: *You do not undertake to instruct Scouts, in any formalized manner, in the subject of sex and family life. The reasons are that it is not construed to be Scouting's proper are*a, and that you are probably not well qualified to do this. (Emphasis added.)

II

The Court seeks to fill the void by pointing to a statement of "policies and procedures relating to homosexuality and Scouting" signed by BSA's President and Chief Scout Executive in 1978 and addressed to the members of the Executive Committee of the national organization. The letter says that the BSA does "not believe that homosexuality and leadership in Scouting are appropriate." But when the *entire* 1978 letter is read, BSA's position is far more equivocal:

> 4. Q. May an individual who openly declares himself to be a homosexual be employed by the Boy Scouts of America as a professional or non-professional?
> A. Boy Scouts of America does not knowingly employ homosexuals as professionals or non-professionals. We are unaware of any present laws which would prohibit this policy.
> 5. Q. Should a professional or non-professional individual who openly declares himself to be a homosexual be terminated?
> A. Yes, *in the absence of any law to the contrary.* ****In the event that such a law was applicable, it would be necessary for the Boy Scouts of America to obey it, in this case as in Paragraph 4 above.* It is our position, however, that homosexuality and professional or non-professional employment in Scouting are not appropriate. (Emphasis added.)

[A]t most this letter simply adopts an exclusionary membership policy. But simply adopting such a policy has never been considered sufficient, by itself, to prevail on a right to associate claim. Second, the 1978 policy [itself] was never publicly expressed— unlike, for example, the Scout's duty to be "obedient." It was an internal memorandum, never circulated beyond the few members of BSA's

Executive Committee. It remained, in effect, a secret Boy Scouts policy. [T]he 1978 policy appears to be no more than a private statement of a few BSA executives that the organization wishes to exclude gays—and that wish has nothing to do with any expression BSA actually engages in.

The majority also relies on four other policy statements that were issued between 1991 and 1993. All of them were written and issued *after* BSA revoked Dale's membership. Accordingly, they have little, if any, relevance to the legal question before this Court.*** [A]t most the 1991 and 1992 statements declare only that BSA believed "homosexual *conduct* is inconsistent with the requirement in the Scout Oath that a Scout be morally straight and in the Scout Law that a Scout be clean in word and deed." (Emphasis added.) But New Jersey's law prohibits discrimination on the basis of sexual *orientation*. And when Dale was expelled from the Boy Scouts, BSA said it did so because of his sexual orientation, not because of his sexual conduct.[4]

III

Several principles are made perfectly clear by *Jaycees* and *Rotary Club*. First, to prevail on a claim of expressive association in the face of a State's anti-discrimination law, it is not enough simply to engage in *some kind* of expressive activity. Both the Jaycees and the Rotary Club engaged in expressive activity protected by the First Amendment, yet that fact was not dispositive. Second, it is not enough to adopt an openly avowed exclusionary membership policy. Both the Jaycees and the Rotary Club did that as well. Third, it is not sufficient merely to articulate *some* connection between the group's expressive activities and its exclusionary policy.

Rather, in *Jaycees*, we asked whether Minnesota's Human Rights Law requiring the admission of women "impose[d] any *serious burdens*" on the group's "collective effort on behalf of [its] *shared goals*."***The relevant question is whether the mere inclusion of the person at issue would "impose any serious burden," "affect in any significant way," or be "a substantial restraint upon" the organization's "shared goals," "basic goals," or "collective effort to foster beliefs." Accordingly, it is necessary to examine what, exactly, are BSA's shared goals and the degree to which its expressive activities would be burdened, affected, or restrained by including homosexuals.

The evidence before this Court makes it exceptionally clear that BSA has, at most, simply adopted an exclusionary membership policy and has no shared goal of disapproving of homosexuality.*** There is simply no evidence that BSA otherwise teaches anything in this area, or that it instructs Scouts on matters involving

---

4. At oral argument, BSA's counsel was asked: "[W]hat if someone is homosexual in the sense of having a sexual orientation in that direction but does not engage in any homosexual conduct?" Counsel answered: "[I]f that person also were to take the view that the reason they didn't engage in that conduct [was because] it would be morally wrong . . . that person would not be excluded." Tr. of Oral Arg. 8.

homosexuality in ways not conveyed in the Boy Scout or Scoutmaster Handbooks. In short, Boy Scouts of America is simply silent on homosexuality. There is no shared goal or collective effort to foster a belief about homosexuality at all—let alone one that is significantly burdened by admitting homosexuals.

IV

The majority pretermits this entire analysis. It finds that BSA in fact "teach[es] that homosexual conduct is not morally straight." This conclusion, remarkably, rests entirely on statements in BSA's briefs. Moreover, the majority insists that we must "give deference to an association's assertions regarding the nature of its expression" and "we must also give deference to an association's view of what would impair its expression." So long as the record "contains written evidence" to support a group's bare assertion, "[w]e need not inquire further."

[N]othing in our cases calls for this Court to do any such thing. An organization can adopt the message of its choice, and it is not this Court's place to disagree with it. But we must inquire whether the group is, in fact, expressing a message (whatever it may be) and whether that message (if one is expressed) is significantly affected by a State's anti-discrimination law. There is, of course, a valid concern that a court's independent review may run the risk of paying too little heed to an organization's sincerely held views. In this case, no such concern is warranted. It is entirely clear that BSA in fact expresses no clear, unequivocal message burdened by New Jersey's law.

V

Even if BSA's right to associate argument fails, it nonetheless might have a First Amendment right to refrain from including debate and dialogue about homosexuality as part of its mission to instill values in Scouts. It can, for example, advise Scouts who are entering adulthood and have questions about sex to talk "with your parents, religious leaders, teachers, or Scoutmaster," and, in turn, it can direct Scoutmasters who are asked such questions "not undertake to instruct Scouts, in any formalized manner, in the subject of sex and family life" because "it is not construed to be Scouting's proper area."

The majority, though, does not rest its conclusion on the claim that Dale will use his position as a bully pulpit. Rather, it contends that Dale's mere presence among the Boy Scouts will itself force the group to convey a message about homosexuality—even if Dale has no intention of doing so. The majority holds that "[t]he presence of an avowed homosexual and gay rights activist in an assistant scoutmaster's uniform sends a distinc[t] ...message," and, accordingly, BSA is entitled to exclude that message.

The majority's argument relies exclusively on *Hurley* v. *Irish-American Gay, Lesbian and Bisexual Group of Boston, Inc.* Dale's inclusion in the Boy Scouts is nothing like the case in *Hurley*. His participation sends no cognizable message to the Scouts or to the world. Unlike GLIB, Dale did not carry a banner or a sign; he did not distribute any fact sheet; and he expressed no intent to send any message. If there is any kind of message being sent, then, it is by the mere act of joining the Boy Scouts. Such an act does not constitute an instance of symbolic speech under the First Amendment.[5]

Furthermore, it is not likely that BSA would be understood to send any message, either to Scouts or to the world, simply by admitting someone as a member. In 1992 over one million adults were active BSA members. The notion that an organization of that size and enormous prestige implicitly endorses the views that each of those adults may express in a non-Scouting context is simply mind boggling.

VI

Unfavorable opinions about homosexuals "have ancient roots." *Bowers* v. *Hardwick,* 478 U. S. 186, 192 (1986). Like equally atavistic opinions about certain racial groups, those roots have been nourished by sectarian doctrine. That such prejudices are still prevalent and that they have caused serious and tangible harm to countless members of the class New Jersey seeks to protect are established matters of fact that neither the Boy Scouts nor the Court disputes. That harm can only be aggravated by the creation of a constitutional shield for a policy that is itself the product of a habitual way of thinking about strangers. If we would guide by the light of reason, we must let our minds be bold.

I respectfully dissent.

JUSTICE SOUTER, with whom JUSTICE GINSBURG and JUSTICE BREYER join, dissenting.

I join JUSTICE STEVENS's dissent but add this further word on the significance of Part VI of his opinion. The right of expressive association does not, of course, turn on the popularity of the views advanced by a group that claims protection. Whether the group appears to this Court to be in the vanguard or rearguard of social thinking is irrelevant to the group's rights. I conclude that BSA has not made out an expressive association claim, therefore, not because of what BSA may espouse, but because of its failure to make sexual orientation the subject of any unequivocal advocacy, using the channels it customarily employs to state its message. If, on the other hand, an expressive association claim has met the conditions JUSTICE STEVENS describes as necessary, there may well be circumstances in which the antidiscrimination law must yield.

---

5. The majority might have argued (but it did not) that Dale had become so publicly and pervasively identified with a position advocating the moral legitimacy of homosexuality (as opposed to just being an individual who openly stated he is gay) that his leadership position in BSA would necessarily amount to using the organization as a conduit for publicizing his position. But as already noted, when BSA expelled Dale, it had nothing to go on beyond the one newspaper article quoted above, and one newspaper article does not convert Dale into a public symbol for a message. BSA simply has not provided a record that establishes the factual premise for this argument.

Chapter 5

EQUALIZING FREEDOM OF SPEECH BY LEVELING EXPENDITURES AND CONTRIBUTIONS — REGULATING THE USES OF MONEY AND SPEECH

BUCKLEY v. VALEO
424 U.S. 1 (1976)

***

PER CURIAM.

These appeals present constitutional challenges to the key provisions of the Federal Election Campaign Act of 1971, as amended in 1974. *** The statutes at issue contain the following provisions: (a) individual political contributions are limited to $1,000 to any single candidate per election, with an overall annual limitation of $25,000 by any contributor; independent expenditures by individuals and groups "relative to a clearly identified candidate" are limited to $1,000 a year; campaign spending by candidates for various federal offices and spending for national conventions by political parties are subject to prescribed limits; (b) contributions and expenditures above certain threshold levels must be reported and publicly disclosed; (c) a system for public funding of Presidential campaign activities is established by Subtitle H of the Internal Revenue Code; and (d) a Federal Election Commission is established to administer and enforce the legislation.

Plaintiffs included a candidate for the Presidency of the United States, a United States Senator who is a candidate for re-election, a potential contributor, the Committee for a Constitutional Presidency—McCarthy '76, the Conservative Party of the State of New York, the Mississippi Republican Party, the Libertarian Party, the New York Civil Liberties Union, Inc., the American Conservative Union, the Conservative Victory Fund, and Human Events, Inc. On plenary review, a majority of the Court of Appeals rejected, for the most part, appellants' constitutional attacks. [I]n this Court, appellants argue that the Court of Appeals failed to give this legislation the critical scrutiny demanded under accepted First Amendment and equal protection principles. ***

I. CONTRIBUTION AND EXPENDITURE LIMITATIONS

***

A. General Principles

The Act's contribution and expenditure limitations operate in an area of the most fundamental First Amendment activities. Discussion of public issues and de bate on the qualifications of candidates are integral to the operation of the system of government established by our Constitution. The First Amendment affords the broadest protection to such political expression in order "to assure [the] unfettered interchange of ideas for the bringing about of political and social changes desired by the people." Roth v. United States, 354 U.S. 476, 484 (1957). *** In upholding the constitutional validity of the Act's contribution and expenditure provisions on the ground that those provisions should be viewed as regulating conduct, not speech, the Court of Appeals relied upon United States v. O'Brien, 391 U.S. 367 (1968).

We cannot share the view that the present Act's contribution and expenditure limitations are comparable to the restrictions on conduct upheld in *O'Brien*. *** [T]he limitations challenged here would not meet the *O'Brien* test because the governmental interests advanced in support of the Act involve "suppressing communication." Unlike *O'Brien*, where the Selective Service System's administrative interest in the preservation of draft cards was wholly unrelated to their use as a means of communication, it is beyond dispute that the interest in regulating the alleged "conduct" of giving or spending money "arises in some measure because the communication allegedly integral to the conduct is itself thought to be harmful."

The expenditure limitations contained in the Act represent substantial rather than merely theoretical restraints on the quantity and diversity of political speech. The $1,000 ceiling on spending "relative to a clearly identified candidate,"would appear to exclude all citizens and groups except candidates, political parties, and the institutional press from any significant use of the most effective modes of communication.[20] By contrast with a limitation upon expenditures for political expression, a limitation upon the amount that any one person or group may contribute to a candidate or political committee entails only a marginal restriction upon the contributor's ability to engage in free communication. ***

Given the important role of contributions in financing political campaigns, contribution restrictions could have a severe impact on political dialogue if the limitations prevented candidates and political committees from amassing the resources necessary for effective advocacy. There is no indication, however, that the contribution limitations imposed by the Act would have any dramatic adverse effect on the funding of campaigns and political associations. *** And the Act's contribution

---

20. The record indicates that, as of January 1, 1975, one full-page advertisement in a daily edition of a certain metropolitan newspaper cost $6,971.04—almost seven times the annual limit on expenditures "relative to" a particular candidate imposed on the vast majority of individual citizens and associations by § 608 (e)(1).

limitations permit associations and candidates to aggregate large sums of money to promote effective advocacy. By contrast, the Act's $1,000 limitation on independent expenditures "relative to a clearly identified candidate" precludes most associations from effectively amplifying the voice of their adherents, the original basis for the recognition of First Amendment protection of the freedom of association. See NAACP v. Alabama, 357 U.S., at 460. ***

In sum, although the Act's contribution and expenditure limitations both implicate fundamental First Amendment interests, its expenditure ceilings impose significantly more severe restrictions on protected freedoms of political expression and association than do its limitations on financial contributions.

B. Contribution Limitations

Section 608(b) provides, with certain limited exceptions, that "no person shall make contributions to any candidate with respect to any election for Federal office which, in the aggregate, exceed $1,000." The statute defines "person" broadly to include "an individual, partnership, committee, association, corporation or any other organization or group of persons." Appellants contend that the $1,000 contribution ceiling unjustifiably burdens First Amendment freedoms, employs overbroad dollar limits, and discriminates against candidates opposing incumbent officeholders and against minor-party candidates in violation of the Fifth Amendment. We address each of these claims of invalidity in turn. ***

Appellees argue that the Act's restrictions on large campaign contributions are justified by three governmental interests. According to the parties and *amici*, the primary interest served by the limitations and, indeed, by the Act as a whole, is the prevention of corruption and the appearance of corruption spawned by the real or imagined coercive influence of large financial contributions on candidates' positions and on their actions if elected to office. ***

It is unnecessary to look beyond the Act's primary purpose—to limit the actuality and appearance of corruption resulting from large individual financial contributions—in order to find a constitutionally sufficient justification for the $1,000 contribution limitation. To the extent that large contributions are given to secure political *quid pro quo* from current and potential office holders, the integrity of our system of representative democracy is undermined. Although the scope of such pernicious practices can never be reliably ascertained, the deeply disturbing examples surfacing after the 1972 election demonstrate that the problem is not an illusory one.[21] Of almost equal concern as the danger of actual *quid pro quo* arrangements is the impact of the appearance of corruption stemming from public awareness of the opportunities for abuse inherent in a regime of large individual financial contributions.

---

21. The Court of Appeals' opinion in this case discussed a number of the abuses uncovered after the 1972 elections.

Appellants contend that the contribution limitations must be invalidated because bribery laws and narrowly drawn disclosure requirements constitute a less restrictive means of dealing with "proven and suspected *quid pro quo* arrangements." But laws making criminal the giving and taking of bribes deal with only the most blatant and specific attempts of those with money to influence governmental action. And while disclosure requirements serve the many salutary purposes discussed elsewhere in this opinion, Congress was surely entitled to conclude that disclosure was only a partial measure, and that contribution ceilings were a necessary legislative concomitant to deal with the reality or appearance of corruption inherent in a system permitting unlimited financial contributions, even when the identities of the contributors and the amounts of their contributions are fully disclosed. *** We find that, under the rigorous standard of review established by our prior decisions, the weighty interests served by restricting the size of financial contributions to political candidates are sufficient to justify the limited effect upon First Amendment freedoms caused by the $1,000 contribution ceiling.

Apart from these First Amendment concerns, appellants argue that the contribution limitations work such an invidious discrimination between incumbents and challengers that the statutory provisions must be declared unconstitutional on their face. [But] there is no evidence to support the claim that the contribution limitations in themselves discriminate against major-party challengers to incumbents. And, to the extent that incumbents generally are more likely than challengers to attract very large contributions, the Act's $1,000 ceiling has the practical effect of benefitting challengers as a class.[37] ***

The charge of discrimination against minor-party and independent candidates is more troubling, but the record provides no basis for concluding that the Act invidiously disadvantages such candidates. [T]he Act on its face treats all candidates equally with regard to contribution limitations. And the restriction would appear to benefit minor-party and independent candidates relative to their major- party opponents because major-party candidates receive far more money in large contributions.

In view of these considerations, we conclude that the impact of the Act's $1,000 contribution limitation on major-party challengers and on minor-party candidates does not render the provision unconstitutional on its face.

***

C. Expenditure Limitations

The Act's expenditure ceilings impose direct and substantial restraints on the quantity of political speech. The most drastic of the limitations restricts individuals and groups, including political parties that fail to place a candidate on the ballot, to

37. Of the $3,781,254 in contributions raised in 1974 by congressional candidates over and above a $1,000-per-contributor limit, almost twice as much money went to incumbents as to major-party challengers.

an expenditure of $1,000 "relative to a clearly identified candidate during a calendar year." *** The plain effect of § 608(e)(1) is to prohibit all individuals, who are neither candidates nor owners of institutional press facilities, and all groups, except political parties and campaign organizations, from voicing their views "relative to a clearly identified candidate" through means that entail aggregate expenditures of more than $1,000 during a calendar year. The provision, for example, would make it a federal criminal offense for a person or association to place a single one-quarter page advertisement "relative to a clearly identified candidate" in a major metropolitan newspaper.

Before examining the interests advanced in support of § 608(e)(1)'s expenditure ceiling, consideration must be given to appellants' contention that the provision is unconstitutionally vague.

The section prohibits "any expenditure relative to a clearly identified candidate during a calendar year which, *when added to all other expenditures advocating the election or defeat of such candidate,* exceeds $1,000." (Emphasis added.) This context clearly permits, if indeed it does not require, the phrase "relative to" a candidate to be read to mean "advocating the election or defeat of" a candidate.*** We agree that in order to preserve the provision against invalidation on vagueness grounds, § 608(e)(1) must be construed to apply only to expenditures for communications that in express terms advocate the election or defeat of a clearly identified candidate for federal office.[52]

We turn then to the basic First Amendment question—whether § 608(e)(1) even as thus narrowly and explicitly construed, impermissibly burdens the constitutional right of free expression. The Court of Appeals summarily held the provision constitutionally valid on the ground that "section 608(e) is a loophole-closing provision only" that is necessary to prevent circumvention of the contribution limitations. We cannot agree.

The discussion in Part I-A, *supra*, explains why the Act's expenditure limitations impose far greater restraints on the freedom of speech and association than do its contribution limitations. The markedly greater burden on basic freedoms caused by § 608(e)(1) thus cannot be sustained simply by invoking the interest in maximizing the effectiveness of the less intrusive contribution limitations. Rather, the constitutionality of § 608(e)(1) turns on whether the governmental interests advanced in its support satisfy the exacting scrutiny applicable to limitations on core First Amendment rights of political expression.

We find that the governmental interest in preventing corruption and the appearance of corruption is inadequate to justify § 608(e)(1)'s ceiling on independent expenditures. First, assuming, *arguendo*, that large independent expenditures pose

---

52. This construction would restrict the application of § 608 (e)(1) to communications containing express words of advocacy of election or defeat, such as "vote for," "elect," "support," "cast your ballot for," "Smith for Congress," "vote against," "defeat," "reject."

the same dangers of actual or apparent *quid pro quo* arrangements as do large contributions, § 608(e)(1) does not provide an answer that sufficiently relates to the elimination of those dangers. Unlike the contribution limitations' total ban on the giving of large amounts of money to candidates, § 608(e)(1) prevents only some large expenditures. So long as persons and groups eschew expenditures that in express terms advocate the election or defeat of a clearly identified candidate, they are free to spend as much as they want to promote the candidate and his views. The exacting interpretation of the statutory language necessary to avoid unconstitutional vagueness thus undermines the limitation's effectiveness as a loophole-closing provision by facilitating circumvention by those seeking to exert improper influence upon a candidate or officeholder.

Second, quite apart from the shortcomings of § 608(e)(1) in preventing any abuses generated by large independent expenditures, the independent advocacy restricted by the provision does not presently appear to pose dangers of real or apparent corruption comparable to those identified with large campaign contributions. The parties defending § 608(e)(1) contend that it is necessary to prevent would-be contributors from avoiding the contribution limitations by the simple expedient of paying directly for media advertisements or for other portions of the candidate's campaign activities. They argue that expenditures controlled by or coordinated with the candidate and his campaign might well have virtually the same value to the candidate as a contribution and would pose similar dangers of abuse. Yet such controlled or coordinated expenditures are treated as contributions rather than expenditures under the Act. Section 608(b)'s contribution ceilings rather than § 608(e)(1)'s independent expenditure limitation prevent attempts to circumvent the Act through prearranged or coordinated expenditures amounting to disguised contributions. By contrast, § 608(e)(1) limits expenditures for express advocacy of candidates made totally independently of the candidate and his campaign. Rather than preventing circumvention of the contribution limitations, §608 (e)(1) severely restricts all independent advocacy despite its substantially diminished potential for abuse.

While the independent expenditure ceiling thus fails to serve any substantial governmental interest in stemming the reality or appearance of corruption in the electoral process, it heavily burdens core First Amendment expression. Advocacy of the election or defeat of candidates for federal office is no less entitled to protection under the First Amendment than the discussion of political policy generally or advocacy of the passage or defeat of legislation.

It is argued, however, that the ancillary governmental interest in equalizing the relative ability of individuals and groups to influence the outcome of elections serves to justify the limitation on express advocacy of the election or defeat of candidates imposed by § 608(e)(1)'s expenditure ceiling. But the concept that government may restrict the speech of some elements of our society in order to enhance the relative voice of others is wholly foreign to the First Amendment, which was designed "to secure 'the widest possible dissemination of information from diverse and antagonistic sources,'" and "'to assure unfettered interchange of ideas for the bringing about of political and social changes desired by the people.'"

*** In *Mills*, the Court addressed the question whether "a State, consistently with the United States Constitution, can make it a crime for the editor of a daily newspaper to write and publish an editorial on *election day* urging people to vote a certain way on issues submitted to them." 384 U.S., at 215 (emphasis in original). We held that "no test of reasonableness can save [such] a state law from invalidation as a violation of the First Amendment." Yet the prohibition of election- day editorials invalidated in *Mills* is clearly a lesser intrusion on constitutional freedom than a $1,000 limitation on the amount of money any person or association can spend *during an entire election year* in advocating the election or defeat of a candidate for public office. More recently in *Tornillo*, the Court held that Florida could not constitutionally require a newspaper to make space available for a political candidate to reply to its criticism. Yet under the Florida statute, every newspaper was free to criticize any candidate as much as it pleased so long as it undertook the modest burden of printing his reply. *** For the reasons stated, we conclude that § 608(e)(1)'s independent expenditure limitation is unconstitutional under the First Amendment.

2. Limitation on Expenditures by Candidates from Personal or Family Resources

The Act also sets limits on expenditures by a candidate "from his personal funds, or the personal funds of his immediate family, in connection with his campaigns during any calendar year." These ceilings vary from $50,000 for Presidential or Vice Presidential candidates to $35,000 for senatorial candidates, and $25,000 for most candidates for the House of Representatives.

The candidate, no less than any other person, has a First Amendment right to engage in the discussion of public issues and vigorously and tirelessly to advocate his own election and the election of other candidates. *** The primary governmental interest served by the Act—the prevention of actual and apparent corruption of the political process—does not support the limitation on the candidate's expenditure of his own personal funds. As the Court of Appeals concluded: "Manifestly, the core problem of avoiding undisclosed and undue influence on candidates from outside interests has lesser application when the monies involved come from the candidate himself or from his immediate family." Indeed, the use of personal funds reduces the candidate's dependence on outside contributions and thereby counteracts the coercive pressures and attendant risks of abuse to which the Act's contribution limitations are directed.

The ancillary interest in equalizing the relative financial resources of candidates competing for elective office, therefore, provides the sole relevant rationale for § 608 (a)'s expenditure ceiling. That interest is clearly not sufficient to justify the provision's infringement of fundamental First Amendment rights. First, the limitation may fail to promote financial equality among candidates. A candidate who spends less of his personal resources on his campaign may nonetheless outspend his rival as a result of more successful fundraising efforts. [A]nd more fundamentally, the First Amendment simply cannot tolerate § 608(a)'s restriction upon the freedom of a candidate to speak without legislative limit on behalf of his own candidacy. We therefore hold that § 608(a)'s restriction on a candidate's personal expenditures is unconstitutional.

3. Limitations on Campaign Expenditures

***

No governmental interest that has been suggested is sufficient to justify the restriction on the quantity of political expression imposed by § 608(c)'s campaign expenditure limitations. The major evil associated with rapidly increasing campaign expenditures is the danger of candidate dependence on large contributions. The interest in alleviating the corrupting influence of large contributions is served by the Act's contribution limitations and disclosure provisions rather than by § 608(c)'s campaign expenditure ceilings. ***

The interest in equalizing the financial resources of candidates competing for federal office is no more convincing a justification for restricting the scope of federal election campaigns. Given the limitation on the size of outside contributions, the financial resources available to a candidate's campaign, like the number of volunteers recruited, will normally vary with the size and intensity of the candidate's support.[63] There is nothing invidious, improper, or unhealthy in permitting such funds to be spent to carry the candidate's message to the electorate.[64] Moreover, the equalization of permissible campaign expenditures might serve not to equalize the opportunities of all candidates but to handicap a candidate who lacked substantial name recognition or exposure of his views before the start of the campaign.

The campaign expenditure ceilings appear to be designed primarily to serve the governmental interests in reducing the allegedly skyrocketing costs of political campaigns. Appellees and the Court of Appeals stressed statistics indicating that spending for federal election campaigns increased almost 300% between 1952 and 1972 in comparison with a 57.6% rise in the consumer price index during the same period. Appellants respond that during these years the rise in campaign spending lagged behind the percentage increase in total expenditures for commercial advertising and the size of the gross national product. In any event, the mere growth in the cost of federal election campaigns in and of itself provides no basis for governmental restrictions on the quantity of campaign spending and the resulting limitation on the scope of federal campaigns. The First Amendment denies government the power to determine that spending to promote one's political views is wasteful, excessive, or

---

63. This normal relationship may not apply where the candidate devotes a large amount of his personal resources to his campaign.

64. As an opinion dissenting in part from decision below noted: "If a senatorial candidate can raise $1 from each voter, what evil is exacerbated by allowing that candidate to use all that money for political communication? I know of none."

unwise. In the free society ordained by our Constitution it is not the government, but the people—individually as citizens and candidates and collectively as associations and political committees—who must retain control over the quantity and range of debate on public issues in a political campaign. For these reasons we hold that § 608(c) is constitutionally invalid.

In sum, the provisions of the Act that impose a $1,000 limitation on contributions to a single candidate, a $5,000 limitation on contributions by a political committee to a single candidate, and a $25,000 limitation on total contributions by an individual during any calendar year, are constitutionally valid. By contrast, the First Amendment requires the invalidation of the Act's independent expenditure ceiling, its limitation on a candidate's expenditures from his own personal funds, and its ceilings on overall campaign expenditures.

II. REPORTING AND DISCLOSURE REQUIREMENTS

Unlike the limitations on contributions and expenditures, the disclosure requirements of the Act are not challenged by appellants as *per se* unconstitutional restrictions on the exercise of First Amendment freedoms of speech and association. The particular requirements embodied in the Act are attacked as overbroad—both in their application to minor-party and independent candidates and in their extension to contributions as small as $11 or $101.

A. General Principles

***

We long have recognized that significant encroachments on First Amendment rights of the sort that compelled disclosure imposes cannot be justified by a mere showing of some legitimate governmental interest. [W]e have required that the subordinating interests of the State must survive exacting scrutiny. This type of scrutiny is necessary even if any deterrent effect on the exercise of First Amendment rights arises, not through direct government action, but indirectly as an unintended but inevitable result of the government's conduct in requiring disclosure.

The strict test *** is necessary because compelled disclosure has the potential for substantially infringing the exercise of First Amendment rights. But we have acknowledged that there are governmental interests sufficiently important to outweigh the possibility of infringement, particularly when the "free functioning of our national institutions" is involved. Communist Party v. Subversive Activities Control Bd., 367 U.S. 1, 97 (1961).

The governmental interests sought to be vindicated by the disclosure requirements are of this magnitude. They fall into three categories. First, disclosure provides the electorate with information "as to where political campaign money comes from and how it is spent by the candidate" in order to aid the voters in evaluating those who seek federal office. *** Second, disclosure requirements deter actual corruption and avoid the appearance of corruption by exposing large contributions and expenditures to the light of publicity. This exposure may discourage those who would use money for improper purposes either before or after the election. ***

Third, and not least significant, recordkeeping, reporting, and disclosure requirements are an essential means of gathering the data necessary to detect violations of the contribution limitations described above.

It is undoubtedly true that public disclosure of contributions to candidates and political parties will deter some individuals who otherwise might contribute. In some instances, disclosure may even expose contributors to harassment or retaliation. These are not insignificant burdens on individual rights, and they must be weighed carefully against the interests which Congress has sought to promote by this legislation. In this process, we note and agree with appellants' concession that disclosure requirements— certainly in most applications—appear to be the least restrictive means of curbing the evils of campaign ignorance and corruption that Congress found to exist. Appellants argue, however, that the balance tips against disclosure when it is required of contributors to certain parties and candidates. We turn now to this contention.

B. Application to Minor Parties and Independents

***

It is true that the governmental interest in disclosure is diminished when the contribution in question is made to a minor party with little chance of winning an election. As minor parties usually represent definite and publicized viewpoints, there may be less need to inform the voters of the interests that specific candidates represent. Major parties encompass candidates of greater diversity. In many situations the label "Republican" or "Democrat" tells a voter little. The candidate who bears it may be supported by funds from the far right, the far left, or any place in between on the political spectrum. It is less likely that a candidate of, say, the Socialist Labor Party will represent interests that cannot be discerned from the party's ideological position. ***

We are not unmindful that the damage done by disclosure to the associational interests of the minor parties and their members and to supporters of independents could be significant. These movements are less likely to have a sound financial base and thus are more vulnerable to falloffs in contributions. In some instances fears of reprisal may deter contributions to the point where the movement cannot survive. The public interest also suffers if that result comes to pass, for there is a consequent reduction in the free circulation of ideas both within and without the political arena. ***

Appellants agree that "the record here does not reflect the kind of focused and insistent harassment of contributors and members that existed in the NAACP cases." They argue, however, that a blanket exemption for minor parties is necessary lest irreparable injury be done before the required evidence can be gathered. ***

We recognize that unduly strict requirements of proof could impose a heavy burden, but it does not follow that a blanket exemption for minor parties is necessary. Minor parties must be allowed sufficient flexibility in the proof of injury to assure a fair consideration of their claim. The evidence offered need show only a reasonable probability that the compelled disclosure of a party's contributors' names will subject them to threats, harassment, or reprisals from either Government officials or private parties. The proof may include, for example, specific evidence of past or present harassment of members due to their associational ties, or of harassment directed against the organization itself. A pattern of threats or specific manifestations of public hostility may be sufficient. New parties that have no history upon which to draw may be able to offer evidence of reprisals and threats directed against individuals or organizations holding similar views.*

C. Section 434(e)

Section 434(e) requires "[e]very person (other than a political committee or candidate) who makes contributions or expenditures" aggregating over $100 in a calendar year "other than by contribution to a political committee or candidate" to file a statement with the Commission. Unlike the other disclosure provisions, this section does not seek the contribution list of any association. Instead, it requires direct disclosure of what an individual or group contributes or spends. ***

To insure that the reach of § 434(e) is not impermissibly broad, we construe "expenditure" for purposes of that section in the same way we construed the terms of § 608(e)—to reach only funds used for communications that expressly advocate the election or defeat of a clearly identified candidate. This reading is directed precisely to that spending that is unambiguously related to the campaign of a particular federal candidate. ***

The $10 and $100 thresholds are indeed low. Contributors of relatively small amounts are likely to be especially sensitive to recording or disclosure of their political preferences. These strict requirements may well discourage participation by some citizens in the political process, a result that Congress hardly could have intended. *** But we cannot require Congress to establish that it has chosen the highest reasonable threshold. The line is necessarily a judgmental decision, best left in the context of this complex legislation to congressional discretion. We cannot say, on this bare record, that the limits designated are wholly without rationality. ***

III. PUBLIC FINANCING OF PRESIDENTIAL ELECTION CAMPAIGNS

***

A. Summary of Subtitle H

Section 9006 establishes a Presidential Election Campaign Fund (Fund), financed from general revenues in the aggregate amount designated by individual taxpayers, under § 6096, who on their income tax returns may authorize payment to the Fund of one dollar of their tax liability in the case of an individual return or two dollars in the case of a joint return. The Fund consists of three separate accounts to

---

*. **[Ed. Note.** See, e.g., Brown v. Socialist Workers '74 Campaign Committee, 459 U.S. 87 (1982) (disclosure requirements of Ohio law could not constitutionally be applied to Socialist Workers Party).]

finance (1) party nominating conventions, (2) general election campaigns, and (3) primary campaigns.

Chapter 95 of Title 26, which concerns financing of party nominating conventions and general election campaigns, distinguishes among "major," "minor," and "new" parties. A major party is defined as a party whose candidate for President in the most recent election received 25% more of the popular vote. A minor party is defined as a party whose candidate received at least 5% but less than 25% the vote at the most recent election. All other parties are new parties, including both newly created parties and those receiving less than 5% the vote in the last election.

Major parties are entitled to $2,000,000 to defray their national committee Presidential nominating convention expenses, must limit total expenditures to that amount, and may not use any of this money to benefit a particular candidate or delegate. A minor party receives a portion of the major-party entitlement determined by the ratio of the votes received by the party's candidate in the last election to the average of the votes received by the major-parties' candidates. The amounts given to the parties and the expenditure limit are adjusted for inflation, using 1974 as the base year. No financing is provided for new parties, nor is there any express provision for financing independent candidates or parties not holding a convention.

For expenses in the general election campaign, § 9004(a)(1) entitles each major-party candidate to $20,000,000. This amount is also adjusted for inflation. To be eligible for funds the candidate must pledge not to incur expenses in excess of the entitlement under § 9004(a)(1) and not to accept private contributions except to the extent that the fund is insufficient to provide the full entitlement. Minor-party candidates are also entitled to funding, again based on the ratio of the vote received by the party's candidate in the preceding election to the average of the major-party candidates. Minor-party candidates must certify that they will not incur campaign expenses in excess of the major-party entitlement and that they will accept private contributions only to the extent needed to make up the difference between that amount and the public funding grant. New-party candidates receive no money prior to the general election, but any candidate receiving 5% more of the popular vote in the election is entitled to post-election payments according to the formula applicable to minor-party candidates. *** A further eligibility requirement for minor- and new-party candidates is that the candidate's name must appear on the ballot, or electors pledged to the candidate must be on the ballot, in at least 10 States.

Chapter 96 establishes a third account in the Fund, the Presidential Primary Matching Payment Account. This funding is intended to aid campaigns by candidates seeking Presidential nomination "by a political party," in "primary elections." The threshold eligibility requirement is that the candidate raise at least $5,000 in each of 20 States, counting only the first $250 from each person contributing to the candidate. In addition, the candidate must agree to abide by the spending limits in § 9035. Funding is provided according to a matching formula: each qualified candidate is entitled to a sum equal to the total private contributions received, disregarding contributions from any person to the extent that total contributions to the candidate by that person exceed $250. Payments to any candidate under Chapter 96 may not exceed 50% of the overall expenditure ceiling accepted by the candidate.

B. Constitutionality of Subtitle H

Appellants argue that Subtitle H is invalid (1) as "contrary to the 'general welfare,'" Art. I, § 8, (2) because any scheme of public financing of election campaigns is inconsistent with the First Amendment, and (3) because Subtitle H invidiously discriminates against certain interests in violation of the Due Process Clause of the Fifth Amendment. We find no merit in these contentions.

Appellants' "general welfare" contention erroneously treats the General Welfare Clause as a limitation upon congressional power. It is rather a grant of power, the scope of which is quite expansive, particularly in view of the enlargement of power by the Necessary and Proper Clause.

Appellants' challenge to the dollar check-off provision (§ 6096) fails for the same reason. They maintain that Congress is required to permit taxpayers to designate particular candidates or parties as recipients of their money. But the appropriation to the Fund in § 9006 is like any other appropriation from the general revenue except that its amount is determined by reference to the aggregate of the one-and two-dollar authorization on taxpayers' income tax returns. This detail does not constitute the appropriation any less an appropriation by Congress.[124] The fallacy of appellants' argument is therefore apparent; every appropriation made by Congress uses public money in a manner to which some taxpayers object.

Appellants next argue that "by analogy" to the Religion Clauses of the First Amendment public financing of election campaigns, however meritorious, violates the First Amendment. We have, of course, held that the Religion Clauses—"Congress shall make no law respecting an establishment of religion, or prohibiting the free exercise thereof"—require Congress, and the States through the Fourteenth Amendment, to remain neutral in matters of religion. *E.g.*, Abington School Dist. v. Schempp, 374 U.S. 203, 222-226 (1963). The government may not aid one religion to the detriment of others or impose a burden on one religion that is not imposed on others, and may not even aid all religions. *E.g.*, Everson v. Board of Education, 330 U.S. 1, 15-16 (1947). See Kurland, Of Church and State and the Supreme Court, 29 U. Chi. L. Rev. 1, 96 (1961). But the analogy is patently inapplicable to our issue here. Although "Congress shall make no law *** abridging the freedom of speech, or of the press," Subtitle H is a congressional effort, not to abridge, restrict, or censor speech, but rather to use public money to facilitate and enlarge public discussion and

---

124. The scheme involves no compulsion upon individuals to finance the dissemination of ideas with which they disagree, Lathrop v. Donohue, 367 U.S. 820, 871, 882 (1961) (Black, J., dissenting); *** Machinists v. Street, 367 U.S. 740, 778 (1961) (Douglas, J., concurring); *id.*, at 788-792 (Black, J. dissenting). The § 6096 check-off is simply the means by which Congress determines the amount of its appropriation.

participation in the electoral process, goals vital to a self-governing people.[125] Thus, Subtitle H furthers, not abridges, pertinent First Amendment values.[126] Appellants argue, however, that as constructed public financing invidiously discriminates in violation of the Fifth Amendment. We turn therefore to that argument.

*** Any disadvantage suffered by operation of the eligibility formulae under Subtitle H is thus limited to the claimed denial of the enhancement of opportunity to communicate with the electorate that the formulae afford eligible candidates. But eligible candidates suffer a countervailing denial. As we more fully develop later, acceptance of public financing entails voluntary acceptance of an expenditure ceiling. Noneligible candidates are not subject to that limitation. Accordingly, we conclude that public financing is generally less restrictive of access to the electoral process than the ballot-access regulations dealt with in prior cases. ***

CONCLUSION

In summary, we sustain the individual contribution limits, the disclosure and reporting provisions, and the public financing scheme. We conclude, however, that the limitations on campaign expenditures, on independent expenditures by individuals and groups, and on expenditures by a candidate from his personal funds are constitutionally infirm. ***

MR. CHIEF JUSTICE BURGER, concurring in part and dissenting in part.

For reasons set forth more fully later, I dissent from those parts of the Court's holding sustaining the statutory provisions (a) for disclosure of small contributions, (b) for limitations on contributions, and (c) for public financing of Presidential campaigns. In my view, the Act's disclosure scheme is impermissibly broad and violative of the First Amendment as it relates to reporting contributions in excess of $10

---

125. Appellants voice concern that public funding will lead to governmental control of the internal affairs of political parties, and thus to a significant loss of political freedom. The concern is necessarily wholly speculative and hardly a basis for invalidation of the public financing scheme on its face. Congress has expressed its determination to avoid the possibility. S. Rep. No. 93-689, pp. 9-10 (1974).

126. The historical bases of the Religion and Speech Clauses are markedly different. Intolerable persecutions throughout history led to the Framers' firm determination that religious worship—both in method and belief—must be strictly protected from government intervention. "Another purpose of the Establishment Clause rested upon an awareness of the historical fact that governmentally established religions and religious persecutions go hand in hand." Engel v. Vitale, 370 U.S. 421, 432 (1962) (footnote omitted). See Everson v. Board of Education, 330 U.S. 1, 8-15 (1947). But the central purpose of the Speech and Press Clauses was to assure a society in which "uninhibited, robust, and wide-open" public debate concerning matters of public interest would thrive, for only in such a society can a healthy representative democracy flourish. New York Times Co. v. Sullivan, 376 U.S. 254, 270 (1964). Legislation to enhance these First Amendment values is the rule, not the exception. Our statute books are replete with laws providing financial assistance to the exercise of free speech, such as aid to public broadcasting and other forms of educational media, 47 U.S.C. §§ 390-399, and preferential postal rates and antitrust exemptions for newspapers, 39 CFR § 132.2 (1975); 15 U.S.C. §§ 1801-1804.

and $100. The contribution limitations infringe on First Amendment liberties and suffer from the same infirmities that the Court correctly sees in the expenditure ceilings. The system for public financing of Presidential campaigns is, in my judgment, an impermissible intrusion by the Government into the traditionally private political process.

(1)
DISCLOSURE PROVISIONS

***

The public right to know ought not be absolute when its exercise reveals private political convictions. Secrecy, like privacy, is not *per se* criminal. On the contrary, secrecy and privacy as to political preferences and convictions are fundamental in a free society. For example, one of the great political reforms was the advent of the secret ballot as a universal practice. Similarly, the enlightened labor legislation of our time has enshrined the secrecy of choice of a bargaining representative for workers. In other contexts, this Court has seen to it that governmental power cannot be used to force a citizen to disclose his private affiliations, NAACP v. Button, 371 U.S. 415 (1963), even without a record reflecting any systematic harassment or retaliation, as in Shelton v. Tucker, 364 U.S. 479 (1960). For me it is far too late in the day to recognize an ill-defined "public interest" to breach the historic safeguards guaranteed by the First Amendment. ***

In light of these views, it seems to me that the threshold limits fixed at $10 and $100 for anonymous contributions are constitutionally impermissible on their face. As the Court's opinion notes, Congress gave little or no thought, one way or the other, to these limits, but rather lifted figures out of a 65-year-old statute. *** To argue that a 1976 contribution of $10 or $100 entails a risk of corruption or its appearance is simply too extravagant to be maintained. ***

Finally, no legitimate public interest has been shown in forcing the disclosure of modest contributions that are the prime support of new, unpopular, or unfashionable political causes. There is no realistic possibility that such modest donations will have a corrupting influence especially on parties that enjoy only "minor" status. Major parties would not notice them; minor parties need them. Furthermore, as the Court candidly recognizes, minor parties and new parties tend to be sharply ideological in character, and the public can readily discern where such parties stand, without resorting to the indirect device of recording the names of financial supporters. To hold, as the Court has, that privacy must sometimes yield to congressional investigations of alleged subversion, is quite different from making domestic political partisans give up privacy. ***

I would therefore hold unconstitutional the provisions requiring reporting of contributions of more than $10 and to make a public record of the name, address, and occupation of a contributor of more than $100.

(2)
CONTRIBUTION AND EXPENDITURE

I agree fully with that part of the Court's opinion that holds unconstitutional the limitations the Act puts on campaign expenditures which "place substantial and direct restrictions on the ability of candidates, citizens, and associations to engage in protected political expression, restrictions that the First Amendment cannot tolerate." *** Yet when it approves similarly stringent limitations on contributions, the Court ignores the reasons it finds so persuasive in the context of expenditures. For me contributions and expenditures are two sides of the same First Amendment coin. ***

*** I see only two possible ways in which money differs from volunteer work, endorsements, and the like. Money can be used to buy favors, because an unscrupulous politician can put it to personal use; second, giving money is a less visible form of associational activity. With respect to the first problem, the Act does not attempt to do any more than the bribery laws to combat this sort of corruption. In fact, the Act does not reach at all, and certainly the contribution limits do not reach, forms of "association" that can be fully as corrupt as a contribution intended as a *quid pro quo* —such as the eleventh-hour endorsement by a former rival, obtained for the promise of a federal appointment. This underinclusiveness is not a constitutional flaw, but it demonstrates that the contribution limits do not clearly focus on this first distinction. To the extent Congress thought that the second problem, the lesser visibility of contributions, required that money be treated differently from other forms of associational activity, disclosure laws are the simple and wholly efficacious answer; they make the invisible apparent.

(3)
PUBLIC FINANCING

I dissent from Part III sustaining the constitutionality of the public financing provisions of Subtitle H. ***

I agree with MR. JUSTICE REHNQUIST that the scheme approved by the Court today invidiously discriminates against minor parties. Assuming, *arguendo*, the constitutionality of the overall scheme, there is a legitimate governmental interest in requiring a group to make a "preliminary showing of a significant modicum of support." Jenness v. Fortson, 403 U.S. 431, 442 (1971). But the present system could preclude or severely hamper access to funds before a given election by a group or an individual who might, at the time of the election, reflect the views of a major segment or even a majority of the electorate. The fact that there have been few drastic realignments in our basic two-party structure in 200 years is no constitutional justification for freezing the status quo of the present major parties at the expense of such future political movements. ***

I would also find unconstitutional the system of matching grants which makes a candidate's ability to amass private funds the sole criterion for eligibility for public funds. Such an arrangement can put at serious disadvantage a candidate with a potentially large, widely diffused—but poor—constituency. The ability of a candidate's supporters to help pay for his campaign cannot be equated with their willingness to cast a ballot for him. See Lubin v. Panish, 415 U.S. 709 (1974); Bullock v. Carter, 405 U.S. 134 (1972). ***

MR. JUSTICE WHITE, concurring in part and dissenting in part.

***

*** I dissent, from the Court's view that the expenditure limitations of 18 U.S.C. §§ 608 (c) and (e) (1970 ed., Supp. IV) violate the First Amendment. ***

Let us suppose that each of two brothers spends $1 million on TV spot announcements that he has individually prepared and in which he appears, urging the election of the same named candidate in identical words. One brother has sought and obtained the approval of the candidate; the other has not. The former may validly be prosecuted under § 608(e); under the Court's view, the latter may not, even though the candidate could scarcely help knowing about and appreciating the expensive favor. For constitutional purposes it is difficult to see the difference between the two situations. I would take the word of those who know—that limiting independent expenditures is essential to prevent transparent and widespread evasion of the contribution limits.

It is also important to restore and maintain public confidence in federal elections. It is critical to obviate or dispel the impression that federal elections are purely and simply a function of money, that federal offices are bought and sold or that political races are reserved for those who have the facility—and the stomach— for doing whatever it takes to bring together those interests, groups, and individuals that can raise or contribute large fortunes in order to prevail at the polls.

The ceiling on candidate expenditures represents the considered judgment of Congress that elections are to be decided among candidates none of whom has overpowering advantage by reason of a huge campaign war chest. ***

I also disagree with the Court's judgment that § 608(a), which limits the amount of money that a candidate or his family may spend on his campaign, violates the Constitution. Although it is true that this provision does not promote any interest in preventing the corruption of candidates, the provision does, nevertheless, serve salutary purposes related to the integrity of federal campaigns. By limiting the importance of personal wealth, § 608(a) helps to assure that only individuals with a modicum of support from others will be viable candidates. This in turn would tend to discourage any notion that the outcome of elections is primarily a function of money. Similarly, § 608(a) tends to equalize access to the political arena, encouraging the less wealthy, unable to bankroll their own campaigns, to run for political office.

As with the campaign expenditure limits, Congress was entitled to determine that personal wealth ought to play a less important role in political campaigns than it has in the past. Nothing in the First Amendment stands in the way of that determination. ***

MR. JUSTICE MARSHALL, concurring in part and dissenting in part.

*** The Court invalidates § 608(a) as violative of the candidate's First Amendment rights. "[T]he First Amendment," the Court explains, "simply cannot tolerate § 608(a)'s restriction upon the freedom of a candidate to speak without legislative limit on behalf of his own candidacy." *** I disagree.

To be sure, § 608(a) affects the candidate's exercise of his First Amendment rights. But unlike the other expenditure limitations contained in the Act and invalidated by the Court—the limitation on independent expenditures relative to a clearly identified candidate, § 608(e), and the limitations on overall candidate expenditures, § 608(c)—the limitations on expenditures by candidates from personal resources contained in § 608(a) need never prevent the speaker from spending another dollar to communicate his ideas. Section 608(a) imposes no overall limit on the amount a candidate can spend; it simply limits the "contribution" a candidate may make to his own campaign. The candidate remains free to raise an unlimited amount in contributions from others. So long as the candidate does not contribute to his campaign more than the amount specified in § 608(a), and so long as he does not accept contributions from others in excess of the limitations imposed by § 608(b), he is free to spend without limit on behalf of his campaign. *** The Court views "[t]he ancillary interest in equalizing the relative financial resources of candidates" as the relevant rationale for § 608(a), and deems that interest insufficient to justify § 608(a). *** In my view the interest is more precisely the interest in promoting the reality and appearance of equal access to the political arena. ***

MR. JUSTICE BLACKMUN, concurring in part and dissenting in part.

I am not persuaded that the Court makes, or indeed is able to make, a principled constitutional distinction between the contribution limitations, on the one hand, and the expenditure limitations, on the other, that are involved here. I therefore do not join Part I-B of the Court's opinion or those portions of Part I-A that are consistent with Part I-B. As to those, I dissent. ***

MR. JUSTICE REHNQUIST, concurring in part and dissenting in part.

I concur in Parts I, II, and IV of the Court's opinion. I concur in so much of Part III of the Court's opinion as holds that the public funding of the cost of a Presidential election campaign is a permissible exercise of congressional authority under the power to tax and spend granted by Art. I, but dissent from Part III-B-1 of the Court's opinion, which holds that certain aspects of the statutory treatment of minor parties and independent candidates are constitutionally valid. I state as briefly as possible my reasons for so doing. *** I would hold that, as to general election financing, Congress has not merely treated the two major parties differently from minor parties and independents, but has discriminated in favor of the former in such a way as to run afoul of the Fifth and First Amendments to the United States Constitution.

CITIZENS AGAINST RENT CONTROL v. BERKELEY
454 U.S. 290 (1981)

CHIEF JUSTICE BURGER delivered the opinion of the Court.

The issue on appeal is whether a limitation of $ 250 on contributions to committees formed to support or oppose ballot measures violates the First Amendment.

I

The voters of Berkeley, Cal., adopted the Election Reform Act of 1974, Ord. No. 4700-N.S., by initiative. *** Section 602 of the ordinance provides:

> "No person shall make, and no campaign treasurer shall solicit or accept, any contribution which will cause the total amount contributed by such person with respect to a single election in support of or in opposition to a measure to exceed two hundred and fifty dollars ($250)."

Appellant Citizens Against Rent Control is an unincorporated association formed to oppose a ballot measure at issue in the April 19, 1977, election. The ballot measure would have imposed rent control on many of Berkeley's rental units. To make its views on the ballot measure known, Citizens Against Rent Control raised more than $108,000 from approximately 1,300 contributors. It accepted nine contributions over the $250 limit. Those nine contributions totaled $20,850, or $18,600 more than if none of the contributions exceeded $250. Pursuant to § 604 of the ordinance,[3] appellee Berkeley Fair Campaign Practices Commission, 20 days before the election, ordered appellant Citizens Against Rent Control to pay $18,600 into the city treasury.

Two weeks before the election, Citizens Against Rent Control sought and obtained a temporary restraining order prohibiting enforcement of §§ 602 and 604. The ballot measure relating to rent control was defeated. The Superior Court subsequently granted Citizens Against Rent Control's motion for summary judgment, declaring that § 602 was invalid on its face because it violated the First Amendment of the United States Constitution and Art. I, § 2, of the California Constitution. A panel of the California Court of Appeal unanimously affirmed that conclusion.

The California Supreme Court, dividing 4-3, reversed. We noted probable jurisdiction, and we reverse. ***

There are, of course, some activities, legal if engaged in by one, yet illegal if performed in concert with others, but political expression is not one of them. To place a Spartan limit—or indeed any limit—on individuals wishing to band together

---

3. Section 604 states: "If any person is found guilty of violating the terms of this chapter, each campaign treasurer who received part or all of the contribution or contributions which constitute the violation shall pay promptly, from available campaign funds, if any, the amount received from such persons in excess of the amount permitted by this chapter to the City Auditor for deposit in the General fund of the City."

to advance their views on a ballot measure, while placing none on individuals acting alone, is clearly a restraint on the right of association. Section 602 does not seek to mute the voice of one individual, and it cannot be allowed to hobble the collective expressions of a group.

Buckley identified a single narrow exception to the rule that limits on political activity were contrary to the First Amendment. The exception relates to the perception of undue influence of large contributors to a *candidate*. Federal Courts of Appeals have recognized that Buckley does not support limitations on contributions to committees formed to favor or oppose *ballot measures*. ***

Whatever may be the state interest or degree of that interest in regulating and limiting contributions to or expenditures of a candidate or a candidate's committees there is no significant state or public interest in curtailing debate and discussion of a ballot measure. Placing limits on contributions which in turn limit expenditures plainly impairs freedom of expression. The integrity of the political system will be adequately protected if contributors are identified in a public filing revealing the amounts contributed; if it is thought wise, legislation can outlaw anonymous contributions. *** Reversed and remanded.

JUSTICE REHNQUIST, concurring. [Omitted.]

JUSTICE MARSHALL, concurring in the judgment.

The Court today holds that a local ordinance restricting the amount of money that an individual can contribute to a committee organized to support or oppose a ballot measure violates the right to freedom of speech and association guaranteed by the First Amendment. In reaching this conclusion, however, the Court fails to indicate whether or not it attaches any constitutional significance to the fact that the Berkeley ordinance seeks to limit *contributions* as opposed to direct *expenditures.* *** If I found that the record before the California Supreme Court disclosed sufficient evidence to justify the conclusion that large contributions to ballot measure committees undermined the "confidence of the citizenry in government," First National Bank of Boston v. Bellotti, 435 U.S. 765, 790 (1978), I would join JUSTICE WHITE in dissent on the ground that the State had demonstrated a sufficient governmental interest to sustain the indirect infringement on First Amendment interests resulting from the operation of the Berkeley ordinance. Like JUSTICES BLACKMUN and O'CONNOR, however, I find no such evidentiary support in this record. I therefore concur in the judgment.

JUSTICE BLACKMUN and JUSTICE O'CONNOR, concurring in the judgment. [Omitted.]

JUSTICE WHITE, dissenting.

*** [T]he ordinance regulates contributions but not expenditures and does not prohibit corporate spending. ***

The Court reaches the conclusion that the ordinance is unconstitutional only by giving *Buckley* the most extreme reading and by essentially giving the Berkeley ordinance no reading at all. It holds that the contributions involved here are "beyond question a very significant form of political expression." *** Yet in *Buckley* the Court found that contribution limitations "entai[l] only a marginal restriction upon the contributor's ability to engage in free communication." As with contributions to candidates, ballot measure contributions "involv[e] speech by someone other than the contributor" and a limitation on such donations "does not in any way infringe the contributor's freedom to discuss candidates and issues."

It is bad enough that the Court overstates the extent to which First Amendment interests are implicated. But the Court goes on to assert that the ordinance furthers no legitimate public interest and cannot survive "any degree of scrutiny." Apparently the Court assumes this to be so because the ordinance is not directed at *quid pro quos* between large contributors and candidates for office, "the single narrow exception" for regulation that it viewed Buckley as endorsing. ***

By restricting the size of contributions, the Berkeley ordinance requires major contributors to communicate directly with the voters. *** Of course, entities remain free to make major direct expenditures. But because political communications must state the source of funds, voters will be able to identify the source of such messages and recognize that the communication reflects, for example, the opinion of a single powerful corporate interest rather than the views of a large number of individuals. *** When the infringement is as slight and ephemeral as it is here, the requisite state interest to justify the regulation need not be so high.

FEDERAL ELECTION COMMISSION v. NATIONAL CONSERVATIVE POLITICAL ACTION COMMITTEE

470 U.S. 480 (1985)

JUSTICE REHNQUIST delivered the opinion of the Court.*

The Presidential Election Campaign Fund Act (Fund Act), 26 U.S.C. § 9001 *et seq.*, offers the Presidential candidates of major political parties the option of receiving public financing for their general election campaigns. If a Presidential candidate elects public financing, § 9012(f) makes it a criminal offense for independent "political committees," such as appellees National Conservative Political Action Committee (NCPAC) and Fund For A Conservative Majority (FCM), to expend more than $1,000 to further that candidate's election. A three-judge District Court for the Eastern District of Pennsylvania, in companion lawsuits brought respectively by the Federal Election Commission (FEC) and by the Democratic Party of the United States and the Democratic National Committee (DNC), held § 9012(f)

*JUSTICE BRENNAN joins only Part II of this opinion.

unconstitutional on its face because it violated the First Amendment to the United States Constitution. *** [W]e turn to the merits of the FEC's appeal of its unsuccessful declaratory judgment action against the PACs.

II

NCPAC is a nonprofit, nonmembership corporation formed under the District of Columbia Nonprofit Corporation Act in August 1975 and registered with the FEC as a political committee. Its primary purpose is to attempt to influence directly or indirectly the election or defeat of candidates for federal, state, and local offices by making contributions and by making its own expenditures. It is governed by a three-member board of directors which is elected annually by the existing board. The board's chairman and the other two members make all decisions concerning which candidates to support or oppose, the strategy and methods to employ, and the amounts of money to spend. Its contributors have no role in these decisions. It raises money by general and specific direct mail solicitations. It does not maintain separate accounts for the receipts from its general and specific solicitations, nor is it required by law to do so.

FCM is incorporated under the laws of Virginia and is registered with the FEC as a multicandidate political committee. In all material respects it is identical to NCPAC.

Both NCPAC and FCM are self-described ideological organizations with a conservative political philosophy. They solicited funds in support of President Reagan's 1980 campaign, and they spent money on such means as radio and television advertisements to encourage voters to elect him President. On the record before us, these expenditures were "independent" in that they were not made at the request of or in coordination with the official Reagan election campaign committee or any of its agents. Indeed, there are indications that the efforts of these organizations were at times viewed with disfavor by the official campaign as counterproductive to its chosen strategy. NCPAC and FCM expressed their intention to conduct similar activities in support of President Reagan's reelection in 1984, and we may assume that they did so. ***

In these cases we consider provisions of the Fund Act that make it a criminal offense for political committees such as NCPAC and FCM to make independent expenditures in support of a candidate who has elected to accept public financing. Specifically, § 9012(f) provides:

> "(1) *** it shall be unlawful for any political committee which is not an authorized committee with respect to the eligible candidates of a political party for President and Vice President in a presidential election knowingly and willfully to incur expenditures to further the election of such candidates, which would constitute qualified campaign expenses if incurred by an authorized committee of such candidates, in an aggregate amount exceeding $1,000."

***

*** [T]he PACs independent expenditures at issue in this case are squarely prohibited by § 9012(f), and we proceed to consider whether that prohibition violates the First Amendment.

There can be no doubt that the expenditures at issue in this case produce speech at the core of the First Amendment. ***

The PACs in this case, of course, are not lone pamphleteers or street corner orators in the Tom Paine mold; they spend substantial amounts of money in order to communicate their political ideas through sophisticated media advertisements. And of course the criminal sanction in question is applied to the expenditure of money to propagate political views, rather than to the propagation of those views unaccompanied by the expenditure of money. But for purposes of presenting political views in connection with a nationwide Presidential election, allowing the presentation of views while forbidding the expenditure of more than $1,000 to present them is much like allowing a speaker in a public hall to express his views while denying him the use of an amplifying system. The Court said in *Buckley v. Valeo*:

> "A restriction on the amount of money a person or group can spend on political communication during a campaign necessarily reduces the quantity of expression by restricting the number of issues discussed, the depth of their exploration, and the size of the audience reached. This is because virtually every means of communicating ideas in today's mass society requires the expenditure of money. The distribution of the humblest handbill or leaflet entails printing, paper, and circulation costs. Speeches and rallies generally necessitate hiring a hall and publicizing the event. The electorate's increasing dependence on television, radio, and other mass media for news and information has made these expensive modes of communication indispensable instruments of effective political speech."

We also reject the notion that the PACs' form of organization or method of solicitation diminishes their entitlement to First Amendment protection. The First Amendment freedom of association is squarely implicated in these cases. NCPAC and FCM are mechanisms by which large numbers of individuals of modest means can join together in organizations which serve to "amplif[y] the voice of their adherents." *** It is significant that in 1979-1980 approximately 101,000 people contributed an average of $75 each to NCPAC and in 1980 approximately 100,000 people contributed an average of $25 each to FCM.

The FEC urges that these contributions do not constitute individual speech, but merely "speech by proxy," see California Medical Assn. v. FEC, 453 U.S. 182, 196 (1981) (Marshall, J.) (plurality opinion), because the contributors do not control or decide upon the use of the funds by the PACs or the specific content of the PACs' advertisements and other speech. The plurality emphasized in that case, however, that nothing in the statutory provision in question "limits the amount [an unincorporated association] or any of its members may independently expend in order to advocate political views," but only the amount it may contribute to a multicandidate political committee. Unlike *California Medical Assn.*, the present cases involve limitations on expenditures by PACs, not on the contributions they receive; and in any event these contributions are predominantly small and thus do not raise the same concerns as the sizable contributions involved in *California Medical Assn.*

Another reason the "proxy speech" approach is not useful in this case is that the contributors obviously like the message they are bearing from these organizations and want to add their voices to that message; otherwise they would not part with their money. To say that their collective action in pooling their resources to amplify their voices is not entitled to full First Amendment protection would subordinate the voices of those of modest means as opposed to those sufficiently wealthy to be able to buy expensive media ads with their own resources. ***

We held in *Buckley* and reaffirmed in *Citizens Against Rent Control* that preventing corruption or the appearance of corruption are the only legitimate and compelling government interests thus far identified for restricting campaign finances. In *Buckley* we struck down the FECA's limitation on individuals' independent expenditures because we found no tendency in such expenditures, uncoordinated with the candidate or his campaign, to corrupt or to give the appearance of corruption. ***

We think the same conclusion must follow here. It is contended that, because the PACs may by the breadth of their organizations spend larger amounts than the individuals in *Buckley*, the potential for corruption is greater. But precisely what the "corruption" may consist of we are never told with assurance. The fact that candidates and elected officials may alter or reaffirm their own positions on issues in response to political messages paid for by the PACs can hardly be called corruption, for one of the essential features of democracy is the presentation to the electorate of varying points of view. It is of course hypothetically possible here, as in the case of the independent expenditures forbidden in *Buckley*, that candidates may take notice of and reward those responsible for PAC expenditures by giving official favors to the latter in exchange for the supporting messages. But here, as in *Buckley*, the absence of prearrangement and coordination undermines the value of the expenditure to the candidate, and thereby alleviates the danger that expenditures will be given as a *quid pro quo* for improper commitments from the candidate. On this record, such an exchange of political favors for uncoordinated expenditures remains a hypothetical possibility and nothing more.

Even were we to determine that the large pooling of financial resources by NCPAC and FCM did pose a potential for corruption or the appearance of corruption, § 9012(f) is a fatally overbroad response to that evil. It is not limited to multimillion dollar war chests; its terms apply equally to informal discussion groups that solicit neighborhood contributions to publicize their views about a particular Presidential candidate. ***

[I]t has been suggested that § 9012(f) could be narrowed by limiting its prohibition to political committees in which the contributors have no voice in the use to which the contributions are put. Again, there is no indication in the statute or the legislative history that Congress would be content with such a construction. More importantly, as observed by the District Court, such a construction is intolerably vague. At what point, for example, does a neighborhood group that solicits some outside contributions fall within § 9012(f)? How active do the group members have to be in setting policy to satisfy the control test? Moreover, it is doubtful that the members of a large association in which each have a vote on policy have substantially more control in practice than the contributors to NCPAC and FCM: the latter will surely cease contributing when the message those organizations deliver ceases to please them. *** In *NRWC*, 459 U.S., at 210, we stated:

> "While [2 U.S.C.] § 441b restricts the solicitation of corporations and labor unions without great financial resources, as well as those more fortunately situated, we accept Congress' judgment that it is the potential for such influence that demands regulation. Nor will we second-guess a legislative determination as to the need for prophylactic measures where corruption is the evil feared."

Here, however, the groups and associations in question, designed expressly to participate in political debate, are quite different from the traditional corporations organized for economic gain. In *NRWC* we rightly concluded that Congress might include, along with labor unions and corporations traditionally prohibited from making contributions to political candidates, membership corporations, though contributions by the latter might not exhibit all of the evil that contributions by traditional economically organized corporations exhibit. But this proper deference to a congressional determination of the need for a prophylactic rule where the evil of potential corruption had long been recognized does not suffice to establish the validity of § 9012(f), which indiscriminately lumps with corporations any "committee, association or organization." Indeed, the FEC in its briefs to this Court does not even make an effort to defend the statute under a construction limited in reach to corporations. ***

JUSTICE STEVENS, concurring in part and dissenting in part. [Omitted.]

JUSTICE WHITE dissenting.

***

I continue to believe that Buckley v. Valeo, 424 U.S. 1 (1976), was wrongly decided. *** As in *Buckley*, I am convinced that it is pointless to limit the amount that can be contributed to a candidate or spent with his approval without also limiting the amounts that can be spent on his behalf. In the Fund Act, Congress limited contributions, direct or coordinated, to zero. It is nonsensical to allow the purposes of this limitation to be entirely defeated by allowing the sort of "independent" expenditures at issue here, and the First Amendment does not require us to do so.

Even if I accepted *Buckley* as binding precedent, I nonetheless would uphold § 9012(f). Buckley distinguished "direct political expression," which could not be curtailed, from financial contributions, which could. Limitations on expenditures were considered direct restraints on the right to speak one's mind on public issues and to engage in advocacy protected by the First Amendment. The majority views the challenged provision as being in that category. I disagree. *** [C]ontributors are not engaging in speech; at least, they are not engaging in speech to any greater extent than are those who contribute directly to political campaigns. *Buckley* explicitly distinguished between, on the one hand, using one's own money to express one's views, and, on the other, giving money to someone else in the expectation that that person will use the money to express views with which one is in agreement. This case falls within the latter category. As the *Buckley* Court stated with regard to contributions to campaigns, "the transformation of contributions into political debate involves speech by someone other than the contributor." The majority does not explain the metamorphosis of donated dollars from money into speech by virtue of the identity of the donee. ***

Because it is an indispensable component of the public funding scheme, § 9012(f) is supported by governmental interests absent in *Buckley*. Rather than forcing Congress to abandon public financing because it is unworkable without constitutionally prohibited restrictions on independent spending, I would hold that § 9012(f) is permissible precisely because it is a necessary, narrowly drawn means to a constitutional end. The need to make public financing, with its attendant benefits, workable is a constitutionally sufficient additional justification for the burden on First Amendment rights. ***

JUSTICE MARSHALL, dissenting.

*** Relying on *Buckley*, the Court today strikes down a limitation on expenditures by "political committees." Although I joined the portion of the *Buckley per curiam* that distinguished contributions from independent expenditures for First Amendment purposes, I now believe that the distinction has no constitutional significance. ***

Undoubtedly, when an individual interested in obtaining the proverbial ambassadorship had the option of either contributing directly to a candidate's campaign or doing so indirectly through independent expenditures, he gave money directly. It does not take great imagination, however, to see that, when the possibility for direct financial assistance is severely limited, as it is in light of *Buckley*'s decision to uphold the contribution limitation, such an individual will find other ways to financially benefit the candidate's campaign. It simply belies reality to say that a campaign will not reward massive financial assistance provided in the only way that is legally available. And the possibility of such a reward provides a powerful incentive to channel an independent expenditure into an area that a candidate will appreciate. Surely an eager supporter will be able to discern a candidate's needs and desires; similarly, a willing candidate will notice the supporter's efforts. To the extent that individuals are able to make independent expenditures as part of a *quid pro quo*, they succeed in undermining completely the first rationale for the distinction made in *Buckley*. ***

NOTE

In the last case, *FEC v. NCPAC*, the Court sustained the first amendment claim of independent political action committees (PACs) to operate as nonprofit, nonmembership corporations, soliciting funds from others to be spent as the directors of the Political Action Committee approve for media advertising urging the election or defeat of presidential candidates, including candidates already receiving federal funds. As in *Buckley v. Valeo*, in the Court's review of expenditure restrictions on individuals and political advocacy associations (e.g., the ACLU), the fact that these expenditures were not subject to the direction, control, or coordination of the candidate or of his or her campaign supplied the distinguishing key. Third party first amendment rights cannot be made to turn on whether a given candidate accepts or does not accept public funds.[151]

Would it make any constitutional difference if the limit on such candidate-specific expenditures were applied only to ordinary business corporations, e.g., publicly traded common stock companies primarily in business to produce or sell certain goods or services—such as General Motors or AT&T? Even assuming no public funding of candidates, might a state statute restricting ordinary commercial corporations from authorizing their boards of directors to use general corporate funds[152] to buy media advertisements to support or oppose any candidate for local or state elected office be valid despite *Buckley* and *NCPAC*?[153]

If the Supreme Court upheld the corporation's first amendment claim in respect to such expenditures when directed to advertising campaigns urging the adoption or defeat of a ballot measure,[154] would you expect the result to be any different in

---

151. Consistent with the reasoning in *Buckley*, the candidate can decide whether he or she is better off by accepting public campaign funds and accepting limits on spending his or her own funds (and those of any committee working with the candidate); whatever the candidate's calculus, however, it cannot act to limit the independent first amendment rights of others to "speak" as they wish.

152. As distinct from such funds as the company may gain by means of specially soliciting shareholders to contribute to a segregated corporate fund.

153. Is there a constitutionally-viable distinction insofar as the corporation is a for-profit, commercially owned company, owned by multitudes of shareholders who buy and sell principally (perhaps solely) for investment reasons and not for any reason of political interest? Even though the corporation's articles of incorporation permit the directors to make decisions of this sort, and even though any shareholder personally offended by the corporation's choice of candidates to support or oppose in this way, may sell his or her shares and take their money elsewhere at any time? See Victor Brudney, Association, Advocacy, and the First Amendment, 4 Wm. & Mary Bill of Rts.J. 1, 62-74, and references at 64 n.159 (1995). Compare a nonprofit, ideological corporation; see, e.g., Federal Election Comm'n v. Massachussetts for Citizens for Life, 479 U.S. 238 (1986).

154. See First Nat'l Bank of Boston v. Bellotti, 435 U.S. 765 (1978). And consider also Citizens Against Rent Control v. Berkeley, 454 U.S. 290 (1981).

respect to such expenditures relative to identified candidates for office instead?[155] Though these pro- or anti-candidate expenditures are wholly independent of any expenditures made by the candidate or the candidate's campaign committee? If the outcome were different, on what basis, if any, could such a difference be proposed?[156]

COLORADO REPUBLICAN FEDERAL CAMPAIGN COMMITTEE v. FEDERAL ELECTION COMMISSION

518 U.S. 604 (1996)

JUSTICE BREYER announced the judgment of the Court and delivered an opinion, in which JUSTICE O'CONNOR and JUSTICE SOUTER join.

In April 1986, before the Colorado Republican Party had selected its senatorial candidate for the fall's election, that Party's Federal Campaign Committee bought radio advertisements attacking Timothy Wirth, the Democratic Party's likely candidate. The Federal Election Commission (FEC) charged that this "expenditure" exceeded the dollar limits that a provision of the Federal Election Campaign Act of 1971 (FECA) imposes upon political party "expenditure[s] in connection with" a "general election campaign" for congressional office. This case focuses upon the constitutionality of those limits as applied to this case. We conclude that the First Amendment prohibits the application of this provision to the kind of expenditure at issue here — an expenditure that the political party has made independently, without coordination with any candidate.

I

To understand the issues and our holding, one must begin with FECA as it emerged from Congress in 1974. ***

---

155. Suppose the for-profit, large corporation is itself a "media" company, e.g., a newspaper such as the Miami Herald, devoting free space in its own publications to express its endorsement for candidates it wants to see elected. (The outcome here is quite clear, is it not?)

156. See Austin v. Michigan Chamber of Commerce, 494 U.S. 652 (1990) (sustaining such a limit). For a useful critical review of *Austin*, see Larry E. Ribstein, Corporate Political Speech, 49 Wash. & Lee L.Rev. 109 (1992). For two (of many) substantial and contrasting reviews on the general questions raised in the *Buckley* line of cases (i.e. various bills on public financing, election "reform," and limitations on money and speech), compare J. Skelly Wright, Money and the Pollution of Politics: Is the First Amendment an Obstacle to Political Equality?, 82 Colum.L.Rev. 609 (1982), with Joel L. Fleischman & Pope McCorkle, Level-Up Rather Than Level-Down: Toward a New Theory of Campaign Finance Reform, 1 J.Law & Pol. 211 (1984). See also Lillian R. BeVier, Money and Politics: A Perspective on the First Amendment and Campaign Finance Reform, 73 Cal.L.Rev. 1045 (1985); Lillian R. BeVier, Campaign Finance Reform: Specious Arguments, Intractable Dilemmas, 94 Colum.L.Rev. 1258 (1994); Victor Blasi, Free Speech and the Widening Gyre of Fund-Raising: Why Campaign Spending Limits May Not Violate the First Amendment After All, 94 Colum.L.Rev. 1281 (1994); Jamin Raskin & John Bonifaz, The Constitutional Imperative and Practical Superiority of Democratically Financed Elections, 94 Colum.L.Rev. 1160 (1994).

Most of the provisions this Court found unconstitutional imposed expenditure limits. *** The provisions that the Court found constitutional mostly imposed contribution limits — limits that apply both when an individual or political committee contributes money directly to a candidate and also when they indirectly contribute by making expenditures that they coordinate with the candidate. See *Buckley*, [424 U.S.] at 23-36. See also *California Medical Assn. [v. Federal Election Comm'n*, 453 U.S.], at 193-199 (limits on contributions to political committees). Consequently, for present purposes, the Act now prohibits individuals and political committees from making direct, or indirect, contributions that exceed the [specified] limits.

FECA also has a special provision, directly at issue in this case, that governs contributions and expenditures by political parties. After exempting political parties from the general contribution and expenditure limitations of the statute, the Party Expenditure Provision then imposes a substitute limitation upon party "expenditures" in a senatorial campaign equal to the greater of $20,000 or "2 cents multiplied by the voting age population of the State," § 441a(d)(3)(A)(I), adjusted for inflation since 1974, § 441a(c). The Provision permitted a political party in Colorado in 1986 to spend about $103,000 in connection with the general election campaign of a candidate for the United States Senate. ***

II

The summary judgment record indicates that the expenditure in question is what this Court in Buckley called an "independent" expenditure, not a "coordinated" expenditure that other provisions of FECA treat as a kind of campaign "contribution." The record describes how the expenditure was made. In a deposition, the Colorado Party's Chairman, Howard Callaway, pointed out that, at the time of the expenditure, the Party had not yet selected a senatorial nominee from among the three individuals vying for the nomination. He added that he arranged for the development of the script at his own initiative, that he, and no one else, approved it, that the only other politically relevant individuals who might have read it were the party's executive director and political director, and that all relevant discussions took place at meetings attended only by party staff. *** We can find no "genuine" issue of fact in this respect. And we therefore treat the expenditure, for constitutional purposes, as an "independent" expenditure, not an indirect campaign contribution.

So treated, the expenditure falls within the scope of the Court's precedents that extend First Amendment protection to independent expenditures. Beginning with *Buckley*, the Court's cases have found a "fundamental constitutional difference between money spent to advertise one's views independently of the candidate's campaign and money contributed to the candidate to be spent on his campaign." At the same time, reasonable contribution limits directly and materially advance the Government's interest in preventing exchanges of large financial contributions for political favors. ***

Given these established principles, we do not see how a provision that limits a political party's independent expenditures can escape their controlling effect. A political party's independent expression not only reflects its members' views about the philosophical and governmental matters that bind them together, it also seeks to convince others to join those members in a practical democratic task, the task of creating a government that voters can instruct and hold responsible for subsequent success or failure. The independent expression of a political party's views is "core" First Amendment activity no less than is the independent expression of individuals, candidates, or other political committees. ***

We recognize that FECA permits individuals to contribute more money ($20,000) to a party than to a candidate ($1,000) or to other political committees ($5,000). We also recognize that FECA permits unregulated "soft money" contributions to a party for certain activities, such as electing candidates for state office, or for voter registration and "get out the vote" drives, see § 431(8)(B)(xii). But the opportunity for corruption posed by these greater opportunities for contributions is, at best, attenuated. If anything, an independent expenditure made possible by a $20,000 donation, but controlled and directed by a party rather than the donor, would seem less likely to corrupt than the same (or a much larger) independent expenditure made directly by that donor. In any case, the constitutionally significant fact, present equally in both instances, is the lack of coordination between the candidate and the source of the expenditure.

The Government does not point to record evidence or legislative findings suggesting any special corruption problem in respect to independent party expenditures. In fact, rather than indicating a special fear of the corruptive influence of political parties, the legislative history demonstrates Congress' general desire to enhance what was seen as an important and legitimate role for political parties in American elections.

We therefore believe that this Court's prior case law controls the outcome here. We do not see how a Constitution that grants to individuals, candidates, and ordinary political committees the right to make unlimited independent expenditures could deny the same right to political parties.

IV

The Colorado Party and supporting *amici* have argued a broader question than we have decided, for they have claimed that, in the special case of political parties, the First Amendment forbids congressional efforts to limit coordinated expenditures as well as independent expenditures. Because the expenditure before us is an independent expenditure we have not reached this broader question in deciding the Party's "as applied" challenge.* ***

---

*. [**Ed. Note**. The Court did reach this question, however, in 2001. Following the Court's remand, the court of appeals held that even closely coordinated party expenditures could not be limited by Congress. The Supreme Court reversed. Thus, the feature of the federal statute limiting the amount of party expenditures in coordination with a candidate, like the limit on party contributions to a candidate or his committee, was upheld. (See Federal Election Commission v. Colorado Republican Federal Campaign Committee,121 S. Ct. 2351 (June 25, 2001) (Opinion for the Court by Souter, J., in

[T]he judgment of the Court of Appeals is vacated, and the case is remanded for further proceedings.

JUSTICE KENNEDY, with whom THE CHIEF JUSTICE and JUSTICE SCALIA join, concurring in the judgment and dissenting in part.

In agreement with JUSTICE THOMAS, I would hold that the Colorado Republican Party, in its pleadings in the District Court and throughout this litigation, has preserved its claim that the constraints imposed by the Federal Election Campaign Act of 1971 (FECA), both on its face and as interpreted by the Federal Elections Commission (FEC), violate the First Amendment. ***

The central holding in *Buckley v. Valeo*, 424 U.S. 1 (1976), is that spending money on one's own speech must be permitted, and this is what political parties do when they make the expenditures FECA restricts. FECA calls spending of this nature a "contribution," § 441a(a)(7)(B)(I), and it is true that contributions can be restricted consistent with *Buckley*. *** In my view, we should not transplant the reasoning of cases upholding ordinary contribution limitations to a case involving FECA's restrictions on political party spending.

The First Amendment embodies a "profound national commitment to the principle that debate on public issues should be uninhibited, robust, and wide- open." *New York Times Co. v. Sullivan*, 376 U.S. 254, 270 (1964). Political parties have a unique role in serving this principle; they exist to advance their members' shared political beliefs. *** Having identified its members, however, a party can give effect to their views only by selecting and supporting candidates. A political party has its own traditions and principles that transcend the interests of individual candidates and campaigns; but in the context of particular elections, candidates are necessary to make the party's message known and effective, and vice versa.

It makes no sense, therefore, to ask, as FECA does, whether a party's spending is made "in cooperation, consultation, or concert with" its candidate. The answer in most cases will be yes, but that provides more, not less, justification for holding unconstitutional the statute's attempt to control this type of party spending, which bears little resemblance to the contributions discussed in *Buckley*. Party spending "in cooperation, consultation, or concert with" its candidates of necessity "communicate[s] the underlying basis for the support," i.e., the hope that he or she will be elected and will work to further the party's political agenda.

The problem is not just the absence of a basis in our First Amendment cases for treating the party's spending as contributions. The greater difficulty posed by the statute is its stifling effect on the ability of the party to do what it exists to do. *** Congress may have authority, consistent with the First Amendment, to restrict undifferentiated political party contributions which satisfy the constitutional criteria we

---

which Stevens, O'Connor, Ginsberg, and Breyer, JJ., joined; dissent by Thomas, J., in which Scalia and Kennedy, JJ., and Rehnquist, C.J., joined).)

discussed in *Buckley*, but that type of regulation is not at issue here. ***

JUSTICE THOMAS, concurring in the judgment and dissenting in part, with whom THE CHIEF JUSTICE and JUSTICE SCALIA join in Parts I and III.

I agree that petitioners' rights under the First Amendment have been violated, but I think we should reach the facial challenge in this case in order to make clear the circumstances under which political parties may engage in political speech without running afoul of 2 U.S.C. § 441a(d)(3). In resolving that challenge, I would reject the framework established by *Buckley v. Valeo*, 424 U.S. 1 (1976), for analyzing the constitutionality of campaign finance laws and hold that § 441a(d)(3)'s limits on independent and coordinated expenditures fail strict scrutiny. But even under *Buckley*, § 441a(d)(3) cannot stand, because the anti-corruption rationale that we have relied upon in sustaining other campaign finance laws is inapplicable where political parties are the subject of such regulation. ***

II

[U]nlike the *Buckley* Court, I believe that contribution limits infringe as directly and as seriously upon freedom of political expression and association as do expenditure limits. The protections of the First Amendment do not depend upon so fine a line as that between spending money to support a candidate or group and giving money to the candidate or group to spend for the same purpose. In principle, people and groups give money to candidates and other groups for the same reason that they spend money in support of those candidates and groups: because they share social, economic, and political beliefs and seek to have those beliefs affect governmental policy. I think that the *Buckley* framework for analyzing the constitutionality of campaign finance laws is deeply flawed. Accordingly, I would not employ it, as JUSTICE BREYER and JUSTICE KENNEDY do.

***

Instead, I begin with the premise that there is no constitutionally significant difference between campaign contributions and expenditures: both forms of speech are central to the First Amendment. Curbs on protected speech, we have repeatedly said, must be strictly scrutinized. ***

The formula for strict scrutiny is, of course, well-established. It requires both a compelling governmental interest and legislative means narrowly tailored to serve that interest. *** In my opinion, FECA's monetary caps fail the narrow tailoring test. Addressing the constitutionality of FECA's contribution caps, the *Buckley* appellants argued:

> "If a small minority of political contributions are given to secure appointments for the donors or some other quid pro quo, that cannot serve to justify prohibiting all large contributions, the vast majority of which are given not for any such purpose but to further the expression of political views which the

> candidate and donor share. Where First Amendment rights are involved, a blunderbuss approach which prohibits mostly innocent speech cannot be held a means narrowly and precisely directed to the governmental interest in the small minority of contributions that are not innocent." ***

*** As one commentator has observed, "it must not be forgotten that a large number of contributions are made without any hope of specific gain: for the promotion of a program, because of enthusiasm for a candidate, or to promote what the giver vaguely conceives to be the national interest." L. Overacker, Money in Elections 192 (1974).

In contrast, federal bribery laws are designed to punish and deter the corrupt conduct the Government seeks to prevent under FECA, and disclosure laws work to make donors and donees accountable to the public for any questionable financial dealings in which they may engage. In light of these alternatives, wholesale limitations that cover contributions having nothing to do with bribery — but with speech central to the First Amendment — are not narrowly tailored. ***

III

Were I convinced that the *Buckley* framework rested on a principled distinction between contributions and expenditures, which I am not, I would nevertheless conclude that § 441a(d)(3)'s limits on political parties violate the First Amendment. *** [A]s long as the Court continues to permit Congress to subject individuals to limits on the amount they can give to parties, and those limits are uniform as to all donors, there is little risk that an individual donor could use a party as a conduit for bribing candidates.

*** And insofar as it appears that Congress did not actually enact § 441a(d)(3) in order to stop corruption by political parties "but rather for the constitutionally insufficient purpose of reducing what it saw as wasteful and excessive campaign spending," [*ante* citing *Buckley*] the statute's ceilings on coordinated expenditures are as unwarranted as the caps on independent expenditures.

In sum, there is only a minimal threat of "corruption," as we have understood that term, when a political party spends to support its candidate or to oppose his competitor, whether or not that expenditure is made in concert with the candidate. Parties and candidates have traditionally worked together to achieve their common goals, and when they engage in that work, there is no risk to the Republic. To the contrary, the danger to the Republic lies in Government suppression of such activity. ***

JUSTICE STEVENS, with whom JUSTICE GINSBURG joins, dissenting.

In my opinion, all money spent by a political party to secure the election of its candidate for the office of United States Senator should be considered a "contribution" to his or her campaign. I therefore disagree with the conclusion reached in Part III of the Court's opinion.

I am persuaded that three interests provide a constitutionally sufficient predicate for federal limits on spending by political parties. First, such limits serve the interest in avoiding both the appearance and the reality of a corrupt political process. A party shares a unique relationship with the candidate it sponsors because their political fates are inextricably linked. That interdependency creates a special danger that the party — or the persons who control the party — will abuse the influence it has over the candidate by virtue of its power to spend. The provisions at issue are appropriately aimed at reducing that threat. ***

Second, these restrictions supplement other spending limitations embodied in the Act, which are likewise designed to prevent corruption. Individuals and certain organizations are permitted to contribute up to $1,000 to a candidate. Since the same donors can give up to $5,000 to party committees, § 441a(a)(1)(C), if there were no limits on party spending, their contributions could be spent to benefit the candidate and thereby circumvent the $1,000 cap. We have recognized the legitimate interest in blocking similar attempts to undermine the policies of the Act. See *California Medical Assn. v. Federal Election Comm'n.*, 453 U.S. 182, 197-199 (1981) (plurality opinion) (approving ceiling on contributions to political action committees to prevent circumvention of limitations on individual contributions to candidates).

Finally, I believe the Government has an important interest in leveling the electoral playing field by constraining the cost of federal campaigns. As Justice White pointed out in his opinion in *Buckley*, "money is not always equivalent to or used for speech, even in the context of political campaigns." It is quite wrong to assume that the net effect of limits on contributions and expenditures — which tend to protect equal access to the political arena, to free candidates and their staffs from the interminable burden of fund-raising, and to diminish the importance of repetitive 30-second commercials — will be adverse to the interest in informed debate protected by the First Amendment.***

Accordingly, I would affirm the judgment of the Court of Appeals.

NOTE

In 1999, the Court granted certiorari in a case involving the constitutionality of a state limit on contributions to candidates for state political office, set at $1000 in 1996 (and adjusted for inflation, since then, to $1075). Although the contribution limit was set to equal the limit sustained (in 1976) in *Buckley*, counsel for a candidate and a PAC successfully argued before the United States Court of Appeals for the Eighth Circuit that the State of Missouri had not justified the burden imposed by the limit. *See Shrink Missouri Government PAC v. Nixon*, 161 F.3d 519 (8th Cir. 1998) (striking contribution limit). The Supreme Court reversed. *See Nixon v. Shrink Missouri Government PAC*, 528 U.S. 377 120 S.Ct. 897 (2000) (opinion of the court by Souter, J., dissent by Justices Kennedy, Scalia, and Thomas.)

Chapter 6

ANONYMITY AND THE FIRST AMENDMENT

INTRODUCTORY NOTE

In Buckley v. Valeo, 42 4 U.S. 1 (1976), while the Supreme Court upheld the requirement of the Federal Election Campaign Act of 1974 requirement that political parties disclose the identities of their contributors, it carved out an exemption for "minor" political parties able to show "a reasonable probability that the compelled disclosure of a party's contributors' names will subject them to threats, harassment, or reprisals from either Government officials or private parties."[1] Even earlier, the Court had found the first amendment precludes a state from forcing disclosure of NAACP membership lists—at least when the state's justification for forced disclosure is ultimately unrelated to the information sought (for example, in one case, a municipal licensing scheme).[2] These cases suggest that *ordinarily* an organization may not be forced to disclose its membership lists *if* to do so would subject its members to private (or government) harassment (i.e. which might target political beliefs or deter protected activity). These organizations will instead be permitted to guard the anonymity of their sustaining members.[3] The first amendment thus includes some sort of privilege to keep one's ideas and beliefs private.[4]

Of course, it is not only to avoid harassment that an individual might choose anonymity. She might do so to evade criminal prosecution (or civil suit).[5] When anonymously communicated words make *clear* that grounds lie for criminal prose-

---

1. 424 U.S. at 74.

2. Bates v. City of Little Rock, 361 U.S. 516 (1960); NAACP v. Alabama, 357 U.S. 449 (1958).

3. See Brown v. Socialist Workers '74 Campaign, 459 U.S. 87 (1982) (granting the Socialist Party an exemption to the Ohio Campaign Expense Reporting Law on the strength of a *Buckley* showing).

4. See also Wilkinson v. United States, 365 U.S. 399 (1961) and its companion case Braden v. United States, 365 U.S. 431 (1961). The Court sustained Wilkinson's conviction under 2 U.S.C. § 192 for failure to answer questions put to him, about his political beliefs, by the House Committee on Un-American Activities. (The *Braden* decision was roughly the same.) The justices dissenting in both cases construed the first amendment as forbidding "any agency of the Federal Government *** to harass or punish people for their beliefs, or for their speech about, or public criticism of, laws and public officials." *Braden*, 365 U.S. at 445 (Black, J., dissenting). See also Gibson v. Florida Legis. Investigative Comm., 372 U.S. 539 (1963) (finding the first amendment precludes forced disclosure of NAACP membership list, which the Committee sought in order to determine if certain suspected Communists were members).

5. Recall, for example, that in the *Abrams* case, the five Russian immigrants prosecuted under the Espionage Act had distributed pseudonymous circulars (signed "The Rebels") critical of the American government and war effort. See p. 45, *supra*. One might similarly recall that James Madison and Thomas Jefferson *anonymously* drafted responses to the Alien and Sedition Acts (the Virginia and Kentucky Resolutions), which were then pushed through their respective state legislatures without authorial identity attached.

cution, the government may call on others to identify the speaker: for example, even a reporter who promises source confidentiality in return for a confession of illegal conduct evidently may not guard the anonymity of his informant in the face of a bona fide grand jury investigation—indeed, despite any injury to the free flow of information to the press.[6] And might the government in behalf of serving the public interest of generally facilitating valid criminal prosecutions or valid civil suits which might result from speech (e.g., a suit for libel), enact a general ban on *all* anonymous handbills? Apparently not. In *Talley v. California*,[7] the Supreme Court invalidated a Los Angeles ordinance which had banned the distribution of anonymous handbills in order to prevent fraud, false advertising, and libel.

Although the *Talley* Court held that a broad ban on all anonymous pamphlets could not be squared with the first amendment,[8] it did not rule on the constitutionality of a narrower disclosure requirement (pertaining not to *all* handbills, but some subset thereof). Such statutes do exist—for example, in the election codes of most states. Indeed, by 1994, nearly every state (and the federal government[9]) had passed statutes requiring the disclosure of some party's identity on political literature pertaining to elections. The most common explanations given for those statutes were that they deter fraud and libel in the election arena and that they provide valuable information to the voters. With respect to the former justifications, it would seem such a statute would fall squarely under the *Talley* decision. But with respect to the latter justification, the question would turn on the strength of the interest in anonymity identified in *Buckley* and the *NAACP* cases. The Court faced the issue in its 1994 term, in the case which follows.

---

6. See Branzburg v. Hayes, 408 U.S. 665 (1972) (reporter who promised source confidentiality for story on conversion of marijuana into hashish could be compelled to identify his informants to the grand jury). Suppose, however, the anonymously spoken words indicated conduct only *potentially* illegal (i.e. the news story was not sufficiently informative on the point), and suppose the grand jury investigation seemed perhaps not in good faith? Must the reporter still reveal his informant? Might he at least put the state to a greater showing? See 408 U.S. at 710 (Powell, J., concurring) (suggesting a qualified reporter's privilege); see also Zurcher v. Stanford Daily, 436 U.S. 547 (1978).

7. 362 U.S. 60 (1960).

8. Id. at 64-65 ("Anonymous pamphlets, leaflets, brochures and even books have played an important role in the progress of mankind *** [continuing to give many historical examples]. It is plain that anonymity has sometimes been assumed for the most constructive of reasons.").

9. See 2 U.S.C. § 441d (1988).

McINTYRE v. OHIO ELECTIONS COMMISSION
514 U.S. 334 (1995)

JUSTICE STEVENS delivered the opinion of the Court.

The question presented is whether an Ohio statute that prohibits the distribution of anonymous campaign literature is a "law *** abridging the freedom of speech" within the meaning of the First Amendment.

I

On April 27, 1988, Margaret McIntyre distributed leaflets to persons attending a public meeting at the Blendon Middle School in Westerville, Ohio. At this meeting, the superintendent of schools planned to discuss an imminent referendum on a proposed school tax levy. The leaflets expressed Mrs. McIntyre's opposition to the levy. There is no suggestion that the text of her message was false, misleading, or libelous. She had composed and printed it on her home computer and had paid a professional printer to make additional copies. Some of the handbills identified her as the author; others merely purported to express the views of "CONCERNED PARENTS AND TAX PAYERS." Except for the help provided by her son and a friend, who placed some of the leaflets on car windshields in the school parking lot, Mrs. McIntyre acted independently.

While Mrs. McIntyre distributed her handbills, an official of the school district, who supported the tax proposal, advised her that the unsigned leaflets did not conform to the Ohio election laws. *** The proposed school levy was defeated at the next two elections, but it finally passed on its third try in November 1988. Five months later, the same school official filed a complaint with the Ohio Elections Commission charging that Mrs. McIntyre's distribution of unsigned leaflets violated § 3599.09(A) of the Ohio Code.[3] ***

II

***

"Anonymous pamphlets, leaflets, brochures and even books have played an important role in the progress of mankind." Talley v. California, 362 U.S. 60, 64 (1960). Great works of literature have frequently been produced by authors writing

---

3. Ohio Rev.Code Ann. § 3599.09(A) (1988) provides: "No person shall write, print, post, or distribute, or cause to be written, printed, posted, or distributed, a notice, placard, dodger, advertisement, sample ballot, or any other form of general publication which is designed to promote the nomination or election or defeat of a candidate, or to promote the adoption or defeat of any issue, or to influence the voters in any election, or make an expenditure for the purpose of financing political communications through newspapers, magazines, outdoor advertising facilities, direct mailings, or other similar types of general public political advertising, or through flyers, handbills, or other nonperiodical printed matter, unless there appears on such form of publication in a conspicuous place or is contained within said statement the name and residence or business address of the chairman, treasurer, or secretary of the organization issuing the same, or the person who issues, makes, or is responsible therefor. ***"

under assumed names.[4] *** The decision in favor of anonymity may be motivated by fear of economic or official retaliation, by concern about social ostracism, or merely by a desire to preserve as much of one's privacy as possible. Whatever the motivation may be, at least in the field of literary endeavor, the interest in having anonymous works enter the marketplace of ideas unquestionably outweighs any public interest in requiring disclosure as a condition of entry.[5] Accordingly, an author's decision to remain anonymous, like other decisions concerning omissions or additions to the content of a publication, is an aspect of the freedom of speech protected by the First Amendment.

The freedom to publish anonymously extends beyond the literary realm. In *Talley*, the Court held that the First Amendment protects the distribution of unsigned handbills urging readers to boycott certain Los Angeles merchants who were allegedly engaging in discriminatory employment practices. Writing for the Court, Justice Black noted that "[p]ersecuted groups and sects from time to time throughout history have been able to criticize oppressive practices and laws either anonymously or not at all." On occasion, quite apart from any threat of persecution, an advocate may believe her ideas will be more persuasive if her readers are unaware of her identity. Anonymity thereby provides a way for a writer who may be personally unpopular to ensure that readers will not prejudge her message simply because they do not like its proponent. The specific holding in *Talley* related to advocacy of an economic boycott, but the Court's reasoning embraced a respected tradition of anonymity in the advocacy of political causes.[6] ***

III

California had defended the Los Angeles ordinance at issue in *Talley* as a law "aimed at providing a way to identify those responsible for fraud, false advertising and libel." We rejected that argument because nothing in the text or legislative history of the ordinance limited its application to those evils. *** The Ohio statute likewise contains no language limiting its application to fraudulent, false, or libelous statements; to the extent, therefore, that Ohio seeks to justify § 3599.09(A) as a means to prevent the dissemination of untruths, its defense must fail for the same rea-

---

4. American names such as Mark Twain (Samuel Langhorne Clemens) and O. Henry (William Sydney Porter) come readily to mind. Benjamin Franklin employed numerous different pseudonyms. Distinguished French authors such as Voltaire (Francois Marie Arouet) and George Sand (Amandine Aurore Lucie Dupin), and British authors such as George Eliot (Mary Ann Evans), Charles Lamb (sometimes wrote as "Elia"), and Charles Dickens (sometimes wrote as "Boz"), also published under assumed names. ***

5. Though such a requirement might provide assistance to critics in evaluating the quality and significance of the writing, it is not indispensable. *** [S]uch evaluations are possible—indeed, perhaps more reliable—when any bias associated with the author's identity is prescinded.

6. That tradition is most famously embodied in the Federalist Papers, authored by James Madison, Alexander Hamilton, and John Jay, but signed "Publius." Publius's opponents, the Anti-Federalists, also tended to publish under pseudonyms. ***

son given in *Talley*. As the facts of this case demonstrate, the ordinance plainly applies even when there is no hint of falsity or libel.

Ohio's statute does, however, contain a different limitation: It applies only to unsigned documents designed to influence voters in an election. We must, therefore, decide whether and to what extent the First Amendment's protection of anonymity encompasses documents intended to influence the electoral process.

Ohio places its principal reliance on cases such as Anderson v. Celebrezze, 460 U.S. 780 (1983); Storer v. Brown, 415 U.S. 724 (1974); and Burdick v. Takushi, 504 U.S. 428 (1992), in which we reviewed election code provisions governing the voting process itself. ***

*** § 3599.09(A) of the Ohio Code does not control the mechanics of the electoral process. It is a regulation of pure speech. Moreover, even though this provision applies evenhandedly to advocates of differing viewpoints, it is a direct regulation of the content of speech. Every written document covered by the statute must contain "the name and residence or business address of the chairman, treasurer, or secretary of the organization issuing the same, or the person who issues, makes, or is responsible therefor." Furthermore, the category of covered documents is defined by their content—only those publications containing speech designed to influence the voters in an election need bear the required markings. Consequently, we are not faced with an ordinary election restriction; this case "involves a limitation on political expression subject to exacting scrutiny."

Indeed, as we have explained on many prior occasions, the category of speech regulated by the Ohio statute occupies the core of the protection afforded by the First Amendment: *** Of course, core political speech need not center on a candidate for office. The principles enunciated in *Buckley* extend equally to issue-based elections such as the school-tax referendum that Mrs. McIntyre sought to influence through her handbills. ***

Nevertheless, the State argues that even under the strictest standard of review, the disclosure requirement in § 3599.09(A) is justified by two important and legitimate state interests. Ohio judges its interest in preventing fraudulent and libelous statements and its interest in providing the electorate with relevant information to be sufficiently compelling to justify the anonymous speech ban.

Insofar as the interest in informing the electorate means nothing more than the provision of additional information that may either buttress or undermine the argument in a document, we think the identity of the speaker is no different from other components of the document's content that the author is free to include or exclude. Moreover, in the case of a handbill written by a private citizen who is not known to the recipient, the name and address of the author adds little, if anything, to the reader's ability to evaluate the document's message. Thus, Ohio's informational interest is plainly insufficient to support the constitutionality of its disclosure requirement.

The state interest in preventing fraud and libel stands on a different footing. We agree with Ohio's submission that this interest carries special weight during election campaigns when false statements, if credited, may have serious adverse consequences for the public at large. Ohio does not, however, rely solely on § 3599.09(A) to protect that interest. Its Election Code includes detailed and specific prohibitions against making or disseminating false statements during political campaigns. Thus, Ohio's prohibition of anonymous leaflets plainly is not its principal weapon against fraud.[13]

As this case demonstrates, the prohibition encompasses documents that are not even arguably false or misleading. It applies not only to the activities of candidates and their organized supporters, but also to individuals acting independently and using only their own modest resources. It applies not only to elections of public officers, but also to ballot issues that present neither a substantial risk of libel nor any potential appearance of corrupt advantage. It applies not only to leaflets distributed on the eve of an election, when the opportunity for reply is limited, but also to those distributed months in advance. We recognize that a State's enforcement interest might justify a more limited identification requirement, but Ohio has shown scant cause for inhibiting the leafletting at issue here.

V

Finally, Ohio vigorously argues that our opinions in First Nat. Bank of Boston v. Bellotti, 435 U.S. 765 (1978), and Buckley v. Valeo, 424 U.S. 1 (1976), amply support the constitutionality of its disclosure requirement. In *Bellotti*, we reversed a judgment of the Supreme Judicial Court of Massachusetts sustaining a state law that prohibited corporate expenditures designed to influence the vote on referendum proposals. [A]lthough we commented in dicta on the prophylactic effect of requiring identification of the source of corporate advertising, that footnote did not necessarily apply to independent communications by an individual like Mrs. McIntyre.

[I]n *Buckley*, we stressed the importance of providing "the electorate with information 'as to where political campaign money comes from and how it is spent by the candidate.'" Those comments concerned contributions to the candidate or expenditures authorized by the candidate or his responsible agent. They had no reference to the kind of independent activity pursued by Mrs. McIntyre.

VI

Under our Constitution, anonymous pamphleteering is not a pernicious, fraudulent practice, but an honorable tradition of advocacy and of dissent. Anonymity is a shield from the tyranny of the majority. *** It thus exemplifies the purpose behind the Bill of Rights, and of the First Amendment in particular: to protect unpopular

---

13. The same can be said with regard to "libel," as many of the election code provisions prohibit false statements about candidates. To the extent those provisions may be underinclusive, Ohio courts also enforce the common-law tort of defamation.

individuals from retaliation—and their ideas from suppression—at the hand of an intolerant society. The right to remain anonymous may be abused when it shields fraudulent conduct. But political speech by its nature will sometimes have unpalatable consequences, and, in general, our society accords greater weight to the value of free speech than to the dangers of its misuse. *** Ohio has not shown that its interest in preventing the misuse of anonymous election-related speech justifies a prohibition of all uses of that speech. ***

The judgment of the Ohio Supreme Court is reversed.

JUSTICE GINSBURG, concurring.

*** The Court's decision finds unnecessary, overintrusive, and inconsistent with American ideals the State's imposition of a fine on an individual leafleteer who, within her local community, spoke her mind, but sometimes not her name. We do not thereby hold that the State may not in other, larger circumstances, require the speaker to disclose its interest by disclosing its identity.***

JUSTICE THOMAS, concurring in the judgment. [Omitted.]

JUSTICE SCALIA, with whom THE CHIEF JUSTICE joins, dissenting.

[T]he Court invalidates a species of protection for the election process that exists, in a variety of forms, in every State except California, and that has a pedigree dating back to the end of the 19th century. *** A governmental practice that has become general throughout the United States, and particularly one that has the validation of long, accepted usage, bears a strong presumption of constitutionality. And that is what we have before us here. Such a universal and long established American legislative practice must be given precedence, I think, over historical and academic speculation regarding a restriction that assuredly does not go to the heart of free speech. ***

I respectfully dissent.

QUESTION

Would *McIntyre* bring into question state laws or local ordinances that forbid wearing masks in public to disguise one's identity? Such laws might well inhibit people from participating in demonstrations where they have reason to fear repercussions if personally recognized. Those repercussions might include the loss of one's job, acts of arson, or personal acts of retaliation—precisely the sorts of things feared by the NAACP members who (successfully) challenged forced disclosure of membership lists in the 1960s. Does the validity of such an ordinance depend upon the person to whom it is applied—for example, a "civil rights" demonstrator as opposed to a member of the Ku Klux Klan?[14]

In the 1998 Term, the Supreme Court again addressed the effect of the First Amendment on balancing claims of anonymity against state interests in the fair regulation of elections and public referenda ballot measures. It did so in the following case, discussing and applying *McIntyre* along the way.

BUCKLEY V. AMERICAN CONSTITUTIONAL LAW FOUNDATION, INC.
525 U.S. 182 (1999)

JUSTICE GINSBURG delivered the opinion of the Court.

I-II

Colorado allows its citizens to make laws directly through initiatives placed on election ballots. We review in this case three conditions Colorado places on the ballot-initiative process: (1) the requirement that initiative-petition circulators be registered voters; (2) the requirement that they wear an identification badge bearing the circulator's name; and (3) the requirement that proponents of an initiative report the names and addresses of all paid circulators and the amount paid to each circulator.

In *Meyer v. Grant*, 486 U.S. 414 (1988), we struck down Colorado's prohibition of payment for the circulation of ballot-initiative petitions.[*] We have also

---

14. For lower court cases reaching quite different results, compare Hernandez v. Commonwealth, 406 S.E.2d 398 (Va. Ct. App. 1991), and State v. Miller, 398 S.Ed.2d 547 (Ga. 1990), with Ryan v. Mackey, 462 F.Supp. 90 (N.D. Tex. 1978), and Ghafari v. Municipal Court, 150 Cal.Rptr. 813 (Cal. Ct. App. 1978). See also Wayne R. Allen, Note, Klan, Cloth and Constitution: Anti-Mask Laws and the First Amendment, 25 Ga.L.Rev. 819 (1991); Oskar E. Rey, Note, Antimask Laws: Exploring the Outer Bounds of Protected Speech Under the First Amendment, 66 Wash.L.Rev. 1139 (1991).

*. **[Ed. Note**: The decision in *Meyer v. Grant* was unanimous. The Court held that the state had no credible evidence that *paid* petition circulators were per se more likely than *volunteer* circulators to falsify voter signatures, or mislead those asked to sign the petition re the nature of the proposed measure; moreover, the Court noted, alternative means of policing the integrity of such soliciting (e.g, felony penalties for falsification, disclosure requirements on the petition itself) were readily available to the states insofar as there was some bona fide concern.

Note, too, however, that the Court has not held that "the right of the people...to petition the Government for a redress of grievances" (as provided in the First Amendment) requires the national government—or any state government—to provide *any* kind of initiative-and-referendum mechanism by means of which laws may be made directly "by the people" rather than solely through some elected, legislative branch of government. (Indeed, far from the First Amendent or any other clause having been construed to guarantee some form of direct law-making power in "the people," as through an initiative-and-referendum mechanism, it has been vigorously argued that the Constitution forbids, rather than requires (or even permits) direct law-making "by the people" as such. *See*, e.g., *Pacific States Tel. Co.*

recognized, however, that "there must be a substantial regulation of elections if they are to be fair and honest and if some sort of order, rather than chaos, is to accompany the democratic processes." *Storer v. Brown*, 415 U.S. 724, 730 (1974). Taking careful account of these guides, the Court of Appeals for the Tenth Circuit upheld some of the State's regulations, but found the three controls at issue excessively restrictive of political speech, and therefore declared them invalid. [We] now affirm that judgment. ***

We [shall] therefore detail why we are satisfied that, as in *Meyer*, the restrictions in question significantly inhibit communication with voters about proposed political change, and are not warranted by the state interests (administrative efficiency, fraud detection, informing voters) alleged to justify those restrictions.[12] Our judgment is informed by other means Colorado employs to accomplish its regulatory purposes.

III

When this case was before the District Court, registered voters in Colorado numbered approximately 1.9 million. At least 400,000 persons eligible to vote were not registered. *** The Tenth Circuit reasoned that the registration requirement placed on Colorado's voter-eligible population produces a speech diminution of the very kind produced by the ban on paid circulators at issue in *Meyer*. We agree. The requirement that circulators be not merely voter eligible, but registered voters, decreases the pool of potential circulators as certainly as that pool is decreased by the prohibition of payment to circulators. Both provisions "limi[t] the number of voices who will convey [the initiative proponents'] message" and, consequently, cut down "the size of the audience [proponents] can reach." In this case, as in *Meyer*, the requirement "imposes a burden on political expression that the State has failed to justify."***

---

v. Oregon, 223 U.S. 118 (1912) (argument that the provision in Art. I, § 4 ("The United States shall guarantee to every State in this Union a *Republican* Form of Government") distinguishes republican (representative) government from direct democracies, and therefore only laws made by representative bodies—not by the indiscriminate citizenry at large—should be accepted as valid by courts). *But see* William Mayton, *Direct Democracy, Federalism and the Guarantee Clause*, 2 The Green Bag 269 (1999) (Art. I, § 4 does not prohibit a state, rather, it guarantees to every state, a prerogative to provide means for direct law-making by the people of that state, insofar as a state may wish so to provide). *Query*: At the national level, were Congress to authorize some form of citizen initiative-and-referendum mechanism, to enable "the people" to make laws for the United States. Would it be sustainable pursuant to the "necessary and proper" clause in Article I, § 8, or is it forbidden by Art. I, §1 ("All legislative Powers herein granted shall be vested in a Congress of the United States")?]

12. Our decision is entirely in keeping with the "now-settled approach" that state regulations "impos[ing] 'severe burdens' on speech ... [must] be narrowly tailored to serve a compelling state interest." See post, at 649 (THOMAS, J., concurring in judgment).

The State's dominant justification appears to be its strong interest in policing lawbreakers among petition circulators. Colorado seeks to ensure that circulators will be amenable to the Secretary of State's subpoena power, which in these matters does not extend beyond the State's borders. ACLF did not challenge Colorado's right to require that all circulators be residents, a requirement that, the Tenth Circuit said, "more precisely achieved" the State's subpoena service objective. Colorado maintains that it is more difficult to determine who is a state resident than it is to determine who is a registered voter. The force of that argument is diminished, however, by the affidavit attesting to residence that each circulator must submit with each petition section.

In sum, assuming that a residence requirement would be upheld as a needful integrity-policing measure — a question we, like the Tenth Circuit, have no occasion to decide because the parties have not placed the matter of residence at issue — the added registration requirement is not warranted. That requirement cuts down the number of message carriers in the ballot-access arena without impelling cause.

IV

Colorado enacted the provision requiring initiative-petition circulators to wear identification badges in 1993, five years after our decision in *Meyer*. The Tenth Circuit held the badge requirement invalid insofar as it requires circulators to display their names. The Court of Appeals did not rule on the constitutionality of other elements of the badge provision, namely the "requirements that the badge disclose whether the circulator is paid or a volunteer, and if paid, by whom." Nor do we.

The badge requirement, a veteran ballot-initiative-petition organizer stated, "very definitely limited the number of people willing to work for us and the degree to which those who were willing to work would go out in public." Another witness told of harassment he personally experienced as circulator of a hemp initiative petition. He also testified to the reluctance of potential circulators to face the recrimination and retaliation that bearers of petitions on "volatile" issues sometimes encounter: "[W]ith their name on a badge, it makes them afraid." Other petition advocates similarly reported that "potential circulators were not willing to wear personal identification badges."

Colorado urges that the badge enables the public to identify, and the State to apprehend, petition circulators who engage in misconduct. Here again, the affidavit requirement, unsuccessfully challenged below, is responsive to the State's concern. This notarized submission, available to law enforcers, renders less needful the State's provision for personal names on identification badges. *** As the Tenth Circuit explained, the name badge requirement "forces circulators to reveal their identities at the same time they deliver their political message"; it operates when reaction to the circulator's message is immediate and "may be the most intense, emotional, and unreasoned." The affidavit, in contrast, does not expose the circulator to the risk of "heat of the moment" harassment. *** In sum, we conclude, as did the Court of Appeals, that Colorado's current badge requirement discourages participation in the petition circulation process by forcing name identification without sufficient cause.

V

Like the badge requirement, Colorado's disclosure provisions were enacted post-*Meyer* in 1993. The Tenth Circuit trimmed these provisions. Colorado requires ballot-initiative proponents who pay circulators to file both a final report when the initiative petition is submitted to the Secretary of State, and monthly reports during the circulation period. The Tenth Circuit invalidated the[se] report provision[s] only insofar as [they] compelled disclosure of information specific to each paid circulator, in particular, the circulators' names and addresses and the total amount paid to each circulator.***

Through the disclosure requirements that remain in place, voters are informed of the source and amount of money spent by proponents to get a measure on the ballot; in other words, voters will be told who has proposed a measure, and who has provided funds for its circulation. The added benefit of revealing the names of paid circulators and amounts paid to each circulator, the lower courts fairly determined from the record as a whole, is hardly apparent and has not been demonstrated.[22]

In addition, as we stated in *Meyer*, absent evidence to the contrary, "we are not prepared to assume that a professional circulator — whose qualifications for similar future assignments may well depend on a reputation for competence and integrity — is any more likely to accept false signatures than a volunteer who is motivated entirely by an interest in having the proposition placed on the ballot."[23]

In sum, we agree with the Court of Appeals appraisal: Listing paid circulators and their income from circulation "forc[es] paid circulators to surrender the anonymity enjoyed by their volunteer counterparts"; no more than tenuously related

---

22. JUSTICE O'CONNOR states that "[k]nowing the names of paid circulators and the amounts paid to them [will] allo[w] members of the public to evaluate the sincerity or, alternatively, the potential bias of any circulator that approaches them." It is not apparent why or how this is so, for the reports containing the names of paid circulators would be filed with the Secretary of State and would not be at hand at the moment the circulators approach.

23. *** Far from making any ultimate finding to that effect, the District Court determined that neither the State's interest in preventing fraud, nor its interest in informing the public concerning the "financial resources ... available to [initiative proponents]" or the "special interests" supporting a ballot measure, is "significantly advanced by disclosure of the names and addresses of each person paid to circulate any section of [a] petition." Such disclosure in proponents' reports, the District Court also observed, risked exposing the paid circulators "to intimidation, harassment and retribution in the same manner as the badge requirement."

to the substantial interests disclosure serves, Colorado's reporting requirements, to the extent that they target paid circulators, fail exacting scrutiny." *** Affirmed.*

---

*. **[Ed. Note.** Thomas, J., concurred in the judgment, but wrote separately. O'Connor and Breyer, JJ., dissented in part as did Rehnquist, C.J., in a separate opinion. They voted to sustain the reporting requirements imposed upon proponents disclosing all paid circulators' names and addresses, both in the required monthly and their final reports, as serving legitimate public interests to determine who such persons were and how much each was paid. They voted also to sustain the registered voter requirement. But they agreed with the Court's application of *McIntyre* in invalidating the badge information requirement — as failing "strict scrutiny" re the protection of anonymity from forced disclosure in direct political speech. (The Court was thus unanimous in holding the badge-disclosure provision invalid on First Amendment grounds, applying and extending *McIntyre*.)]

Chapter 7

THE FIRST AMENDMENT AND THE LESSER PROTECTION OF NONPOLITICAL SPEECH IN THE UNITED STATES

A. COMMERCIAL SPEECH

The extent to which advertising is assimilated within ordinary standards of economic due process review and the uncertainties of distinguishing what is or is not "commercial speech."

"Commercial Speech" in the Supreme Court

In an early footnote tucked away in the Introduction to these materials,[1] an example of "commercial speech" was used to check one's impulse to adhere to an absolute view of free speech (i.e. the view that Congress is forbidden to enact *any* restriction of free speech in the United States). The example was one of commercial fraud involving an interstate seller of pork bellies who deliberately misstates the nutritional value of his product, and a Federal Trade Commission cease-and-desist order banning the misleading advertisement following a full, fair, adversary proceeding, complete with clear and convincing evidence establishing the factual falsity of the advertiser's profit-seeking misrepresentations. We now return to the general area represented by that hypothetical, to review it in greater detail with more discernment and case-by-case care.

I

The original case was put in the setting of an FTC false advertising, cease-and-desist proceeding, in order to relate the case to congressional powers of regulation, as distinct from those severally possessed by the states. But, now noting that, generally speaking the Supreme Court does not significantly distinguish the application of the first amendment via the fourteenth amendment in respect to such subjects as the states have power to regulate pursuant to their conventional police power interests, here we can generalize the example, can we not? So, the case could as easily be simply a case of a local drug store *truthfully* advertising cut-rate prescription retail drug prices, and a state law or local ordinance either regulating or even prohibiting such advertisements altogether, and a fourteenth amendment challenge to that state or local law. How should the fourteenth amendment question be addressed? More specifically, should it be addressed (merely) in terms of fourteenth amendment,

1. See *supra note* 29, page 18, Chapter 1.

"economic substantive due process" judicial review, or should it be addressed as a case of free speech?

In the FTC case, as we first proposed it, what was forbidden was solely advertising that was alleged to be false or at least highly misleading. And we imagined a carefully wrought administrative procedure (for responding to consumer concerns), a fair hearing, a heavy burden-of-proof on the government, etc.—all suggesting that first amendment concerns, such as they might be, have all been duly fitted into place. But our case need not have been modeled in this way. Rather, the case may in fact be one in which Congress enacts a ban on advertising a given service or product, whether through the mails or in any interstate medium, period. In such a case, from the congressional view, the absence of falsehood in the advertisement would make no difference at all. (Indeed, the truth of the advertisement might make it "worse").[2] Does the first amendment permit Congress to keep consumers ignorant of services and products otherwise available to them? Even when trade in those products or services is itself wholly lawful? If so, why, and to what extent? (And, moreover, just what shall be deemed to be "commercial" speech?) Would it matter that the advertisement might be one placed by an attorney? An advertisement drawing attention to his or her specialty as a "personal injury" lawyer, and advertising copy explaining that he or she is available on the basis of a purely contingent fee ("no success, no charge!")?

II

Among the most notable early cases touching on this subject was *Railway Express Agency v. New York.*[3] The *Railway Express Agency* case sustained a prohibition of advertising vehicles on the streets of New York City, exempting only business delivery vehicles advertising the "usual business" of the owner, thus disallowing an REA vehicle otherwise lawfully on the city streets from substituting poster ads for a local radio station (WOR) and for Camel Cigarettes, for poster ads for REA itself. The Supreme Court was unanimous in finding no (economic) substantive due process violation insofar as REA complained that the restriction was an unconstitutional re-

---

2. For example, suppose this case: Widgets, a handy item one might find in many homes, formerly cost $3 to produce. X Corp. has discovered a way to manufacture widgets for $1, and is eager to promote sales by truthfully advertising the new reduced price at which it will sell widgets. Congress, however, does not favor any increased consumption of widgets, and has by statute already forbidden "*any* advertisement of widgets in any medium affecting commerce." Obviously X Corp. cannot (consistent with this act of Congress) advertise the new and much lower price of its product. The very *truthfulness* of X Corp.'s proposed advertisements makes the "danger" identified by Congress (the purchase and use of widgets) greater than would be the case if the proposed ads were utterly false. Consumers are kept ignorant of the newly available lower price of widgets solely by the act of Congress. They are misled (by that act) to believe widgets may still sell at $3, and they are thus deceived (as a consequence of the act) about a matter of interest to them—on a matter X Corp. *would* bring to their attention (by truthful informational advertising) but for the act of Congress that threatens X Corp. with heavy fines.

3. 336 U.S. 106 (1949).

straint of its liberty and property interests as a commercial enterprise. Justice Jackson wrote a famous, barely concurring, opinion as to REA's equal protection complaint.[4] Even so, no "*heightened scrutiny*" was given either to REA's due process claim or to REA's equal protection claim. No distinctive first amendment review was even implied in the opinions at the time. Indeed, in the *Railway Express Agency* case, it appears to have been taken for granted that "advertising-as-an-incident-of-commerce" is *wholly* subsumed in mere economic substantive due process (and mere economic equal protection) review.[5] In brief, the framework yielded *nothing* identified to the first amendment, though advertising is certainly "speech" of a sort.

III

The *Railway Express Agency* decision is representative of "commercial speech" cases in general. The latitude of regulatory state power in respect to commercial speech or commercial advertising generally was treated by the Supreme Court as an included part of the latitude of regulatory state power over the general "liberty" (and "property") freedoms of entrepreneurs, following the repudiation of *Lochner v. New York.* The Supreme Court had freely sustained that larger field of substantive regulation, with minimal substantive review in respect to the states, beginning with *Nebbia v. New York*, in 1934. (It did likewise, in *United States v. Carolene Products*, vis-à-vis Congress, in 1938.) In brief, commercial speech was, as well illustrated by *Railway Express* itself, treated mostly as "commerce," and little (if at all) as "speech," for purposes of substantive constitutional review. In textual Bill of Rights terms, the dispositive clause was the fifth amendment (substantive) due process clause—not the first amendment free speech clause. Commercial speech was thus principally a subset of economic due process, rather than a subset of (first amendment) free speech, review.

The cases immediately ahead in these materials begin from this point. But, just as with the assumptions prior to (but not after) *New York Times v. Sullivan*, in respect to libel—that "libel" raises no first amendment questions (yet today "libel" bristles with first amendment questions)—commercial speech has become an intermingled,

---

4. The ordinance did not equally restrict *fixed* display advertisements for the same products, though these (much more garish) displays fronted on the same city streets. In other words, fixed advertisements were *not* restricted to advertisements for the usual business of the owner of the business premises on which the advertisements were displayed. As between an ad carried for Camel Cigarettes on an REA truck, the same ad carried on a Reynolds Tobacco delivery vehicle, and the same ad on a fixed display, REA argued there was no rational distinction to be made.

5. Substantive due process review of economic legislation is highly deferential; if the means selected have a reasonable relation to a proper legislative purpose, and are neither arbitrary nor discriminatory, the requirements of substantive due process are satisfied. See Ferguson v. Skrupa, 372 U.S. 726 (1963) (sustaining Kansas statute limiting the business of debt adjusting to lawyers); Nebbia v. New York, 291 U.S. 502 (1934) (sustaining New York minimum price law for milk); William Cohen & Jonathan D. Varat, Constitutional Law: Cases and Materials 535 (11th ed. 2001) ("No economic regulatory statute has been held invalid under due process since 1937.").

specialized subset of first amendment case law as well. The principal cases we examine here, moving from *Valentine v. Chrestensen*, are meant to describe these developments up to date.

VALENTINE v. CHRESTENSEN

316 U.S. 52 (1942)

MR. JUSTICE ROBERTS delivered the opinion of the Court.

The respondent, a citizen of Florida, owns a former United States Navy submarine which he exhibits for profit. In 1940 he brought it to New York City and moored it at a State pier in the East River. He prepared and printed a handbill advertising the boat and soliciting visitors for a stated admission fee. On his attempting to distribute the bill in the city streets, he was advised by the petitioner, as Police Commissioner, that this activity would violate § 318 of the Sanitary Code, which forbids distribution in the streets of commercial and business advertising matter, but was told that he might freely distribute handbills solely devoted to "information or a public protest."

Respondent thereupon prepared and showed to the petitioner, in proof form, a double-faced handbill. On one side was a revision of the original, altered by the removal of the statement as to admission fee but consisting only of commercial advertising. On the other side was a protest against the action of the City Dock Department in refusing the respondent wharfage facilities at a city pier for the exhibition of his submarine, but no commercial advertising. The Police Department advised that distribution of a bill containing only the protest would not violate § 318, and would not be restrained, but that distribution of the double-faced bill was prohibited. The respondent, nevertheless, proceeded with the printing of his proposed bill and started to distribute it. He was restrained by the police.

Respondent then brought this suit to enjoin the petitioner from interfering with the distribution. In his complaint he alleged a violation of § 1 of the Fourteenth Amendment of the Constitution; and prayed an injunction. The District Court granted an interlocutory injunction, and after trial on a stipulation from which the facts appear as above recited, granted a permanent injunction. The Circuit Court of Appeals, by a divided court, affirmed.

The question is whether the application of the ordinance to the respondent's activity was, in the circumstances, an unconstitutional abridgement of the freedom of the press and of speech.

1. This court has unequivocally held that the streets are proper places for the exercise of the freedom of communicating information and disseminating opinion and that, though the states and municipalities may appropriately regulate the privilege in the public interest, they may not unduly burden or proscribe its employment in these public thoroughfares. We are equally clear that the Constitution imposes no such restraint on government as respects purely commercial advertising. Whether,

and to what extent, one may promote or pursue a gainful occupation in the streets, to what extent such activity shall be adjudged a derogation of the public right of user, are matters for legislative judgment. The question is not whether the legislative body may interfere with the harmless pursuit of a lawful business, but whether it must permit such pursuit by what it deems an undesirable invasion of, or interference with, the full and free use of the highways by the people in fulfillment of the public use to which streets are dedicated. If the respondent was attempting to use the streets of New York by distributing commercial advertising, the prohibition of the code provision was lawfully invoked against his conduct.

2. The respondent contends that, in truth, he was engaged in the dissemination of matter proper for public information, none the less so because there was inextricably attached to the medium of such dissemination commercial advertising matter. The court below appears to have taken this view, since it adverts to the difficulty of apportioning, in a given case, the contents of the communication as between what is of public interest and what is for private profit. We need not indulge nice appraisal based upon subtle distinctions in the present instance nor assume possible cases not now presented. It is enough for the present purpose that the stipulated facts justify the conclusion that the affixing of the protest against official conduct to the advertising circular was with the intent, and for the purpose, of evading the prohibition of the ordinance. If that evasion were successful, every merchant who desires to broadcast advertising leaflets in the streets need only append a civic appeal, or a moral platitude, to achieve immunity from the law's command.

The decree is Reversed.

BIGELOW v. VIRGINIA

421 U.S. 809 (1975)

MR. JUSTICE BLACKMUN delivered the opinion of the Court.

The Virginia Weekly was a newspaper published by the Virginia Weekly Associates of Charlottesville. It was issued in that city and circulated in Albemarle County, with particular focus on the campus of the University of Virginia. Appellant, Jeffrey C. Bigelow, was a director and the managing editor and responsible officer of the newspaper.[1]

On February 8, 1971, the Weekly was published and circulated under the direct responsibility of the appellant. On page 2 of that issue was the following advertisement:

---

1. His brief describes the publication as an "underground newspaper." The appellee states that there is no evidence in the record to support that description.

"UNWANTED PREGNANCY
LET US HELP YOU
Abortions are now legal in New York.
There are no residency requirements.
FOR IMMEDIATE PLACEMENT IN ACCREDITED
HOSPITALS AND CLINICS AT LOW COST
Contact
WOMEN'S PAVILION
515 Madison Avenue
New York, N.Y. 10022
or call any time
(212) 371-6670 or (212) 371-6650
AVAILABLE 7 DAYS A WEEK
STRICTLY CONFIDENTIAL. We will make
all arrangements for you and help you
with information and counseling."

On May 13 Bigelow was charged with violating Va. Code Ann. § 18.1-63 (1960). The statute at that time read:

> "If any person, by publication, lecture, advertisement, or by the sale or circulation of any publication, or in any other manner, encourage or prompt the procuring of abortion or miscarriage, he shall be guilty of a misdemeanor."

The Supreme Court of Virginia by a 4-2 vote, affirmed Bigelow's conviction. The court first rejected the appellant's claim that the advertisement was purely informational and thus was not within the "encourage or prompt" language of the statute. It held, instead, that the advertisement "clearly exceeded an informational status" and "constituted an active offer to perform a service, rather than a passive statement of fact." It then rejected Bigelow's First Amendment claim. This, the court said, was a "commercial advertisement" and, as such, "may be constitutionally prohibited by the state," particularly "where, as here, the advertising relates to the medical-health field." The issue, in the court's view, was whether the statute was a valid exercise of the State's police power. It answered this question in the affirmative, noting that the statute's goal was "to ensure that pregnant women in Virginia who decided to have abortions come to their decisions without the commercial advertising pressure usually incidental to the sale of a box of soap powder." The court then turned to Bigelow's claim of overbreadth. It held that because the appellant himself lacked a legitimate First Amendment interest, inasmuch as his activity "was of a purely commercial nature," he had no "standing to rely upon the hypothetical rights of those in the non-commercial zone." ***

Bigelow took a timely appeal to this Court. During the pendency of his appeal, Roe v. Wade, 410 U.S. 113 (1973), and Doe v. Bolton, 410 U.S. 179 (1973), were decided. We subsequently vacated Bigelow's judgment of conviction and remanded the case for further consideration in the light of *Roe* and *Doe*. ***

The Supreme Court of Virginia, again affirmed appellant's conviction, observing that neither *Roe* nor *Doe* "mentioned the subject of abortion advertising" and finding nothing in those decisions "which in any way affects our earlier view."[5] Once again, Bigelow appealed. We noted probable jurisdiction in order to review the important First Amendment issue presented.

In view of the statute's amendment since Bigelow's conviction in such a way as "effectively to repeal" its prior application, there is no possibility now that the statute's pre-1972 form will be applied again to appellant or will chill the rights of others. *** We therefore decline to rest our decision on overbreadth and we pass on to the further inquiry, of greater moment not only for Bigelow but for others, whether the statute as applied to appellant infringed constitutionally protected speech. ***

The appellee, as did the Supreme Court of Virginia, relies on Valentine v. Chrestensen, 316 U.S. 52 (1942), where a unanimous Court, in a brief opinion, sustained an ordinance which had been interpreted to ban the distribution of a handbill advertising the exhibition of a submarine. The handbill solicited customers to tour the ship for a fee. The promoter-advertiser had first attempted to distribute a single-faced handbill consisting only of the advertisement, and was denied permission to do so. He then had printed, on the reverse side of the handbill, a protest against official conduct refusing him the use of wharfage facilities. The Court found that the message of asserted "public interest" was appended solely for the purpose of evading the ordinance and therefore did not constitute an "exercise of the freedom of communicating information and disseminating opinion." It said:

> "We are equally clear that the Constitution imposes no such restraint on government as respects purely commercial advertising."

But the holding is distinctly a limited one: the ordinance was upheld as a reasonable regulation of the manner in which commercial advertising could be distributed. The fact that it had the effect of banning a particular handbill does not mean that *Chrestensen* is authority for the proposition that all statutes regulating commercial advertising are immune from constitutional challenge. The case obviously does not support any sweeping proposition that advertising is unprotected *per se*. ***

The legitimacy of appellant's First Amendment claim in the present case is demonstrated by the important differences between the advertisement presently at issue and those involved in *Chrestensen* ***. The advertisement published in appellant's newspaper did more than simply propose a commercial transaction. It contained factual material of clear "public interest." Portions of its message, most prominently

---

5. Virginia asserts, rightfully we feel, that this is "a First Amendment case" and "not an abortion case."

the lines, "Abortions are now legal in New York. There are no residency requirements," involve the exercise of the freedom of communicating information and disseminating opinion.

Viewed in its entirety, the advertisement conveyed information of potential interest and value to a diverse audience—not only to readers possibly in need of the services offered, but also to those with a general curiosity about, or genuine interest in, the subject matter or the law of another State and its development, and to readers seeking reform in Virginia. The mere existence of the Women's Pavilion in New York City, with the possibility of its being typical of other organizations there, and the availability of the services offered, were not unnewsworthy. Also, the activity advertised pertained to constitutional interests. See Roe v. Wade, 410 U.S. 113 (1973), and Doe v. Bolton, 410 U.S. 179 (1973). Thus, in this case, appellant's First Amendment interests coincided with the constitutional interests of the general public.

Moreover, the placement services advertised in appellant's newspaper were legally provided in New York at that time. The Virginia Legislature could not have regulated the advertiser's activity in New York, and obviously could not have proscribed the activity in that State. Neither could Virginia prevent its residents from traveling to New York to obtain those services or, as the State conceded, prosecute them for going there. Doe v. Bolton, 410 U.S., at 200. Virginia possessed no authority to regulate the services provided in New York—the skills and credentials of the New York physicians and of the New York professionals who assisted them, the standards of the New York hospitals and clinics to which patients were referred, or the practices and charges of the New York referral services.

A State does not acquire power or supervision over the internal affairs of another State merely because the welfare and health of its own citizens may be affected when they travel to that State. It may seek to disseminate information so as to enable its citizens to make better informed decisions when they leave. But it may not, under the guise of exercising internal police powers, bar a citizen of another State from disseminating information about an activity that is legal in that State.

We conclude, therefore, that the Virginia courts erred in their assumptions that advertising, as such, was entitled to no First Amendment protection and that appellant Bigelow had no legitimate First Amendment interest. We need not decide in this case the precise extent to which the First Amendment permits regulation of advertising that is related to activities the State may legitimately regulate or even prohibit. ***

We conclude that Virginia could not apply Va. Code Ann. § 18.1-63 (1960), as it read in 1971, to appellant's publication of the advertisement in question without unconstitutionally infringing upon his First Amendment rights. The judgment of the Supreme Court of Virginia is therefore reversed.

MR. JUSTICE REHNQUIST, with whom MR. JUSTICE WHITE joins, dissenting.

The Court's opinion does not confront head-on the question which this case poses, but makes contact with it only in a series of verbal sideswipes. The result is the fashioning of a doctrine which appears designed to obtain reversal of this judgment, but at the same time to save harmless from the effects of that doctrine the many prior cases of this Court which are inconsistent with it.

I am in agreement with the Court, that Virginia's statute cannot properly be invalidated on grounds of overbreadth,[1] given that the sole prosecution which has ever been brought under this now substantially altered statute is that now in issue.

If the Court's decision does, indeed, turn upon its conclusion that the advertisement here in question was protected by the First and Fourteenth Amendments, the subject of the advertisement ought to make no difference. It will not do to say, as the Court does, that this advertisement conveyed information about the "subject matter or the law of another State and its development" to those "seeking reform in Virginia," and that it related to abortion, as if these factors somehow put it on a different footing from other commercial advertising. This was a proposal to furnish services on a commercial basis, and since we have always refused to distinguish for First Amendment purposes on the basis of content, it is no different from an advertisement for a bucket shop operation or a Ponzi scheme which has its headquarters in New York. If Virginia may not regulate advertising of commercial abortion agencies because of the interest of those seeking to reform Virginia's abortion laws, it is difficult to see why it is not likewise precluded from regulating advertising for an out-of-state bucket shop on the ground that such information might be of interest to those interested in repealing Virginia's "blue sky" laws.

Beginning at least with our decision in Delamater v. South Dakota, 205 U.S. 93, 100 (1907), we have consistently recognized that irrespective of a State's power to regulate extraterritorial commercial transactions in which its citizens participate it retains an independent power to regulate the business of commercial solicitation and advertising within its borders. Thus, for example, in Head v. New Mexico Board, 374 U.S. 424 (1963), we upheld the power of New Mexico to prohibit commercial advertising by a New Mexico radio station of optometric services provided in Texas.

Were the Court's statements taken literally, they would presage a standard of the lowest common denominator for commercial ethics and business conduct. Securities issuers could circumvent the established blue-sky laws of States which had carefully drawn such laws for the protection of their citizens by establishing as a situs for transactions those States without such regulations, while spreading offers throughout the country. Loan sharks might well choose States with unregulated small loan industries, luring the unwary with immune commercial advertisements. And imagination would place the only limit on the use of such an *** artificially created territorial contacts to bilk the public and circumvent long-established state schemes of regulation.

---

1. The Court states that the Virginia Supreme Court placed no limiting interpretation on its statute and that it implied that the statute might apply to doctors, husbands, and lecturers. The Court is in error: the Virginia Supreme Court stated that it would not interpret the statute to encompass such situations.

Since the Court saves harmless from its present opinion our prior cases in this area, it may be fairly inferred that it does not intend the results which might otherwise come from a literal reading of its opinion. But solely on the facts before it, I think the Court today simply errs in assessing Virginia's interest in its statute because it does not focus on the impact of the practices in question on the State. Although the commercial referral agency, whose advertisement in Virginia was barred, was physically located outside the State, this physical contact says little about Virginia's concern for the touted practices. Virginia's interest in this statute lies in preventing commercial exploitation of the health needs of its citizens. So long as the statute bans commercial advertising by publications within the State, the extraterritorial location at which the services are actually provided does not diminish that interest.

Since the statute in question is a "reasonable regulation that serves a legitimate public interest," I would affirm the judgment of the Supreme Court of Virginia.

VIRGINIA STATE BOARD OF PHARMACY v. VIRGINIA CITIZENS CONSUMER COUNCIL

425 U.S. 748 (1976)

MR. JUSTICE BLACKMUN delivered the opinion of the Court.

The plaintiff-appellees in this case attack § 54-524.35 of Va. Code Ann. (1974), which provides that a pharmacist licensed in Virginia is guilty of unprofessional conduct if he "(3) publishes, advertises or promotes, directly or indirectly, in any manner whatsoever, any amount, price, fee, premium, discount, rebate or credit terms for any drugs which may be dispensed only by prescription."[2] The three- judge District Court declared the quoted portion of the statute "void and of no effect." We noted probable jurisdiction of the appeal.

I

The "practice of pharmacy" is statutorily declared to be "a professional practice affecting the public health, safety and welfare," and to be "subject to regulation and control in the public interest." Indeed, the practice is subject to extensive regulation aimed at preserving high professional standards. The regulatory body is the appellant Virginia State Board of Pharmacy. *** It may issue a license, necessary for the practice of pharmacy in the State, only upon evidence that the applicant is "of good moral character," is a graduate in pharmacy of a school approved by the Board, and has had "a suitable period of experience [the period required not to exceed 12

---

2. Section 54-524.35 provides [that]: "Any pharmacist shall be considered guilty of unprofessional conduct who *** (3) publishes, advertises or promotes, directly or indirectly, in any manner whatsoever, any amount, price, fee, premium, discount, rebate or credit terms for professional services or for drugs containing narcotics or for any drugs which may be dispensed only by prescription."

months] acceptable to the Board." The applicant must pass the examination prescribed by the Board. ***

Once licensed, a pharmacist is subject to a civil monetary penalty, or to revocation or suspension of his license, if the Board finds that he "is not of good moral character," or *** is guilty of "unprofessional conduct."

Inasmuch as only a licensed pharmacist may dispense prescription drugs in Virginia, § 54-524.48,[5] advertising or other affirmative dissemination of prescription drug price information is effectively forbidden in the State. Some pharmacies refuse even to quote prescription drug prices over the telephone. The Board's position, however, is that this would not constitute an unprofessional publication. It is clear, nonetheless, that all advertising of such prices, in the normal sense, is forbidden. The prohibition does not extend to nonprescription drugs, but neither is it confined to prescriptions that the pharmacist compounds himself. Indeed, about 95% of all prescriptions now are filled with dosage forms prepared by the pharmaceutical manufacturer.

II - III

* * *

The present attack on the statute is one made not by one directly subject to its prohibition, that is, a pharmacist, but by prescription drug consumers who claim that they would greatly benefit if the prohibition were lifted and advertising freely allowed. The plaintiffs are an individual Virginia resident who suffers from diseases that require her to take prescription drugs on a daily basis, and two nonprofit organizations.[10] Their claim is that the First Amendment entitles the user of prescription drugs to receive information that pharmacists wish to communicate to them through advertising and other promotional means, concerning the prices of such drugs.

Certainly that information may be of value. Drug prices in Virginia, for both prescription and nonprescription items, strikingly vary from outlet to outlet even within the same locality. It is stipulated, for example, that in Richmond "the cost of 40 Achromycin tablets ranges from $2.59 to $6.00, a difference of 140% [*sic*]," and that in the Newport News-Hampton area the cost of tetracycline ranges from $1.20 to $9.00, a difference of 650%. *** The question first arises whether, even assuming that First Amendment protection attaches to the flow of drug price information, it is a protection enjoyed by the appellees as recipients of the information, and not solely, if at all, by the advertisers themselves who seek to disseminate that information.

---

5. Exception is made for "legally qualified" practitioners of medicine, dentistry, osteopathy, chiropody, and veterinary medicine.

10. The organizations are the Virginia Citizens Consumer Council, Inc., and the Virginia State AFL-CIO. Each has a substantial membership (approximately 150,000 and 69,000, respectively) many of whom are users of prescription drugs. *** The American Association of Retired Persons and the National Retired Teachers Association, also claiming many members who "depend substantially on prescription drugs for their well-being," are among those who have filed briefs *amici curiae* in support of the appellees.

Freedom of speech presupposes a willing speaker. But where a speaker exists, as is the case here,[14] the protection afforded is to the communication, to its source and to its recipients both. ***

IV

The appellants contend that the advertisement of prescription drug prices is outside the protection of the First Amendment because it is "commercial speech." There can be no question that in past decisions the Court has given some indication that commercial speech is unprotected. ***

Last Term, in Bigelow v. Virginia, 421 U.S. 809 (1975), the notion of unprotected "commercial speech" all but passed from the scene. *** The advertisement in question, in addition to announcing that abortions were legal in New York, offered the services of a referral agency in that State. We rejected the contention that the publication was unprotected because it was commercial. *** We concluded that "the Virginia courts erred in their assumptions that advertising, as such, was entitled to no First Amendment protection," and we observed that the "relationship of speech to the marketplace of products or of services does not make it valueless in the marketplace of ideas."

Some fragment of hope for the continuing validity of a "commercial speech" exception arguably might have persisted because of the subject matter of the advertisement in *Bigelow*. We noted that in announcing the availability of legal abortions in New York, the advertisement "did more than simply propose a commercial transaction. It contained factual material of clear 'public interest.'" And, of course, the advertisement related to activity with which, at least in some respects, the State could not interfere. See Roe v. Wade, 410 U.S. 113 (1973); Doe v. Bolton, 410 U.S. 179 (1973). Indeed, we observed: "We need not decide in this case the precise extent to which the First Amendment permits regulation of advertising that is related to activities the State may legitimately regulate or even prohibit."

Here, in contrast, the question whether there is a First Amendment exception for "commercial speech" is squarely before us. Our pharmacist does not wish to editorialize on any subject, cultural, philosophical, or political. He does not wish to report any particularly newsworthy fact, or to make generalized observations even about commercial matters. The "idea" he wishes to communicate is simply this: "I will sell you the X prescription drug at the Y price." Our question, then, is whether this communication is wholly outside the protection of the First Amendment.

V

We begin with several propositions that already are settled or beyond serious dispute. It is clear, for example, that speech does not lose its First Amendment protection because money is spent to project it, as in a paid advertisement of one form or another. Speech likewise is protected even though it is carried in a form that is

---

14. "In the absence of Section 54-524.35 (3), some pharmacies in Virginia would advertise, publish and promote price information regarding prescription drugs." Stipulation of Facts ¶ 26, App. 15.

"sold" for profit, Smith v. California, 361 U.S. 147, 150 (1959) (books); Joseph Burstyn, Inc. v. Wilson, 343 U.S. 495, 501 (1952) (motion pictures); Murdock v. Pennsylvania, 319 U.S., at 111 (religious literature), and even though it may involve a solicitation to purchase or otherwise pay or contribute money. *New York Times Co. v. Sullivan*, [376 U.S. 254 (1964)].

If there is a kind of commercial speech that lacks all First Amendment protection, therefore, it must be distinguished by its content. Yet the speech whose content deprives it of protection cannot simply be speech on a commercial subject. No one would contend that our pharmacist may be prevented from being heard on the subject of whether, in general, pharmaceutical prices should be regulated, or their advertisement forbidden.

Our question is whether speech which does "no more than propose a commercial transaction" is so removed from any "exposition of ideas," Chaplinsky v. New Hampshire, 315 U.S. 568, 572 (1942), that it lacks all protection. Our answer is that it is not.

Focusing first on the individual parties to the transaction that is proposed in the commercial advertisement, we may assume that the advertiser's interest is a purely economic one. That hardly disqualifies him from protection under the First Amendment. The interests of the contestants in a labor dispute are primarily economic, but it has long been settled that both the employee and the employer are protected by the First Amendment when they express themselves on the merits of the dispute in order to influence its outcome.

As to the particular consumer's interest in the free flow of commercial information, that interest may be as keen, if not keener by far, than his interest in the day's most urgent political debate. Appellees' case in this respect is a convincing one. Those whom the suppression of prescription drug price information hits the hardest are the poor, the sick, and particularly the aged. A disproportionate amount of their income tends to be spent on prescription drugs; yet they are the least able to learn, by shopping from pharmacist to pharmacist, where their scarce dollars are best spent.

Generalizing, society also may have a strong interest in the free flow of commercial information. Even an individual advertisement, though entirely "commercial," may be of general public interest. The facts of decided cases furnish illustrations: advertisements stating that referral services for legal abortions are available; that a manufacturer of artificial furs promotes his product as an alternative to the extinction by his competitors of fur-bearing mammals; and that a domestic producer advertises his product as an alternative to imports that tend to deprive American residents of their jobs, cf. Chicago Joint Board v. Chicago Tribune Co., 435 F. 2d 470 (CA7 1970), cert. denied, 402 U.S. 973 (1971). Obviously, not all commercial messages contain the same or even a very great public interest element. There are few to which such an element, however, could not be added. Our pharmacist, for example, could cast himself as a commentator on store-to-store disparities in drug prices, giving his own and those of a competitor as proof. We see little point in requiring him to do so, and little difference if he does not.

Moreover, there is another consideration that suggests that no line between publicly "interesting" or "important" commercial advertising and the opposite kind could ever be drawn. Advertising, however tasteless and excessive it sometimes may seem, is nonetheless dissemination of information as to who is producing and selling what product, for what reason, and at what price. So long as we preserve a predominantly free enterprise economy, the allocation of our resources in large measure will be made through numerous private economic decisions. It is a matter of public interest that those decisions, in the aggregate, be intelligent and well informed. To this end, the free flow of commercial information is indispensable. *** And if it is indispensable to the proper allocation of resources in a free enterprise system, it is also indispensable to the formation of intelligent opinions as to how that system ought to be regulated or altered. Therefore, even if the First Amendment were thought to be primarily an instrument to enlighten public decisionmaking in a democracy, we could not say that the free flow of information does not serve that goal.[20]

Arrayed against these substantial individual and societal interests are a number of justifications for the advertising ban. These have to do principally with maintaining a high degree of professionalism on the part of licensed pharmacists.[21] Indisputably, the State has a strong interest in maintaining that professionalism. It is exercised in a number of ways for the consumer's benefit. There is the clinical skill involved in the compounding of drugs, although, as has been noted, these now make up only a small percentage of the prescriptions filled. Yet, even with respect to manufacturer-prepared compounds, there is room for the pharmacist to serve his customer well or badly. Drugs kept too long on the shelf may lose their efficacy or become adulterated. They can be packaged for the user in such a way that the same results occur. The expertise of the pharmacist may supplement that of the prescrib-

---

20. Pharmaceuticals themselves provide a not insignificant illustration. The parties have stipulated that expenditures for prescription drugs in the United States in 1970 were estimated at $9.14 billion. *** The task of predicting the effect that a free flow of drug price information would have on the production and consumption of drugs obviously is a hazardous and speculative one. It was recently undertaken, however, by the staff of the Federal Trade Commission in the course of its report on the merits of a possible Commission rule that would outlaw drug price advertising restrictions. The staff concluded that consumer savings would be "of a very substantial magnitude, amounting to many millions of dollars per year."

21. An argument not advanced by the Board, either in its brief or in the testimony proffered prior to summary judgment, but which on occasion has been made to other courts is that the advertisement of low drug prices will result in overconsumption and in abuse of the advertised drugs. The argument prudently has been omitted. By definition, the drugs at issue here may be sold only on a physician's prescription. We do not assume, as apparently the dissent does, that simply because low prices will be freely advertised, physicians will overprescribe, or that pharmacists will ignore the prescription requirement.

ing physician, if the latter has not specified the amount to be dispensed or the directions that are to appear on the label. ***

Price advertising, it is argued, will place in jeopardy the pharmacist's expertise and, with it, the customer's health. It is claimed that the aggressive price competition that will result from unlimited advertising will make it impossible for the pharmacist to supply professional services in the compounding, handling, and dispensing of prescription drugs. Such services are time consuming and expensive; if competitors who economize by eliminating them are permitted to advertise their resulting lower prices, the more painstaking and conscientious pharmacist will be forced either to follow suit or to go out of business. It is also claimed that prices might not necessarily fall as a result of advertising. If one pharmacist advertises, others must, and the resulting expense will inflate the cost of drugs.

It appears to be feared that if the pharmacist who wishes to provide low cost, and assertedly low quality, services is permitted to advertise, he will be taken up on his offer by too many unwitting customers. They will choose the low-cost, low- quality service and drive the "professional" pharmacist out of business. They will respond only to costly and excessive advertising, and end up paying the price. They will go from one pharmacist to another, following the discount, and destroy the pharmacist-customer relationship. They will lose respect for the profession because it advertises. All this is not in their best interests, and all this can be avoided if they are not permitted to know who is charging what.

There is, of course, an alternative to this highly paternalistic approach. That alternative is to assume that this information is not in itself harmful, that people will perceive their own best interests if only they are well enough informed, and that the best means to that end is to open the channels of communication rather than to close them. If they are truly open, nothing prevents the "professional" pharmacist from marketing his own assertedly superior product, and contrasting it with that of the low-cost, high-volume prescription drug retailer. But the choice among these alternative approaches is not ours to make or the Virginia General Assembly's. It is precisely this kind of choice, between the dangers of suppressing information, and the dangers of its misuse if it is freely available, that the First Amendment makes for us. Virginia is free to require whatever professional standards it wishes of its pharmacists; it may subsidize them or protect them from competition in other ways. Cf. Parker v. Brown, 317 U.S. 341 (1943). But it may not do so by keeping the public in ignorance of the entirely lawful terms that competing pharmacists are offering. In this sense, the justifications Virginia has offered for suppressing the flow of prescription drug price information, far from persuading us that the flow is not protected by the First Amendment, have reinforced our view that it is. We so hold.

VI

In concluding that commercial speech, like other varieties, is protected, we of course do not hold that it can never be regulated in any way. Some forms of commercial speech regulation are surely permissible. We mention a few only to make clear that they are not before us and therefore are not foreclosed by this case. There is no claim, for example, that the prohibition on prescription drug price advertising is a mere time, place, and manner restriction. We have often approved restrictions of that kind provided that they are justified without reference to the content of the regulated speech, that they serve a significant governmental interest, and that in so doing they leave open ample alternative channels for communication of the information. ***

Nor is there any claim that prescription drug price advertisements are forbidden because they are false or misleading in any way. Untruthful speech, commercial or otherwise, has never been protected for its own sake. Obviously, much commercial speech is not provably false, or even wholly false, but only deceptive or misleading. We foresee no obstacle to a State's dealing effectively with this problem.[24] The First Amendment, as we construe it today, does not prohibit the State from insuring that the stream of commercial information flow cleanly as well as freely. ***

Also there is no claim that the transactions proposed in the forbidden advertisements are themselves illegal in any way.

Finally, the special problems of the electronic broadcast media are likewise not in this case. *** What is at issue is whether a State may completely suppress the dissemination of concededly truthful information about entirely lawful activity, fearful of that information's effect upon its disseminators and its recipients.

---

24. In concluding that commercial speech enjoys First Amendment protection, we have not held that it is wholly undifferentiable from other forms. There are common sense differences between speech that does "no more than propose a commercial transaction," and other varieties. Even if the differences do not justify the conclusion that commercial speech is valueless, and thus subject to complete suppression by the State, they nonetheless suggest that a different degree of protection is necessary to insure that the flow of truthful and legitimate commercial information is unimpaired. The truth of commercial speech, for example, may be more easily verifiable by its disseminator than, let us say, news reporting or political commentary, in that ordinarily the advertiser seeks to disseminate information about a specific product or service that he himself provides and presumably knows more about than anyone else. Also, commercial speech may be more durable than other kinds. Since advertising is the *sine qua non* of commercial profits, there is little likelihood of its being chilled by proper regulation and forgone entirely.

Attributes such as these, the greater objectivity and hardiness of commercial speech, may make it less necessary to tolerate inaccurate statements for fear of silencing the speaker. Compare New York Times Co. v. Sullivan, 376 U.S. 254 (1964), with Dun & Bradstreet, Inc. v. Grove, 404 U.S. 898 (1971). They may also make it appropriate to require that a commercial message appear in such a form, or include such additional information, warnings, and disclaimers, as are necessary to prevent its being deceptive. Compare Miami Herald Publishing Co. v. Tornillo, 418 U.S. 241 (1974), with Banzhaf v. FCC, 132 U.S.App.D.C. 14, 405 F. 2d 1082 (1968), cert. denied sub nom. Tobacco Institute, Inc. v. FCC, 396 U.S. 842 (1969). Cf. United States v. 95 Barrels of Vinegar, 265 U.S. 438, 443 (1924) ("It is not difficult to choose statements, designs and devices which will not deceive"). They may also make inapplicable the prohibition against prior restraints. Compare New York Times Co. v. United States, 403 U.S. 713 (1971), with Donaldson v. Read Magazine, 333 U.S. 178, 189-191 (1948); FTC v. Standard Education Society, 302 U.S. 112 (1937); E.F. Drew & Co. v. FTC, 235 F. 2d 735, 739-740 (CA2 1956), cert. denied, 352 U.S. 969 (1957).

Reserving other questions,[25] we conclude that the answer to this one is in the negative.

The judgment of the District Court is affirmed.

MR. JUSTICE STEVENS took no part in the consideration or decision of this case.

MR. CHIEF JUSTICE BURGER, concurring. [Omitted.]

MR. JUSTICE STEWART, concurring.

* * *

Today the Court ends the anomalous situation created by *Chrestensen* and holds that a communication which does no more than propose a commercial transaction is not "wholly outside the protection of the First Amendment." *** But since it is a cardinal principle of the First Amendment that "government has no power to restrict expression because of its message, its ideas, its subject matter, or its content," the Court's decision calls into immediate question the constitutional legitimacy of every state and federal law regulating false or deceptive advertising. I write separately to explain why I think today's decision does not preclude such governmental regulation. ***

The principles recognized in the libel decisions suggest that government may take broader action to protect the public from injury produced by false or deceptive price or product advertising than from harm caused by defamation. In contrast to the press, which must often attempt to assemble the true facts from sketchy and sometimes conflicting sources under the pressure of publication deadlines, the commercial advertiser generally knows the product or service he seeks to sell and is in a position to verify the accuracy of his factual representations before he disseminates them. The advertiser's access to the truth about his product and its price substantially eliminates any danger that governmental regulation of false or misleading price or product advertising will chill accurate and nondeceptive commercial expression. There is, therefore, little need to sanction "some falsehood in order to protect speech that matters." *** Indeed, the elimination of false and deceptive claims serves to promote the one facet of commercial price and product advertising that warrants First Amendment protection — its contribution to the flow of accurate and reliable information relevant to public and private decisionmaking.

MR. JUSTICE REHNQUIST, dissenting.

---

25. We stress that we have considered in this case the regulation of commercial advertising by pharmacists. Although we express no opinion as to other professions, the distinctions, historical and functional, between professions, may require consideration of quite different factors. Physicians and lawyers, for example, do not dispense standardized products; they render professional services of almost infinite variety and nature, with the consequent enhanced possibility for confusion and deception if they were to undertake certain kinds of advertising.

The logical consequences of the Court's decision in this case, a decision which elevates commercial intercourse between a seller hawking his wares and a buyer seeking to strike a bargain to the same plane as has been previously reserved for the free marketplace of ideas, are far reaching indeed. Under the Court's opinion the way will be open not only for dissemination of price information but for active promotion of prescription drugs, liquor, cigarettes, and other products the use of which it has previously been thought desirable to discourage. Now, however, such promotion is protected by the First Amendment so long as it is not misleading or does not promote an illegal product or enterprise. *** This effort to reach a result which the Court obviously considers desirable is a troublesome one, for two reasons. It extends standing to raise First Amendment claims beyond the previous decisions of this Court. It also extends the protection of that Amendment to purely commercial endeavors which its most vigorous champions on this Court had thought to be beyond its pale.

I

I do not find the question of the appellees' standing to urge the claim which the Court decides quite as easy as the Court does. The Court finds standing on the part of the consumer appellees based upon a "right to 'receive information.'" *** Yet it has been stipulated in this case that the challenged statute does not prohibit anyone from receiving this information either in person or by phone. *** The statute forbids "only publish[ing], advertis[ing] or promot[ing]" prescription drugs.

The statute, in addition, only forbids *pharmacists* to publish this price information. There is no prohibition against a consumer group, such as appellees, collecting and publishing comparative price information as to various pharmacies in an area. Indeed they have done as much in their briefs in this case. Yet, though appellees could both receive and publish the information in question the Court finds that they have standing to protest that pharmacists are not allowed to advertise. Thus, contrary to the assertion of the Court, appellees are not asserting their "right to receive information" at all but rather the right of some third party to publish. In the cases relied upon by the Court, the plaintiffs asserted their right to receive information which would not be otherwise reasonably available to them. They did not seek to assert the right of a third party, not before the Court, to disseminate information. Here, the only group truly restricted by this statute, the pharmacists, have not even troubled to join in this litigation and may well feel that the expense and competition of advertising is not in their interest.

II

Thus the issue on the merits is not, as the Court phrases it, whether "[o]ur pharmacist" may communicate the fact that he "will sell you the X prescription drug at the Y price." No pharmacist is asserting any such claim to so communicate. The issue is rather whether appellee consumers may override the legislative determination that pharmacists should not advertise even though the pharmacists themselves do not object. In deciding that they may do so, the Court necessarily adopts a rule which cannot be limited merely to dissemination of price alone, and which cannot possibly be confined to pharmacists but must likewise extend to lawyers, doctors, and all other professions. ***

The Court insists that the rule it lays down is consistent even with the view that the First Amendment is "primarily an instrument to enlighten public decisionmaking in a democracy." *** I had understood this view to relate to public decisionmaking as to political, social, and other public issues, rather than the decision of a particular individual as to whether to purchase one or another kind of shampoo. It is undoubtedly arguable that many people in the country regard the choice of shampoo as just as important as who may be elected to local, state, or national political office, but that does not automatically bring information about competing shampoos within the protection of the First Amendment. It is one thing to say that the line between strictly ideological and political commentaries and other kinds of commentary is difficult to draw, and that the mere fact that the former may have in it an element of commercialism does not strip it of First Amendment protection. See New York Times Co. v. Sullivan, 376 U.S. 254 (1964). But it is another thing to say that because that line is difficult to draw, we will stand at the other end of the spectrum and reject out of hand the observation of so dedicated a champion of the First Amendment as Mr. Justice Black that the protections of that Amendment do not apply to a "'merchant' who goes from door to door 'selling pots.'" Breard v. City of Alexandria, 341 U.S. 622, 650 (1951) (dissenting).

In the case of "our" hypothetical pharmacist, he may now presumably advertise not only the prices of prescription drugs, but may attempt to energetically promote their sale so long as he does so truthfully. Quite consistently with Virginia law requiring prescription drugs to be available only through a physician, "our" pharmacist might run any of the following representative advertisements in a local newspaper:

> "Pain getting you down? Insist that your physician prescribe Demerol. You pay a little more than for aspirin, but you get a lot more relief."
> "Can't shake the flu? Get a prescription for Tetracycline from your doctor today."
> "Don't spend another sleepless night. Ask your doctor to prescribe Seconal without delay."

Unless the State can show that these advertisements are either actually untruthful or misleading, it presumably is not free to restrict in any way commercial efforts on the part of those who profit from the sale of prescription drugs to put them in the widest possible circulation. But such a line simply makes no allowance whatever for what appears to have been a considered legislative judgment in most States that while prescription drugs are a necessary and vital part of medical care and treatment, there are sufficient dangers attending their widespread use that they simply may not be promoted in the same manner as hair creams, deodorants, and toothpaste. ***

Both Congress and state legislatures have by law sharply limited the permissible dissemination of information about some commodities because of the potential harm resulting from those commodities, even though they were not thought to be sufficiently demonstrably harmful to warrant outright prohibition of their sale. Current prohibitions on television advertising of liquor and cigarettes are prominent in this category, but apparently under the Court's holding so long as the advertisements are not deceptive they may no longer be prohibited. ***

CENTRAL HUDSON GAS & ELECTRIC CORPORATION v. PUBLIC SERVICE COMMISSION OF NEW YORK

447 U.S. 557 (1980)

MR. JUSTICE POWELL delivered the opinion of the Court.

This case presents the question whether a regulation of the Public Service Commission of the State of New York violates the First and Fourteenth Amendments because it completely bans promotional advertising by an electrical utility.

I

In December 1973, the Commission, appellee here, ordered electric utilities in New York State to cease all advertising that "promot[es] the use of electricity." The order was based on the Commission's finding that "the interconnected utility system in New York State does not have sufficient fuel stocks or sources of supply to continue furnishing all customer demands for the 1973-1974 winter."

The Policy Statement divided advertising expenses "into two broad categories: promotional—advertising intended to stimulate the purchase of utility services—and institutional and informational, a broad category inclusive of all advertising not clearly intended to promote sales." The Commission declared all promotional advertising contrary to the national policy of conserving energy. It acknowledged that the ban is not a perfect vehicle for conserving energy. For example, the Commission's order prohibits promotional advertising to develop consumption during periods when demand for electricity is low. By limiting growth in "off-peak" consumption, the ban limits the "beneficial side effects" of such growth in terms of more efficient use of existing powerplants. *** And since oil dealers are not under the Commission's jurisdiction and thus remain free to advertise, it was recognized that the ban can achieve only "piecemeal conservationism." Still, the Commission adopted the restriction because it was deemed likely to "result in some dampening of unnecessary growth" in energy consumption. ***

Appellant challenged the order in state court, arguing that the Commission had restrained commercial speech in violation of the First and Fourteenth Amendments. The Commission's order was upheld by the trial court and at the intermediate appellate level. The New York Court of Appeals affirmed. We noted probable jurisdiction, and now reverse.

II

The Commission's order restricts only commercial speech, that is, expression related solely to the economic interests of the speaker and its audience. The First Amendment, as applied to the States through the Fourteenth Amendment, protects commercial speech from unwarranted governmental regulation. *Virginia Pharmacy Board*, 425 U.S., at 761-762. Commercial expression not only serves the economic interest of the speaker, but also assists consumers and furthers the societal interest in the fullest possible dissemination of information. In applying the First Amendment to this area, we have rejected the "highly paternalistic" view that government has complete power to suppress or regulate commercial speech. ***

Nevertheless, our decisions have recognized "the 'commonsense' distinction between speech proposing a commercial transaction, which occurs in an area traditionally subject to government regulation, and other varieties of speech."[5] The Constitution therefore accords a lesser protection to commercial speech than to other constitutionally guaranteed expression. ***

The First Amendment's concern for commercial speech is based on the informational function of advertising. See First National Bank of Boston v. Bellotti, 435 U.S. 765, 783 (1978). Consequently, there can be no constitutional objection to the suppression of commercial messages that do not accurately inform the public about lawful activity. The government may ban forms of communication more likely to deceive the public than to inform it, or commercial speech related to illegal activity, Pittsburgh Press Co. v. Human Relations Comm'n, 413 U.S. 376, 388 (1973).

If the communication is neither misleading nor related to unlawful activity, the government's power is more circumscribed. The State must assert a substantial interest to be achieved by restrictions on commercial speech. Moreover, the regulatory technique must be in proportion to that interest. The limitation on expression must

---

5. In an opinion concurring in the judgment, MR. JUSTICE STEVENS suggests that the Commission's order reaches beyond commercial speech to suppress expression that is entitled to the full protection of the First Amendment. *** We find no support for this claim in the record of this case. The Commission's Policy Statement excluded "institutional and informational" messages from the advertising ban, which was restricted to all advertising "clearly intended to promote sales." *** Nevertheless, the concurring opinion of MR. JUSTICE STEVENS views the Commission's order as suppressing more than commercial speech because it would outlaw, for example, advertising that promoted electricity consumption by touting the environmental benefits of such uses. *** Apparently the opinion would accord full First Amendment protection to all promotional advertising that includes claims "relating to *** questions frequently discussed and debated by our political leaders." ***

Although this approach responds to the serious issues surrounding our national energy policy as raised in this case, we think it would blur further the line the Court has sought to draw in commercial speech cases. It would grant broad constitutional protection to any advertising that links a product to a current public debate. But many, if not most, products may be tied to public concerns with the environment, energy, economic policy, or individual health and safety. We rule today in *Consolidated Edison Co. v. Public Service Comm'n,*, that utilities enjoy the full panoply of First Amendment protections for their direct comments on public issues. There is no reason for providing similar constitutional protection when such statements are made only in the context of commercial transactions. ***

be designed carefully to achieve the State's goal. Compliance with this requirement may be measured by two criteria. First, the restriction must directly advance the state interest involved; the regulation may not be sustained if it provides only ineffective or remote support for the government's purpose. Second, if the governmental interest could be served as well by a more limited restriction on commercial speech, the excessive restrictions cannot survive.

Under the first criterion, the Court has declined to uphold regulations that only indirectly advance the state interest involved. *** The Court noted in *Virginia Pharmacy Board* that "[t]he advertising ban does not directly affect professional standards one way or the other." ***

The second criterion recognizes that the First Amendment mandates that speech recognizes that the First Amendment mandates that speech restrictions be "narrowly drawn." *In re* Primus, 436 U.S. 412, 438 (1978).[8] The regulatory technique may extend only as far as the interest it serves. The State cannot regulate speech that poses no danger to the asserted state interest, nor can it completely suppress information when narrower restrictions on expression would serve its interest as well. For example, in *Bates* the Court explicitly did not "foreclose the possibility that some limited supplementation, by way of warning or disclaimer or the like, might be required" in promotional materials. 433 U.S., at 384. See *Virginia Pharmacy Board,* at 773. And in Carey v. Population Services International, 431 U.S. 678, 701-702 (1977), we held that the State's "arguments *** do not justify the total suppression of advertising concerning contraceptives." This holding left open the possibility that the State could implement more carefully drawn restrictions. See *id.*, at 712 (POWELL, J., concurring in part and in judgment); *id.*, at 716-717 (STEVENS, J., concurring in part and in judgment).[9]

---

8. This analysis is not an application of the "overbreadth" doctrine. The latter theory permits the invalidation of regulations on First Amendment grounds even when the litigant challenging the regulation has engaged in no constitutionally protected activity. E.g., Kunz v. New York, 340 U.S. 290 (1951). The overbreadth doctrine derives from the recognition that unconstitutional restriction of expression may deter protected speech by parties not before the court and thereby escape judicial review. Broadrick v. Oklahoma, 413 U.S. 601, 612-613 (1973); see Note, The First Amendment Overbreadth Doctrine, 83 Harv. L. Rev. 844, 853-858 (1970). This restraint is less likely where the expression is linked to "commercial well-being" and therefore is not easily deterred by "overbroad regulation." *Bates v. State Bar of Arizona*, [433 U.S.] at 381.

In this case, the Commission's prohibition acts directly against the promotional activities of Central Hudson, and to the extent the limitations are unnecessary to serve the State's interest, they are invalid.

9. We review with special care regulations that entirely suppress commercial speech in order to pursue a nonspeech-related policy. In those circumstances, a ban on speech could screen from public view the underlying governmental policy. See *Virginia Pharmacy Board*, 425 U.S., at 780, n. 8 (STEWART, J., concurring). Indeed, in recent years this Court has not approved a blanket ban on commercial speech unless the expression itself was flawed in some way, either because it was deceptive or related to unlawful activity.

In commercial speech cases, then, a four-part analysis has developed. At the outset, we must determine whether the expression is protected by the First Amendment. For commercial speech to come within that provision, it at least must concern lawful activity and not be misleading. Next, we ask whether the asserted governmental interest is substantial. If both inquiries yield positive answers, we must determine whether the regulation directly advances the governmental interest asserted, and whether it is not more extensive than is necessary to serve that interest.

III

We now apply this four-step analysis for commercial speech to the Commission's arguments in support of its ban on promotional advertising.

A

The Commission does not claim that the expression at issue either is inaccurate or relates to unlawful activity. Yet the New York Court of Appeals questioned whether Central Hudson's advertising is protected commercial speech. Because appellant holds a monopoly over the sale of electricity in its service area, the state court suggested that the Commission's order restricts no commercial speech of any worth. *** Monopoly over the supply of a product provides no protection from competition with substitutes for that product. Electric utilities compete with suppliers of fuel oil and natural gas in several markets, such as those for home heating and industrial power. *** For consumers in those competitive markets, advertising by utilities is just as valuable as advertising by unregulated firms.

Even in monopoly markets, the suppression of advertising reduces the information available for consumer decisions and thereby defeats the purpose of the First Amendment. The New York court's argument appears to assume that the providers of a monopoly service or product are willing to pay for wholly ineffective advertising. *** A consumer may need information to aid his decision whether or not to use the monopoly service at all, or how much of the service he should purchase. In the absence of factors that would distort the decision to advertise, we may assume that the willingness of a business to promote its products reflects a belief that consumers are interested in the advertising.[11] Since no such extraordinary conditions have been identified in this case, appellant's monopoly position does not alter the First Amendment's protection for its commercial speech.

---

11. There may be a greater incentive for a utility to advertise if it can use promotional expenses in determining its rate of return, rather than pass those costs on solely to shareholders. That practice, however, hardly distorts the economic decision whether to advertise. Unregulated businesses pass on promotional costs to consumers, and this Court expressly approved the practice for utilities in West Ohio Gas Co. v. Public Utilities Comm'n, 294 U.S. 63, 72 (1935).

B

The Commission offers two state interests as justifications for the ban on promotional advertising. The first concerns energy conservation. Any increase in demand for electricity—during peak or off-peak periods—means greater consumption of energy. The Commission argues, and the New York court agreed, that the State's interest in conserving energy is sufficient to support suppression of advertising designed to increase consumption of electricity. In view of our country's dependence on energy resources beyond our control, no one can doubt the importance of energy conservation. Plainly, therefore, the state interest asserted is substantial.

The Commission also argues that promotional advertising will aggravate inequities caused by the failure to base the utilities' rates on marginal cost. The utilities argued to the Commission that if they could promote the use of electricity in periods of low demand, they would improve their utilization of generating capacity. The Commission responded that promotion of off-peak consumption also would increase consumption during peak periods. If peak demand were to rise, the absence of marginal cost rates would mean that the rates charged for the additional power would not reflect the true costs of expanding production. Instead, the extra costs would be borne by all consumers through higher overall rates. Without promotional advertising, the Commission stated, this inequitable turn of events would be less likely to occur. The choice among rate structures involves difficult and important questions of economic supply and distributional fairness. The State's concern that rates be fair and efficient represents a clear and substantial governmental interest.

C

Next, we focus on the relationship between the State's interests and the advertising ban. Under this criterion, the Commission's laudable concern over the equity and efficiency of appellant's rates does not provide a constitutionally adequate reason for restricting protected speech. The link between the advertising prohibition and appellant's rate structure is, at most, tenuous. The impact of promotional advertising on the equity of appellant's rates is highly speculative. Advertising to increase off-peak usage would have to increase peak usage, while other factors that directly affect the fairness and efficiency of appellant's rates remained constant. Such conditional and remote eventualities simply cannot justify silencing appellant's promotional advertising.

In contrast, the State's interest in energy conservation is directly advanced by the Commission order at issue here. There is an immediate connection between advertising and demand for electricity. Central Hudson would not contest the advertising ban unless it believed that promotion would increase its sales. Thus, we find a direct link between the state interest in conservation and the Commission's order.

D

We come finally to the critical inquiry in this case: whether the Commission's complete suppression of speech ordinarily protected by the First Amendment is no more extensive than necessary to further the State's interest in energy conservation. The Commission's order reaches all promotional advertising, regardless of the impact of the touted service on overall energy use. But the energy conservation rationale, as important as it is, cannot justify suppressing information about electric devices or services that would cause no net increase in total energy use. In addition, no showing has been made that a more limited restriction on the content of promotional advertising would not serve adequately the State's interests.

Appellant insists that but for the ban, it would advertise products and services that use energy efficiently. These include the "heat pump," which both parties acknowledge to be a major improvement in electric heating, and the use of electric heat as a "backup" to solar and other heat sources. Although the Commission has questioned the efficiency of electric heating before this Court, neither the Commission's Policy Statement nor its order denying rehearing made findings on this issue. In the absence of authoritative findings to the contrary, we must credit as within the realm of possibility the claim that electric heat can be an efficient alternative in some circumstances.

The Commission's order prevents appellant from promoting electric services that would reduce energy use by diverting demand from less efficient sources, or that would consume roughly the same amount of energy as do alternative sources. In neither situation would the utility's advertising endanger conservation or mislead the public. To the extent that the Commission's order suppresses speech that in no way impairs the State's interest in energy conservation, the Commission's order violates the First and Fourteenth Amendments and must be invalidated. ***

The Commission also has not demonstrated that its interest in conservation cannot be protected adequately by more limited regulation of appellant's commercial expression. To further its policy of conservation, the Commission could attempt to restrict the format and content of Central Hudson's advertising. It might, for example, require that the advertisements include information about the relative efficiency and expense of the offered service, both under current conditions and for the foreseeable future.[13] ***

IV

Our decision today in no way disparages the national interest in energy conservation. *** When, however, such action involves the suppression of speech, the First and Fourteenth Amendments require that the restriction be no more extensive than

---

13. The Commission also might consider a system of previewing advertising campaigns to insure that they will not defeat conservation policy. It has instituted such a program for approving "informational" advertising under the Policy Statement challenged in this case. *** We have observed that commercial speech is such a sturdy brand of expression that traditional prior restraint doctrine may not apply to it. Virginia Pharmacy Board v. Virginia Citizens Consumer Council, 425 U.S., at 771-772, n.24. And in other area of speech regulation, such as obscenity, we have recognized that a prescreening arrangement can pass constitutional muster if it includes adequate procedural safeguards. Freedman v. Maryland, 380 U.S. 51 (1965).

is necessary to serve the state interest. In this case, the record before us fails to show that the total ban on promotional advertising meets this requirement.

Accordingly, the judgment of the New York Court of Appeals is Reversed.

MR. JUSTICE BRENNAN, concurring in the judgment. [Omitted]

MR. JUSTICE BLACKMUN, with whom MR. JUSTICE BRENNAN joins, concurring in the judgment.

*** I concur only in the Court's judgment because I believe the test now evolved and applied by the Court is not consistent with our prior cases and does not provide adequate protection for truthful, nonmisleading, noncoercive commercial speech.

*** I agree with the Court that this level of intermediate scrutiny is appropriate for a restraint on commercial speech designed to protect consumers from misleading or coercive speech, or a regulation related to the time, place, or manner of commercial speech. I do not agree, however, that the Court's four-part test is the proper one to be applied when a State seeks to suppress information about a product in order to manipulate a private economic decision that the State cannot or has not regulated or outlawed directly. ***

The Court recognizes that we have never held that commercial speech may be suppressed in order to further the State's interest in discouraging purchases of the underlying product that is advertised. Permissible restraints on commercial speech have been limited to measures designed to protect consumers from fraudulent, misleading, or coercive sales techniques. Those designed to deprive consumers of information about products or services that are legally offered for sale consistently have been invalidated.

I seriously doubt whether suppression of information concerning the availability and price of a legally offered product is ever a permissible way for the State to "dampen" demand for or use of the product. Even though "commercial" speech is involved, such a regulatory measure strikes at the heart of the First Amendment. This is because it is a covert attempt by the State to manipulate the choices of its citizens, not by persuasion or direct regulation, but by depriving the public of the information needed to make a free choice. As the Court recognizes, the State's policy choices are insulated from the visibility and scrutiny that direct regulation would entail and the conduct of citizens is molded by the information that government chooses to give them. ***

*** No differences between commercial speech and other protected speech justify suppression of commercial speech in order to influence public conduct through manipulation of the availability of information. ***

It appears that the Court would permit the State to ban all direct advertising of air conditioning, assuming that a more limited restriction on such advertising would not effectively deter the public from cooling its homes. In my view, our cases do not support this type of suppression. If a governmental unit believes that use or overuse of air conditioning is a serious problem, it must attack that problem directly, by prohibiting air conditioning or regulating thermostat levels. Just as the Commonwealth of Virginia may promote professionalism of pharmacists directly, so too New York may *not* promote energy conservation "by keeping the public in ignorance." *Virginia Pharmacy Board*, 425 U.S., at 770.

MR. JUSTICE STEVENS, with whom MR. JUSTICE BRENNAN joins, concurring in the judgment. [Omitted.]

MR. JUSTICE REHNQUIST, dissenting.

* * *

The Court's analysis in my view is wrong in several respects. Initially, I disagree with the Court's conclusion that the speech of a state-created monopoly, which is the subject of a comprehensive regulatory scheme, is entitled to protection under the First Amendment. ***

The state-created monopoly status of a utility arises from the unique characteristics of the services that a utility provides. As recognized in Cantor v. Detroit Edison Co., 428 U.S. 579, 595-596 (1976), "public utility regulation typically assumes that the private firm is a natural monopoly and that public controls are necessary to protect the consumer from exploitation." The consequences of this natural monopoly in my view justify much more wide-ranging supervision and control of a utility under the First Amendment than this Court held in *Bellotti* to be permissible with regard to ordinary corporations. [T]he extensive regulations governing decisionmaking by public utilities suggest that for purposes of First Amendment analysis, a utility is far closer to a state- controlled enterprise than is an ordinary corporation. Accordingly, I think a State has broad discretion in determining the statements that a utility may make in that such statements emanate from the entity created by the State to provide important and unique public services. ***

The Court today holds not only that commercial speech is entitled to First Amendment protection, but also that when it is protected a State may not regulate it unless its reason for doing so amounts to a "substantial" governmental interest, its regulation "directly advances" that interest, and its manner of regulation is "not more extensive than necessary" to serve the interest. *** The test adopted by the Court thus elevates the protection accorded commercial speech that falls within the scope of the First Amendment to a level that is virtually indistinguishable from that of noncommercial speech. I think the Court in so doing has effectively accomplished the "devitalization" of the First Amendment that it counseled against in *Ohralik*. I think it has also, by labeling economic regulation of business conduct as a restraint on "free speech," gone far to resurrect the discredited doctrine of cases such as *Lochner* and Tyson & Brother v. Banton, 273 U.S. 418 (1927). New York's order here is in my view more akin to an economic regulation to which virtually complete deference should be accorded by this Court. ***

While it is true that an important objective of the First Amendment is to foster the free flow of information, identification of speech that falls within its protection is not aided by the metaphorical reference to a "marketplace of ideas." There is no reason for believing that the marketplace of ideas is free from market imperfections any more than there is to believe that the invisible hand will always lead to optimum economic decisions in the commercial market. See, e.g., Baker, Scope of the First Amendment, Freedom of Speech, 25 UCLA L. Rev. 964, 967-981 (1978). ***

*** Nor do I think there is any basis for concluding that individual citizens of the State will recognize the need for and act to promote energy conservation to the extent the government deems appropriate, if only the channels of communication are left open. Thus, even if I were to agree that commercial speech is entitled to some First Amendment protection, I would hold here that the State's decision to ban promotional advertising, in light of the substantial state interest at stake, is a constitutionally permissible exercise of its power to adopt regulations designed to promote the interests of its citizens. ***

I remain of the view that the Court unlocked a Pandora's Box when it "elevated" commercial speech to the level of traditional political speech by according it First Amendment protection in Virginia Pharmacy Board v. Virginia Citizens Consumer Council, 425 U.S. 748 (1976). The line between "commercial speech," and the kind of speech that those who drafted the First Amendment had in mind, may not be a technically or intellectually easy one to draw, but it surely produced far fewer problems than has the development of judicial doctrine in this area since *Virginia Pharmacy Board.* For in the world of political advocacy and its marketplace of ideas, there is no such thing as a "fraudulent" idea: there may be useless proposals, totally unworkable schemes, as well as very sound proposals that will receive the imprimatur of the "marketplace of ideas" through our majoritarian system of election and representative government. The free flow of information is important in this context not because it will lead to the discovery of any objective "truth," but because it is essential to our system of self-government. ***

The Court concedes that the state interest in energy conservation is plainly substantial, as is the State's concern that its rates be fair and efficient. It also concedes that there is a direct link between the Commission's ban on promotional advertising and the State's interest in conservation. The Court nonetheless strikes down the ban on promotional advertising because the Commission has failed to demonstrate, under the final part of the Court's four-part test, that its regulation is no more extensive than necessary to serve the State's interest. ***

*** The Court's analysis in this regard is in my view fundamentally misguided because it fails to recognize that the beneficial side effects of "more efficient use" may be inconsistent with the goal of energy conservation. Indeed, the Commission explicitly found that the promotion of off-peak consumption would impair conservation efforts.

The Court concludes that the Commission's ban on promotional advertising must be struck down because it is more extensive than necessary: it may result in the suppression of advertising by utilities that promotes the use of electrical devices or services that cause no net increase in total energy use. *** The New York Public Service Commission, however, considered the merits of the heat pump and concluded that it would most likely result in an overall increase in electric energy consumption. The Commission stated:

> "[I]nstallation of a heat pump means also installation of central air-conditioning. To this extent, promotion of off-peak electric space heating involves promotion of on-peak summer air-conditioning as well as on-peak usage of electricity for water heating. And the price of electricity to most consumers in the State does not now fully reflect the much higher marginal costs of on-peak consumption in summer peaking markets. In these circumstances, there would be a subsidization of consumption on-peak, and consequently, higher rates for all consumers."

For the foregoing reasons, I would affirm the judgment of the New York Court of Appeals.

BOLGER v. YOUNGS DRUGS PRODUCTS CORPORATION
463 U.S. 60 (1983)

JUSTICE MARSHALL delivered the opinion of the Court.

Title 39 U.S.C. § 3001(e)(2) prohibits the mailing of unsolicited advertisements for contraceptives. The District Court held that, as applied to appellee's mailings, the statute violates the First Amendment. We affirm.

I

Section 3001(e)(2) states that "[a]ny unsolicited advertisement of matter which is designed, adapted, or intended for preventing conception is nonmailable matter, shall not be carried or delivered by mail, and shall be disposed of as the Postal Service directs ***."[1] As interpreted by Postal Service regulations, the statutory provision does not apply to unsolicited advertisements in which the mailer has no commercial interest.

Appellee Youngs Drug Products Corp. (Youngs) is engaged in the manufacture, sale, and distribution of contraceptives. Youngs markets its products primarily through sales to chain warehouses and wholesale distributors, who in turn sell contraceptives to retail pharmacists, who then sell those products to individual customers. Appellee publicizes the availability and desirability of its products by various methods. This litigation resulted from Youngs' decision to undertake a cam-

1. Section 3001(e)(2) contains express limitations. In particular, an advertisement is not deemed unsolicited "if it is contained in a publication for which the addressee has paid or promised to pay a consideration or which he has otherwise indicated he desires to receive." In addition, the provision does not apply to advertisements mailed to certain recipients such as a manufacturer of contraceptives, a licensed physician, or a pharmacist.

paign of unsolicited mass mailings to members of the public. In conjunction with its wholesalers and retailers, Youngs seeks to mail to the public on an unsolicited basis three types of materials:

—multi-page, multi-item flyers promoting a large variety of products available at a drugstore, including prophylactics;

—flyers exclusively or substantially devoted to promoting prophylactics;

—informational pamphlets discussing the desirability and availability of prophylactics in general or Youngs' products in particular.[4]***

The District Court determined that § 3001(e)(2), by its plain language, prohibited all three types of proposed mailings. The court then addressed the constitutionality of the statute as applied to these mailings. Finding all three types of materials to be commercial solicitations, the court considered the constitutionality of the statute within the framework established by this Court for analyzing restrictions imposed on commercial speech. The court concluded that the statutory prohibition was more extensive than necessary to the interests asserted by the Government, and it therefore held that the statute's absolute ban on the three types of mailings violated the First Amendment. ***

II

Beginning with Bigelow v. Virginia, 421 U.S. 809 (1975), this Court extended the protection of the First Amendment to commercial speech. Nonetheless, our decisions have recognized "the 'common-sense' distinction between speech proposing a commercial transaction, which occurs in an area traditionally subject to government regulation, and other varieties of speech." Ohralik v. Ohio State Bar Assn., 436 U.S. 447, 455-456 (1978). Thus, we have held that the Constitution accords less protection to commercial speech than to other constitutionally safeguarded forms of expression. Because the degree of protection afforded by the First Amendment depends on whether the activity sought to be regulated constitutes commercial or noncommercial speech, we must first determine the proper classification of the mailings at issue here.

Most of appellee's mailings fall within the core notion of commercial speech—"speech which does 'no more than propose a commercial transaction.'" *Virginia Pharmacy Board v. Virginia Citizens Consumer Council, Inc.*, [425 U.S.], at 762,

4. In the District Court, Youngs offered two examples of informational pamphlets. The first, entitled "Condoms and Human Sexuality," is a 12-page pamphlet describing the use, manufacture, desirability, and availability of condoms, and providing detailed descriptions of various Trojan-brand condoms manufactured by Youngs. The second, entitled "Plain Talk about Venereal Disease," is an eight-page pamphlet discussing at length the problem of venereal disease and the use and advantages of condoms in aiding the prevention of venereal disease. The only identification of Youngs or its products is at the bottom of the last page of the pamphlet, which states that the pamphlet has been contributed as a public service by Youngs, the distributor of Trojan-brand prophylactics.

quoting Pittsburgh Press Co. v. Human Relations Comm'n, 3 U.S. 376, 385 (1973).[12] Youngs' informational pamphlets, however, cannot be characterized merely as proposals to engage in commercial transactions. Their proper classification as commercial or noncommercial speech thus presents a closer question. The mere fact that these pamphlets are conceded to be advertisements clearly does not compel the conclusion that they are commercial speech. See New York Times Co. v. Sullivan, 376 U.S. 254, 265-266 (1964). Similarly, the reference to a specific product does not by itself render the pamphlets commercial speech.[13] *** Finally, the fact that Youngs has an economic motivation for mailing the pamphlets would clearly be insufficient by itself to turn the materials into commercial speech. See Bigelow v. Virginia, 421 U.S., at 818; Ginzburg v. United States, 383 U.S. 463, 474 (1966); Thornhill v. Alabama, 310 U.S. 88 (1940).

The combination of *all* these characteristics, however, provides strong support for the District Court's conclusion that the informational pamphlets are properly characterized as commercial speech. The mailings constitute commercial speech notwithstanding the fact that they contain discussions of important public issues such as venereal disease and family planning. We have made clear that advertising which "links a product to a current public debate" is not thereby entitled to the constitutional protection afforded noncommercial speech. Central Hudson Gas & Electric Corp. v. Public Service Comm'n of New York, 447 U.S., at 563, n. 5. A company has the full panoply of protections available to its direct comments on public issues, so there is no reason for providing similar constitutional protection when such statements are made in the context of commercial transactions. ***

We conclude, therefore, that all of the mailings in this case are entitled to the qualified but nonetheless substantial protection accorded to commercial speech.

III

*** In *Central Hudson* we adopted a four-part analysis for assessing the validity of restrictions on commercial speech. First, we determine whether the expression is

---

12. For example, the drugstore flyer consists primarily of price and quantity information.

13. One of the informational pamphlets, "Condoms and Human Sexuality," specifically refers to a number of Trojan-brand condoms manufactured by appellee and describes the advantages of each type.

The other informational pamphlet, "Plain Talk about Venereal Disease," repeatedly discusses condoms without any specific reference to those manufactured by appellee. The only reference to appellee's products is contained at the very bottom of the last page, where appellee is identified as the distributor of Trojan-brand prophylactics. That a product is referred to generically does not, however, remove it from the realm of commercial speech. For example, a company with sufficient control of the market for a product may be able to promote the product without reference to its own brand names. Or a trade association may make statements about a product without reference to specific brand names. See, e.g., National Comm'n on Egg Nutrition v. FTC, 570 F.2d 157 (CA7 1977) (enforcing in part a Federal Trade Commission order prohibiting false and misleading advertising by an egg industry trade association concerning the relationship between cholesterol, eggs, and heart disease). In this case, Youngs describes itself as "the leader in the manufacture and sale" of contraceptives.

constitutionally protected. For commercial speech to receive such protection, "it at least must concern lawful activity and not be misleading." Second, we ask whether the governmental interest is substantial. If so, we must then determine whether the regulation directly advances the government interest asserted, and whether it is not more extensive than necessary to serve that interest. Applying this analysis, we conclude that § 3001(e)(2) is unconstitutional as applied to appellee's mailings.

We turn first to the protection afforded by the First Amendment. The State may deal effectively with false, deceptive, or misleading sales techniques. *** In this case, however, appellants have never claimed that Youngs' proposed mailings fall into any of these categories. To the contrary, advertising for contraceptives not only implicates "'substantial individual and societal interests'" in the free flow of commercial information, but also relates to activity which is protected from unwarranted state interference. ***

We must next determine whether the Government's interest in prohibiting the mailing of unsolicited contraceptive advertisements is a substantial one. The prohibition in § 3001(e)(2) originated in 1873 as part of the Comstock Act, a criminal statute designed "for the suppression of Trade in and Circulation of obscene Literature and Articles of immoral Use." *** Appellants do not purport to rely on justifications for the statute offered during the 19th Century.[20] Instead, they advance interests that concededly were not asserted when the prohibition was enacted into law. This reliance is permissible since the insufficiency of the original motivation does not diminish other interests that the restriction may now serve. ***

In particular, appellants assert that the statute (1) shields recipients of mail from materials that they are likely to find offensive and (2) aids parents' efforts to control the manner in which their children become informed about sensitive and important subjects such as birth control. The first of these interests carries little weight. *** At least where obscenity is not involved, we have consistently held that the fact that protected speech may be offensive to some does not justify its suppression. We specifically declined to recognize a distinction between commercial and noncommercial speech that would render this interest a sufficient justification for a prohibition of commercial speech. ***

Recognizing that their reliance on this interest is "problematic," appellants attempt to avoid the clear import of *Carey* by emphasizing that § 3001(e)(2) is aimed at the mailing of materials to the home. We have, of course, recognized the important interest in allowing addressees to give notice to a mailer that they wish no further mailings which, in their sole discretion, they believe to be erotically arousing or sexually provocative. *** But we have never held that the Government itself can shut off the flow of mailings to protect those recipients who might potentially be of-

20. The party seeking to uphold a restriction on commercial speech carries the burden of justifying it. See Central Hudson Gas & Electric Corp. v. Public Service Comm'n of New York, 447 U.S. 557, 570 (1980); *Linmark Associates, Inc. v. Willingboro*, [431 U.S.] at 95.

fended. *** Consequently, the "short, though regular, journey from mail box to trash can *** is an acceptable burden, at least so far as the Constitution is concerned." Lamont v. Commissioner of Motor Vehicles, 269 F. Supp. 880, 883 (SDNY), summarily aff'd, 386 F.2d 449 (CA2 1967), cert. denied, 391 U.S. 915 (1968).

The second interest asserted by appellants—aiding parents' efforts to discuss birth control with their children—is undoubtedly substantial. "[P]arents have an important "guiding role" to play in the upbringing of their children *** which presumptively includes counseling them on important decisions." H.L. v. Matheson, 450 U.S. 398, 410 (1981), quoting Bellotti v. Baird, 443 U.S. 622, 637 (1979). As a *means* of effectuating this interest, however, § 3001(e)(2) fails to withstand scrutiny.

To begin with, § 3001(e)(2) provides only the most limited incremental support for the interest asserted. We can reasonably assume that parents already exercise substantial control over the disposition of mail once it enters their mailboxes. Under 39 U.S.C. § 3008, parents can also exercise control over information that flows into their mailboxes. And parents must already cope with the multitude of external stimuli that color their children's perception of sensitive subjects.[26] Under these circumstances, a ban on unsolicited advertisements serves only to assist those parents who desire to keep their children from confronting such mailings, who are otherwise unable to do so, and whose children have remained relatively free from such stimuli.

This marginal degree of protection is achieved by purging all mailboxes of unsolicited material that is entirely suitable for adults. We have previously made clear that a restriction of this scope is more extensive than the Constitution permits, for the government may not "reduce the adult population *** to reading only what is fit for children." Butler v. Michigan, 352 U.S. 380, 383 (1957).[27] The level of discourse reaching a mailbox simply cannot be limited to that which would be suitable for a sandbox. ***

IV

We thus conclude that the justifications offered by appellants are insufficient to warrant the sweeping prohibition on the mailing of unsolicited contraceptive advertisements. As applied to appellee's mailings, § 3001(e)(2) is unconstitutional. The judgment of the District Court is therefore [a]ffirmed.

JUSTICE BRENNAN took no part in the decision of this case.

---

26. For example, many magazines contain advertisements for contraceptives. See M. Redford, G. Duncan, & D. Prager, The Condom: Increasing Utilization in the United States 145 (1974) (ads accepted in Family Health, Psychology Today, and Ladies' Home Journal in 1970). Section 3001(e)(2) itself permits the mailing of publications containing contraceptive advertisements to subscribers. Similarly, drugstores commonly display contraceptives. And minors taking a course in sex education will undoubtedly be exposed to the subject of contraception.

27. In *Butler* this Court declared unconstitutional a Michigan statute that banned reading materials inappropriate for children. The legislation was deemed not "reasonably restricted" to the evil it sought to address; rather, the effect of the statute was "to burn the house to roast the pig."

JUSTICE REHNQUIST, with whom JUSTICE O'CONNOR joins, concurring in the judgment. [Omitted]

JUSTICE STEVENS, concurring in the judgment.

***

It matters whether a law regulates communications for their ideas or for their style. Governmental suppression of a specific point of view strikes at the core of First Amendment values. In contrast, regulations of form and context may strike a constitutionally appropriate balance between the advocate's right to convey a message and the recipient's interest in the quality of his environment ***

> "The fact that the advertising of a particular subject matter is *sometimes* offensive does not deprive all such advertising of First Amendment protection; but it is equally clear to me that the existence of such protection does not deprive the State of all power to regulate such advertising in order to minimize its offensiveness. A picture which may appropriately be included in an instruction book may be excluded from a billboard." Carey v. Population Services International, 431 U.S. 678, 717 (1977) (opinion of STEVENS, J.).

The statute at issue in this case censors ideas, not style. It prohibits appellee from mailing any unsolicited advertisement of contraceptives, no matter how unobtrusive and tactful; yet it permits anyone to mail unsolicited advertisements of devices intended to facilitate conception, no matter how coarse or grotesque. It thus excludes one advocate from a forum to which adversaries have unlimited access. I concur in the Court's judgment that the First Amendment prohibits the application of the statute to these materials.

ZAUDERER v. OFFICE OF DISCIPLINARY COUNCIL OF THE SUPREME COURT OF OHIO

471 U.S. 626 (1985)

JUSTICE WHITE delivered the opinion of the Court.

* * *

Appellant is an attorney practicing in Columbus, Ohio. In the spring of 1982, appellant placed an advertisement in 36 Ohio newspapers publicizing his willingness to represent women who had suffered injuries resulting from their use of a contraceptive device known as the Dalkon Shield Intrauterine Device. The advertisement featured a line drawing of the Dalkon Shield accompanied by the question, "DID YOU USE THIS IUD?" The advertisement then related the following information:

> "The Dalkon Shield Interuterine [sic] Device is alleged to have caused serious pelvic infections resulting in hospitalizations, tubal damage, infertility, and hysterectomies. It is also alleged to have caused unplanned pregnancies ending

> in abortions, miscarriages, septic abortions, tubal or ectopic pregnancies, and full-term deliveries. If you or a friend have had a similar experience do not assume it is too late to take legal action against the Shield's manufacturer. Our law firm is presently representing women on such cases. The cases are handled on a contingent fee basis of the amount recovered. If there is no recovery, no legal fees are owed by our clients."

The ad concluded with the name of appellant's law firm, its address, and a phone number that the reader might call for "free information."

The advertisement was successful in attracting clients: appellant received well over 200 inquiries regarding the advertisement, and he initiated lawsuits on behalf of 106 of the women who contacted him as a result of the advertisement. The ad, however, also aroused the interest of the Office of Disciplinary Counsel. ***

The complaint alleged that in running the ad and accepting employment by women responding to it, appellant had violated the following Disciplinary Rules: DR 2-101(B), which prohibits the use of illustrations in advertisements run by attorneys, requires that ads by attorneys be "dignified," and limits the information that may be included in such ads to a list of 20 items; DR 2-103(A), which prohibits an attorney from "recommend[ing] employment, as a private practitioner, of himself, his partner, or associate to a non-lawyer who has not sought his advice regarding employment of a lawyer;" and DR 2-104(A), which provides (with certain exceptions not applicable here) that "[a] lawyer who has given unsolicited advice to a layman that he should obtain counsel or take legal action shall not accept employment resulting from that advice."

The complaint also alleged that the advertisement violated DR 2-101(B)(15), which provides that any advertisement that mentions contingent-fee rates must "disclos[e] whether percentages are computed before or after deduction of court costs and expenses," and that the ad's failure to inform clients that they would be liable for costs (as opposed to legal fees) even if their claims were unsuccessful rendered the advertisement "deceptive" in violation of DR 2-101(A). The complaint did not allege that the Dalkon Shield advertisement was false or deceptive in any respect other than its omission of information relating to the contingent-fee arrangement; indeed, the Office of Disciplinary Counsel stipulated that the information and advice regarding Dalkon Shield litigation was not false, fraudulent, misleading, or deceptive and that the drawing was an accurate representation of the Dalkon Shield.

The charges against appellant were heard by a panel of the Board of Commissioners on Grievances and Discipline of the Supreme Court of Ohio. *** The panel found that the use of an illustration in appellant's Dalkon Shield advertisement violated DR 2-101(B), that the ad's failure to disclose the client's potential liability for costs even if her suit were unsuccessful violated both DR 2-101(A) and DR 2-101(B)(15), that the advertisement constituted self-recommendation in violation of DR 2-103(A), and that appellant's acceptance of offers of employment resulting from the advertisement violated DR 2-104(A).[5]

Contending that Ohio's Disciplinary Rules violate the First Amendment insofar as they authorize the State to discipline him for the content of his Dalkon Shield advertisement, appellant filed this appeal. We noted probable jurisdiction, and now affirm in part and reverse in part.

II

There is no longer any room to doubt that what has come to be known as "commercial speech" is entitled to the protection of the First Amendment, albeit to protection somewhat less extensive than that afforded "noncommercial speech." More subject to doubt, perhaps, are the precise bounds of the category of expression that may be termed commercial speech, but it is clear enough that the speech at issue in this case—advertising pure and simple—falls within those bounds.

Our general approach to restrictions on commercial speech is also by now well settled. The States and the Federal Government are free to prevent the dissemination of commercial speech that is false, deceptive, or misleading, see Friedman v. Rogers, 440 U.S. 1 (1979), or that proposes an illegal transaction, see Pittsburgh Press Co. v. Human Relations Comm'n, 413 U.S. 376 (1973). Commercial speech that is not false or deceptive and does not concern unlawful activities, however, may be restricted only in the service of a substantial governmental interest, and only through means that directly advance that interest. *Central Hudson Gas & Electric*, [447 U.S.] at 566. Our application of these principles to the commercial speech of attorneys has led us to conclude that blanket bans on price advertising by attorneys and rules preventing attorneys from using nondeceptive terminology to describe their fields of practice are impermissible, see Bates v. State Bar of Arizona, 433 U.S. 350 (1977); but that rules prohibiting in-person solicitation of clients by attorneys are, at least under some circumstances, permissible, see Ohralik v. Ohio State Bar Assn., 436 U.S. 447 (1978). To resolve this appeal, we must apply the teachings of these cases to three separate forms of regulation Ohio has imposed on advertising by its attorneys: prohibitions on soliciting legal business through advertisements containing advice and information regarding specific legal problems; restrictions on the use of illustrations in advertising by lawyers; and disclosure requirements relating to the terms of contingent fees.

III

* * *

The advertisement's information and advice concerning the Dalkon Shield were, as the Office of Disciplinary Counsel stipulated, neither false nor deceptive: in fact, they were entirely accurate. The advertisement did not promise readers that lawsuits alleging injuries caused by the Dalkon Shield would be successful, nor did it suggest that appellant had any special expertise in handling such lawsuits other than his

5. The panel did not find that the advertisement's alleged lack of "dignity" or its inclusion of information not allowed by DR 2-101(B)(1)-(20) constituted an independent violation.

employment in other such litigation. Rather, the advertisement reported the indisputable fact that the Dalkon Shield has spawned an impressive number of lawsuits[10] and advised readers that appellant was currently handling such lawsuits and was willing to represent other women asserting similar claims. In addition, the advertisement advised women that they should not assume that their claims were time-barred— advice that seems completely unobjectionable in light of the trend in many States toward a "discovery rule" for determining when a cause of action for latent injury or disease accrues. The State's power to prohibit advertising that is "inherently misleading," see *In re* R.M.J., 455 U.S., at 203, thus cannot justify Ohio's decision to discipline appellant for running advertising geared to persons with a specific legal problem.

Because appellant's statements regarding the Dalkon Shield were not false or deceptive, our decisions impose on the State the burden of establishing that prohibiting the use of such statements to solicit or obtain legal business directly advances a substantial governmental interest. *** Our decision in *Ohralik* was largely grounded on the substantial differences between face-to-face solicitation and the advertising we had held permissible in *Bates*. In-person solicitation by a lawyer, we concluded, was a practice rife with possibilities for overreaching, invasion of privacy, the exercise of undue influence, and outright fraud. In addition, we noted that in-person solicitation presents unique regulatory difficulties because it is "not visible or otherwise open to public scrutiny." ***

It is apparent that the concerns that moved the Court in *Ohralik* are not present here. Although some sensitive souls may have found appellant's advertisement in poor taste, it can hardly be said to have invaded the privacy of those who read it. *** In addition, a printed advertisement, unlike a personal encounter initiated by an attorney, is not likely to involve pressure on the potential client for an immediate yes-or-no answer to the offer of representation. Thus, a printed advertisement is a means of conveying information about legal services that is more conducive to reflection and the exercise of choice on the part of the consumer than is personal solicitation by an attorney. Accordingly, the substantial interests that justified the ban on in-person solicitation upheld in *Ohralik* cannot justify the discipline imposed on appellant for the content of his advertisement.

Nor does the traditional justification for restraints on solicitation—the fear that lawyers will "stir up litigation"—justify the restriction imposed in this case. In evaluating this proffered justification, it is important to think about what it might mean to say that the State has an interest in preventing lawyers from stirring up litigation. It is possible to describe litigation itself as an evil that the State is entitled

---

10. By 1979, it was "estimated that 2500 claims [had] been made *** for injuries allegedly caused by [the Dalkon Shield]." Van Dyke, The Dalkon Shield: A "Primer" in IUD Liability, 6 West. St. U.L. Rev. 1, 3, n. 7 (1978). By mid-1980, the number of lawsuits had risen to 4,000. Bamford, Dalkon Shield Starts Losing in Court, 2 American Lawyer 31 (July 1980).

to combat: after all, litigation consumes vast quantities of social resources to produce little of tangible value but much discord and unpleasantness. "[A]s a litigant," Judge Learned Hand once observed, "I should dread a lawsuit beyond almost anything else short of sickness and death." L. Hand, The Deficiencies of Trials to Reach the Heart of the Matter, in 3 Association of the Bar of the City of New York, Lectures on Legal Topics 89, 105 (1926).

But we cannot endorse the proposition that a lawsuit, as such, is an evil. Over the course of centuries, our society has settled upon civil litigation as a means for redressing grievances, resolving disputes, and vindicating rights when other means fail. There is no cause for consternation when a person who believes in good faith and on the basis of accurate information regarding his legal rights that he has suffered a legally cognizable injury turns to the courts for a remedy: "we cannot accept the notion that it is always better for a person to suffer a wrong silently than to redress it by legal action." Bates v. State Bar of Arizona, 433 U.S., at 376. The State is not entitled to interfere with that access by denying its citizens accurate information about their legal rights. Accordingly, it is not sufficient justification for the discipline imposed on appellant that his truthful and nondeceptive advertising had a tendency to or did in fact encourage others to file lawsuits. ***

The State's argument proceeds from the premise that it is intrinsically difficult to distinguish advertisements containing legal advice that is false or deceptive from those that are truthful and helpful, much more so than is the case with other goods or services.[12] This notion is belied by the facts before us: appellant's statements regarding Dalkon Shield litigation were in fact easily verifiable and completely accurate. Nor is it true that distinguishing deceptive from nondeceptive claims in advertising involving products other than legal services is a comparatively simple and straightforward process. ***

*** The First Amendment protections afforded commercial speech would mean little indeed if such arguments were allowed to prevail. Our recent decisions involving commercial speech have been grounded in the faith that the free flow of commercial information is valuable enough to justify imposing on would-be regulators the costs of distinguishing the truthful from the false, the helpful from the misleading, and the harmless from the harmful. *** An attorney may not be disciplined

12. The State's argument may also rest in part on a suggestion that even completely accurate advice regarding the legal rights of the advertiser's audience may lead some members of the audience to initiate meritless litigation against innocent defendants. To the extent that this is the State's contention, it is unavailing. To be sure, some citizens, accurately informed of their legal rights, may file lawsuits that ultimately turn out not to be meritorious. But the State is not entitled to prejudge the merits of its citizens' claims by choking off access to information that may be useful to its citizens in deciding whether to press those claims in court. As we observed in Bates v. State Bar of Arizona, 433 U.S., at 375, n. 31, if the State's concern is with abuse of process, it can best achieve its aim by enforcing sanctions against vexatious litigation.

for soliciting legal business through printed advertising containing truthful and nondeceptive information and advice regarding the legal rights of potential clients.

IV

The application of DR 2-101(B)'s restriction on illustrations in advertising by lawyers to appellant's advertisement fails for much the same reasons as does the application of the self-recommendation and solicitation rules. The use of illustrations or pictures in advertisements serves important communicative functions: it attracts the attention of the audience to the advertiser's message, and it may also serve to impart information directly. *** Because the illustration for which appellant was disciplined is an accurate representation of the Dalkon Shield and has no features that are likely to deceive, mislead, or confuse the reader, the burden is on the State to present a substantial governmental interest justifying the restriction as applied to appellant and to demonstrate that the restriction vindicates that interest through the least restrictive available means. *** [A]ppellant may not be disciplined for his use of an accurate and nondeceptive illustration.

V

In requiring attorneys who advertise their willingness to represent clients on a contingent-fee basis to state that the client may have to bear certain expenses even if he loses, Ohio has not attempted to prevent attorneys from conveying information to the public; it has only required them to provide somewhat more information than they might otherwise be inclined to present. We have, to be sure, held that in some instances compulsion to speak may be as violative of the First Amendment as prohibitions on speech. See, e.g., Wooley v. Maynard, 430 U.S. 705 (1977); Miami Herald Publishing Co. v. Tornillo, 418 U.S. 241 (1974). Indeed, in West Virginia State Bd. of Ed. v. Barnette, 319 U.S. 624 (1943), the Court went so far as to state that "involuntary affirmation could be commanded only on even more immediate and urgent grounds than silence."

But the interests at stake in this case are not of the same order as those discussed in *Wooley, Tornillo*, and *Barnette*. Ohio has not attempted to "prescribe what shall be orthodox in politics, nationalism, religion, or other matters of opinion or force citizens to confess by word or act their faith therein." The State has attempted only to prescribe what shall be orthodox in commercial advertising, and its prescription has taken the form of a requirement that appellant include in his advertising purely factual and uncontroversial information about the terms under which his services will be available. [I]n virtually all our commercial speech decisions to date, we have emphasized that because disclosure requirements trench much more narrowly on an advertiser's interests than do flat prohibitions on speech, "warning[s] or disclaimer[s] might be appropriately required *** in order to dissipate the possibility of consumer confusion or deception."

We do not suggest that disclosure requirements do not implicate the advertiser's First Amendment rights at all. We recognize that unjustified or unduly burdensome disclosure requirements might offend the First Amendment by chilling protected commercial speech. But we hold that an advertiser's rights are adequately protected as long as disclosure requirements are reasonably related to the State's interest in preventing deception of consumers.[14]

*** The State's position that it is deceptive to employ advertising that refers to contingent-fee arrangements without mentioning the client's liability for costs is reasonable enough to support a requirement that information regarding the client's liability for costs be disclosed. ***

JUSTICE POWELL took no part in the decision of this case.

JUSTICE BRENNAN, with whom JUSTICE MARSHALL joins, concurring in part, concurring in the judgment in part, and dissenting in part. [Omitted.]

JUSTICE O'CONNOR [with whom THE CHIEF JUSTICE and JUSTICE REHNQUIST join], dissenting in part.

*** I dissent from Part III of the Court's opinion. In my view, the use of unsolicited legal advice to entice clients poses enough of a risk of overreaching and undue influence to warrant Ohio's rule. *** Because I would defer to the judgment of the States that have chosen to preclude use of unsolicited legal advice to entice clients, I respectfully dissent from Part III of the Court's opinion.[*]

---

14. We reject appellant's contention that we should subject disclosure requirements to a strict "least restrictive means" analysis under which they must be struck down if there are other means by which the State's purposes may be served. Although we have subjected outright prohibitions on speech to such analysis, all our discussions of restraints on commercial speech have recommended disclosure requirements as one of the acceptable less restrictive alternatives to actual suppression of speech.

*. **[Ed. Note**: In *Zauderer*, the Court distinguished its earlier decision in Ohralik v. Ohio State Bar Ass'n, 436 U.S. 447 (1978), in which it had upheld a state bar regulation forbidding "in-person" solicitation by attorneys. Later, however, the Court struck down a Florida law prohibiting uninvited direct in-person solicitation of business by certified public accountants. Edenfield v. Fane, 507 U.S. 761 (1993) (holding that the state had not demonstrated that the "harms" it alleged to accompany such direct uninvited overtures were realistic, or that the ban was a sufficiently direct means of alleviating such few speculative abuses as against its First Amendment interference). The Court also limited *Ohralik*, describing *Zauderer* as one of several cases making clear "that *Ohralik*'s holding was narrow and depended upon certain 'unique features of in-person solicitation by lawyers' that were present in the circumstances of that case.") 507 U.S., at 774. But that disclaimer proved to be premature. See Florida Bar v. Went For It, Inc., 515 U.S. 618 (1995) (state bar regulation forbidding direct mail solicitation of personal injury victims within 30 days of an accident or injury-producing event, sustained, five-to-four, as a defensible limited time and manner commercial speech restriction: (a) to protect accident victim privacy from predatory intrusion during immediate post-accident period of uncertainty and suffering; and (b) to prevent undermining public confidence in the professional standards of the bar.)]

POSADAS DE PUERTO RICO ASSOCIATES v. TOURISM COMPANY OF PUERTO RICO
478 U.S. 328 (1986)

JUSTICE REHNQUIST delivered the opinion of the Court.

***

In 1948, the Puerto Rico Legislature legalized certain forms of casino gambling. The Games of Chance Act of 1948, authorized the playing of roulette, dice, and card games in licensed "gambling rooms." Bingo and slot machines were later added to the list of authorized games of chance under the Act. The legislature's intent was set forth in the Act's Statement of Motives:

> "The purpose of this Act is to contribute to the development of tourism by means of the authorization of certain games of chance which are customary in the recreation places of the great tourist centers of the world, and by the establishment of regulations for and the strict surveillance of said games by the government, in order to ensure for tourists the best possible safeguards, while at the same time opening for the Treasurer of Puerto Rico an additional source of income." Games of Chance Act of 1948, Act No. 221 of May 15, 1948, §1.

The Act also provided that "[n]o gambling room shall be permitted to advertise or otherwise offer their facilities to the public of Puerto Rico." Regulation 76a-1(7), as amended in 1971, provides in pertinent part:

> "No concessionaire, nor his agent or employee is authorized to advertise the gambling parlors to the public in Puerto Rico. The advertising of our games of chance is hereby authorized through newspapers, magazines, radio, television and other publicity media outside Puerto Rico subject to the prior editing and approval by the Tourism Development Company of the advertisement to be submitted in draft to the Company."

In 1975, appellant Posadas de Puerto Rico Associates, a partnership organized under the laws of Texas, obtained a franchise to operate a gambling casino and began doing business under the name Condado Holiday Inn Hotel and Sands Casino. In 1978, appellant was twice fined by the Tourism Company for violating the advertising restrictions in the Act and implementing regulations.

Appellant filed a declaratory judgment action against the Tourism Company in the Superior Court of Puerto Rico, San Juan Section, seeking a declaration that the Act and implementing regulations, both facially and as applied by the Tourism Company, violated appellant's commercial speech rights under the United States Constitution. [T]he court issued a narrowing construction of the statute, declaring that "the only advertisement prohibited by the law originally is that which is contracted with an advertising agency, for consideration, to attract the resident to bet at the dice, card, roulette and bingo tables." The court also issued the following narrowing construction of Regulation 76a-1(7): "Advertisements of the casinos in Puerto Rico are prohibited in the local publicity media addressed to inviting the residents of Puerto Rico to visit the casinos.

* * * * *

> "We hereby allow, within the jurisdiction of Puerto Rico, advertising by the casinos addressed to tourists, provided they do not invite the residents of Puerto Rico to visit the casino, even though said announcements may incidentally reach the hands of a resident. Within the ads of casinos by this regulation figure *** the ads of casinos in magazines for distribution primarily in Puerto Rico to the tourist, including the official guide of the Tourism Company 'Que Pasa in Puerto Rico' and any other tourist facility guide in Puerto Rico, even though said magazines may be available to the residents and in movies, television, radio, newspapers and trade magazines which may be published, taped, or filmed in the exterior for tourism promotion in the exterior even though they may be exposed or incidentally circulated in Puerto Rico. For example: an advertisement in the New York Times, an advertisement in CBS which reaches us through Cable TV,

whose main objective is to reach the potential tourist. *** "The direct promotion of the

Under *Central Hudson*, commercial speech receives a limited form of First Amendment protection so long as it concerns a lawful activity and is not misleading or fraudulent. Once it is determined that the First Amendment applies to the particular kind of commercial speech at issue, then the speech may be restricted only if the government's interest in doing so is substantial, the restrictions directly advance the government's asserted interest, and the restrictions are no more extensive than necessary to serve that interest. ***

The particular kind of commercial speech at issue here, namely, advertising of casino gambling aimed at the residents of Puerto Rico, concerns a lawful activity and is not misleading or fraudulent, at least in the abstract. We must therefore proceed to the three remaining steps of the *Central Hudson* analysis in order to determine whether Puerto Rico's advertising restrictions run afoul of the First Amendment. The first of these three steps involves an assessment of the strength of the government's interest in restricting the speech. The interest at stake in this case, as determined by the Superior Court, is the reduction of demand for casino gambling by the residents of Puerto Rico. The Tourism Company's brief before this Court explains the legislature's belief that "[e]xcessive casino gambling among local residents *** would produce serious harmful effects on the health, safety and welfare of the Puerto Rican citizens, such as the disruption of moral and cultural patterns, the increase in local crime, the fostering of prostitution, the development of corruption, and the infiltration of organized crime." These are some of the very same concerns, of course, that have motivated the vast majority of the 50 States to prohibit casino gambling. We have no difficulty in concluding that the Puerto Rico Legislature's interest in the health, safety, and welfare of its citizens constitutes a "substantial" governmental interest.

The last two steps of the *Central Hudson* analysis basically involve a consideration of the "fit" between the legislature's ends and the means chosen to accomplish those ends. Step three asks the question whether the challenged restrictions on commercial speech "directly advance" the government's asserted interest. In the instant case, the answer to this question is clearly "yes." The Puerto Rico Legislature obviously believed, when it enacted the advertising restrictions at issue here, that advertising of casino gambling aimed at the residents of Puerto Rico would serve to increase the demand for the product advertised. We think the legislature's belief is a reasonable one, and the fact that appellant has chosen to litigate this case all the way to this Court indicates that appellant shares the legislature's view.***

We also think it clear beyond peradventure that the challenged statute and regulations satisfy the fourth and last step of the *Central Hudson* analysis, namely, whether the restrictions on commercial speech are no more extensive than necessary to serve the government's interest. The narrowing constructions of the advertising restrictions announced by the Superior Court ensure that the restrictions will not affect advertising of casino gambling aimed at tourists, but will apply only to such advertising when aimed at the residents of Puerto Rico. ***

In short, we conclude that the statute and regulations at issue in this case, as construed by the Superior Court, pass muster under each prong of the *Central Hudson* test. We therefore hold that the Supreme Court of Puerto Rico properly rejected appellant's First Amendment claim.

Appellant argues, however, that the challenged advertising restrictions are constitutionally defective under our decisions in Carey v. Population Services International, 431 U.S. 678 (1977), and Bigelow v. Virginia, 421 U.S. 809 (1975). In *Carey*, this Court struck down a ban on any "advertisement or display" of contraceptives, and in *Bigelow*, we reversed a criminal conviction based on the advertisement of an abortion clinic. We think appellant's argument ignores a crucial distinction between the *Carey* and *Bigelow* decisions and the instant case. In *Carey* and *Bigelow*, the underlying conduct that was the subject of the advertising restrictions was constitutionally protected and could not have been prohibited by the State. Here, on the other hand, the Puerto Rico Legislature surely could have prohibited casino gambling by the residents of Puerto Rico altogether. In our view, the greater power to completely ban casino gambling necessarily includes the lesser power to ban advertising of casino gambling, and *Carey* and *Bigelow* are hence inapposite.

Appellant also makes the related argument that, having chosen to legalize casino gambling for residents of Puerto Rico, the legislature is prohibited by the First Amendment from using restrictions on advertising to accomplish its goal of reducing demand for such gambling. We disagree. In our view, appellant has the argument backwards. As we noted in the preceding paragraph, it is precisely *because* the government could have enacted a wholesale prohibition of the underlying conduct that it is permissible for the government to take the less intrusive step of allowing the conduct, but reducing the demand through restrictions on advertising. It would surely be a Pyrrhic victory for casino owners such as appellant to gain recognition of a First Amendment right to advertise their casinos to the residents of Puerto Rico, only to thereby force the legislature into banning casino gambling by residents altogether. It would just as surely be a strange constitutional doctrine which would concede to the legislature the authority to totally ban a product or activity, but deny to the legislature the authority to forbid the stimulation of demand for the product or activity through advertising on behalf of those who would profit from such increased demand. Legislative regulation of products or activities deemed harmful, such as cigarettes, alcoholic beverages, and prostitution, has varied from outright prohibition on the one hand, to legalization of the product or activity with restrictions on stimulation of its demand on the other hand, see, e.g., Nev. Rev. Stat. §§ 244.345(1), (8) (1986) (authorizing licensing of houses of prostitution except in counties with more than 250,000 population), §§ 201.430, 201.440 (prohibiting advertising of houses of prostitution "[i]n any public theater, on the public streets of any city or town, or on any public highway," or "in [a] place of business").[10] To rule out the latter, intermediate kind of response would require more than we find in the First Amendment.

***[W]ith the interpretive assistance of the implementing regulations as modified by the Superior Court, we do not find the statute unconstitutionally vague.

For the foregoing reasons, the decision of the Supreme Court of Puerto Rico that, as construed by the Superior Court, § 8 of the Games of Chance Act of 1948 and the implementing regulations do not facially violate the First Amendment or the due process or equal protection guarantees of the Constitution, is affirmed.[11]

JUSTICE BRENNAN, with whom JUSTICE MARSHALL and JUSTICE BLACKMUN join, dissenting.

*** I do not believe that Puerto Rico constitutionally may suppress truthful commercial speech in order to discourage its residents from engaging in lawful activity.

It is well settled that the First Amendment protects commercial speech from unwarranted governmental regulation. ***

The Court asserts that the Commonwealth has a legitimate and substantial interest in discouraging its residents from engaging in casino gambling. *** Neither

---

10. See also 15 U.S.C. § 1335 (prohibiting cigarette advertising "on any medium of electronic communication subject to the jurisdiction of the Federal Communications Commission"), upheld in Capital Broadcasting Co. v. Mitchell, 333 F. Supp. 582 (DC 1971), summarily aff'd sub nom. Capital Broadcasting Co. v. Acting Attorney General, 405 U.S. 1000 (1972); Fla. Stat. § 561.42(10)-(12) (1985) (prohibiting all signs except for one sign per product in liquor store windows).

11. JUSTICE STEVENS claims that the Superior Court's narrowing construction creates an impermissible "prior restraint" on protected speech, because that court required the submission of certain casino advertising to appellee for its prior approval. *** This argument was not raised by appellant either below or in this Court, and we therefore express no view on the constitutionality of the particular portion of the Superior Court's narrowing construction cited by JUSTICE STEVENS.

the statute on its face nor the legislative history indicates that the Puerto Rico Legislature thought that serious harm would result if residents were allowed to engage in casino gambling; indeed, the available evidence suggests exactly the opposite. Puerto Rico has legalized gambling casinos, and permits its residents to patronize them. *** Residents of Puerto Rico are also permitted to engage in a variety of other gambling activities—including horse racing, "picas," cockfighting, and the Puerto Rico lottery—all of which are allowed to advertise freely to residents. Indeed, it is surely not farfetched to suppose that the legislature chose to restrict casino advertising not because of the "evils" of casino gambling, but because it preferred that Puerto Ricans spend their gambling dollars on the Puerto Rico lottery. In any event, in light of the legislature's determination that serious harm will*not* result if residents are permitted and *encouraged* to gamble, I do not see how Puerto Rico's interest in discouraging its residents from engaging in casino gambling can be characterized as "substantial," even if the legislature had actually asserted such an interest which, of course, it has not. ***

The Court nevertheless sustains Puerto Rico's advertising ban because the legislature *could* have determined that casino gambling would seriously harm the health, safety, and welfare of the Puerto Rican citizens. ***[4] This reasoning is contrary to this Court's long-established First Amendment jurisprudence. When the government seeks to place restrictions upon commercial speech, a court may not, as the Court implies today, simply speculate about valid reasons that the government might have for enacting such restrictions. Rather, the government ultimately bears the burden of justifying the challenged regulation, and it is incumbent upon the government to *prove* that the interests it seeks to further are real and substantial. See *Zauderer*, 471 U.S., at 641; *In re R.M.J.*, 455 U.S., at 205-206; *Friedman*, 440 U.S., at 15. In this case, appellee has not shown that "serious harmful effects" will result if Puerto Rico residents gamble in casinos, and the legislature's decision to legalize such activity suggests that it believed the opposite to be true. In short, appellees have failed to show that a substantial government interest supports Puerto Rico's ban on protected expression.

Even assuming that appellee could show that the challenged restrictions are supported by a substantial governmental interest, this would not end the inquiry into

---

4. The Court reasons that because Puerto Rico could legitimately decide to prohibit casino gambling entirely, it may also take the "less intrusive step" of legalizing casino gambling but restricting speech. *** According to the Court, it would "surely be a strange constitutional doctrine which would concede to the legislature the authority to totally ban [casino gambling] but deny to the legislature the authority to forbid the stimulation of demand for [casino gambling]" by banning advertising. I do not agree that a ban on casino advertising is "less intrusive" than an outright prohibition of such activity. A majority of States have chosen not to legalize casino gambling, and we have never suggested that this might be unconstitutional. However, having decided to legalize casino gambling, Puerto Rico's decision to ban truthful speech concerning entirely lawful activity raises serious First Amendment problems. Thus, the "constitutional doctrine" which bans Puerto Rico from banning advertisements concerning lawful casino gambling is not so strange a restraint—it is called the First Amendment.

their constitutionality. See *Linmark Associates*, 431 U.S., at 94; *Virginia Pharmacy Board*, 425 U.S., at 766. Appellee must still demonstrate that the challenged advertising ban directly advances Puerto Rico's interest in controlling the harmful effects allegedly associated with casino gambling. *Central Hudson*, 447 U.S., at 564. The Court proclaims that Puerto Rico's legislature "obviously believed *** that advertising of casino gambling aimed at the residents of Puerto Rico would serve to increase the demand for the product advertised." *** However, even assuming that an advertising ban would effectively reduce residents' patronage of gambling casinos,[5] it is not clear how it would directly advance Puerto Rico's interest in controlling the "serious harmful effects" the Court associates with casino gambling. In particular, it is unclear whether banning casino advertising aimed at residents would affect local crime, prostitution, the development of corruption, or the infiltration of organized crime. Because Puerto Rico actively promotes its casinos to tourists, these problems are likely to persist whether or not residents are also encouraged to gamble. Absent some showing that a ban on advertising aimed only at residents will directly advance Puerto Rico's interest in controlling the harmful effects allegedly associated with casino gambling, Puerto Rico may not constitutionally restrict protected expression in that way.

Finally, appellees have failed to show that Puerto Rico's interest in controlling the harmful effects allegedly associated with casino gambling "cannot be protected adequately by more limited regulation of appellant's commercial expression." *Central Hudson*, at 570. Rather than suppressing constitutionally protected expression, Puerto Rico could seek directly to address the specific harms thought to be associated with casino gambling. Thus, Puerto Rico could continue carefully to monitor casino operations to guard against "the development of corruption, and the infiltration of organized crime." *** It could vigorously enforce its criminal statutes to combat "the increase in local crime [and] the fostering of prostitution." It could establish limits on the level of permissible betting, or promulgate additional speech designed to discourage casino gambling among residents, in order to avoid the "disruption of moral and cultural patterns," that might result if residents were to engage in excessive casino gambling. Such measures would directly address the problems appellee associates with casino gambling, while avoiding the First Amendment problems raised where the government seeks to ban constitutionally protected speech. ***

The Court believes that Puerto Rico constitutionally may prevent its residents from obtaining truthful commercial speech concerning otherwise lawful activity because of the effect it fears this information will have. However, "[i]t is precisely this kind of choice between the dangers of suppressing information, and the dangers of

5. Unlike the Court, I do not read the fact that appellant has chosen to litigate the case here to necessarily indicate that appellant itself believes that Puerto Rico residents would respond to casino advertising. In light of appellees' arbitrary and capricious application of § 8, appellant could justifiably have believed that, notwithstanding the Superior Court's "narrowing" construction, its First Amendment rights could be safeguarded effectively only if the Act was invalidated on its face.

its misuse if it is freely available, that the First Amendment makes for us." *Virginia Pharmacy Board*, 425 U.S., at 770. *** Accordingly, I would hold that Puerto Rico may not suppress the dissemination of truthful information about entirely lawful activity merely to keep its residents ignorant. The Court, however, would allow Puerto Rico to do just that, thus dramatically shrinking the scope of First Amendment protection available to commercial speech, and giving government officials unprecedented authority to eviscerate constitutionally protected expression. I respectfully dissent.

JUSTICE STEVENS, with whom JUSTICE MARSHALL and JUSTICE BLACKMUN join, dissenting. [Omitted.]

NOTE

I. Suppose in New York where casino gambling is not permitted, that Acme Casino, a company profitably operating casinos in New Jersey (where such casinos are lawful), buys ad space in the New York Times, in which it says:

"Let's vote to make casino gambling lawful in New York."

Would a state law forbidding the Times to carry such an advertisement be subject to the *Posadas* rationale?

II. What are the ramifications of the Court's view in *Posadas* that to the extent a state legislature could constitutionally restrict or eliminate a particular kind of commercial service (e.g., gambling) or product (e.g., tobacco), it may do the "lesser" thing of restricting or eliminating advertisements of that service or product?

A. Suppose in a jurisdiction where casino gambling is lawful, the Acme Company takes out the following advertisement in a newspaper of general circulation:

> As residents of this state already know, casino gambling is lawful for everyone over the age of eighteen. What you may not know is this. Standardly, in casino establishments the roulette wheel odds in rouge et noir (i.e. betting on red or betting on black) favor the house by four percent. At Acme, however, the roulette wheel odds in rouge et noir favor the house by only half as much, i.e. by a mere two percent. For better value, consider the odds and consider ACME.

Would a state law forbidding any such notice be valid under the *Posadas* case? Assuming you conclude that it might be valid, would it also be valid as applied to a news story in the same newspaper, i.e. a news story reporting on rouge et noir odds at the various casinos, reporting that only at Acme is the house favored by a mere two percent? Would it (should it) make any difference whether the newspaper published the information: (a) because it regarded the furnishing of such information of news interest and of consumer interest in the same fashion as information (it might from time to time publish) of which gas stations were selling gasoline at prices lower than at other stations; (b) because by publishing such information it believed it would sell more newspapers (and thus also more advertising, the rates of which are driven by its circulation figures); (c) because of a combination of (a) and (b)?

B. If, consistent with *Posadas*, you think the commercial advertisement placed by Acme could be forbidden (because clearly the state could forbid commercial gambling itself), what distinctions, if any, can you propose for the following variations:

1. Suppose that a state could, consistent with the fourteenth amendment economic substantive due process,[5] forbid the sale of prescription drugs at a discount. Suppose, however, that the state legislature has not in fact done so. Instead, it forbids any *advertisement* of prescription drugs at discounted prices. Is the measure: (a) invalid under *Virginia State Board of Pharmacy*; (b) valid under *Posadas*; (c) controlled instead by *Central Hudson*?

2. In *Posadas*, Justice Rehnquist distinguished between commercial speech about products/services the legislatures *may not* disallow (for example, contraceptive devices or medically safe abortion services), and commercial speech about products/services the legislature *may* disallow (e.g., gambling, or maybe sale of tobacco products). Presumably the rationale of *Posadas* would not apply to state regulation of the former.

So, for example, the state could not forbid publication, distribution or sale of Marx's *Das Kapital*; correspondingly, it could not regulate commercial speech pertaining to this book, except narrowly in ways consistent with *Central Hudson* (and related cases). Similarly, the state could not forbid the rendering legal professional services (consistent with the due process clause and the right to counsel furnished by the Constitution). Accordingly, the lawyer advertising cases (e.g., *Bates, Ohralik, Zauderer*) would appear to be governed by the *Central Hudson* formula and not by the *Posadas* rationale.

Consider, however, a prohibition on lawyer advertising of legal services available on a contingent fee basis. Would such a prohibition be (a) invalid under *Zauderer*;[6] (b) valid under *Posadas*?[7] To what extent does the *Posadas* test require a threshold inquiry: a determination of the extent to which the legislature may, in fact, outlaw a particular kind of product, service, or commercial practice, so as to determine which commercial speech doctrine applies? Where *Posadas* applies, to what

---

5. See, e.g., Nebbia v. New York, 291 U.S. 502 (1934) (sustaining state law which forbade sale of milk at less than nine cents a quart, as applied to small grocer who sold two quarts for eighteen cents but included a "free" loaf of bread).

6. Assume that the prohibition applies even to clear, accurate advertisements which contain no misleading omissions. (In *Zauderer*, of course, the Ohio Supreme Court had disciplined an attorney for failure to disclose that, despite a contingent fee arrangement, a client might be liable for significant costs after an unsuccessful lawsuit.)

7. Perhaps the state might constitutionally forbid this form of legal services; the contingent fee arrangement is generally disallowed in England, as well as in other countries, as a form of barratry, champerty, or maintenance.

extent does it affect a return to the 1942 *Valentine v. Chrestensen* approach to constitutional protection of commercial speech?[8]

3. Suppose one went back to the original ordinance at issue in *Valentine v. Chrestensen*—a ban only on commercial leaflets in downtown streets. Similarly, consider a ban on purely commercial sound trucks—vehicles on the streets solely to move about to broadcast ordinary commercial messages. In each of these cases, might not the avoidance of clutter, litter, noise, and further congestion be regarded as a "substantial" enough public interest to meet the first part of the *Central Hudson* three-part test (the test applicable to commercial speech neither soliciting an unlawful transaction nor false or misleading)? Would one concede also that the regulation at issue "directly" (rather than only indirectly) advances these interests, thus sufficiently satisfying that part of the test was well? If, moreover, the regulations are content neutral insofar as they show no favoritism toward certain commercial messages but apply uniformly, may they also be deemed to meet the third part as well, i.e. as no "more extensive than is necessary" to serve those interests efficiently as well?

A number of cities have acted on the assumption that regulations of this sort are valid under *Central Hudson*, and not merely under *Valentine v. Chrestensen.* How secure is that assumption?[9] Consider the following decision by the Supreme Court.

CITY OF CINCINNATI v. DISCOVERY NETWORK INC.
(507 U.S. 410 (1993)

JUSTICE STEVENS delivered the opinion of the Court.

Motivated by its interest in the safety and attractive appearance of its streets and sidewalks, the city of Cincinnati has refused to allow respondents to distribute their commercial publications through freestanding newsracks located on public property. The question presented is whether this refusal is consistent with the First Amendment. In agreement with the District Court and the Court of Appeals, we hold that it is not.

---

8. For several critical reviews of *Posadas* and of the commercial speech cases generally, see Edward L. Barrett, Jr., "The Unchartered Area"—Commercial Speech and the First Amendment, 13 U.C. Davis L.Rev. 175 (1980); Daniel A. Farber, Commercial Speech and First Amendment Theory, 74 Nw. U.L.Rev. 372 (1979); Thomas H. Jackson & John Calvin Jeffries, Jr., Commercial Speech: Economic Due Process and the First Amendment, 65 Va L.Rev. 1 (1979); David F. McGowan, A Critical Analysis of Commercial Speech, 78 Cal.L.Rev. 359 (1990); Frederick Schauer, Commercial Speech and the Architecture of the First Amendment, 56 U.Cin.L.Rev. 1181 (1988); Steven H. Shiffrin, the First Amendment and Economic Regulation: Away from a General Theory of the First Amendment, 78 Nw.U.L.Rev. 1212 (1983). For a more sympathetic review see Robert Post, The Constitutional Status of Commercial Speech, 48 U.C.L.A. L. Rev. 1 (2000).

9. For the New York Court of Appeals decision following relitigation of the New York ordinance at issue in *Valentine v. Chrestensen*, see People v. Remeny, 355 N.E.2d 375 (N.Y. 1976).

I

Respondent, Discovery Network, Inc., is engaged in the business of providing adult educational, recreational, and social programs to individuals in the Cincinnati area. It advertises those programs in a free magazine that it publishes nine times a year. Although these magazines consist primarily of promotional material pertaining to Discovery's courses, they also include some information about current events of general interest. Approximately one third of these magazines are distributed through the 38 newsracks that the city authorized Discovery to place on public property in 1989.

Respondent, Harmon Publishing Company, Inc., publishes and distributes a free magazine that advertises real estate for sale at various locations throughout the United States. In 1989 Harmon received the city's permission to install 24 newsracks at approved locations. About 15% of its distribution in the Cincinnati area is through those devices.

In March 1990, the city's Director of Public Works notified each of the respondents that its permit to use dispensing devices on public property was revoked, and ordered the newsracks removed within 30 days. Each notice explained that respondent's publication was a "commercial handbill" within the meaning of § 714-1-C of the Municipal Code[10] and therefore § 714-23 of the Code[11] prohibited its distribution on public property. ***

After an evidentiary hearing the District Court concluded that "the regulatory scheme advanced by the City of Cincinnati completely prohibiting the distribution of commercial handbills on the public right of way violates the First Amendment." The city had the burden of establishing "a reasonable 'fit' between the legislature's ends and the means chosen to accomplish those ends." *** It explained that the "fit" in this case was unreasonable because the number of news racks dispensing commercial handbills was "minute" compared with the total number (1,500-2,000) on the public right of way, and because they affected public safety in only a minimal

---

10. That section provides: "'Commercial Handbill' shall mean any printed or written matter, dodger, circular, leaflet, pamphlet, paper, booklet or any other printed or otherwise reproduced original or copies of any matter of literature:

"(a) Which advertises for sale any merchandise, product, commodity or thing; or

"(b) Which directs attention to any business or mercantile or commercial establishment, or other activity, for the purpose of directly promoting the interest thereof by sales; or

"(c) Which directs attention to or advertises any meeting, theatrical performance, exhibition or event of any kind for which an admission fee is charged for the purpose of private gain or profit." ***

11. That section provides: "No person shall throw or deposit any commercial or non-commercial handbill in or upon any sidewalk, street or other public place within the city. Nor shall any person hand out or distribute or sell any commercial handbill in any public place. Provided, however, that it shall not be unlawful on any sidewalk, street or other public place within the city for any person to hand out or distribute, without charge to the receiver thereof, any non-commercial handbill to any person willing to accept it, except within or around the city hall building."

way. Moreover, the practices in other communities indicated that the City's safety and esthetic interests could be adequately protected "by regulating the size, shape, number or placement of such devices."

On appeal, the city argued that since a number of courts had held that a complete ban on the use of newsracks dispensing traditional newspapers would be unconstitutional,[7] and that the "Constitution accords a lesser protection to commercial speech than to other constitutionally guaranteed expression," Central Hudson Gas & Electric Corp. v. Public Service Comm'n of New York, 447 U.S. 557, 563 (1980), its preferential treatment of newspapers over commercial publications was a permissible method of serving its legitimate interest in ensuring safe streets and regulating visual blight. The Court of Appeals disagreed, holding that the lesser status of commercial speech is relevant only when its regulation was designed either to prevent false or misleading advertising, or to alleviate distinctive adverse effects of the specific speech at issue. *** The importance of the Court of Appeals decision, together with the dramatic growth in the use of newsracks throughout the country,[10] prompted our grant of certiorari. ***

II

There is no claim in this case that there is anything unlawful or misleading about the contents of respondents' publications. Moreover, respondents do not challenge their characterization as "commercial speech." Nor do respondents question the substantiality of the city's interest in safety and esthetics. It was, therefore, proper for the District Court and the Court of Appeals to judge the validity of the city's prohibition under the standard we set forth in *Central Hudson* and State Univ. of New York v. Fox, 492 U.S. 469 (1989). It was the city's burden to establish a "reasonable fit" between its legitimate interests in safety and esthetics and its choice of a limited and selective prohibition of newsracks as the means chosen to serve those interests.[12]

---

7. See Sentinel Communications Co. v. Watts, 936 F. 2d 1189, 1196-1197 (CA11 1991), and cases cited therein.

10. We are advised that almost half of the single copy sales of newspapers are now distributed through newsracks. See Brief for the American Newspaper Publishers Association et al. as Amici Curiae 2.

12. As we stated in *Fox*:

> "[W]hile we have insisted that the free flow of commercial information is valuable enough to justify imposing on would-be regulators the costs of distinguishing *** the harmless from the harmful, we have not gone so far as to impose upon them the burden of demonstrating that the distinction is 100% complete, or that the manner of restriction is absolutely the least severe that will achieve the desired end. What our decisions require is a 'fit' between the legislature's ends and the means chosen to accomplish those ends—a fit that is not necessarily perfect, but reasonable; that represents not necessarily the single best disposition but one whose scope is in proportion to the interest served; that employs not necessarily the least restrictive means but, as we have put it in the other contexts discussed above, a means narrowly tailored to achieve the desired objective. Within those bounds we leave it to governmental decision-makers to judge what manner of regulation may best be employed. ***

There is ample support in the record for the conclusion that the city did not "establish the reasonable fit we require." *Fox*, 492 U.S., at 480. The ordinance on which it relied was an outdated prohibition against the distribution of any commercial handbills on public property. The fact that the city failed to address its recently developed concern about newsracks by regulating their size, shape, appearance, or number indicates that it has not "carefully calculated" the costs and benefits associated with the burden on speech imposed by its prohibition.[13] The benefit to be derived from the removal of 62 newsracks while about 1,500-2,000 remain in place was considered "minute" by the District Court and "paltry" by the Court of Appeals. We share their evaluation of the "fit" between the city's goal and its method of achieving it. ***

III

[F]or the purpose of deciding this case, we assume that all of the speech barred from Cincinnati's sidewalks is what we have labeled "core" commercial speech and that no such speech is found in publications that are allowed to use newsracks. We nonetheless agree with the Court of Appeals that Cincinnati's actions in this case run afoul of the First Amendment. Not only does Cincinnati's categorical ban on commercial newsracks place too much importance on the distinction between commercial and noncommercial speech, but in this case, the distinction bears no relationship *whatsoever* to the particular interests that the city has asserted. It is therefore an impermissible means of responding to the city's admittedly legitimate interests. ***

The city has asserted an interest in esthetics, but respondent publishers' newsracks are no greater an eyesore than the newsracks permitted to remain on Cincinnati's sidewalks. Each newsrack, whether containing "newspapers" or "commercial handbills," is equally unattractive. *** As we have explained, the city's primary concern, as argued to us, is with the aggregate number of newsracks on its streets. On that score, however, all newsracks, regardless of whether they contain commercial or noncommercial publications, are equally at fault. In fact, the newspapers are arguably the greater culprit because of their superior number.

"Here we require the government goal to be substantial, and the cost to be carefully calculated. Moreover, since the State bears the burden of justifying its restrictions, it must affirmatively establish the reasonable fit we require."

13. We reject the city's argument that the lower courts' and our consideration of alternative, less drastic measures by which the city could effectuate its interests in safety and esthetics somehow violates *Fox*'s holding that regulations on commercial speech are not subject to "least-restrictive-means" analysis. To repeat, see n. 12, *supra*, while we have rejected the "least-restrictive-means" test for judging restrictions on commercial speech, so too have we rejected mere rational basis review. A regulation need not be "absolutely the least severe that will achieve the desired end," *Fox*, 492 U.S. at 480, but if there are numerous and obvious less-burdensome alternatives to the restriction on commercial speech, that is certainly a relevant consideration in determining whether the "fit" between ends and means is reasonable.

Cincinnati has not asserted an interest in preventing commercial harms by regulating the information distributed by respondent publishers' newsracks, which is, of course, the typical reason why commercial speech can be subject to greater governmental regulation than noncommercial speech. ***

A closer examination of one of the cases we have mentioned, *Bolger v. Youngs Drug Products*, demonstrates the fallacy of the city's argument that a reasonable fit is established by the mere fact that the entire burden imposed on commercial speech by its newsrack policy may in some small way limit the total number of newsracks on Cincinnati's sidewalks. Here, the city contends that safety concerns and visual blight may be addressed by a prohibition that distinguishes between commercial and noncommercial publications that are equally responsible for those problems. In *Bolger*, however, in rejecting the Government's reliance on its interest in protecting the public from "offensive" speech, "[we] specifically declined to recognize a distinction between commercial and noncommercial speech that would render this interest a sufficient justification for a prohibition of commercial speech." Moreover, the fact that the regulation "provide[d] only the most limited incremental support for the interest asserted,"—that it achieved only a "marginal degree of protection," for that interest—supported our holding that the prohibition was invalid. Finally, in *Bolger*, as in this case, the burden on commercial speech was imposed by denying the speaker access to one method of distribution—there the United States mails, and here the placement of newsracks on public property—without interfering with alternative means of access to the audience. As then JUSTICE REHNQUIST explained in his separate opinion, that fact did not minimize the significance of the burden:

> "[T]he Postal Service argues that Youngs can communicate with the public otherwise than through the mail. [This argument falls] wide of the mark. A prohibition on the use of the mails is a significant restriction of First Amendment rights. We have noted that '"[t]he United States may give up the Post Office when it sees fit, but while it carries it on the use of the mails is as much a part of free speech as the right to use our tongues."' Blount v. Rizzi, 400 U.S., at 416, quoting Milwaukee Social Democratic Publishing Co. v. Burleson, 255 U.S. 407, 437 (1921) (Holmes, J., dissenting)." ***

In a similar vein, even if we assume, *arguendo*, that the city might entirely prohibit the use of newsracks on public property, as long as this avenue of communication remains open, these devices continue to play a significant role in the dissemination of protected speech.

In the absence of some basis for distinguishing between "newspapers" and "commercial handbills" that is relevant to an interest asserted by the city, we are unwilling to recognize Cincinnati's bare assertion that the "low value" of commercial speech is a sufficient justification for its selective and categorical ban on newsracks dispensing "commercial handbills." Our holding, however, is narrow. As should be clear from the above discussion, we do not reach the question whether, given certain facts and under certain circumstances, a community might be able to justify differential treatment of commercial and noncommercial newsracks. We simply hold that on this record Cincinnati has failed to make such a showing. ***

IV

By the same reasoning, the city's heavy reliance on Renton v. Playtime Theatres, Inc., 475 U.S. 41 (1986), is misplaced. In *Renton*, a city ordinance imposed particular zoning regulations on movie theaters showing adult films. The Court recognized that the ordinance did not fall neatly into the "content-based" or "content-neutral" category in that "the ordinance treats theaters that specialize in adult films differently from other kinds of theaters." *** We upheld the regulation, however, largely because it was justified not by an interest in suppressing adult films, but by the city's concern for the "secondary effects" of such theaters on the surrounding neighborhoods. *** In contrast to the speech at issue in *Renton*, there are no secondary effects attributable to respondent publishers' newsracks that distinguish them from the newsracks Cincinnati permits to remain on its sidewalks.

In sum, the city's newsrack policy is neither content-neutral nor, as demonstrated in Part III, *supra*, "narrowly tailored." Thus, regardless of whether or not it leaves open ample alternative channels of communication, it cannot be justified as a legitimate time, place, or manner restriction on protected speech. ***

The judgment of the Court of Appeals is [a]ffirmed.

JUSTICE BLACKMUN, concurring. [Omitted.]

CHIEF JUSTICE REHNQUIST, with whom JUSTICE WHITE and JUSTICE THOMAS join, dissenting.

*** Because the city chose to address its newsrack problem by banning only those newsracks that disseminate commercial handbills, rather than regulating all newsracks (including those that disseminate traditional newspapers) alike, the Court holds that its actions violate the First Amendment to the Constitution. I believe this result is inconsistent with prior precedent.

"Our jurisprudence has emphasized that" commercial speech [enjoys] a limited measure of protection, commensurate with its subordinate position in the scale of First Amendment values, "and is subject to modes of regulation that might be impermissible in the realm of noncommercial expression." We have advanced several reasons for this treatment, among which is that commercial speech is more durable than other types of speech, since it is "the offspring of economic self-interest." Commercial speech is also "less central to the interests of the First Amendment" than other types of speech, such as political expression. Finally, there is an inherent danger that conferring equal status upon commercial speech will erode the First Amendment protection accorded noncommercial speech, "simply by a leveling process of the force of the Amendment's guarantee with respect to the latter kind of speech." ***

I agree with the Court that the city's prohibition against respondents' newsracks is properly analyzed under *Central Hudson*, but differ as to the result this analysis should produce.

Although the Court does not say so, there can be no question that Cincinnati's prohibition against respondents' newsracks "directly advances" its safety and esthetic interests because, if enforced, the city's policy will decrease the number of newsracks on its street corners. *** This conclusion is not altered by the fact that the city has chosen to address its problem by banning only those newsracks that disseminate commercial speech, rather than regulating all newsracks alike. ***

If (as I am certain) Cincinnati may regulate newsracks that disseminate commercial speech based on the interests it has asserted, I am at a loss as to why its scheme is unconstitutional because it does not also regulate newsracks that disseminate noncommercial speech. One would have thought that the city, perhaps even following the teachings of our commercial speech jurisprudence, could have decided to place the burden of its regulatory scheme on less protected speech (*i.e.*, commercial handbills) without running afoul of the First Amendment. Today's decision, though, places the city in the position of having to decide between restricting more speech—fully protected speech—and allowing the proliferation of newsracks on its street corners to continue unabated. It scarcely seems logical that the First Amendment compels such a result. In my view, the city may order the removal of *all* newsracks from its public right-of-ways if it so chooses. But however it decides to address its newsrack problem, it should be allowed to proceed in the manner and scope it sees fit so long as it does not violate established First Amendment principles, such as the rule against discrimination on the basis of content. ***

*** I dissent.

Questions And Notes

1. If commercial newsracks[10] had composed a greater proportion of all the newsracks in Cincinnati (so the degree of gain in the avoidance of growing newsrack congestion would have been far greater than in the actual case), would the ordinance *then* have satisfied the "reasonable fit" requirement in the Court's test evidently requires?

2. Or must *any* distinction in the city's regulation of commercial newsracks (as compared with its regulation of ordinary newsracks) rest on some distinction fairly related to a kind of hazard more characteristic of the latter?[11] If the extent to which

---

10. "Commercial newsracks" meaning newsracks containing only advertiser newspapers (for example, "*The Cincinnati Real Estate Advertiser*").

11. See, e.g., the Court's discussion, in *Cincinnati Discovery*, of the zoning regulation in *Renton v. Playtime Theatres, Inc.*, 475 U.S. 41 (1986) (sustaining a content-specific zoning regulation that more severely restricted locations of adult movie theaters than other businesses, where the alleged concern

one kind of newsrack contributes to the problem of clutter is no greater than the extent to which another kind contributes to that same problem, the city may not treat them differently? The city may not forbid (or limit the number of) commercial newsracks, while not forbidding (or equally limiting the number of) noncommercial newsracks? But why should this be so?[12]

3. Suppose the problem of newsrack congestion has become a substantial problem partly *because of* the proliferation of *commercial* newsracks. May the city, in these circumstances, elect to prefer noncommercial over purely commercial newsracks—to disallow the one without otherwise restricting the other?

4. Also in 1993, the Court decided *United States v. Edge Broadcasting Co.*[13] Federal law generally prohibits the broadcast of lottery advertisements. An exception is allowed for states with state-run lotteries: a broadcast station licensed to a location in such a state may advertise the state-run lottery in question. North Carolina is a "non-lottery state"; Virginia is a "lottery state." Edge Broadcasting, a North Carolina station near the border with Virginia, had a listening audience composed mostly (90%) of Virginia residents. At the same time, Edge Broadcasting reached listeners in nine North Carolina Counties. Evidence suggested that these North Carolina listeners were inundated with Virginia lottery advertisements from other media sources (for example, newspapers). (Moreover, Virginia stations advertising the Virginia lottery could reach well within North Carolina.) Thus, preventing Edge Broadcasting from broadcasting lottery ads would not, in fact, shield those North Carolina citizens from lottery ads. It would, however, somewhat reduce the amount of such advertising reaching them. Edge Broadcasting challenged the federal statute which prohibited it from running ads for the Virginia lottery. The Court sustained the federal law (7 to 2).

Is the "fit" any better in *Edge* than in *Cincinnati Discovery*? If not, how is this case distinguishable from *Cincinnati Discovery*? Is it that gambling is not only not protected (cf. *Bigelow*), but something of a "vice" (cf. *Posadas*)?[14] Might the Court have been moved by federalism concerns? (It characterized the substantial state interest—the second prong of *Central Hudson*—as a "congressional policy of balancing the interests of lottery and non-lottery states.")

---

of the ordinance was not the content of the films but rather the adverse "secondary effects" of adult theaters, and where other feasible sites for such theaters were not foreclosed).

12. Is it not assumed about commercial speech that it is "hardy," that it will tend to find alternative routes for advertising ordinary commercial goods and services, unlike a great deal of noncommercial speech?

13. U.S. & F.E.C. v. Edge Broadcasting, 509 U.S. 418

14. Suppose the state has a substantial interest in discouraging cigarette smoking. What of a state statute banning the placement of cigarette advertising in sports stadiums and sports facilities? (Assume that sports spectators would still encounter cigarette advertisements in magazines and newspapers.)

44 LIQUORMART, INC. V. RHODE ISLAND
517 U.S. 484 (1996)

[JUSTICE STEVENS announced the judgment of the Court and delivered the opinion of the Court with respect to Parts I, II, VII, and VIII.]

I

In 1956, the Rhode Island Legislature enacted two separate prohibitions against advertising the retail price of alcoholic beverages. The first applies to vendors licensed in Rhode Island as well as to out-of-state manufacturers, wholesalers, and shippers. It prohibits them from "advertising in any manner whatsoever" the price of any alcoholic beverage offered for sale in the State; the only exception is for price tags or signs displayed with the merchandise within licensed premises and not visible from the street. The second statute applies to the Rhode Island news media. It contains a categorical prohibition against the publication or broadcast of any advertisements—even those referring to sales in other States—that "make reference to the price of any alcoholic beverages." ***

II

Petitioners 44 Liquormart, Inc. (44 Liquormart), and Peoples Super Liquor Stores, Inc. (Peoples), are licensed retailers of alcoholic beverages. Petitioner 44 Liquormart operates a store in Rhode Island and petitioner Peoples operates several stores in Massachusetts that are patronized by Rhode Island residents. Peoples uses alcohol price advertising extensively in Massachusetts, where such advertising is permitted, but Rhode Island newspapers and other media outlets have refused to accept such ads.

44 Liquormart, joined by Peoples, filed this action against the administrator in the Federal District Court seeking a declaratory judgment that the two statutes and the administrator's implementing regulations violate the First Amendment. The Rhode Island Liquor Stores Association was allowed to intervene as a defendant and in due course the State of Rhode Island replaced the administrator as the principal defendant. The parties stipulated that the price advertising ban is vigorously enforced, that Rhode Island permits "all advertising of alcoholic beverages excepting references to price outside the licensed premises," and that petitioners' proposed ads do not concern an illegal activity and presumably would not be false or misleading. The parties disagreed, however, about the impact of the ban on the promotion of temperance in Rhode Island.

In his findings of fact, the District Judge first noted that there was a pronounced lack of unanimity among researchers who have studied the impact of advertising on the level of consumption of alcoholic beverages. He referred to a 1985 Federal Trade Commission study that found no evidence that alcohol advertising significantly affects alcohol abuse. *** After summarizing the testimony of the expert witnesses for both parties, he found "as a fact that Rhode Island's off-premises liquor price advertising ban has no significant impact on levels of alcohol consumption in Rhode

Island." *** Acknowledging that it might have been reasonable for the state legislature to "assume a correlation between the price advertising ban and reduced consumption," he held that more than a rational basis was required to justify the speech restriction, and that the State had failed to demonstrate a reasonable "fit" between its policy objectives and its chosen means.

The Court of Appeals reversed. It found "inherent merit" in the State's submission that competitive price advertising would lower prices and that lower prices would produce more sales. Moreover, it agreed with the reasoning of the Rhode Island Supreme Court that the Twenty-first Amendment gave the statutes an added presumption of validity. *** We granted certiorari [and now reverse the Court of Appeals].

III*

Virginia Pharmacy Bd. reflected the conclusion that the *** interest that supports regulation of potentially misleading advertising, namely the public's interest in receiving accurate commercial information, also supports an interpretation of the First Amendment that provides constitutional protection for the dissemination of accurate and nonmisleading commercial messages. *** [O]ur early cases uniformly struck down several broadly based bans on truthful, nonmisleading commercial speech, each of which served ends unrelated to consumer protection.***

In *Central Hudson*, we took stock of our developing commercial speech jurisprudence. [W]e considered a regulation "completely" banning all promotional advertising by electric utilities. Our decision acknowledged the special features of commercial speech but identified the serious First Amendment concerns that attend blanket advertising prohibitions that do not protect consumers from commercial harms.

Five Members of the Court recognized that the state interest in the conservation of energy was substantial, and that there was "an immediate connection between advertising and demand for electricity." Nevertheless, they concluded that the regulation was invalid because the Commission had failed to make a showing that a more limited speech regulation would not have adequately served the State's interest.[9]

In reaching its conclusion, the majority explained that although the special nature of commercial speech may require less than strict review of its regulation, special concerns arise from "regulations that entirely suppress commercial speech in order to pursue a nonspeech-related policy." As a result, the Court concluded that "special care" should attend the review of such blanket bans, and it pointedly remarked that "in recent years this Court has not approved a blanket ban on

---

*. **[Ed. Note.** Stevens, Kennedy, Souter, Ginsburg, JJ.]

9. In other words, the regulation failed the fourth step in the four-part inquiry that the majority announced in its opinion. ***

commercial speech unless the speech itself was flawed in some way, either because it was deceptive or related to unlawful activity."[10]

IV*

As our review of the case law reveals, Rhode Island errs in concluding that all commercial speech regulations are subject to a similar form of constitutional review simply because they target a similar category of expression.

*** When a State regulates commercial messages to protect consumers from misleading, deceptive, or aggressive sales practices, or requires the disclosure of beneficial consumer information, the purpose of its regulation is consistent with the reasons for according constitutional protection to commercial speech and therefore justifies less than strict review. However, when a State entirely prohibits the dissemination of truthful, nonmisleading commercial messages for reasons unrelated to the preservation of a fair bargaining process, there is far less reason to depart from the rigorous review that the First Amendment generally demands. ***

It is the State's interest in protecting consumers from "commercial harms" that provides "the typical reason why commercial speech can be subject to greater governmental regulation than noncommercial speech." Cincinnati v. Discovery Network, Inc., 507 U.S. 410, 426 (1993). Yet bans that target truthful, nonmisleading commercial messages rarely protect consumers from such harms. Instead, such bans often serve only to obscure an "underlying governmental policy" that could be implemented without regulating speech. In this way, these commercial speech bans not only hinder consumer choice, but also impede debate over central issues of public policy.

Precisely because bans against truthful, nonmisleading commercial speech rarely seek to protect consumers from either deception or overreaching, they usually rest solely on the offensive assumption that the public will respond "irrationally" to the truth. The First Amendment directs us to be especially skeptical of regulations that seek to keep people in the dark for what the government perceives to be their own good. ***

V*

The State argues that the price advertising prohibition should nevertheless be upheld because it directly advances the State's substantial interest in promoting temperance, and because it is no more extensive than necessary. Although there is some

10. The Justices concurring in the judgment adopted a somewhat broader view. They expressed "doubt whether suppression of information concerning the availability and price of a legally offered product is ever a permissible way for the State to 'dampen' the demand for or use of the product." Indeed, Justice Blackmun believed that even "though 'commercial' speech is involved, such a regulation strikes at the heart of the First Amendment."

*. **[Ed. Note.** Stevens, Kennedy, Ginsburg, JJ.]

*. **[Ed. Note.** Stevens, Kennedy, Souter, Ginsburg, JJ.]

confusion as to what Rhode Island means by temperance, we assume that the State asserts an interest in reducing alcohol consumption.

We can agree that common sense supports the conclusion that a prohibition against price advertising, like a collusive agreement among competitors to refrain from such advertising, will tend to mitigate competition and maintain prices at a higher level than would prevail in a completely free market. Despite the absence of proof on the point, we can even agree with the State's contention that it is reasonable to assume that demand, and hence consumption throughout the market, is somewhat lower whenever a higher, noncompetitive price level prevails. However, without any findings of fact, or indeed any evidentiary support whatsoever, we cannot agree with the assertion that the price advertising ban will significantly advance the State's interest in promoting temperance.

Although the record suggests that the price advertising ban may have some impact on the purchasing patterns of temperate drinkers of modest means, the State has presented no evidence to suggest that its speech prohibition will significantly reduce market-wide consumption.[16] Indeed, the District Court's considered and uncontradicted finding on this point is directly to the contrary. Moreover, the evidence suggests that the abusive drinker will probably not be deterred by a marginal price increase, and that the true alcoholic may simply reduce his purchases of other necessities.[17] ***

The State also cannot satisfy the requirement that its restriction on speech be no more extensive than necessary. It is perfectly obvious that alternative forms of regulation that would not involve any restriction on speech would be more likely to achieve the State's goal of promoting temperance. As the State's own expert conceded, higher prices can be maintained either by direct regulation or by increased taxation. Per capita purchases could be limited as is the case with prescription drugs. Even educational campaigns focused on the problems of excessive, or even moderate, drinking might prove to be more effective.

As a result, even under the less than strict standard that generally applies in commercial speech cases, the State has failed to establish a "reasonable fit" between its abridgment of speech and its temperance goal. It necessarily follows that the price advertising ban cannot survive the more stringent constitutional review that *Central Hudson* itself concluded was appropriate for the complete suppression of truthful, nonmisleading commercial speech.

---

16. The appellants' stipulation that they each expect to realize a $100,000 benefit per year if the ban is lifted is not to the contrary. The stipulation shows only that the appellants believe they will be able to compete more effectively for existing alcohol consumers if there is no ban on price advertising. It does not show that they believe either the number of alcohol consumers, or the number of purchases by those consumers, will increase in the ban's absence. ***

17. Although the Court of Appeals concluded that the regulation directly advanced the State's interest, it did not dispute the District Court's conclusion that the evidence suggested that, at most, a price advertising ban would have a marginal impact on overall alcohol consumption.

VI*

The State responds by arguing that it merely exercised appropriate "legislative judgment" in determining that a price advertising ban would best promote temperance. Relying on the *Central Hudson* analysis set forth in Posadas de Puerto Rico Associates v. Tourism Co. of P. R., 478 U.S. 328 (1986),*** Rhode Island argues that, because expert opinions as to the effectiveness of the price advertising ban "go both ways," the Court of Appeals correctly concluded that the ban constituted a "reasonable choice" by the legislature. The State next contends that precedent requires us to give particular deference to that legislative choice because the State could, if it chose, ban the sale of alcoholic beverages outright. ***

The reasoning in *Posadas* does support the State's argument, but, on reflection, we are now persuaded that *Posadas* erroneously performed the First Amendment analysis. The casino advertising ban was designed to keep truthful, nonmisleading speech from members of the public for fear that they would be more likely to gamble if they received it. As a result, the advertising ban served to shield the State's anti-gambling policy from the public scrutiny that more direct, nonspeech regulation would draw. ***

Because the 5-to-4 decision in *Posadas* marked such a sharp break from our prior precedent, and because it concerned a constitutional question about which this Court is the final arbiter, we decline to give force to its highly deferential approach.

Instead, in keeping with our prior holdings, we conclude that a state legislature does not have the broad discretion to suppress truthful, nonmisleading information for paternalistic purposes that the *Posadas* majority was willing to tolerate. ***

We also cannot accept the State's second contention, which is premised entirely on the "greater-includes-the-lesser" reasoning endorsed toward the end of the majority's opinion in *Posadas*. ***

Although we do not dispute the proposition that greater powers include lesser ones, we fail to see how that syllogism requires the conclusion that the State's power to regulate commercial activity is "greater" than its power to ban truthful, nonmisleading commercial speech. Contrary to the assumption made in *Posadas*, we think it quite clear that banning speech may sometimes prove far more intrusive than banning conduct. *** In short, we reject the assumption that words are necessarily less vital to freedom than actions, or that logic somehow proves that the power to prohibit an activity is necessarily "greater" than the power to suppress speech about it.

As a matter of First Amendment doctrine, the *Posadas* syllogism is even less defensible. The text of the First Amendment makes clear that the Constitution presumes that attempts to regulate speech are more dangerous than attempts to regulate conduct. That presumption accords with the essential role that the free flow of information plays in a democratic society. As a result, the First Amendment directs that government may not suppress speech as easily as it may suppress conduct, and that

---

*. **[Ed. Note.** Stevens, Kennedy, Thomas, Ginsburg, JJ.]

speech restrictions cannot be treated as simply another means that the government may use to achieve its ends.

These basic First Amendment principles clearly apply to commercial speech; indeed, the *Posadas* majority impliedly conceded as much by applying the *Central Hudson* test. Thus, it is no answer that commercial speech concerns products and services that the government may freely regulate. Our decisions from *Virginia Pharmacy Bd.* on have made plain that a State's regulation of the sale of goods differs in kind from a State's regulation of accurate information about those goods. The distinction that our cases have consistently drawn between these two types of governmental action is fundamentally incompatible with the absolutist view that the State may ban commercial speech simply because it may constitutionally prohibit the underlying conduct.[20] *** As the entire Court apparently now agrees, the statements in the *Posadas* opinion on which Rhode Island relies are no longer persuasive.

Finally, we find unpersuasive the State's contention that, under *Posadas* and *Edge*, the price advertising ban should be upheld because it targets commercial speech that pertains to a "vice" activity. *** [T]he scope of any "vice" exception to the protection afforded by the First Amendment would be difficult, if not impossible, to define. Almost any product that poses some threat to public health or public morals might reasonably be characterized by a state legislature as relating to "vice activity." *** [A] "vice" label that is unaccompanied by a corresponding prohibition against the commercial behavior at issue fails to provide a principled justification for the regulation of commercial speech about that activity.

VII

[A]lthough the Twenty-first Amendment limits the effect of the dormant Commerce Clause on a State's regulatory power over the delivery or use of intoxicating beverages within its borders, "the Amendment does not license the States to ignore their obligations under other provisions of the Constitution." That general conclusion reflects our specific holdings that the Twenty-first Amendment does not in any way diminish the force of the Supremacy Clause, the Establishment Clause, or the Equal Protection Clause. We see no reason why the First Amendment should not also be included in that list. *** The Twenty-first Amendment, therefore, cannot save Rhode Island's ban on liquor price advertising.

---

20. It is also no answer to say that it would be "strange" if the First Amendment tolerated a seemingly "greater" regulatory measure while forbidding a "lesser" one. We recently held that although the government had the power to proscribe an entire category of speech, such as obscenity or so-called fighting words, it could not limit the scope of its ban to obscene or fighting words that expressed a point of view with which the government disagrees. R.A.V. v. St. Paul, 505 U.S. 377 (1992). Similarly, in Cincinnati v. Discovery Network, Inc., 507 U.S. 410 (1993), we assumed that States could prevent all newsracks from being placed on public sidewalks, but nevertheless concluded that they could not ban only those newsracks that contained certain commercial publications.

VIII

Because Rhode Island has failed to carry its heavy burden of justifying its complete ban on price advertising, we conclude that R.I. Gen. Laws §§ 3-8-7 and 3-8-8.1, as well as Regulation 32 of the Rhode Island Liquor Control Administration, abridge speech in violation of the First Amendment as made applicable to the States by the Due Process Clause of the Fourteenth Amendment. The judgment of the Court of Appeals is therefore reversed. ***

JUSTICE SCALIA, concurring in part and concurring in the judgment.

I share JUSTICE THOMAS's discomfort with the *Central Hudson* test, which seems to me to have nothing more than policy intuition to support it. I also share JUSTICE STEVENS' aversion towards paternalistic governmental policies that prevent men and women from hearing facts that might not be good for them. ***

Since I do not believe we have before us the wherewithal to declare *Central Hudson* wrong—or at least the wherewithal to say what ought to replace it—I must resolve this case in accord with our existing jurisprudence, which all except JUSTICE THOMAS agree would prohibit the challenged regulation. I am not disposed to develop new law, or reinforce old, on this issue, and accordingly I merely concur in the judgment of the Court. ***

JUSTICE THOMAS, concurring in Parts I, II, VI, and VII, and concurring in the judgment.

In cases such as this, in which the government's asserted interest is to keep legal users of a product or service ignorant in order to manipulate their choices in the marketplace, the balancing test adopted in *Central Hudson* should not be applied, in my view. ***

I do not join the principal opinion's application of the *Central Hudson* balancing test because I do not believe that such a test should be applied to a restriction of "commercial" speech, at least when, as here, the asserted interest is one that is to be achieved through keeping would-be recipients of the speech in the dark.[5] Application of the advancement-of-state-interest prong of *Central Hudson* makes little sense to me in such circumstances. Faulting the State for failing to show that its price advertising ban decreases alcohol consumption "significantly," as JUSTICE STEVENS does, seems to imply that if the State had been more successful at keeping consumers ignorant and thereby decreasing their consumption, then the restriction might have been upheld. This contradicts *Virginia Pharmacy Bd.*'s rationale for protecting "commercial" speech in the first instance.

---

5. In other words, I do not believe that a *Central Hudson*-type balancing test should apply when the asserted purpose is like the one put forth by the government in *Central Hudson* itself. Whether some type of balancing test is warranted when the asserted state interest is of a different kind is a question that I do not consider here.

Both JUSTICE STEVENS and JUSTICE O'CONNOR appear to adopt a stricter, more categorical interpretation of the fourth prong of *Central Hudson* than that suggested in some of our other opinions, one that could, as a practical matter, go a long way toward the position I take. *** In their application of the fourth prong, both JUSTICE STEVENS and JUSTICE O'CONNOR hold that because the State can ban the sale of lower priced alcohol altogether by instituting minimum prices or levying taxes, it cannot ban advertising regarding lower priced liquor. Although the tenor of JUSTICE O'CONNOR's opinion (and, to a lesser extent, that of JUSTICE STEVENS's opinion) might suggest that this is just another routine case-by-case application of *Central Hudson*'s fourth prong, the Court's holding will in fact be quite sweeping if applied consistently in future cases. The opinions would appear to commit the courts to striking down restrictions on speech whenever a direct regulation (i.e., a regulation involving no restriction on speech regarding lawful activity at all) would be an equally effective method of dampening demand by legal users. But it would seem that directly banning a product (or rationing it, taxing it, controlling its price, or otherwise restricting its sale in specific ways) would virtually always be at least as effective in discouraging consumption as merely restricting advertising regarding the product would be, and thus virtually all restrictions with such a purpose would fail the fourth prong of the *Central Hudson* test. This would be so even if the direct regulation is, in one sense, more restrictive of conduct generally. ***

The upshot of the application of the fourth prong in the opinions of JUSTICE STEVENS and of JUSTICE O'CONNOR seems to be that the government may not, for the purpose of keeping would-be consumers ignorant and thus decreasing demand, restrict advertising regarding commercial transactions—or at least that it may not restrict advertising regarding commercial transactions except to the extent that it outlaws or otherwise directly restricts the same transactions within its own borders.[7] I welcome this outcome; but, rather than "applying" the fourth prong of *Central Hudson* to reach the inevitable result that all or most such advertising restrictions must

---

7. The two most obvious situations in which no equally effective direct regulation will be available for discouraging consumption (and thus, the two situations in which the Court and I might differ on the outcome) are: (1) When a law directly regulating conduct would violate the Constitution (e.g., because the item is constitutionally protected), or (2) when the sale is to occur outside the State's borders. As to the first situation: Although the Court's application of the fourth prong today does not specifically foreclose regulations or bans of advertising regarding items that cannot constitutionally be banned, it would seem strange to hold that the government's power to interfere with transmission of information regarding these items, in order to dampen demand for them, is more extensive than its power to restrict, for the same purpose, advertising of items that are not constitutionally protected. As to the second situation: When a State seeks to dampen consumption by its citizens of products or services outside its borders, it does not have the option of direct regulation. *** Perhaps JUSTICE STEVENS and JUSTICE O'CONNOR would distinguish a situation in which a State had actually banned sales of lower priced alcohol within the State and had then, through a ban of advertising by out-of-state sellers, sought to keep residents ignorant of the fact that lower priced alcohol was legally available in other States. The outcome in *Edge* may well be in conflict with the principles espoused in *Virginia Pharmacy Bd.* and ratified by me today.

be struck down, I would adhere to the doctrine adopted in *Virginia Pharmacy Bd.* and in Justice Blackmun's *Central Hudson* concurrence, that all attempts to dissuade legal choices by citizens by keeping them ignorant are impermissible. ***

JUSTICE O'CONNOR, with whom THE CHIEF JUSTICE, JUSTICE SOUTER, and JUSTICE BREYER join, concurring in the judgment. ***

Both parties agree that the first two prongs of the *Central Hudson* test are met. Even if we assume arguendo that Rhode Island's regulation also satisfies the requirement that it directly advance the governmental interest, Rhode Island's regulation fails the final prong; that is, its ban is more extensive than necessary to serve the State's interest. ***

Rhode Island offers one, and only one, justification for its ban on price advertising. Rhode Island says that the ban is intended to keep alcohol prices high as a way to keep consumption low. *** The fit between Rhode Island's method and this particular goal is not reasonable. If the target is simply higher prices generally to discourage consumption, the regulation imposes too great, and unnecessary, a prohibition on speech in order to achieve it. The State has other methods at its disposal— methods that would more directly accomplish this stated goal without intruding on sellers' ability to provide truthful, nonmisleading information to customers. *** The ready availability of such alternatives—at least some of which would far more effectively achieve Rhode Island's only professed goal, at comparatively small additional administrative cost— demonstrates that the fit between ends and means is not narrowly tailored. ***

Respondents point for support to *Posadas* where, applying the *Central Hudson* test, we upheld the constitutionality of a Puerto Rico law that prohibited the advertising of casino gambling aimed at residents of Puerto Rico, but permitted such advertising aimed at tourists. *** The Court accepted without question Puerto Rico's account of the effectiveness and reasonableness of its speech restriction. Respondents ask us to make a similar presumption here to uphold the validity of Rhode Island's law.

It is true that Posadas accepted as reasonable, without further inquiry, Puerto Rico's assertions that the regulations furthered the government's interest and were no more extensive than necessary to serve that interest. Since *Posadas*, however, this Court has examined more searchingly the State's professed goal, and the speech restriction put into place to further it, before accepting a State's claim that the speech restriction satisfies First Amendment scrutiny. In *** these cases we declined to accept at face value the proffered justification for the State's regulation, but examined carefully the relationship between the asserted goal and the speech restriction used to reach that goal. The closer look that we have required since *Posadas* comports better with the purpose of the analysis set out in *Central Hudson*, by requiring the State to show that the speech restriction directly advances its interest and is narrowly tailored. Under such a closer look, Rhode Island's price-advertising ban clearly fails to pass muster.

Because Rhode Island's regulation fails even the less stringent standard set out in *Central Hudson*, nothing here requires adoption of a new analysis for the evaluation of commercial speech regulation. The principal opinion acknowledges that "even under the less than strict standard that generally applies in commercial speech cases, the State has failed to establish a reasonable fit between its abridgement of speech and its temperance goal." Because we need go no further, I would not here undertake the question whether the test we have employed since *Central Hudson* should be displaced.

NOTES

1. Does *Liquormart* stand for the proposition that a "lesser" restriction is invalid where a "greater" restriction would serve the end to be achieved with equal (or, indeed, with far greater) direct effect? Is this also Justice Thomas's summary of the majority opinion? Is it correct?

2. Note that in *Liquormart* promotional advertising was not forbidden— to the contrary, only price terms were forbidden. Neither was there any dollar restriction on how much money might be spent on promotional advertising, whether to encourage general consumer awareness of liquor's ready availability, or of particular brands, or of particular stores. Doesn't the effect of *failing* to limit or forbid promotional advertising make the mere ban on *price* terms sufficiently problematic (in terms of having a "substantial" effect to reduce intemperance) to raise a fair question whether "temperance" as such was, after all, really the main object of this law? Or does nothing turn on this?

3. Suppose, to follow up on the implications of the preceding question, the state defended the ban on price advertising not on the basis of encouraging "temperance."[17] Suppose, rather, Rhode Island defended the ban on liquor price advertising as part of a legislative policy "to favor small retailers as such."[18] — And suppose the evidence were compelling that it had just that effect (albeit, to be sure, as any such legislative preference may tend to do, at consumer expense). *Now* will the ban be sustained? Why or why not? (Is the "governmental interest" in the maintenance of small retailers permissible? May it also be "substantial?" (Who says it cannot be said

---

17. How direct was the ban in relation to encouraging "temperance" as the desired end? Very direct? Or only highly indirect, and even then additionally attenuated (note the ban on price advertising does not in so many words, or otherwise, affirmatively encourage "temperance" in any way; note, too, that the least temperate are among the least likely to be affected (i.e. least "in the dark" about price)).

18. May it not in fact have a far closer fit with this objective (the product of successful lobbying by a trade association of small retail liquor stores) than with the objective of "temperance"?

to be a "substantial" interest of the state?) Is it "directly" advanced? Does the price advertising ban have a "reasonable fit" to *that* end?)

GREATER NEW ORLEANS BROADCASTING ASS'N INC. v. UNITED STATES

527 U.S. 173 (1999)

JUSTICE STEVENS delivered the opinion of the Court.

I

Through most of the 19th and the first half of the 20th centuries, Congress adhered to a policy that not only discouraged the operation of lotteries and similar schemes, but forbade the dissemination of information concerning such enterprises by use of the mails, even when the lottery in question was chartered by a state legislature. Consistent with this Court's earlier view that commercial advertising was unprotected by the First Amendment, see *Valentine v. Chrestensen*, 316 U.S. 52, 54 (1942), we found that the notion that "lotteries ... are supposed to have a demoralizing influence upon the people" provided sufficient justification for excluding circulars concerning such enterprises from the federal postal system. *Ex parte Jackson*, 96 U.S. 727, 736-737 (1878). We likewise deferred to congressional judgment in upholding the similar exclusion for newspapers that contained either lottery advertisements or prize lists.

[In 1934,] Congress extended its restrictions on lottery-related information to broadcasting. Now codified at 18 U.S.C. § 1304, the statute prohibits radio and television broadcasting, by any station for which a license is required, of "any advertisement of or information concerning any lottery, gift enterprise, or similar scheme, offering prizes dependent in whole or in part upon lot or chance, or any list of the prizes drawn or awarded by means of any such lottery, gift enterprise, or scheme." ***

During the second half of this century, Congress dramatically narrowed the scope of the broadcast prohibition in § 1304. [In 1975], advertisements of State-conducted lotteries [were exempted] from the nationwide postal restrictions and from the broadcast restriction, when "broadcast by a radio or television station licensed to a location in...a State which conducts such a lottery."***In 1988, 25 U.S.C. § 2701 et seq., authorized Native American tribes to conduct various forms of gambling — including casino gambling — [and] exempted any gaming conducted by an Indian tribe pursuant to the Act from both the postal and transportation restrictions in 18 U.S.C. §§ 1301-1302, and the broadcast restriction in § 1304. [And] 18 U.S.C. §1307(a(2)] extended the exemption from §§ 1301-1304 for state-run lotteries to include any other lottery, gift enterprise, or similar scheme — not prohibited by the law of the State in which it operates — when conducted by: (I) any governmental organization; (ii) any not-for-profit organization; or (iii) a commercial organization as a promotional activity "clearly occasional and ancillary to the primary business of that organization." *** [T]he exemptions in both of these 1988 statutes are not geographically limited; they shield messages from § 1304's reach in States that do not authorize such gambling as well as those that do.***

III

In a number of cases involving restrictions on speech that is "commercial" in nature, we have employed *Central Hudson*'s four-part test to resolve First Amendment challenges[.] ***Partly because of [its] intricacies, petitioners as well as certain judges, scholars, and amici curiae have advocated repudiation of the *Central Hudson* standard and implementation of a more straightforward and stringent test for assessing the validity of governmental restrictions on commercial speech. As the opinions in *44 Liquormart* demonstrate, reasonable judges may disagree about the merits of such proposals. It is, however, an established part of our constitutional jurisprudence that we do not ordinarily reach out to make novel or unnecessarily broad pronouncements on constitutional issues when a case can be fully resolved on a narrower ground. In this case, there is no need to break new ground. *Central Hudson,* as applied in our more recent commercial speech cases, provides an adequate basis for decision.

IV

All parties to this case agree that the messages petitioners wish to broadcast constitute commercial speech, and that these broadcasts would satisfy the first part of the *Central Hudson* test: Their content is not misleading and concerns lawful activities, i.e., private casino gambling in Louisiana and Mississippi. As well, the proposed commercial messages would convey information — whether taken favorably unfavorably by the audience — about an activity that is the subject of intense public debate in many communities. In addition, petitioners' broadcasts presumably would disseminate accurate information as to the operation of market competitors, such as pay-out ratios, which can benefit listeners by informing their consumption choices and fostering price competition. Thus, even if the broadcasters' interest in conveying these messages is entirely pecuniary, the interests of, and benefit to, the audience may be broader.

The second part of the *Central Hudson* test asks whether the asserted governmental interest served by the speech restriction is substantial. The Solicitor General identifies two such interests: (1) reducing the social costs associated with "gambling" or "casino gambling," and (2) assisting States that "restrict gambling" or "prohibit casino gambling" within their own borders. Underlying Congress' statutory scheme, the Solicitor General contends, is the judgment that gambling contributes to corruption and organized crime; underwrites bribery, narcotics trafficking, and other illegal conduct; imposes a regressive tax on the poor; and "offers a false but sometimes irresistible hope of financial advancement."

We can accept the characterization of these two interests as "substantial," but that conclusion is by no means self-evident. No one seriously doubts that the Federal Government may assert a legitimate and substantial interest in alleviating the societal ills recited above, or in assisting like-minded States to do the same. But in the judgment of both the Congress and many state legislatures, the social costs that support the suppression of gambling are offset, and sometimes outweighed, by countervailing policy considerations, primarily in the form of economic benefits.[5] Despite its awareness of the potential social costs, Congress has not only sanctioned casino gambling for Indian tribes through tribal-state compacts, but has enacted other statutes that reflect approval of state legislation that authorizes a host of public and private gambling activities.*** Whatever its character in 1934 when §1304 was adopted, the federal policy of discouraging gambling in general, and casino gambling in particular, is now decidedly equivocal.***[W]e cannot ignore Congress' unwillingness to adopt a single national policy that consistently endorses either interest asserted by the Solicitor General. Even though the Government has identified substantial interests, when we consider both their quality and the information sought to be suppressed, the crosscurrents in the scope and application of §1304 become more difficult for the Government to defend.

V

The third part of the *Central Hudson* test asks whether the speech restriction directly and materially advances the asserted governmental interest. "This burden is not satisfied by mere speculation or conjecture; rather, a governmental body seeking to sustain a restriction on commercial speech must demonstrate that the harms it recites are real and that its restriction will in fact alleviate them to a material degree." *Edenfield v. Fane*, 507 U.S. 761, 770-71 (1993). Consequently, "the regulation may not be sustained if it provides only ineffective or remote support for the government's purpose." *Central Hudson*, 447 U.S., at 564. We have observed that "this requirement is critical; otherwise, 'a State could with ease restrict commercial speech in the service of other objectives that could not themselves justify a burden on commercial expression.'" *Rubin*, 514 U.S., at 487, quoting *Edenfield*, 507 U.S., at 771.

The fourth part of the test complements the direct-advancement inquiry of the third, asking whether the speech restriction is not more extensive than necessary to serve the interests that support it. The Government is not required to employ the least restrictive means conceivable, but it must demonstrate narrow tailoring of the

5. Some form of gambling is legal in nearly every State. 37 States and the District of Columbia operate lotteries. As of 1997, commercial casino gambling existed in 11 States, and at least 5 authorize state-sponsored video gambling. About half the States in the Union host Class III Indian gaming (which may encompass casino gambling), including Louisiana, Mississippi, and four other States that had private casinos. One count by the Bureau of Indian Affairs tallied 60 tribes that advertise their casinos on television and radio. By the mid-1990's, tribal casino-style gambling generated over $3 billion in gaming revenue — increasing its share to 18% of all casino gaming revenue, matching the total for the casinos in Atlantic City, New Jersey, and reaching about half the figure for Nevada's casinos. ***

challenged regulation to the asserted interest — "a fit that is not necessarily perfect, but reasonable; that represents not necessarily the single best disposition but one whose scope is in proportion to the interest served." *Fox*, 492 U.S. at 480. [T]he challenged regulation should indicate that its proponent "'carefully calculated' the costs and benefits associated with the burden on speech imposed by its prohibition." *Discovery Network*, 507 U.S. at 417 (1993).

As applied to petitioners' case, § 1304 cannot satisfy these standards. With regard to the first asserted interest — alleviating the social costs of casino gambling by limiting demand — the Government contends that its broadcasting restrictions directly advance that interest because "promotional" broadcast advertising concerning casino gambling increases demand for such gambling, which in turn increases the amount of casino gambling that produces those social costs. Additionally, the Government believes that compulsive gamblers are especially susceptible to the pervasiveness and potency of broadcast advertising. Assuming the accuracy of this causal chain, it does not necessarily follow that the Government's speech ban has directly and materially furthered the asserted interest. While it is no doubt fair to assume that more advertising would have some impact on overall demand for gambling, it is also reasonable to assume that much of that advertising would merely channel gamblers to one casino rather than another. More important, any measure of the effectiveness of the Government's attempt to minimize the social costs of gambling cannot ignore Congress' simultaneous encouragement of tribal casino gambling, which may well be growing at a rate exceeding any increase in gambling or compulsive gambling that private casino advertising could produce.

We need not resolve the question whether any lack of evidence in the record fails to satisfy the standard of proof under *Central Hudson*, however, because the flaw in the Government's case is more fundamental: The operation of § 1304 and its attendant regulatory regime is so pierced by exemptions and inconsistencies that the Government cannot hope to exonerate it. Under current law, a broadcaster may not carry advertising about privately operated commercial casino gambling, regardless of the location of the station or the casino. On the other hand, advertisements for tribal casino gambling authorized by state compacts — whether operated by the tribe or by a private party pursuant to a management contract — are subject to no such broadcast ban, even if the broadcaster is located in or broadcasts to a jurisdiction with the strictest of antigambling policies. Government-operated, nonprofit, and "occasional and ancillary" commercial casinos are likewise exempt.***

Even putting aside the broadcast exemptions for arguably distinguishable sorts of gambling that might also give rise to social costs about which the Federal Government is concerned — such as state lotteries and parimutuel betting on horse and dog races, the Government presents no convincing reason for pegging its speech ban to the identity of the owners or operators of the advertised casinos. The Government***admits that tribal casinos offer precisely the same types of gambling as private casinos. Further, the Solicitor General does not maintain that government-operated casino gaming is any different, that States cannot derive revenue from taxing private casinos, or that any one class of casino operators is likely to advertise in a meaningfully distinct manner than the others.

Ironically, the most significant difference identified by the Government between tribal and other classes of casino gambling is that the former are "heavily regulated." If such direct regulation provides a basis for believing that the social costs of gambling in tribal casinos are sufficiently mitigated to make their advertising tolerable, one would have thought that Congress might have at least experimented with comparable regulation before abridging the speech rights of federally unregulated casinos. While Congress' failure to institute such direct regulation of private casino gambling does not necessarily compromise the constitutionality of § 1304, it does undermine the asserted justifications for the restriction before us. There surely are practical and nonspeech-related forms of regulation — including a prohibition or supervision of gambling on credit; limitations on the use of cash machines on casino premises; controls on admissions; pot or betting limits; location restrictions; and licensing requirements — that could more directly and effectively alleviate some of the social costs of casino gambling.***

Given the special federal interest in protecting the welfare of Native Americans, we recognize that there may be valid reasons for imposing commercial regulations on non-Indian businesses that differ from those imposed on tribal enterprises. It does not follow, however, that those differences also justify abridging non-Indians' freedom of speech more severely than the freedom of their tribal competitors. For the power to prohibit or to regulate particular conduct does not necessarily include the power to prohibit or regulate speech about that conduct. It is well settled that the First Amendment mandates closer scrutiny of government restrictions on speech than of its regulation of commerce alone. And to the extent that the purpose and operation of federal law distinguishes among information about tribal, governmental, and private casinos based on the identity of their owners or operators, the Government presents no sound reason why such lines bear any meaningful relationship to the particular interest asserted: minimizing casino gambling and its social costs by way of a (partial) broadcast ban. [D]ecisions that select among speakers conveying virtually identical messages are in serious tension with the principles undergirding the First Amendment.

The second interest asserted by the Government — the derivative goal of "assisting" States with policies that disfavor private casinos — adds little to its case. We cannot see how this broadcast restraint, ambivalent as it is, might directly and adequately further any *state* interest in dampening consumer demand for casino gambling if it cannot achieve the same goal with respect to the similar *federal* interest.***[T]he Government's second asserted interest provides no more convincing basis for upholding the regulation than the first.

VI

Accordingly, respondents cannot overcome the presumption that the speaker and the audience, not the Government, should be left to assess the value of accurate and nonmisleading information about lawful conduct. Had the Federal Government adopted a more coherent policy, or accommodated the rights of speakers in States that have legalized the underlying conduct, this might be a different case. But under current federal law, as applied to petitioners and the messages that they wish to convey, the broadcast prohibition in 18 U.S.C. §1304 and 47 CFR §73.1211 (1998) violates the First Amendment. The judgment of the Court of Appeals is therefore reversed.

CHIEF JUSTICE REHNQUIST, concurring.

I agree with the Court that "[t]he operation of § 1304 and its attendant regulatory regime is so pierced by exemptions and inconsistencies," that it violates the First Amendment.***

Were Congress to undertake substantive regulation of the gambling industry, rather than simply the manner in which it may broadcast advertisements, "exemptions and inconsistencies" such as those in §1304 might well prove constitutionally tolerable.*** But when Congress regulates commercial speech, the *Central Hudson* test imposes a more demanding standard of review. I agree with the Court that that standard has not been met here and I join its opinion.

JUSTICE THOMAS, concurring in the judgment.

I continue to adhere to my view that "[i]n cases such as this, in which the government's asserted interest is to keep legal users of a product or service ignorant in order to manipulate their choices in the marketplace," the *Central Hudson* test should not be applied because "such an 'interest' is per se illegitimate and can no more justify regulation of 'commercial speech' than it can justify regulation of 'noncommercial' speech." *44 Liquormart, Inc. v. Rhode Island*, 517 U.S. 484, 518 (1996) (concurring in part and concurring in the judgment). Accordingly, I concur only in the judgment.

LORILLARD TOBACCO COMPANY v. REILLY

121 S. Ct. 2404 (2001)

JUSTICE O'CONNOR delivered the opinion of the Court.

In January 1999, the Attorney General of Massachusetts promulgated comprehensive regulations governing the advertising and sale of cigarettes, smokeless tobacco, and cigars. *** Regulations being challenged before this Court provide:

(2) **Retail Outlet Sales Practices.** [I]t shall be an unfair or deceptive act or practice for any person who sells or distributes cigarettes, cigars, or smokeless tobacco products through a retail outlet located within Massachusetts to ***

(c) Us[e] self-service displays of cigarettes or smokeless tobacco products;

(d) Fail to place cigarettes and smokeless tobacco products out of the reach of all consumers, and in a location accessible only to outlet personnel.

(5) **Advertising Restrictions.** [I]t shall be an unfair or deceptive act or practice for any manufacturer, distributor or retailer to engage in any of the following practices:

(a) Outdoor advertising, including advertising in enclosed stadiums and advertising from within a retail establishment that is directed toward or visible from the outside of the establishment, in any location that is within a 1,000 foot radius of any public playground, playground area in a public park, elementary school or secondary school;

(b) Point-of-sale advertising of cigarettes, cigars, or smokeless tobacco products any portion of which is placed lower than five feet from the floor of any retail establishment which is located within a one thousand foot radius of any public playground, playground area in a public park, elementary school or secondary school, and which is not an adult-only retail establishment.

The term "advertisement" is defined as:

any oral, written, graphic, or pictorial statement or representation, made by, or on behalf of, any person who manufactures, packages, imports for sale, distributes or sells [tobacco products] within Massachusetts, the purpose or effect of which is to promote the use or sale of the product. ***

III

Petitioners urge us to reject the Central Hudson analysis and apply strict scrutiny. They are not the first litigants to do so. See , *e.g.*, *Greater New Orleans Broadcasting Assn., Inc. v. United States*, 527 U.S. 173, 184 (1999). Admittedly, several Members of the Court have expressed doubts about the Central Hudson analysis and whether it should apply in particular cases. *** But here, as in Greater New Orleans, we see "no need to break new ground. Central Hudson, as applied in our more recent commercial speech cases, provides an adequate basis for decision."

Only the last two steps of Central Hudson's four-part analysis are at issue here. The Attorney General has assumed for purposes of summary judgment that petitioners' speech is entitled to First Amendment protection. With respect to the second step, none of the petitioners contests the importance of the State's interest in preventing the use of tobacco products by minors.

The third step of Central Hudson concerns the relationship between the harm that underlies the State's interest and the means identified by the State to advance that interest. It requires that

> "the speech restriction directly and materially advance the asserted governmental interest. 'This burden is not satisfied by mere speculation or conjecture; rather, a governmental body seeking to sustain a restriction on commercial speech must demonstrate that the harms it recites are real and that its restriction will in fact alleviate them to a material degree.'" Greater New Orleans, supra, at 188.

We do not, however, require that "empirical data come . . . accompanied by a surfeit of background information . . ."

The last step of the Central Hudson analysis "complements" the third step, "asking whether the speech restriction is not more extensive than necessary to serve the interests that support it." Greater New Orleans, supra, at 188. We have made it clear that "the least restrictive means" is not the standard; instead, the case law requires a reasonable "'fit between the legislature's ends and the means chosen to accomplish those ends, . . . a means narrowly tailored to achieve the desired objective.'" Focusing on the third and fourth steps of the Central Hudson analysis, we first address the outdoor advertising and point-of-sale advertising regulations. We then address the sales practices regulations.

B

The outdoor advertising regulations prohibit smokeless tobacco or cigar advertising within a 1,000-foot radius of a school or playground. *** The smokeless tobacco and cigar petitioners contend that the Attorney General's regulations do not satisfy Central Hudson's third step. They maintain that although the Attorney General may have identified a problem with underage cigarette smoking, he has not identified an equally severe problem with respect to underage use of smokeless tobacco or cigars. *** Our review of the record reveals that the Attorney General has provided ample documentation of the problem with underage use of smokeless tobacco and cigars. In addition, we disagree with petitioners' claim that there is no evidence that preventing targeted campaigns and limiting youth exposure to advertising will decrease underage use of smokeless tobacco and cigars. On this record and in the posture of summary judgment, we are unable to conclude that the Attorney General's decision to regulate advertising of smokeless tobacco and cigars in an effort to combat the use of tobacco products by minors was based on mere "speculation [and] conjecture."

2

Whatever the strength of the Attorney General's evidence to justify the outdoor advertising regulations, however, we conclude that the regulations do not satisfy the fourth step of the Central Hudson analysis. The final step of the Central Hudson analysis, the "critical inquiry in this case," requires a reasonable fit between the means and ends of the regulatory scheme. 447 U.S. at 569. The Attorney General's regulations do not meet this standard. The broad sweep of the regulations indicates that the Attorney General did not "carefully calculate the costs and benefits associated with the burden on speech imposed" by the regulations. Cincinnati v. Discovery Network, Inc., 507 U.S. 410, (1993).

The outdoor advertising regulations prohibit any such advertising within 1,000 feet of schools or playgrounds. In the District Court, petitioners maintained that this prohibition would prevent advertising in 87% to 91% of Boston, Worchester, and Springfield, Massachusetts. The 87% to 91% figure appears to include not only the effect of the regulations, but also the limitations imposed by other generally applicable zoning restrictions.

The substantial geographical reach of the Attorney General's outdoor advertising regulations is compounded by other factors. "Outdoor" advertising includes not only advertising located outside an establishment, but also advertising inside a store if that advertising is visible from outside the store. The regulations restrict advertisements of any size and the term advertisement also includes oral statements.

In some geographical areas, these regulations would constitute nearly a complete ban on the communication of truthful information about smokeless tobacco and cigars to adult consumers. The breadth and scope of the regulations, and the process by which the Attorney General adopted the regulations, do not demonstrate a careful calculation of the speech interests involved.

First, the Attorney General did not seem to consider the impact of the 1,000-foot restriction on commercial speech in major metropolitan areas. [T]he effect of the Attorney General's speech regulations will vary based on whether a locale is rural, suburban, or urban. The uniformly broad sweep of the geographical limitation demonstrates a lack of tailoring.

In addition, the range of communications restricted seems unduly broad. For instance, it is not clear from the regulatory scheme why a ban on oral communications is necessary to further the State's interest. Apparently that restriction means that a retailer is unable to answer inquiries about its tobacco products if that communication occurs outdoors. Similarly, a ban on all signs of any size seems ill suited to target the problem of highly visible billboards, as opposed to smaller signs. To the extent that studies have identified particular advertising and promotion practices that appeal to youth, tailoring would involve targeting those practices while permitting others. As crafted, the regulations make no distinction among practices on this basis.

The State's interest in preventing underage tobacco use is substantial, and even compelling, but it is no less true that the sale and use of tobacco products by adults is a legal activity. We must consider that tobacco retailers and manufacturers have an interest in conveying truthful information about their products to adults, and adults have a corresponding interest in receiving truthful information about tobacco products.*** Butler v. Michigan, 352 U.S. 380, 383, (1957) ("The incidence of this enactment is to reduce the adult population . . . to reading only what is fit for children"). As the State protects children from tobacco advertisements, tobacco manufacturers and retailers and their adult consumers still have a protected interest in communication.

In addition, a retailer in Massachusetts may have no means of communicating to passersby on the street that it sells tobacco products because alternative forms of advertisement, like newspapers, do not allow that retailer to propose an instant transaction in the way that onsite advertising does. The ban on any indoor advertising that is visible from the outside also presents problems in establishments like convenience stores, which have unique security concerns that counsel in favor of full visibility of the store from the outside. It is these sorts of considerations that the Attorney General failed to incorporate into the regulatory scheme.

We conclude that the Attorney General has failed to show that the outdoor advertising regulations are not more extensive than necessary to advance the State's substantial interest in preventing underage tobacco use. ***

A careful calculation of the costs of a speech regulation does not mean that a State must demonstrate that there is no incursion on legitimate speech interests, but a speech regulation cannot unduly impinge on the speaker's ability to propose a commercial transaction and the adult listener's opportunity to obtain information about products. After reviewing the outdoor advertising regulations, we find the calculation in this case insufficient for purposes of the First Amendment.

C

Massachusetts has also restricted indoor, point-of-sale advertising. Advertising cannot be "placed lower than five feet from the floor of any retail establishment which is located within a one thousand foot radius of" any school or playground. ***

We conclude that the point-of-sale advertising regulations fail both the third and fourth steps of the Central Hudson analysis. A regulation cannot be sustained if it "'provides only ineffective or remote support for the government's purpose,'" The 5 foot rule does not seem to advance that goal. Not all children are less than 5 feet tall, and those who are certainly have the ability to look up and take in their surroundings. ***

Massachusetts may wish to target tobacco advertisements and displays that entice children, much like floor-level candy displays in a convenience store, but the blanket height restriction does not constitute a reasonable fit with that goal. The Court of Appeals recognized that the efficacy of the regulation was questionable, but decided that "in any event, the burden on speech imposed by the provision is very limited." 218 F.3d at 51. There is no de minimis exception for a speech restriction that lacks sufficient tailoring or justification. We conclude that the restriction on the height of indoor advertising is invalid under Central Hudson's third and fourth prongs.

D

The Attorney General also promulgated a number of regulations that restrict sales practices by cigarette, smokeless tobacco, and cigar manufacturers and retailers. Among other restrictions, the regulations bar the use of self-service displays and require that tobacco products be placed out of the reach of all consumers in a location accessible only to salespersons.

Petitioners devoted little of their briefing to the sales practices regulations, and our understanding of the regulations is accordingly limited by the parties' submissions. As we read the regulations, they basically require tobacco retailers to place tobacco products behind counters and require customers to have contact with a salesperson before they are able to handle a tobacco product.

The *** petitioners contend that "the same First Amendment principles that require invalidation of the outdoor and indoor advertising restrictions require invalidation of the display regulations at issue in this case." We reject these contentions. ***

Massachusetts' sales practices provisions regulate conduct that may have a communicative component, but Massachusetts seeks to regulate the placement of tobacco products for reasons unrelated to the communication of ideas. See United States v. O'Brien, 391 U.S. 367 (1968).. We conclude that the State has demonstrated a substantial interest in preventing access to tobacco products by minors and has adopted an appropriately narrow means of advancing that interest. See O'Brien, supra, at 382.

The regulations do not significantly impede adult access to tobacco products. Moreover, retailers have other means of exercising any cognizable speech interest in the presentation of their products. We presume that vendors may place empty tobacco packaging on open display, and display actual tobacco products so long as that display is only accessible to sales personnel.

We conclude that the sales practices regulations withstand First Amendment scrutiny. The means chosen by the State are narrowly tailored to prevent access to tobacco products by minors, are unrelated to expression, and leave open alternative avenues for vendors to convey information about products and for would-be customers to inspect products before purchase.

IV

We have observed that "tobacco use, particularly among children and adolescents, poses perhaps the single most significant threat to public health in the United States." FDA v. Brown & Williamson Tobacco Corp., 529 U.S. at 161. *** [But] the First Amendment also constrains state efforts to limit advertising of tobacco products, because so long as the sale and use of tobacco is lawful for adults, the tobacco industry has a protected interest in communicating information about its products and adult customers have an interest in receiving that information. *** The judgment of the United States Court of Appeals for the First Circuit is therefore affirmed in part and reversed in part, and the cases are remanded for further proceedings consistent with this opinion.

JUSTICE KENNEDY, with whom JUSTICE SCALIA joins, concurring in part and concurring in the judgment.

The obvious overbreadth of the outdoor advertising restrictions suffices to invalidate them under the fourth part of the test in Central Hudson Gas & Elec. Corp. v. Public Serv. Comm'n of N. Y., 447 U.S. 557, (1980). As a result, in my view, there is no need to consider whether the restrictions satisfy the third part of the test, a proposition about which there is considerable doubt. Cf. post, THOMAS, J., concurring in part and concurring in judgment. Neither are we required to consider whether Central Hudson should be retained in the face of the substantial objections that can be made to it. See post opinion of THOMAS, J. My continuing concerns that the test gives insufficient protection to truthful, nonmisleading commercial speech require me to refrain from expressing agreement with the Court's application of the third part of *Central Hudson*.

JUSTICE THOMAS, concurring in part and concurring in the judgment.

I continue to believe that when the government seeks to restrict truthful speech in order to suppress the ideas it conveys, strict scrutiny is appropriate, whether or not the speech in question may be characterized as "commercial." See 44 Liquormart, Inc. v. Rhode Island, 517 U.S. 484, 518, (1996) (THOMAS, J., concurring in part and concurring in judgment). I would subject all of the advertising restrictions to strict scrutiny and would hold that they violate the First Amendment.

I

Respondents suggest in passing that the regulations are "zoning-type restrictions" that should receive "the intermediate level of scrutiny traditionally associated with various forms of 'time, place, and manner' regulations." We have indeed upheld time, place, and manner regulations that prohibited certain kinds of outdoor signs, [b]ut the abiding characteristic of valid time, place, and manner regulations is their content neutrality. See Ward v. Rock Against Racism, 491 U.S. 781, 791-796, (1989).

The regulations here are very different. Massachusetts is not concerned with any "secondary effects" of tobacco advertising -- it is concerned with the advertising's primary effect, which is to induce those who view the advertisements to purchase and use tobacco products. In other words, it seeks to suppress speech about tobacco because it objects to the content of that speech. We have consistently applied strict scrutiny to such content-based regulations of speech. See, e.g., Turner Broadcasting System, Inc. v. FCC, 512 U.S. 622, (1994).

In 44 Liquormart, several Members of the Court said much the same thing:

> "When a State entirely prohibits the dissemination of truthful, nonmisleading commercial messages for reasons unrelated to the preservation of a fair bargaining process, there is far less reason to depart from the rigorous review that the First Amendment generally demands." 517 U.S. at 501 (opinion of STEVENS, J., joined by KENNEDY and GINSBURG, JJ.).

Whatever power the State may have to regulate commercial speech, it may not use that power to limit the content of commercial speech, as it has done here, "for reasons unrelated to the preservation of a fair bargaining process." Such content-discriminatory regulation -- like all other content-based regulation of speech -- must be subjected to strict scrutiny.

C

***

Viewed as an effort to proscribe solicitation to unlawful conduct, these regulations clearly fail the Brandenburg test. A State may not "forbid or proscribe advocacy of the use of force or of law violation except where such advocacy is directed to inciting or producing imminent lawless action and is likely to incite or produce such action." Brandenburg, at 447. Even if Massachusetts could prohibit advertisements reading, "Hey kids, buy cigarettes here," these regulations sweep much more broadly than that. They cover "any . . . statement or representation . . . the purpose or effect of which is to promote the use or sale" of tobacco products, whether or not the statement is directly or indirectly addressed to minors. On respondents' theory, all tobacco advertising may be limited because some of its viewers may not legally act on it.

It is difficult to see any stopping point to a rule that would allow a State to prohibit all speech in favor of an activity in which it is illegal for minors to engage. Presumably, the State could ban car advertisements in an effort to enforce its restrictions on underage driving. It could regulate advertisements urging people to vote, because children are not permitted to vote. And, although the Solicitor General resisted this implication of her theory, see Tr. of Oral Arg. 55-56, the State could prohibit advertisements for adult businesses, which children are forbidden to patronize. ***

II

Under strict scrutiny, the advertising ban may be saved only if it is narrowly tailored to promote a compelling government interest. If that interest could be served by an alternative that is less restrictive of speech, then the State must use that alternative instead. Applying this standard, the regulations here must fail. ***

The regulations fail the narrow tailoring inquiry for another, more fundamental reason. In addition to examining a narrower advertising ban, the State should have examined ways of advancing its interest that do not require limiting speech at all. Here, respondents had several alternatives. Most obviously, they could have directly regulated the conduct with which they were concerned. See, *e.g., Rubin v. Coors Brewing Co.*, 514 U.S. 476, 490-491, (1995) (invalidating ban on disclosure of alcohol content on beer labels, in part because the Government could have pursued alternatives such as "directly limiting the alcohol content of beers"); see also *44 Liquormart*, 517 U.S. at 524 (THOMAS, J., concurring in part and concurring in judgment) ("[I]t would seem that directly banning a product (or . . . otherwise restricting its sale in specific ways) would virtually always be at least as effective in discouraging consumption as merely restricting advertising"). Massachusetts already prohibits the sale of tobacco to minors, but it could take steps to enforce that prohibition more vigorously. It also could enact laws prohibiting the purchase, possession, or use of tobacco by minors. And, if its concern is that tobacco advertising communicates a message with which it disagrees, it could seek to counteract that message with "more speech, not enforced silence," *Whitney v. California*, 274 U.S. 357, 377, (1927) (Brandeis, J., concurring).

III

Underlying many of the arguments of respondents and their amici is the idea that tobacco is in some sense *sui generis* -- that it is so special, so unlike any other object of regulation, that application of normal First Amendment principles should be suspended. ***

No legislature has ever sought to restrict speech about an activity it regarded as harmless and inoffensive. Calls for limits on expression always are made when the specter of some threatened harm is looming. The identity of the harm may vary. People will be inspired by totalitarian dogmas and subvert the Republic. They will be inflamed by racial demagoguery and embrace hatred and bigotry. Or they will be enticed by cigarette advertisements and choose to smoke, risking disease. It is therefore no answer for the State to say that the makers of cigarettes are doing harm: perhaps they are. But in that respect they are no different from the purveyors of other harmful products, or the advocates of harmful ideas. When the State seeks to silence them, they are all entitled to the protection of the First Amendment.

JUSTICE SOUTER, concurring in part and dissenting in part. [Omitted.]

JUSTICE STEVENS, with whom JUSTICE GINSBURG and JUSTICE BREYER join. ***

II-III

On the First Amendment issues raised by petitioners, I *** reach [a] different dispositions [than the Court] as to the 1,000-foot rule and the height restrictions for indoor advertising, and my evaluation of the sales practice restrictions differs from the Court's.

THE 1,000-FOOT RULE

I am in complete accord with the Court's analysis of the importance of the interests served by the advertising restrictions. As the Court lucidly explains, few interests are more "compelling," than ensuring that minors do not become addicted to a dangerous drug before they are able to make a mature and informed decision as to the health risks associated with that substance. Unlike other products sold for human consumption, tobacco products are addictive and ultimately lethal for many long-term users. When that interest is combined with the State's concomitant concern for the effective enforcement of its laws regarding the sale of tobacco to minors, it becomes clear that Massachusetts' regulations serve interests of the highest order and are, therefore, immune from any ends-based challenge, whatever level of scrutiny one chooses to employ.

Nevertheless, noble ends do not save a speech-restricting statute whose means are poorly tailored. Such statutes may be invalid for two different reasons. First, the means chosen may be insufficiently related to the ends they purportedly serve. See, *e.g., Rubin v. Coors Brewing Co.*, 514 U.S. 476, (1995) (striking a statute prohibiting beer labels from displaying alcohol content because the provision did not significantly forward the government's interest in the health, safety, and welfare of its citizens). Alternatively, the statute may be so broadly drawn that, while effectively achieving its ends, it unduly restricts communications that are unrelated to its policy aims.

To my mind, the 1,000-foot rule does not present a tailoring problem of the first type. *** However, I share the majority's concern as to whether the 1,000-foot rule unduly restricts the ability of cigarette manufacturers to convey lawful information to adult consumers. ***

Finding the appropriate balance is no easy matter. Though many factors plausibly enter the equation when calculating whether a child-directed location restriction goes too far in regulating adult speech, one crucial question is whether the regulatory scheme leaves available sufficient "alternative avenues of communication." *Renton v. Playtime Theatres, Inc.*, 475 U.S. 41, 50, (1986); *Members of City Council of Los Angeles v. Taxpayers for Vincent*, 466 U.S. 789, 819, (1984) (BRENNAN, J., dissenting). Because I do not think the record contains sufficient information to enable us to answer that question, I would vacate the award of summary judgment upholding the 1,000-foot rule and remand for trial on that issue.*** The fact that 80% or 90% of an urban area is unavailable to tobacco advertisements may be constitutionally irrelevant if the available areas are so heavily trafficked or so central to the city's cultural life that they provide a sufficient forum for the propagation of a manufacturer's message. One electric sign in Times Square or at the foot of the Golden Gate Bridge may be seen by more potential customers than a hundred signs dispersed in residential neighborhoods.

Finally, the Court lacks information as to other avenues of communication available to cigarette manufacturers and retailers. For example, depending on the answers to empirical questions on which we lack data, the ubiquity of print advertisements hawking particular brands of cigarettes might suffice to inform adult consumers of the special advantages of the respective brands. Similarly, print advertisements, circulars mailed to people's homes, word of mouth, and general information may or may not be sufficient to imbue the adult population with the knowledge that particular stores, chains of stores, or types of stores sell tobacco products. ***

THE SALES PRACTICE RESTRICTIONS

After addressing petitioners' challenge to the sales practice restrictions imposed by the Massachusetts statute, the Court concluded that these provisions did not violate the First Amendment. I concur in that judgment, but write separately on this issue to make two brief points.

First, I agree with the District Court and the Court of Appeals that the sales practice restrictions are best analyzed as regulating conduct, not speech.. Restrictions as to the accessibility of dangerous or legally-restricted products are a common feature of the regulatory regime governing American retail stores. I see nothing the least bit constitutionally problematic in requiring individuals to ask for the assistance of a salesclerk in order to examine or purchase a handgun, a bottle of penicillin, or a package of cigarettes.

*** Though I agree with much of what the Court has to say about the First Amendment, I ultimately disagree with its disposition or its reasoning on each of the regulations before us.

GLICKMAN V. WILEMAN BROTHERS & ELLIOTT, INC.*

521 U.S. 457 (1997)

JUSTICE STEVENS delivered the opinion of the Court.

A number of growers, handlers, and processors of California tree fruits (respondents) brought this proceeding to challenge the validity of various regulations contained in marketing orders promulgated by the Secretary of Agriculture. The orders impose assessments that cover the cost of generic advertising of California nectarines, plums, and peaches. The question presented is whether the requirement that respondents finance such generic advertising is a law "abridging the freedom of speech" within the meaning of the First Amendment.

I

Congress enacted the Agricultural Marketing Agreement Act of 1937 in order to establish and maintain orderly marketing conditions and fair prices for agricultural commodities. Marketing orders promulgated pursuant to the AMAA are a species of economic regulation that has displaced competition in a number of discrete markets; they are expressly exempted from the antitrust laws. Marketing orders must be approved by either two-thirds of the affected producers or by producers who market at least two-thirds of the volume of the commodity.

---

*. **[Ed. Note**: This recent "commercial speech" case concerns forced financial contributions for promotional advertising. It is thus also closely related to the cases and materials in ch. 3, at pp. 550-567 ("The First Amendment in Specific Environments— Coerced Expression and Freedom Not to Speak"), and particularly to *Abood v. Detroit Bd. of Educ.* (p. 561). The Court acknowledges the connection of this case with these earlier cases which the reader may wish to review. Because the case is also treated as a "commercial speech" case which allegedly should therefore also be reviewed under the *Central Hudson* standards for commercial speech (rather than under *Abood*), however, the case appears here. (As the reader will see, the Court sharply contests the applicability of *Central Hudson* to the case— albeit, assuredly, a case of "commercial" speech).

Among the collective activities that Congress authorized for certain specific commodities is "any form of marketing promotion including paid advertising." The central message of the generic advertising at issue in this case is that "California Summer Fruits" are wholesome, delicious, and attractive to discerning shoppers.

[II-V]

Respondent Wileman Bros. & Elliott, Inc., is a large producer of these fruits that packs and markets its own output as well as that grown by other farmers. [Wileman, along with 15 other handlers] challenged the generic advertising provisions of the orders as violative of the First Amendment. ***

In challenging the constitutionality of the generic advertising program in the Court of Appeals, respondents relied, in part, on their claimed disagreement with the content of some of the generic advertising. The District Court had found no merit to this aspect of their claim,[10] and the Court of Appeals did not rely on it for its conclusion that the program was unconstitutional. Rather, the Court of Appeals invalidated the entire program on the theory that the program could not survive *Central Hudson* because the Government had failed to prove that generic advertising was more effective than individual advertising in increasing consumer demand for California nectarines, plums, and peaches. *** Although respondents have continued in this Court to argue about their disagreement with particular messages, those arguments, while perhaps calling into question the administration of portions of the program, have no bearing on the validity of the entire program.

For purposes of our analysis, we neither accept nor reject the factual assumption underlying the Court of Appeals' invalidation of the program-namely that generic advertising may not be the most effective method of promoting the sale of these commodities. The legal question that we address is whether being compelled to fund this advertising raises a First Amendment issue for us to resolve, or rather is simply a question of economic policy for Congress and the Executive to resolve. ***

The Court of Appeals apparently accepted respondents' argument that the assessments infringe First Amendment rights because they constitute compelled speech. Our compelled speech case law, however, is clearly inapplicable to the regulatory scheme at issue here. The use of assessments to pay for advertising does not require respondents to repeat an objectional message out of their own mouths, cf. *West Virginia Bd. of Ed. v. Barnette*, require them to use their own property to convey an antagonistic ideological message, cf. *Wooley v. Maynard*, or require them to

---

10. The District Court stated: "Scattered throughout plaintiffs' briefs are additional objections which are difficult to characterize or quantify. They assert that the advertising condones 'lying' in that it promotes the 'lie' that red colored fruit is superior, that it rewards mediocrity by advertising all varieties of California fruit to be of equal quality, that it promotes sexually subliminal messages as evidenced by an ad depicting a young girl in a wet bathing suit, and that it promotes the 'socialistic programs' of the Secretary. It is impossible from these 'vague claims' to determine that plaintiffs' first amendment rights have been significantly infringed."

be publicly identified or associated with another's message, cf.*PruneYard Shopping Center v. Robins*. Respondents are not required themselves to speak, but are merely required to make contributions for advertising. [T]he advertising is attributed not to them, but to the California Tree Fruit Agreement or "California Summer Fruits."

*** However, *Abood*, and the cases that follow it, did not announce a broad First Amendment right not to be compelled to provide financial support for any organization that conducts expressive activities. Rather, *Abood* merely recognized a First Amendment interest in not being compelled to contribute to an organization whose expressive activities conflict with one's "freedom of belief."

*** Here, however, requiring respondents to pay the assessments cannot be said to engender any crisis of conscience. None of the advertising in this record promotes any particular message other than encouraging consumers to buy California tree fruit. Neither the fact that respondents may prefer to foster that message independently in order to promote and distinguish their own products, nor the fact that they think more or less money should be spent fostering it, makes this case comparable to those in which an objection rested on political or ideological disagreement with the content of the message. ***

Moreover, rather than suggesting that mandatory funding of expressive activities always constitutes compelled speech in violation of the First Amendment, our cases provide affirmative support for the proposition that assessments to fund a lawful collective program may sometimes be used to pay for speech over the objection of some members of the group. Thus, in *Lehnert v. Ferris Faculty Assn.*, while we held that the cost of certain publications that were not germane to collective- bargaining activities could not be assessed against dissenting union members, we squarely held that it was permissible to charge them for those portions of "the Teachers' Voice that concern teaching and education generally, professional development, unemployment, job opportunities, award programs, and other miscellaneous matters." That holding was an application of the rule announced in *Abood* and further refined in *Keller v. State Bar of Cal.*, a case involving bar association activities.

As we pointed out in *Keller*, "*Abood* held that a union could not expend a dissenting individual's dues for ideological activities not 'germane' to the purpose for which compelled association was justified: collective bargaining. Here the compelled association and integrated bar are justified by the State's interest in regulating the legal profession and improving the quality of legal services. The State Bar may therefore constitutionally fund activities germane to those goals out of the mandatory dues of all members. It may not, however, in such manner fund activities of an ideological nature which fall outside of those areas of activity." This test is clearly satisfied in this case because (1) the generic advertising of California peaches and nectarines is unquestionably germane to the purposes of the marketing orders and, (2) in any event, the assessments are not used to fund ideological activities.

We are not persuaded that any greater weight should be given to the fact that some producers do not wish to foster generic advertising than to the fact that many of them may well object to the marketing orders themselves because they might earn more money in an unregulated market. Similar criticisms might be directed at other features of the regulatory orders that impose restraints on competition that arguably disadvantage particular producers for the benefit of the entire market. Although one may indeed question the wisdom of such a program, its debatable features are insufficient to warrant special First Amendment scrutiny. It was therefore error for the Court of Appeals to rely on *Central Hudson* for the purpose of testing the constitutionality of market order assessments for promotional advertising.[18]

The Court of Appeals' decision to apply the *Central Hudson* test is inconsistent with the very nature and purpose of the collective action program at issue here. *** If there were no marketing orders at all to set maturity levels, size, quantity and other features, competition might well generate greater production of nectarines, peaches, and plums. It may also be true that if there were no generic advertising, competition would generate even more advertising and an even larger consumer demand than does the cooperative program. But the potential benefits of individual advertising do not bear on the question whether generic advertising directly advances the statute's collectivist goals. *** While the First Amendment unquestionably protects the individual producer's right to advertise its own brands, the statute is designed to further the economic interests of the producers as a group. *** Appropriate respect for the power of Congress to regulate commerce among the States provides abundant support for the constitutionality of these marketing orders on the following reasoning.

Generic advertising is intended to stimulate consumer demand for an agricultural product in a regulated market. That purpose is legitimate and consistent with the regulatory goals of the overall statutory scheme. At least a majority of the producers in each of the markets in which such advertising is authorized must be persuaded that it is effective, or presumably the programs would be discontinued. Whether the benefits from the advertising justify its cost is a question that not only might be answered differently in different markets, but also involves the exercise of policy judgments that are better made by producers and administrators than by judges.

*** In sum, what we are reviewing is a species of economic regulation that should enjoy the same strong presumption of validity that we accord to other policy judgments made by Congress.

The judgment of the Court of Appeals is reversed.

JUSTICE SOUTER, with whom THE CHIEF JUSTICE and JUSTICE SCALIA join, and with whom JUSTICE THOMAS joins except as to Part II, dissenting.

---

18. The Court of Appeals fails to explain why the *Central Hudson* test, which involved a restriction on commercial speech, should govern a case involving the compelled funding of speech. Given the fact that the Court of Appeals relied on *Abood* for the proposition that the program implicates the First Amendment, it is difficult to understand why the Court of Appeals did not apply *Abood*'s "germaneness" test.

The Court today finds no First Amendment right to be free of coerced subsidization of commercial speech, for two principal reasons. First, the Court finds no discernible element of speech in the implementation of the Government's marketing orders, beyond what it sees as "germane" to the undoubtedly valid, nonspeech elements of the orders. Second, the Court in any event takes the position that a person who is neither barred from saying what he wishes, nor subject to personal attribution of speech he dislikes, has no First Amendment objection to mandatory subsidization of speech unless it is ideological or political or contains a message with which the objecting person disagrees. I part company with the Court on each of these closely related points. The legitimacy of governmental regulation does not validate coerced subsidies for speech that the government cannot show to be reasonably necessary to implement the regulation, and the very reasons for recognizing that commercial speech falls within the scope of First Amendment protection likewise justifies the protection of those who object to subsidizing it against their will. I therefore conclude that forced payment for commercial speech should be subject to the same level of judicial scrutiny as any restriction on communications in that category. Because I believe that the advertising scheme here fails that test, I respectfully dissent.

[I-II]

*** Since commercial speech is not subject to any categorical exclusion from First Amendment protection, and indeed is protectible as a speaker's chosen medium of commercial enterprise, it becomes subject to a second First Amendment principle: that compelling cognizable speech officially is just as suspect as suppressing it, and is typically subject to the same level of scrutiny.

As a familiar corollary to the principle that what may not be suppressed may not be coerced, we have recognized (thus far, outside the context of commercial speech) that individuals have a First Amendment interest in freedom from compulsion to subsidize speech and other expressive activities undertaken by private and quasi-private organizations.[2] We first considered this issue in *Abood v. Detroit Bd. of Ed.* [As] in this case, the sole imposition upon nonmembers was the assessment to help pay for the union's activities. And yet, purely financial as the imposition was, we held that the union's use of dissenters' service fees for expressive purposes unrelated to collective bargaining violated the First Amendment rights of those employees. ***

Decisions postdating *Abood* have made clear that its limited sanction for laws affecting First Amendment interests may not be expanded to cover every imposition that is in some way "germane" to a regulatory program in the sense of relating sympathetically to it. Rather, to survive scrutiny under *Abood*, a mandatory fee must not only be germane to some otherwise legitimate regulatory scheme; it must also be

---

2. The Secretary of Agriculture does not argue that the advertisements at issue represent so-called "government speech," with respect to which the government may have greater latitude in selecting content than otherwise permissible under the First Amendment.

justified by vital policy interests of the government and not add significantly to the burdening of free speech inherent in achieving those interests. *Lehnert v. Ferris Faculty Assn.* [500 U.S. 507 (1991)].

Thus, in *Lehnert* eight Justices concluded that a teachers' union could not constitutionally charge objecting employees for a public relations campaign meant to raise the esteem for teachers in the public mind and so increase the public's willingness to pay for public education. The advertising campaigns here suffer from the same defect as the public relations effort to stimulate demand for the teachers' product. *** Thus, the *Abood* line does not permit this program merely because it is germane to the marketing orders.

The Court's second misemployment of *Abood* and its successors is its reliance on them for the proposition that when government neither forbids speech nor attributes it to an objector, it may compel subsidization for any objectionable message that is not political or ideological. But this, of course, is entirely at odds with the principle that speech significant enough to be protected at some level is outside the government's power to coerce or to support by mandatory subsidy without further justification. Since a commercial speaker (who does not mislead) may generally promote commerce as he sees fit, the government requires some justification (such as its necessity for otherwise valid regulation) before it may force him to subsidize commercial speech to which he objects. ***

An apparent third ground for the Court's conclusion that the First Amendment is not implicated here is its assumption that respondents do not disagree with the advertisements they object to subsidizing. But this assumption is doubtful and would be beside the point even if true. [R]espondents do claim to disagree with the messages of some promotions they are being forced to fund. *** In any event, the requirement of disagreement finds no legal warrant in our compelled-speech cases. *** What counts here, then, is not whether respondents fail to disagree with the generalized message of the generic ads that California fruit is good, but that they do indeed deny that the general message is as valuable and worthy of their support as more particular claims about the merits of their own brands. One need not "disagree" with an abstractionist when buying a canvas from a representational painter; one merely wishes to support a different act of expression. ***

For the reasons discussed above, none of the Court's grounds suffices for discounting respondents' interests in expression here and treating these compelled advertising schemes as regulations of purely economic conduct instead of commercial speech. I would therefore adhere to the principle laid down in our compelled-speech cases: laws requiring an individual to engage in or pay for expressive activities are reviewed under the same standard that applies to laws prohibiting one from engaging in or paying for such activities. Under the test for commercial speech, the law may be held constitutional only if (1) the interest being pursued by the government is substantial, (2) the regulation directly advances that interest and (3) is narrowly tailored to serve it. *** In this case, the Secretary has failed to establish that the challenged advertising programs satisfy any of these three prongs of the *Central Hudson* test. ***

*** The record indicates merely that numerous commodity groups have come to the Congress and asked for authority to provide for [market development and advertising] activities under the terms of their agreement and it has always been granted. *** [T]he most reasonable inference is not of a substantial government interest, but effective politics on the part of producers who see the chance to spread their advertising costs. Nothing more appears. ***

Even if the Secretary could establish a sufficiently substantial interest, he would need also to show how the compelled advertising programs directly advance that interest, that is, how the schemes actually contribute to stabilizing agricultural markets and maintaining farm income by stimulating consumer demand. *** The Secretary argues that though respondents have voiced the desire to do more individual advertising if the system of mandatory assessments were ended, other handlers who benefit from the Government's program might well become "free riders" if promotion were to become wholly voluntary, to the point of cutting the sum total of advertising done. That might happen. It is also reasonably conceivable, though, that pure self-interest would keep the level of voluntary advertising high enough that the mandatory program could only be seen as affecting the details of the ads or shifting their costs, in either event without effect on market stability or income to producers as a group. We, of course, do not know, but these possibilities alone should be fatal to the Government here, which has the burden to establish the factual justification for ordering a subsidy for commercial speech.***

Finally, a regulation of commercial speech must be narrowly tailored to achieving the government's interests; there must be a "'fit' between the legislature's ends and the means chosen to accomplish those ends,—a fit *** that represents not necessarily the single best disposition but one whose scope is in proportion to the interest served." Respondents argue that the mandatory advertising schemes for California peaches, plums, and nectarines fail this narrow tailoring requirement, because they deny handlers any credit toward their assessments for some or all of their individual advertising expenditures. The point is well-taken. *** Indeed, the remarkable thing is that the AMAA itself provides for exactly such credits for individual advertising expenditures under marketing orders for almonds, filberts, raisins, walnuts, olives, and Florida Indian River grapefruit, but not for other commodities. ***

Although the government's obligation is not a heavy one in *Central Hudson* and the cases that follow it, we have understood it to call for some showing beyond plausibility, and there has been none here. I would accordingly affirm the judgment of the Ninth Circuit.

JUSTICE THOMAS, with whom JUSTICE SCALIA joins as to Part II, dissenting.

I write separately to note my disagreement with the majority's conclusion that coerced funding of advertising by others does not involve "speech" at all and does not even raise a First Amendment "issue." ***

In numerous cases, this Court has recognized that paying money for the purposes of advertising involves speech. The Court also has recognized that compelling speech raises a First Amendment issue just as much as restricting speech. Given these two elemental principles of our First Amendment jurisprudence, it is incongruous to suggest that forcing fruit-growers to contribute to a collective advertising campaign does not even involve speech, while at the same time effectively conceding that forbidding a fruit-grower from making those same contributions voluntarily would violate the First Amendment. ***

What we are now left with, if we are to take the majority opinion at face value, is one of two disturbing consequences: Either (1) paying for advertising is not speech at all, while such activities as draft card burning, flag burning, armband wearing, public sleeping, and nude dancing are, or (2) compelling payment for third party communication does not implicate speech, and thus the Government would be free to force payment for a whole variety of expressive conduct that it could not restrict. In either case, surely we have lost our way.

NOTES

1. Does the Court hold that Wileman's claim fails because the AMAA provision for forced contributions to generic advertising satisfies *Central Hudson*'s first amendment standards and does not transgress *Abood*'s first amendment limitations? Or does it hold, rather, that the provision is merely an "economic" regulation not even subject to First Amendment review?*

2. If, pursuant to an authorizing act of Congress, the Department of Agriculture itself spent funds from its budget to buy radio and tv ads promoting California peaches and nectarines, would Wileman (or anyone else) have a first amendment claim? If not according to the majority in *Glickman*, then according to the dissent? If not (i.e. if not even according to the dissent in *Glickman*), why not? How is this different from the situation in *Glickman* itself? (See n.2 of the dissent.)

3. In *Abood*, suppose a portion of the teachers' union dues (which nonmembers were also required to pay pursuant to the agency shop provision of the collective bar-

---

*. [**Ed. Note**: Despite the (five/four) decision in *Wileman*, the Court subsequently held that where there is no overall regulatory scheme pursuant to a valid act of Congress (i.e., a comprehensive scheme that organizes producers into groups defined by agricultural product, with group-benefitting marketing orders controlling how much, when and how a given agricultural product shall be brought to market, all undertaken for the "collective" benefit of the producers), the First Amendment *will* apply to an act that forces producers to contribute to a mere free-standing "generic" advertising scheme. *See* United States v. United Foods, Inc., 121 S. Ct. 2334 (June 25, 2001) (Objection on First Amendment grounds by major mushroom producer who preferred to advertise his own "brand" in his own way, objecting to forced contribution to pay generic mushroom promotional advertising as determined by mushroom grower association under government sanction, *sustained*, six -to-three, applying *Abood* and *Central Hudson* rigorously...).

gaining contract) were spent on advertisements to promote public confidence in teachers, e.g., to pay for bumper strips, declaring: "Teachers Are Our Children's Most Precious Resource." How, if at all, would this differ from an advertising campaign approved by the designated producers group in *Glickman*, paying for and distributing bumper strips declaring: "Hardly Anything Is Sweeter than a California Peach"?

4. In *Glickman*, the Court reversed the court of appeals in its holding that "the entire program" was invalid (i.e. that it failed to meet the requirements of *Central Hudson*, and that Wileman could thus not be made to contribute to it *at all*). Insofar as Wileman also objected to *particular* advertisements on the basis that they conveyed messages contrary to his own beliefs, the Court acknowledged the point but observed that "those arguments, while perhaps calling into question the administration of portions of the program, have no bearing on the validity of the entire program."

However, might they have a bearing were Wileman now not to attack "the *entire* program," but to seek to be excused only from that portion of the advertising assessment representing *merely* the fraction of the advertising devoted to such messages as he declares to be "false" in his own view, or "offensive to" his beliefs? Suppose, in the previous hypothetical involving the bumper strip declaring that "Hardly Anything is Sweeter than a California Peach," Wileman objects, declaring: "Here, again, just as in the ad depicting a young girl in a wet bathing suit [see n.10 in majority opinion], this ad carries a prurient sexualized suggestion I resent, reject, and find humiliating." May he successfully demand a rebate from his advertising assessment in fair proportion to the costs of these kinds of ads as a fraction of the whole?

B. The Uncertainties of Regulating or Criminalizing the "Obscene"

1. "Obscenity"[19] and the First Amendment: An Introduction and Background

In a 1942 case previously noted in these materials, *Chaplinsky v. New Hampshire*,[20] the Supreme Court sustained the conviction of a Jehovah's Witness for addressing a police officer as a "God damned racketeer" and "a damned fascist," in the heat of being led away from a spot on the public street where he had been aggressively trying to proselytize passersby. The charge against Chaplinsky was not based

---

19. "*Obscene*: 1. Offensive to accepted standards of decency or modesty. 2. Inciting lustful feelings; indecent; lewd. 3. Offensive or repulsive to the senses; loathsome. [Old French, from Latin *obscenus, obscaenus*, ill-boding, inauspicious, repulsive.]" (American Heritage Dictionary, 1971 ed.). (Cf. "*pornographic*: written or graphic forms of communication intended to excite lascivious feelings. [From Greek *pornographos*, writing about prostitutes.]")

20. 315 U.S. 568 (1942).

on his annoyance of the pedestrians,[21] but on his use of epithets, face-to-face, addressed to the policeman. It was not brought under a state anti-obscenity statute, but under an act forbidding anyone to address "any offensive, derisive or annoying word to any other person" lawfully in a public place. Nevertheless, in the course of his opinion for the Court upholding the statute as applied in this case, Justice Murphy also included the following, much more general paragraph:

> There are certain well-defined and narrowly limited classes of speech, the prevention and punishment of which have never been thought to raise any Constitutional problem. *These include the lewd and obscene*, the profane, the libelous, and the insulting or "fighting" words—those which by their very utterance inflict injury or tend to incite an immediate breach of the peace. [S]uch utterances are no essential part of any exposition of ideas, and are of such slight social value as a step to truth that any benefit that may be derived from them is clearly outweighed by the social interest in order and morality.[22]

To be sure, other portions of the Court's opinion in the case suggested that this paragraph might not mean literally what it appeared to say.[23] But it has been taken to say that certain named categories of speech are wholly excluded from the first amendment. "Lewd and obscene" speech are examples of such excluded categories, "the prevention and punishment of which have never been thought to raise any Constitutional problem," *Chaplinsky* declares. Accordingly, if that is so, the correct approach to this subject would be a one-step approach, nothing more, because insofar as the speech in question were either lewd or obscene, the government could enter

---

21. Cantwell v. Connecticut, 310 U.S. 296 (1940), overturned a conviction in just such a case, sheltering street proselytizing in accordance with the felt obligations of one's religion, even when conducted aggressively, and with condemnation of other faiths. *Cantwell* is significant aside from its general usefulness as a strong first amendment case. It is the first case holding that the free exercise of religion clause of the first amendment fully applies—via the due process clause—to the states. Several earlier cases had presaged that holding, e.g., Pierce v. Society of Sisters, 268 U.S. 510 (1925) ("liberty" in the fourteenth amendment's due process clause includes freedom of religion).

22. 315 U.S. at 571-72 (emphasis added). See also Cantwell v. Connecticut, 310 U.S. 296 (1940) (dictum); Zechariah Chafee, Free Speech in the United States 149-150 (1942) ("[O]bscenity, profanity, and gross libels of individuals *** fall outside the protection of the free speech clauses as I have defined them.")

23. Much of the balance of the full opinion, as well as one not unreasonable reading of this excerpt, is approximately consistent with a Learned Hand style of general first amendment test, rather than with the view that the first amendment has no application at all. The Court noted that the words were not part of the defendant's street corner remarks; rather, they were addressed personally and directly to the arresting officer, away from the forum, and spoken as words of immediate personal abuse. The case might have been reasoned in terms of whether police officers must accept an unmitigated amount of verbal abuse as part of their work and must refrain from striking back, or whether the avoidance of provoking the arresting officer or subjecting him to personal humiliation in the circumstances would justify the restriction on the citizen under the circumstances, rather than on the theory that the first amendment has no application at all.

a demurrer to any claim of first amendment protection in respect to such speech, and thereby prevail in the case at hand even with no showing of danger or of evil or of harm. The state would but cite *Chaplinsky* in support of its demurrer. Once it is determined that the speech was "obscene" speech, the defendant cannot invoke the first amendment (for this is just what is meant in saying that a given class of utterances is excluded from the first amendment, is it not?).

We have seen this approach in several earlier areas of our first amendment investigations, but in each previous instance in which we encountered it, it did not long endure. In the just completed section of our work on "commercial" speech, for instance, we noted that the same thing was once also said to be true there as well. *Valentine v. Chrestensen*, coincidentally also decided in 1942, conveyed such a suggestion respecting ordinary commercial advertising. Any such advertising was treated as but an incident of the ordinary trade or business practice of the entrepreneur and, as such, it was deemed equally subject to such regulation as the state might choose to impose consistent solely with a "minimum rationality," substantive due process test, with no special first amendment claim at all. *Railway Express Agency v. New York* (1949) likewise treated commercial advertising as merely an incident of economic activity protected by mere minimum, substantive due process review. But as we learned, beginning not later than the *Virginia State Board of Pharmacy* decision, in 1976, no such exclusionary first amendment boundary now cordons off commercial speech. Rather, as we have noted in the previous section of our work, the first amendment now applies to this field generally, pursuant to the four-part *Central Hudson* test.

Similarly, prior to *New York Times v. Sullivan* (1964), the whole class of utterances called "libel" was allegedly outside the first amendment—just as the quoted paragraph from *Chaplinsky* declared. Yet, beginning with *New York Times v. Sullivan*, the view has become altogether different with respect to criminal or civil actions for libel, as well as in respect to commercial speech.[24] "Libel," we have seen, even as "commercial" speech, is now understood to embrace quite a complex first amendment subject.[25]

Indeed, on reflection, the evolved, specialized first amendment treatment of each of those subjects has but mirrored the consistent pattern of nearly every other subject we have reviewed in this course. That pattern has become virtually a matter of pre-

---

24. To recall the critical quotation from *New York Times v. Sullivan*, "*[L]ibel can claim no talismanic immunity from constitutional limitations*. It must be measured by standards that satisfy the First Amendment." (emphasis added). To recall the parallel observation in the *Virginia Pharmacy* case, "Last term, in *Bigelow v. Virginia*, the notion of unprotected 'commercial speech' all but passed from the scene."

25. E.g., it now matters to ask: "Libel" of whom? (A public figure, limited public figure, nonpublic figure?) "Libel" in reference to what kind of subject? (A subject of public interest or not?) "Libel" in what manner of medium? "Libel" with *what degree of scienter*, with *what kind of damages* in mind, etc., are all now regarded as highly pertinent questions driven by first amendment concerns.

dictable routine. It has run pretty much in the following way. First, at "time one," a subject is said not to raise first amendment problems at all.[26] Somewhat later, that categorical denial is withdrawn.[27] Eventually the first amendment becomes systematically applied, i.e. applied to the once-orphaned field, albeit with a particular contour of doctrine somewhat formulaically shaped.[28] And so it has gone for us, at every stage of our unhurried first amendment review.

In keeping with these other developments that we have already traced, e.g., on commercial speech and on libel, as we begin our work here one might expect to see a parallel development in the case law of "obscenity." In brief, one might expect that sometime after 1942,[29] the Court would certainly find that "obscenity" is not unprotected by the first amendment but, rather, the first amendment *extent* of protection (as with libel or as with commercial speech) would be worked out on a case by case basis, perhaps in keeping with time, place, and manner doctrines we have examined in related areas, but presumably not much more.[30] Surprisingly, however, that has not in fact happened. Surprisingly, in a literal sense the *Chaplinsky* dictum is still the law. Narrowly speaking, the first amendment law of obscenity, 1942-2002, can be summarized in the following way.

---

26. The first cases we examined appeared to take this view with respect to restrictions on public employees. See McAuliffe v. Mayor of New Bedford, 29 N.E. 517 (1892); Scopes v. State, 289 S.W. 363 (Tenn. 1927); Bailey v. Richardson, 341 U.S. 918 (1951). Likewise the first cases we examined appeared to take the very same view respecting restrictive uses of publicly-owned property. See Davis v. Massachusetts, 167 U.S. (1897). Each of these subjects, like "libel," and like "commercial speech," had no significant first amendment standing, though each is now a principal source of ongoing dispute.

27. See, e.g., Pickering v. Board of Educ., 391 U.S. 563 (1967) (in respect to public employees); Hague v. CIO, 307 U.S. 954 (1939) (in respect to publicly-owned parks).

28. For example, the "four part" (commercial) speech test of *Central Hudson*, the *Pickering-Connick-Mt. Healthy* "test" (of public employee speech), the "forum" (public property) analysis outlined in the *Cornelius* case, and the four-part *O'Brien* "test," and the complex web of libel analysis.

29. The date of the oft-repeated *Chaplinsky* dictum.

30. So, even as to "fighting words" themselves (the immediate subject of the Supreme Court's pronouncements in *Chaplinsky*), it is an oversimplification to regard such speech as "excluded" from the first amendment. Crude, insulting speech, including a great deal that may stir others to anger, is not now excluded from full first amendment protection, depending upon the place where it occurs, whether it has an ideological content, how captive the persons subjected to it may or may not be, and a variety of other things as well. See, e.g., Hustler Magazine v. Falwell, 485 U.S. 46 (1988) (disallowing personal tort remedy for intentional infliction of emotional distress); People v. Cohen, 403 U.S. 15 (1971) (disallowing disorderly conduct charge for failure on officer's request to remove jacket with "Fuck The Draft" within courthouse corridors trafficked by women and children); Kunz v. New York, 340 U.S. 290 (1951), reviewed in these materials previously. See also Rosenfield v. New Jersey, 408 U.S. 901 (1972); Lewis v. New Orleans, 408 U.S. 913 (1972); Brown v. Oklahoma, 408 U.S. 914 (1972); Gooding v. Wilson, 405 U.S. 518 (1972); Terminiello v. Chicago, 337 U.S. 1 (1949); Cantwell v. Connecticut, 310 U.S. 296 (1940); Harry Kalven, A Worthy Tradition 80-118 (1988). An especially strong state case disallowing a "fighting words" rationale even in circumstances of extreme provocation and targeted insult, despite *Chaplinsky*, is Skokie v. National Socialist Party, 373 N.E.2d 21 (Ill. 1978). For two additional cases further limiting the "fighting words" doctrine, see R.A.V. v. City of St. Paul, 505 U.S. 377 (1992); City of Houston v. Hill, 482 U.S. 452 (1982).

2. An Overview and Summary of Supreme Court Responses

In 1958, sixteen years after *Chaplinsky*, the Supreme Court again held that "obscenity" derives *no* protection from the first amendment. It did so on the basis of its conclusion that the first amendment deemed such speech to have no value at all.[31] Nine years later, in 1967, the Court concluded that obscenity still derives no protection from the first amendment, but only if it has no redeeming value, a requirement moreover, the government must establish affirmatively in each case.[32] Otherwise, it then held, that which may well be "obscene" (in the ordinary dictionary sense) may nonetheless be protected by the first amendment, albeit still subject to some degree of social control principally according to time, place, manner, and age.[33]

This shift *de facto*, although not *de jure*,[34] obviously was a very major shift indeed. For without repudiating the general position (i.e. that "obscenity" has no first amendment protection), practically speaking the first amendment was brought into the field through a back door. The back door approach was to admit at least some relevance of standard first amendment review via the three-part special definition of "obscenity" the Court deemed somehow required by the strictures of the first amendment itself, despite what it had previously declared (i.e. that implicit in the

---

31. *Roth-Alberts*: "[I]mplicit in the history of the first amendment is the rejection of obscenity as utterly without redeeming social importance. *** [We] hold that obscenity is not within the area of constitutionally protected speech or press." Compare, however, what might equally be said of "libel" or of "fighting words" (e.g., "Implicit in the history of the first amendment is the rejection of libel as utterly without redeeming social importance. *** [We] hold that libel is not within the area of constitutionally protected speech or press"). The latter sentence reads as compellingly as the former, surely. Why, then, is "libel" often within—rather than never within—the area of constitutionally protected speech or press? Why, correspondingly, may not "obscenity" at least be sometimes within, rather than never within, the first amendment? According to the general view of the first amendment, moreover, *who decides* whether certain speech may or may not have some kind of "value," the founding fathers, today's legislators, the Supreme Court, or each individual for himself or herself? Is it the lack of alleged value that subjects speech to regulation consistent with the first amendment, or, rather, the felt need to avoid or redress certain harms? In the case of "obscenity," (as compared with "libel," "criminal solicitation," and "advocacy of violence") what *is* the alleged harm? Surely these are not idle questions; but, note, insofar as "obscenity" is regarded as excluded from the first amendment, they evidently need not even be addressed.

32. *Memoirs*: "[In order for published material to be treated as obscene and therefore excluded from the protection of the first amendment] it must be established that (a) the dominant theme of the material taken as a whole appeals to a prurient interest in sex; (b) the material is patently offensive because it affronts contemporary community standards relating to the description or representation of sexual matters; *and* (c) the material is utterly without redeeming social value." The emphasis added is meant to highlight the Court's departure respecting its definition of "obscenity" from the ordinary dictionary definition (p. 726 note 19 *supra*). The dictionary definition is unconcerned with the personal or "social value" of obscenity, such as such value may or may not be, i.e. the dictionary definition has nothing resembling part (c) of the Supreme Court's *Memoirs* test.

33. See, e.g., Redrup v. New York, 386 U.S. 767 (1967); Stanley v. Georgia, 394 U.S. 557 (1969).

34. I.e. *de jure* it remained at all times true that if the utterance, speech, or other material were "obscene," then it received no first amendment protection.

history of the first amendment was the rejection of obscenity as of so little value as to require no weighing or balancing at all), with the Court itself undertaking to monitor the manner in which that three-part definition was applied by judges and juries, virtually from case to case. By 1969, a majority of the Court appeared to be ready to abandon the position that "obscenity" has no first amendment protection; moreover, the issue, as with libel, the uses of public property, etc., would then become not *whether*, but, rather, *how much*?[35]

In 1973, however, the Court backed away. It concluded again that obscenity derives no protection from the first amendment, and this time it held that that is so even assuming there may be *some* redeeming value of some sort.[36] In doing so, it substantially reversed the contrary trend of the decisional law that had occurred during the previous fifteen years. And, briefly, this has since remained the prevailing view within the Supreme Court. We shall examine several cases to help determine how the current standard actually works. Here, in completing an introductory overview of the field, we shall note but a few features along the way.

First, the evident reason for the principal 1973 modification (namely, that some slight modicum of alleged literary, artistic, political, or scientific value may not be enough to pull otherwise-obscene material within the protection of the first amendment), may come from the concerns reflected in the *Ginzburg* case (presented *infra*). The marketing of the particular magazine involved in the case emphasized its promise of prurient content. Included within the magazine, however, were some few features and reprinted bawdy literary tales such that at least *those* parts of the magazine could fairly be said by reliable experts on literature to have redeeming literary value. The Court's decision, sustaining Ginzburg's conviction, obviously meant to permit the government to head off what it (the Court as well as the government) regarded as mere evasions of otherwise valid anti-obscenity laws by entrepreneurs who would take due commercial care to pad the publication with some passing gesture to a serious idea, discussion, editorial, etc., to frustrate any prosecutorial attempt.

The *Miller* modification of the *Memoirs* standard (requiring the prosecution to convince judge and jury the material is "utterly" lacking in redeeming literary, artistic, political, or scientific value) was almost certainly made largely to bring this sort of commercial charade to an end; but it may apply even when, in contrast to

---

35. See Stanley v. Georgia, 394 U.S. 557 (1969). The Court accepted the government's view that the material in question was "obscene" even according to its own, three-part test, yet reversed the conviction of the accused.

36. *Miller*: "A state offense must *** be limited to works which, taken as a whole, appeal to the prurient interest in sex, which portray sexual conduct in a patently offensive way, and which, taken as a whole, do not have *serious* literary, artistic, political, or scientific value." (emphasis added). (A modicum of literary, artistic, political, or scientific value may not suffice.) Moreover, evidently some *other* kind of "value" (e.g., value personal to the consumer?) may not count, if the material is otherwise "obscene," though the Court is unclear why this is so.

Ginzburg, the facts show no deliberate deviousness on the producer's or exhibitor's part.[37]

Second, even the *Miller-Slaton* standard, announced in 1973, is itself not conclusive as to material that may be found obscene. So, for example, even if the material in question would *not* be obscene as a general matter,[38] it may still be regulated as such, and successful criminal prosecutions brought, if found obscene (by the *Miller-Slaton* test) in terms of some targeted subset of the population to whom it is sent for its appeal. For example, if obscene "for children" (though not for adults), the material may be criminalized as to its distribution to children.[39] If obscene "for homosexuals" (though not for others),[40] it may evidently be criminalized as to that targeted market.[41]

Conversely, however, the fact that material may be obscene (*but only as to juveniles*) will not sustain a regulation banning the material from others on that account.[42] In other words, a general ban may not be sustained by a "most vulnerable

---

37. Note, also, that the *Miller* standard makes one other change of the same kind; it speaks of "works *** taken as a whole," rather than (as in both *Roth* and *Memoirs*) of "*the dominant theme* of the material taken as a whole" (emphasis added). The shift may seem trivial, but it is meant to cope with a defense strategy similar to the strategy (some redeeming value) in *Ginzburg*. That strategy was keyed to using a moral theme, as it were, as the dominant theme of the obscene work, i.e. to suggest in the text accompanying the otherwise obscene film, magazine, etc., that the dissolute, wayward, free-wheeling sexual promiscuity of the described (fictitious) characters was, in the end, their undoing. So, the "theme" was that the depicted licentiousness reaped a bad outcome, after all. *Miller* is meant to cut off this device for salvaging an otherwise "obscene" cheaply-produced commercial flick or sex magazine.

38. It might not be obscene even under *Miller-Slaton*, because, for example, so far as the average adult person in the relevant contemporary community may be concerned, taken as a whole the film or magazine does not engender a prurient response; alternatively, though it evokes a prurient response, the particular portrayal of sexual conduct might not flunk the "patently offensive," independent, second part of the test.

39. Ginsberg v. New York, 390 U.S. 629 (1968). This issue is separate and additional to the criminalization of the use of minors even in the production of nonobscene, but sexually explicit, materials, sustained in New York v. Ferber, 458 U.S. 747 (1982). The basis of the *Ferber* decision was the protection of minors from "exploitation" as such (akin to a child labor law) but the *Ferber* doctrine does not sanction laws outlawing pedophilia material *per se*. Such material remains subject to prohibition only if it is obscene under the *Miller-Slaton* standards, adjusted by the targeted-audience rationale we have already noted.

40. Because, for instance, it lacks capacity to stimulate in nonhomosexual persons any erotic response (and thus, while still possibly patently offensive as to them, it has no prurient appeal for them).

41. Mishkin v. New York, 383 U.S. 502 (1966).

42. Butler v. Michigan, 352 U.S. 380 (1957) (The state may not reduce the adult population to reading only what is fit for children). See also Sable Communications of California, Inc. v. FCC, 492 U.S. 115 (1989) (Congressional ban on "indecent" dial-a-porn telephone services, to protect children, held invalid as unconstitutionally overbroad, because the ban affected adults and was not limited to such dial-a-porn messages as would satisfy the *Miller-Slaton* test) (but see dicta suggesting that if the total ban were the only efficient way such calls could be made unavailable to juveniles, then it might be sustained *despite its invasion of adult first amendment rights*).

member(s) of the community" test.[43] This much was itself settled originally in *Roth-Alberts*, rejecting the *Regina v. Hicklin* most-vulnerable-member-of-the community standard of the older common law. Rather, differentiating statutes (e.g., disallowing commercial motion picture exhibitors to admit persons under 17 to films "obscene" for minors, but not otherwise forbidding the films to be shown) may be permitted and applied.[44]

Mere parity of reasoning would suggest that specialized audiences (such as personnel of the Kinsey Institute or users of Masters & Johnson) should be able to invoke a successful first amendment claim even with regard to material which otherwise fails the *Miller-Slaton* test. In other words: in the environment in question, the material *has* "serious redeeming value," and it accordingly qualifies for first amendment protection *in that environment* (but not in the general commercial market). There appears to be no direct Supreme Court decision on the point, but it is strongly arguable that even producers or senders of "obscene" materials should be fully protected insofar as the delivery were limited to such "redeeming-use" audiences as those just described.[45]

These sorts of special problems aside, moreover, because of the still-prevailing majority view (i.e. that if the material is "obscene" it receives no first amendment protection—thus no usual first amendment proof of actual harm need be met by the

---

43. See also Pinkus v. United States, 436 U.S. 293 (1978) (*Butler v. Michigan* applied); Reno v. American Civil Liberties Union, 521 U.S. 824 (1997).

44. This may be a suitable place to note (and distinguish), the "rating" system (P, PG, PG-13, R, NC-17) the film industry uses. These ratings are *not* ratings based on first amendment criteria. The fact that a film may have a PG-13 rating does not mean that it could not therefore be seen by youngsters under thirteen, a film rated NC-17 does not mean that it would necessarily be subject to successful criminal prosecution even assuming persons under the age of seventeen may be admitted. Thus a state law presuming to mimic the rating system would not *necessarily* be constitutional. (It is nonetheless true that the rating system practically affects which films are available (exhibitors are very chary of taking X-rated films, partly from fear of inviting criminal prosecution), so its *de facto* influence is quite strong.) (Note, however, there is no obligation on a film producer to submit its film to the rating system; accordingly, a number of films will carry no rating at all.)

45. An interesting variation of the example might be one we ourselves could provide: to distribute within this classroom examples of work otherwise held to be suppressible (because found to be "obscene"), in order that, as lawyers in training, one be able to compare material which has been upheld with material that has not been upheld in the courts. *Query*, whether a criminal prosecution for such limited use of the materials, in this class, could, consistent with the first amendment, be sustained. Assuming it could not be sustained, to what extent might one extend the example itself? (E.g., if one is free to inspect and discuss such material in a first amendment law school course, ought not one also be able to secure a copy of such material from a willing supplier, with the supplier equally being protected in having made it available for such classroom use, with reliance upon the first amendment as against any attempt to prosecute the supplier himself? Cf. Lamont v. Postmaster General, 381 U.S. 301 (1965).)

state),[46] some real strains are felt at the margin of uncertainty as to whether particular works are obscene. Since so much rides on the right guess respecting the nonobscenity of the material in question, one's uncertainty may *per se* produce a large chilling effect.[47]

Two principal cases in the following materials illustrate the problem (and the Supreme Court's response) in the obscenity area: *Freedman v. Maryland* (1965) and *Smith v. California* (1959). The *Smith* case holds that in order that one be criminally accountable under an anti-obscenity law, one must at least know or have reason to know the content of the books or journals comprising the inventory of one's retail shop. The scienter requirement of the *Smith* case lifts the chilling effect that might otherwise result from being unable to stock any larger assortment of printed materials that one had the time (or the means of paying employees) to read.[48]

Freedman v. Maryland, relatedly, is twice significant. First, it is a "hostile" case insofar as the Court approved a form of prior restraint: it held that requiring

---

46. Though note, again, that whether particular material is "obscene" is not a function inherent in the material itself but is, rather, partly contingent upon the community in which it appears (e.g., the film *The Devil in Miss Jones* may be obscene in one state or one town, but not obscene in a different state or a different town, although, to be found obscene even in the most restrictive community the material must separately meet the minimum qualifications of "obscene" speech as set in *Miller-Slaton.* (See, e.g., Jenkins v. Georgia, 418 U.S. 153 (1974) (film *Carnal Knowledge*, judged by Georgia jury to be obscene pursuant to *Miller-Slaton* jury instruction, held not obscene as a matter of constitutional law, because the manner in which intimate erotic sexual acts were depicted lacked sufficient coarseness to be deemed patently offensive as a matter of law).)

47. The problem has an obvious kinship with the overbreadth doctrine we have encountered before, i.e. speech-specific statutes on their face forbidding speech not within the constitutional authority of the state to forbid, are subject to attack even by a party whose speech could clearly have been reached under a more narrowly drawn statute. (The "guilty" go free in order that the "innocent" not be unduly "chilled.") The problem has an obvious kinship, as well, with the chilling effect rationale for protecting libel as strongly as it is protected under the *New York Times v. Sullivan* rule. (Newspapers are given a first amendment immunity for public figure libel even when false and damaging statements are *negligently* researched and published, in order that there be adequate "breathing space" for publishers who might otherwise be too fearful to publish critical stories.)

48. If *Smith* imports a special scienter requirement (as it does) in order that protected materials not be suppressed, might it not likewise be argued that the first amendment may require some limitation on the magnitude of penalty or punishment the state may impose, since at least as chilling an effect inhibiting book sellers to carry close-to-the-edge books (or film exhibitors carrying close-to-the-edge films), must surely result when the criminal sanction for an obscenity law violation is very great (e.g., up to five years in prison, or forfeiture of one's store—for having sold "criminal contraband")? Bearing in mind that, consistent with *Roth-Alberts-Miller* doctrine, "obscenity" having been formally excluded from the first amendment (such that the state need make no conventional showing of any strong reason for disallowing it in the first place), with the result that so much is made to depend upon sorting the "obscene" from the "nonobscene" in terms of one's liability, a strong argument along these lines would seem to be sound. Thus far, however, a majority of the Supreme Court has *not* accepted such an argument. Fort Wayne Books, Inc. v. Indiana, 489 U.S. 46 (1989). Correspondingly, some states have strengthened their anti-obscenity laws in recent years, with very heavy sanctions (as has been done vis-à-vis dealing in drugs).

submission of commercial films to some kind of local film clearance board may not *per se* violate the first amendment, though a strong contrary argument can surely be made that it does.[49] (One might plausibly have thought that such preview clearance boards would be prohibited,[50] given the usual first amendment presumption against a regime of prior restraint.) Second, however, because the orientation of the censor is presumed to be such that in close cases he or she will be prone to err in favor of protecting the public rather than the exhibitor, *Freedman* mandates special safeguards insofar as film clearance procedures are used at all. Specifically, it requires that the relevant standards be both specifically and narrowly defined; that the time within which the censor must decide (or failing which, the film may be shown) be short, and if the censorship decision is adverse to the film, an expeditious review must be provided in the courts, in which it is the censor's burden to sustain the adverse censorship decision (not the film exhibitor's burden to show the decision was in error). The *Freedman* standards, moreover, have been carried over into other prior restraints environments, noted in our previous work.[51]

Finally, within the most recent decade (1990-2000), there have been new problems and subtleties to confront in this unruly field, for example, the proliferation of accessible websites virtually worldwide and interactive transmissions, of nearly every imaginable sort. Whether cases and doctrines developed more in the age of the Post Office will work in the age of the Internet, however, remains to be seen....

ROTH v. UNITED STATES
ALBERTS v. CALIFORNIA
354 U.S. 476 (1957)

MR. JUSTICE BRENNAN delivered the opinion of the Court.

The constitutionality of a criminal obscenity statute is the question in each of these cases. In *Roth*, the primary constitutional question is whether the federal obscenity statute[1] violates the provision of the First Amendment that "Congress shall

---

49. *Freedman* was not new in this respect. See Times Film Corp. v. Chicago, 365 U.S. 43 (1961) (film clearance municipal ordinance sustained as not invalid *per se*, five-to-four) (Warren, Black, Douglas, Brennan, JJ., dissenting).

50. See, e.g., Bantam Books, Inc. v. Sullivan, 372 U.S. 58 (1963) (prior restraint systems are presumed to be invalid). (And see prior discussion, beginning even with Blackstone, all the way through *Pentagon Papers* and *Nebraska Press*.)

51. See, e.g., Carroll v. President and Comm'rs of Princess Anne, 393 U.S. 174 (1968) (ten-day ex parte injunction against imminent public political meeting held void for failure to satisfy *Freedman* standards). For a general review, see Henry P. Monaghan, First Amendment Due Process, 83 Harv.L.Rev. 518 (1970).

1. The federal obscenity statute provided, in pertinent part:

"Every obscene, lewd, lascivious, or filthy book, pamphlet, picture, paper, letter, writing, print, or other publication of an indecent character; and—

make no law abridging the freedom of speech, or of the press." In *Alberts*, the primary constitutional question is whether the obscenity provisions of the California Penal Code[2] invade the freedoms of speech and press as they may be incorporated in the liberty protected from state action by the Due Process Clause of the Fourteenth Amendment.

Roth conducted a business in New York in the publication and sale of books, photographs and magazines. He used circulars and advertising matter to solicit sales. He was convicted by a jury in the District Court for the Southern District of New York upon 4 counts of a 26-count indictment charging him with mailing obscene circulars and advertising, and an obscene book, in violation of the federal obscenity statute. His conviction was affirmed by the Court of Appeals for the Second Circuit. We granted certiorari.

Alberts conducted a mail-order business from Los Angeles. He was convicted under a misdemeanor complaint which charged him with lewdly keeping for sale obscene and indecent books, and with writing, composing and publishing an obscene advertisement of them, in violation of the California Penal Code. The conviction was affirmed by the Appellate Department of the Superior Court of the State of California. We noted probable jurisdiction.

I

The dispositive question is whether obscenity is utterance within the area of protected speech and press.[8] Although this is the first time the question has been squarely presented to this Court, either under the First Amendment or under the Fourteenth Amendment, expressions found in numerous opinions indicate that this

---

"Every written or printed card, letter, circular, book, pamphlet, advertisement, or notice of any kind giving information, directly or indirectly, where, or how, or from whom, or by what means any of such mentioned matters, articles, or things may be obtained or made, whether sealed or unsealed ***

"Is declared to be nonmailable matter and shall not be conveyed in the mails or delivered from any post office or by any letter carrier.

"Whoever knowingly deposits for mailing or delivery, anything declared by this section to be nonmailable, or knowingly takes the same from the mails for the purpose of circulating or disposing thereof, or of aiding in the circulation or disposition thereof, shall be fined not more than $5,000 or imprisoned not more than five years, or both."

2. The California Penal Code provides, in pertinent part:

"Every person who wilfully and lewdly, either: ***

"3. Writes, composes, stereotypes, prints, publishes, sells, distributes, keeps for sale, or exhibits any obscene or indecent writing, paper, or book; or designs, copies, draws, engraves, paints, or otherwise prepares any obscene or indecent picture or print; or molds, cuts, casts, or otherwise makes any obscene or indecent figure; or,

"4. Writes, composes, or publishes any notice or advertisement of any such writing, paper, book, picture, print or figure; is guilty of a misdemeanor.

8. No issue is presented in either case concerning the obscenity of the material involved.

Court has always assumed that obscenity is not protected by the freedoms of speech and press.

The guaranties of freedom of expression in effect in 10 of the 14 States which by 1792 had ratified the Constitution, gave no absolute protection for every utterance. Thirteen of the 14 States provided for the prosecution of libel, and all of those States made either blasphemy or profanity, or both, statutory crimes. As early as 1712, Massachusetts made it criminal to publish "any filthy, obscene, or profane song, pamphlet, libel or mock sermon" in imitation or mimicking of religious services. ***

In light of this history, it is apparent that the unconditional phrasing of the First Amendment was not intended to protect every utterance. This phrasing did not prevent this Court from concluding that libelous utterances are not within the area of constitutionally protected speech. At the time of the adoption of the First Amendment, obscenity law was not as fully developed as libel law, but there is sufficiently contemporaneous evidence to show that obscenity, too, was outside the protection intended for speech and press.

The protection given speech and press was fashioned to assure unfettered interchange of ideas for the bringing about of political and social changes desired by the people. *** All ideas having even the slightest redeeming social importance—unorthodox ideas, controversial ideas, even ideas hateful to the prevailing climate of opinion— have the full protection of the guaranties, unless excludable because they encroach upon the limited area of more important interests. But implicit in the history of the First Amendment is the rejection of obscenity as utterly without redeeming social importance. This rejection for that reason is mirrored in the universal judgment that obscenity should be restrained, reflected in the international agreement of over 50 nations, in the obscenity laws of all of the 48 States, and in the 20 obscenity laws enacted by the Congress from 1842 to 1956. This is the same judgment expressed by this Court in Chaplinsky v. New Hampshire, 315 U.S. 568, 571-572:

> "*** There are certain well-defined and narrowly limited classes of speech, the prevention and punishment of which have never been thought to raise any Constitutional problem. *These include the lewd and obscene ***. It has been well observed that such utterances are no essential part of any exposition of ideas, and are of such slight social value as a step to truth that any benefit that may be derived from them is clearly outweighed by the social interest in order and morality.* ***" (Emphasis added.)

We hold that obscenity is not within the area of constitutionally protected speech or press.

It is strenuously urged that these obscenity statutes offend the constitutional guaranties because they punish incitation to impure sexual *thoughts*, not shown to be related to any overt antisocial conduct which is or may be incited in the persons stimulated to such *thoughts*. In *Roth*, the trial judge instructed the jury: "The words 'obscene, lewd and lascivious' as used in the law, signify that form of immorality which has relation to sexual impurity and has a tendency to excite lustful *thoughts*." (Emphasis added.) In *Alberts*, the trial judge applied the test laid down in People v. Wepplo, 178 P.2d 853, namely, whether the material has "a substantial tendency to deprave or corrupt its readers by inciting lascivious *thoughts* or arousing lustful desires." (Emphasis added.) It is insisted that the constitutional guaranties are violated because convictions may be had without proof either that obscene material will perceptibly create a clear and present danger of anti-social conduct, or will probably induce its recipients to such conduct. But, in light of our holding that obscenity is not protected speech, the complete answer to this argument is in the holding of this Court in Beauharnais v. Illinois, [343 U.S.] at 266:

> "Libelous utterances not being within the area of constitutionally protected speech, it is unnecessary, either for us or for the State courts, to consider the issues behind the phrase 'clear and present danger.' Certainly no one would contend that obscene speech, for example, may be punished only upon a showing of such circumstances. Libel, as we have seen, is in the same class."

II

However, sex and obscenity are not synonymous. Obscene material is material which deals with sex in a manner appealing to prurient interest.[20] The portrayal of sex, *e.g.*, in art, literature and scientific works, is not itself sufficient reason to deny material the constitutional protection of freedom of speech and press. Sex, a great and mysterious motive force in human life, has indisputably been a subject of absorbing interest to mankind through the ages; it is one of the vital problems of human interest and public concern.

The fundamental freedoms of speech and press have contributed greatly to the development and well-being of our free society and are indispensable to its continued growth. Ceaseless vigilance is the watchword to prevent their erosion by Congress or by the States. The door barring federal and state intrusion into this area cannot be left ajar; it must be kept tightly closed and opened only the slightest crack necessary to prevent encroachment upon more important interests. It is therefore vital that the

---

20. *I.e.*, material having a tendency to excite lustful thoughts. Webster's New International Dictionary (Unabridged, 2d ed., 1949) defines *prurient*, in pertinent part, as follows:

> "*** Itching; longing; uneasy with desire or longing; of persons, having itching, morbid, or lascivious longings; of desire, curiosity, or propensity, lewd. ***"

Pruriency is defined, in pertinent part, as follows:

> "*** Quality of being prurient; lascivious desire or thought. ***"

* * *

We perceive no significant difference between the meaning of obscenity developed in the case law and the definition of the A.L.I., Model Penal Code, § 207.10 (2) (Tent. Draft No. 6, 1957), *viz.*:

> "*** A thing is obscene if, considered as a whole, its predominant appeal is to prurient interest, i.e., a shameful or morbid interest in nudity, sex, or excretion, and if it goes substantially beyond customary limits of candor in description or representation of such matters. ***"

standards for judging obscenity safeguard the protection of freedom of speech and press for material which does not treat sex in a manner appealing to prurient interest.

The early leading standard of obscenity allowed material to be judged merely by the effect of an isolated excerpt upon particularly susceptible persons. Regina v. Hicklin, [1868] L.R. 3 Q.B. 360. Some American courts adopted this standard but later decisions have rejected it and substituted this test: whether to the average person, applying contemporary community standards, the dominant theme of the material taken as a whole appeals to prurient interest. The *Hicklin* test, judging obscenity by the effect of isolated passages upon the most susceptible persons, might well encompass material legitimately treating with sex, and so it must be rejected as unconstitutionally restrictive of the freedoms of speech and press. On the other hand, the substituted standard provides safeguards adequate to withstand the charge of constitutional infirmity.

Both trial courts below sufficiently followed the proper standard. Both courts used the proper definition of obscenity. ***

It is argued that the statutes do not provide reasonably ascertainable standards of guilt and therefore violate the constitutional requirements of due process. Winters v. People of State of New York, 333 U.S. 507. The federal obscenity statute makes punishable the mailing of material that is "obscene, lewd, lascivious, or filthy *** or other publications of an indecent character."[28] The California statute makes punishable, *inter alia*, the keeping for sale or advertising material that is "obscene or indecent." The thrust of the argument is that these words are not sufficiently precise because they do not mean the same thing to all people, all the time, everywhere.

Many decisions have recognized that these terms of obscenity statutes are not precise. This Court, however, has consistently held that lack of precision is not itself offensive to the requirements of due process. "[T]he Constitution does not require impossible standards"; all that is required is that the language "conveys sufficiently definite warning as to the proscribed conduct when measured by common understanding and practices ***." United States v. Petrillo, 332 U.S. 1, 7-8. These words, applied according to the proper standard for judging obscenity, already discussed, give adequate warning of the conduct proscribed and mark boundaries sufficiently distinct for judges and juries fairly to administer the law.

III

In summary, then, we hold that these statutes, applied according to the proper standard for judging obscenity, do not offend constitutional safeguards against convictions based upon protected material, or fail to give men in acting adequate notice of what is prohibited.

---

28. This Court, as early as 1896, said of the federal obscenity statute:

"*** Every one who uses the mails of the United States for carrying papers or publications must take notice of what, in this enlightened age, is meant by decency, purity, and chastity in social life, and what must be deemed obscene, lewd, and lascivious." ***

Roth's argument that the federal obscenity statute unconstitutionally encroaches upon the powers reserved by the Ninth and Tenth Amendments to the States and to the people to punish speech and press where offensive to decency and morality is hinged upon his contention that obscenity is expression not excepted from the sweep of the provision of the First Amendment that "*Congress* shall make *no law* abridging the freedom of speech, or of the press" (Emphasis added.) That argument falls in light of our holding that obscenity is not expression protected by the First Amendment.[31] We therefore hold that the federal obscenity statute punishing the use of the mails for obscene material is a proper exercise of the postal power delegated to Congress by Art. I, § 8, cl. 7. ***

The judgments are [a]ffirmed.

MR. CHIEF JUSTICE WARREN, concurring in the result.

I agree with the result reached by the Court in these cases, but, because we are operating in a field of expression and because broad language used here may eventually be applied to the arts and sciences and freedom of communication generally, I would limit our decision to the facts before us and to the validity of the statutes in question as applied. ***

The line dividing the salacious or pornographic from literature or science is not straight and unwavering. Present laws depend largely upon the effect that the materials may have upon those who receive them. It is manifest that the same object may have a different impact, varying according to the part of the community it reached. But there is more to these cases. It is not the book that is on trial; it is a person. The conduct of the defendant is the central issue, not the obscenity of a book or picture. The nature of the materials is, of course, relevant as an attribute of the defendant's conduct, but the materials are thus placed in context from which they draw color and character. A wholly different result might be reached in a different setting.

The personal element in these cases is seen most strongly in the requirement of *scienter*. Under the California law, the prohibited activity must be done "wilfully and lewdly." The federal statute limits the crime to acts done "knowingly." In his charge to the jury, the district judge stated that the matter must be "calculated" to corrupt or debauch. The defendants in both these cases were engaged in the business of purveying textual or graphic matter openly advertised to appeal to the erotic interest of their customers. They were plainly engaged in the commercial exploitation of the morbid and shameful craving for materials with prurient effect. I believe that the State and Federal Governments can constitutionally punish such conduct. That is all that these cases present to us, and that is all we need to decide.

---

31. For the same reason, we reject, in this case, the argument that there is greater latitude for state action under the word "liberty" under the Fourteenth Amendment than is allowed to Congress by the language of the First Amendment.

I agree with the Court's decision in its rejection of the other contentions raised by these defendants.

MR. JUSTICE HARLAN, concurring in the result in No. 61 [*Alberts*], and dissenting in No. 582 [*Roth*].

I regret not to be able to join the Court's opinion. I cannot do so because I find lurking beneath its disarming generalizations a number of problems which not only leave me with serious misgivings as to the future effect of today's decisions, but which also, in my view, call for different results in these two cases.

I

In final analysis, the problem presented by these cases is how far, and on what terms, the state and federal governments have power to punish individuals for disseminating books considered to be undesirable because of their nature or supposed deleterious effect upon human conduct. Proceeding from the premise that "no issue is presented in either case, concerning the obscenity of the material involved," the Court finds the "dispositive question" to be "whether obscenity is utterance within the area of protected speech and press," and then holds that "obscenity" is not so protected because it is "utterly without redeeming social importance." This sweeping formula appears to me to beg the very question before us. The Court seems to assume that "obscenity" is a peculiar *genus* of "speech and press," which is as distinct, recognizable, and classifiable as poison ivy is among other plants. On this basis the *constitutional* question before us simply becomes, as the Court says, whether "obscenity," as an abstraction, is protected by the First and Fourteenth Amendments, and the question whether a *particular* book may be suppressed becomes a mere matter of classification, of "fact," to be entrusted to a fact-finder and insulated from independent constitutional judgment. But surely the problem cannot be solved in such a generalized fashion. Every communication has an individuality and "value" of its own. The suppression of a particular writing or other tangible form of expression is, therefore, an *individual* matter, and in the nature of things every such suppression raises an individual constitutional problem, in which a reviewing court must determine for *itself* whether the attacked expression is suppressible within constitutional standards. Since those standards do not readily lend themselves to generalized definitions, the constitutional problem in the last analysis becomes one of particularized judgments which appellate courts must make for themselves.

I do not think that reviewing courts can escape this responsibility by saying that the trier of the facts, be it a jury or a judge, has labeled the questioned matter as "obscene," for, if "obscenity" is to be suppressed, the question whether a particular work is of that character involves not really an issue of fact but a question of constitutional *judgment* of the most sensitive and delicate kind. Many juries might find that Joyce's "Ulysses" or Bocaccio's "Decameron" was obscene, and yet the conviction of a defendant for selling either book would raise, for me, the gravest constitutional problems, for no such verdict could convince me, without more, that these books are "utterly without redeeming social importance." In short, I do not understand how the Court can resolve the constitutional problems now before it without making its own independent judgment upon the character of the material upon which these convictions were based. ***

[T]he Court has not been bothered by the fact that the two cases involve different statutes. In California the book must have a "tendency to deprave or corrupt its readers"; under the federal statute it must tend "to stir sexual impulses and lead to sexually impure thoughts." The two statutes do not seem to me to present the same problems. Yet the Court compounds confusion when it superimposes on these two statutory definitions a third, drawn from the American Law Institute's Model Penal Code, Tentative Draft No. 6: "A thing is obscene if, considered as a whole, its predominant appeal is to prurient interest." The bland assurance that this definition is the same as the ones with which we deal flies in the face of the authors' express rejection of the "deprave and corrupt" and "sexual thoughts" tests:

> "Obscenity [in the Tentative Draft] is defined in terms of material which appeals predominantly to prurient interest in sexual matters and which goes beyond customary freedom of expression in these matters. We reject the prevailing test of tendency to arouse lustful thoughts or desires because it is unrealistically broad for a society that plainly tolerates a great deal of erotic interest in literature, advertising, and art, and because regulation of thought or desire, unconnected with overt misbehavior, raises the most acute constitutional as well as practical difficulties. We likewise reject the common definition of obscene as that which 'tends to corrupt or debase.' If this means anything different from tendency to arouse lustful thought and desire, it suggests that change of character or actual misbehavior follows from contact with obscenity. Evidence of such consequences is lacking. *** On the other hand, 'appeal to prurient interest' refers to qualities of the material itself: the capacity to attract individuals eager for a forbidden look ***."

As this passage makes clear, there is a significant distinction between the definitions used in the prosecutions before us, and the American Law Institute formula. If, therefore, the latter is the correct standard, as my Brother BRENNAN elsewhere intimates, then these convictions should surely be reversed. Instead, the Court merely assimilates the various tests into one indiscriminate potpourri.

I now pass to the consideration of the two cases before us.

II

I concur in the judgment of the Court in No. 61, *Alberts v. California*. The question in this case is whether the defendant was deprived of liberty without due process of law when he was convicted for selling certain materials found by the judge to be obscene because they would have a "tendency to deprave or corrupt its readers by exciting lascivious thoughts or arousing lustful desire."

In judging the constitutionality of this conviction, we should remember that our function in reviewing state judgments under the Fourteenth Amendment is a narrow one. We do not decide whether the policy of the State is wise, or whether it is based on assumptions scientifically substantiated. We can inquire only whether the state action so subverts the fundamental liberties implicit in the Due Process Clause that it cannot be sustained as a rational exercise of power. See Jackson, J., dissenting in Beauharnais v. Illinois, 343 U.S. 250, 287. The States' power to make printed words criminal is, of course, confined by the Fourteenth Amendment, but only insofar as such power is inconsistent with our concepts of "ordered liberty." Palko v. Connecticut, 302 U.S. 319, 324-325.

What, then, is the purpose of this California statute? Clearly the state legislature has made the judgment that printed words *can* "deprave or corrupt" the reader—that words can incite to antisocial or immoral action. The assumption seems to be that the distribution of certain types of literature will induce criminal or immoral sexual conduct. It is well known, of course, that the validity of this assumption is a matter of dispute among critics, sociologists, psychiatrists, and penologists. There is a large school of thought, particularly in the scientific community, which denies any causal connection between the reading of pornography and immorality, crime, or delinquency. Others disagree. Clearly it is not our function to decide this question. That function belongs to the state legislature. Nothing in the Constitution requires California to accept as truth the most advanced and sophisticated psychiatric opinion. It seems to me clear that it is not irrational, in our present state of knowledge, to consider that pornography can induce a type of sexual conduct which a State may deem obnoxious to the moral fabric of society. In fact the very division of opinion on the subject counsels us to respect the choice made by the State.

Furthermore, even assuming that pornography cannot be deemed ever to cause, in an immediate sense, criminal sexual conduct, other interests within the proper cognizance of the States may be protected by the prohibition placed on such materials. The State can reasonably draw the inference that over a long period of time the indiscriminate dissemination of materials, the essential character of which is to degrade sex, will have an eroding effect on moral standards. And the State has a legitimate interest in protecting the privacy of the home against invasion of unsolicited obscenity.

Above all stands the realization that we deal here with an area where knowledge is small, data are insufficient, and experts are divided. Since the domain of sexual morality is pre-eminently a matter of state concern, this Court should be slow to interfere with state legislation calculated to protect that morality. It seems to me that nothing in the broad and flexible command of the Due Process Clause forbids California to prosecute one who sells books whose dominant tendency might be to "deprave or corrupt" a reader. I agree with the Court, of course, that the books must be judged as a whole and in relation to the normal adult reader.

What has been said, however, does not dispose of the case. It still remains for us to decide whether the state court's determination that this material should be suppressed is consistent with the Fourteenth Amendment; and that, of course, presents a federal question as to which we, and not the state court, have the ultimate responsibility. And so, in the final analysis, I concur in the judgment because, upon an independent perusal of the material involved, and in light of the considerations discussed above, I cannot say that its suppression would so interfere with the communication of "ideas" in any proper sense of that term that it would offend the Due Process Clause. I therefore agree with the Court that appellant's conviction must be affirmed.

III

I dissent in No. 582, *Roth v. United States*.

We are faced here with the question whether the federal obscenity statute, as construed and applied in this case, violates the First Amendment to the Constitution. To me, this question is of quite a different order than one where we are dealing with state legislation under the Fourteenth Amendment. I do not think it follows that state and federal powers in this area are the same, and that just because the State may suppress a particular utterance, it is automatically permissible for the Federal Government to do the same. ***

The Constitution differentiates between those areas of human conduct subject to the regulation of the States and those subject to the powers of the Federal Government. The substantive powers of the two governments, in many instances, are distinct. And in every case where we are called upon to balance the interest in free expression against other interests, it seems to me important that we should keep in the forefront the question of whether those other interests are state or federal.

The Federal Government has, for example, power to restrict seditious speech directed against it, because that Government certainly has the substantive authority to protect itself against revolution. But in dealing with obscenity we are faced with the converse situation, for the interests which obscenity statutes purportedly protect are primarily entrusted to the care, not of the Federal Government, but of the States. Congress has no substantive power over sexual morality. Such powers as the Federal Government has in this field are but incidental to its other powers, here the postal power, and are not of the same nature as those possessed by the States, which bear direct responsibility for the protection of the local moral fabric.[5] ***

Not only is the federal interest in protecting the Nation against pornography attenuated, but the dangers of federal censorship in this field are far greater than anything the States may do. It has often been said that one of the great strengths of our federal system is that we have, in the forty-eight States, forty-eight experimental

5. The hoary dogma of *Ex parte* Jackson, 96 U.S. 727, and Public Clearing House v. Coyne, 194 U.S. 497, that the use of the mails is a privilege on which the Government may impose such conditions as it chooses, has long since evaporated. See Brandeis, J., dissenting, in Milwaukee Social Democratic Publishing Co. v. Burleson, 255 U.S. 407, 430-433 ***.

social laboratories. *** Different States will have different attitudes toward the same work of literature. The same book which is freely read in one State might be classed as obscene in another.[7] And it seems to me that no overwhelming danger to our freedom to experiment and to gratify our tastes in literature is likely to result from the suppression of a borderline book in one of the States, so long as there is no uniform nation-wide suppression of the book, and so long as other States are free to experiment with the same or bolder books.

Quite a different situation is presented, however, where the Federal Government imposes the ban. The danger is perhaps not great if the people of one State, through their legislature, decide that "Lady Chatterley's Lover" goes so far beyond the acceptable standards of candor that it will be deemed offensive and non-sellable, for the State next door is still free to make its own choice. At least we do not have one uniform standard. But the dangers to free thought and expression are truly great if the Federal Government imposes a blanket ban over the Nation on such a book. The prerogative of the States to differ on their ideas of morality will be destroyed, the ability of States to experiment will be stunted. The fact that the people of one State cannot read some of the works of D.H. Lawrence seems to me, if not wise or desirable, at least acceptable. But that no person in the United States should be allowed to do so seems to me to be intolerable, and violative of both the letter and spirit of the First Amendment.

I judge this case, then, in view of what I think is the attenuated federal interest in this field, in view of the very real danger of a deadening uniformity which can result from nation-wide federal censorship, and in view of the fact that the constitutionality of this conviction must be weighed against the First and not the Fourteenth Amendment. So viewed, I do not think that this conviction can be upheld. The petitioner was convicted under a statute which, under the judge's charge, makes it criminal to sell books which "tend to stir sexual impulses and lead to sexually impure thoughts." *** Not only did this charge fail to measure up to the standards which I understand the Court to approve, but as far as I can see, much of the great literature of the world could lead to conviction under such a view of the statute. Moreover, in no event do I think that the limited federal interest in this area can extend to mere "thoughts." The Federal Government has no business, whether under the postal or commerce power, to bar the sale of books because they might lead to any kind of "thoughts."

It is no answer to say, as the Court does, that obscenity is not protected speech. The point is that this statute, as here construed, defines obscenity so widely that it encompasses matters which might very well be protected speech. I do not think that

---

7. To give only a few examples: Edmund Wilson's "Memoirs of Hecate County" was found obscene in New York, see Doubleday & Co. v. New York, 335 U.S. 848; a bookseller indicted for selling the same book was acquitted in California. "God's Little Acre" was held to be obscene in Massachusetts, not obscene in New York and Pennsylvania.

the federal statute can be constitutionally construed to reach other than what the Government has termed as "hard-core" pornography. Nor do I think the statute can fairly be read as directed only at *persons* who are engaged in the business of catering to the prurient minded, even though their wares fall short of hard-core pornography. Such a statute would raise constitutional questions of a different order. That being so, and since in my opinion the material here involved cannot be said to be hard-core pornography, I would reverse this case with instructions to dismiss the indictment.

MR. JUSTICE DOUGLAS, with whom MR. JUSTICE BLACK concurs, dissenting.

When we sustain these convictions, we make the legality of a publication turn on the purity of thought which a book or tract instills in the mind of the reader. I do not think we can approve that standard and be faithful to the command of the First Amendment, which by its terms is a restraint on Congress and which by the Fourteenth is a restraint on the States.

In the *Roth* case the trial judge charged the jury that the statutory words "obscene, lewd and lascivious" describe "that form of immorality which has relation to sexual impurity and has a tendency to excite lustful thoughts."

*** The trial judge who, sitting without a jury, heard the *Alberts* case and the appellate court that sustained the judgment of conviction, took California's definition of "obscenity" from People v. Wepplo, 178 P. 2d 853, 855. That case held that a book is obscene "if it has a substantial tendency to deprave or corrupt its readers by inciting lascivious thoughts or arousing lustful desire."

By these standards punishment is inflicted for thoughts provoked, not for overt acts nor antisocial conduct. This test cannot be squared with our decisions under the First Amendment. Even the ill-starred *Dennis* case conceded that speech to be punishable must have some relation to action which could be penalized by government. Dennis v. United States, 341 U.S. 494, 502- 511. *** This issue cannot be avoided by saying that obscenity is not protected by the First Amendment. The question remains, what is the constitutional test of obscenity?

The tests by which these convictions were obtained require only the arousing of sexual thoughts. Yet the arousing of sexual thoughts and desires happens every day in normal life in dozens of ways. Nearly 30 years ago a questionnaire sent to college and normal school women graduates asked what things were most stimulating sexually. Of 409 replies, 9 said "music"; 18 said "pictures"; 29 said "dancing"; 40 said "drama"; 95 said "books"; and 218 said "man." Alpert, Judicial Censorship of Obscene Literature, 52 Harv. L. Rev. 40, 73.

The test of obscenity the Court endorses today gives the censor free range over a vast domain. To allow the State to step in and punish mere speech or publication that the judge or the jury thinks has an *undesirable* impact on thoughts but that is not shown to be a part of unlawful action is drastically to curtail the First Amendment. As recently stated by two of our outstanding authorities on obscenity, "The danger of influencing a change in the current moral standards of the community, or of shocking or offending readers, or of stimulating sex thoughts or desires apart from objective conduct, can never justify the losses to society that result from interference with literary freedom." Lockhart & McClure, Literature, The Law of Obscenity, and the Constitution, 38 Minn. L. Rev. 295, 387. ***

[T]he trial judge in the *Roth* case charged the jury in the alternative that the federal obscenity statute outlaws literature dealing with sex which offends "the common conscience of the community." That standard is, in my view, more inimical still to freedom of expression. *** Certainly that standard would not be an acceptable one if religion, economics, politics or philosophy were involved. How does it become a constitutional standard when literature treating with sex is concerned?

Any test that turns on what is offensive to the community's standards is too loose, too capricious, too destructive of freedom of expression to be squared with the First Amendment. *** This is community censorship in one of its worst forms. It creates a regime where in the battle between the literati and the Philistines, the Philistines are certain to win. If experience in this field teaches anything, it is that "censorship of obscenity has almost always been both irrational and indiscriminate." Lockhart & McClure, at 371. The test adopted here accentuates that trend. ***

I can understand (and at times even sympathize) with programs of civic groups and church groups to protect and defend the existing moral standards of the community. I can understand the motives of the Anthony Comstocks who would impose Victorian standards on the community. When speech alone is involved, I do not think that government, consistently with the First Amendment, can become the sponsor of any of these movements. I do not think that government, consistently with the First Amendment, can throw its weight behind one school or another. ***

The Court today suggests a third standard. It defines obscene material as that "which deals with sex in a manner appealing to prurient interest." Like the standards applied by the trial judges below, that standard does not require any nexus between the literature which is prohibited and action which the legislature can regulate or prohibit. Under the First Amendment, that standard is no more valid than those which the courts below adopted. ***

Freedom of expression can be suppressed if, and to the extent that, it is so closely brigaded with illegal action as to be an inseparable part of it. *** As a people, we cannot afford to relax that standard. For the test that suppresses a cheap tract today can suppress a literary gem tomorrow. All it need do is to incite a lascivious thought or arouse a lustful desire. The list of books that judges or juries can place in that category is endless.

I would give the broad sweep of the First Amendment full support. I have the same confidence in the ability of our people to reject noxious literature as I have in their capacity to sort out the true from the false in theology, economics, politics, or any other field.

SMITH v. CALIFORNIA
361 U.S. 147 (1959)

MR. JUSTICE BRENNAN delivered the opinion of the Court.

Appellant, the proprietor of a bookstore, was convicted in a California Municipal Court under a Los Angeles City ordinance which makes it unlawful "for any person to have in his possession any obscene or indecent writing, [or] book *** [in] any place of business where *** books *** are sold or kept for sale." The offense was defined by the Municipal Court, and by the Appellate Department of the Superior Court, which affirmed the Municipal Court judgment imposing a jail sentence on appellant, as consisting solely of the possession, in the appellant's bookstore, of a certain book found upon judicial investigation to be obscene. The definition included no element of scienter—knowledge by appellant of the contents of the book —and thus the ordinance was construed as imposing a "strict" or "absolute" criminal liability. ***

We have held that obscene speech and writings are not protected by the constitutional guarantees of freedom of speech and the press. Roth v. United States, 354 U.S. 476. The ordinance here in question, to be sure, only imposes criminal sanctions on a bookseller if in fact there is to be found in his shop an obscene book. But our holding in *Roth* does not recognize any state power to restrict the dissemination of books which are not obscene; and we think this ordinance's strict liability feature would tend seriously to have that effect, by penalizing booksellers, even though they had not the slightest notice of the character of the books they sold. The appellee and the court below analogize this strict liability penal ordinance to familiar forms of penal statutes which dispense with any element of knowledge on the part of the person charged, food and drug legislation being a principal example. We find the analogy instructive in our examination of the question before us. The usual rationale for such statutes is that the public interest in the purity of its food is so great as to warrant the imposition of the highest standard of care on distributors—in fact an absolute standard which will not hear the distributor's plea as to the amount of care he has used. *** His ignorance of the character of the food is irrelevant. There is no specific constitutional inhibition against making the distributors of food the strictest censors of their merchandise, but the constitutional guarantees of the freedom of speech and of the press stand in the way of imposing a similar requirement on the bookseller. By dispensing with any requirement of knowledge of the contents of the book on the part of the seller, the ordinance tends to impose a severe limitation on the public's access to constitutionally protected matter. *** It has been well observed of a statute construed as dispensing with any requirement of scienter that: "Every bookseller would be placed under an obligation to make himself aware of the contents of every book in his shop. It would be altogether unreasonable to demand so near an approach to omniscience." The King v. Ewart, 25 N.Z.L.R. 709, 729 (C.A.). And the bookseller's burden would become the public's burden, for by restricting him the public's access to reading matter would be restricted. ***

It is argued that unless the scienter requirement is dispensed with, regulation of the distribution of obscene material will be ineffective, as booksellers will falsely disclaim knowledge of their books' contents or falsely deny reason to suspect their obscenity. We might observe that it has been some time now since the law viewed itself as impotent to explore the actual state of a man's mind. See Pound, The Role of the Will in Law, 68 Harv. L. Rev. 1. Cf. American Communications Assn. v. Douds, 339 U.S. 382, 411. Eyewitness testimony of a bookseller's perusal of a book hardly need be a necessary element in proving his awareness of its contents. The circumstances may warrant the inference that he was aware of what a book contained, despite his denial.

We need not and most definitely do not pass today on what sort of mental element is requisite to a constitutionally permissible prosecution of a bookseller for carrying an obscene book in stock; whether honest mistake as to whether its contents in fact constituted obscenity need be an excuse; whether there might be circumstances under which the State constitutionally might require that a bookseller investigate further, or might put on him the burden of explaining why he did not, and what such circumstances might be. Doubtless any form of criminal obscenity statute applicable to a bookseller will induce some tendency to self-censorship and have some inhibitory effect on the dissemination of material not obscene, but we consider today only one which goes to the extent of eliminating all mental elements from the crime.

Reversed.

MR. JUSTICE BLACK, concurring.

The appellant was sentenced to prison for possessing in his bookstore an "obscene" book in violation of a Los Angeles city ordinance. I concur in the judgment holding that ordinance unconstitutional, but not for the reasons given in the Court's opinion.

*** The Court's opinion correctly points out how little extra burden will be imposed on prosecutors by requiring proof that a bookseller was aware of a book's contents when he possessed it. And if the Constitution's requirement of knowledge is so easily met, the result of this case is that one particular bookseller gains his freedom, but the way is left open for state censorship and punishment of all other booksellers by merely adding a few new words to old censorship laws. Our constitutional safeguards for speech and press therefore gain little. Their victory, if any, is a Pyrrhic one. Cf. Beauharnais v. Illinois, 343 U.S. 250, 267, at 275 (dissenting opinion).***

MR. JUSTICE FRANKFURTER, concurring. [Omitted]

MR. JUSTICE DOUGLAS, concurring.

I need not repeat here all I said in my dissent in Roth v. United States, 354 U.S. 476, 508, to underline my conviction that neither the author nor the distributor of this book can be punished under our Bill of Rights for publishing or distributing it. ***

Yet my view is in the minority; and rather fluid tests of obscenity prevail which require judges to read condemned literature and pass judgment on it. This role of censor in which we find ourselves is not an edifying one. But since by the prevailing school of thought we must perform it, I see no harm, and perhaps some good, in the rule fashioned by the Court which requires a showing of scienter. ***

MR. JUSTICE HARLAN, concurring in part and dissenting in part. [Omitted.]

KINGSLEY INTERNATIONAL PICTURES CORPORATION v. REGENTS OF THE UNIVERSITY OF THE STATE OF NEW YORK

360 U.S. 684 (1959)

MR. JUSTICE STEWART delivered the opinion of the Court.

The New York statute makes it unlawful "to exhibit, or to sell, lease or lend for exhibition at any place of amusement for pay or in connection with any business in the state of New York, any motion picture film or reel [with certain exceptions not relevant here], unless there is at the time in full force and effect a valid license or permit therefor of the education department." The law provides that a license shall issue "unless such film or a part thereof is obscene, indecent, immoral, inhuman, sacrilegious, or is of such a character that its exhibition would tend to corrupt morals or incite to crime." A recent statutory amendment provides that, "the term 'immoral' and the phrase 'of such a character that its exhibition would tend to corrupt morals' shall denote a motion picture film or part thereof, the dominant purpose or effect of which is erotic or pornographic; or which portrays acts of sexual immorality, perversion, or lewdness, or which expressly or impliedly presents such acts as desirable, acceptable or proper patterns of behavior."

As the distributor of a motion picture entitled "Lady Chatterley's Lover," the appellant Kingsley submitted that film to the Motion Picture Division of the New York Education Department for a license. Finding three isolated scenes in the film "'immoral' within the intent of our Law," the Division refused to issue a license until the scenes in question were deleted. The distributor petitioned the Regents of the University of the State of New York for a review of that ruling. The Regents upheld the denial of a license, but on the broader ground that "the whole theme of this motion picture is immoral under said law, for that theme is the presentation of adultery as a desirable, acceptable and proper pattern of behavior."

The Court of Appeals unanimously and explicitly rejected any notion that the film is obscene. Rather, the court found that the picture as a whole "alluringly portrays adultery as proper behavior." As Chief Judge Conway's prevailing opinion emphasized, therefore, the only portion of the statute involved in this case is that part of §§ 122 and 122-a of the Education Law requiring the denial of a license to motion pictures "which are immoral in that they portray 'acts of sexual immorality *** as desirable, acceptable or proper patterns of behavior.'"

That construction, we emphasize, gives to the term "sexual immorality" a concept entirely different from the concept embraced in words like "obscenity" or "pornography." Moreover, it is not suggested that the film would itself operate as an incitement to illegal action. Rather, the New York Court of Appeals tells us that the relevant portion of the New York Education Law requires the denial of a license to any motion picture which approvingly portrays an adulterous relationship, quite without reference to the manner of its portrayal. ***

It is contended that the State's action was justified because the motion picture attractively portrays a relationship which is contrary to the moral standards, the religious precepts, and the legal code of its citizenry. This argument misconceives what it is that the Constitution protects. Its guarantee is not confined to the expression of ideas that are conventional or shared by a majority. It protects advocacy of the opinion that adultery may sometimes be proper, no less than advocacy of socialism or the single tax. And in the realm of ideas it protects expression which is eloquent no less than that which is unconvincing.

Advocacy of conduct proscribed by law is not, as Mr. Justice Brandeis long ago pointed out, "a justification for denying free speech where the advocacy falls short of incitement and there is nothing to indicate that the advocacy would be immediately acted on." Whitney v. California, 274 U.S. 357, at 376 (concurring opinion).

The inflexible command which the New York Court of Appeals has attributed to the State Legislature thus cuts so close to the core of constitutional freedom as to make it quite needless in this case to examine the periphery. Specifically, there is no occasion to consider the appellant's contention that the State is entirely without power to require films of any kind to be licensed prior to their exhibition. Nor need we here determine whether, despite problems peculiar to motion pictures, the controls which a State may impose upon this medium of expression are precisely coextensive with those allowable for newspapers, books, or individual speech. It is enough for the present case to reaffirm that motion pictures are within the First and Fourteenth Amendments' basic protection. Joseph Burstyn, Inc. v. Wilson, 343 U.S. 495.

Reversed. [Concurring opinions omitted.]

A BOOK NAMED "JOHN CLELAND'S MEMOIRS OF A WOMAN WOMAN OF PLEASURE" v. ATTORNEY GENERAL OF MASSACHUSETTS

383 U.S. 413 (1966)

MR. JUSTICE BRENNAN announced the judgment of the Court and delivered an opinion in which THE CHIEF JUSTICE and MR. JUSTICE FORTAS join.

This is an obscenity case in which *Memoirs of a Woman of Pleasure* (commonly known as *Fanny Hill*), written by John Cleland in about 1750, was adjudged obscene in a proceeding that put on trial the book itself, and not its publisher or distributor. The proceeding was a civil equity suit brought by the Attorney General of Massachusetts, pursuant to General Laws of Massachusetts, Chapter 272, §§ 28C-28H, to have the book declared obscene. Section 28C requires that the petition commencing the suit be "directed against [the] book by name" and that an order to show cause "why said book should not be judicially determined to be obscene" be published in a daily newspaper and sent by registered mail "to all persons interested in the publication." Publication of the order in this case occurred in a Boston daily newspaper, and a copy of the order was sent by registered mail to G.P. Putnam's Sons, alleged to be the publisher and copyright holder of the book.

As authorized by § 28D, G.P. Putnam's Sons intervened in the proceedings in behalf of the book, but it did not claim the right provided by that section to have the issue of obscenity tried by a jury. At the hearing before a justice of the Superior Court, which was conducted, under § 28F, "in accordance with the usual course of proceedings in equity," the court received the book in evidence and also, as allowed by the section, heard the testimony of experts[2] and accepted other evidence, such as book reviews, in order to assess the literary, cultural, or educational character of the book. This constituted the entire evidence, as neither side availed itself of the opportunity provided by the section to introduce evidence "as to the manner and form of its publication, advertisement, and distribution." The trial justice entered a final decree, which adjudged *Memoirs* obscene and declared that the book "is not entitled to the protection of the First and Fourteenth Amendments to the Constitution of the United States against action by the Attorney General or other law enforcement officer pursuant to the provisions of *** § 28B, or otherwise." The Massachusetts Supreme Judicial Court affirmed the decree. *** We noted probable jurisdiction. We reverse.

I

* * *

We defined obscenity in *Roth* in the following terms: "[Whether] to the average person, applying contemporary community standards, the dominant theme of the material taken as a whole appeals to prurient interest." Under this definition, as elaborated in subsequent cases, three elements must coalesce: it must be established that

---

2. *** "In the view of one or another or all of the following viz., the chairman of the English department at Williams College, a professor of English at Harvard College, an associate professor of English literature at Boston University, an associate professor of English at Massachusetts Institute of Technology, and an assistant professor of English and American literature at Brandeis University, the book is a minor 'work of art' having 'literary merit' and 'historical value' and containing a good deal of 'deliberate, calculated comedy.' It is a piece of 'social history of interest to anyone who is interested in fiction as a way of understanding society in the past.' *** In the opinion of the other academic witness, the headmaster of a private school, whose field is English literature, the book is without literary merit and is obscene, impure, hard core pornography, and is patently offensive."

(a) the dominant theme of the material taken as a whole appeals to a prurient interest in sex; (b) the material is patently offensive because it affronts contemporary community standards relating to the description or representation of sexual matters; and (c) the material is utterly without redeeming social value.

The Supreme Judicial Court purported to apply the *Roth* definition of obscenity and held all three criteria satisfied. We need not consider the claim that the court erred in concluding that *Memoirs* satisfied the prurient appeal and patent offensiveness criteria; for reversal is required because the court misinterpreted the social value criterion. The court applied the criterion in this passage:

> "It remains to consider whether the book can be said to be 'utterly without social importance.' We are mindful that there was expert testimony, much of which was strained, to the effect that Memoirs is a structural novel with literary merit; that the book displays a skill in characterization and a gift for comedy; that it plays a part in the history of the development of the English novel; and that it contains a moral, namely, that sex with love is superior to sex in a brothel. But the fact that the testimony may indicate this book has some minimal literary value does not mean it is of any social importance. We do not interpret the 'social importance' test as requiring that a book which appeals to prurient interest and is patently offensive must be unqualifiedly worthless before it can be deemed obscene." ***

The Supreme Judicial Court erred in holding that a book need not be "unqualifiedly worthless before it can be deemed obscene." A book cannot be proscribed unless it is found to be *utterly* without redeeming social value. This is so even though the book is found to possess the requisite prurient appeal and to be patently offensive. Each of the three federal constitutional criteria is to be applied independently; the social value of the book can neither be weighed against nor canceled by its prurient appeal or patent offensiveness. Hence, even on the view of the court below that *Memoirs* possessed only a modicum of social value, its judgment must be reversed as being founded on an erroneous interpretation of a federal constitutional standard.

II

It does not necessarily follow from this reversal that a determination that *Memoirs* is obscene in the constitutional sense would be improper under all circumstances. On the premise, which we have no occasion to assess, that *Memoirs* has the requisite prurient appeal and is patently offensive, but has only a minimum of social value, the circumstances of production, sale, and publicity are relevant in determining whether or not the publication or distribution of the book is constitutionally protected. Evidence that the book was commercially exploited for the sake of prurient appeal, to the exclusion of all other values, might justify the conclusion that the book was utterly without redeeming social importance. It is not that in such a setting the social value test is relaxed so as to dispense with the requirement that a book be utterly devoid of social value, but rather that, as we elaborate in *Ginzburg v. United*

States, where the purveyor's sole emphasis is on the sexually provocative aspects of his publications, a court could accept his evaluation at its face value. In this proceeding, however, the courts were asked to judge the obscenity of *Memoirs* in the abstract, and the declaration of obscenity was neither aided nor limited by a specific set of circumstances of production, sale, and publicity. All possible uses of the book must therefore be considered, and the mere risk that the book might be exploited by panderers because it so pervasively treats sexual matters cannot alter the fact—given the view of the Massachusetts court attributing to *Memoirs* a modicum of literary and historical value—that the book will have redeeming social importance in the hands of those who publish or distribute it on the basis of that value.

Reversed.

MR. JUSTICE DOUGLAS, concurring in the judgment.

Memoirs of a Woman of Pleasure, or, as it is often titled, *Fanny Hill,* concededly is an erotic novel. It was first published in about 1749 and has endured to this date, despite periodic efforts to suppress it.[3] In 1963, an American publishing house undertook the publication of *Memoirs*. The record indicates that an unusually large number of orders were placed by universities and libraries; the Library of Congress requested the right to translate the book into Braille. But the Commonwealth of Massachusetts instituted the suit that ultimately found its way here, praying that the book be declared obscene so that the citizens of Massachusetts might be spared the necessity of determining for themselves whether or not to read it. ***

The censor is always quick to justify his function in terms that are protective of society. But the First Amendment, written in terms that are absolute, deprives the States of any power to pass on the value, the propriety, or the morality of a particular expression. *** Perhaps the most frequently assigned justification for censorship is the belief that erotica produce antisocial sexual conduct. But that relationship has yet to be proven. Indeed, if one were to make judgments on the basis of speculation, one might guess that literature of the most pornographic sort would, in many cases, provide a substitute—not a stimulus—for antisocial sexual conduct. See Murphy, The Value of Pornography, 10 Wayne L. Rev. 655, 661 and n. 19 (1964). As I read the First Amendment, judges cannot gear the literary diet of an entire nation to whatever tepid stuff is incapable of triggering the most demented mind. The First Amendment demands more than a horrible example or two of the perpetrator of a crime of sexual

3. *Memoirs* was the subject of what is generally regarded as the first recorded suppression of a literary work in this country on grounds of obscenity. See Commonwealth v. Holmes, 17 Mass. 336 (1821). The edition there condemned differed from the present volume in that it contained apparently erotic illustrations.

violence, in whose pocket is found a pornographic book, before it allows the Nation to be saddled with a regime of censorship.[11]

Whatever may be the reach of the power to regulate *conduct*, I stand by my view in *Roth v. United States*, that the First Amendment leaves no power in government over *expression of ideas*. ***

MR. JUSTICE CLARK, dissenting.

It is with regret that I write this dissenting opinion. However, the public should know of the continuous flow of pornographic material reaching this Court and the increasing problem States have in controlling it. *Memoirs of a Woman of Pleasure*, the book involved here, is typical. I have "stomached" past cases for almost 10 years without much outcry. *** In order to give my remarks the proper setting I have been obliged to portray the book's contents, which causes me embarrassment. However, quotations from typical episodes would so debase our Reports that I will not follow that course. ***

Memoirs is nothing more than a series of minutely and vividly described sexual episodes. The book starts with Fanny Hill, a young 15-year-old girl, arriving in London to seek household work. She goes to an employment office where through happenstance she meets the mistress of a bawdy house. This takes 10 pages. The remaining 200 pages of the book detail her initiation into various sexual experiences, from a lesbian encounter with a sister prostitute to all sorts and types of sexual debauchery in bawdy houses and as the mistress of a variety of men. This is presented to the reader through an uninterrupted succession of descriptions by Fanny, either as an observer or participant, of sexual adventures so vile that one of the male expert witnesses in the case was hesitant to repeat any one of them in the courtroom. These scenes run the gamut of possible sexual experience such as lesbianism, female masturbation, homosexuality between young boys, the destruction of a maidenhead with consequent gory descriptions, the seduction of a young virgin boy, the flagellation

---

11. It would be a futile effort even for a censor to attempt to remove all that might possibly stimulate antisocial sexual conduct:

"The majority [of individuals], needless to say, are somewhere between the over-scrupulous extremes of excitement and frigidity ***. Within this variety, it is impossible to define 'hard-core' pornography, as if there were some singly lewd concept from which all profane ideas passed by imperceptible degrees into that sexuality called holy. But there is no 'hard-core.' Everything, every idea, is capable of being obscene if the personality perceiving it so apprehends it.

"It is for this reason that books, pictures, charades, ritual, the spoken word, *can* and *do* lead directly to conduct harmful to the self indulging in it and to others. Heinrich Pommerenke, who was a rapist, abuser, and mass slayer of women in Germany, was prompted to his series of ghastly deeds by Cecil B. DeMille's *The Ten Commandments*. During the scene of the Jewish women dancing about the Golden Calf, all the doubts of his life came clear: Women were the source of the world's trouble and it was his mission to both punish them for this and to execute them. Leaving the theater, he slew his first victim in a park nearby. ***" Murphy, *supra*, at 668.

of male by female, and vice versa, followed by fervid sexual engagement, and other abhorrent acts, including over two dozen separate bizarre descriptions of different sexual intercourses between male and female characters. In one sequence four girls in a bawdy house are required in the presence of one another to relate the lurid details of their loss of virginity and their glorification of it. This is followed the same evening by "publick trials" in which each of the four girls engages in sexual intercourse with a different man while the others witness, with Fanny giving a detailed description of the movement and reaction of each couple. ***

*** In my view, the book's repeated and unrelieved appeals to the prurient interest of the average person leave it utterly without redeeming social importance.

In his separate concurrence, my Brother DOUGLAS asserts there is no proof that obscenity produces antisocial conduct. *** [T]here are medical experts who believe that such stimulation frequently manifests itself in criminal sexual behavior or other antisocial conduct. For example, Dr. George W. Henry of Cornell University has expressed the opinion that obscenity, with its exaggerated and morbid emphasis on sex, particularly abnormal and perverted practices, and its unrealistic presentation of sexual behavior and attitudes, may induce antisocial conduct by the average person. A number of sociologists think that this material may have adverse effects upon individual mental health, with potentially disruptive consequences for the community. ***

MR. JUSTICE HARLAN, dissenting.

My premise is that in the area of obscenity the Constitution does not bind the States and the Federal Government in precisely the same fashion. This approach is plainly consistent with the language of the First and Fourteenth Amendments and, in my opinion, more responsive to the proper functioning of a federal system of government in this area. Federal suppression of allegedly obscene matter should, in my view, be constitutionally limited to that often described as "hard-core pornography." To me it is plain, for instance, that *Fanny Hill* does not fall within this class and could not be barred from the federal mails. ***

State obscenity laws present problems of quite a different order. The varying conditions across the country, the range of views on the need and reasons for curbing obscenity, and the traditions of local self-government in matters of public welfare all favor a far more flexible attitude in defining the bounds for the States. From my standpoint, the Fourteenth Amendment requires of a State only that it apply criteria rationally related to the accepted notion of obscenity and that it reach results not wholly out of step with current American standards. *** I think it more satisfactory to acknowledge that on this record the book has been shown to have some quantum of social value, that it may at the same time be deemed offensive and salacious, and that the State's decision to weigh these elements and to ban this particular work does not exceed constitutional limits.

MR. JUSTICE WHITE, dissenting. [Omitted]

GINZBURG v. UNITED STATES
383 U.S. 463 (1966)

MR. JUSTICE BRENNAN delivered the opinion of the Court.

A judge sitting without a jury in the District Court for the Eastern District of Pennsylvania convicted petitioner Ginzburg and three corporations controlled by him upon all 28 counts of an indictment charging violation of the federal obscenity statute, 18 U.S.C. § 3237 (1964 ed.). ***

In the cases in which this Court has decided obscenity questions since *Roth*, it has regarded the materials as sufficient in themselves for the determination of the question. In the present case, however, the prosecution charged the offense in the context of the circumstances of production, sale, and publicity and assumed that, standing alone, the publications themselves might not be obscene. We agree that the question of obscenity may include consideration of the setting in which the publications were presented as an aid to determining the question of obscenity, and assume without deciding that the prosecution could not have succeeded otherwise.

The three publications were EROS, a hard-cover magazine of expensive format; Liaison, a bi-weekly newsletter; and *The Housewife's Handbook on Selective Promiscuity* (hereinafter the *Handbook*), a short book. The issue of EROS, contains 15 articles and photo-essays on the subject of love, sex, and sexual relations. The specified issue of Liaison, Vol. 1, No. 1, contains a prefatory "letter from the Editors" announcing its dedication to "keeping sex an art and preventing it from becoming a science." The remainder of the issue consists of digests of two articles concerning sex and sexual relations which had earlier appeared in professional journals and a report of an interview with a psychotherapist who favors the broadest license in sexual relationships. As the trial judge noted, "[w]hile the treatment is largely superficial, it is presented entirely without restraint of any kind. According to defendants' own expert, it is entirely without literary merit." The *Handbook* purports to be a sexual autobiography detailing with compete candor the author's sexual experiences from age 3 to age 36. The text includes, and prefatory and concluding sections of the book elaborate, her views on such subjects as sex education of children, laws regulating private consensual adult sexual practices, and the equality of women in sexual relationships. It was claimed at trial that women would find the book valuable, for example as a marriage manual or as an aid to the sex education of their children.

Besides testimony as to the merit of the material, there was abundant evidence to show that each of the accused publications was originated or sold as stock in trade of the sordid business of pandering—"the business of purveying textual or graphic matter openly advertised to appeal to the erotic interest of their customers." EROS early sought mailing privileges from the postmasters of Intercourse and Blue Ball,

Pennsylvania. The trial court found the obvious, that these hamlets were chosen only for the value their names would have in furthering petitioners' efforts to sell their publications on the basis of salacious appeal; the facilities of the post offices were inadequate to handle the anticipated volume of mail, and the privileges were denied. Mailing privileges were then obtained from the postmaster of Middlesex, New Jersey.

The "leer of the sensualist" also permeates the advertising for the three publications. The circulars sent for EROS and Liaison stressed the sexual candor of the respective publications, and openly boasted that the publishers would take full advantage of what they regarded as an unrestricted license allowed by law in the expression of sex and sexual matters. ***

This evidence, in our view, was relevant in determining the ultimate question of obscenity and, in the context of this record, serves to resolve all ambiguity and doubt. The deliberate representation of petitioners' publications as erotically arousing, for example, stimulated the reader to accept them as prurient; he looks for titillation, not for saving intellectual content. Where the purveyors sole emphasis is on the sexually provocative aspects of his publications, that fact may be decisive in the determination of obscenity.

We perceive no threat to First Amendment guarantees in thus holding that in close cases evidence of pandering may be probative with respect to the nature of the material in question and thus satisfy the *Roth* test. No weight is ascribed to the fact that petitioners have profited from the sale of publications which we have assumed but do not hold cannot themselves be adjudged obscene in the abstract; to sanction consideration of this fact might indeed induce self-censorship, and offend the frequently stated principle that commercial activity, in itself, is no justification for narrowing the protection of expression secured by the First Amendment. Rather, the fact that each of these publications was created or exploited entirely on the basis of its appeal to prurient interests strengthens the conclusion that the transactions here were sales of illicit merchandise, not sales of constitutionally protected matter.

Affirmed.

MR. JUSTICE BLACK, dissenting.

I agree with part II of the dissent of my Brother DOUGLAS in this case, and I would reverse Ginzburg's conviction on this ground alone.

I agree with my Brother HARLAN that the Court has in effect rewritten the federal obscenity statute and thereby imposed on Ginzburg standards and criteria that Congress never thought about; or if it did think about them, certainly it did not adopt them. Consequently, Ginzburg is, as I see it, having his conviction and sentence affirmed upon the basis of a statute amended by this Court for violation of which amended statute he was not charged in the courts below. Such an affirmance we have said violates due process. ***

MR. JUSTICE DOUGLAS, dissenting.

Today's condemnation of the use of sex symbols to sell literature engrafts another exception on First Amendment rights that is as unwarranted as the judge-made exception concerning obscenity. This new exception condemns an advertising technique as old as history. The advertisements of our best magazines are chock-full of thighs, ankles, calves, bosoms, eyes, and hair, to draw the potential buyer's attention to lotions, tires, food, liquor, clothing, autos, and even insurance policies. The sexy advertisement neither adds to nor detracts from the quality of the merchandise being offered for sale. And I do not see how it adds to or detracts one whit from the legality of the book being distributed. A book should stand on its own, irrespective of the reasons why it was written or the wiles used in selling it. I cannot imagine any promotional effort that would make chapters 7 and 8 of the Song of Solomon any less or any more worthy of First Amendment protection than does their unostentatious inclusion in the average edition of the Bible. ***

Some of the tracts for which publishers go to prison concern normal sex, some homosexuality, some the masochistic yearning that is probably present in everyone and dominant in some. Masochism is a desire to be punished or subdued. In the broad frame of reference the desire may be expressed in the longing to be whipped and lashed, bound and gagged, and cruelly treated. Why is it unlawful to cater to the needs of this group? They are, to be sure, somewhat offbeat, nonconformist, and odd. But we are not in the realm of criminal conduct, only ideas and tastes. Some like Chopin, others like "rock and roll." ***

II

This leads me to the conclusion, previously noted, that the First Amendment allows all ideas to be expressed—whether orthodox, popular, offbeat, or repulsive. I do not think it permissible to draw lines between the "good" and the "bad" and be true to the constitutional mandate to let all ideas alone. If our Constitution permitted "reasonable" regulation of freedom of expression, as do the constitutions of some nations, we would be in a field where the legislative and the judiciary would have much leeway. But under our charter all regulation or control of expression is barred. Government does not sit to reveal where the "truth" is. People are left to pick and choose between competing offerings. There is no compulsion to take and read what is repulsive any more than there is to spend one's time poring over government bulletins, political tracts, or theological treatises. ***

I think this is the ideal of the Free Society written into our Constitution. We have no business acting as censors or endowing any group with censorship powers. It is shocking to me for us to send to prison anyone for publishing anything, especially tracts so distant from any incitement to action as the ones before us. ***

MR. JUSTICE HARLAN, dissenting.

I would reverse the convictions of Ginzburg and his three corporate co-defendants.

Although it is not clear whether the majority views the panderer test as a statutory gloss or as constitutional doctrine, I read the opinion to be in the latter category. The First Amendment, in the obscenity area, no longer fully protects material on its face nonobscene, for such material must now also be examined in the light of the defendant's conduct, attitude, motives. This seems to me a mere euphemism for allowing punishment of a person who mails otherwise constitutionally protected material just because a jury or a judge may not find him or his business agreeable. Were a State to enact a "panderer" statute under its police power, I have little doubt that—subject to clear drafting to avoid attacks on vagueness and equal protection grounds —such a statute would be constitutional. Possibly the same might be true of the Federal Government acting under its postal or commerce powers. What I fear the Court has done to day is in effect to write a new statute, but without the sharply focused definitions and standards necessary in such a sensitive area. Casting dubious gloss over a straightforward 101-year old statute is for me an astonishing piece of judicial improvisation. ***

*** In addition, I think such a test for obscenity is impermissibly vague, and unwarranted by anything in the First Amendment or in 18 U.S.C. § 1461.

I would reverse the judgments below.

MR. JUSTICE STEWART, dissenting.

***

The Court today appears to concede that the materials Ginzburg mailed were themselves protected by the First Amendment. But, the Court says, Ginzburg can still be sentenced to five years in prison for mailing them. Why? Because, says the Court, he was guilty of "commercial exploitation," of "pandering," and of "titillation." But Ginzburg was not charged with "commercial exploitation"; he was not charged with "pandering"; he was not charged with "titillation." Therefore, to affirm his conviction now on any of those grounds, even if otherwise valid, is to deny him due process of law. ***

For me, however, there is another aspect of the Court's opinion in this case that is even more regrettable. Today the Court assumes the power to deny Ralph Ginzburg the protection of the First Amendment because it disapproves of his "sordid business." That is a power the Court does not possess. For the First Amendment protects us all with an even hand. It applies to Ralph Ginzburg with no less completeness and force than to G. P. Putnam's Sons. In upholding and enforcing the Bill of Rights, this Court has no power to pick or to choose. When we lose sight of that fixed star of constitutional adjudication, we lose our way. For then we forsake a government of law and are left with government by Big Brother.

I dissent.

MISHKIN v. NEW YORK
383 U.S. 502 (1966)

MR. JUSTICE BRENNAN delivered the opinion of the Court.

This case, like *Ginzburg v. United States*, also decided today, involves convictions under a criminal obscenity statute. A panel of three judges of the Court of Special Sessions of the City of New York found appellant guilty of violating § 1141 of the New York Penal Law[1] by hiring others to prepare obscene books with intent to sell them. ***

Appellant was not prosecuted for anything he said or believed, but for what he did, for his dominant role in several enterprises engaged in producing and selling allegedly obscene books. Fifty books are involved in this case. They portray sexuality in many guises. Some depict relatively normal heterosexual relations, but more depict such deviations as sado-masochism, fetishism, and homosexuality. Many have covers with drawings of scantily clad women being whipped, beaten, tortured, or abused. *** Typical of appellant's instructions was that related by one author who testified that appellant insisted that the books be "full of sex scenes and lesbian scenes. *** [T]he sex had to be very strong, it had to be rough, it had to be clearly spelled out. *** I had to write sex very bluntly, make the sex scenes between men and women, and women and women, and men and men. *** [A]nd there were spankings and scenes—sex in an abnormal and irregular fashion." Another author testified that appellant instructed him "to deal very graphically with the darkening of the flesh under flagellation." Artists testified in similar vein as to appellant's instructions regarding illustrations and covers for the books. All the books are cheaply prepared paperbound "pulps" with imprinted sales prices that are several thousand percent above costs.

*** [A]ppellant's sole contention regarding the nature of the material is that some of the books involved in this prosecution, those depicting various deviant sexual practices, such as flagellation, fetishism, and lesbianism, do not satisfy the prurient-appeal requirement because they do not appeal to a prurient interest of the "average person" in sex, that "instead of stimulating the erotic, they disgust and sicken." We reject this argument as being founded on an unrealistic interpretation of the prurient- appeal requirement.

---

1. Section 1141 of the Penal Law, in pertinent part, reads as follows:

"1. A person who *** has in his possession with intent to sell, lend, distribute *** any obscene, lewd, lascivious, filthy, indecent, sadistic, masochistic or disgusting book *** or who *** prints, utters, publishes, or in any manner manufactures, or prepares any such book *** or who

"2. In any manner, hires, employs, uses or permits any person to do or assist in doing any act or thing mentioned in this section, or any of them,

"Is guilty of a misdemeanor. ***

Where the material is designed for and primarily disseminated to a clearly defined deviant sexual group, rather than the public at large, the prurient-appeal requirement of the *Roth* test is satisfied if the dominant theme of the material taken as a whole appeals to the prurient interest in sex of the members of that group. The reference to the "average" or "normal" person in *Roth*, does not foreclose this holding. In regard to the prurient-appeal requirement, the concept of the "average" or "normal" person was employed in *Roth* to serve the essentially negative purpose of expressing our rejection of that aspect of the *Hicklin* test, Regina v. Hicklin, [1868] L.R. 3. Q.B. 360, that made the impact on the most susceptible person determinative. We adjust the prurient-appeal requirement to social realities by permitting the appeal of this type of material to be assessed in terms of the sexual interests of its intended and probable recipient group; and since our holding requires that the recipient group be defined with more specificity than in terms of sexually immature persons, it also avoids the inadequacy of the most-susceptible-person facet of the *Hicklin* test.

No substantial claim is made that the books depicting sexually deviant practices are devoid of prurient appeal to sexually deviant groups. The evidence fully establishes that these books were specifically conceived and marketed for such groups. *** Affirmed.

[The concurring opinion of MR. JUSTICE HARLAN, and dissenting opinion of JUSTICES BLACK, DOUGLAS and STEWART, have been omitted.]

REDRUP v. NEW YORK

386 U.S. 767 (1967)

PER CURIAM.

These three cases arise from a recurring conflict—the conflict between asserted state power to suppress the distribution of books and magazines through criminal or civil proceedings, and the guarantees of the First and Fourteenth Amendments of the United States Constitution.

I

In No. 3, *Redrup v. New York*, the petitioner was a clerk at a New York City newsstand. A plainclothes patrolman approached the newsstand, saw two paperback books on a rack—Lust Pool, and Shame Agent—and asked for them by name. The petitioner handed him the books and collected the price of $1.65. As a result of this transaction, the petitioner was charged in the New York City Criminal Court with violating a state criminal law. He was convicted, and the conviction was affirmed on appeal.

In No. 16, *Austin v. Kentucky*, the petitioner owned and operated a retail bookstore and newsstand in Paducah, Kentucky. A woman resident of Paducah purchased two magazines from a salesgirl in the petitioner's store, after asking for them by name—High Heels, and Spree. As a result of this transaction the petitioner stands convicted in the Kentucky courts for violating a criminal law of that State.

In No. 50, *Gent v. Arkansas*, the prosecuting attorney of the Eleventh Judicial District of Arkansas brought a civil proceeding under a state statute to have certain issues of various magazines declared obscene, to enjoin their distribution and to obtain a judgment ordering their surrender and destruction. The magazines proceeded against were: Gent, Swank, Bachelor, Modern Man, Cavalcade, Gentleman, Ace, and Sir. The County Chancery Court entered the requested judgment after a trial with an advisory jury, and the Supreme Court of Arkansas affirmed, with minor modifications.

In none of the cases was there a claim that the statute in question reflected a specific and limited state concern for juveniles. See Prince v. Massachusetts, 321 U.S. 158; cf. Butler v. Michigan, 352 U.S. 380. In none was there any suggestion of an assault upon individual privacy by publication in a manner so obtrusive as to make it impossible for an unwilling individual to avoid exposure to it. *** And in none was there evidence of the sort of "pandering" which the Court found significant in Ginzburg v. United States, 383 U.S. 463.

II

The Court originally limited review in these cases to certain particularized questions, upon the hypothesis that the material involved in each case was of a character described as "obscene in the constitutional sense" in Memoirs v. Massachusetts, 383 U.S. 413, 418. But we have concluded that the hypothesis upon which the Court originally proceeded was invalid, and accordingly that the cases can and should be decided upon a common and controlling fundamental constitutional basis, without prejudice to the questions upon which review was originally granted. We have concluded, in short, that the distribution of the publications in each of these cases is protected by the First and Fourteenth Amendments from governmental suppression, whether criminal or civil, *in personam* or *in rem*.

Two members of the Court have consistently adhered to the view that a State is utterly without power to suppress, control, or punish the distribution of any writings or pictures upon the ground of their "obscenity." A third has held to the opinion that a State's power in this area is narrowly limited to a distinct and clearly identifiable class of material. Others have subscribed to a not dissimilar standard, holding that a State may not constitutionally inhibit the distribution of literary material as obscene unless "(a) the dominant theme of the material taken as a whole appeals to a prurient interest in sex; (b) the material is patently offensive because it affronts contemporary community standards relating to the description or representation of sexual matters; and (c) the material is utterly without redeeming social value," emphasizing that the "three elements must coalesce," and that no such material can "be proscribed unless it is found to be utterly without redeeming social value." Memoirs v. Massachusetts, 383 U.S. 413, 418-419. Another Justice has not viewed the "social value" element as an independent factor in the judgment of obscenity.

Whichever of these constitutional views is brought to bear upon the cases before us, it is clear that the judgments cannot stand. Accordingly, the judgment in each case is reversed.

It is so ordered.

MR. JUSTICE HARLAN, whom MR. JUSTICE CLARK joins, dissenting. [Omitted.]

STANLEY v. GEORGIA
394 U.S. 557 (1969)

MR. JUSTICE MARSHALL delivered the opinion of the Court.

An investigation of appellant's alleged bookmaking activities led to the issuance of a search warrant for appellant's home. Under authority of this warrant, federal and state agents secured entrance. They found very little evidence of bookmaking activity, but while looking through a desk drawer in an upstairs bedroom, one of the federal agents, accompanied by a state officer, found three reels of eight-millimeter film. Using a projector and screen found in an upstairs living room, they viewed the films. The state officer concluded that they were obscene and seized them. Since a further examination of the bedroom indicated that appellant occupied it, he was charged with possession of obscene matter and placed under arrest. He was later indicted for "knowingly [having] possession of *** obscene matter" in violation of Georgia law. Appellant was tried before a jury and convicted. The Supreme Court of Georgia affirmed.

Appellant raises several challenges to the validity of his conviction.[2] We find it necessary to consider only one. Appellant argues here, and argued below, that the Georgia obscenity statute, insofar as it punishes mere private possession of obscene matter, violates the First Amendment, as made applicable to the States by the Fourteenth Amendment. For reasons set forth below, we agree that the mere private possession of obscene matter cannot constitutionally be made a crime.

The court below saw no valid constitutional objection to the Georgia statute, even though it extends further than the typical statute forbidding commercial sales of obscene material. It held that "[it] is not essential to an indictment charging one with possession of obscene matter that it be alleged that such possession was 'with intent to sell, expose or circulate the same.'" The State and appellant both agree that the question here before us is whether "a statute imposing criminal sanctions upon the mere [knowing] possession of obscene matter" is constitutional. In this context, Georgia concedes that the present case appears to be one of "first impression on this

---

2. Appellant does not argue that the films are not obscene. For the purpose of this opinion, we assume that they are obscene under any of the tests advanced by members of this Court. See Redrup v. New York, 386 U.S. 767 (1967).

exact point," but contends that since "obscenity is not within the area of constitutionally protected speech or press," Roth v. United States, 354 U.S. 476, 485 (1957), the States are free, subject to the limits of other provisions of the Constitution, to deal with it any way deemed necessary, just as they may deal with possession of other things thought to be detrimental to the welfare of their citizens. If the State can protect the body of a citizen, may it not, argues Georgia, protect his mind?

It is true that *Roth* does declare, seemingly without qualification, that obscenity is not protected by the First Amendment. That statement has been repeated in various forms in subsequent cases. *** However, neither *Roth* nor any subsequent decision of this Court dealt with the precise problem involved in the present case. Roth was convicted of mailing obscene circulars and advertising, and an obscene book, in violation of a federal obscenity statute. The defendant in a companion case, Alberts v. California, 354 U.S. 476 (1957), was convicted of "lewdly keeping for sale obscene and indecent books, and [of] writing, composing and publishing an obscene advertisement of them. ***" Those cases dealt with the power of the State and Federal Governments to prohibit or regulate certain public actions taken or intended to be taken with respect to obscene matter. Indeed, with one exception, we have been unable to discover any case in which the issue in the present case has been fully considered.

In this context, we do not believe that this case can be decided simply by citing *Roth. Roth* and its progeny certainly do mean that the First and Fourteenth Amendments recognize a valid governmental interest in dealing with the problem of obscenity. *** *Roth* and the cases following it discerned such an "important interest" in the regulation of commercial distribution of obscene material. That holding cannot foreclose an examination of the constitutional implications of a statute forbidding mere private possession of such material.

It is now well established that the Constitution protects the right to receive information and ideas. "This freedom [of speech and press] *** necessarily protects the right to receive ***." Martin v. City of Struthers, 319 U.S. 141, 143 (1943); see Griswold v. Connecticut, 381 U.S. 479, 482 (1965); Lamont v. Postmaster General, 381 U.S. 301, 307-308 (1965) (BRENNAN, J., concurring); cf. Pierce v. Society of Sisters, 268 U.S. 510 (1925). This right to receive information and ideas, regardless of their social worth, see Winters v. New York, 333 U.S. 507, 510 (1948), is fundamental to our free society. Moreover, in the context of this case—a prosecution for mere possession of printed or filmed matter in the privacy of a person's own home—that right takes on an added dimension. For also fundamental is the right to be free, except in very limited circumstances, from unwanted governmental intrusions into one's privacy. See *Griswold v. Connecticut*; cf. NAACP v. Alabama, 357 U.S. 449, 462 (1958).

These are the rights that appellant is asserting in the case before us. He is asserting the right to read or observe what he pleases—the right to satisfy his intellectual and emotional needs in the privacy of his own home. He is asserting the right to be free from state inquiry into the contents of his library. Georgia contends that appellant does not have these rights, that there are certain types of materials that the individual may not read or even possess. Georgia justifies this assertion by arguing that the films in the present case are obscene. But we think that mere categorization of these films as "obscene" is insufficient justification for such a drastic invasion of personal liberties guaranteed by the First and Fourteenth Amendments. Whatever may be the justifications for other statutes regulating obscenity, we do not think they reach into the privacy of one's own home. If the First Amendment means anything, it means that a State has no business telling a man, sitting alone in his own house, what books he may read or what films he may watch. Our whole constitutional heritage rebels at the thought of giving government the power to control men's minds.

And yet, in the face of these traditional notions of individual liberty, Georgia asserts the right to protect the individual's mind from the effects of obscenity. We are not certain that this argument amounts to anything more than the assertion that the State has the right to control the moral content of a person's thoughts. To some, this may be a noble purpose, but it is wholly inconsistent with the philosophy of the First Amendment. *** Whatever the power of the state to control public dissemination of ideas inimical to the public morality, it cannot constitutionally premise legislation on the desirability of controlling a person's private thoughts.

Perhaps recognizing this, Georgia asserts that exposure to obscene materials may lead to deviant sexual behavior or crimes of sexual violence. There appears to be little empirical basis for that assertion. But more important, if the State is only concerned about printed or filmed materials inducing antisocial conduct, we believe that in the context of private consumption of ideas and information we should adhere to the view that "[among] free men, the deterrents ordinarily to be applied to prevent crime are education and punishment for violations of the law ***." Whitney v. California, 274 U.S. 357, 378 (1927) (Brandeis, J., concurring). See Emerson, Toward a General Theory of the First Amendment, 72 Yale L.J. 877, 938 (1963). Given the present state of knowledge, the State may no more prohibit mere possession of obscene matter on the ground that it may lead to antisocial conduct than it may prohibit possession of chemistry books on the ground that they may lead to the manufacture of homemade spirits.

It is true that in *Roth* this Court rejected the necessity of proving that exposure to obscene material would create a clear and present danger of antisocial conduct or would probably induce its recipients to such conduct. But that case dealt with public distribution of obscene materials and such distribution is subject to different objections. For example, there is always the danger that obscene material might fall into the hands of children, see *Ginsberg v. New York,* or that it might intrude upon the sensibilities or privacy of the general public. See Redrup v. New York, 386 U.S. 767, 769 (1967). No such dangers are present in this case.

Finally, we are faced with the argument that prohibition of possession of obscene materials is a necessary incident to statutory schemes prohibiting distribution.

That argument is based on alleged difficulties of proving an intent to distribute or in producing evidence of actual distribution. We are not convinced that such difficulties exist, but even if they did we do not think that they would justify infringement of the individual's right to read or observe what he pleases. Because that right is so fundamental to our scheme of individual liberty, its restriction may not be justified by the need to ease the administration of otherwise valid criminal laws. See Smith v. California, 361 U.S. 147 (1959).

We hold that the First and Fourteenth Amendments prohibit making mere private possession of obscene material a crime.[11] *Roth* and the cases following that decision are not impaired by today's holding. As we have said, the States retain broad power to regulate obscenity; that power simply does not extend to mere possession by the individual in the privacy of his own home. Accordingly, the judgment of the court below is reversed and the case is remanded for proceedings not inconsistent with this opinion.

It is so ordered.

MR. JUSTICE BLACK, concurring.

I agree with the Court that the mere possession of reading matter or movie films, whether labeled obscene or not, cannot be made a crime by a State without violating the First Amendment, made applicable to the States by the Fourteenth. ***

MR. JUSTICE STEWART, with whom MR. JUSTICE BRENNAN and MR. JUSTICE WHITE join, concurring in the result.

* * *

Because the films were seized in violation of the Fourth and Fourteenth Amendments, they were inadmissible in evidence at the appellant's trial. Mapp v. Ohio, 367 U.S. 643. Accordingly, the judgment of conviction must be reversed.

---

11. What we have said in no way infringes upon the power of the State or Federal Government to make possession of other items, such as narcotics, firearms, or stolen goods, a crime. Our holding in the present case turns upon the Georgia statute's infringement of fundamental liberties protected by the First and Fourteenth Amendments. No First Amendment rights are involved in most statutes making mere possession criminal.

Nor do we mean to express any opinion on statutes making criminal possession of other types of printed, filmed, or recorded materials. See, e.g., 18 U.S.C. § 793 (d), which makes criminal the otherwise lawful possession of materials which "the possessor has reason to believe could be used to the injury of the United States or to the advantage of any foreign nation ***." In such cases, compelling reasons may exist for overriding the right of the individual to possess those materials.

MILLER v. CALIFORNIA

413 U.S. 15 (1973)

MR. CHIEF JUSTICE BURGER delivered the opinion of the Court.

* * *

Appellant conducted a mass mailing campaign to advertise the sale of illustrated books, euphemistically called "adult" material. After a jury trial, he was convicted of violating California Penal Code § 311.2 (a), a misdemeanor, by knowingly distributing obscene matter, and the Appellate Department, Superior Court of California, County of Orange, summarily affirmed the judgment without opinion. Appellant's conviction was specifically based on his conduct in causing five unsolicited advertising brochures to be sent through the mail in an envelope addressed to a restaurant in Newport Beach, California. The envelope was opened by the manager of the restaurant and his mother. They had not requested the brochures; they complained to the police.

The brochures advertise four books entitled "Intercourse," "Man-Woman," "Sex Orgies Illustrated," and "An Illustrated History of Pornography," and a film entitled "Marital Intercourse." While the brochures contain some descriptive printed material, primarily they consist of pictures and drawings very explicitly depicting men and women in groups of two or more engaging in a variety of sexual activities, with genitals often prominently displayed.

I

This case involves the application of a State's criminal obscenity statute to a situation in which sexually explicit materials have been thrust by aggressive sales action upon unwilling recipients who had in no way indicated any desire to receive such materials. This Court has recognized that the States have a legitimate interest in prohibiting dissemination or exhibition of obscene material[2] when the mode of

---

2. This Court has defined "obscene material" as "material which deals with sex in a manner appealing to prurient interest," *Roth v. United States*, but the *Roth* definition does not reflect the precise meaning of "obscene" as traditionally used in the English language. Derived from the Latin *obscaenus*, *ob*, to, plus *caenum*, filth, "obscene" is defined in the Webster's Third New International Dictionary (Unabridged 1969) as "1a: disgusting to the senses *** b: grossly repugnant to the generally accepted notions of what is appropriate *** 2: offensive or revolting as countering or violating some ideal or principle." The Oxford English Dictionary (1933 ed.) gives a similar definition, "[o]ffensive to the senses, or to taste or refinement; disgusting, repulsive, filthy, foul, abominable, loathsome."

The material we are discussing in this case is more accurately defined as "pornography" or "pornographic material." "Pornography" derives from the Greek (*porne*, harlot, and *graphos*, writing). The word now means "1: a description of prostitutes or prostitution 2: a depiction (as in writing or painting) of licentiousness or lewdness: a portrayal of erotic behavior designed to cause sexual excitement." Webster's Third New International Dictionary, *supra*. Pornographic material which is obscene forms a sub- group of all "obscene" expression, but not the whole, at least as the word "obscene" is now used in our language. We note, therefore, that the words "obscene material," as used in this case, have a specific judicial meaning which derives from the *Roth* case, *i.e.*, obscene material "which deals with sex." See also ALI Model Penal Code § 251.4 (l) "Obscene Defined." (Official Draft 1962.)

dissemination carries with it a significant danger of offending the sensibilities of unwilling recipients or of exposure to juveniles. *** It is in this context that we are called on to define the standards which must be used to identify obscene material that a State may regulate without infringing on the First Amendment as applicable to the States through the Fourteenth Amendment.

The dissent of Mr. Justice Brennan reviews the background of the obscenity problem, but since the Court now undertakes to formulate standards more concrete than those in the past, it is useful for us to focus on two of the landmark cases in the somewhat tortured history of the Court's obscenity decisions. In Roth v. United States, 354 U.S. 476 (1957), the Court sustained a conviction under a federal statute punishing the mailing of "obscene, lewd, lascivious or filthy ***" materials. The key to that holding was the Court's rejection of the claim that obscene materials were protected by the First Amendment. ***

Nine years later, in Memoirs v. Massachusetts, 383 U.S. 413 (1966), the Court veered sharply away from the *Roth* concept and, with only three Justices in the plurality opinion, articulated a new test of obscenity. The plurality held that under the *Roth* definition

> "as elaborated in subsequent cases, three elements must coalesce: it must be established that (a) the dominant theme of the material taken as a whole appeals to a prurient interest in sex; (b) the material is patently offensive because it affronts contemporary community standards relating to the description or representation of sexual matters; and (c) the material is utterly without redeeming social value." ***

While *Roth* presumed "obscenity" to be "utterly without redeeming social importance," *Memoirs* required that to prove obscenity it must be affirmatively established that the material is "*utterly* without redeeming social value." Thus, even as they repeated the words of *Roth*, the *Memoirs* plurality produced a drastically altered test that called on the prosecution to prove a negative, *i.e.*, that the material was "*utterly* without redeeming social value"—a burden virtually impossible to discharge under our criminal standards of proof. ***

The case we now review was tried on the theory that the California Penal Code § 311 approximately incorporates the three-stage *Memoirs* test. But now the *Memoirs* test has been abandoned as unworkable by its author,[4] and no Member of the Court today supports the *Memoirs* formulation.

II

This much has been categorically settled by the Court, that obscene material is unprotected by the First Amendment. We acknowledge, however, the inherent dangers of undertaking to regulate any form of expression. State statutes designed

4. See the dissenting opinion of Mr. Justice Brennan in Paris Adult Theatre I v. Slaton, [413 U.S. 49].

to regulate obscene materials must be carefully limited. As a result, we now confine the permissible scope of such regulation to works which depict or describe sexual conduct. That conduct must be specifically defined by the applicable state law, as written or authoritatively construed.[6] A state offense must also be limited to works which, taken as a whole, appeal to the prurient interest in sex, which portray sexual conduct in a patently offensive way, and which, taken as a whole, do not have serious literary, artistic, political, or scientific value.

The basic guidelines for the trier of fact must be: (a) whether "the average person, applying contemporary community standards" would find that the work, taken as a whole, appeals to the prurient interest; (b) whether the work depicts or describes, in a patently offensive way, sexual conduct specifically defined by the applicable state law; and (c) whether the work, taken as a whole, lacks serious literary, artistic, political, or scientific value. We do not adopt as a constitutional standard the "*utterly* without redeeming social value" test of *Memoirs v. Massachusetts*; that concept has never commanded the adherence of more than three Justices at one time.[7] If a state law that regulates obscene material is thus limited, as written or construed, the First Amendment values applicable to the States through the Fourteenth Amendment are adequately protected by the ultimate power of appellate courts to conduct an independent review of constitutional claims when necessary. ***

*** It is possible, to give a few plain examples of what a state statute could define for regulation under part (b) of the standard announced in this opinion, *supra*:

(a) Patently offensive representations or descriptions of ultimate sexual acts, normal or perverted, actual or simulated.

(b) Patently offensive representations or descriptions of masturbation, excretory functions, and lewd exhibition of the genitals.

Sex and nudity may not be exploited without limit by films or pictures exhibited or sold in places of public accommodation any more than live sex and nudity can be exhibited or sold without limit in such public places.[8] At a minimum, prurient, patently offensive depiction or description of sexual conduct must have serious literary,

6. See, *e.g.*, Oregon Laws 1971, c. 743, Art. 29, §§ 255-262, and Hawaii Penal Code, Tit. 37, §§ 1210-1216, 1972 Hawaii Session Laws, Act 9, c. 12, pt. II, pp. 126-129, as examples of state laws directed at depiction of defined physical conduct, as opposed to expression. Other state formulations could be equally valid in this respect. In giving the Oregon and Hawaii statutes as examples, we do not wish to be understood as approving of them in all other respects nor as establishing their limits as the extent of state power.

We do not hold, as MR. JUSTICE BRENNAN intimates, that all States other than Oregon must now enact new obscenity statutes. Other existing state statutes, as construed heretofore or hereafter, may well be adequate. ***

7. *** We also reject, as a constitutional standard, the ambiguous concept of "social importance." ***

8. Although we are not presented here with the problem of regulating lewd public conduct itself, the States have greater power to regulate nonverbal, physical conduct than to suppress depictions or descriptions of the same behavior. ***

artistic, political, or scientific value to merit First Amendment protection. For example, medical books for the education of physicians and related personnel necessarily use graphic illustrations and descriptions of human anatomy. In resolving the inevitably sensitive questions of fact and law, we must continue to rely on the jury system, accompanied by the safeguards that judges, rules of evidence, presumption of innocence, and other protective features provide, as we do with rape, murder, and a host of other offenses against society and its individual members.[9]

Under the holdings announced today, no one will be subject to prosecution for the sale or exposure of obscene materials unless these materials depict or describe patently offensive "hard core" sexual conduct specifically defined by the regulating state law, as written or construed. We are satisfied that these specific prerequisites will provide fair notice to a dealer in such materials that his public and commercial activities may bring prosecution.

It is certainly true that the absence, since *Roth,* of a single majority view of this Court as to proper standards for testing obscenity has placed a strain on both state and federal courts. But today, for the first time since *Roth* was decided in 1957, a majority of this Court has agreed on concrete guidelines to isolate "hard core" pornography from expression protected by the First Amendment. Now we may abandon the casual practice of Redrup v. New York, 386 U.S. 767 (1967), and attempt to provide positive guidance to federal and state courts alike. ***

III

Under a National Constitution, fundamental First Amendment limitations on the powers of the States do not vary from community to community, but this does not mean that there are, or should or can be, fixed, uniform national standards of precisely what appeals to the "prurient interest" or is "patently offensive." These are essentially questions of fact, and our Nation is simply too big and too diverse for this Court to reasonably expect that such standards could be articulated for all 50 States in a single formulation, even assuming the prerequisite consensus exists. When triers of fact are asked to decide whether "the average person, applying contemporary community standards" would consider certain materials "prurient," it would be unrealistic to require that the answer be based on some abstract formulation. The adversary system, with lay jurors as the usual ultimate factfinders in criminal prosecutions, has historically permitted triers of fact to draw on the standards of their community, guided always by limiting instructions on the law. To require a State to structure obscenity proceedings around evidence of a *national* "community standard" would be an exercise in futility.

As noted before, this case was tried on the theory that the California obscenity statute sought to incorporate the tripartite test of *Memoirs.* *** The jury, however, was explicitly instructed that, in determining whether the "dominant theme of the

---

9. The mere fact juries may reach different conclusions as to the same material does not mean that constitutional rights are abridged. ***

material as a whole *** appeals to the prurient interest" and in determining whether the material "goes substantially beyond customary limits of candor and affronts contemporary community standards of decency," it was to apply "contemporary community standards of the State of California." ***

We conclude that neither the State's alleged failure to offer evidence of "national standards," nor the trial court's charge that the jury consider state community standards, were constitutional errors. Nothing in the First Amendment requires that a jury must consider hypothetical and unascertainable "national standards" when attempting to determine whether certain materials are obscene as a matter of fact. *** It is neither realistic nor constitutionally sound to read the First Amendment as requiring that the people of Maine or Mississippi accept public depiction of conduct found tolerable in Las Vegas, or New York City.[13] ***

IV

***

In sum, we (a) reaffirm the *Roth* holding that obscene material is not protected by the First Amendment; (b) hold that such material can be regulated by the States, subject to the specific safeguards enunciated above, without a showing that the material is "*utterly* without redeeming social value"; and (c) hold that obscenity is to be determined by applying "contemporary community standards," *** not "national standards." The judgment of the Appellate Department of the Superior Court, Orange County, California, is vacated and the case remanded to that court for further proceedings not inconsistent with the First Amendment standards established by this opinion. ***

MR. JUSTICE DOUGLAS, dissenting.

* * *

Today the Court retreats from the earlier formulations of the constitutional test and undertakes to make new definitions. This effort, like the earlier ones, is earnest and well intentioned. The difficulty is that we do not deal with constitutional terms, since "obscenity" is not mentioned in the Constitution or Bill of Rights. And the First

---

13. In Jacobellis v. Ohio, 378 U.S. 184 (1964), two Justices argued that application of "local" community standards would run the risk of preventing dissemination of materials in some places because sellers would be unwilling to risk criminal conviction by testing variations in standards from place to place. *Id.*, at 193-195 (opinion of BRENNAN, J., joined by Goldberg, J.). The use of "national" standards, however, necessarily implies that materials found tolerable in some places, but not under the "national" criteria, will nevertheless be unavailable where they are acceptable. Thus, in terms of danger to free expression, the potential for suppression seems at least as great in the application of a single nationwide standard as in allowing distribution in accordance with local tastes, a point which Mr. Justice Harlan often emphasized. ***

Appellant also argues that adherence to a "national standard" is necessary "in order to avoid unconscionable burdens on the free flow of interstate commerce." *** Appellant's argument would appear without substance in any event. Obscene material may be validly regulated by a State in the exercise of its traditional local power to protect the general welfare of its population despite some possible incidental effect on the flow of such materials across state lines. ***

Amendment makes no such exception from "the press" which it undertakes to protect nor, as I have said on other occasions, is an exception necessarily implied, for there was no recognized exception to the free press at the time the Bill of Rights was adopted which treated "obscene" publications differently from other types of papers, magazines, and books. So there are no constitutional guidelines for deciding what is and what is not "obscene." ***

We deal with highly emotional, not rational, questions. To many the Song of Solomon is obscene. I do not think we, the judges, were ever given the constitutional power to make definitions of obscenity. If it is to be defined, let the people debate and decide by a constitutional amendment what they want to ban as obscene and what standards they want the legislatures and the courts to apply. Perhaps the people will decide that the path towards a mature, integrated society requires that all ideas competing for acceptance must have no censor. Perhaps they will decide otherwise. Whatever the choice, the courts will have some guidelines. Now we have none except our own predilections.

MR. JUSTICE BRENNAN, with whom MR. JUSTICE STEWART and MR. JUSTICE MARSHALL join, dissenting. [Omitted.]

PARIS ADULT THEATRE I v. SLATON

413 U.S. 49 (1973)

MR. CHIEF JUSTICE BURGER delivered the opinion of the Court.

Petitioners are two Atlanta, Georgia, movie theaters and their owners and managers, operating in the style of "adult" theaters. On December 28, 1970, respondents, the local state district attorney and the solicitor for the local state trial court, filed civil complaints in that court alleging that petitioners were exhibiting to the public for paid admission two allegedly obscene films, contrary to Georgia Code Ann. § 26-2101.[1] The two films in question, "Magic Mirror" and "It All Comes Out in the End," depict sexual conduct characterized by the Georgia Supreme Court as "hard core pornography" leaving "little to the imagination." ***

On January 13, 1971, 15 days after the proceedings began, the films were produced by petitioners at a jury-waived trial. Certain photographs, also produced at trial, were stipulated to portray the single entrance to both Paris Adult Theatre I and Paris Adult Theatre II as it appeared at the time of the complaints. These photographs show a conventional, inoffensive theater entrance, without any pictures, but with signs indicating the theaters exhibit "Atlanta's Finest Mature Feature Films."

---

1. This is a civil proceeding. Georgia Code Ann. § 26-2101 defines a criminal offense, but the exhibition of materials found to be "obscene" as defined by that statute may be enjoined in a civil proceeding under Georgia law. ***

On the door itself is a sign saying: "Adult Theatre—You must be 21 and able to prove it. If viewing the nude body offends you. Please Do Not Enter."

The two films were exhibited to the trial court. The only other state evidence was testimony by criminal investigators that they had paid admission to see the films and that nothing on the outside of the theater indicated the full nature of what was shown. In particular, nothing indicated that the films depicted—as they did—scenes of simulated fellatio, cunnilingus, and group sex intercourse. There was no evidence presented that minors had ever entered the theaters. Nor was there evidence presented that petitioners had a systematic policy of barring minors, apart from posting signs at the entrance. On April 12, 1971, the trial judge dismissed respondents' complaints. He assumed "that obscenity is established," but stated:

> "It appears to the Court that the display of these films in a commercial theatre, when surrounded by requisite notice to the public of their nature and by reasonable protection against the exposure of these films to minors, is constitutionally permissible."

On appeal, the Georgia Supreme Court unanimously reversed. It assumed that the adult theaters in question barred minors and gave a full warning to the general public of the nature of the films shown, but held that the films were without protection under the First Amendment. ***

It should be clear from the outset that we do not undertake to tell the States what they must do, but rather to define the area in which they may chart their own course in dealing with obscene material. This Court has consistently held that obscene material is not protected by the First Amendment as a limitation on the state police power by virtue of the Fourteenth Amendment. *** Today, in *Miller v.* California, we have sought to clarify the constitutional definition of obscene material subject to regulation by the States, and we vacate and remand this case for reconsideration in light of *Miller*.

We categorically disapprove the theory, apparently adopted by the trial judge, that obscene, pornographic films acquire constitutional immunity from state regulation simply because they are exhibited for consenting adults only. This holding was properly rejected by the Georgia Supreme Court.

In particular, we hold that there are legitimate state interests at stake in stemming the tide of commercialized obscenity, even assuming it is feasible to enforce effective safeguards against exposure to juveniles and to passersby. These include the interest of the public in the quality of life and the total community environment, the tone of commerce in the great city centers, and, possibly, the public safety itself. The Hill-Link Minority Report of the Commission on Obscenity and Pornography indicates that there is at least an arguable correlation between obscene material and crime. *** It is not for us to resolve empirical uncertainties underlying state legislation, save in the exceptional case where that legislation plainly impinges upon rights protected by the Constitution itself. ***

Finally, petitioners argue that conduct which directly involves "consenting adults" only has, for that sole reason, a special claim to constitutional protection. Our Constitution establishes a broad range of conditions on the exercise of power by the States, but for us to say that our Constitution incorporates the proposition that conduct involving consenting adults only is always beyond state regulation,[14] is a step we are unable to take.[15] Commercial exploitation of depictions, descriptions, or exhibitions of obscene conduct on commercial premises open to the adult public falls within a State's broad power to regulate commerce and protect the public environment. The issue in this context goes beyond whether someone, or even the majority, considers the conduct depicted as "wrong" or "sinful." The States have the power to make a morally neutral judgment that public exhibition of obscene material, or commerce in such material, has a tendency to injure the community as a whole, to endanger the public safety, or to jeopardize in Mr. Chief Justice Warren's words, the States' "right *** to maintain a decent society." Jacobellis v. Ohio, 378 U.S., at 199 (dissenting opinion).

To summarize, we have today reaffirmed the basic holding of *Roth v. United States,* that obscene material has no protection under the First Amendment. *** We have directed our holdings, not at thoughts or speech, but at depiction and description of specifically defined sexual conduct that States may regulate within limits designed to prevent infringement of First Amendment rights. We have also reaffirmed the holdings of *United States v. Reidel,* [402 U.S. 351], and *United States v. Thirty-Seven Photographs,* [402 U.S. 363], that commerce in obscene material is unprotected by any constitutional doctrine of privacy. *** In this case we hold that the States have a legitimate interest in regulating commerce in obscene material and in regulating exhibition of obscene material in places of public accommodation, including so-called "adult" theaters from which minors are excluded. In light of these holdings, nothing precludes the State of Georgia from the regulation of the allegedly obscene material exhibited in Paris Adult Theatre I or II, provided that the applicable Georgia law, as written or authoritatively interpreted by the Georgia courts, meets the First Amendment standards set forth in Miller v. California, 413 U.S., at 23-25. ***

Vacated and remanded.

MR. JUSTICE DOUGLAS, dissenting. [Omitted.]

MR. JUSTICE BRENNAN, with whom MR. JUSTICE STEWART and MR. JUSTICE MARSHALL join, dissenting.

---

14. Cf. J. Mill, On Liberty 13 (1955 ed.).

15. The state statute books are replete with constitutionally unchallenged laws against prostitution, suicide, voluntary self-mutilation, brutalizing "bare fist" prize fights, and duels, although these crimes may only directly involve "consenting adults." Statutes making bigamy a crime surely cut into an individual's freedom to associate but few today seriously claim such statutes violate the First Amendment or any other constitutional provision.

*** I am convinced that the approach initiated 16 years ago in Roth v. United States, 354 U.S. 476 (1957), and culminating in the Court's decision today, cannot bring stability to this area of the law without jeopardizing fundamental First Amendment values, and I have concluded that the time has come to make a significant departure from that approach. ***

Our experience since *Roth* requires us not only to abandon the effort to pick out obscene materials on a case-by-case basis, but also to reconsider a fundamentally postulate of *Roth*: that there exists a definable class of sexually oriented expression that may be totally suppressed by the Federal and State Governments. Assuming that such a class of expression does in fact exist, I am forced to conclude that the concept of "obscenity" cannot be defined with sufficient specificity and clarity to provide fair notice to persons who create and distribute sexually oriented materials, to prevent substantial erosion of protected speech as a byproduct of the attempt to suppress unprotected speech, and to avoid very costly institutional harms.

*** I would hold *** that at least in the absence of distribution to juveniles or obtrusive exposure to unconsenting adults, the First and Fourteenth Amendments prohibit the State and Federal Governments from attempting wholly to suppress sexually oriented materials on the basis of their allegedly "obscene" contents. Nothing in this approach precludes those governments from taking action to serve what may be strong and legitimate interests through regulation of the manner of distribution of sexually oriented material.

*** Since the Supreme Court of Georgia erroneously concluded that the State has power to suppress sexually oriented material even in the absence of distribution to juveniles or exposure to unconsenting adults, I would reverse that judgment and remand the case to that court for further proceedings not inconsistent with this opinion.

NEW YORK v. FERBER

458 U.S. 747 (1982)

JUSTICE WHITE delivered the opinion of the Court.

I

In recent years, the exploitive use of children in the production of pornography has become a serious national problem.[1] The Federal Government and 47 States

---

1. "[C]hild pornography and child prostitution have become highly organized, multimillion dollar industries that operate on a nationwide scale." S. Rep. No. 95-438, p. 5 (1977). One researcher has documented the existence of over 260 different magazines which depict children engaging in sexually explicit conduct. *Ibid.* "Such magazines depict children, some as young as three to five years of age. *** The activities featured range from lewd poses to intercourse, fellatio, cunnilingus, masturbation, rape, incest and sado-masochism." *Id.*, at 6. In Los Angeles alone, police reported that 30,000 children have been sexually exploited. Sexual Exploitation of Children, Hearings before the Subcommittee on Select Education of the House Committee on Education and Labor, 95th Cong., 1st Sess., 41-42 (1977).

have sought to combat the problem with statutes specifically directed at the production of child pornography. At least half of such statutes do not require that the materials produced be legally obscene. Thirty-five States and the United States Congress have also passed legislation prohibiting the distribution of such materials; 20 States prohibit the distribution of material depicting children engaged in sexual conduct without requiring that the material be legally obscene.

New York is one of the 20. Section 263.05 criminalizes as a class C felony the use of a child in a sexual performance. A "[s]exual performance" is defined as "any performance or part thereof which includes sexual conduct by a child less than sixteen years of age." "Sexual conduct" is in turn defined in § 263.00(3):

> "'Sexual conduct' means actual or simulated sexual intercourse, deviate sexual intercourse, sexual bestiality, masturbation, sado-masochistic abuse, or lewd exhibition of the genitals."

A performance is defined as "any play, motion picture, photograph or dance" or "any other visual representation exhibited before an audience." § 263.00(4).

At issue in this case is § 263.15, defining a class D felony:[3]

> "A person is guilty of promoting a sexual performance by a child when, knowing the character and content thereof, he produces, directs or promotes any performance which includes sexual conduct by a child less than sixteen years of age."

To "promote" is also defined:

> "'Promote' means to procure, manufacture, issue, sell, give, provide, lend, mail, deliver, transfer, transmute, publish, distribute, circulate, disseminate, present, exhibit or advertise, or to offer or agree to do the same."

A companion provision bans only the knowing dissemination of obscene material.

This case arose when Paul Ferber, the proprietor of a Manhattan bookstore specializing in sexually oriented products, sold two films to an undercover police officer. The films are devoted almost exclusively to depicting young boys masturbating. Ferber was indicted on two counts of violating § 263.10 and two counts of violating § 263.15, the two New York laws controlling dissemination of child pornography. After a jury trial, Ferber was acquitted of the two counts of promoting an obscene sexual performance, but found guilty of the two counts under § 263.15, which did not require proof that the films were obscene.

The New York Court of Appeals reversed, holding that § 263.15 violated the First Amendment. We granted the State's petition for certiorari, presenting the single question:

---

3. Class D felonies carry a maximum punishment for up to seven years as to individuals, and as to corporations a fine of up to $10,000. N.Y. Penal Law §§ 70.00, 80.10 (McKinney 1975). Respondent Ferber was sentenced to 45 days in prison.

"To prevent the abuse of children who are made to engage in sexual conduct for commercial purposes, could the New York State Legislature, consistent with the First Amendment, prohibit the dissemination of material which shows children engaged in sexual conduct, regardless of whether such material is obscene?"

II

The Court of Appeals proceeded on the assumption that the standard of obscenity incorporated in § 263.10, which follows the guidelines enunciated in Miller v. California, 413 U.S. 15 (1973), constitutes the appropriate line dividing protected from unprotected expression by which to measure a regulation directed at child pornography. The Court of Appeals' assumption was not unreasonable in light of our decisions. *** For the following reasons, however, we are persuaded that the States are entitled to greater leeway in the regulation of pornographic depictions of children.

First. The prevention of sexual exploitation and abuse of children constitutes a government objective of surpassing importance. *** *Second*. The distribution of photographs and films depicting sexual activity by juveniles is intrinsically related to the sexual abuse of children in at least two ways. First, the materials produced are a permanent record of the children's participation and the harm to the child is exacerbated by their circulation. Second, the distribution network for child pornography must be closed if the production of material which requires the sexual exploitation of children is to be effectively controlled. *** While the production of pornographic materials is a low-profile, clandestine industry, the need to market the resulting products requires a visible apparatus of distribution. The most expeditious if not the only practical method of law enforcement may be to dry up the market for this material by imposing severe criminal penalties on persons selling, advertising, or otherwise promoting the product. ***

Third. The advertising and selling of child pornography provide an economic motive for and are thus an integral part of the production of such materials, an activity illegal throughout the Nation. *** *Fourth*. The value of permitting live performances and photographic reproductions of children engaged in lewd sexual conduct is exceedingly modest, if not *de minimis*. We consider it unlikely that visual depictions of children performing sexual acts or lewdly exhibiting their genitals would often constitute an important and necessary part of a literary performance or scientific or educational work. As a state judge in this case observed, if it were necessary for literary or artistic value, a person over the statutory age who perhaps looked younger could be utilized. Simulation outside of the prohibition of the statute could provide another alternative. Nor is there any question here of censoring a particular literary theme or portrayal of sexual activity. The First Amendment interest is limited to that of rendering the portrayal somewhat more "realistic" by utilizing or photographing children.

Fifth. Recognizing and classifying child pornography as a category of material outside the protection of the First Amendment is not incompatible with our earlier decisions.*** [I]t is not rare that a content-based classification of speech has been accepted because it may be appropriately generalized that within the confines of the given classification, the evil to be restricted so overwhelmingly outweighs the expressive interests, if any, at stake, that no process of case-by-case adjudication is required. When a definable class of material, such as that covered by § 263.15, bears so heavily and pervasively on the welfare of children engaged in its production, we think the balance of competing interests is clearly struck and that it is permissible to consider these materials as without the protection of the First Amendment.

There are, of course, limits on the category of child pornography which, like obscenity, is unprotected by the First Amendment. As with all legislation in this sensitive area, the conduct to be prohibited must be adequately defined by the applicable state law, as written or authoritatively construed. Here the nature of the harm to be combated requires that the state offense be limited to works that *visually* depict sexual conduct by children below a specified age.[17] The category of "sexual conduct" proscribed must also be suitably limited and described.

The test for child pornography is separate from the obscenity standard enunciated in *Miller*, but may be compared to it for purpose of clarity. The *Miller* formulation is adjusted in the following respects: A trier of fact need not find that the material appeals to the prurient interest of the average person; it is not required that sexual conduct portrayed be done so in a patently offensive manner; and the material at issue need not be considered as a whole. We note that the distribution of descriptions or other depictions of sexual conduct, not otherwise obscene, which do not involve live performance or photographic or other visual reproduction of live performances, retains First Amendment protection. As with obscenity laws, criminal responsibility may not be imposed without some element of scienter on the part of the defendant. Smith v. California, 361 U.S. 147 (1959); Hamling v. United States, 418 U.S. 87 (1974).[*] ***

III

It remains to address the claim that the New York statute is unconstitutionally overbroad because it would forbid the distribution of material with serious literary, scientific, or educational value or material which does not threaten the harms sought to be combated by the State. Respondent prevailed on that ground below, and it is to that issue that we now turn.

The New York Court of Appeals recognized that overbreadth scrutiny has been limited with respect to conduct-related regulation, Broadrick v. Oklahoma, 413 U.S. 601 (1973), but it did not apply the test enunciated in *Broadrick* because the challenged statute, in its view, was directed at "pure speech." The court went on to find

---

17. Sixteen States define a child as a person under age 18. Four States define a child as under 17 years old. The federal law and 16 States, including New York, define a child as under 16. ***

*. **[Ed. Note**. See United States v. X-Citement Video, Inc., 513 U.S. 64 (1994), for further clarification of the scienter requirement.]

that § 263.15 was fatally overbroad: "[T]he statute would prohibit the showing of any play or movie in which a child portrays a defined sexual act, real or simulated, in a nonobscene manner. It would also prohibit the sale, showing, or distributing of medical or educational materials containing photographs of such acts. Indeed, by its terms, the statute would prohibit those who oppose such portrayals from providing illustrations of what they oppose." ***

The scope of the First Amendment overbreadth doctrine, like most exceptions to established principles, must be carefully tied to the circumstances in which facial invalidation of a statute is truly warranted. Because of the wide-reaching effects of striking down a statute on its face at the request of one whose own conduct may be punished despite the First Amendment, we have recognized that the overbreadth doctrine is "strong medicine" and have employed it with hesitation, and then "only as a last resort." *Broadrick*, 413 U.S., at 613. We have, in consequence, insisted that the overbreadth involved be "substantial" before the statute involved will be invalidated on its face.[24] ***

Applying these principles, we hold that § 263.15 is not substantially overbroad. We consider this the paradigmatic case of a state statute whose legitimate reach dwarfs its arguably impermissible applications. New York, as we have held, may constitutionally prohibit dissemination of material specified in § 263.15. While the reach of the statute is directed at the hard core of child pornography, the Court of Appeals was understandably concerned that some protected expression, ranging from medical textbooks to pictorials in the National Geographic would fall prey to the statute. How often, if ever, it may be necessary to employ children to engage in conduct clearly within the reach of § 263.15 in order to produce educational, medical, or artistic works cannot be known with certainty. Yet we seriously doubt, and it has not been suggested, that these arguably impermissible applications of the statute amount to more than a tiny fraction of the materials within the statute's reach. Nor will we assume that the New York courts will widen the possibly invalid reach of the statute by giving an expansive construction to the proscription on "lewd exhibition[s] of the genitals." Under these circumstances, § 263.15 is "not substantially overbroad and *** whatever overbreadth may exist should be cured through case-by-case analysis of the fact situations to which its sanctions, assertedly, may not be applied." Broadrick v. Oklahoma, 413 U.S., at 615-616.***

---

24. When a federal court is dealing with a federal statute challenged as overbroad, it should, of course, construe the statute to avoid constitutional problems, if the statute is subject to such a limiting construction. *** Furthermore, if the federal statute is not subject to a narrowing construction and is impermissibly overbroad, it nevertheless should not be stricken down on its face; if it is severable, only the unconstitutional portion is to be invalidated. United States v. Thirty-seven Photographs, 402 U.S. 363 (1971). A state court is also free to deal with a state statute in the same way. If the invalid reach of the law is cured, there is no longer reason for proscribing the statute's application to unprotected conduct. Here, of course, we are dealing with a state statute on direct review of a state-court decision that has construed the statute. Such a construction is binding on us.

The decision of the New York Court of Appeals is reversed, and the case is remanded to that court for further proceedings not inconsistent with this opinion.

JUSTICE O'CONNOR, concurring.

Although I join the Court's opinion, I write separately to stress that the Court does not hold that New York must except "material with serious literary, scientific, or educational value," from its statute. The Court merely holds that, even if the First Amendment shelters such material, New York's current statute is not sufficiently overbroad to support respondent's facial attack. The compelling interests identified in today's opinion suggest that the Constitution might in fact permit New York to ban knowing distribution of works depicting minors engaged in explicit sexual conduct, regardless of the social value of the depictions. ***

On the other hand, it is quite possible that New York's statute is overbroad because it bans depictions that do not actually threaten the harms identified by the Court. For example, clinical pictures of adolescent sexuality, such as those that might appear in medical textbooks, might not involve the type of sexual exploitation and abuse targeted by New York's statute. Nor might such depictions feed the poisonous "kiddie porn" market that New York and other States have attempted to regulate. Similarly, pictures of children engaged in rites widely approved by their cultures, such as those that might appear in issues of the National Geographic, might not trigger the compelling interests identified by the Court. It is not necessary to address these possibilities further today, however, because this potential overbreadth is not sufficiently substantial to warrant facial invalidation of New York's statute.

JUSTICE BRENNAN, with whom JUSTICE MARSHALL joins, concurring in the judgment. [Omitted.]

JUSTICE STEVENS, concurring in the judgment.

Two propositions seem perfectly clear to me. First, the specific conduct that gave rise to this criminal prosecution is not protected by the Federal Constitution; second, the state statute that respondent violated prohibits some conduct that is protected by the First Amendment. The critical question, then, is whether this respondent, to whom the statute may be applied without violating the Constitution, may challenge the statute on the ground that it conceivably may be applied unconstitutionally to others in situations not before the Court. I agree with the Court's answer to this question but not with its method of analyzing the issue. ***

A holding that respondent may be punished for selling these two films does not require us to conclude that other users of these very films, or that other motion pictures containing similar scenes, are beyond the pale of constitutional protection. Thus, the exhibition of these films before a legislative committee studying a proposed amendment to a state law, or before a group of research scientists studying human behavior, could not, in my opinion, be made a crime. Moreover, it is at least conceivable that a serious work of art, a documentary on behavioral problems, or a medical or psychiatric teaching device, might include a scene from one of these films and, when viewed as a whole in a proper setting, be entitled to constitutional protection. The question whether a specific act of communication is protected by the First Amendment always requires some consideration of both its content and its context.

The Court's holding that this respondent may not challenge New York's statute as overbroad follows its discussion of the contours of the category of nonobscene child pornography that New York may legitimately prohibit. Having defined that category in an abstract setting,[3] the Court makes the empirical judgment that the arguably impermissible application of the New York statute amounts to only a "tiny fraction of the materials within the statute's reach." *** Even assuming that the Court's empirical analysis is sound,[4] I believe a more conservative approach to the issue would adequately vindicate the State's interest in protecting its children and cause less harm to the federal interest in free expression.

A hypothetical example will illustrate my concern. Assume that the operator of a New York motion picture theater specializing in the exhibition of foreign feature films is offered a full-length movie containing one scene that is plainly lewd if viewed in isolation but that nevertheless is part of a serious work of art. If the child actor resided abroad, New York's interest in protecting its young from sexual exploitation would be far less compelling than in the case before us. The federal interest in free expression would, however, be just as strong as if an adult actor had been used. I would postpone decision of my hypothetical case until it actually arises. Advocates of a liberal use of overbreadth analysis could object to such postponement on the ground that it creates the risk that the exhibitor's uncertainty may produce self-censorship. But that risk obviously interferes less with the interest in free expression than does an abstract, advance ruling that the film is simply unprotected whenever it contains a lewd scene, no matter how brief.

---

3. "The test for child pornography is separate from the obscenity standard enunciated in *Miller*, but may be compared to it for purpose of clarity. The *Miller* formulation is adjusted in the following respects: A trier of fact need not find that the material appeals to the prurient interest of the average person; it is not required that sexual conduct portrayed be done so in a patently offensive manner; and the material at issue need not be considered as a whole." ***

4. The Court's analysis is directed entirely at the permissibility of the statute's coverage of non-obscene material. Its empirical evidence, however, is drawn substantially from congressional Committee Reports that ultimately reached the conclusion that a prohibition against *obscene* child pornography— coupled with sufficiently stiff sanctions—is an adequate response to this social problem. The Senate Committee on the Judiciary concluded that "virtually all of the materials that are normally considered child pornography are obscene under the current standards," and that "[i]n comparison with this blatant pornography, non-obscene materials that depict children are very few and very inconsequential." ***

*** Although I disagree with the Court's position that such speech is totally without First Amendment protection, I agree that generally marginal speech does not warrant the extraordinary protection afforded by the overbreadth doctrine.

Because I have no difficulty with the statute's application in this case, I concur in the Court's judgment.

NOTES, DEVELOPMENTS, AND QUESTIONS SUBSEQUENT TO *NEW YORK V. FERBER*

1. As noted in *Ferber*, "[t]hirty-five States and the United States Congress" have enacted statutes forbidding the production, reproduction, distribution, dissemination or (under some of these laws) possession of any visual depiction of an underage person taking part in some described act (e.g. "actual or simulated sexual intercourse"), or depicted in some sexually explicit way (e.g., with "lewd exhibition of genitals"). That the performance or visual depiction — or the work of which it is a part — is not "obscene"[1]is treated as irrelevant. It is the "exploitation" of youngsters featured in sexual performances or pictures with which these laws is concerned — a concern the Court agrees a legislature may conclude may not be adequately met by forbidding their use only in such depictions as would also qualify as "obscene."[2] In keeping with that rationale, however, the Court also notes that none of these statutes applies where the depicted persons are not in fact underage, however they may have been selected and featured for their very youthful look.[3]

2. As noted also in *Ferber*, there is a parallel act of Congress, 18 U.S.C.§ 2252. Titled "The Protection of Children Against Sexual Exploitation Act of 1977," the federal statute differs from the New York statute principally in extending the critical

---

1. [i.e. that it does not meet the *Roth-Miller-Slayton-Ginsberg-Mishkin* standards of obscenity]

2. Note, nevertheless, the Court's admission these laws are facially directed to "speech" (pictures, visual depictions) and, on their face, bring within immediate threat of severe criminal sanction some material which the First Amendment may well protect despite the sexually explicit (but nonobscene) manner in which a particular young person may be shown (e.g., in a particular issue of National Geographic). Moreover, the Court sustained the New York statute despite the absence of any provision providing for *any* exceptions, dismissing the "unconstitutional chilling effect" complaint. (By denying that the degree of facial overbreadth was "substantial," it disallowed a "void on its face" challenge, even while reserving an "as applied" challenge as it might arise in a case suitably presenting the question in a specific factual context.)

3. As might be the case, for example, in casting the lead female role in a stage or film version of Vladimir Nabokov's Lolita, or in preparing copy for a magazine apparently featuring prepubescent girls and boys in various sexually explicit depictions. (If "obscene," such depictions might put the producer, distributor or buyer at risk but, if so, presumably only under the more stringent requirements of being "obscene"). Nor do these statutes apply to essays, novels, or other forms of speech describing, whether clinically or alluringly, varieties or qualities of sexuality or sensuality of the young, nor to "visual depictions" that are themselves graphic illustrations but of no actual underage person (i.e., an artist's imaginative renderings are not reached). So, "ideological pedophilia" (books, films, plays, etc., presenting the "affirmative case" for "freer sexual liberality involving pubescent or prepubescent 'minors'") is not, as such, affected by the New York law. (See and compare *Kingsley International Pictures Corp. v. Regents of The University of The State of New York*, casebook at p. 750.)

age of any "performer" forbidden to be featured in any visual depiction of "sexually explicit conduct" to anyone under eighteen (rather than only to those under sixteen). In this respect, the federal statute does sweep more widely than the New York act. (Additionally, the sanctions for violations of this federal act are quite severe — up to fifteen years imprisonment for a single offense, up to thirty years for two or more.)[4]

This 1977 federal act was initially held unconstitutional, however, for lack of any scienter requirement respecting the age of the person or persons depicted in the sexually explicit material. That is, as the ninth circuit understood the matter, this act (unlike the New York statute upheld in *Ferber*) applied whether or not one charged under the act neither knew or had reason to know that anyone featured in any of the sexually explicit visual depictions was in fact under eighteen.[5] The Supreme Court reversed this ninth circuit decision, but only after it substantially narrowed the statute by implying a scienter requirement. According to the Court's ruling, to pursue a successful prosecution under § 2252, the government must in each case prove — by evidence convincing to a jury beyond reasonable doubt — that: (a) the defendant was aware of the sexually explicit nature of the material; and (b) was also aware that one or more of the persons depicted in the material was underage (i.e., under eighteen years of age).[6] And so matters stood, as of 1994.

---

4. The 1977 act was enacted by Congress pursuant to its express power to "regulate Commerce...among the several states" (U.S. Const. Art. I §8, cl. 3). Note, however, under the 1977 act, it is not necessary that there be any sale, or purchase, or commercial exchange — whether in interstate commerce or otherwise — to trigger the act. Rather, the act applies in respect to any visual depiction of the described forbidden kind (i.e., of a person under eighteen depicted in certain sexually-explicit acts or poses) produced (or intended to be produced) for distribution via any medium of interstate commerce, as it likewise applies to any such depiction distributed or received by means of any such medium (including receiving by computer). Moreover, the act also applies if the visual depiction of the described forbidden kind is produced (whether "produced" by the sender or "produced" by the receiver) by means merely "*using* materials that have been mailed or shipped or transported in interstate or foreign commerce by any means." In brief, the federal statute is extremely far-reaching in its application and effect, substantially overlapping most of the state laws of the same general kind. (For example, a lower federal court has held that the statute applies even if the only connection with interstate commerce is that the camera (or some component thereof) used to produce the picture, or the film, or the photographic paper used to print the picture, had an out-of-state origin; nor is it consequential that the defendant did not know the statute would thus apply.)

5. Applying the Supreme Court's earlier decision in *Smith v. California* (casebook at p. 777), the ninth circuit held the act to be "void on its face."

6. *See United States v. X-Citement Video, Inc.*, 513 U.S. 64, 78 (1994) (emphasis added) ("[W]e conclude that the term 'knowingly' in § 2252 extends *both* to the sexually explicit nature of the material *and to the age of the performers.*") (*Query* whether actual knowledge, rather than some lesser scienter standard (e.g., "reason to know") is constitutionally required of such statutes according to *Smith.*)

3. Shortly thereafter, however, Congress enacted an additional measure, 18 U.S.C. § 2252A.[7] Dissatisfied with the limited reach of the 1977 Act insofar as it only reached sexually explicit visual depictions (or "performances") of actual minors (i.e., of persons under eighteen), Congress extended the definition of "child pornography" in a new section (§2256), to include any visual depiction[8] where

> (A) the production of such visual depiction involves the use of a minor engaging in sexually explicit conduct;[9] [or]
> (B) such visual depiction is, or appears to be, of a minor engaging in sexually explicit conduct;[10]
> (C) such visual depiction has been created, adapted, or modified to appear that an identifiable

---

7. The 1977 Act was enacted to halt the use of underage persons in the production and circulation of sexually explicit performances or material depicting such performances, on a finding by Congress like that relied upon by New York in *Ferber* — that "the use of children as subjects of pornographic materials is harmful to the physiological, emotional, and mental health of the child," i.e. the health of the child or children *thus used* or identifiably featured in the production. (Thus the very title of the 1977 Act as "The Protection of Children Against Sexual Exploitation Act of 1977.") The 1996 additions include this concern, but go well beyond, even as made quite clear by the much blunter title of the 1996 Act ("The Child Pornography Prevention Act"). What is sought to be "prevented" is "child pornography," neither more nor less. The phrase refers to a certain kind of material (just as the phrase "racist speech" refers to a certain kind of speech). Such material may typically involve underage persons in its presentation but need not involve any such person still to *be* "child pornography" in Congress's view.

Indeed, the phrase "child pornography" has been used from time to time to describe three different things, although some who use the term may think it properly applies (or should be applied) to all three of the varieties hereinafter described. For purposes of first amendment analysis in the assessment of different particular statutes, however, it may be useful to distinguish or separate these several strands: (a) "child pornography" as sexually explicit suggestive material *meant to appeal to minors* (see, e.g., *Ginsberg v. New York*, 390 U.S. 629 (1968) (sustaining restrictions on sales or distributions to minors of sexually explicit material the first amendment protects in respect to adults), and compare *Butler v. Michigan* (casebook at p. 760 n. 40), *Reno v. American Civil Liberties Union* (the next principal case) ; (b) "child pornography" as sexually explicit materials not particularly (and sometimes not at all) *meant to appeal to minors*, but *using* minors as performers, or *using* minors in sexually explicit depictions (e.g., as reviewed in *Ferber*); (c) "child pornography" as any sexually explicit material *conducive to exciting, promoting, encouraging, or gratifying a sexual interest in children.*

8. [Including "undeveloped film and videotape, and data stored on computer disk or by electronic means which is capable of conversion into a visual image."] (Note, however, that "*verbal depictions*" are evidently excluded from the act, e.g., alluring, even graphic, sexual descriptions of minors as willing and/or desirable objects of sexual desire, are per se not subject to the act.) (Cf. The Indianapolis ordinance in *American Booksellers v. Hudnut*, casebook at p. 222 (actionable "pornography" defined as "the graphic sexually explicit subordination of women, whether in pictures or in words...." [etc.].)

9. [This part may be but a restatement from the pre-existing statute.]

10. [I.e. "*appears* to be...of a minor," though it is not, rather, it is actually of one who is eighteen or older. (Additionally, this part of the act may reach any such visual depiction even if it is of no real or actual person at all, as would be true, for example, of a graphic artist's imaginative drawings of prepubescent minors engaged in sexually-explicit conduct or poses)].

> minor is engaging in sexually explicit conduct; [or]
> (D) such visual depiction is advertised, promoted, presented, described, or distributed in such a manner that conveys the impression that the material is or contains [such a visual depiction].

Under new subsections (B) and (D) of § 2252A, even if the "performer" (i.e., the person visually depicted as engaged in "sexually explicit conduct") is an adult and *not* a person under eighteen, if the visual depiction "appears" to be of such a person, or if the material is presented *so to suggest* it is (though it is not), the producer (including as a "producer" any distributor or exhibitor) is subject to conviction — *unless* in the case of a producer,[11] the defendant can and does prove the following to be true, in which case only shall he or she have an affirmative defense:

(1) the alleged child pornography was produced using an *actual* person or persons engaging in sexually explicit conduct; [*and*]

(2) each such person was an adult at the time the material was produced; [*and*]

(3) the defendant did not advertise, promote, present, describe, or distribute the material in such a manner as to convey the impression it is or contains a visual depiction of a minor engaging in sexually explicit conduct.

These 1996 additions to the federal act clearly carry quite far beyond the original, limited design of 18 U.S.C. §2252. Even so, can these provisions also be squared with the first amendment? If so, on what possible rationale(s), and to what extent?[12]

---

11. (But evidently *not* in the case of one who knowingly receives and has in their possession three or more such visual depictions, i.e., the "affirmative defense" as immediately described in the text (and as set forth in § 2252A(c) of the Act), is evidently *not* available to one who "knowingly possesses any book, magazine periodical, film, videotape, computer disk, or any other material that contains 3 or more images of child pornography that has been...transported in interstate or foreign commerce by any means...or that was produced using materials that have been [so transported]." (See 18 U.S.C. § 2256(8) (defining "child pornography"), and compare § 2252A(a) describing who is subject to criminal prosecution for producing, distributing, or possessing such material), and §2252A(c) (describing who may and may not present an affirmative defense, and describing the necessary elements of such defense).)

12. For two recent — but far from conclusive — lower court opinions, *see The Free Speech Coalition v. Reno*, 1997 U.S. Dist. Lexis 12212/25 Media L. Rep. 2305 (N.D. Cal.) (sustaining the act against first amendment "overbreadth" objections); *United States v. Hilton*, 999 F. Supp. 131 (D. Me. 1998) (voiding the act on first amendment "vagueness" grounds), *reversed*, 167 F.3d 61 (1st Cir. 1999), *petition for certiorari filed. See also American Booksellers Ass'n v. Hudnut* (casebook at 252); *Ginsberg v. United States* (casebook at 790); *Mishkin v. New York* (Casebook at 797). (Recall still again that there is, in respect to what is covered in these provisions, just as in *Ferber*, no requirement that the material be "obscene.")

JENKINS v. GEORGIA
418 U.S. 153 (1974)

MR. JUSTICE REHNQUIST delivered the opinion of the Court.

Appellant was convicted in Georgia of the crime of distributing obscene material. His conviction, in March 1972, was for showing the film "Carnal Knowledge" in a movie theater in Albany, Georgia. ***

*** We conclude here that the film "Carnal Knowledge" is not obscene under the constitutional standards announced in Miller v. California, 413 U.S. 15 (1973), and that the First and Fourteenth Amendments therefore require that the judgment of the Supreme Court of Georgia affirming appellant's conviction be reversed. ***

We agree with the Supreme Court of Georgia's implicit ruling that the Constitution does not require that juries be instructed in state obscenity cases to apply the standards of a hypothetical statewide community. *Miller* approved the use of such instructions; it did not mandate their use. What *Miller* makes clear is that state juries need not be instructed to apply "national standards." We also agree with the Supreme Court of Georgia's implicit approval of the trial court's instructions directing jurors to apply "community standards" without specifying what "community." *Miller* held that it was constitutionally permissible to permit juries to rely on the understanding of the community from which they came as to contemporary community standards, and the States have considerable latitude in framing statutes under this element of the *Miller* decision. A State may choose to define an obscenity offense in terms of "contemporary community standards" as defined in *Miller* without further specification, as was done here, or it may choose to define the standards in more precise geographic terms, as was done by California in *Miller*.

We now turn to the question of whether appellant's exhibition of the film was protected by the First and Fourteenth Amendments. ***

There is little to be found in the record about the film "Carnal Knowledge" other than the film itself.[5] However, appellant has supplied a variety of information and critical commentary, the authenticity of which appellee does not dispute. The film appeared on many "Ten Best" lists for 1971, the year in which it was released. Many but not all of the reviews were favorable. ***

Appellee contends essentially that under *Miller* the obscenity *vel non* of the film "Carnal Knowledge" was a question for the jury, and that the jury having resolved the question against appellant, and there being some evidence to support its findings, the judgment of conviction should be affirmed. We turn to the language of *Miller* to evaluate appellee's contention.

---

5. Appellant testified that the film was "critically acclaimed as one of the ten best pictures of 1971 and Ann Margaret has received an Academy Award nomination for her performance in the picture." He further testified that "Carnal Knowledge" had played in 29 towns in Georgia and that it was booked in 50 or 60 more theaters for spring and summer showing.

Miller states that the questions of what appeals to the "prurient interest" and what is "patently offensive" under the obscenity test which it formulates are "essentially questions of fact." "When triers of fact are asked to decide whether 'the average person, applying contemporary community standards' would consider certain materials 'prurient' it would be unrealistic to require that the answer be based on some abstract formulation. *** To require a State to structure obscenity proceedings around evidence of a national 'community standard' would be an exercise in futility." We held in Paris Adult Theatre I v. Slaton, 413 U.S. 49 (1973), decided on the same day, that expert testimony as to obscenity is not necessary when the films at issue are themselves placed in evidence.

But all of this does not lead us to agree with the Supreme Court of Georgia's apparent conclusion that the jury's verdict against appellant virtually precluded all further appellate review of appellant's assertion that his exhibition of the film was protected by the First and Fourteenth Amendments. Even though questions of appeal to the "prurient interest" or of patent offensiveness are "essentially questions of fact," it would be a serious misreading of *Miller* to conclude that juries have unbridled discretion in determining what is "patently offensive." Not only did we there say that "the First Amendment values applicable to the State through the Fourteenth Amendment are adequately protected by the ultimate power of appellate courts to conduct an independent review of constitutional claims when necessary," but we made it plain that under that holding "no one will be subject to prosecution for the sale or exposure of obscene materials unless these materials depict or describe patently offensive 'hard core' sexual conduct ***."

We also took pains in *Miller* to "give a few plain examples of what a state statute could define for regulation under part (b) of the standard announced," that is, the requirement of patent offensiveness. These examples included "representations or descriptions of ultimate sexual acts, normal or perverted, actual or simulated," and "representations or descriptions of masturbation, excretory functions, and lewd exhibition of the genitals." While this did not purport to be an exhaustive catalog of what juries might find patently offensive, it was certainly intended to fix substantive constitutional limitations, deriving from the First Amendment, on the type of material subject to such a determination. It would be wholly at odds with this aspect of *Miller* to uphold an obscenity conviction based upon a defendant's depiction of a woman with a bare midriff, even though a properly charged jury unanimously agreed on a verdict of guilty.

Our own viewing of the film satisfies us that "Carnal Knowledge" could not be found under the *Miller* standards to depict sexual conduct in a patently offensive way. Nothing in the movie falls within either of the two examples given in *Miller* of material which may constitutionally be found to meet the "patently offensive" element of those standards, nor is there anything sufficiently similar to such material to justify similar treatment. While the subject matter of the picture is, in a broader sense, sex, and there are scenes in which sexual conduct including "ultimate sexual acts" is to be understood to be taking place, the camera does not focus on the bodies of the actors at such times. There is no exhibition whatever of the actors' genitals, lewd or otherwise, during these scenes. There are occasional scenes of nudity, but nudity alone is not enough to make material legally obscene under the *Miller* standards.

Appellant's showing of the film "Carnal Knowledge" is simply not the "public portrayal of hard core sexual conduct for its own sake, and for the ensuing commercial gain" which we said was punishable in *Miller*. We hold that the film could not, as a matter of constitutional law, be found to depict sexual conduct in a patently offensive way, and that it is therefore not outside the protection of the First and Fourteenth Amendments because it is obscene. No other basis appearing in the record upon which the judgment of conviction can be sustained, we reverse the judgment of the Supreme Court of Georgia.

MR. JUSTICE DOUGLAS, being of the view that any ban on obscenity is prohibited by the First Amendment, made applicable to the States through the Fourteenth, concurs in the reversal of this conviction.

MR. JUSTICE BRENNAN, with whom MR. JUSTICE STEWART and MR. JUSTICE MARSHALL join, concurring in the result.

Today's decision confirms my observation in Paris Adult Theatre I v. Slaton, 413 U.S. 49 (1973), that the Court's new formulation does not extricate us from the mire of case-by-case determinations of obscenity. ***

After the Court's decision today, there can be no doubt that *Miller* requires appellate courts—including this Court—to review independently the constitutional fact of obscenity. Moreover, the Court's task is not limited to reviewing a jury finding under part (c) of the *Miller* test that "the work, taken as a whole, lack[ed] serious literary, artistic, political, or scientific value." *Miller* also requires independent review of a jury's determination under part (b) of the *Miller* test that "the work depicts or describes, in a patently offensive way, sexual conduct specifically defined by the applicable state law."

In order to make the review mandated by *Miller*, the Court was required to screen the film "Carnal Knowledge" and make an independent determination of obscenity *vel non*. Following that review, the Court holds that "Carnal Knowledge" "could not, as a matter of constitutional law, be found to depict sexual conduct in a patently offensive way, and that it is therefore not outside the protection of the First and Fourteenth Amendments because it is obscene."

Thus, it is clear that as long as the *Miller* test remains in effect "one cannot say with certainty that material is obscene until at least five members of this Court, applying inevitably obscure standards, have pronounced it so." Paris Adult Theatre I v. Slaton, 413 U.S., at 92 (BRENNAN, J., dissenting). Because of the attendant uncertainty of such a process and its inevitable institutional stress upon the judiciary, I continue to adhere to my view that, "at least in the absence of distribution to juveniles or obstrusive exposure to unconsenting adults, the First and Fourteenth Amendments prohibit the State and Federal Governments from attempting wholly to suppress sexually oriented materials on the basis of their allegedly 'obscene' contents." *Id.*, at 113. It is clear that, tested by that constitutional standard, the Georgia obscenity statutes under which appellant Jenkins was convicted are constitutionally overbroad and therefore facially invalid. I therefore concur in the result in the Court's reversal of Jenkins' conviction.

CONCLUDING NOTE: EXCERPTS FROM CERTAIN BAWDY VERSES

Your rounded thighs are like jewels,
the work of a master hand.
Your navel is a rounded bowl
that never lacks mixed wine.
Your belly is a heap of wheat,
encircled with lilies.
Your two breasts are like two fawns,
twins of a gazelle.

* * *

How fair and pleasant you are,
O loved one, delectable maiden!
You are stately as a palm tree,
and your breasts are like its clusters.
I say I will climb the palm tree
and lay hold of its branches.
Oh, may your breasts be like
clusters of the vine,
and the scent of your breath like apples,
and your kisses like the best wine
that goes down smoothly
gliding over lips and teeth.

* * *

O that you were like a brother to me,
that nursed at my mother's breast!
I would give you spiced wine to drink
the juice of my pomegranates.
Make haste, my beloved,
and be like a gazelle
or a young stag
upon the mountain of spices.

---

1. Are these verses "obscene"?[1] What is the proper test to be applied—What part of that test (*Miller-Slaton-Jenkins*) necessarily precludes the conclusion that these verses can be found "obscene"?

2. Suppose these verses are accompanied by illustrations graphically depicting the artist's rendering of these verses; at least *then* may the work "as a whole," inclusive of these verses, be "obscene"?[2]

3. If, with accompanying illustrations, these and similar bawdy verses are collected in a slick commercial magazine featuring the lurid magazine title,*Concupiscent Sex*, and the magazine is ordered from a New York mailhouse by a postal inspector in Provo, Utah, responding to a mailed leaflet soliciting orders for the magazine for $3.50, could a federal criminal conviction for mailing nonmailable material be sustained?[3] *Whose* "contemporary community" standards apply? New York (the state in which the magazine was put into the mail)? *Utah* (the state in which it is taken from the mail and read)? *Provo* (the immediate community to which the magazine was directed and in which it was taken from the mail)? The *United States* overall (because it was a federal statute, and not a state statute or local ordinance)?[4]

4. Suppose these verses were spoken in heavy rhythm, accented with strong body movements and accompanied by evocative sounds ("rap" fashion). Would a criminal prosecution for exhibiting "obscenity" be sustainable against first amendment objections, under a state or local anti-obscenity law as applied to a nightclub or

---

1. Alternatively (by way of review), might they be suppressible:

(a) by public school board decision disallowing their inclusion in any book or written material used in grades K through 12?

(b) pursuant to a public university anti-harassment rule as applied to a student with these verses printed on a t-shirt (s)he wears on campus or in class?

(c) pursuant to a Title VII action brought by a female co-worker or the EEOC to enjoin workplace discrimination against the company failing to discipline a male co-worker for the display of these verses in large print on a poster above his desk in an office she also shares?

2. To what extent, if any, may it matter that the "artist" providing the graphics is famous or not famous? Suppose the illustrations are crude but the artist is nonetheless famous. What difference may it make? (Should a famous illustrator's signature provide a first amendment safe harbor? How famous, in his day, was Van Gogh?)

3. See Ginzburg v. United States, 383 U.S. 463 (1966).

4. For a decision by the Court that the "literary, artistic, political, or scientific value" factor is not to be measured by local community standards but by "whether a reasonable person would find such value in the material, taken as a whole," see Pope v. Illinois, 481 U.S. 497, 501 (1987). Given that that may be so, is it a question of fact for the jury to determine whether a reasonable person would so conclude, a question of law addressed to the trial (and appellate) court, or a mixed question of law and fact, or a question of constitutional fact? Compare the Court's treatment of the second factor ("patent offensiveness") on this question, in Jenkins v. Georgia, 418 U.S. 153 (1974). (Note that in Miller v. California, 413 U.S. 15, 25 n.7 (1973), Chief Justice Burger excluded the consideration of "social importance" as distinct from literary, artistic, political, or scientific value, under part three of the test. Why is that?)

cabaret?[5] Would the result be different if the same performance were instead rendered in Carnegie Hall?[6]

5. Of what consequence would it be were these verses not described as "bawdy" verses? Would it make any difference if instead one described them as "prurient" or "lewd"—or as an example of "pandering to male stereotype" (i.e. sexual images of women as erotic objects craving to be possessed)?[7]

However they strike you on first impression, is it of any consequence to learn that they are in fact verses from Holy Scripture, passages from the Old Testament, and thus (?) not bawdy verses at all?[8] Would this datum make any difference in respect to the proper outcome of any of the cases hypothesized *supra*? Why?

6. If in one or more of the above settings a prosecution or a civil action for injunction were brought not under an anti-*obscenity* law but instead under an anti-*blasphemy* law,[9] how would you expect the first amendment to be applied?[10]

7. Given that the various proceedings hypothesized *supra*, were not brought under an anti-blasphemy law, but under an anti-obscenity law, even so, why should the outcome be different? What is the "governmental interest" (i.e. the "harm" to be avoided) sufficient to override the first amendment claims ?[11]

---

5. As a variation, would such a prosecution be upheld insofar as the statute or ordinance is limited to such establishments as are licensed to serve alcoholic beverages? (See City of Newport v. Iacobucci, 479 U.S. 92 (1986); New York State Liquor Auth. v. Bellanca, 452 U.S. 714 (1981); California v. LaRue, 409 U.S. 109 (1972).) As a further variation, would such a prosecution be upheld insofar as the statute or ordinance is limited to such establishments admitting persons under the age of seventeen? (See Ginsburg v. New, York 390 U.S. 629 (1968).)

6. If so, why? Because the booking of the act at Carnegie Hall *per se* proves "serious *** artistic *** value?"

7. See Susan Brownmiller, Against Our Will: Men, Women and Rape 394 (1975); Catherine A. MacKinnon, Feminism Unmodified 146-228 (1987) ("Pornography is the undiluted essence of anti-female propaganda."); Cass R. Sunstein, Pornography and the First Amendment, 1986 Duke L.J. 589 (1986). Cf. Kingsley Int'l Pictures Corp. v. Regents of State Univ. of N.Y., 360 U.S. 684 (1959); American Booksellers Ass'n v. Hudnut, 771 F.2d 323 (7th Cir. 1985), summarily aff'd, 475 U.S. 1001 (1986).

8. Old Testament, The Song of Solomon, chapters 7 & 8. (See the opinions by Douglas, J., dissenting in Ginzburg v. United States, 383 U.S. at 482-492, and in Miller v. California, 413 U.S. at 34-47, providing references to these passages.)

9. The point of this alternative prosection being that a recognized religion's verses or religious scripture are used in a manner or setting that distorts them and makes a vile, inflammatory misappropriation belittling their sacredness and profaning their true meaning, presenting a false image of holy text. (Cf. the call for the death of Salman Rushdie, following publication of *The Satanic Verses*.)

10. See Burstyn, Inc. v. Wilson, 343 U.S. 495 (1952). See also Kingsley Int'l Pictures Corp. v. Regents of S.U.N.Y., 360 U.S. 684 (1959) (ideological obscenity fully protected).

11. Is the thought that pornography (i.e. "true" pornography) acts not on the mind even in the usual way of highly affective speech (e.g., Cohen v. California, 403 U.S. 15 (1971) ("Fuck the Draft"), or on the mind even as dangerous ideological speech, but rather that it acts—and is *meant* to act—much more directly on the senses in the manner of an injected chemical stimulus or as a product made and marketed for stimulative sexual use? So that it ought, therefore, to be treated for purposes of constitutional analysis essentially as regulable as "nonspeech," i.e. on the same terms as sexual products

Question 4 *supra* asked whether an eroticized, set-to-rap-music rhythm, body undulating performance of "The Song of Solomon" in a closely packed nightclub may be obscene although the identical performance rendered the same way, but rendered in Carnegie Hall, would not. The following case may also help one think about the question (among others). The case, *Barnes v. Glen Theatre*, does not involve an obscenity prosecution nor even a law directed to obscenity as such. Nevertheless, it – and the next two cases – should provide an excellent postscript to this subject and to the Supreme Court's own ongoing internal doctrinal disagreements in applying the first amendment to expressive conduct and sex.

BARNES v. GLEN THEATRE, INC.
501 U.S. 560 (1991)

CHIEF JUSTICE REHNQUIST announced the judgment of the Court and delivered an opinion, in which JUSTICE O'CONNOR and JUSTICE KENNEDY join.

Respondents are two establishments in South Bend, Indiana, that wish to provide totally nude dancing as entertainment, and individual dancers who are employed at these establishments. They claim that the First Amendment's guarantee of freedom of expression prevents the State of Indiana from enforcing its public indecency law to prevent this form of dancing. We reject their claim.

The Kitty Kat Lounge, Inc. (Kitty Kat), is located in the city of South Bend. It sells alcoholic beverages and presents "go-go dancing." Its proprietor desires to present "totally nude dancing," but an applicable Indiana statute regulating public nudity requires that the dancers wear "pasties" and a "G-string" when they dance.

---

may be regulated, or as prescription or nonprescription drugs may be regulated, rather than as "speech"? (Compare Mishkin v. New York, 383 U.S. 502 (1966) with Bowers v. Hardwick, 478 U.S. 186 (1986). But see Stanley v. Georgia, 394 U.S. 557 (1969).)

For development of arguments of this sort (generally, and with reference to obscenity specifically), see Frederick Schauer, Speech and "Speech"— Obscenity and "Obscenity": An Exercise in the Interpretation of Constitutional Language, 67 Geo.L.J. 899 (1979); Frederick Schauer, Response: Pornography and the First Amendment, 40 U.Pitt.L.Rev. 605 (1979). But if the "harm" to be avoided is sexual excitement *per se*, then even assuming that *other* modes of stimulating such excitement may be regulated or forbidden (e.g., vibrators, dildos, and aphrodisiacs), presumably it is so *only* because they are not speech but rather are nonspeech products subject only to extremely weak substantive fifth and fourteenth amendment ("commercial products") due process review. Is Professor Schauer's point that the Song of Solomon, Eros, Lust Pool, or Shame Agent, may not be speech, and not products of a free press? If not, what are they? Is this an area where one can attempt to apply even the reasoning derived from United States v. O'Brien, 391 U.S. 370 (1968)? (Is reading even a thoroughly "hard core" pornographic book "the same" as tearing or burning or rubbing against the pages of that book?) As a general alternative to the Court's current approach, see also Redrup v. New York, 386 U.S. 767 (1967) (*supra*). (Some state supreme courts do not now exclude "obscene" speech from ordinary first amendment review pursuant to state constitutional free speech provisions. See, e.g., State v. Henry, 732 P.2d 9 (Or. 1987).))

Respondent Glen Theatre, Inc., is an Indiana corporation with a place of business in South Bend. Its primary business is supplying so-called adult entertainment through written and printed materials, movie showings, and live entertainment at an enclosed "bookstore." The live entertainment at the "bookstore" consists of nude and seminude performances and showings of the female body through glass panels. Customers sit in a booth and insert coins into a timing mechanism that permits them to observe the live nude and seminude dancers for a period of time. One of Glen Theatre's dancers, Gayle Ann Marie Sutro, has danced, modeled, and acted professionally for more than 15 years, and in addition to her performances at the Glen Theatre, can be seen in a pornographic movie at a nearby theater.

*** The District Court originally granted respondents' prayer for an injunction, finding that the statute was facially overbroad. The Court of Appeals for the Seventh Circuit reversed, deciding that previous litigation with respect to the statute in the Supreme Court of Indiana and this Court precluded the possibility of such a challenge,[1] and remanded to the District Court in order for the plaintiffs to pursue their claim that the statute violated the First Amendment as applied to their dancing. On remand, the District Court concluded that "the type of dancing these plaintiffs wish to perform is not expressive activity protected by the Constitution of the United States," and rendered judgment in favor of the defendants. The case was again appealed to the Seventh Circuit, and *** that court reversed the District Court, holding that the nude dancing involved here was expressive conduct protected by the First Amendment.

Several of our cases contain language suggesting that nude dancing of the kind involved here is expressive conduct protected by the First Amendment. In Doran v. Salem Inn, Inc., 422 U.S. 922, 932 (1975), we said: "[A]lthough the customary 'barroom' type of nude dancing may involve only the barest minimum of protected expression, we recognized in California v. LaRue, 409 U.S. 109, 118 (1972), that this form of entertainment might be entitled to First and Fourteenth Amendment protection under some circumstances." *** These statements support the conclusion of the Court of Appeals that nude dancing of the kind sought to be performed here is expressive conduct within the outer perimeters of the First Amendment, though we view it as only marginally so. This, of course, does not end our inquiry. We must determine the level of protection to be afforded to the expressive conduct at issue,

1. The Indiana Supreme Court appeared to give the public indecency statute a limiting construction to save it from a facial overbreadth attack:

> "There is no right to appear nude in public. Rather, it *may* be constitutionally required to tolerate or to allow some nudity as a part of some larger form of expression meriting protection, when the communication of ideas is involved." State v. Baysinger, 272 Ind. 236, 247, 397 N.E.2d 580, 587 (1979) (emphasis added) ***.
>
> *** [T]he Indiana Supreme Court did not affirmatively limit the reach of the statute in *Baysinger*, but merely said that to the extent the First Amendment would require it, the statute might be unconstitutional as applied to some activities.

and must determine whether the Indiana statute is an impermissible infringement of that protected activity.

Indiana has not banned nude dancing as such, but has proscribed public nudity across the board. The Supreme Court of Indiana has construed the Indiana statute to preclude nudity in what are essentially places of public accommodation such as the Glen Theatre and the Kitty Kat Lounge. [M]inors are excluded and there are no nonconsenting viewers. Respondents contend that while the State may license establishments such as the ones involved here, and limit the geographical area in which they do business, it may not in any way limit the performance of the dances within them without violating the First Amendment. The petitioners contend, on the other hand, that Indiana's restriction on nude dancing is a valid "time, place or manner" restriction under cases such as Clark v. Community for Creative Non-Violence, 468 U.S. 288 (1984).

The "time, place, or manner" test was developed for evaluating restrictions on expression taking place on public property which had been dedicated as a "public forum," Ward v. Rock Against Racism, 491 U.S. 781, 791 (1989), although we have on at least one occasion applied it to conduct occurring on private property. See Renton v. Playtime Theatres, Inc., 475 U.S. 41 (1986). In *Clark* we observed that this test has been interpreted to embody much the same standards as those set forth in United States v. O'Brien, 391 U.S. 367 (1968), and we turn, therefore, to the rule enunciated in *O'Brien*.

Applying the four-part *O'Brien* test we find that Indiana's public indecency statute is justified despite its incidental limitations on some expressive activity. The public indecency statute is clearly within the constitutional power of the State and furthers substantial governmental interests. [S]tatutes of this sort are of ancient origin, and presently exist in at least 47 States. Public indecency statutes such as the one before us reflect moral disapproval of people appearing in the nude among strangers in public places.

This interest is unrelated to the suppression of free expression. Some may view restricting nudity on moral grounds as necessarily related to expression. We disagree. It can be argued, of course, that almost limitless types of conduct—including appearing in the nude in public—are "expressive," and in one sense of the word this is true. People who go about in the nude in public may be expressing something about themselves by so doing. But the court rejected this expansive notion of "expressive conduct" in *O'Brien* ***. And in Dallas v. Stanglin, 490 U.S. 19, we further observed:

> "It is possible to find some kernel of expression in almost every activity a person undertakes—for example, walking down the street or meeting one's friends at a shopping mall—but such a kernel is not sufficient to bring the activity within the protection of the First Amendment. We think the activity of these dance-hall patrons coming together to engage in recreational dancing—is not protected by the First Amendment." ***

Respondents contend that even though prohibiting nudity in public generally may not be related to suppressing expression, prohibiting the performance of nude dancing is related to expression because the state seeks to prevent its erotic message. ***

But we do not think that when Indiana applies its statute to the nude dancing in these nightclubs it is proscribing nudity because of the erotic message conveyed by the dancers. Presumably numerous other erotic performances are presented at these establishments and similar clubs without any interference from the State, so long as the performers wear a scant amount of clothing. Likewise, the requirement that the dancers don pasties and a G-string does not deprive the dance of whatever erotic message it conveys; it simply makes the message slightly less graphic. The perceived evil that Indiana seeks to address is not erotic dancing, but public nudity. The appearance of people of all shapes, sizes and ages in the nude at a beach, for example, would convey little if any erotic message, yet the State still seeks to prevent it. Public nudity is the evil the State seeks to prevent, whether or not it is combined with expressive activity.

This conclusion is buttressed by a reference to the facts of *O'Brien*. *** It was assumed that O'Brien's act in burning the certificate had a communicative element in it sufficient to bring into play the First Amendment, but it was for the noncommunicative element that he was prosecuted. So here with the Indiana statute; while the dancing to which it was applied had a communicative element, it was not the dancing that was prohibited, but simply its being done in the nude.

The fourth part of the *O'Brien* test requires that the incidental restriction on First Amendment freedom be no greater than is essential to the furtherance of the governmental interest. As indicated in the discussion above, the governmental interest served by the text of the prohibition is societal disapproval of nudity in public places and among strangers. The statutory prohibition is not a means to some greater end, but an end in itself. It is without cavil that the public indecency statute is "narrowly tailored"; Indiana's requirement that the dancers wear at least pasties and a G-string is modest, and the bare minimum necessary to achieve the state's purpose.

The judgment of the Court of Appeals accordingly is Reversed.

JUSTICE SCALIA, concurring in the judgment.

I agree that the judgment of the Court of Appeals must be reversed. In my view, however, the challenged regulation must be upheld, not because it survives some lower level of First-Amendment scrutiny, but because, as a general law regulating conduct and not specifically directed at expression, it is not subject to First-Amendment scrutiny at all.

I

Indiana's public indecency statute provides:

"(a) A person who knowingly or intentionally, in a public place:

"(1) engages in sexual intercourse;

"(2) engages in deviate sexual conduct;

"(3) appears in a state of nudity; or
"(4) fondles the genitals of himself or another person;
commits public indecency, a Class A misdemeanor.

On its face, this law is not directed at expression in particular. As Judge Easterbrook put it in his dissent below: "Indiana does not regulate dancing. It regulates public nudity. Almost the entire domain of Indiana's statute is unrelated to expression, unless we view nude beaches and topless hot dog vendors as speech." The intent to convey a "message of eroticism" (or any other message) is not a necessary element of the statutory offense of public indecency; nor does one commit that statutory offense by conveying the most explicit "message of eroticism," so long as he does not commit any of the four specified acts in the process.

The dissent confidently asserts that the purpose of restricting nudity in public places in general is to protect nonconsenting parties from offense; and argues that since only consenting, admission-paying patrons see respondents dance, that purpose cannot apply and the only remaining purpose must relate to the communicative elements of the performance. Perhaps the dissenters believe that "offense to others" *ought* to be the only reason for restricting nudity in public places generally, but there is no basis for thinking that our society has ever shared that Thoreauvian "you-may-do-what-you-like-so-long-as-it-does-not-injure-someone-else" beau ideal—much less for thinking that it was written into the Constitution. The purpose of Indiana's nudity law would be violated, I think, if 60,000 fully consenting adults crowded into the Hoosierdome to display their genitals to one another, even if there were not an offended innocent in the crowd. Our society prohibits, and all human societies have prohibited, certain activities not because they harm others but because they are considered, in the traditional phrase, "*contra bonos mores*," *i.e.*, immoral. *** The purpose of the Indiana statute, as both its text and the manner of its enforcement demonstrate, is to enforce the traditional moral belief that people should not expose their private parts indiscriminately, regardless of whether those who see them are disedified. Since that is so, the dissent has no basis for positing that, where only thoroughly edified adults are present, the purpose must be repression of communication.[2]

II

Since the Indiana regulation is a general law not specifically targeted at expressive conduct, its application to such conduct does not in my view implicate the First

2. The dissent *** also misunderstands what is meant by the term "general law." I do not mean that the law restricts the targeted conduct in all places at all times. A law is "general" for the present purposes if it regulates conduct without regard to whether that conduct is expressive. Concededly, Indiana bans nudity in public places, but not within the privacy of the home. (That is not surprising, since the common law offense, and the traditional moral prohibition, runs against *public* nudity, not against all nudity. ***) But that confirms, rather than refutes, the general nature of the law: One may not go nude in public, whether or not one intends thereby to convey a message, and similarly one *may* go nude in private, again whether or not that nudity is expressive.

Amendment. *** This is not to say that the First Amendment affords no protection to expressive conduct. Where the government prohibits conduct *precisely because of its communicative attributes*, we hold the regulation unconstitutional. See, e.g., United States v. Eichman, 496 U.S. 310 (1990) (burning flag); Texas v. Johnson, 491 U.S. 397 (1989) (same); Spence v. Washington, 418 U.S. 405 (1974) (defacing flag); Tinker v. Des Moines Independent Community School District, 393 U.S. 503 (1969) (wearing black arm bands); Brown v. Louisiana, 383 U.S. 131 (1966) (participating in silent sit-in); Stromberg v. California, 283 U.S. 359 (1931) (flying a red flag).[4] In each of the foregoing cases, we explicitly found that suppressing communication was the object of the regulation of conduct. Where that has not been the case, however —where suppression of communicative use of the conduct was merely the incidental effect of forbidding the conduct for other reasons—we have allowed the regulation to stand. ***

III

While I do not think the plurality's conclusions differ greatly from my own, I cannot entirely endorse its reasoning. The plurality purports to apply to this general law, insofar as it regulates this allegedly expressive conduct, an intermediate level of First Amendment scrutiny: the government interest in the regulation must be "'important or substantial,'" *** quoting *O'Brien*, [391 U.S.], at 377. As I have indicated, I do not believe such a heightened standard exists. I think we should avoid wherever possible, moreover, a method of analysis that requires judicial assessment of the "importance" of government interests—and especially of government interests in various aspects of morality.

*** In *Bowers*, we held that since homosexual behavior is not a fundamental right, a Georgia law prohibiting private homosexual intercourse needed only a rational basis in order to comply with the Due Process Clause. Moral opposition to homosexuality, we said, provided that rational basis. I would uphold the Indiana statute on precisely the same ground: moral opposition to nudity supplies a rational basis for its prohibition, and since the First Amendment has no application to this case no more than that is needed. ***

JUSTICE SOUTER, concurring in the judgment.

Not all dancing is entitled to First Amendment protection as expressive activity. This Court has previously categorized ballroom dancing as beyond the Amendment's protection, Dallas v. Stanglin, 490 U.S. 19, 24-25 (1989), and dancing as aerobic

---

4. It is easy to conclude that conduct has been forbidden because of its communicative attributes when the conduct in question is what the Court has called "inherently expressive," and what I would prefer to call "conventionally expressive"—such as flying a red flag. I mean by that phrase (as I assume the Court means by "inherently expressive") conduct that is normally engaged in for the purpose of communicating an idea, or perhaps an emotion, to someone else. I am not sure whether dancing fits that description ***. But even if it does, this law is directed against nudity, not dancing. Nudity is *not* normally engaged in for the purpose of communicating an idea or an emotion.

exercise would likewise be outside the First Amendment's concern. But dancing as a performance directed to an actual or hypothetical audience gives expression at least to generalized emotion or feeling, and where the dancer is nude or nearly so the feeling expressed, in the absence of some contrary clue, is eroticism, carrying an endorsement of erotic experience. Such is the expressive content of the dances described in the record. *** Thus I agree with the plurality and the dissent that an interest in freely engaging in the nude dancing at issue here is subject to a degree of First Amendment protection.

I also agree with the plurality that the appropriate analysis to determine the actual protection required by the First Amendment is the four-part enquiry described in United States v. O'Brien, 391 U.S. 367 (1968), for judging the limits of appropriate state action burdening expressive acts as distinct from pure speech or representation. I nonetheless write separately to rest my concurrence in the judgment, not on the possible sufficiency of society's moral views to justify the limitations at issue, but on the State's substantial interest in combating the secondary effects of adult entertainment establishments of the sort typified by respondents' establishments. ***

In Renton v. Playtime Theatres, Inc., 475 U.S. 41 (1986), we upheld a city's zoning ordinance designed to prevent the occurrence of harmful secondary effects, including the crime associated with adult entertainment, by protecting approximately 95% of the city's area from the placement of motion picture theaters emphasizing "'matter depicting, describing or relating to "specified sexual activities" or "specified anatomical areas" *** for observation by patrons therein.'" *** In light of*Renton*'s recognition that legislation seeking to combat the secondary effects of adult entertainment need not await localized proof of those effects, the State of Indiana could reasonably conclude that forbidding nude entertainment of the type offered at the Kitty Kat Lounge and the Glen Theatre's "bookstore" furthers its interest in preventing prostitution, sexual assault, and associated crimes. The statute as applied to nudity of the sort at issue here therefore satisfies the second prong of *O'Brien*.[2]

The third *O'Brien* condition is that the governmental interest be "unrelated to the suppression of free expression," 391 U.S., at 377, and, on its face, the governmental interest in combating prostitution and other criminal activity is not at all inherently related to expression. *** Because the State's interest in banning nude dancing results from a simple correlation of such dancing with other evils, rather than from

2. Because there is no overbreadth challenge before us, we are not called upon to decide whether the application of the statute would be valid in other contexts. It is enough, then, to say that the secondary effects rationale on which I rely here would be open to question if the State were to seek to enforce the statute by barring expressive nudity in classes of productions that could not readily be analogized to the adult films at issue in Renton v. Playtime Theatres, Inc., 475 U.S. 41 (1986). It is difficult to see, for example, how the enforcement of Indiana's statute against nudity in a production of "Hair" or "Equus" somewhere other than an "adult" theater would further the State's interest in avoiding harmful secondary effects, in the absence of evidence that expressive nudity outside the context of *Renton*-type adult entertainment was correlated with such secondary effects.

a relationship between the other evils and the expressive component of the dancing, the interest is unrelated to the suppression of free expression. *Renton* is again persuasive in support of this conclusion. ***

The fourth *O'Brien* condition, that the restriction be no greater than essential to further the governmental interest, requires little discussion. Pasties and a G-string moderate the expression to some degree, to be sure, but only to a degree. Dropping the final stitch is prohibited, but the limitation is minor when measured against the dancer's remaining capacity and opportunity to express the erotic message. Nor, so far as we are told, is the dancer or her employer limited by anything short of obscenity laws from expressing an erotic message by articulate speech or representational means; a pornographic movie featuring one of respondents, for example, was playing nearby without any interference from the authorities at the time these cases arose.

Accordingly, I find *O'Brien* satisfied and concur in the judgment.

JUSTICE WHITE, with whom JUSTICE MARSHALL, JUSTICE BLACKMUN, and JUSTICE STEVENS join, dissenting.

The first question presented to us in this case is whether nonobscene nude dancing performed as entertainment is expressive conduct protected by the First Amendment. The Court of Appeals held that it is, observing that our prior decisions permit no other conclusion. Not surprisingly, then, the plurality now concedes that "nude dancing of the kind sought to be performed here is expressive conduct within the outer perimeters of the First Amendment ***." This is no more than recognizing, as the Seventh Circuit observed, that dancing is an ancient art form and "inherently embodies the expression and communication of ideas and emotions."[1]

As Judge Posner argued in his thoughtful concurring opinion in the Court of Appeals, the nudity of the dancer is an integral part of the emotions and thoughts that a nude dancing performance evokes. *** The sight of a fully clothed, or even a partially clothed, dancer generally will have a far different impact on a spectator than that of a nude dancer, even if the same dance is performed. The nudity is itself an expressive component of the dance, not merely incidental "conduct." ***

This being the case, it cannot be that the statutory prohibition is unrelated to expressive conduct. Since the State permits the dancers to perform if they wear pas-

---

1. JUSTICE SCALIA suggests that performance dancing is not inherently expressive activity, but the Court of Appeals has the better view: "Dance has been defined as 'the art of moving the body in a rhythmical way, usually to music, to express an emotion or idea, to narrate a story, or simply to take delight in the movement itself.' 16 The New Encyclopedia Britannica 935 (1989). Inherently, it is the communication of emotion or ideas." *** JUSTICE SCALIA cites Dallas v. Stanglin, 490 U.S. 19 (1989), but that decision dealt with social dancing, not performance dancing; and the submission in that case, which we rejected, was not that social dancing was an expressive activity but that plaintiff's *associational* rights were violated by restricting admission to dance halls on the basis of age. The Justice also asserts that even if dancing is inherently expressive, nudity is not. The statement may be true, but it tells us nothing about dancing in the nude.

ties and G-strings but forbids nude dancing, it is precisely because of the distinctive, expressive content of the nude dancing performances at issue in this case that the State seeks to apply the statutory prohibition. It is only because nude dancing performances may generate emotions and feelings of eroticism and sensuality among the spectators that the State seeks to regulate such expressive activity, apparently on the assumption that creating or emphasizing such thoughts and ideas in the minds of the spectators may lead to increased prostitution and the degradation of women. But generating thoughts, ideas, and emotions is the essence of communication. The nudity element of nude dancing performances cannot be neatly pigeonholed as mere "conduct" independent of any expressive component of the dance.[2] ***

That the performances in the Kitty Kat Lounge may not be high art, to say the least, and may not appeal to the Court, is hardly an excuse for distorting and ignoring settled doctrine. The Court's assessment of the artistic merits of nude dancing performances should not be the determining factor in deciding this case. In the words of Justice Harlan, "[I]t is largely because governmental officials cannot make principled decisions in this area that the Constitution leaves matters of taste and style so largely to the individual." Cohen v. California, 403 U.S. 15, 25 (1971). "[W]hile the entertainment afforded by a nude ballet at Lincoln Center to those who can pay the price may differ vastly in content (as viewed by judges) or in quality (as viewed by critics), it may not differ in substance from the dance viewed by the person who *** wants some 'entertainment' with his beer or shot of rye." Salem Inn, Inc. v. Frank, 501 F.2d 18, 21, n.3 (CA2 1974), aff'd in part, Doran v. Salem Inn, Inc., 422 U.S. 922 (1975). ***

As I see it, our cases require us to affirm absent a compelling state interest supporting the statute. Neither the Court nor the State suggest that the statute could withstand scrutiny under that standard. Accordingly, I would affirm the judgment of the Court of Appeals, and dissent from this Court's judgment.[3]

---

2. JUSTICE SOUTER agrees with the Court that the third requirement of the *O'Brien* test is satisfied, but only because he is not certain that there is a causal connection between the message conveyed by nude dancing and the evils which the State is seeking to prevent. *** JUSTICE SOUTER's analysis is at least as flawed as that of the plurality. If JUSTICE SOUTER is correct that there is no causal connection between the message conveyed by the nude dancing at issue here and the negative secondary effects that the State desires to regulate, the State does not have even a rational basis for its absolute prohibition on nude dancing that is admittedly expressive. Furthermore, if the real problem is the "concentration of crowds of men predisposed to the" designated evils, then the First Amendment requires that the State address that problem in a fashion that does not include banning an entire category of expressive activity. See *Renton v. Playtime Theatres, Inc.*, 475 U.S. 41 (1986).

3. [**Ed. Note** For virtual reprise of *Barnes v. Glen Theatre, Inc.*, *see* City of Erie v. Pap's A.M., 529 U.S. 277.(2000). (City ordinance banning "public nudity" including "nude erotic dancing," and requiring minimum "pasties" and "G-string" on adult performers; *sustained*, six-to-three). Judgment of Court in an Opinion by O'Connor, J., joined by Rehnquist, C.J., Kennedy and Breyer, JJ., applying *O'Brien* to sustain the ordinance; separate opinion by Scalia, J., which Thomas, J. joined, finding no First Amendment question. Souter, J., dissented, finding *O'Brien* appropriate but faulting majority's application (and retracting parts of his *Barnes* concurrence); Stevens and Ginsburg, JJ., separately

RENO V. AMERICAN CIVIL LIBERTIES UNION
521U.S.844 (1997)

JUSTICE STEVENS delivered the opinion of the Court.

At issue is the constitutionality of two statutory provisions enacted to protect minors from "indecent" and "patently offensive" communications on the Internet. Notwithstanding the legitimacy and importance of the congressional goal of protecting children from harmful materials, we agree with the three-judge District Court that the statute abridges "the freedom of speech" protected by the First Amendment.

I
The Internet

The Internet is the outgrowth of what began in 1969 as a military program called "ARPANET," which was designed to enable computers operated by the military, defense contractors, and universities conducting defense-related research to communicate with one another by redundant channels even if some portions of the network were damaged in a war. While ARPANET no longer exists, it provided an example for the development of a number of civilian networks that, eventually linking with each other, now enable tens of millions of people to communicate with one another and to access vast amounts of information from around the world. The Internet is "a unique and wholly new medium of worldwide human communication."

The number of "host" computers—those that store information and relay communications—increased from about 300 in 1981 to approximately 9,400,000 by the time of the trial in 1996. Roughly 60% of these hosts are located in the United States. About 40 million people used the Internet at the time of trial, a number that is expected to mushroom to 200 million by 1999.

Individuals can obtain access to the Internet from many different sources, generally hosts themselves or entities with a host affiliation. Most universities provide access for their students and faculty; many corporations provide their employees with access through an office network; many communities and local libraries provide free access; and an increasing number of storefront "computer coffee shops" provide access for a small hourly fee. Several major national "online services" offer access to their own extensive proprietary networks as well as a link to the much larger resources of the Internet. These commercial online services had almost 12 million individual subscribers at the time of trial.

Anyone with access to the Internet may take advantage of a wide variety of communication and information retrieval methods. [T]hose most relevant to this case are electronic mail ("e-mail"), automatic mailing list services ("mail exploders," sometimes referred to as "listservs"), "newsgroups," "chat rooms," and the "World

---

dissented, finding *O'Brien* plainly inapplicable and concluding as had the state supreme court, that the ordinance was not sustainable under *Ward* (i.e., not sustainable as a content-neutral, "time, place, and manner" test).]

Wide Web." All of these methods can be used to transmit text; most can transmit sound, pictures, and moving video images.

E-mail enables an individual to send an electronic message—generally akin to a note or letter—to another individual or to a group of addressees. A mail exploder is a sort of e-mail group. Subscribers can send messages to a common e-mail address, which then forwards the message to the group's other subscribers. Newsgroups also serve groups of regular participants, but these postings may be read by others as well. There are thousands of such groups, each serving to foster an exchange of information or opinion on a particular topic running the gamut from, say, the music of Wagner to Balkan politics to AIDS prevention to the Chicago Bulls.

The best known category of communication over the Internet is the World Wide Web, which allows users to search for and retrieve information stored in remote computers, as well as, in some cases, to communicate back to designated sites. *** The Web is comparable, from the readers' viewpoint, to both a vast library including millions of readily available and indexed publications and a sprawling mall offering goods and services.

From the publishers' point of view, it constitutes a vast platform from which to address and hear from a world-wide audience of millions of readers, viewers, researchers, and buyers. Any person or organization with a computer connected to the Internet can "publish" information. Publishers may either make their material available to the entire pool of Internet users, or confine access to a selected group, such as those willing to pay for the privilege. No single organization controls any membership in the Web, nor is there any centralized point from which individual Web sites or services can be blocked from the Web.

Sexually Explicit Material

Sexually explicit material on the Internet includes text, pictures, and chat and extends from the modestly titillating to the hardest-core. These files are created, named, and posted in the same manner as material that is not sexually explicit, and may be accessed either deliberately or unintentionally during the course of an imprecise search. Thus, for example,

> "when the UCR/California Museum of Photography posts to its Web site nudes by Edward Weston and Robert Mapplethorpe to announce that its new exhibit will travel to Baltimore and New York City, those images are available not only in Los Angeles, Baltimore, and New York City, but also in Cincinnati, Mobile, or Beijing—wherever Internet users live. Similarly, the safer sex instructions that Critical Path posts to its Web site, written in street language so that the teenage receiver can understand them, are available not just in Philadelphia, but also in Provo and Prague."

Though such material is widely available, users seldom encounter such content accidentally. Almost all sexually explicit images are preceded by warnings as to the content. Unlike communications received by radio or television, the receipt of information on the Internet requires a series of affirmative steps more deliberate and directed than merely turning a dial. A child requires some sophistication and some ability to read to retrieve material and thereby to use the Internet unattended.

Systems have been developed to help parents control the material that may be available on a home computer with Internet access. Although parental control software currently can screen for certain suggestive words or for known sexually explicit sites, it cannot now screen for sexually explicit images." ***

Age Verification

The problem of age verification differs for different uses of the Internet. The District Court categorically determined that there "is no effective way to determine the identity or the age of a user who is accessing material through e-mail, mail exploders, newsgroups or chat rooms." The Government offered no evidence that there was a reliable way to screen recipients and participants in such fora for age.

Technology exists by which an operator of a Web site may condition access on the verification of requested information such as a credit card number or an adult password. Using credit card possession as a surrogate for proof of age would impose costs on non-commercial Web sites that would require many of them to shut down. For that reason, at the time of the trial, credit card verification was "effectively unavailable to a substantial number of Internet content providers." Moreover, the imposition of such a requirement "would completely bar adults who do not have a credit card and lack the resources to obtain one from accessing any blocked material."

Commercial pornographic sites that charge their users for access have assigned them passwords as a method of age verification. The record does not contain any evidence concerning the reliability of these technologies. [T]he District Court found that an adult password requirement would impose significant burdens on noncommercial sites, both because they would discourage users from accessing their sites and because the cost of creating and maintaining such screening systems would be "beyond their reach."

II

The [primary purpose of the] Telecommunications Act of 1996 was to reduce regulation and encourage "the rapid deployment of new telecommunications technologies." An amendment offered in the Senate was the source of the two statutory provisions challenged in this case. The first [§ 223(a)] prohibits the knowing transmission of obscene or indecent messages to any recipient under 18 years of age. It provides in pertinent part:

> "(a) Whoever [by means of any telecommunications device] knowingly—
>
> "(1) initiates the transmission of any comment, request, suggestion, proposal, image, or other communication which is obscene or indecent, knowing that the recipient of the communication is under 18 years of age, [or]
>
> "(2) knowingly permits any telecommunications facility under his control to be used for any activity prohibited by paragraph (1) with the intent that it be used for such activity—

—shall be fined under Title 18, or imprisoned not more than two years, or both.

The second provision [§ 223(d)] prohibits the knowing sending or displaying of patently offensive messages in a manner that is available to a person under 18 years of age. It provides:

> Whoever— ***
>
> (1) knowingly uses any interactive computer service to display in a manner available to a person under 18 years of age, any comment, request, suggestion, proposal, image, or other communication that, in context, depicts or describes, in terms patently offensive as measured by contemporary community standards, sexual or excretory activities or organs, [or]
>
> "(2) knowingly permits any telecommunications facility under such person's control to be used for an activity prohibited by paragraph (1) with the intent that it be used for such activity—
>
> —shall be fined under Title 18, United States Code, or imprisoned not more than two years, or both.

The breadth of these prohibitions is qualified by two affirmative defenses. One covers those who take "good faith, reasonable, effective, and appropriate actions" to restrict access by minors to the prohibited communications. The other covers those who restrict access to covered material by requiring certain designated forms of age proof, such as a verified credit card or an adult identification number or code.

[III - XI]

[T]he Government contends that the CDA is plainly constitutional under three of our prior decisions: (1) *Ginsberg v. New York*; (2) *FCC v. Pacifica Foundation*; and (3) *Renton v. Playtime Theatres, Inc.* ***

In four important respects, the statute upheld in *Ginsberg* was narrower than the CDA. First, we noted in *Ginsberg* that "the prohibition against sales to minors does not bar parents who so desire from purchasing the magazines for their children." Under the CDA, by contrast, neither the parents' consent—nor even their participation—in the communication would avoid the application of the statute. Second, the New York statute applied only to commercial transactions, whereas the CDA contains no such limitation. Third, the New York statute cabined its definition of material that is harmful to minors with the requirement that it be "utterly without redeeming social importance for minors." The CDA fails to provide us with any definition of the term "indecent" as used in § 223(a)(1) and, importantly, omits any requirement that the "patently offensive" material covered by § 223(d) lack serious literary, artistic, political, or scientific value. ***

*** [T]here are [likewise] significant differences between the order upheld in *Pacifica* and the CDA. First, the order in *Pacifica*, issued by an agency that had been regulating radio stations for decades, targeted a specific broadcast that represented a rather dramatic departure from traditional program content in order to designate when—rather than whether—it would be permissible to air such a program in that particular medium. The CDA's broad categorical prohibitions are not limited to particular times and are not dependent on any evaluation by an agency familiar with the unique characteristics of the Internet. Second, the Commission's declaratory order was not punitive; we expressly refused to decide whether the indecent broadcast "would justify a criminal prosecution." Finally, the Commission's order applied to a medium which as a matter of history had "received the most limited First Amendment protection," in large part because warnings could not adequately protect the listener from unexpected program content. The Internet, however, has no comparable history. Moreover, the District Court found that the risk of encountering indecent material by accident is remote because a series of affirmative steps is required to access specific material.

In *Renton*, we upheld a zoning ordinance that kept adult movie theatres out of residential neighborhoods. According to the Government, the CDA is constitutional because it constitutes a sort of "cyberzoning" on the Internet. But the CDA applies broadly to the entire universe of cyberspace. And the purpose of the CDA is to protect children from the primary effects of "indecent" and "patently offensive" speech, rather than any "secondary" effect of such speech. Thus, the CDA is a content-based blanket restriction on speech, and, as such, cannot be "properly analyzed as a form of time, place, and manner regulation." ***

Finally, unlike the conditions that prevailed when Congress first authorized regulation of the broadcast spectrum, the Internet can hardly be considered a "scarce" expressive commodity. [O]ur cases provide no basis for qualifying the level of First Amendment scrutiny that should be applied to this medium.

Regardless of whether the CDA is so vague that it violates the Fifth Amendment, the many ambiguities concerning the scope of its coverage render it problematic for purposes of the First Amendment. For instance, each of the two parts of the CDA uses a different linguistic form. The first uses the word "indecent," while the second speaks of material that "in context, depicts or describes, in terms patently offensive as measured by contemporary community standards, sexual or excretory activities or organs." Given the absence of a definition of either term, this difference in language will provoke uncertainty among speakers about how the two standards relate to each other and just what they mean.[37] ***

We are persuaded that the CDA lacks the precision that the First Amendment requires when a statute regulates the content of speech. In order to deny minors access to potentially harmful speech, the CDA effectively suppresses a large amount of speech that adults have a constitutional right to receive and to address to one another. *** In arguing that the CDA does not so diminish adult communication, the Government relies on the incorrect factual premise that prohibiting a transmission

37. The statute does not indicate whether the "patently offensive" and "indecent" determinations should be made with respect to minors or the population as a whole.

whenever it is known that one of its recipients is a minor would not interfere with adult-to- adult communication. [T]his premise is untenable. Knowledge that, for instance, one or more members of a 100-person chat group will be minor—and therefore that it would be a crime to send the group an indecent message—would surely burden communication among adults.[42] The District Court found that at the time of trial existing technology did not include any effective method for a sender to prevent minors from obtaining access to its communications on the Internet without also denying access to adults. ***

The breadth of the CDA's coverage is wholly unprecedented. Unlike the regulations upheld in *Ginsberg* and *Pacifica*, the scope of the CDA is not limited to commercial speech or commercial entities. Its open-ended prohibitions embrace all non-profit entities and individuals posting indecent messages or displaying them on their own computers in the presence of minors. The general, undefined terms "indecent" and "patently offensive" cover large amounts of nonpornographic material with serious educational or other value.[44] Moreover, the "community standards" criterion as applied to the Internet means that any communication available to a nation-wide audience will be judged by the standards of the community most likely to be offended by the message. The regulated subject matter includes any of the seven "dirty words" used in the *Pacifica* monologue, the use of which the Government's expert acknowledged could constitute a felony. It may also extend to discussions about prison rape or safe sexual practices, artistic images that include nude subjects, and arguably the card catalogue of the Carnegie Library. ***

The Government also asserts that the "knowledge" requirement of both §§ 223(a) and (d), especially when coupled with the "specific child" element found in § 223(d), saves the CDA from overbreadth. This argument ignores the fact that most Internet fora—including chat rooms, newsgroups, mail exploders, and the Web—are open to all comers. Even the strongest reading of the "specific person" requirement of § 223(d) cannot save the statute. It would confer broad powers of censorship, in the form of a "heckler's veto," upon any opponent of indecent speech who might simply log on and inform the would-be discoursers that his 17-year-old child —a "specific person under 18 years of age,"—would be present.

The Government's three remaining arguments focus on the defenses provided in § 223(e)(5). First, relying on the "good faith, reasonable, effective, and appropriate actions" provision, the Government suggests that "tagging" provides a defense that saves the constitutionality of the Act. The Government recognizes that its proposed screening software does not currently exist. Even if it did, there is no way to know

---

42. The Government agrees that these provisions are applicable whenever "a sender transmits a message to more than one recipient, knowing that at least one of the specific persons receiving the message is a minor."

44. Transmitting obscenity and child pornography, whether via the Internet or other means, is already illegal under federal law for both adults and juveniles. See 18 U.S.C. §§ 1464-1465 (criminalizing obscenity); § 2251 (criminalizing child pornography).

whether a potential recipient will actually block the encoded material. Without the impossible knowledge that every guardian in America is screening for the "tag," the transmitter could not reasonably rely on its action to be "effective."

For its second and third arguments concerning defenses—which we can consider together—the Government relies on the latter half of § 223(e)(5), which applies when the transmitter has restricted access by requiring use of a verified credit card or adult identification. [T]his defense would not significantly narrow the statute's burden on noncommercial speech. Even with respect to the commercial pornographers that would be protected by the defense, the Government failed to adduce any evidence that these verification techniques actually preclude minors from posing as adults.[47] *** For the foregoing reasons, the judgment of the district court is affirmed. ***

JUSTICE O'CONNOR, with whom THE CHIEF JUSTICE joins, concurring in the judgment in part and dissenting in part.

I write separately to explain why I view the Communications Decency Act of 1996 (CDA) as little more than an attempt by Congress to create "adult zones" on the Internet. The Court has previously sustained such zoning laws, but only if they respect the First Amendment rights of adults and minors. That is to say, a zoning law is valid if (i) it does not unduly restrict adult access to the material; and (ii) minors have no First Amendment right to read or view the banned material.

The Court in *Ginsberg* did not question—and therefore necessarily assumed—that an adult zone, once created, would succeed in preserving adults' access while denying minors' access to the regulated speech. Before today, there was no reason to question this assumption, for the Court has previously only considered laws that operated in the physical world, a world that with two characteristics that make it possible to create "adult zones": geography and identity.

Although the prospects for the eventual zoning of the Internet appear promising, I agree with the Court that we must evaluate the constitutionality of the CDA as it applies to the Internet as it exists today. Given the present state of cyberspace, I agree with the Court that the "display" provision cannot pass muster. Until gateway technology is available throughout cyberspace, and it is not in 1997, a speaker cannot be reasonably assured that the speech he displays will reach only adults because it is impossible to confine speech to an "adult zone." *** As a result, the "display" provision cannot withstand scrutiny.

The "indecency transmission" and "specific person" provisions present a closer issue, for they are not unconstitutional in all of their applications. [T]he "indecency transmission" provision makes it a crime to transmit knowingly an indecent message to a person the sender knows is under 18 years of age. The "specific person"

---

47. Thus, ironically, this defense may significantly protect commercial purveyors of obscene postings while providing little (or no) benefit for transmitters of indecent messages that have significant social or artistic value.

provision proscribes the same conduct, although it does not as explicitly require the sender to know that the intended recipient of his indecent message is a minor. Appellant urges the Court to construe the provision to impose such a knowledge requirement, and I would do so. ***

*** Because the rights of adults are infringed only by the "display" provision and by the "indecency transmission" and "specific person" provisions as applied to communications involving more than one adult, I would invalidate the CDA only to that extent. Insofar as the "indecency transmission" and "specific person" provisions prohibit the use of indecent speech in communications between an adult and one or more minors, however, they can and should be sustained. The Court reaches a contrary conclusion, and from that holding that I respectfully dissent.

NOTES AND RECENT DEVELOPMENTS PERTINENT TO *RENO* AND THE INTERNET

1. After the Court decided *Reno v. ACLU,* Congress enacted the Child Online Protection Act ("COPA"), 47 U.S.C.§ 231. The statute (with emphasis added) provides that whoever "knowingly and with knowledge of the character of the material, in interstate or foreign commerce by means of the World Wide Web, makes any communication for *commercial* purposes that is available to any minor and that includes any material that is harmful to minors shall be fined not more than $50,000 . . . ." Section 431(e)(6) defines material that is "harmful to minors" as material

— that is obscene *or* that

> (A) the average person, applying contemporary community standards, would find, taking the material as a whole and with respect to minors, is designed to appear to, or is designed to pander to, the prurient interest;
>
> (B) depicts, describes, or represents, in a manner patently offensive with respect to minors, an actual or simulated sexual act or sexual contact, an actual or simulated normal or perverted sexual act, or a lewd exhibition of the genitals or post-pubescent female breast; and
>
> (C) taken as a whole, lacks serious literary, artistic, political, or scientific value for minors.

Has Congress remedied the problem(s), or is this susceptible to the same sort of challenge as that brought by plaintiffs in *Reno v. ACLU*? See *ACLU v. Reno*, 31 F. Supp.2d 473 (E.D. Pa. 1999), aff'd. 217 F.3d 162 (3d Cir. Pa. 2000), cert. granted, Ashcroft v. ACLU, 149 L. Ed. 2d 1001, 121 S. Ct. 1997 (2001).

2. A different section of the Communications Decency Act, not involved in *Reno*, relieves providers or users of any "interactive computer service"[61] of liability for *declining* to carry any material the provider or user of such a service finds objectionable. 47 U.S.C.§ 230(c) is captioned: "Protection for "good samaritan" blocking and screening of offensive material." Subsection (2) of § 230(c) provides:

> Civil Liability. No provider or user of an interactive computer service shall be held liable on account of —
>
> (A) Any action voluntarily in good faith to restrict access to or availability of material that the provider or user considers to be obscene, lewd, lascivious, filthy, excessively violent, harassing, or otherwise objectionable, whether or not such material is constitutionally protected...

On its face this section would appear to apply to *any* provider or to any user of such a service, including "providers" or "users" operating under state and local government authority. Even so, it probably does not do so.[62] Section 230 itself is captioned: "Protection for *private* blocking and screening of offensive material," and the few courts thus far addressing the section have construed it to reflect a policy by Congress merely (if significantly) to insulate *private* parties and companies from possible tort or other state-law based suits by persons seeking legal recourse against them for blocking access to material they wish to receive.[63]

---

61. The phrase "interactive computer service" is defined in the same section (§ 230(e)) as follows: "any information service, system, or access software provider that provides or enables computer access by multiple users to a computer server, including specifically a service or system that provides access to the Internet and such systems operated or services offered by libraries or educational institutions."

62. Were it to do so, the first amendment issues confronted in *Reno* would be obvious (i.e., to grant a virtual censorship power to units of state and local government in the sweeping terms of this section, is a near-certain formula to insure the act would not be sustained).

63. *See, e.g., Zeran v. America Online Inc.*, 129 F.3d 327 (4th Cir. 1997), *cert. denied*, 118 S. Ct. 2341 (1998); *Mainstream Loudoun v. Bd. Of Trustees of Loudoun Cty Library*, 2 F. Supp.2d 783 (E.D. Va. 1998) (both cases construing § 230(c)(2) this way). Section 230(d) lends some support to this interpretation. [Section] 230(d)(3) is captioned "Effect on ... State law," and provides that "No cause of action may be brought and no liability may be imposed under any State or local law that is inconsistent with this section." A "state or local law" would presumably be "inconsistent" with § 230(c)(2) insofar as it would provide a cause of action against a provider or user of an interactive computer service screening, or blocking, or refusing access in any manner § 230 expressly permits them "voluntarily" so to choose to do. (Given this understanding of the act, note its similarly to the provisions of the cablevision act reviewed in *Denver Area*, p. 502, *supra*, which expressly permit cable companies to block access to "indecent" material on leased access and public access channels, sustained in part, held unconstitutional in part.) (Recall from *PruneYard Shopping Center*, casebook at p. 537, that some states, e.g., California, have constitutional provisions protecting freedom of speech from private abridgment and not merely from abridgment by government. Section 230(d)(3) would appear to preclude the California Supreme Court from applying any such provision against any private party

Even so, some government entities *have* mandated the installation of software blocking programs on their own government initiative, on computer terminals maintained under their authority, limiting what adults as well as "children" (minors) are able to access. And some have done so, even in a manner as broad (or broader) than the restriction imposed by Congress held void for overbreadth, in *Reno*.

For example, pursuant to a general Virginia statute authorizing local public library boards to adopt regulations for "the government of the free public library system as may be expedient," a county library board in Virginia directed that site-blocking software be installed in *each* branch library on computers, effective to block material deemed harmful to juveniles. To implement the policy, the county library board chose "X-Stop," a commercial software product which, as installed, blocked access to sites local library patrons would otherwise be able to access from computer terminals at the public library, but were no longer able so to do because of the X-Stop screening. Local resident adult library users finding Internet access sites blocked by the X-Stop software, when they came to the library and attempted to use the public library computer terminals, filed suit in federal district court to have the board enjoined from maintaining the system.[64] Considering the case in light of *Reno*, how might one expect the court to rule?[65]

---

acting within the scope of § 230(c)(2)(A).

The legislative history accompanying § 230(c) also suggests it is meant to protect interactive computer service providers, such as AOL and Compuserve, from becoming liable, as publishers, to persons suing for defamation, for digitalized statements sent over the service provider's system, merely because they presume to screen some of the material accessed through their systems, but do not presume to act as "editors" in any general sense. Generally, commercial information service providers who merely provide the interactive connecting and transmission service for paying users are not regarded as "publishers" of the information carried by means of their service (and thus are not liable themselves for libelous statements others originate and send or retransmit through their system). *See* discussion in *Cubby, Inc. v. Compuserve, Inc.*, 776 F. Supp. 135 (S.D.N.Y. 1991); *see also* Michael Hadley, Note, *The Gertz Doctrine and Internet Defamation,* 84 Va. L. Rev. 477 (1998). Where such a company assumes responsibility for "editing" what comes through its system, however, it may be sued as a (re)publisher of a libelous statement. *See, e.g., Stratton Oakmont, Inc. v. Prodigy Services Co.*, 1995 WL 323710 (N.Y.S.Ct.). What § 230(d)(3) does is to make clear that a commercial private service provider shall *not* become liable in libel for acting as an "editor" in the manner Congress expressly authorizes in § 230(c).

64. The case in this respect is similar to *Board of Educ. v. Pico*, casebook at p. 347 (suit by students to enjoin removal of books from public school library), and to *Lamont v. Postmaster General*, 381 U.S. 301 (1965) (noted in casebook at p.380, n. 65) (suit by postal addressee of intercepted mail).

65. *See Mainstream Loudoun v. Bd. of Trustees of Loudoun Cty. Library*, 2 F. Supp.2d 783 (E.D. Va. 1998). See also, Bernard W. Bell, *Filth, Filtering & The First Amendment: Ruminations on Public Libraries Use of Internet Filtering Software*, 53 Fed. Comm. L.J. 191 (2001).

NATIONAL ENDOWMENT FOR THE ARTS v. FINLEY
524 U.S. 569 (1998)

JUSTICE O'CONNOR delivered the opinion of the Court.

I (A)

[In 1965, an] enabling statute vest[ed] the NEA with substantial discretion to award grants; it identifie[d] only the broadest funding priorities, including "artistic and cultural significance, giving emphasis to American creativity and cultural diversity," "professional excellence," and the encouragement of "public knowledge, education, understanding, and appreciation of the arts." Since 1965, the NEA has distributed over three billion dollars in grants to individuals and organizations, funding that has served as a catalyst for increased state, corporate, and foundation support for the arts.

Throughout the NEA's history, only a handful of the agency's roughly 100,000 awards have generated formal complaints about misapplied funds or abuse of the public's trust. Two provocative works, however, prompted public controversy. The Institute of Contemporary Art at the University of Pennsylvania had used $30,000 of a visual arts grant it received from the NEA to fund a 1989 retrospective of photographer Robert Mapplethorpe's work. The exhibit included homoerotic photographs that several Members of Congress condemned as pornographic. Members also denounced artist Andres Serrano's work Piss Christ, a photograph of a crucifix immersed in urine.

In the 1990 appropriations bill, Congress adopted a bipartisan compromise between Members opposing any funding restrictions and those favoring some guidance to the agency. The Amendment became § 954(d)(1), which directs the Chairperson, in establishing procedures to judge the artistic merit of grant applications, to "take into consideration general standards of decency and respect for the diverse beliefs and values of the American public."[1]

The NEA has not promulgated any official interpretation of the provision, but in December 1990, the Council unanimously adopted a resolution to implement § 954(d)(1) merely by ensuring that the members of the advisory panels that conduct the initial review of grant applications represent geographic, ethnic, and aesthetic

---

1. Title 20 U.S.C.§ 954 (d) provides that:

"No payment shall be made under this section except upon application therefor which is submitted to the National Endowment for the Arts in accordance with regulations issued and procedures established by the Chairperson. In establishing such regulations and procedures, the Chairperson shall ensure that

(1) artistic excellence and artistic merit are the criteria by which applications are judged, taking into consideration general standards of decency and respect for the diverse beliefs and values of the American public; and

(2) applications are consistent with the purposes of this section. Such regulations and procedures shall clearly indicate that obscenity is without artistic merit, is not protected speech, and shall not be funded."]

diversity. John Frohnmayer, then Chairperson of the NEA, also declared that he would "count on [the] procedures" ensuring diverse membership on the peer review panels to fulfill Congress' mandate.

B

The four individual respondents in this case, Karen Finley, John Fleck, Holly Hughes, and Tim Miller, are performance artists who applied for NEA grants before § 954(d)(1) was enacted. When Congress enacted § 954(d)(1), respondents, now joined by the National Association of Artists' Organizations (NAAO), amended their complaint to challenge the provision as void for vagueness and impermissibly viewpoint based.*** Respondents raise a facial constitutional challenge to § 954(d)(1), and consequently they confront "a heavy burden" in advancing their claim. Facial invalidation "is, manifestly, strong medicine" that "has been employed by the Court sparingly and only as a last resort." *Broadrick v. Oklahoma*, 413 U.S. 601, 613 (1973). To prevail, respondents must demonstrate a substantial risk that application of the provision will lead to the suppression of speech.

Respondents argue that the provision is a paradigmatic example of viewpoint discrimination because it rejects any artistic speech that either fails to respect mainstream values or offends standards of decency. The NEA, however, reads the provision as merely hortatory, and contends that it stops well short of an absolute restriction. *** We do not decide whether the NEA's view — that the formulation of diverse advisory panels is sufficient to comply with Congress' command — is in fact a reasonable reading of the statute. It is clear, however, that the text of § 954(d)(1) imposes no categorical requirement. The advisory language stands in sharp contrast to congressional efforts to prohibit the funding of certain classes of speech. See § 954(d)(2) ("Obscenity is without artistic merit, is not protected speech, and shall not be funded").

That § 954(d)(1) admonishes the NEA merely to take "decency and respect" into consideration, and that the legislation was aimed at reforming procedures rather than precluding speech, undercut respondents' argument that the provision inevitably will be utilized as a tool for invidious viewpoint discrimination. In cases where we have struck down legislation as facially unconstitutional, the dangers were both more evident and more substantial. In *R.A.V. v. St. Paul*, 505 U.S. 377 (1992), for example, we invalidated on its face a municipal ordinance that defined as a criminal offense the placement of a symbol on public or private property "'which one knows or has reasonable grounds to know arouses anger, alarm, or resentment in others on the basis of race, color, creed, religion, or gender.'" That provision set forth a clear penalty, proscribed views on particular "disfavored subjects," and suppressed "distinctive ideas, conveyed by a distinctive message." ***

The NEA's enabling statute contemplates a number of indisputably constitutional applications for both the "decency" prong of § 954(d)(1) and its reference to "respect for the diverse beliefs and values of the American public." Educational programs are central to the NEA's mission. And it is well established that "decency" is a permissible factor where "educational suitability" motivates its consideration. *Board of Ed., Island Trees Union Free School Dist. No. 26 v. Pico*, 457 U.S. 853, 871 (1982); see also *Bethel School Dist. No. 403 v. Fraser*, 478 U.S. 675, 683 (1986) ("Surely it is a highly appropriate function of public school education to prohibit the use of vulgar and offensive terms in public discourse").

Permissible applications of the mandate to consider "respect for the diverse beliefs and values of the American public" are also apparent. The agency expressly takes diversity into account, giving special consideration to "projects and productions ... that reach, or reflect the culture of, a minority, inner city, rural, or tribal community." ***

We recognize, of course, that reference to these permissible applications would not alone be sufficient to sustain the statute against respondents' First Amendment challenge. But neither are we persuaded that, in other applications, the language of § 954(d)(1) itself will give rise to the suppression of protected expression. The agency may decide to fund particular projects for a wide variety of reasons, "such as the technical proficiency of the artist, the creativity of the work, the anticipated public interest in or appreciation of the work, the work's contemporary relevance, its educational value, its suitability for or appeal to special audiences (such as children or the disabled), its service to a rural or isolated community, or even simply that the work could increase public knowledge of an art form." Brief for Petitioners 32.

Respondents do not allege discrimination in any particular funding decision. (In fact, after filing suit to challenge § 954(d)(1), two of the individual respondents received NEA grants.) If the NEA were to leverage its power to award subsidies on the basis of subjective criteria into a penalty on disfavored viewpoints, then we would confront a different case. *** Unless and until § 954(d)(1) is applied in a manner that raises concern about the suppression of disfavored viewpoints, however, we uphold the constitutionality of the provision.

B[1]

Finally, although the First Amendment certainly has application in the subsidy context, we note that the Government may allocate competitive funding according to criteria that would be impermissible were direct regulation of speech or a criminal penalty at stake. So long as legislation does not infringe on other constitutionally protected rights, Congress has wide latitude to set spending priorities. In the 1990 Amendments that incorporated § 954(d)(1), Congress modified the declaration of purpose in the NEA's enabling act to provide that arts funding should "contribute to public support and confidence in the use of taxpayer funds," and that "public funds ... must ultimately serve public purposes the Congress defines." § 951(5). And as we held in *Rust*, Congress may "selectively fund a program to encourage certain activities it believes to be in the public interest, without at the same time funding an alternative program which seeks to deal with the problem in another way."

---

1. [Ginsburg, J., did not join this portion of the opinion.]

III

The lower courts also erred in invalidating § 954(d)(1) as unconstitutionally vague. The terms of the provision are undeniably opaque, and if they appeared in a criminal statute or regulatory scheme, they could raise substantial vagueness concerns. It is unlikely, however, that speakers will be compelled to steer too far clear of any "forbidden area" in the context of grants of this nature. We recognize, as a practical matter, that artists may conform their speech to what they believe to be the decision-making criteria in order to acquire funding. But when the Government is acting as patron rather than as sovereign, the consequences of imprecision are not constitutionally severe.

In the context of selective subsidies, it is not always feasible for Congress to legislate with clarity. Indeed, if this statute is unconstitutionally vague, then so too are all government programs awarding scholarships and grants on the basis of subjective criteria such as "excellence." See, e.g., 2 U.S.C. § 802 (establishing the Congressional Award Program to "promote initiative, achievement, and excellence among youths in the areas of public service, personal development, and physical *** fitness"); 20 U.S.C. § 956(c)(1) (providing funding to the National Endowment for the Humanities to promote "progress and scholarship in the humanities"). *** To accept respondents' vagueness argument would be to call into question the constitutionality of these valuable government programs and countless others like them.***

Section 954(d)(1) merely adds some imprecise considerations to an already subjective selection process. It does not, on its face, impermissibly infringe on First or Fifth Amendment rights. Accordingly, the judgment of the Court of Appeals is reversed and the case is remanded for further proceedings consistent with this opinion.

JUSTICE SCALIA, with whom JUSTICE THOMAS joins, concurring in the judgment.

"The operation was a success, but the patient died." What such a procedure is to medicine, the Court's opinion in this case is to law. It sustains the constitutionality of 20 U.S.C. § 954(d)(1) by gutting it. *** I write separately because, unlike the Court, I think that § 954(d)(1) must be evaluated as written, rather than as distorted by the agency it was meant to control. By its terms, it establishes content- and viewpoint-based criteria upon which grant applications are to be evaluated. And that is perfectly constitutional.

I-II

I agree with the Court that § 954(d)(1) "imposes no categorical requirement," in the sense that it does not require the denial of all applications that violate general standards of decency or exhibit disrespect for the diverse beliefs and values of Americans. Compare § 954(d)(2) ("Obscenity ... shall not be funded"). But the factors need not be conclusive to be discriminatory. To the extent a particular applicant exhibits disrespect for the diverse beliefs and values of the American public or fails to comport with general standards of decency, the likelihood that he will receive a grant diminishes. ***

This unquestionably constitutes viewpoint discrimination.[1] That conclusion is not altered by the fact that the statute does not "compel" the denial of funding, any more than a provision imposing a five-point handicap on all black applicants for civil service jobs is saved from being race discrimination by the fact that it does not compel the rejection of black applicants. If viewpoint discrimination in this context is unconstitutional (a point I shall address anon), the law is invalid unless there are some situations in which the decency and respect factors do not constitute viewpoint discrimination. And there is none. *** And the conclusion of viewpoint discrimination is not affected by the fact that what constitutes "decency" or "the diverse beliefs and values of the American people" is difficult to pin down, any more than a civil-service preference in favor of those who display "Republican-party values" would be rendered nondiscriminatory by the fact that there is plenty of room for argument as to what Republican-party values might be.

III

The Court devotes so much of its opinion to explaining why this statute means something other than what it says that it neglects to cite the constitutional text governing our analysis. The First Amendment reads: "Congress shall make no law ... *abridging* the freedom of speech." To abridge is "to contract, to diminish; to deprive of." T. Sheridan, A Complete Dictionary of the English Language (6th ed. 1796). With the enactment of § 954(d)(1), Congress did not abridge the speech of those who disdain the beliefs and values of the American public, nor did it abridge indecent speech. Those who wish to create indecent and disrespectful art are as unconstrained now as they were before the enactment of this statute. Avant-garde artistes such as respondents remain entirely free to epater les bourgeois;[2] they are merely deprived of the additional satisfaction of having the bourgeoisie taxed to pay for it.***

The nub of the difference between me and the Court is that I regard the distinction between "abridging" speech and funding it as a fundamental divide, on this side of which the First Amendment is inapplicable. The Court, by contrast, seems

---

1. If there is any uncertainty on the point, it relates to the adjective, which is not at issue in the current discussion. That is, one might argue that the decency and respect factors constitute content discrimination rather than viewpoint discrimination, which would render them easier to uphold. Since I believe this statute must be upheld in either event, I pass over this conundrum and assume the worst.

2. Which they do quite well. The oeuvres d'art for which the four individual plaintiffs in this case sought funding have been described as follows: "Finley's controversial show, 'We Keep Our victims Ready,' contains three segments. In the second segment, Finley visually recounts a sexual assault by stripping to the waist and smearing chocolate on her breasts and by using profanity to describe the assault. Fleck appears dressed as a mermaid, urinates on the stage and creates an altar out of a toilet by putting a photograph of Jesus Christ on the lid."

to believe that the First Amendment, despite its words, has some ineffable effect upon funding, imposing constraints of an indeterminate nature which it announces (without troubling to enunciate any particular test) are not violated by the statute here — or, more accurately, are not violated by the quite different, emasculated statute that it imagines.*** It is no secret that the provision was prompted by, and directed at, the funding of such offensive productions. Instead of banning the funding of such productions absolutely, which I think would have been entirely constitutional, Congress took the lesser step of requiring them to be disfavored in the evaluation of grant applications. The Court's opinion today renders even that lesser step a nullity. For that reason, I concur only in the judgment.

JUSTICE SOUTER, dissenting

The question here is whether the italicized segment of this statute is unconstitutional on its face: "artistic excellence and artistic merit are the criteria by which applications [for grants from the National Endowment for the Arts] are judged, *taking into consideration general standards of decency and respect for the diverse beliefs and values of the American public.*" It is.

The decency and respect proviso mandates viewpoint-based decisions in the disbursement of government subsidies, and the Government has wholly failed to explain why the statute should be afforded an exemption from the fundamental rule of the First Amendment that viewpoint discrimination in the exercise of public authority over expressive activity is unconstitutional. *** Nor may the question raised be answered in the Government's favor on the assumption that some constitutional applications of the statute are enough to satisfy the demand of facial constitutionality[.] This assumption is irreconcilable with our long standing and sensible doctrine of facial overbreadth, applicable to claims brought under the First Amendment's speech clause. I respectfully dissent.

I

"If there is a bedrock principle underlying the First Amendment, it is that the government may not prohibit the expression of an idea simply because society finds the idea itself offensive or disagreeable." *Texas v. Johnson*, 491 U.S. 397, 414 (1989). *** Because this principle applies not only to affirmative suppression of speech, but also to disqualification for government favors, Congress is generally not permitted to pivot discrimination against otherwise protected speech on the offensiveness or unacceptability of the views it expresses.

It goes without saying that artistic expression lies within this First Amendment protection. The constitutional protection of artistic works turns not on the political significance that may be attributable to such productions, though they may indeed comment on the political,[1] but simply on their expressive character, which falls within a spectrum of protected "speech" extending outward from the core of overtly political declarations. Put differently, art is entitled to full protection because our "cultural life," just like our native politics, "rests upon [the] ideal" of governmental viewpoint neutrality. *Turner Broadcasting System, Inc. v. FCC*, 512 U.S. 622, 641 (1994).

When called upon to vindicate this ideal, we characteristically begin by asking "whether the government has adopted a regulation of speech because of disagreement with the message it conveys. The government's purpose is the controlling consideration." *Ward v. Rock Against Racism.* The answer in this case is damning. One need do nothing more than read the text of the statute to conclude that Congress's purpose in imposing the decency and respect criteria was to prevent the funding of art that conveys an offensive message; the decency and respect provision on its face is quintessentially viewpoint based, and quotations from the Congressional Record merely confirm the obvious legislative purpose. In the words of the cosponsor of the bill enacted the proviso, "works which deeply offend the sensibilities of significant portions of the public ought not to be supported with public funds."[2]

II

In the face of such clear legislative purpose, so plainly expressed, the Court has its work cut out for it in seeking a constitutional reading of the statute.

A

The Court says, first, that because the phrase "general standards of decency and respect for the diverse beliefs and values of the American public" is imprecise and capable of multiple interpretations, "the considerations that the provision introduces, by their nature, do not engender the kind of directed viewpoint discrimination that would prompt this Court to invalidate a statute on its face." Unquestioned case law, however, is clearly to the contrary. *** Except when protecting children from exposure to indecent material, see *FCC v. Pacifica Foundation*, 438 U.S. 726 (1978), the First Amendment has never been read to allow the government to rove around imposing general standards of decency, see, e.g., *Reno v. American Civil Liberties Union*, 521 U.S. ___ (1997) (striking down on its face a statute that regulated "indecency" on the Internet). ***

---

1. Art "may affect public attitudes and behavior in a variety of ways, ranging from direct espousal of a political or social doctrine to the subtle shaping of thought which characterizes all artistic expression."*Joseph Burstyn, Inc. v. Wilson*, 343 U.S. 495, 501 (1952).

2. There is, of course, nothing whatsoever unconstitutional about this view as a general matter. Congress has no obligation to support artistic enterprises that many people detest. The First Amendment speaks up only when Congress decides to participate in the Nation's artistic life by legal regulation, as it does through a subsidy scheme like the NEA. If Congress does choose to spend public funds in this manner, it may not discriminate by viewpoint in deciding who gets the money.

Just as self-evidently, a statute disfavoring speech that fails to respect America's "diverse beliefs and values" is the very model of viewpoint discrimination; it penalizes any view disrespectful to any belief or value espoused by someone in the American populace. Boiled down to its practical essence, the limitation obviously means that art that disrespects the ideology, opinions, or convictions of a significant segment of the American public is to be disfavored, whereas art that reinforces those values is not. After all, the whole point of the proviso was to make sure that works like Serrano's ostensibly blasphemous portrayal of Jesus would not be funded, while a reverent treatment, conventionally respectful of Christian sensibilities, would not run afoul of the law. Nothing could be more viewpoint based than that. ***

III

*** Our most thorough statement of these principles is found in the recent case of *Rosenberger v. Rector and Visitors of Univ. of Va.*, 515 U.S. 819,(1995), which held that the University of Virginia could not discriminate on viewpoint in underwriting the speech of student-run publications. *** *Rosenberger* controls here. The NEA, like the student activities fund in *Rosenberger*, is a subsidy scheme created to encourage expression of a diversity of views from private speakers. *** The NEA's purpose is to "support new ideas" and "to help create and sustain ... a climate encouraging freedom of thought, imagination, and inquiry." §§ 951(10),(7). Given this congressional choice to sustain freedom of expression, *Rosenberger* teaches that the First Amendment forbids decisions based on viewpoint popularity. So long as Congress chooses to subsidize expressive endeavors at large, it has no business requiring the NEA to turn down funding applications of artists and exhibitors who devote their "freedom of thought, imagination, and inquiry" to defying our tastes, our beliefs, or our values. ***

IV

Although I, like the Court, recognize that "facial challenges to legislation are generally disfavored," the proviso is the type of statute that most obviously lends itself to such an attack. The NEA does not offer a list of reasons when it denies a grant application, and an artist or exhibitor whose subject raises a hint of controversy can never know for sure whether the decency and respect criteria played a part in any decision by the NEA to deny funding. *** In the world of NEA funding, this is so because the makers or exhibitors of potentially controversial art will either trim their work to avoid anything likely to offend, or refrain from seeking NEA funding altogether. Either way, to whatever extent NEA eligibility defines a national mainstream, the proviso will tend to create a timid esthetic. *** The Court does not strike down the proviso, however. Instead, it preserves the irony of a statutory mandate to deny recognition to virtually any expression capable of causing offense in any quarter as the most recent manifestation of a scheme enacted to "create and sustain ... a climate encouraging freedom of thought, imagination, and inquiry." § 951(7).

Part II

THE ESTABLISHMENT AND FREE EXERCISE CLAUSES

Chapter 8

AN INTRODUCTION TO THE CHURCH-STATE CLAUSES OF THE FIRST AMENDMENT

A. THE PROBLEM OF STANDING

We began coverage of the free speech and free press clauses, in the introductory materials of this book, with the reminder that students enrolled in this course may have already been introduced to the first amendment indirectly, in a general constitutional law course.[1] We begin coverage of the free exercise and establishment clauses of the first amendment in exactly the same fashion.

In a general constitutional law course, the church-state clauses may have been introduced indirectly through discussion of Article III of the Constitution and the requirements for standing to sue. To review briefly: the judicial power of Article III courts extends only to "cases" and "controversies." In other words, in order to have standing to sue in an Article III court, one must present a "case or controversy." The question of standing, then, involves a constitutional inquiry respecting what constitutes a "case or controversy," as such.

1. Case or Controversy

The Article III idea of "case or controversy" generally requires: (a) two or more parties who are genuinely adverse; (b) a concrete set of facts; (c) some kind of injury-in-fact either threatened or already inflicted; and (d) a request for a form of relief that would lift the threat of injury or provide adequate redress. The deter-

---

1. As to the free speech and free press clauses, the refresher from constitutional law was, roughly, this: cases such as *Griswold v. Connecticut*, 381 U.S. 479 (1965), analyzed certain substantive due process claims in a special way ("strict scrutiny" judicial review). They proceeded by way of analogy to certain specially favored rights, such as those of freedom of speech and of the press, explicitly protected by the first amendment itself. In offering the analogy, the Court adverted to the "penumbra" of first amendment protection and proceeded from there. For example: one's interest in the privacy of one's *political* affiliations, the Court noted in *Griswold*, is protected by the first amendment from compulsory disclosure in certain circumstances. This observation served in *Griswold* as a point of departure for developing a more general thesis of privacy rights. Even in a general constitutional law course, thus, one might have been made aware of the fact that express first amendment rights would not be subjected to mere "rationality" review. By way of another example: coverage of Article III concepts of standing in a basic constitutional law course may have adverted to the exceptional treatment of standing to bring first amendment claims: that standing is available to challenge an act as facially invalid on grounds of overbreadth or vagueness, despite the standard rule applicable to *ius tertii* claims. Thus even before reading the introductory materials in Chapter 1, students enrolled in this course may have been "on notice" that laws adversely affecting freedom of speech and freedom of the press are treated under much more rigorous standards of judicial review than are other sorts of constitutional claims.

mination of the case, moreover, must be final and not merely advisory to the parties or to someone else. Indeed, early on, the Supreme Court declared the merely *advisory* opinion *beyond* the Article III authority of federal courts. (It was a service proposed for, but expressly rejected for, federal courts.)[2]

By moving through a variety of pertinent Supreme Court cases, between the extremes of a "purely advisory opinion" on the one hand,[3] and the tightest example of a "litigable case" on the other hand,[4] a student of constitutional law gradually comes to terms with virtually all of the more particularized requirements of an Article III "case." These requirements, of course, include such elements as "ripeness"[5] and "lack of mootness,"[6] as well as such refinements as "independent and adequate state grounds."[7]

In respect to the Article III requirement of standing to sue, one will recall that the general Article III rule is that one must assert some kind of injury that is *definite*,

---

2. The point was itself interestingly involved in the presidential campaign of 1988, between Governor Michael Dukakis of Massachusetts and Vice President George Bush. Mr. Bush faulted Mr. Dukakis for declining to sign an act of the Massachusetts legislature requiring all public school teachers to lead a recitation of the Pledge of Allegiance at the beginning of each day's opening class. The Governor had declined to do so after the Massachusetts Supreme Court rendered an advisory opinion that such a requirement would not be enforceable in light of the United States Supreme Court's rulings in cases such as West Virginia Bd. of Education v. Barnette, 319 U.S. 624 (1943), and Wooley v. Maynard, 430 U.S. 705 (1977), and in light of several lower federal court decisions. See Opinion of the Justices to the Governor, 363 N.E.2d 251 (Mass. 1977). The Governor returned the bill to the legislature for reconsideration in light of the state supreme court's five-to-two ruling. The state supreme court's ruling, of course, was itself not subject to further review in the U.S. Supreme Court—since it arose under a procedure not satisfying the Article III "case or controversy" requirements. Critics of Dukakis noted that he was legally free to sign the law, despite the state supreme court's advisory opinion. Others strongly defended his decision. (*Query*, incidentally: was the Massachusetts Supreme Court correct, or incorrect, on the substantive first amendment point?)

3. For example, an individual legislator, lobbyist, citizen, or President who is interested in drafting and submitting some sort of bill, who desires expert judicial assistance in drafting it, and who writes an Article III court to ask how it might best be done, *but who* (assuming the court complies with the request) might nonetheless change his mind and give the matter no further thought.

4. For example, a person about to be executed for an alleged crime, with no hope other than his pending habeas petition in federal court, alleging that the lethal injection is about to be administered although no trial has been held to determine his guilt.

5. A case prematurely brought may resemble the solicitation of an advisory opinion, to the extent that there is no demonstration that plaintiff will suffer *imminent and certain* injury unless a court intervenes and adjudicates the plaintiff's questions of law.

6. That is: the more obvious it is that the once-threatened injury is no longer imminent nor likely to be renewed, or the more obvious it is that in light of the relief originally requested it is now too late, so also the clearer it becomes that an adjudication can now furnish no more than the satisfaction of the plaintiff's (moot) interest in the legal question as such.

7. Specifically: if the injury the plaintiff seeks to avert cannot be avoided even assuming the lower court utterly erred in ruling against him on his constitutional objection—because the decision against the plaintiff rested additionally on a consideration of state law he is unable to show to be erroneous on federal grounds—then, again, deciding the federal constitutional question would do no more than satisfy the plaintiff's curiosity. It would not affect the outcome of the case.

material, and *particular to oneself* (i.e. that it is not merely an injury to another— unless one is able to assert some sort of special legal relationship enabling one to sue on the other's behalf). Nor may it merely be an injury of a *de minimis* sort, or of a kind indiscriminately borne by others such that the grievance sounds more frankly political than legal (at least as Article III courts are likely to hold).

2. *Frothingham v. Mellon*

Distinctions of this last sort, between injuries cognizable for Article III standing purposes and either injuries of a *de minimis* sort or injuries of a kind indiscriminately borne by others, are not always clear. Nonetheless, a leading example was provided by the 1923 case of *Frothingham v. Mellon*.[8] The *Frothingham* case involved an individual federal taxpayer's suit against the Secretary of the Treasury, challenging the constitutionality of certain congressionally authorized expenditures of federal funds.[9] The Supreme Court held that it had no authority to address the plaintiff's claims. Specifically, the taxpayer's claim of injury was thought too attenuated (her objection was not to the tax imposed on her, but to the expenditure subsequent), perhaps too minuscule (no more than pennies of hers could be involved), and in any event too indifferent to distinguish her from countless other taxpayers. The Court apparently regarded Mrs. Frothingham as wanting to settle the substantive constitutionality of an Act of Congress not really differentially affecting her in any significant (i.e. not *de minimis*) way. The Court declined to hear the case, remanding her instead to the political process where, it implied, such general objections to certain expenditures properly belonged.

3. *Flast v. Cohen*

In 1968, however, despite *Frothingham v. Mellon*, a different result was reached on the standing of an otherwise identically situated mere taxpayer. In this later case, *Flast v. Cohen*,[10] there was little to help one see how Mr. Flast was, in any important way, distinguishable from Mrs. Frothingham (both being ordinary general income taxpayers). Nonetheless, Mr. Flast was found to have standing to challenge proposed disbursements made by the Secretary of Health, Education, and Welfare— including disbursements inclusive of certain parochial schools and church related activities.

---

8. 262 U.S. 447 (1923).

9. The expenditures were challenged on the basis that: (a) they were not within the enumerated objects listed in Article I, Section 8, of the federal constitution, pursuant to which Congress was authorized to make expenditures from taxes levied by the United States; (b) since they were not authorized by the Constitution, the taxes from which the expenditures were appropriated were not levied lawfully, but were rather a taking of property invalid under the fifth amendment; and (c) the expenditures were not merely constitutionally unauthorized, but they also sought to interfere with subjects reserved solely to the states by the tenth amendment. On all three grounds, the complaint averred, the Secretary of the Treasury should be enjoined.

10. 392 U.S. 83 (1968).

The question, then, was what distinction might be drawn between *Frothingham* and *Flast.* Why was Flast allowed to proceed in an Article III court against Secretary Cohen, when Mrs. Frothingham (who in her day certainly paid more in taxes than had Mr. Flast in his day) had been barred against Secretary Mellon?

What the Warren Court appeared to hold, in *Flast v. Cohen,* was that a federal[11] taxpayer's standing to seek injunctive relief against a proposed federal expenditure depended not on the amount he or she may have personally paid in taxes, *but on which constitutional clause the plaintiff relied* in framing the complaint. If the complaint were framed in terms of "specific constitutional limitations imposed upon the exercise of the congressional taxing and spending power and not simply that the enactment is generally beyond the powers delegated to Congress by Art. I, Section 8,"[12] then the plaintiff's standing *qua* taxpayer might suffice. The Court viewed the clause relied upon by Flast as such a clause, but the clauses invoked by Frothingham were not viewed as such clauses. Accordingly, Mr. Flast succeeded in his claim of standing to sue, even though Mrs. Frothingham had not.

4. The Church-State Clauses and Standing to Sue

For many, however, the distinction drawn by the Supreme Court between *Flast* and *Frothingham,* seemed difficult to comprehend. The problem was not so much an intellectual problem with the basic idea, which is to relate the kind of injury one relies upon for standing (injury to one *as a taxpayer*) to some clause evidently specifically meant to protect one *as a taxpayer* (even if the protection is protection from certain *uses* of the funds coerced by way of taxation, rather than protection from anything else).[13] Rather, the problem lay in the seeming arbitrariness of the Court's disposition to say which clauses were clauses imposing "specific" limitations on taxing and spending, as distinct from other clauses (such as those on which Mrs. Frothingham relied) that do not meet that test.[14] What made the Court treat the clause

---

11. The rule pertinent to standing may be somewhat different in the case of a state or local taxpayer, but that need not trouble us here.

12. *Flast,* 392 U.S. at 102.

13. Suppose a clause in the constitution that provided that "no person shall be taxed in order to support another person's religious practices." And suppose that Congress proposed to use tax monies to subsidize religious practices. The standing of the taxpayer would be clear, would it not? The clause just quoted describes as an injury to a taxpayer the "injury" of having such money as may be collected from him as taxes given to subsidize someone else's religion. Suing to restrain the disbursing agent from making any such payment is, accordingly, just what one would expect.

14. The Supreme Court subsequently limited the reach of *Flast v. Cohen* in Valley Forge College v. Americans United, 454 U.S. 464 (1982) (no taxpayer standing where the allegedly improper government assistance to a religious organization inheres in the proposed giveaway of federal property, rather than the disbursement of funds to which the plaintiff taxpayer may have been compelled to contribute). As of 2001, moreover, except for the very narrow exception represented by *Flast v. Cohen* itself, the Court has declined to find any other exception to *Frothingham.* Only the establishment clause has been identified as sufficient to anchor taxpayer standing to litigate expenditures not provided for within the same statute levying the tax. (*Query*: Would a taxpayer suit to enjoin spending measures objected to

relied upon by Flast as more of a specific limitation on expenditures than any of the several clauses relied upon by Frothingham?

In framing her objections to the proposed expenditures by Secretary Mellon, Mrs Frothingham had relied upon three clauses: (1) the tax-and-spend clause in Article I, (2) the tenth amendment, and (3) the fifth amendment due process clause. Mr. Flast, on the other hand, relied merely upon this clause in the first amendment:

> Congress shall make no law respecting an establishment of religion.[15]

In what special way, if any, was this clause a special *taxpayer* protection clause? Nothing on its face suggests that it is. Yet, the Warren Court treated it as such, and made that treatment *the* critical distinction for the purpose of Flast's standing to sue. On what basis did the Warren Court presume to do so? The Warren Court relied on some few earlier cases that had previously engaged the same clause in the Supreme Court, cases that in turn relied upon statements identified to church-state controversies in which James Madison and Thomas Jefferson had been engaged near in time to the proposal of the first amendment. The Warren Court believed that that history was germane to an understanding of the establishment clause, and accordingly germane to Flast's theory of standing.

In 1777, the Court noted, Jefferson had drafted A Bill for Establishing Religious Freedom in Virginia. Among its passages were several directed to the impropriety of government coercing any person's financial support of a religion, whether his own or one with whose doctrines he disagreed:

> [T]o compel a man to furnish contributions of money for the propagation of opinions he disbelieves, is sinful and tyrannical; *** even *** forcing him to support this or that teacher of his own religious persuasion [is wrong].[16]

---

on free speech grounds be treated more like *Flast* than like *Frothingham*? Suppose an act of Congress authorized the Pentagon to spend $100 million to buy television network advertising slots to press the alleged need for invading Iraq. Who, if anyone, would have standing to sue to enjoin the Pentagon on a first amendment claim that the first amendment disallows the government to attempt to influence the direction or outcome of political debate in the United States by harnessing the tax-and-spend powers to generate domestic partisan political propaganda?) (And what of the substantive first amendment question in this hypothetical? To be sure, as we saw in *Buckley v. Valeo*, the Court has held that private persons cannot be limited in spending as much as they may have the personal means and personal will to spend, to speak for or against such issues or candidates as they wish. But does the basis of that decision apply also to allow *the government* to spend as much coercively-collected taxpayer money as it wishes, to try to influence the direction of political discussion? That important question is not foreclosed by the *Buckley* case, is it?)

15. The full clause is, of course, more inclusive: "Congress shall make no law respecting an establishment of religion, or prohibiting the free exercise thereof *** ." But Flast did not rely on the latter part of the clause.

16. Virginia Bill for Religious Liberty, 12 Hening, Statutes of Virginia 84 (1823).

In Jefferson's view, financial support of religion should be forthcoming from *voluntary* contributions alone—from those devoted to its particular creed, theology, and ministers—rather than furnished by the state.

Likewise, in remonstrating in Virginia against a proposed bill to provide tax support for religious teachers, a bill ultimately abandoned under protest, Madison had taken the view that no matter how small the tax, its imposition was objectionable in principle:

> Who does not see *** [t]hat the same authority which can force a citizen to contribute three pence only of his property for the support of any one establishment, may force him to conform to any other establishment in all cases whatsoever?[17]

The balance of Madison's Memorial and Remonstrance went on to criticize the effects, historically, of linking *any* church or religion with state fiscal supports, claiming that it at once made those thus supported both dependent on, as well as forever entangled with, the state—consequences in Madison's view fraught with disaster for the freedom of religion as well as the neutrality of civil government.[18]

Believing this history to be germane, the Court in *Flast* identified the "no-law-respecting-an-establishment-of-religion" clause as a clause meant for protection of taxpayers, as such, against any form of national religious assistance from national taxes. No amount would be *de minimis*—not even "three pence." The proposed (forbidden) use was the injury which Flast, as a taxpayer, had standing to challenge.

5. The Court's Interpretive Stance With Respect to the Church-State Clauses

The larger proposition implicit in *Flast v. Cohen* is that the Supreme Court generally accepts the first amendment's church-state clauses with an orientation derived

---

17. Memorial and Remonstrance Against Religious Assessments, 2 Writings of James Madison 183, 186 (G. Hunt ed., 1901).

18. After leaving the Presidency, Madison reflected the following thoughts on the appointment, use, and payment of national chaplains:

> Is the appointment of Chaplains to the two Houses of Congress consistent with the Constitution and with the pure principles of religious freedom? *** In strictness the answer on both points must be in the negative. The Constitution *** forbids everything like an establishment of a national religion. The law appointing Chaplains establishes a religious worship for the national representatives, to be performed by Ministers of religion, elected by a majority of them; and these are to be paid out of the national taxes. *** If Religion consists in voluntary acts of individuals, singly, or voluntarily associated, and [if] it be proper that public functionaries, as well as their Constituents should discharge their religious duties, let them like their Constituents, do so at their own expense.

Madison, Aspects of Monopoly One Hundred Years Ago, Harper's Mag. 489, 493 (1914), quoted in Ansen Phelps Stokes, Church and State in the United States 346-47 (1950). Cf. Marsh v. Chambers, 463 U.S. 783 (1983) (sustaining use of tax funds to pay state legislative chaplains).

from James Madison's and Thomas Jefferson's views, rather than the views of those clauses others might think to be preferable or more correct.[19]

This interpretive stance of the Court is of no small moment. The phrasing of this part of the first amendment is somewhat awkward and ambiguous (i.e. not "no law respecting religion," but "no law respecting *an establishment of* religion"). A wide range of very different interpretations are compatible with the text.[20] The states did not all treat religion in the same separationist manner as was settled in Virginia in the 1780s—several maintained subsidies of various substantial types, and some states were virtually founded by religions.[21]

There was virtually no useful discussion of the establishment clause at all, in 1789, when Madison submitted his original draft of the Bill of Rights in Congress. Not until 1947, in *Everson v. Board of Education*,[22] did the Supreme Court provide any serious direct address to the clause. *Everson* will be the first principal case with which we begin our work on the church-state clauses (see Chapter 9). It is *Everson*

---

19. Many are inclined to read the establishment clause as merely interdicting the establishment of a national religion, or a single nationally-preferred religion, a reading the clause will of course bear. See, for example, Wallace v. Jaffree, 472 U.S. 38 (1985) (Rehnquist, J., dissenting) (the establishment clause is concerned with "the establishment of a national church, and perhaps the preference of one religious sect over another"). (See also Justice Thomas, concurring, in Rosenberger v. Rector and Visitors of the University of Virginia, 1995 WL 38206 (S.Ct. 1995); but see the opinion in the same case by Justice Souter.) For a work strongly supporting this view (cited and relied upon by Justice Rehnquist), see Robert L. Cord, Separation of Church and State: Historical Fact and Current Fiction (1982). For some contrary views, however, see Thomas J. Curry, The First Freedoms: Church and State in America to the Passage of the First Amendment (1986); Leonard W. Levy, The Establishment Clause: Religion and the First Amendment (1986); William L. Miller, The First Liberty: Religion and The American Republic (1985). For another discussion of the strong separationist approach, see Edward J. Eberle, *Roger Williams' Gift: Religious Freedom in America*, 4 Roger Williams Univ. L. Rev. 425 (1999).

20. See, e.g., Joseph Story, II Commentaries on the Constitution of the United States 627-34 (5th ed. 1891) ("[I]t is impossible for those who believe in the truth of Christianity as a divine revelation to doubt that it is the especial duty of government to foster and encourage it among all the citizens and subjects. *** The real difficulty lies in ascertaining the limits to which government may rightfully go in fostering and encouraging religion. *** The real object of the amendment was not to countenance, much less to advance, Mahometanism, or Judaism, or infidelity, by prostrating Christianity; but to exclude all rivalry among Christian sects, and to prevent any national ecclesiastical establishment which should give to a hierarchy the exclusive patronage of the national government.").

21. Indeed, it is arguable in part that the first amendment was agreeable to these states that did maintain religious establishment laws, because it would bar Congress from interfering with their own state constitutional treatment of religion—just as it would bar Congress from interfering with the different arrangement reached in every other state. See William Van Alstyne, Trends in the Supreme Court: Mr Jefferson's Crumbling Wall—A Comment on *Lynch v. Donnelly*, 1984 Duke L.J. 770, 772-29; Jed Rubenfeld, Anti-establishmentarianism: Why RFRA Really was Unconstitutional, 95 Mich. L. Rev. 2347 (1999).

22. 330 U.S. 1 (1947) (see *infra* p. 834).

(1947) that provided the constitutional theory of *Flast v. Cohen* (1968).

B. OTHER CLAUSES RESPECTING RELIGION

Aside from the first amendment, the Constitution makes reference to religion in several *other* clauses. The other clauses include the following:

> Article VI, cl. 3:
>
> The Senators and Representatives before mentioned, and the Members of the several State Legislatures, and all executive and judicial Officers, both of the United States and of the several States, shall be bound by *Oath or Affirmation*, to support this Constitution; *but no religious Test shall ever be required as a Qualification to any Office or public Trust under the United States*.
>
> Article II, § 1, cl. 8:
>
> Before [the President] enters the Execution of his Office, he shall take the following *Oath or Affirmation*:—"I do solemnly *swear (or affirm)* that I will faithfully execute the Office of President of the United States, and will to the best of my Ability, preserve, protect, and defend the Constitution of the United States."[23]
>
> Article I, § 3, cl. 6:
>
> The Senate shall have the sole Power to try all Impeachments. When sitting for that purpose, they shall be on *Oath or Affirmation*.
>
> Fourth Amendment:
>
> *** and no Warrants shall issue, but upon probable cause, supported by *Oath or affirmation*, and particularly describing the place to be searched and the persons or things to be seized.

Note that these quoted passages seem to indicate some sort of effort to provide for a neutral civil national government[24] quite distinct from the various church-state arrangements within the several states forming the United States.[25] So, for example:

---

23. Note that here (as in Article VI) the alternative of affirming (rather than subscribing by "oath") is provided for. Note also that there is no "so help me God" feature in the sentence the President is expected to say.

24. See also Article XI of the Treaty of Peace and Friendship, Nov 4, 1796 - Jan. 3, 1797, United States-Tripoli, 8 Stat. 154, 155, T.S. No. 358 ("As the government of the United States of America is not in any sense founded on the Christian religion—as it has in itself no character of enmity against the laws, religion, or tranquility of Musselmen * * * it is declared by the parties, that no pretext arising from religious opinions shall ever produce an interruption of the harmony existing between the two countries.").

25. Similarly, the original motto of the United States was "E Pluribus Unum" (and *not* "In God We Trust"). "In God We Trust" did not appear on American currency until the Lincoln administration

(1) Article VI disallows any religious test for holding office under the authority of the United States; (2) the oath or affirmation provided for the President is itself civil; (3) the several clauses otherwise providing for "oath"[26] provide the alternative of a mere affirmation; and (4) the Preamble to the Constitution is itself civil and secular, rather than religious.[27]

C. THE INCORPORATION QUESTION: THE BLAINE AMENDMENT, CONTROVERSY RESPECTING THE FOURTEENTH AMENDMENT, AND STATE CONSTITUTIONS

1. The Fourteenth Amendment and the Blaine Amendment

In *Everson* (the first principal case, *infra* chapter 9), the Supreme Court was not dealing with the first amendment; rather it was dealing with the fourteenth amendment, which has no express church-state clauses at all. We examined the relationship between the fourteenth and first amendments with respect to free speech in Chapter 2,[28] but the same question is even muddier where the church-state clauses are concerned, partly because of the failed Blaine amendment of 1875. In 1875, James Blaine, Representative from Maine, introduced the following amendment in House of Representatives (on the suggestion of President Ulysses S. Grant):

> No state shall make any law respecting an establishment of religion or prohibiting the free exercise thereof; and, no money raised by taxation in any state for the support of public schools, or derived from any public fund therefore, nor any public lands devoted thereto, shall ever be under the control of

---

and the Civil War, and it did not become standard on all currency until the 1950s. In this same decade (the period of the Cold War with the Soviet Union), Congress changed the national motto to "In God We Trust," and "under God" was added to the Pledge of Allegiance.

26. "Oath: A formal declaration or promise to fulfill a pledge, often calling upon God or some other sacred object as witness." American Heritage Dictionary 904 (W. Morris ed. 1971).

27. But see the theistic references in the Declaration of Independence ("to assume among the powers of the earth the separate and equal station to which the laws of nature and of nature's God entitle them *** endowed by their Creator with certain inalienable rights *** "). And consider Art. I § 7, cl. 2 ("If any Bill shall not be returned by the President within ten Days (*Sundays excepted*) after it shall have been presented to him, the Same shall be a Law, in like Manner as if he had signed it, unless the Congress by their Adjournment prevent its Return, in which Case it shall not be a Law.") Why "*Sundays excepted*"? Note, also, that at the end of Article VII, the final sentence memorializing the date of the Constitution's own completion reads in the following way: "done in Convention by the Unanimous Consent of the States present the Seventeenth Day of September *in the Year of our Lord* one thousand seven hundred and Eighty seven ***." See also Zorach v. Clauson, 343 U.S. 306 (1952) (Douglas, J., concurring) ("We are a religious people whose institutions presuppose a Supreme Being.").

28. See *supra* pp. 56-70

> any religious sect, nor shall any money so raised or lands so devoted be divided between religious sects or denominations.[29]

The Blaine amendment passed in the House 180 to 7 (98 not voting). Following discussion and some changes in the Senate, it failed to garner the two-thirds vote necessary (28 to 16, 27 not voting).

The failure of the Blaine amendment in Congress is often offered as evidence of a contemporary understanding in Congress that the fourteenth amendment did *not* "incorporate" the establishment clause of the first amendment. If it did, why the proposal for an additional amendment, the entire first phrase of which is verbatim the same as the first amendment—except that it speaks to what "no state" (rather than no "Congress") may do? The force of this argument has been discounted on several grounds:

a. Prior to the Blaine amendment, but subsequent to the fourteenth amendment, the Supreme Court decided the *Slaughterhouse Cases*.[30] That decision had eviscerated the privileges and immunities clause—the clause actually relied upon in Congress for the incorporation thesis. Insofar as the Court subsequently merely corrected its own error—albeit through the due process clause rather than the privileges and immunities clauses—the matter has simply come out approximately in the right way.
b. The form the Blaine amendment ultimately assumed in Congress was more detailed and complex than the first amendment's more succinct and simpler provision; the resistance it encountered in the Senate was due partly to uncertainty respecting the appropriateness and consequences of the added provisions which were controversial in their sheer detail.
c. The free exercise clause of the first amendment, like the establishment clause, is also reproduced verbatim in the Blaine amendment. Parity of reasoning would suggest that the fourteenth amendment thus does not propose any protection for the free exercise of religion from state abridgment—but far fewer persons believe this to be the case.
d. An argument that the free exercise part of the first amendment is nonetheless picked up by the "liberty" portion of the due process clause, while the establishment clause is allegedly not similarly incorporated, has no confirming support either in the associated history of the fourteenth amendment or in the treatment and fate of the Blaine amendment as such.

---

29. The antecedent address by Grant on September 29, 1875, in Des Moines, Iowa, provided: "Let us all labor to add all needful guarantees for the security of free thought, free speech, a free press, pure morals, unfettered religious sentiments, and of equal right and privileges to all men, irrespective of nationality, color, or religion. *** Leave the matter of religion to the family altar, the church, and the private school, supported entirely by private contributions. Keep the church and the state forever separate."

30. 83 U.S. 36 (1872).

It is true, nonetheless, that the modern Court's continuing reliance solely on the due process clause (rather than on the privileges and immunities clause) gives Court critics a textual basis for arguing that the fourteenth amendment only forbids those state practices regarding establishment of religion as might be inconsistent with the "liberty" of religion.[31] Indeed, several Justices subscribe to this view.[32]

2. State Constitutions

A version of the Blaine amendment was adopted in a number of states. The state supreme courts in some of those states have construed the state constitutional clause as a more complete and more stringent restriction on the state's use of tax revenue than the United States Supreme Court construed the first amendment in its first serious discussion of the establishment clause.[33]

D. SELECTED BIBLIOGRAPHY OF RECENT BOOK-LENGTH TREATMENTS OF THE FREE EXERCISE AND ESTABLISHMENT CLAUSES

Boston, Rob, and Lynn, Barry W., Why the Religious Right Is Wrong: About Separation of Church and State (1994).

Carter, Stephen, The Culture of Disbelief: How American Law and Politics Trivalize Religious Devotion (1993).

Choper, Jesse H., Securing Religious Liberty: Principles for Judicial Interpretation of the Religion Clauses (1995).

Cord, Robert L., Separation of Church and State: Historical Fact and Current Fiction (1982).

Curry, Thomas J., The First Freedoms: Church and State in America to the Passage of the First Amendment (1986).

Dreisbach, Daniel L., Real Threat and Mere Shadow: Religious Liberty and the First Amendment (1987).

Epps, Garrett, To an Unknown God (2001).

Feldman, Stephen M. (ed.) Law and Religion : A Critical Anthology (2000).

---

31. In brief, this view puts the dominant stress on the free exercise of religion. It reads the prohibition on laws respecting an establishment of religion as a restriction on such laws as may impair the free exercise of religion, but not otherwise. For a recent Note also arguing that the establishment clause was not a contemplated element of the fourteenth amendment and that the fourteenth amendment incorporates only the free exercise portion of the first amendment, see Note, Rethinking the Incorporation of the Establishment Clause: A Federalist View, 105 Harv.L.Rev. 1700 (1992).

32. See, e.g., County of Allegheny v. ACLU, 429 U.S. 573 (1989). For a recent effort to work through the incorporation issue discussed in these pages, see Kurt T. Lash, *The Second Adoption of the Establishment Clause: The Rise of the Nonestablishment Principle*, 27 Ariz. St. L. J. 1085 (1995).

33. See Everson v. Board of Education, 330 U.S. 1 (1947). For a fuller discussion, see Chester J. Antieau, et al., Religion Under the State Constitutions (1965).

Feldman, Stephen M. Please Don't Wish Me a Merry Christmas : A Critical History of the Separation of Church and State (1997).

Greenawalt, Kent, Private Conscience and Public Reasons (1995).

Greenawalt, Kent, Religious Convictions and Political Choices (1988).

Hall, TimothyJ., Separating Church and State: Roger Williams and Religious Liberty (1998)

Haas, Carol. Engel V. Vitale: Separation of Church and State (1994).

Levy, Leonard W., The Establishment Clause: Religion and the First Amendment (2d ed. 1994).

McBrien, Richard P., Caesar's Coin: Religion and Politics in America (1987).

McWhirter, Darien A. The Separation of Church and State (1994).

Miller, W., The First Liberty: Religion and the First Amendment (1985).

Owen, J. Judd. Religion and the Demise of Liberal Rationalism : The Foundational Crisis of the Separation of Church and State (2001).

Pfeffer, Leo, Religion, State, and the Burger Court (1985).

Segers, Mary, Jelen, Ted G., and Cochran, Clarke E. A Wall of Separation?: Debating the Public Role of Religion (1999).

Smith, Steven R., Public Prayer and the Constitution (1987).

Smith, Steven R., Foreordained Failure: The Quest for a Constitutional Principle of Religious Freedom (1995).

Swomley, John M., Religious Liberty and the Secular State: The Constitutional Context (1987).

Thiemann, Ronald, Religion in Public Life: A Dilemma for Democracy (1996).

Weber, Paul J. (ed.) Equal Separation (1990).

Weldon, Mark Whitten, The Myth of Christian America: What You Need to Know about the Separation of Church and State (1999).

Chapter 9

"CONGRESS SHALL MAKE NO LAW RESPECTING AN ESTABLISHMENT OF RELIGION ***"

A. THE GENERAL TEST(S)

EVERSON v. BOARD OF EDUCATION
330 U.S. 1 (1947)

MR. JUSTICE BLACK delivered the opinion of the Court.

A New Jersey statute authorizes its local school districts to make rules and contracts for the transportation of children to and from schools.[1] The appellee, a township board of education, acting pursuant to this statute, authorized reimbursement to parents of money expended by them for the bus transportation of their children on regular busses operated by the public transportation system. Part of this money was for the payment of transportation of some children in the community to Catholic parochial schools. These church schools give their students, in addition to secular education, regular religious instruction conforming to the religious tenets and modes of worship of the Catholic Faith. The superintendent of these schools is a Catholic priest.

The appellant, in his capacity as a district taxpayer, filed suit in a state court challenging the right of the Board to reimburse parents of parochial school students. He contended that the statute and the resolution passed pursuant to it violated both the State and the Federal Constitutions. ***

The only contention here is that the state statute and the resolution, insofar as they authorized reimbursement to parents of children attending parochial schools, violate the Federal Constitution in these two respects, which to some extent overlap. *First*. They authorize the State to take by taxation the private property of some and bestow it upon others, to be used for their own private purposes. This, it is alleged, violates the due process clause of the Fourteenth Amendment. *Second*. The statute and the resolution forced inhabitants to pay taxes to help support and maintain

---

1. "Whenever in any district there are children living remote from any schoolhouse, the board of education of the district may make rules and contracts or the transportation of such children to and from school, including the transportation of school children to and from school other than a public school, except such school as is operated for profit in whole or in part.

"When any school district provides any transportation for public school children to and from school, transportation from any point in such established school route to any other point in such established school route shall be supplied to school children residing in such school district in going to and from school other than a public school, except such school as is operated for profit in whole or in part." New Jersey Laws, 1941, c. 191, p. 581; N.J.R.S. Cum. Supp., tit. 18, c. 14, § 8.

schools which are dedicated to, and which regularly teach, the Catholic Faith. This is alleged to be a use of state power to support church schools contrary to the prohibition of the First Amendment which the Fourteenth Amendment made applicable to the states. ***

It is much too late to argue that legislation intended to facilitate the opportunity of children to get a secular education serves no public purpose. *** The same thing is no less true of legislation to reimburse needy parents, or all parents, for payment of the fares of their children so that they can ride in public busses to and from schools rather than run the risk of traffic and other hazards incident to walking or "hitch-hiking."***

Insofar as the second phase of the due process argument may differ from the first, it is by suggesting that taxation for transportation of children to church schools constitutes support of a religion by the State. But if the law is invalid for this reason, it is because it violates the First Amendment's prohibition against the establishment of religion by law. This is the exact question raised by appellant's second contention, to consideration of which we now turn.

*** The First Amendment, as made applicable to the states by the Fourteenth, Murdock v. Pennsylvania, 319 U.S. 105, commands that a state "shall make no law respecting an establishment of religion, or prohibiting the free exercise thereof. ***" These words of the First Amendment reflected in the minds of early Americans a vivid mental picture of conditions and practices which they fervently wished to stamp out in order to preserve liberty for themselves and for their posterity. Doubtless their goal has not been entirely reached; but so far has the Nation moved toward it that the expression "law respecting an establishment of religion," probably does not so vividly remind present-day Americans of the evils, fears, and political problems that caused that expression to be written into our Bill of Rights. Whether this New Jersey law is one respecting an "establishment of religion" requires an understanding of the meaning of that language, particularly with respect to the imposition of taxes. Once again,[2] therefore, it is not inappropriate briefly to review the background and environment of the period in which that constitutional language was fashioned and adopted.

A large proportion of the early settlers of this country came here from Europe to escape the bondage of laws which compelled them to support and attend government-favored churches. The centuries immediately before and contemporaneous with the colonization of America had been filled with turmoil, civil strife, and persecutions, generated in large part by established sects determined to maintain their absolute political and religious supremacy. With the power of government supporting them, at various times and places, Catholics had persecuted Protestants, Protestants had persecuted Catholics, Protestant sects had persecuted other Protestant sects, Catholics of one shade of belief had persecuted Catholics of another shade of belief,

2. See Reynolds v. United States, 98 U.S. 145, 162 ***.

and all of these had from time to time persecuted Jews. In efforts to force loyalty to whatever religious group happened to be on top and in league with the government of a particular time and place, men and women had been fined, cast in jail, cruelly tortured, and killed. Among the offenses for which these punishments had been inflicted were such things as speaking disrespectfully of the views of ministers of government-established churches, non-attendance at those churches, expressions of non-belief in their doctrines, and failure to pay taxes and tithes to support them.[3]

These practices of the old world were transplanted to and began to thrive in the soil of the new America. The very charters granted by the English Crown to the individuals and companies designated to make the laws which would control the destinies of the colonials authorized these individuals and companies to erect religious establishments which all, whether believers or non-believers, would be required to support and attend.[4] ***

These practices became so commonplace as to shock the freedom-loving colonials into a feeling of abhorrence.[9] The imposition of taxes to pay ministers' salaries and to build and maintain churches and church property aroused their indignation. It was these feelings which found expression in the First Amendment. No one locality and no one group throughout the Colonies can rightly be given entire credit for having aroused the sentiment that culminated in adoption of the Bill of Rights' provisions embracing religious liberty. But Virginia, where the established church had achieved a dominant influence in political affairs and where many excesses attracted wide public attention, provided a great stimulus and able leadership for the movement. ***

The movement toward this end reached its dramatic climax in Virginia in 1785-86 when the Virginia legislative body was about to renew Virginia's tax levy for the support of the established church. Thomas Jefferson and James Madison led the fight against this tax. Madison wrote his great Memorial and Remonstrance against the law. In it, he eloquently argued that a true religion did not need the support of

---

3. See, e.g., Macaulay, History of England (1849) I, cc. 2, 4; The Cambridge Modern History (1908) V, cc. V, IX, XI; Beard, Rise of American Civilization (1933) I, 60; Cobb, Rise of Religious Liberty in America (1902) c. II; Sweet, The Story of Religion in America (1939) c. II; Sweet, Religion in Colonial America (1942) 320-322.

4. See, *e.g.*, the charter of the colony of Carolina which gave the grantees the right of "patronage and advowsons of all the churches and chapels *** together with licence and power to build and found churches, chapels and oratories *** and to cause them to be dedicated and consecrated, according to the ecclesiastical laws of our kingdom of England." ***

9. Madison wrote to a friend in 1774: "That diabolical, hell-conceived principle of persecution rages among some *** This vexes me the worst of anything whatever. There are at this time in the adjacent country not less than five or six well-meaning men in close jail for publishing their religious sentiments, which in the main are very orthodox. I have neither patience to hear, talk, or think of anything relative to this matter; for I have squabbled and scolded, abused and ridiculed, so long about it to little purpose, that I am without common patience. So I must beg you to pity me, and pray for liberty of conscience to all." I Writings of James Madison (1900) 18, 21.

law; that no person, either believer or non-believer, should be taxed to support a religious institution of any kind; that the best interest of a society required that the minds of men always be wholly free; and that cruel persecutions were the inevitable result of government-established religions. Madison's Remonstrance received strong support throughout Virginia, and the Assembly postponed consideration of the proposed tax measure until its next session. When the proposal came up for consideration at that session, it not only died in committee, but the Assembly enacted the famous "Virginia Bill for Religious Liberty" originally written by Thomas Jefferson. ***

This Court has previously recognized that the provisions of the First Amendment, in the drafting and adoption of which Madison and Jefferson played such leading roles, had the same objective and were intended to provide the same protection against governmental intrusion on religious liberty as the Virginia statute. *Reynolds v. United States, supra* at 164 ***. Prior to the adoption of the Fourteenth Amendment, the First Amendment did not apply as a restraint against the state. Most of them did soon provide similar constitutional protections for religious liberty. But some states persisted for about half a century in imposing restraints upon the free exercise of religion and in discriminating against particular religious groups. In recent years, so far as the provision against the establishment of a religion is concerned, the question has most frequently arisen in connection with proposed state aid to church schools and efforts to carry on religious teachings in the public schools in accordance with the tenets of a particular sect. *** The state courts, in the main, have remained faithful to the language of their own constitutional provisions designed to protect religious freedom and to separate religions and governments. Their decisions, however, show the difficulty in drawing the line between tax legislation which provides funds for the welfare of the general public and that which is designed to support institutions which teach religion.

The meaning and scope of the First Amendment, preventing establishment of religion or prohibiting the free exercise thereof, in the light of its history and the evils it was designed forever to suppress, have been several times elaborated by the decisions of this Court prior to the application of the First Amendment to the states by the Fourteenth. The broad meaning given the Amendment by these earlier cases has been accepted by this Court in its decisions concerning an individual's religious freedom rendered since the Fourteenth Amendment was interpreted to make the prohibitions of the First applicable to state action abridging religious freedom. There is every reason to give the same application and broad interpretation to the "establishment of religion" clause. The interrelation of these complementary clauses was well summarized in a statement of the Court of Appeals of South Carolina,[23] quoted with approval by this Court in Watson v. Jones, 13 Wall. 679, 730: "The structure of our government has, for the preservation of civil liberty, rescued the temporal institutions

23. Harmon v. Dreher, Speer's Equity Reports (S.C., 1843), 87, 120.

from religious interference. On the other hand, it has secured religious liberty from the invasion of the civil authority."

The "establishment of religion" clause of the First Amendment means at least this: Neither a state nor the Federal Government can set up a church. Neither can pass laws which aid one religion, aid all religions, or prefer one religion over another. Neither can force nor influence a person to go to or to remain away from church against his will or force him to profess a belief or disbelief in any religion. No person can be punished for entertaining or professing religious beliefs or disbeliefs, for church attendance or non-attendance. No tax in any amount, large or small, can be levied to support any religious activities or institutions, whatever they may be called, or whatever form they may adopt to teach or practice religion. Neither a state nor the Federal Government can, openly or secretly, participate in the affairs of any religious organizations or groups and vice versa. In the words of Jefferson, the clause against establishment of religion by law was intended to erect "a wall of separation between church and State." *Reynolds v. United States, supra* at 164.

We must consider the New Jersey statute in accordance with the foregoing limitations imposed by the First Amendment. But we must not strike that state statute down if it is within the State's constitutional power even though it approaches the verge of that power. *** New Jersey cannot consistently with the "establishment of religion" clause of the First Amendment contribute tax-raised funds to the support of an institution which teaches the tenets and faith of any church. On the other hand, other language of the amendment commands that New Jersey cannot hamper its citizens in the free exercise of their own religion. Consequently, it cannot exclude individual Catholics, Lutherans, Mohammedans, Baptists, Jews, Methodists, Non-believers, Presbyterians, or the members of any other faith, *because of their faith, or lack of it*, from receiving the benefits of public welfare legislation. While we do not mean to intimate that a state could not provide transportation only to children attending public schools, we must be careful, in protecting the citizens of New Jersey against state-established churches, to be sure that we do not inadvertently prohibit New Jersey from extending its general state law benefits to all its citizens without regard to their religious belief.

Measured by these standards, we cannot say that the First Amendment prohibits New Jersey from spending tax-raised funds to pay the bus fares of parochial school pupils as a part of a general program under which it pays the fares of pupils attending public and other schools. It is undoubtedly true that children are helped to get to church schools. There is even a possibility that some of the children might not be sent to the church schools if the parents were compelled to pay their children's bus fares out of their own pockets when transportation to a public school would have been paid for by the State. The same possibility exists where the state requires a local transit company to provide reduced fares to school children including those attending parochial schools,[24] or where a municipally owned transportation system undertakes to carry all school children free of charge. Moreover, state-paid policemen, detailed to protect children going to and from church schools from the very real hazards of traffic, would serve much the same purpose and accomplish much the same result as state provisions intended to guarantee free transportation of a kind which the state deems to be best for the school children's welfare. And parents might refuse to risk their children to the serious danger of traffic accidents going to and from parochial schools, the approaches to which were not protected by policemen. Similarly, parents might be reluctant to permit their children to attend schools which the state had cut off from such general government services as ordinary police and fire protection, connections for sewage disposal, public highways and sidewalks. Of course, cutting off church schools from these services, so separate and so indisputably marked off from the religious function, would make it far more difficult for the schools to operate. But such is obviously not the purpose of the First Amendment. That Amendment requires the state to be a neutral in its relations with groups of religious believers and non-believers; it does not require the state to be their adversary. State power is no more to be used so as to handicap religions than it is to favor them.

This Court has said that parents may, in the discharge of their duty under state compulsory education laws, send their children to a religious rather than a public school if the school meets the secular educational requirements which the state has power to impose. See Pierce v. Society of Sisters, 268 U.S. 510. It appears that these parochial schools meet New Jersey's requirements. The State contributes no money to the schools. It does not support them. Its legislation, as applied, does no more than provide a general program to help parents get their children, regardless of their religion, safely and expeditiously to and from accredited schools.

The First Amendment has erected a wall between church and state. That wall must be kept high and impregnable. We could not approve the slightest breach. New Jersey has not breached it here.

Affirmed.

MR. JUSTICE JACKSON, dissenting.

I find myself, contrary to first impressions, unable to join in this decision. I have a sympathy, though it is not ideological, with Catholic citizens who are compelled by law to pay taxes for public schools, and also feel constrained by conscience and discipline to support other schools for their own children. Such relief to them as this

---

24. New Jersey long ago permitted public utilities to charge school children reduced rates. See Public S.R. Co. v. Public Utility Comm'rs, 81 N.J.L. 363, 80 A. 27 (1911); see also *Interstate Ry. v. Massachusetts*, [207 U.S. 79]. The District of Columbia Code requires that the new charter of the District public transportation company provide a three-cent fare "for school children *** going to and from public, parochial, or like schools. ***" 47 Stat. 752, 759.

case involves is not in itself a serious burden to taxpayers and I had assumed it to be as little serious in principle. Study of this case convinces me otherwise. The Court's opinion marshals every argument in favor of state aid and puts the case in its most favorable light, but much of its reasoning confirms my conclusions that there are no good grounds upon which to support the present legislation. In fact, the undertones of the opinion, advocating complete and uncompromising separation of Church from State, seem utterly discordant with its conclusion yielding support to their commingling in educational matters. The case which irresistibly comes to mind as the most fitting precedent is that of Julia who, according to Byron's reports, "whispering 'I will ne'er consent,'—consented."

I-II

The Court sustains this legislation by assuming two deviations from the facts of this particular case; first, it assumes a state of facts the record does not support, and secondly, it refuses to consider facts which are inescapable on the record. ***

The Township of Ewing is not furnishing transportation to the children in any form; it is not operating school busses itself or contracting for their operation; and it is not performing any public service of any kind with this taxpayer's money. All school children are left to ride as ordinary paying passengers on the regular busses operated by the public transportation system. What the Township does, and what the taxpayer complains of, is at stated intervals to reimburse parents for the fares paid, provided the children attend either public schools or Catholic Church schools. ***

The New Jersey Act in question makes the character of the school, not the needs of the children, determine the eligibility of parents to reimbursement. ***

Of course, this case is not one of a Baptist or a Jew or an Episcopalian or a pupil of a private school complaining of discrimination. It is one of a taxpayer urging that he is being taxed for an unconstitutional purpose. I think he is entitled to have us consider the Act just as it is written. *** As applied to this taxpayer by the action he complains of, certainly the Act does not authorize reimbursement to those who choose any alternative to the public school except Catholic Church schools.

If we are to decide this case on the facts before us, our question is simply this: Is it constitutional to tax this complainant to pay the cost of carrying pupils to Church schools of one specified denomination?

Whether the taxpayer constitutionally can be made to contribute aid to parents of students because of their attendance at parochial schools depends upon the nature of those schools and their relation to the Church. ***

*** Under the rubric "Catholic Schools," the Canon Law of the Church, by which all Catholics are bound, provides:

> 1215. Catholic children are to be educated in schools where not only nothing contrary to Catholic faith and morals is taught, but rather in schools where religious and moral training occupy the first place. ***
>
> 1217. Catholic children shall not attend non-Catholic, indifferent, schools

> that are mixed, that is to say, schools open to Catholics and non- Catholics alike. The bishop of the diocese only has the right, in harmony with the instructions of the Holy See, to decide under what circumstances, and with what safeguards to prevent loss of faith, it may be tolerated that Catholic children go to such schools. (Canon 1374.) ***

I should be surprised if any Catholic would deny that the parochial school is a vital, if not the most vital, part of the Roman Catholic Church. If put to the choice, that venerable institution, I should expect, would forego its whole service for mature persons before it would give up education of the young, and it would be a wise choice. Its growth and cohesion, discipline and loyalty, spring from its schools. Catholic education is the rock on which the whole structure rests, and to render tax aid to its Church school is indistinguishable to me from rendering the same aid to the Church itself.

III

It is of no importance in this situation whether the beneficiary of this expenditure of tax-raised funds is primarily the parochial school and incidentally the pupil, or whether the aid is directly bestowed on the pupil with indirect benefits to the school. The state cannot maintain a Church and it can no more tax its citizens to furnish free carriage to those who attend a Church. The prohibition against establishment of religion cannot be circumvented by a subsidy, bonus or reimbursement of expense to individuals for receiving religious instruction and indoctrination.

*** Of course, the state may pay out tax-raised funds to relieve pauperism, but it may not under our Constitution do so to induce or reward piety. It may spend funds to secure old age against want, but it may not spend funds to secure religion against skepticism. It may compensate individuals for loss of employment, but it cannot compensate them for adherence to a creed.

It seems to me that the basic fallacy in the Court's reasoning, which accounts for its failure to apply the principles it avows, is in ignoring the essentially religious test by which beneficiaries of this expenditure are selected. A policeman protects a Catholic, of course—but not because he is a Catholic; it is because he is a man and a member of our society. The fireman protects the Church school—but not because it is a Church school; it is because it is property, part of the assets of our society. Neither the fireman nor the policeman has to ask before he renders aid "Is this man or building identified with the Catholic Church?" But before these school authorities draw a check to reimburse for a student's fare they must ask just that question, and if the school is a Catholic one they may render aid because it is such, while if it is of any other faith or is run for profit, the help must be withheld. To consider the converse of the Court's reasoning will best disclose its fallacy. That there is no parallel between police and fire protection and this plan of reimbursement is apparent from the incongruity of the limitation of this Act if applied to police and fire service. Could we sustain an Act that said the police shall protect pupils on the way to or from public schools and Catholic schools but not while going to and coming from other schools, and firemen shall extinguish a blaze in public or Catholic school buildings but shall not put out a blaze in Protestant Church schools or private schools operated for profit? That is the true analogy to the case we have before us and I should think it pretty plain that such a scheme would not be valid.

*** There is no answer to the proposition, more fully expounded by MR. JUSTICE RUTLEDGE, that the effect of the religious freedom Amendment to our Constitution was to take every form of propagation of religion out of the realm of things which could directly or indirectly be made public business and thereby be supported in whole or in part at taxpayers' expense. That is a difference which the Constitution sets up between religion and almost every other subject matter of legislation, a difference which goes to the very root of religious freedom and which the Court is overlooking today. This freedom was first in the Bill of Rights because it was first in the forefathers' minds; it was set forth in absolute terms, and its strength is its rigidity. It was intended not only to keep the states' hands out of religion, but to keep religion's hands off the state, and, above all, to keep bitter religious controversy out of public life by denying to every denomination any advantage from getting control of public policy or the public purse. Those great ends I cannot but think are immeasurably compromised by today's decision.

This policy of our Federal Constitution has never been wholly pleasing to most religious groups. They all are quick to invoke its protections; they all are irked when they feel its restraints. This Court has gone a long way, if not an unreasonable way, to hold that public business of such paramount importance as maintenance of public order, protection of the privacy of the home, and taxation may not be pursued by a state in a way that even indirectly will interfere with religious proselyting. See dissent in Douglas v. Jeannette, 319 U.S. 157, 166; Murdock v. Pennsylvania, 319 U.S. 105; Martin v. Struthers, 319 U.S. 141; Jones v. Opelika, 316 U.S. 584, reversed on rehearing, 319 U.S. 103.

But we cannot have it both ways. Religious teaching cannot be a private affair when the state seeks to impose regulations which infringe on it indirectly, and a public affair when it comes to taxing citizens of one faith to aid another, or those of no faith to aid all. If these principles seem harsh in prohibiting aid to Catholic education, it must not be forgotten that it is the same Constitution that alone assures Catholics the right to maintain these schools at all when predominant local sentiment would forbid them. Pierce v. Society of Sisters, 268 U.S. 510. Nor should I think that those who have done so well without this aid would want to see this separation between Church and State broken down. If the state may aid these religious schools, it may herefore regulate them. ***

MR. JUSTICE FRANKFURTER joins in this opinion.

MR. JUSTICE RUTLEDGE, with whom MR. JUSTICE FRANKFURTER, MR. JUSTICE JACKSON and MR. JUSTICE BURTON agree, dissenting.

This case forces us to determine squarely for the first time what was "an establishment of religion" in the First Amendment's conception; and by that measure to decide whether New Jersey's action violates its command. The facts may be stated shortly, to give setting and color to the constitutional problem. ***

Named parents have paid the cost of public conveyance of their children from their homes in Ewing to three public high schools and four parochial schools outside the district. Semiannually the Board has reimbursed the parents from public school funds raised by general taxation. Religion is taught as part of the curriculum in each of the four private schools, as appears affirmatively by the testimony of the superintendent of parochial schools in the Diocese of Trenton. ***

I

Not simply an established church, but any law respecting an establishment of religion is forbidden. The Amendment was broadly but not loosely phrased. It is the compact and exact summation of its author's views formed during his long struggle for religious freedom. In Madison's own words characterizing Jefferson's Bill for Establishing Religious Freedom, the guaranty he put in our national charter, like the bill he piloted through the Virginia Assembly, was "a Model of technical precision, and perspicuous brevity." Madison could not have confused "church" and "religion," or "an established church" and "an establishment of religion."

The Amendment's purpose was not to strike merely at the official establishment of a single sect, creed or religion, outlawing only a formal relation such as had prevailed in England and some of the colonies. Necessarily it was to uproot all such relationships. But the object was broader than separating church and state in this narrow sense. It was to create a complete and permanent separation of the spheres of religious activity and civil authority by comprehensively forbidding every form of public aid or support for religion. In proof the Amendment's wording and history unite with this Court's consistent utterances whenever attention has been fixed directly upon the question.

"Religion" appears only once in the Amendment. But the word governs two prohibitions and governs them alike. It does not have two meanings, one narrow to forbid "an establishment" and another, much broader, for securing "the free exercise thereof." "Thereof" brings down "religion" with its entire and exact content, no more and no less, from the first into the second guaranty, so that Congress and now the states are as broadly restricted concerning the one as they are regarding the other. ***

"Religion" has the same broad significance in the twin prohibition concerning "an establishment." The Amendment was not duplicitous. "Religion" and "establishment" were not used in any formal or technical sense. The prohibition broadly forbids state support, financial or other, of religion in any guise, form or degree. It outlaws all use of public funds for religious purposes.

II

No provision of the Constitution is more closely tied to or given content by its generating history than the religious clause of the First Amendment. It is at once the refined product and the terse summation of that history. The history includes not only Madison's authorship and the proceedings before the First Congress, but also the long and intensive struggle for religious freedom in America, more especially in Virginia, of which the Amendment was the direct culmination. ***

The climax came in the legislative struggle of 1784-1785 over the Assessment Bill. *** This was nothing more nor less than a taxing measure for the support of religion, designed to revive the payment of tithes suspended since 1777. So long as it singled out a particular sect for preference it incurred the active and general hostility of dissentient groups. It was broadened to include them, with the result that some subsided temporarily in their opposition. As altered, the bill gave to each taxpayer the privilege of designating which church should receive his share of the tax. In default of designation the legislature applied it to pious uses. But what is of the utmost significance here, "in its final form the bill left the taxpayer the option of giving his tax to education."

Madison was unyielding at all times, opposing with all his vigor the general and nondiscriminatory as he had the earlier particular and discriminatory assessments proposed. *** And before the Assembly reconvened in the fall he issued his historic Memorial and Remonstrance.

*** [T]he Remonstrance is at once the most concise and the most accurate statement of the views of the First Amendment's author concerning what is "an establishment of religion." ***

As the Remonstrance discloses throughout, Madison opposed every form and degree of official relation between religion and civil authority. For him religion was a wholly private matter beyond the scope of civil power either to restrain or to support. Denial or abridgment of religious freedom was a violation of rights both of conscience and of natural equality. State aid was no less obnoxious or destructive to freedom and to religion itself than other forms of state interference. "Establishment" and "free exercise" were correlative and coextensive ideas, representing only different facets of the single great and fundamental freedom. The Remonstrance, following the Virginia statute's example, referred to the history of religious conflicts and the effects of all sorts of establishments, current and historical, to suppress religion's free exercise. With Jefferson, Madison believed that to tolerate any fragment of establishment would be by so much to perpetuate restraint upon that freedom. Hence he sought to tear out the institution not partially but root and branch, and to bar its return forever.

In no phase was he more unrelentingly absolute than in opposing state support or aid by taxation. Not even "three pence" contribution was thus to be exacted from any citizen for such a purpose. ***

III

* * *

Does New Jersey's action furnish support for religion by use of the taxing power? Certainly it does, if the test remains undiluted as Jefferson and Madison made it, that money taken by taxation from one is not to be used or given to support another's religious training or belief, or indeed one's own. ***

*** Here parents pay money to send their children to parochial schools and funds raised by taxation are used to reimburse them. This not only helps the children to get to school and the parents to send them. It aids them in a substantial way to get the very thing which they are sent to the particular school to secure, namely, religious training and teaching.

Believers of all faiths, and others who do not express their feeling toward ultimate issues of existence in any creedal form, pay the New Jersey tax. When the money so raised is used to pay for transportation to religious schools, the Catholic taxpayer to the extent of his proportionate share pays for the transportation of Lutheran, Jewish and otherwise religiously affiliated children to receive their non-Catholic religious instruction. Their parents likewise pay proportionately for the transportation of Catholic children to receive Catholic instruction. Each thus contributes to "the propagation of opinions which he disbelieves" in so far as their religions differ, as do others who accept no creed without regard to those differences. Each thus pays taxes also to support the teaching of his own religion, an exaction equally forbidden since it denies "the comfortable liberty" of giving one's contribution to the particular agency of instruction he approves.

New Jersey's action therefore exactly fits the type of exaction and the kind of evil at which Madison and Jefferson struck. Under the test they framed it cannot be said that the cost of transportation is no part of the cost of education or of the religious instruction given. That it is a substantial and a necessary element is shown most plainly by the continuing and increasing demand for the state to assume it. *** And the very purpose of the state's contribution is to defray the cost of conveying the pupil to the place where he will receive not simply secular, but also and primarily religious, teaching and guidance. ***

Finally, transportation, where it is needed, is as essential to education as any other element. Its cost is as much a part of the total expense, except at times in amount, as the cost of textbooks, of school lunches, of athletic equipment, of writing and other materials; indeed of all other items composing the total burden. ***

For me, therefore, the feat is impossible to select so indispensable an item from the composite of total costs, and characterize it as not aiding, contributing to, promoting or sustaining the propagation of beliefs which it is the very end of all to bring about. Unless this can be maintained, and the Court does not maintain it, the aid thus given is outlawed. Payment of transportation is no more, nor is it any the less essential to education, whether religious or secular, than payment for tuitions, for teachers' salaries, or buildings, equipment and necessary materials. Nor is it any the less directly related, in a school giving religious instruction, to the primary religious objective all those essential items of cost are intended to achieve. ***

V-VI

No one conscious of religious values can be unsympathetic toward the burden which our constitutional separation puts on parents who desire religious instruction mixed with secular for their children. They pay taxes for others' children's education, at the same time the added cost of instruction for their own. Nor can one happily see benefits denied to children which others receive, because in conscience they or their parents for them desire a different kind of training others do not demand.

But if those feelings should prevail, there would be an end to our historic constitutional policy and command. No more unjust or discriminatory in fact is it to deny attendants at religious schools the cost of their transportation than it is to deny them tuitions, sustenance for their teachers, or any other educational expense which others receive at public cost. Hardship in fact there is which none can blink. But, for assuring to those who undergo it the greater, the most comprehensive freedom, it is one written by design and firm intent into our basic law.

Of course discrimination in the legal sense does not exist. The child attending the religious school has the same right as any other to attend the public school. ***

The problem then cannot be cast in terms of legal discrimination or its absence. This would be true, even though the state in giving aid should treat all religious instruction alike. Thus, if the present statute and its application were shown to apply equally to all religious schools of whatever faith, yet in the light of our tradition it could not stand. For then the adherent of one creed still would pay for the support of another, the childless taxpayer with others more fortunate. Then too there would seem to be no bar to making appropriations for transportation and other expenses of children attending public or other secular schools, after hours in separate places and classes for their exclusively religious instruction. The person who embraces no creed also would be forced to pay for teaching what he does not believe. Again, it was the furnishing of "contributions of money for the propagation of opinions which he disbelieves" that the fathers outlawed. That consequence and effect are not removed by multiplying to all-inclusiveness the sects for which support is exacted. The Constitution requires, not comprehensive identification of state with religion, but complete separation. ***

Two great drives are constantly in motion to abridge, in the name of education, the complete division of religion and civil authority which our forefathers made. One is to introduce religious education and observances into the public schools. The other, to obtain public funds for the aid and support of various private religious schools. *** In my opinion both avenues were closed by the Constitution. Neither should be opened by this Court. ***

NOTE ON THE *EVERSON* OPINIONS

In *Everson,* all nine Justices appear to concur in Justice Black's general explication of the first amendment and its full applicability to the states, in keeping with his understanding of the Madison-Jefferson view:

> The "establishment of religion" clause of the First Amendment means at least this: Neither a state nor the Federal Government can set up a church. Neither can pass laws which *aid one religion, aid all religions, or prefer one religion over another*. Neither can force nor influence a person to go to or to remain away from church against his will or force him to profess a belief or disbelief in any religion. No person can be punished for entertaining or professing religious beliefs or disbeliefs, for church attendance or non-attendance. *No tax in any amount, large or small, can be levied to support any religious activities or institutions, whatever they may be called, or whatever form they may adopt to teach or practice religion.* Neither a state nor the Federal Government can, openly or secretly, participate in the affairs of any religious organizations or groups and vice versa. In the words of Jefferson, the clause against establishment of religion by law was intended to "erect a wall of separation between church and State."

Given its unanimous agreement on this meaning of the "no establishment" clause, why (i.e. on what basis) does the Court nonetheless divide, five-to-four? More specifically:

1. In light of the italicized portions of the paragraph from Justice Black's opinion, how does he nonetheless conclude that no tax herein involved provides support for any "religious institution?" (The parochial schools are surely religious institutions, are they not?)
   (i) Had the buses used for the parochial school students been owned and operated by those schools, with payment to the parents to reimburse them for such fares as the parochial school children might be required to pay to ride the parochial school buses (though not in excess of such fares as the regular buses might charge public school riders), would the result have been the same? What difference, if any, would there be?
   (ii) Had the parochial schools operated their own buses to insure the safe transport of parochial school children to travel to and from those schools at the beginning and close of each school day, with Ewing Township agreeing by contract to reimburse the schools for the cost of defraying such means of transportation, what difference then, if any?

2. What distinction, if any, underlies Justice Jackson's agreement that furnishing police protection inclusive of children en route to parochial school, or fire protection inclusive of churches and parochial schools, presents no issue under the establishment clause? How does he characterize the actual reimbursement plan adopted by the Township Board of Education? What is Justice Black's

treatment of that complaint?

3. The Court does not particularly note the extent to which the tax revenues used to support the reimbursement plan were contributed equally by those with children enrolled in parochial school. Assuming (as the Court appears to) that they are fully included in the tax base, is it arguable that failure to include them in the bus fare reimbursement plan would be invalid, either as a denial of equal protection or as a violation of the "free exercise" clause? All nine members of the Court appear to agree that no such question would arise. Do you agree? Why or why not?

Responding to *Everson* and other cases treated by the Supreme Court under the church-state clauses of the first amendment, Professor Philip Kurland proposed the following synthesis of the two clauses in 1961:[1]

> [T]he thesis proposed here as the proper construction of the religion clause of the first amendment is that the freedom and separation clauses should be read as a single precept that government cannot utilize religion as a standard for action or inaction because these clauses prohibit classification in terms of religion either to confer a benefit or to impose a burden.

1. Is *Everson* consistent with this view?
2. What kinds of laws or practices might not be valid if this view were to be followed?[2]

In a recent discussion of Professor Kurland's proposal ("religion blindness"), Professor Jesse Choper argues that while it eliminates the need to define "religion," it suffers from two significant drawbacks. First, he says, it "produces results hostile to religious liberty without serving nonestablishment values." In other words, it would prohibit *any* religious exemptions from general regulations. Second, it "permits forms of aid that subvert historical and contemporary aims of the Establishment Clause." That is, churches and synagogues would be entitled to precisely the same disbursements of general tax funds as other private voluntary organizations (e.g., if a state used tax funds to support buildings for the United Way, the Kurland proposal would require the same disbursements to religious organizations).

Professor Choper proposes a different solution:

---

1. Philip Kurland, Religion and the Law 18 (1961); Philip Kurland, The Irrelevance of the Constitution: The Religion Clauses of the First Amendment and the Supreme Court, 24 Vill.L.Rev. 3, 24 (1978).

2. E.g., state laws requiring businesses generally to close on Sundays? Draft laws providing for exemption from combatant training and service for those with conscientious objections? State or local laws providing tax exempt status for religiously-held property? Internal Revenue Code provisions providing for tax exempt status of income to churches, and tax deduction treatment of charitable contributions to religious organizations? Excusal from public school attendance of children to attend released time classes in religious instruction?

"I believe that the Constitution calls for religion to be treated *specifically*, and that this means more than that religion must be treated *equally* ***. I believe that under the Free Exercise Clause religion must sometimes be afforded special privilege ('preferred' is not an inaccurate term), and that under the Establishment Clause religion must sometimes be subject to special limits ('disfavored' is not an unfair term). Unfortunately, these principles will generate a tension between the two Religion Clauses that the neutrality approach commendably avoids. But *** resolving the conflict is not an insuperable task. Finally, I agree that our constitutional tradition (and government system) would be well served by moving in the direction of equal treatment of political and religious ideologies."[3]

Do the subsequent cases appear to fulfill Professor Kurland's suggestion, or do they seem more in keeping with Professor Choper's proposal? Or with neither?

ILLINOIS EX REL. MCCOLLUM v. BOARD OF EDUCATION OF SCHOOL DISTRICT NO. 71, CHAMPAIGN COUNTY, ILLINOIS

333 U.S. 203 (1948)

MR. JUSTICE BLACK delivered the opinion of the Court.

This case relates to the power of a state to utilize its tax-supported public school system in aid of religious instruction insofar as that power may be restricted by the First and Fourteenth Amendments to the Federal Constitution.

*** Vashti McCollum began this action for mandamus against the Champaign Board of Education in the Circuit Court of Champaign County, Illinois. Her asserted interest was that of a resident and taxpayer of Champaign and of a parent whose child was then enrolled in the Champaign public schools. Illinois has a compulsory education law which *** requires parents to send their children, aged seven to sixteen, to its tax-supported public schools where the children are to remain in attendance during the hours when the schools are regularly in session. Parents who violate this law commit a misdemeanor punishable by fine unless the children attend private or parochial schools which meet educational standards fixed by the State. ***

Appellant's petition for mandamus alleged that religious teachers, employed by private religious groups, were permitted to come weekly into the school buildings during the regular hours set apart for secular teaching, and then and there for a period of thirty minutes substitute their religious teaching for the secular education provided under the compulsory education law. The petitioner charged that this joint public-school religious-group program violated the First and Fourteenth Amend-

3. See Jesse H. Choper, Securing Religious Liberty: Principles for Judicial Interpretation of the Religion Clauses 19-24 (1995).

ments to the United States Constitution. The prayer of her petition was that the Board of Education be ordered to "adopt and enforce rules and regulations prohibiting all instruction in and teaching of religious education in all public schools in Champaign School District Number 71, *** and in all public school houses and buildings in said district when occupied by public schools." ***

Although there are disputes between the parties as to various inferences that may or may not properly be drawn from the evidence concerning the religious program, the following facts are shown by the record without dispute. In 1940 interested members of the Jewish, Roman Catholic, and a few of the Protestant faiths formed a voluntary association called the Champaign Council on Religious Education. They obtained permission from the Board of Education to offer classes in religious instruction to public school pupils in grades four to nine inclusive. Classes were made up of pupils whose parents signed printed cards requesting that their children be permitted to attend; they were held weekly, thirty minutes for the lower grades, forty-five minutes for the higher. The council employed the religious teachers at no expense to the school authorities, but the instructors were subject to the approval and supervision of the superintendent of schools. The classes were taught in three separate religious groups by Protestant teachers, Catholic priests, and a Jewish rabbi, although for the past several years there have apparently been no classes instructed in the Jewish religion. Classes were conducted in the regular classrooms of the school building. Students who did not choose to take the religious instruction were not released from public school duties; they were required to leave their classrooms and go to some other place in the school building for pursuit of their secular studies. On the other hand, students who were released from secular study for the religious instructions were required to be present at the religious classes. Reports of their presence or absence were to be made to their secular teachers.

The foregoing facts *** show the use of tax-supported property for religious instruction and the close cooperation between the school authorities and the religious council in promoting religious education. The operation of the State's compulsory education system thus assists and is integrated with the program of religious instruction carried on by separate religious sects. Pupils compelled by law to go to school for secular education are released in part from their legal duty upon the condition that they attend the religious classes. This is beyond all question a utilization of the tax-established and tax-supported public school system to aid religious groups to spread their faith. And it falls squarely under the ban of the First Amendment (made applicable to the States by the Fourteenth) as we interpreted it in Everson v. Board of Education, 330 U.S. 1. ***

Here not only are the State's tax-supported public school buildings used for the dissemination of religious doctrines. The State also affords sectarian groups an invaluable aid in that it helps to provide pupils for their religious classes through use of the State's compulsory public school machinery. This is not separation of Church and State.

The cause is reversed and remanded to the State Supreme Court for proceedings not inconsistent with this opinion.

MR. JUSTICE FRANKFURTER delivered the following opinion, in which MR. JUSTICE JACKSON, MR. JUSTICE RUTLEDGE and MR. JUSTICE BURTON join.

* * *

We do not consider, as indeed we could not, school programs not before us which, though colloquially characterized as "released time," present situations differing in aspects that may well be constitutionally crucial. Different forms which "released time" has taken during more than thirty years of growth include programs which, like that before us, could not withstand the test of the Constitution; others may be found unexceptionable. We do not now attempt to weigh in the Constitutional scale every separate detail or various combination of factors which may establish a valid "released time" program. We find that the basic Constitutional principle of absolute Separation was violated when the State of Illinois, speaking through its Supreme Court, sustained the school authorities of Champaign in sponsoring and effectively furthering religious beliefs by its educational arrangement. ***

MR. JUSTICE JACKSON, concurring. [Omitted.]

MR. JUSTICE REED, dissenting.

*** I find it difficult to extract from the opinions any conclusion as to what it is in the Champaign plan that is unconstitutional. Is it the use of school buildings for religious instruction; the release of pupils by the schools for religious instruction during school hours; the so-called assistance by teachers in handing out the request cards to pupils, in keeping lists of them for release and records of their attendance; or the action of the principals in arranging an opportunity for the classes and the appearance of the Council's instructors? None of the reversing opinions say whether the purpose of the Champaign plan for religious instruction during school hours is unconstitutional or whether it is some ingredient used in or omitted from the formula that makes the plan unconstitutional. ***

Mr. Jefferson, as one of the founders of the University of Virginia, a school which from its establishment in 1819 has been wholly governed, managed and controlled by the State of Virginia, was faced with the same problem that is before this Court today: the question of the constitutional limitation upon religious education in public schools. In his annual report as Rector, to the President and Directors of the Literary Fund, dated October 7, 1822, approved by the Visitors of the University of whom Mr. Madison was one, Mr. Jefferson set forth his views at some length. These suggestions of Mr. Jefferson were adopted and ch. II, § 1, of the Regulations of the University of October 4, 1824, provided that:

> "Should the religious sects of this State, or any of them, according to the invitation held out to them, establish within, or adjacent to, the precincts of the University, schools for instruction in the religion of their sect, the students of

the University will be free, and expected to attend religious worship at the establishment of their respective sects, in the morning, and in time to meet their school in the University at its stated hour."

Thus, the "wall of separation between church and State" that Mr. Jefferson built at the University which he founded did not exclude religious education from that school. The difference between the generality of his statements on the separation of church and state and the specificity of his conclusions on education are considerable. A rule of law should not be drawn from a figure of speech. ***

*** Devotion to the great principle of religious liberty should not lead us into a rigid interpretation of the constitutional guarantee that conflicts with accepted habits of our people. This is an instance where, for me, the history of past practices is determinative of the meaning of a constitutional clause, not a decorous introduction to the study of its text. The judgment should be affirmed.*

ZORACH v. CLAUSON

343 U.S. 306 (1952)

MR. JUSTICE DOUGLAS delivered the opinion of the Court.

New York City has a program which permits its public schools to release students during the school day so that they may leave the school buildings and school grounds and go to religious centers for religious instruction or devotional exercises. A student is released on written request of his parents. Those not released stay in the classrooms. The churches make weekly reports to the schools, sending a list of children who have been released from public school but who have not reported for religious instruction.

This "released time" program involves neither religious instruction in public school classrooms nor the expenditure of public funds. All costs, including the application blanks, are paid by the religious organizations. The case is therefore unlike McCollum v. Board of Education, 333 U.S. 203, which involved a "released time" program from Illinois. In that case the classrooms were turned over to religious instructors. We accordingly held that the program violated the First Amendment which (by reason of the Fourteenth Amendment) prohibits the states from establishing religion or prohibiting its free exercise.

---

*. **[Ed. Note**: Suppose the arrangement in McCollum held to be prohibited by the establishment clause was modified in the two following respects: (a) the classrooms were made available for outside groups only before or after regularly scheduled classes were not in session; (b) such outside groups were not limited to religious groups. *See Good News* (etc. *held*, 5/4, the establishment clause does not itself forbid such an accommodation; moreover, the "viewpoint neutrality" requirement of the freedom of speech clause forbids the state thus to permit other nonprofit groups the after-hours use of such classrooms while not permitting their use by religious groups.)

Appellants, who are taxpayers and residents of New York City and whose children attend its public schools, challenge the present law, contending it is in essence not different from the one involved in the *McCollum* case. Their argument *** reduces itself to this: the weight and influence of the school is put behind a program for religious instruction; public school teachers police it, keeping tab on students who are released; the classroom activities come to a halt while the students who are released for religious instruction are on leave; the school is a crutch on which the churches are leaning for support in their religious training; without the cooperation of the schools this "released time" program, like the one in the *McCollum* case, would be futile and ineffective. The New York Court of Appeals sustained the law against this claim of unconstitutionality. The case is here on appeal. ***

There is a suggestion that the system involves the use of coercion to get public school students into religious classrooms. There is no evidence in the record before us that supports that conclusion.[6] The present record indeed tells us that the school authorities are neutral in this regard and do no more than release students whose parents so request. If in fact coercion were used, if it were established that any one or more teachers were using their office to persuade or force students to take the religious instruction, a wholly different case would be presented. Hence we put aside that claim of coercion both as respects the "free exercise" of religion and "an establishment of religion" within the meaning of the First Amendment.

Moreover, apart from that claim of coercion, we do not see how New York by this type of "released time" program has made a law respecting an establishment of religion within the meaning of the First Amendment. ***

We are a religious people whose institutions presuppose a Supreme Being. We guarantee the freedom to worship as one chooses. We make room for as wide a variety of beliefs and creeds as the spiritual needs of man deem necessary. We sponsor an attitude on the part of government that shows no partiality to any one group and that lets each flourish according to the zeal of its adherents and the appeal of its dogma. When the state encourages religious instruction or cooperates with religious authorities by adjusting the schedule of public events to sectarian needs, it follows the best of our traditions. For it then respects the religious nature of our people and accommodates the public service to their spiritual needs. To hold that it may not would be to find in the Constitution a requirement that the government show a callous indifference to religious groups. That would be preferring those who believe in no religion over those who do believe. Government may not finance religious groups nor undertake religious instruction nor blend secular and sectarian education nor use secular institutions to force one or some religion on any person. But we find no constitutional requirement which makes it necessary for government to be hostile to religion and to throw its weight against efforts to widen the effective

---

6. Nor is there any indication that the public schools enforce attendance at religious schools by punishing absentees from the released time programs for truancy.

scope of religious influence. The government must be neutral when it comes to competition between sects. It may not thrust any sect on any person. It may not make a religious observance compulsory. It may not coerce anyone to attend church, to observe a religious holiday, or to take religious instruction. But it can close its doors or suspend its operations as to those who want to repair to their religious sanctuary for worship or instruction. No more than that is undertaken here. ***

MR. JUSTICE BLACK, dissenting.

***

I see no significant difference between the invalid Illinois system and that of New York here sustained. *** Here the sole question is whether New York can use its compulsory education laws to help religious sects get attendants presumably too unenthusiastic to go unless moved to do so by the pressure of this state machinery. That this is the plan, purpose, design and consequence of the New York program cannot be denied. The state thus makes religious sects beneficiaries of its power to compel children to attend secular schools. *** New York is manipulating its compulsory education laws to help religious sects get pupils. This is not separation but combination of Church and State. ***

MR. JUSTICE FRANKFURTER, dissenting.

By way of emphasizing my agreement with MR. JUSTICE JACKSON's dissent, I add a few words. *** There is all the difference in the world between letting the children out of school and letting some of them out of school into religious classes. If every one is free to make what use he will of time wholly unconnected from schooling required by law—those who wish sectarian instruction devoting it to that purpose, those who have ethical instruction at home, to that, those who study music, to that—then of course there is no conflict with the Fourteenth Amendment. The pith of the case is that formalized religious instruction is substituted for other school activity which those who do not participate in the released-time program are compelled to attend. ***

MR. JUSTICE JACKSON, dissenting.

This released time program is founded upon a use of the State's power of coercion, which, for me, determines its unconstitutionality. Stripped to its essentials, the plan has two stages: first, that the State compel each student to yield a large part of his time for public secular education; and, second, that some of it be "released" to him on condition that he devote it to sectarian religious purposes.

No one suggests that the Constitution would permit the State directly to require this "released" time to be spent "under the control of a duly constituted religious body." This program accomplishes that forbidden result by indirection. If public education were taking so much of the pupils' time as to injure the public or the students' welfare by encroaching upon their religious opportunity, simply shortening everyone's school day would facilitate voluntary and optional attendance at Church classes. But that suggestion is rejected upon the ground that if they are made free many students will not go to the Church. Hence, they must be deprived of freedom for this period, with Church attendance put to them as one of the two permissible ways of using it. *** Here schooling is more or less suspended during the "released time" so the nonreligious attendants will not forge ahead of the churchgoing absentees. But it serves as a temporary jail for a pupil who will not go to Church. It takes more subtlety of mind than I possess to deny that this is governmental constraint in support of religion. It is as unconstitutional, in my view, when exerted by indirection as when exercised forthrightly. ***

ENGEL v. VITALE

370 U.S. 421 (1962)

MR. JUSTICE BLACK delivered the opinion of the Court.

The respondent Board of Education of Union Free School District No. 9, New Hyde Park, New York, acting in its official capacity under state law, directed the School District's principal to cause the following prayer to be said aloud by each class in the presence of a teacher at the beginning of each school day:

> "Almighty God, we acknowledge our dependence upon Thee, and we beg Thy blessings upon us, our parents, our teachers and our Country."

This daily procedure was adopted on the recommendation of the State Board of Regents, a governmental agency created by the State Constitution to which the New York Legislature has granted broad supervisory, executive, and legislative powers over the State's public school system. These state officials composed the prayer which they recommended and published as a part of their "Statement on Moral and Spiritual Training in the Schools," saying: "We believe that this Statement will be subscribed to by all men and women of good will, and we call upon all of them to aid in giving life to our program."

*** The New York Court of Appeals, over the dissents of Judges Dye and Fuld, sustained an order of the lower state courts which had upheld the power of New York to use the Regents' prayer as a part of the daily procedures of its public schools so long as the schools did not compel any pupil to join in the prayer over his or his parents' objection. We granted certiorari to review this important decision involving rights protected by the First and Fourteenth Amendments.

We think that by using its public school system to encourage recitation of the Regents' prayer, the State of New York has adopted a practice wholly inconsistent with the Establishment Clause. There can, of course, be no doubt that New York's program of daily classroom invocation of God's blessings as prescribed in the Regents' prayer is a religious activity. It is a solemn avowal of divine faith and supplication for the blessings of the Almighty. ***

The petitioners contend among other things that the state laws requiring or permitting use of the Regents' prayer must be struck down as a violation of the Establishment Clause because that prayer was composed by governmental officials as a part of a governmental program to further religious beliefs. For this reason, petitioners argue, the State's use of the Regents' prayer in its public school system breaches the constitutional wall of separation between Church and State. We agree with that contention since we think that the constitutional prohibition against laws respecting an establishment of religion must at least mean that in this country it is no part of the business of government to compose official prayers for any group of the American people to recite as a part of a religious program carried on by government.

It is a matter of history that this very practice of establishing governmentally composed prayers for religious services was one of the reasons which caused many of our early colonists to leave England and seek religious freedom in America. ***

It is an unfortunate fact of history that when some of the very groups which had most strenuously opposed the established Church of England found themselves sufficiently in control of colonial governments in this country to write their own prayers into law, they passed laws making their own religion the official religion of their respective colonies. *** But the successful Revolution against English political domination was shortly followed by intense opposition to the practice of establishing religion by law. This opposition crystallized rapidly into an effective political force in Virginia where the minority religious groups such as Presbyterians, Lutherans, Quakers and Baptists had gained such strength that the adherents to the established Episcopal Church were actually a minority themselves. In 1785-1786, those opposed to the established Church, led by James Madison and Thomas Jefferson, who, though themselves not members of any of these dissenting religious groups, opposed all religious establishments by law on grounds of principle, obtained the enactment of the famous "Virginia Bill for Religious Liberty" by which all religious groups were placed on an equal footing so far as the State was concerned. ***

*** The First Amendment was added to the Constitution to stand as a guarantee that neither the power nor the prestige of the Federal Government would be used to control, support or influence the kinds of prayer the American people can say—that the people's religions must not be subjected to the pressures of government for change each time a new political administration is elected to office. Under that Amendment's prohibition against governmental establishment of religion, as reinforced by the provisions of the Fourteenth Amendment, government in this country, be it state or federal, is without power to prescribe by law any particular form of prayer which is to be used as an official prayer in carrying on any program of governmentally sponsored religious activity.

There can be no doubt that New York's state prayer program officially establishes the religious beliefs embodied in the Regents' prayer. The respondents' argument to the contrary, which is largely based upon the contention that the Regents' prayer is "non-denominational" and the fact that the program, as modified and approved by state courts, does not require all pupils to recite the prayer but permits those who wish to do so to remain silent or be excused from the room, ignores the essential nature of the program's constitutional defects. Neither the fact that the prayer may be denominationally neutral nor the fact that its observance on the part of the students is voluntary can serve to free it from the limitations of the Establishment Clause, as it might from the Free Exercise Clause, of the First Amendment, both of which are operative against the States by virtue of the Fourteenth Amendment. Although these two clauses may in certain instances overlap, they forbid two quite different kinds of governmental encroachment upon religious freedom. The Establishment Clause, unlike the Free Exercise Clause, does not depend upon any showing of direct governmental compulsion and is violated by the enactment of laws which establish an official religion whether those laws operate directly to coerce nonobserving individuals or not. This is not to say, of course, that laws officially prescribing a particular form of religious worship do not involve coercion of such individuals. When the power, prestige and financial support of government is placed behind a particular religious belief, the indirect coercive pressure upon religious minorities to conform to the prevailing officially approved religion is plain. But the purposes underlying the Establishment Clause go much further than that. Its first and most immediate purpose rested on the belief that a union of government and religion tends to destroy government and to degrade religion. The history of governmentally established religion, both in England and in this country, showed that whenever government had allied itself with one particular form of religion, the inevitable result had been that it had incurred the hatred, disrespect and even contempt of those who held contrary beliefs. That same history showed that many people had lost their respect for any religion that had relied upon the support of government to spread its faith. The Establishment Clause thus stands as an expression of principle on the part of the Founders of our Constitution that religion is too personal, too sacred, too holy, to permit its "unhallowed perversion" by a civil magistrate.[15] ***

The judgment of the Court of Appeals of New York is reversed and the cause remanded for further proceedings not inconsistent with this opinion.

MR. JUSTICE FRANKFURTER took no part in the decision of this case.

MR. JUSTICE WHITE took no part in the consideration or decision of this case.

MR. JUSTICE DOUGLAS, concurring.

It is customary in deciding a constitutional question to treat it in its narrowest form. Yet at times the setting of the question gives it a form and content which no abstract treatment could give. The point for decision is whether the Government can constitutionally finance a religious exercise. Our system at the federal and state

---

15. Memorial and Remonstrance against Religious Assessments, II Writings of Madison, at 187.

levels is presently honeycombed with such financing. Nevertheless, I think it is an unconstitutional undertaking whatever form it takes. ***

Plainly, our Bill of Rights would not permit a State or the Federal Government to adopt an official prayer and penalize anyone who would not utter it. This, however, is not that case, for there is no element of compulsion or coercion in New York's regulation requiring that public schools be opened each day with the following prayer:

> Almighty God, we acknowledge our dependence upon Thee, and we beg Thy blessings upon us, our parents, our teachers and our Country.

*** No student, however, is compelled to take part. The respondents have adopted a regulation which provides that "Neither teachers nor any school authority shall comment on participation or non-participation *** nor suggest or request that any posture or language be used or dress be worn or be not used or not worn." Provision is also made for excusing children, upon written request of a parent or guardian, from the saying of the prayer or from the room in which the prayer is said. A letter implementing and explaining this regulation has been sent to each taxpayer and parent in the school district. As I read this regulation, a child is free to stand or not stand, to recite or not recite, without fear of reprisal or even comment by the teacher or any other school official. In short, the only one who need utter the prayer is the teacher; and no teacher is complaining of it. ***

The question presented by this case is therefore an extremely narrow one. It is whether New York oversteps the bounds when it finances a religious exercise.

What New York does on the opening of its public schools is what we do when we open court. Our Crier has from the beginning announced the convening of the Court and then added "God save the United States and this Honorable Court." That utterance is a supplication, a prayer in which we, the judges, are free to join, but which we need not recite any more than the students need recite the New York prayer.

What New York does on the opening of its public schools is what each House of Congress does at the opening of each day's business. Reverend Frederick B. Harris is Chaplain of the Senate; Reverend Bernard Braskamp is Chaplain of the House. Guest chaplains of various denominations also officiate.

In New York the teacher who leads in prayer is on the public payroll; and the time she takes seems minuscule as compared with the salaries appropriated by state legislatures and Congress for chaplains to conduct prayers in the legislative halls. Only a bare fraction of the teacher's time is given to reciting this short 22-word prayer, about the same amount of time that our Crier spends announcing the opening of our sessions and offering a prayer for this Court. Yet for me the principle is the same, no matter how briefly the prayer is said, for in each of the instances given the person praying is a public official on the public payroll, performing a religious exercise in a governmental institution.[6] ***

MR. JUSTICE STEWART, dissenting.

A local school board in New York has provided that those pupils who wish to do so may join in a brief prayer at the beginning of each school day, acknowledging their dependence upon God and asking His blessing upon them and upon their parents, their teachers, and their country. The Court today decides that in permitting this brief nondenominational prayer the school board has violated the Constitution of the United States. I think this decision is wrong. ***

With all respect, I think the Court has misapplied a great constitutional principle. I cannot see how an "official religion" is established by letting those who want to say a prayer say it. On the contrary, I think that to deny the wish of these school children to join in reciting this prayer is to deny them the opportunity of sharing in the spiritual heritage of our Nation. ***

At the opening of each day's Session of this Court we stand, while one of our officials invokes the protection of God. Since the days of John Marshall our Crier has said, "God save the United States and this Honorable Court." Both the Senate and the House of Representatives open their daily Sessions with prayer. Each of our Presidents, from George Washington to John F. Kennedy, has upon assuming his Office asked the protection and help of God.

*** In 1954 Congress added a phrase to the Pledge of Allegiance to the Flag so that it now contains the words "one Nation *under God*, indivisible, with liberty and justice for all." In 1952 Congress enacted legislation calling upon the President each year to proclaim a National Day of Prayer. Since 1865 the words "IN GOD WE TRUST" have been impressed on our coins.

Countless similar examples could be listed, but there is no need to belabor the obvious.[9] It was all summed up by this Court just ten years ago in a single sentence: "We are a religious people whose institutions presuppose a Supreme Being." Zorach v. Clauson, 343 U.S. 306, 313.

I do not believe that this Court, or the Congress, or the President has by the actions and practices I have mentioned established an "official religion" in violation

---

6. The fact that taxpayers do not have standing in the federal courts to raise the issue (Frothingham v. Mellon, 262 U.S. 447) is of course no justification for drawing a line between what is done in New York on the one hand and on the other what we do and what Congress does in this matter of prayer.

9. I am at a loss to understand the Court's unsupported *ipse dixit* that these official expressions of religious faith in and reliance upon a Supreme Being "bear no true resemblance to the unquestioned religious exercise that the State of New York has sponsored in this instance." *** I can hardly think that the Court means to say that the First Amendment imposes a lesser restriction upon the Federal Government than does the Fourteenth Amendment upon the States. Or is the Court suggesting that the Constitution permits judges and Congressmen and Presidents to join in prayer, but prohibits school children from doing so?

of the Constitution. And I do not believe the State of New York has done so in this case. What each has done has been to recognize and to follow the deeply entrenched and highly cherished spiritual traditions of our Nation—traditions which come down to us from those who almost two hundred years ago avowed their "firm Reliance on the Protection of divine Providence" when they proclaimed the freedom and independence of this brave new world.

I dissent.

B. THE GENERAL TEST REFINED

ABINGTON SCHOOL DISTRICT v. SCHEMPP
374 U.S. 203 (1963)*

MR. JUSTICE CLARK delivered the opinion of the Court.

Once again we are called upon to consider the scope of the provision of the First Amendment to the United States Constitution which declares that "Congress shall make no law respecting an establishment of religion, or prohibiting the free exercise thereof. ***" These companion cases present the issues in the context of state action requiring that schools begin each day with readings from the Bible. ***

The Commonwealth of Pennsylvania by law requires that "At least ten verses from the Holy Bible shall be read, without comment, at the opening of each public school on each school day. Any child shall be excused from such Bible reading, or attending such Bible reading, upon the written request of his parent or guardian." ***

On each school day at the Abington Senior High School between 8:15 and 8:30 a.m., while the pupils are attending their home rooms or advisory sections, opening exercises are conducted pursuant to the statute. The exercises are broadcast into each room in the school building through an intercommunications system and are conducted under the supervision of a teacher by students attending the school's radio and television workshop. Selected students from this course gather each morning in the school's workshop studio for the exercises, which include readings by one of the students of 10 verses of the Holy Bible, broadcast to each room in the building. This is followed by the recitation of the Lord's Prayer, likewise over the intercommunications system, but also by the students in the various classrooms, who are asked to stand and join in repeating the prayer in unison. The exercises are closed with the flag salute and such pertinent announcements as are of interest to the students. Participation in the opening exercises, as directed by the statute, is voluntary. The student reading the verses from the Bible may select the passages and read from any version he chooses, although the only copies furnished by the school are

---

*. **[Ed. Note.** Two cases were consolidated for review by the Court. Only the facts of No. 142, *Abington*, are reproduced here.]

the King James version, copies of which were circulated to each teacher by the school district. During the period in which the exercises have been conducted the King James, the Douay and the Revised Standard versions of the Bible have been used, as well as the Jewish Holy Scriptures. There are no prefatory statements, no questions asked or solicited, no comments or explanations made and no interpretations given at or during the exercises. The students and parents are advised that the student may absent himself from the classroom or, should he elect to remain, not participate in the exercises.

It appears from the record that in schools not having an intercommunications system the Bible reading and the recitation of the Lord's Prayer were conducted by the home-room teacher,[2] who chose the text of the verses and read them herself or had students read them in rotation or by volunteers. This was followed by a standing recitation of the Lord's Prayer, together with the Pledge of Allegiance to the Flag by the class in unison and a closing announcement of routine school items of interest.

At the first trial Edward Schempp and the children testified as to specific religious doctrines purveyed by a literal reading of the Bible "which were contrary to the religious beliefs which they held and to their familial teaching." *** Edward Schempp testified at the second trial that he had considered having Roger and Donna excused from attendance at the exercises but decided against it for several reasons, including his belief that the children's relationships with their teachers and classmates would be adversely affected. ***

The trial court, in striking down the practices and the statute requiring them, made specific findings of fact that the children's attendance at Abington Senior High School is compulsory and that the practice of reading 10 verses from the Bible is also compelled by law. It also found that:

> "The reading of the verses, even without comment, possesses a devotional and religious character and constitutes in effect a religious observance. The devotional and religious nature of the morning exercises is made all the more apparent by the fact that the Bible reading is followed immediately by a recital in unison by the pupils of the Lord's Prayer. The fact that some pupils, or theoretically all pupils, might be excused from attendance at the exercises does not mitigate the obligatory nature of the ceremony for Section 1516 unequivocally requires the exercises to be held every school day in every school in the Commonwealth. The exercises are held in the school buildings and perforce are conducted by and under the authority of the local school authorities and during school sessions. Since the statute requires the reading of the 'Holy Bible,' a Christian document, the practice prefers the Christian religion. ***

---

2. The statute as amended imposes no penalty upon a teacher refusing to obey its mandate. However, it remains to be seen whether one refusing could have his contract of employment terminated for "wilful violation of the school laws." 24 Pa.Stat. (Supp. 1960) § 11-1122.

The wholesome "neutrality" of which this Court's cases speak *** stems from a recognition of the teachings of history that powerful sects or groups might bring about a fusion of governmental and religious functions or a concert or dependency of one upon the other to the end that official support of the State or Federal Government would be placed behind the tenets of one or of all orthodoxies. This the Establishment Clause prohibits. And a further reason for neutrality is found in the Free Exercise Clause, which recognizes the value of religious training, teaching and observance and, more particularly, the right of every person to freely choose his own course with reference thereto, free of any compulsion from the state. This the Free Exercise Clause guarantees. Thus, as we have seen, the two clauses may overlap. As we have indicated, the Establishment Clause has been directly considered by this Court eight times in the past score of years and, with only one Justice dissenting on the point, it has consistently held that the clause withdrew all legislative power respecting religious belief or the expression thereof. The test may be stated as follows: what are the purpose and the primary effect of the enactment? If either is the advancement or inhibition of religion then the enactment exceeds the scope of legislative power as circumscribed by the Constitution. That is to say that to withstand the strictures of the Establishment Clause there must be a secular legislative purpose and a primary effect that neither advances nor inhibits religion. *** [I]t is necessary in a free exercise case for one to show the coercive effect of the enactment as it operates against him in the practice of his religion. The distinction between the two clauses is apparent—a violation of the Free Exercise Clause is predicated on coercion while the Establishment Clause violation need not be so attended.

Applying the Establishment Clause principles to the cases at bar we find that the States are requiring the selection and reading at the opening of the school day of verses from the Holy Bible and the recitation of the Lord's Prayer by the students in unison. These exercises are prescribed as part of the curricular activities of students who are required by law to attend school. They are held in the school buildings under the supervision and with the participation of teachers employed in those schools. None of these factors, other than compulsory school attendance, was present in the program upheld in *Zorach v. Clauson*. The trial court in No. 142 has found that such an opening exercise is a religious ceremony and was intended by the State to be so. We agree with the trial court's finding as to the religious character of the exercises. Given that finding, the exercises and the law requiring them are in violation of the Establishment Clause.

There is no such specific finding as to the religious character of the exercises in No. 119, and the State contends (as does the State in No. 142) that the program is an effort to extend its benefits to all public school children without regard to their religious belief. Included within its secular purposes, it says, are the promotion of moral values, the contradiction to the materialistic trends of our times, the perpetuation of our institutions and the teaching of literature. The case came up on demurrer, of course, to a petition which alleged that the uniform practice under the rule had been to read from the King James version of the Bible and that the exercise was sectarian. The short answer, therefore, is that the religious character of the exercise was admitted by the State. But even if its purpose is not strictly religious, it is sought to be accomplished through readings, without comment, from the Bible. Surely the place of the Bible as an instrument of religion cannot be gainsaid, and the State's recognition of the pervading religious character of the ceremony is evident from the rule's specific permission of the alternative use of the Catholic Douay version as well as the recent amendment permitting nonattendance at the exercises. None of these factors is consistent with the contention that the Bible is here used either as an instrument for nonreligious moral inspiration or as a reference for the teaching of secular subjects.

The conclusion follows that in both cases the laws require religious exercises and such exercises are being conducted in direct violation of the rights of the appellees and petitioners.[9] Nor are these required exercises mitigated by the fact that individual students may absent themselves upon parental request, for that fact furnishes no defense to a claim of unconstitutionality under the Establishment Clause. See *Engel v. Vitale*, [370 U.S.], at 430. Further, it is no defense to urge that the religious practices here may be relatively minor encroachments on the First Amendment. The breach of neutrality that is today a trickling stream may all too soon become a raging torrent and, in the words of Madison, "it is proper to take alarm at the first experiment on our liberties." ***

It is insisted that unless these religious exercises are permitted a "religion of secularism" is established in the schools. We agree of course that the State may not establish a "religion of secularism" in the sense of affirmatively opposing or showing hostility to religion, thus "preferring those who believe in no religion over those who do believe." *Zorach v. Clauson*, [343 U.S.], at 314. We do not agree, however, that this decision in any sense has that effect. In addition, it might well be said that one's education is not complete without a study of comparative religion or the history of religion and its relationship to the advancement of civilization. It certainly may be said that the Bible is worthy of study for its literary and historic qualities. Nothing we have said here indicates that such study of the Bible or of religion, when presented objectively as part of a secular program of education, may not be effected consistently with the First Amendment. But the exercises here do not fall into those categories. They are religious exercises, required by the States in violation of the command of the First Amendment that the Government maintain strict neutrality, neither aiding nor opposing religion. ***

*** Applying that rule to the facts of these cases, we affirm the judgment in No.

---

9. It goes without saying that the laws and practices involved here can be challenged only by persons having standing to complain. But the requirements for standing to challenge state action under the Establishment Clause, unlike those relating to the Free Exercise Clause, do not include proof that particular religious freedoms are infringed.

142. In No. 119, the judgment is reversed and the cause remanded to the Maryland Court of Appeals for further proceedings consistent with this opinion.*

MR. JUSTICE DOUGLAS, concurring.

I join the opinion of the Court and add a few words in explanation.

While the Free Exercise Clause of the First Amendment is written in terms of what the State may not require of the individual, the Establishment Clause, serving the same goal of individual religious freedom, is written in different terms.

Establishment of a religion can be achieved in several ways. The church and state can be one; the church may control the state or the state may control the church; or the relationship may take one of several possible forms of a working arrangement between the two bodies. Under all of these arrangements the church typically has a place in the state's budget, and church law usually governs such matters as baptism, marriage, divorce and separation, at least for its members and sometimes for the entire body politic. Education, too, is usually high on the priority list of church interests. In the past schools were often made the exclusive responsibility of the church. Today in some state-church countries the state runs the public schools, but compulsory religious exercises are often required of some or all students. Thus, under the agreement Franco made with the Holy See when he came to power in Spain, "The Church regained its place in the national budget. It insists on baptizing all children and has made the catechism obligatory in state schools."

The vice of all such arrangements under the Establishment Clause is that the state is lending its assistance to a church's efforts to gain and keep adherents. Under the First Amendment it is strictly a matter for the individual and his church as to what church he will belong to and how much support, in the way of belief, time, activity or money, he will give to it. ***

These regimes violate the Establishment Clause in two different ways. In each case the State is conducting a religious exercise; and, as the Court holds, that cannot be done without violating the "neutrality" required of the State by the balance of power between individual, church and state that has been struck by the First Amendment. But the Establishment Clause is not limited to precluding the State itself from conducting religious exercises. It also forbids the State to employ its facilities or funds in a way that gives any church, or all churches, greater strength in our society than it would have by relying on its members alone. Thus, the present regimes must fall under that clause for the additional reason that public funds, though small in

---

*. **[Ed. Note.** In 1992, the Supreme Court also held it to be inconsistent with the establishment clause for a state legislature to authorize public school principals to provide a religious invocation and benediction as a formal part of the public school graduation exercises. Lee v. Weisman,505 U.S. 577 (1992). But the case (included *infra* at p. 971) is best not considered here for class discussion. Rather, because *Lee v. Weisman* followed two decades of further doctrinal developments after *Schempp*, it is more appropriate to assess its significance after completing the remaining cases and materials in this section.]

amount, are being used to promote a religious exercise. Through the mechanism of the State, all of the people are being required to finance a religious exercise that only some of the people want and that violates the sensibilities of others. ***

Such contributions may not be made by the State even in a minor degree without violating the Establishment Clause. It is not the amount of public funds expended; as this case illustrates, it is the use to which public funds are put that is controlling. For the First Amendment does not say that some forms of establishment are allowed; it says that "no law respecting an establishment of religion" shall be made. What may not be done directly may not be done indirectly lest the Establishment Clause become a mockery.

MR. JUSTICE BRENNAN, concurring.

* * *

When John Locke ventured in 1689, "I esteem it above all things necessary to distinguish exactly the business of civil government from that of religion and to settle the just bounds that lie between the one and the other," he anticipated the necessity which would be thought by the Framers to require adoption of a First Amendment, but not the difficulty that would be experienced in defining those "just bounds." The fact is that the line which separates the secular from the sectarian in American life is elusive. The difficulty of defining the boundary with precision inheres in a paradox central to our scheme of liberty. While our institutions reflect a firm conviction that we are a religious people, those institutions by solemn constitutional injunction may not officially involve religion in such a way as to prefer, discriminate against, or oppress, a particular sect or religion. Equally the Constitution enjoins those involvements of religious with secular institutions which (a) serve the essentially religious activities of religious institutions; (b) employ the organs of government for essentially religious purposes; or (c) use essentially religious means to serve governmental ends where secular means would suffice. ***

I join fully in the opinion and the judgment of the Court. I see no escape from the conclusion that the exercises called in question in these two cases violate the constitutional mandate. The reasons we gave only last Term in Engel v. Vitale, 370 U.S. 421, for finding in the New York Regents' prayer an impermissible establishment of religion, compel the same judgment of the practices at bar. The involvement of the secular with the religious is no less intimate here; and it is constitutionally irrelevant that the State has not composed the material for the inspirational exercises presently involved. *** While it is my view that not every involvement of religion in public life is unconstitutional, I consider the exercises at bar a form of involvement which clearly violates the Establishment Clause.

The importance of the issue and the deep conviction with which views on both sides are held seem to me to justify detailing at some length my reasons for joining the Court's judgment and opinion. [Omitted.]

MR. JUSTICE GOLDBERG, with whom MR. JUSTICE HARLAN joins, concurring.

* * *

The practices here involved do not fall within any sensible or acceptable concept of compelled or permitted accommodation and involve the state so significantly and directly in the realm of the sectarian as to give rise to those very divisive influences and inhibitions of freedom which both religion clauses of the First Amendment preclude. The state has ordained and has utilized its facilities to engage in unmistakably religious exercises—the devotional reading and recitation of the Holy Bible—in a manner having substantial and significant import and impact. That it has selected, rather than written, a particular devotional liturgy seems to me without constitutional import. The pervasive religiosity and direct governmental involvement inhering in the prescription of prayer and Bible reading in the public schools, during and as part of the curricular day, involving young impressionable children whose school attendance is statutorily compelled, and utilizing the prestige, power, and influence of school administration, staff, and authority, cannot realistically be termed simply accommodation, and must fall within the interdiction of the First Amendment. I find nothing in the opinion of the Court which says more than this. ***

MR. JUSTICE STEWART, dissenting. [Omitted.]

WALZ v. TAX COMMISSION OF THE CITY OF NEW YORK

397 U.S. 664 (1970)

MR. CHIEF JUSTICE BURGER delivered the opinion of the Court.

Appellant, owner of real estate in Richmond County, New York, sought an injunction in the New York courts to prevent the New York City Tax Commission from granting property tax exemptions to religious organizations for religious properties used solely for religious worship. The exemption from state taxes is authorized by Art. 16, § 1, of the New York Constitution, which provides in relevant part:

> "Exemptions from taxation may be granted only by general laws. Exemptions may be altered or repealed except those exempting real or personal property used exclusively for religious, educational or charitable purposes as defined by law and owned by any corporation or association organized or conducted exclusively for one or more of such purposes and not operating for profit."

The essence of appellant's contention was that the New York City Tax Commission's grant of an exemption to church property indirectly requires the appellant to make a contribution to religious bodies and thereby violates provisions prohibiting establishment of religion under the First Amendment which under the Fourteenth Amendment is binding on the States. ***

The Court has struggled to find a neutral course between the two Religion Clauses, both of which are cast in absolute terms, and either of which, if expanded to a logical extreme, would tend to clash with the other. ***

Each value judgment under the Religion Clauses must therefore turn on whether particular acts in question are intended to establish or interfere with religious beliefs and practices or have the effect of doing so. Adherence to the policy of neutrality that derives from an accommodation of the Establishment and Free Exercise Clauses has prevented the kind of involvement that would tip the balance toward government control of churches or governmental restraint on religious practice. ***

The legislative purpose of the property tax exemption is neither the advancement nor the inhibition of religion; it is neither sponsorship nor hostility. New York, in common with the other States, has determined that certain entities that exist in a harmonious relationship to the community at large, and that foster its "moral or mental improvement," should not be inhibited in their activities by property taxation or the hazard of loss of those properties for nonpayment of taxes. It has not singled out one particular church or religious group or even churches as such; rather, it has granted exemption to all houses of religious worship within a broad class of property owned by nonprofit, quasi-public corporations which include hospitals, libraries, playgrounds, scientific, professional, historical, and patriotic groups. The State has an affirmative policy that considers these groups as beneficial and stabilizing influences in community life and finds this classification useful, desirable, and in the public interest. Qualification for tax exemption is not perpetual or immutable; some tax-exempt groups lose that status when their activities take them outside the classification and new entities can come into being and qualify for exemption.

Governments have not always been tolerant of religious activity, and hostility toward religion has taken many shapes and forms—economic, political, and sometimes harshly oppressive. Grants of exemption historically reflect the concern of authors of constitutions and statutes as to the latent dangers inherent in the imposition of property taxes; exemption constitutes a reasonable and balanced attempt to guard against those dangers. The limits of permissible state accommodation to religion are by no means co-extensive with the noninterference mandated by the Free Exercise Clause. ***

We find it unnecessary to justify the tax exemption on the social welfare services or "good works" that some churches perform for parishioners and others— family counselling, aid to the elderly and the infirm, and to children. Churches vary substantially in the scope of such services; programs expand or contract according to resources and need. As public-sponsored programs enlarge, private aid from the church sector may diminish. The extent of social services may vary, depending on whether the church serves an urban or rural, a rich or poor constituency. To give emphasis to so variable an aspect of the work of religious bodies would introduce an element of governmental evaluation and standards as to the worth of particular social welfare programs, thus producing a kind of continuing day-to-day relationship which the policy of neutrality seeks to minimize. Hence, the use of a social welfare yardstick as a significant element to qualify for tax exemption could conceivably give rise to confrontations that could escalate to constitutional dimensions.

Determining that the legislative purpose of tax exemption is not aimed at establishing, sponsoring, or supporting religion does not end the inquiry, however. We must also be sure that the end result—the effect—is not an excessive government entanglement with religion. The test is inescapably one of degree. Either course, taxation of churches or exemption, occasions some degree of involvement with religion. Elimination of exemption would tend to expand the involvement of government by giving rise to tax valuation of church property, tax liens, tax foreclosures, and the direct confrontations and conflicts that follow in the train of those legal processes.

Granting tax exemptions to churches necessarily operates to afford an indirect economic benefit and also gives rise to some, but yet a lesser, involvement than taxing them. In analyzing either alternative the questions are whether the involvement is excessive, and whether it is a continuing one calling for official and continuing surveillance leading to an impermissible degree of entanglement. Obviously a direct money subsidy would be a relationship pregnant with involvement and, as with most governmental grant programs, could encompass sustained and detailed administrative relationships for enforcement of statutory or administrative standards, but that is not this case. The hazards of churches supporting government are hardly less in their potential than the hazards of government supporting churches;[3] each relationship carries some involvement rather than the desired insulation and separation. We cannot ignore the instances in history when church support of government led to the kind of involvement we seek to avoid.

The grant of a tax exemption is not sponsorship since the government does not transfer part of its revenue to churches but simply abstains from demanding that the church support the state. No one has ever suggested that tax exemption has converted libraries, art galleries, or hospitals into arms of the state or put employees "on the public payroll." There is no genuine nexus between tax exemption and establishment of religion. As Mr. Justice Holmes commented in a related context "a page of history is worth a volume of logic." New York Trust Co. v. Eisner, 256 U.S. 345, 349 (1921). The exemption creates only a minimal and remote involvement between church and state and far less than taxation of churches. It restricts the fiscal relationship between church and state, and tends to complement and reinforce the desired separation insulating each from the other.

***

All of the 50 States provide for tax exemption of places of worship, most of them doing so by constitutional guarantees. For so long as federal income taxes have had any potential impact on churches—over 75 years—religious organizations have been expressly exempt from the tax. Such treatment is an "aid" to churches no more

---

3. The support of religion with direct allocation of public revenue was a common colonial practice. See C. Antieau, A. Downey, & E. Roberts, Freedom from Federal Establishment cc. 1 and 2 (1964). A general assessment proposed in the Virginia Legislature in 1784 prompted the writing of James Madison's Remonstrance.

and no less in principle than the real estate tax exemption granted by States. Few concepts are more deeply embedded in the fabric of our national life, beginning with pre-Revolutionary colonial times, than for the government to exercise at the very least this kind of benevolent neutrality toward churches and religious exercise generally so long as none was favored over others and none suffered interference. ***

It is obviously correct that no one acquires a vested or protected right in violation of the Constitution by long use, even when that span of time covers our entire national existence and indeed predates it. Yet an unbroken practice of according the exemption to churches, openly and by affirmative state action, not covertly or by state inaction, is not something to be lightly cast aside. Nearly 50 years ago Mr. Justice Holmes stated:

> If a thing has been practised for two hundred years by common consent, it will need a strong case for the Fourteenth Amendment to affect it. *** Jackman v. Rosenbaum Co., 260 U.S. 22, 31 (1922).

Nothing in this national attitude toward religious tolerance and two centuries of uninterrupted freedom from taxation has given the remotest sign of leading to an established church or religion and on the contrary it has operated affirmatively to help guarantee the free exercise of all forms of religious belief. ***

Affirmed.

MR. JUSTICE BRENNAN, concurring.

* * *

Government has two basic secular purposes for granting real property tax exemptions to religious organizations. First, these organizations are exempted because they, among a range of other private, nonprofit organizations contribute to the well-being of the community in a variety of nonreligious ways, and thereby bear burdens that would otherwise either have to be met by general taxation, or be left undone, to the detriment of the community. ***

Second, government grants exemptions to religious organizations because they uniquely contribute to the pluralism of American society by their religious activities. Government may properly include religious institutions among the variety of private, nonprofit groups that receive tax exemptions, for each group contributes to the diversity of association, viewpoint, and enterprise essential to a vigorous, pluralistic society. ***

Against the background of this survey of the history, purpose, and operation of religious tax exemptions, I must conclude that the exemptions do not "serve the essentially religious activities of religious institutions." Their principal effect is to carry out secular purposes—the encouragement of public service activities and of a pluralistic society. During their ordinary operations, most churches engage in activities of a secular nature that benefit the community; and all churches by their existence contribute to the diversity of association, viewpoint, and enterprise so highly valued by all of us. ***

Finally, I do not think that the exemptions "use essentially religious means to serve governmental ends, where secular means would suffice." *** It is true that each church contributes to the pluralism of our society through its purely religious activities, but the state encourages these activities not because it champions religion per se but because it values religion among a variety of private, nonprofit enterprises that contribute to the diversity of the Nation. Viewed in this light, there is no nonreligious substitute for religion as an element in our societal mosaic, just as there is no nonliterary substitute for literary groups. ***

Opinion of MR. JUSTICE HARLAN.

Preliminarily, I think it relevant to face up to the fact that it is far easier to agree on the purpose that underlies the First Amendment's Establishment and Free Exercise Clauses than to obtain agreement on the standards that should govern their application. ***

Two requirements frequently articulated and applied in our cases for achieving this goal are "neutrality" and "voluntarism." E.g., see Abington School Dist. v. Schempp, 374 U.S. 203, 305 (1963) (concurring opinion of Mr. Justice Goldberg); Engel v. Vitale, 370 U.S. 421 (1962). These related and mutually reinforcing concepts are short-form for saying that the Government must neither legislate to accord benefits that favor religion over nonreligion, nor sponsor a particular sect, nor try to encourage participation in or abnegation of religion. Mr. Justice Goldberg's concurring opinion in *Abington* which I joined set forth these principles: "The fullest realization of true religious liberty requires that government neither engage in nor compel religious practices, that it effect no favoritism among sects or between religion and nonreligion, and that it work deterrence of no religious belief." 374 U.S., at 305. The Court's holding in Torcaso v. Watkins, 367 U.S. 488, 495 (1961), is to the same effect: the State cannot "constitutionally pass laws or impose requirements which aid all religions as against non-believers, and neither can [it] aid those religions based on a belief in the existence of God as against those religions founded on different beliefs." In the vast majority of cases the inquiry, albeit an elusive one, can end at this point. Neutrality and voluntarism stand as barriers against the most egregious and hence divisive kinds of state involvement in religious matters.

II

This legislation neither encourages nor discourages participation in religious life and thus satisfies the voluntarism requirement of the First Amendment. Unlike the instances of school prayers, *Abington School Dist. v. Schempp, supra*, and *Engel v. Vitale, supra*, or "released time" programs, Zorach v. Clauson, 343 U.S. 306 (1952), and McCollum v. Board of Education, 333 U.S. 203 (1948), the State is not "utilizing the prestige, power, and influence" of a public institution to bring religion into the lives of citizens. 374 U.S., at 307 (Goldberg, J., concurring).

The statute also satisfies the requirement of neutrality. Neutrality in its application requires an equal protection mode of analysis. The Court must survey meticulously the circumstances of governmental categories to eliminate, as it were, religious gerrymanders. In any particular case the critical question is whether the circumference of legislation encircles a class so broad that it can be fairly concluded that religious institutions could be thought to fall within the natural perimeter.

The statute that implements New York's constitutional provision for tax exemptions to religious organizations has defined a class of nontaxable entities whose common denominator is their nonprofit pursuit of activities devoted to cultural and moral improvement and the doing of "good works" by performing certain social services in the community that might otherwise have to be assumed by government. Included are such broad and divergent groups as historical and literary societies and more generally associations "for the moral or mental improvement of men." The statute by its terms grants this exemption in furtherance of moral and intellectual diversity and would appear not to omit any organization that could be reasonably thought to contribute to that goal.

To the extent that religious institutions sponsor the secular activities that this legislation is designed to promote, it is consistent with neutrality to grant them an exemption just as other organizations devoting resources to these projects receive exemptions. I think, moreover, in the context of a statute so broad as the one before us, churches may properly receive an exemption even though they do not themselves sponsor the secular-type activities mentioned in the statute but exist merely for the convenience of their interested members. As long as the breadth of exemption includes groups that pursue cultural, moral, or spiritual improvement in multifarious secular ways, including, I would suppose, groups whose avowed tenets may be antitheological, atheistic, or agnostic, I can see no lack of neutrality in extending the benefit of the exemption to organized religious groups.[1] ***

MR. JUSTICE DOUGLAS, dissenting.

Petitioner is the owner of real property in New York and is a Christian. But he is not a member of any of the religious organizations, "rejecting them as hostile." The New York statute exempts from taxation real property "owned by a corporation or association organized exclusively for *** religious *** purposes" and used "exclusively for carrying out" such purposes. Yet non-believers who own realty are taxed at the usual rate.

My Brother HARLAN says he "would suppose" that the tax exemption extends to "groups whose avowed tenets may be antitheological, atheistic, or agnostic." ***

---

1. While I would suppose most churches devote part of their resources to secular community projects and conventional charitable activities, it is a question of fact, a fact that would only be relevant if we had before us a statute framed more narrowly to include only "charities" or a limited class of organizations, and churches. In such a case, depending on the administration of the exemption, it might be that the granting of an exemption to religion would turn out to be improper. ***

If it does, then the line between believers and nonbelievers has not been drawn. But, with all respect, there is not even a suggestion in the present record that the statute covers property used exclusively by organizations for "antitheological purposes," "atheistic purposes," or "agnostic purposes."

With all due respect the governing principle is not controlled by *Everson v. Board of Education. Everson* involved the use of public funds to bus children to parochial as well as to public schools. Parochial schools teach religion; yet they are also educational institutions offering courses competitive with public schools. They prepare students for the professions and for activities in all walks of life. Education in the secular sense was combined with religious indoctrination at the parochial schools involved in *Everson*. Even so, the *Everson* decision was five to four and, though one of the five, I have since had grave doubts about it, because I have become convinced that grants to institutions teaching a sectarian creed violate the Establishment Clause. See *Engel v. Vitale, supra*, at 443-444 (DOUGLAS, J., concurring).

This case, however, is quite different. Education is not involved. The financial support rendered here is to the church, the place of worship. A tax exemption is a subsidy. Is my Brother Brennan correct in saying that we would hold that state or federal grants to churches, say, to construct the edifice itself would be unconstitutional? What is the difference between that kind of subsidy and the present subsidy? ***

If believers are entitled to public financial support, so are nonbelievers. A believer and nonbeliever under the present law are treated differently because of the articles of their faith. Believers are doubtless comforted that the cause of religion is being fostered by this legislation. Yet one of the mandates of the First Amendment is to promote a viable, pluralistic society and to keep government neutral, not only between sects, but also between believers and nonbelievers. The present involvement of government in religion may seem *de minimis*. But it is, I fear, a long step down the Establishment path. Perhaps I have been misinformed. But as I have read the Constitution and its philosophy, I gathered that independence was the price of liberty.

I conclude that this tax exemption is unconstitutional.

BOARD OF EDUCATION OF CENTRAL SCHOOL DISTRICT v. ALLEN

392 U.S. 236 (1968)

MR. JUSTICE WHITE delivered the opinion of the Court.

A law of the State of New York requires local public school authorities to lend textbooks free of charge to all students in grades seven through 12; students attending private schools are included. This case presents the question whether this statute is a "law respecting an establishment of religion, or prohibiting the free exercise thereof," and so in conflict with the First and Fourteenth Amendments to the Constitution, because it authorizes the loan of textbooks to students attending parochial schools. We hold that the law is not in violation of the Constitution. ***

Everson v. Board of Education, 330 U.S. 1 (1947), is the case decided by this Court that is most nearly in point for today's problem. *** *Everson* and later cases have shown that the line between state neutrality to religion and state support of religion is not easy to locate. Abington School District v. Schempp, 374 U.S. 203 (1963), fashioned a test subscribed to by eight Justices for distinguishing between forbidden involvements of the State with religion and those contacts which the Establishment Clause permits:

> The test may be stated as follows: what are the purpose and the primary effect of the enactment? If either is the advancement or inhibition of religion then the enactment exceeds the scope of legislative power as circumscribed by the Constitution. That is to say that to withstand the strictures of the Establishment Clause there must be a secular legislative purpose and a primary effect that neither advances nor inhibits religion.***

This test is not easy to apply, but the citation of *Everson* by the *Schempp* Court to support its general standard made clear how the *Schempp* rule would be applied to the facts of *Everson*. The statute upheld in *Everson* would be considered a law having "a secular legislative purpose and a primary effect that neither advances nor inhibits religion." We reach the same result with respect to the New York law requiring school books to be loaned free of charge to all students in specified grades.

Of course books are different from buses. Most bus rides have no inherent religious significance, while religious books are common. However, the language of § 701 does not authorize the loan of religious books, and the State claims no right to distribute religious literature. Although the books loaned are those required by the parochial school for use in specific courses, each book loaned must be approved by the public school authorities; only secular books may receive approval. In judging the validity of the statute on this record we must proceed on the assumption that books loaned to students are books that are not unsuitable for use in the public schools because of religious content.

The major reason offered by appellants for distinguishing free textbooks from free bus fares is that books, but not buses, are critical to the teaching process, and in a sectarian school that process is employed to teach religion. However this Court has long recognized that religious schools pursue two goals, religious instruction and secular education. In the leading case of Pierce v. Society of Sisters, 268 U.S. 510 (1925), the Court held that although it would not question Oregon's power to compel school attendance or require that the attendance be at an institution meeting State-imposed requirements as to quality and nature of curriculum, Oregon had not shown that its interest in secular education required that all children attend publicly operated schools. A premise of this holding was the view that the State's interest in education would be served sufficiently by reliance on the secular teaching that accompanied religious training in the schools maintained by the Society of Sisters. Since*Pierce*, a substantial body of case law has confirmed the power of the States to insist that attendance at private schools, if it is to satisfy state compulsory-attendance laws, be at institutions which provide minimum hours of instruction, employ teachers of specified training, and cover prescribed subjects of instruction. ***

Underlying these cases, and underlying also the legislative judgments that have preceded the court decisions, has been a recognition that private education has played and is playing a significant and valuable role in raising national levels of knowledge, competence, and experience. Americans care about the quality of the secular education available to their children. *** Considering this attitude, the continued willingness to rely on private school systems, including parochial systems, strongly suggests that a wide segment of informed opinion, legislative and otherwise, has found that those schools do an acceptable job of providing secular education to their students. This judgment is further evidence that parochial schools are performing, in addition to their sectarian function, the task of secular education.

Against this background of judgment and experience, unchallenged in the meager record before us in this case, we cannot agree with appellants either that all teaching in a sectarian school is religious or that the processes of secular and religious training are so intertwined that secular textbooks furnished to students by the public are in fact instrumental in the teaching of religion. This case comes to us after summary judgment entered on the pleadings. Nothing in this record supports the proposition that all textbooks, whether they deal with mathematics, physics, foreign languages, history, or literature, are used by the parochial schools to teach religion. No evidence has been offered about particular schools, particular courses, particular teachers, or particular books. We are unable to hold, based solely on judicial notice, that this statute results in unconstitutional involvement of the State with religious instruction or that § 701, for this or the other reasons urged, is a law respecting the establishment of religion within the meaning of the First Amendment. ***

MR. JUSTICE HARLAN, concurring.

Although I join the opinion and judgment of the Court, I wish to emphasize certain of the principles which I believe to be central to the determination of this case, and which I think are implicit in the Court's decision.

The attitude of government toward religion must, as this Court has frequently observed, be one of neutrality. Neutrality is, however, a coat of many colors. It requires that "government neither engage in nor compel religious practices, that it effect no favoritism among sects or between religion and nonreligion, and that it work deterrence of no religious belief." Abington School District v. Schempp, 374 U.S. 203, 305 (concurring opinion of Goldberg, J.). *** I would hold that where the contested governmental activity is calculated to achieve nonreligious purposes otherwise within the competence of the State, and where the activity does not involve the

State "so significantly and directly in the realm of the sectarian as to give rise to *** divisive influences and inhibitions of freedom," it is not forbidden by the religious clauses of the First Amendment.

In my opinion, § 701 of the Education Law of New York does not employ religion as its standard for action or inaction, and is not otherwise inconsistent with these principles.

MR. JUSTICE BLACK, dissenting.

The Court here affirms a judgment of the New York Court of Appeals which sustained the constitutionality of a New York law providing state tax-raised funds to supply school books for use by pupils in schools owned and operated by religious sects. *** For that reason I would reverse the New York Court of Appeals' judgment. This, I am confident, would be in keeping with the deliberate statement we made in Everson v. Board of Education, 330 U.S. 1, 15-16 (1947) ***

The *Everson* and *McCollum* cases plainly interpret the First and Fourteenth Amendments as protecting the taxpayers of a State from being compelled to pay taxes to their government to support the agencies of private religious organizations the taxpayers oppose. ***

As my Brother DOUGLAS, so forcefully shows, in an argument with which I fully agree, upholding a State's power to pay bus or streetcar fares for school children cannot provide support for the validity of a state law using tax-raised funds to buy school books for a religious school. The First Amendment's bar to establishment of religion must preclude a State from using funds levied from all of its citizens to purchase books for use by sectarian schools, which, although "secular," realistically will in some way inevitably tend to propagate the religious views of the favored sect. *** In this sense it is not difficult to distinguish books, which are the heart of any school, from bus fares, which provide a convenient and helpful general public transportation service. With respect to the former, state financial support actively and directly assists the teaching and propagation of sectarian religious viewpoints in clear conflict with the First Amendment's establishment bar; with respect to the latter, the State merely provides a general and nondiscriminatory transportation service in no way related to substantive religious views and beliefs. ***

I still subscribe to the belief that tax-raised funds cannot constitutionally be used to support religious schools, buy their school books, erect their buildings, pay their teachers, or pay any other of their maintenance expenses, even to the extent of one penny. The First Amendment's prohibition against governmental establishment of religion was written on the assumption that state aid to religion and religious schools generates discord, disharmony, hatred, and strife among our people, and that any government that supplies such aids is to that extent a tyranny. And I still believe that the only way to protect minority religious groups from majority groups in this country is to keep the wall of separation between church and state high and impregnable as the First and Fourteenth Amendments provide. The Court's affirmance here bodes nothing but evil to religious peace in this country.

MR. JUSTICE DOUGLAS, dissenting.

* * *

The statute on its face empowers each parochial school to determine for itself which textbooks will be eligible for loans to its students, for the Act provides that the only text which the State may provide is "a book which a pupil is required to use as a text for a semester or more in a particular class in the school he legally attends." This initial and crucial selection is undoubtedly made by the parochial school's principal or its individual instructors, who are, in the case of Roman Catholic schools, normally priests or nuns.

The next step under the Act is an "individual request" for an eligible textbook but the State Education Department has ruled that a pupil may make his request to the local public board of education through a "private school official." Local boards have accordingly provided for those requests to be made by the individual or "by groups or classes." And forms for textbook requisitions to be filled out by the head of the private school are provided.

The role of the local public school board is to decide whether to veto the selection made by the parochial school. This is done by determining first whether the text has been or should be "approved" for use in public schools and second whether the text is "secular," "nonreligious," or "non-sectarian." The local boards apparently have broad discretion in exercising this veto power.

Thus the statutory system provides that the parochial school will ask for the books that it wants. Can there be the slightest doubt that the head of the parochial school will select the book or books that best promote its sectarian creed?

If the board of education supinely submits by approving and supplying the sectarian or sectarian-oriented textbooks, the struggle to keep church and state separate has been lost. If the board resists, then the battle line between church and state will have been drawn and the contest will be on to keep the school board independent or to put it under church domination and control.

Whatever may be said of *Everson*, there is nothing ideological about a bus. There is nothing ideological about a school lunch, or a public nurse, or a scholarship. The constitutionality of such public aid to students in parochial schools turns on considerations not present in this textbook case. The textbook goes to the very heart of education in a parochial school. It is the chief, although not solitary, instrumentality for propagating a particular religious creed or faith. How can we possibly approve such state aid to a religion? A parochial school textbook may contain many, many more seeds of creed and dogma than a prayer. ***

Judge Van Voorhis, joined by Chief Judge Fuld and Judge Breitel, dissenting below, said that the difficulty with the textbook loan program "is that there is no reliable standard by which secular and religious textbooks can be distinguished from each other." *** May John M. Scott's Adventures in Science (1963) be supplied under the textbook loan program? This book teaches embryology in the following manner:

> "To you an animal usually means a mammal, such as a cat, dog, squirrel, or guinea pig. The new animal or embryo develops inside the body of the mother until birth. ***
>
> "The body of a human being grows in the same way, but it is much more remarkable than that of any animal, for the embryo has a human soul infused into the body by God. Human parents are partners with God in creation. They have very great powers and great responsibilities, for through their cooperation with God souls are born for heaven." (At 618-619.)[2]

* * *

MR. JUSTICE FORTAS, dissenting.

The majority opinion of the Court upholds the New York statute by ignoring a vital aspect of it. Public funds are used to buy, for students in sectarian schools, textbooks which are selected and prescribed by the sectarian schools themselves. As my Brother DOUGLAS points out, despite the transparent camouflage that the books are furnished to students, the reality is that they are selected and their use is prescribed by the sectarian authorities. The child must use the prescribed book. He cannot use a different book prescribed for use in the public schools. The State cannot choose the book to be used. It is true that the public school boards must "approve" the book selected by the sectarian authorities; but this has no real significance. The purpose of these provisions is to hold out promise that the books will be "secular" (but cf. Douglas , J., dissenting, ***); but the fact remains that the books are chosen by and for the sectarian schools.

It is misleading to say, as the majority opinion does, that the New York "law merely makes available to all children the benefits of a general program to lend school books free of charge." *** This is not a "general" program. It is a specific program to use state funds to buy books prescribed by sectarian schools which, in New York, are primarily Catholic, Jewish, and Lutheran sponsored schools. It could be called a "general" program only if the school books made available to all children were precisely the same—the books selected for and used in the public schools. But this program is not one in which all children are treated alike, regardless of where they go to school. This program, in its unconstitutional features, is hand-tailored to satisfy the specific needs of sectarian schools. Children attending such schools are given *special* books—books selected by the sectarian authorities. How can this be other than the use of public money to aid those sectarian establishments? ***

This is the feature of the present statute that makes it totally inaccurate to sug-

---

2. Although the author of this textbook is a priest, the text contains no imprimatur and no nihil obstat. Although published by a Catholic press, the Loyola University Press, Chicago, it is not marked in any manner as a "denominational edition," but is simply the general edition of the book. Accordingly, under Opinion of Counsel No. 181, the only document approaching a "regulation" on the issue involved here, Adventures in Science would qualify as "non-sectarian." ***

gest, as the majority does here, that furnishing these specially selected books for use in sectarian schools is like "public provision of police and fire protection, sewage facilities, and streets and sidewalks." *** These are furnished to all alike. They are not selected on the basis of specification by a religious sect. And patrons of any one sect do not receive services or facilities different from those accorded members of other religions or agnostics or even atheists. I would reverse the judgment below.

LEMON v. KURTZMAN

403 U.S. 602 (1971)

MR. CHIEF JUSTICE BURGER delivered the opinion of the Court.

These two appeals raise questions as to Pennsylvania and Rhode Island statutes providing state aid to church-related elementary and secondary schools. Both statutes are challenged as violative of the Establishment and Free Exercise Clauses of the First Amendment and the Due Process Clause of the Fourteenth Amendment.

Pennsylvania has adopted a statutory program that provides financial support to nonpublic elementary and secondary schools by way of reimbursement for the cost of teachers' salaries, textbooks, and instructional materials in specified secular subjects. Rhode Island has adopted a statute under which the State pays directly to teachers in nonpublic elementary schools a supplement of 15% of their annual salary. Under each statute state aid has been given to church-related educational institutions. We hold that both statutes are unconstitutional.

I

The Rhode Island Statute

The Rhode Island Salary Supplement Act was enacted in 1969. It rests on the legislative finding that the quality of education available in nonpublic elementary schools has been jeopardized by the rapidly rising salaries needed to attract competent and dedicated teachers. The Act authorizes state officials to supplement the salaries of teachers of secular subjects in nonpublic elementary schools by paying directly to a teacher an amount not in excess of 15% of his current annual salary. As supplemented, however, a nonpublic school teacher's salary cannot exceed the maximum paid to teachers in the State's public schools, and the recipient must be certified by the state board of education in substantially the same manner as public school teachers. ***

The Act also requires that teachers eligible for salary supplements must teach only those subjects that are offered in the State's public schools. They must use "only teaching materials which are used in the public schools." Finally, any teacher applying for a salary supplement must first agree in writing "not to teach a course in religion for so long as or during such time as he or she receives any salary supplements" under the Act. ***

The Pennsylvania Statute

Pennsylvania has adopted a program that has some but not all of the features of the Rhode Island program. *** The statute authorizes appellee state Superintendent of Public Instruction to "purchase" specified "secular educational services" from nonpublic schools. Under the "contracts" authorized by the statute, the State directly reimburses nonpublic schools solely for their actual expenditures for teachers' salaries, textbooks, and instructional materials. A school seeking reimbursement must maintain prescribed accounting procedures that identify the "separate" cost of the "secular educational service." These accounts are subject to state audit. [T]he Act is now financed by a portion of the state tax on cigarettes.

There are several significant statutory restrictions on state aid. Reimbursement is limited to courses "presented in the curricula of the public schools." It is further limited "solely" to courses in the following "secular" subjects: mathematics, modern foreign languages, physical science, and physical education. Textbooks and instructional materials included in the program must be approved by the state Superintendent of Public Instruction. Finally, the statute prohibits reimbursement for any course that contains "any subject matter expressing religious teaching, or the morals or forms of worship of any sect."

*** It appears that some $5 million has been expended annually under the Act. The State has now entered into contracts with some 1,181 nonpublic elementary and secondary schools with a student population of some 535,215 pupils—more than 20% of the total number of students in the State. More than 96% of these pupils attend church-related schools, and most of these schools are affiliated with the Roman Catholic church. ***

II

In the absence of precisely stated constitutional prohibitions, we must draw lines with reference to the three main evils against which the Establishment Clause was intended to afford protection: "sponsorship, financial support, and active involvement of the sovereign in religious activity." Walz v. Tax Commission, 397 U.S. 664, 668 (1970).

Every analysis in this area must begin with consideration of the cumulative criteria developed by the Court over many years. Three such tests may be gleaned from our cases. First, the statute must have a secular legislative purpose; second, its principal or primary effect must be one that neither advances nor inhibits religion, Board of Education v. Allen, 392 U.S. 236, 243 (1968); finally, the statute must not foster "an excessive government entanglement with religion." *Walz, supra*, at 674.

Inquiry into the legislative purposes of the Pennsylvania and Rhode Island statutes affords no basis for a conclusion that the legislative intent was to advance religion. On the contrary, the statutes themselves clearly state that they are intended to enhance the quality of the secular education in all schools covered by the compulsory attendance laws. There is no reason to believe the legislatures meant anything else. *** The legislatures of Rhode Island and Pennsylvania have concluded that secular and religious education are identifiable and separable. In the abstract we have no quarrel with this conclusion.

The two legislatures, however, have also recognized that church-related elementary and secondary schools have a significant religious mission and that a substantial portion of their activities is religiously oriented. They have therefore sought to create statutory restrictions designed to guarantee the separation between secular and religious educational functions and to ensure that State financial aid supports only the former. All these provisions are precautions taken in candid recognition that these programs approached, even if they did not intrude upon, the forbidden areas under the Religion Clauses. We need not decide whether these legislative precautions restrict the principal or primary effect of the programs to the point where they do not offend the Religion Clauses, for we conclude that the cumulative impact of the entire relationship arising under the statutes in each State involves excessive entanglement between government and religion. ***

In *Allen* the Court refused to make assumptions, on a meager record, about the religious content of the textbooks that the State would be asked to provide. We cannot, however, refuse here to recognize that teachers have a substantially different ideological character from books. In terms of potential for involving some aspect of faith or morals in secular subjects, a textbook's content is ascertainable, but a teacher's handling of a subject is not. We cannot ignore the danger that a teacher under religious control and discipline poses to the separation of the religious from the purely secular aspects of pre-college education. The conflict of functions inheres in the situation.

We need not and do not assume that teachers in parochial schools will be guilty of bad faith or any conscious design to evade the limitations imposed by the statute and the First Amendment. We simply recognize that a dedicated religious person, teaching in a school affiliated with his or her faith and operated to inculcate its tenets, will inevitably experience great difficulty in remaining religiously neutral. Doctrines and faith are not inculcated or advanced by neutrals. With the best of intentions such a teacher would find it hard to make a total separation between secular teaching and religious doctrine. What would appear to some to be essential to good citizenship might well for others border on or constitute instruction in religion. Further difficulties are inherent in the combination of religious discipline and the possibility of disagreement between teacher and religious authorities over the meaning of the statutory restrictions. ***

A comprehensive, discriminating, and continuing state surveillance will inevitably be required to ensure that these restrictions are obeyed and the First Amendment otherwise respected. Unlike a book, a teacher cannot be inspected once so as to determine the extent and intent of his or her personal beliefs and subjective acceptance of the limitations imposed by the First Amendment. These prophylactic contacts will involve excessive and enduring entanglement between state and church. ***

A broader base of entanglement of yet a different character is presented by the divisive political potential of these state programs. In a community where such a large number of pupils are served by church-related schools, it can be assumed that state assistance will entail considerable political activity. Partisans of parochial schools, understandably concerned with rising costs and sincerely dedicated to both the religious and secular educational missions of their schools, will inevitably champion this cause and promote political action to achieve their goals. Those who oppose state aid, whether for constitutional, religious, or fiscal reasons, will inevitably respond and employ all of the usual political campaign techniques to prevail. Candidates will be forced to declare and voters to choose. It would be unrealistic to ignore the fact that many people confronted with issues of this kind will find their votes aligned with their faith. ***

In *Walz* it was argued that a tax exemption for places of religious worship would prove to be the first step in an inevitable progression leading to the establishment of state churches and state religion. That claim could not stand up against more than 200 years of virtually universal practice imbedded in our colonial experience and continuing into the present.

The progression argument, however, is more persuasive here. We have no long history of state aid to church-related educational institutions comparable to 200 years of tax exemption for churches. Indeed, the state programs before us today represent something of an innovation. We have already noted that modern governmental programs have self-perpetuating and self-expanding propensities. These internal pressures are only enhanced when the schemes involve institutions whose legitimate needs are growing and whose interests have substantial political support. Nor can we fail to see that in constitutional adjudication some steps, which when taken were thought to approach "the verge," have become the platform for yet further steps. A certain momentum develops in constitutional theory and it can be a "downhill thrust" easily set in motion but difficult to retard or stop. ***

MR. JUSTICE DOUGLAS, whom MR. JUSTICE BLACK joins, concurring.

* * *

The analysis of the constitutional objections to these two state systems of grants to parochial or sectarian schools must start with the admitted and obvious fact that the *raison d'etre* of parochial schools is the propagation of a religious faith. They also teach secular subjects; but they came into existence in this country because Protestant groups were perverting the public schools by using them to propagate their faith. The Catholics naturally rebelled. If schools were to be used to propagate a particular creed or religion, then Catholic ideals should also be served. Hence the advent of parochial schools. ***

The story of conflict and dissension is long and well known. The result was a state of so-called equilibrium where religious instruction was eliminated from public schools and the use of public funds to support religious schools was deemed to be banned.

But the hydraulic pressures created by political forces and by economic stress were great and they began to change the situation. Laws were passed—state and federal—that dispensed public funds to sustain religious schools and the plea was always in the educational frame of reference: education in all sectors was needed, from languages to calculus to nuclear physics. And it was forcefully argued that a linguist or mathematician or physicist trained in religious schools was just as competent as one trained in secular schools.

And so we have gradually edged into a situation where vast amounts of public funds are supplied each year to sectarian schools.

And the argument is made that the private parochial school system takes about $9 billion a year off the back of government—as if that were enough to justify violating the Establishment Clause.

While the evolution of the public school system in this country marked an escape from denominational control and was therefore admirable as seen through the eyes of those who think like Madison and Jefferson, it has disadvantages. The main one is that a state system may attempt to mold all students alike according to the views of the dominant group and to discourage the emergence of individual idiosyncrasies. Sectarian education, however, does not remedy that condition. The advantages of sectarian education relate solely to religious or doctrinal matters. They give the church the opportunity to indoctrinate its creed delicately and indirectly, or massively through doctrinal courses. ***

When Madison in his Remonstrance attacked a taxing measure to support religious activities, he advanced a series of reasons for opposing it. One that is extremely relevant here was phrased as follows: "[I]t will destroy that moderation and harmony which the forbearance of our laws to intermeddle with Religion, has produced amongst its several sects." Intermeddling, to use Madison's word, or "entanglement," to use what was said in *Walz*, has two aspects. The intrusion of government into religious schools through grants, supervision, or surveillance may result in establishment of religion in the constitutional sense when what the State does enthrones a particular sect for overt or subtle propagation of its faith. Those activities of the State may also intrude on the Free Exercise Clause by depriving a teacher, under threats of reprisals, of the right to give sectarian construction or interpretation of, say, history and literature, or to use the teaching of such subjects to inculcate a religious creed or dogma. ***

In my view the taxpayers' forced contribution to the parochial schools in the present cases violates the First Amendment. ***

MR. JUSTICE BRENNAN. [Omitted.]

MR. JUSTICE WHITE, concurring in the judgments *** and dissenting ***.

* * *

It is enough for me that the States and the Federal Government are financing a separable secular function of overriding importance in order to sustain the legislation here challenged. That religion and private interests other than education may substantially benefit does not convert these laws into impermissible establishments of religion. ***

I do agree, however, that the complaint should not have been dismissed for failure to state a cause of action. [T]he complaint did allege that the schools were operated to fulfill religious purposes and one of the legal theories stated in the complaint was that the Pennsylvania Act "finances and participates in the blending of sectarian and secular instruction." At trial under this complaint, evidence showing such a blend in a course supported by state funds would appear to be admissible and, if credited, would establish financing of religious instruction by the State. Hence, I would reverse the judgment of the District Court and remand the case for trial, thereby holding the Pennsylvania legislation valid on its face but leaving open the question of its validity as applied to the particular facts of this case. *** [2]

TILTON v. RICHARDSON

403 U.S. 672 (1971)

MR. CHIEF JUSTICE BURGER announced the judgment of the Court and an opinion in which MR. JUSTICE HARLAN, MR. JUSTICE STEWART, and MR. JUSTICE BLACKMUN join.

This appeal presents important constitutional questions as to federal aid for church-related colleges and universities under Title I of the Higher Education Facilities Act of 1963, which provides construction grants for buildings and facilities used exclusively for secular educational purposes. We must determine first whether the Act authorizes aid to such church-related institutions, and, if so, whether the Act violates either the Establishment or Free Exercise Clauses of the First Amendment. ***

Appellants are citizens and taxpayers of the United States and residents of Connecticut. They brought this suit for injunctive relief against the officials who administer the Act. Four church- related colleges and universities in Connecticut receiving federal construction grants under Title I were also named as defendants. Federal funds were used for five projects at these four institutions: (1) a library building at Sacred Heart University; (2) a music, drama, and arts building at Annhurst College; (3) a science building at Fairfield University; (4) a library building at Fairfield; and (5) a language laboratory at Albertus Magnus College. ***

---

2. As a postscript I should note that both the federal and state cases are decided on specified Establishment Clause considerations, without reaching the questions that would be presented if the evidence in any of these cases showed that any of the involved schools restricted entry on racial or religious grounds or required all students gaining admission to receive instruction in the tenets of a particular faith. For myself, if such proof were made, the legislation would to that extent be unconstitutional.

II

We are satisfied that Congress intended the Act to include all colleges and universities regardless of any affiliation with or sponsorship by a religious body. ***

Against this background we consider four questions: First, does the Act reflect a secular legislative purpose? Second, is the primary effect of the Act to advance or inhibit religion? Third, does the administration of the Act foster an excessive government entanglement with religion? Fourth, does the implementation of the Act inhibit the free exercise of religion?

The Act itself was carefully drafted to ensure that the federally subsidized facilities would be devoted to the secular and not the religious function of the recipient institutions. It authorizes grants and loans only for academic facilities that will be used for defined secular purposes and expressly prohibits their use for religious instruction, training, or worship. These restrictions have been enforced in the Act's actual administration, and the record shows that some church-related institutions have been required to disgorge benefits for failure to obey them.

Finally, this record fully supports the findings of the District Court that none of the four church-related institutions in this case has violated the statutory restrictions. The institutions presented evidence that there had been no religious services or worship in the federally financed facilities, that there are no religious symbols or plaques in or on them, and that they had been used solely for nonreligious purposes. On this record, therefore, these buildings are indistinguishable from a typical state university facility. Appellants presented no evidence to the contrary.

Appellants instead rely on the argument that government may not subsidize any activities of an institution of higher learning that in some of its programs teaches religious doctrines. This argument rests on *Everson* where the majority stated that the Establishment Clause barred any "tax levied to support any religious institutions whatever form they may adopt to teach or practice religion."

There is no evidence that religion seeps into the use of any of these facilities. Indeed, the parties stipulated in the District Court that courses at these institutions are taught according to the academic requirements intrinsic to the subject matter and the individual teacher's concept of professional standards. Although appellants introduced several institutional documents that stated certain religious restrictions on what could be taught, other evidence showed that these restrictions were not in fact enforced and that the schools were characterized by an atmosphere of academic freedom rather than religious indoctrination. All four institutions, for example, subscribe to the 1940 Statement of Principles on Academic Freedom and Tenure endorsed by the American Association of University Professors and the Association of American Colleges.

Rather than focus on the four defendant colleges and universities involved in this case, however, appellants seek to shift our attention to a "composite profile" that they have constructed of the "typical sectarian" institution of higher education. We are told that such a "composite" institution imposes religious restrictions on admissions, requires attendance at religious activities, compels obedience to the doctrines and dogmas of the faith, requires instruction in theology and doctrine, and does everything it can to propagate a particular religion. Perhaps some church-related schools fit the pattern that appellants describe. Indeed, some colleges have been declared ineligible for aid by the authorities that administer the Act. But appellants do not contend that these four institutions fall within this category. Individual projects can be properly evaluated if and when challenges arise with respect to particular recipients and some evidence is then presented to show that the institution does in fact possess these characteristics. We cannot, however, strike down an Act of Congress on the basis of a hypothetical "profile."

Although we reject appellants' broad constitutional arguments we do perceive an aspect in which the statute's enforcement provisions are inadequate to ensure that the impact of the federal aid will not advance religion. If a recipient institution violates any of the statutory restrictions on the use of a federally financed facility, § 754(b)(2) permits the Government to recover an amount equal to the proportion of the facility's present value that the federal grant bore to its original cost.

This remedy, however, is available to the Government only if the statutory conditions are violated "within twenty years after completion of construction" ***

Limiting the prohibition for religious use of the structure to 20 years obviously opens the facility to use for any purpose at the end of that period. It cannot be assumed that a substantial structure has no value after that period and hence the unrestricted use of a valuable property is in effect a contribution of some value to a religious body. To this extent the Act therefore trespasses on the Religion Clauses. The restrictive obligations of a recipient institution under § 751(a)(2) cannot, compatibly with the Religion Clauses, expire while the building has substantial value. ***

IV

We next turn to the question of whether excessive entanglements characterize the relationship between government and church under the Act. ***

In *DiCenso* the District Court found that the parochial schools in Rhode Island were "an integral part of the religious mission of the Catholic Church." There, the record fully supported the conclusion that the inculcation of religious values was a substantial if not the dominant purpose of the institutions. ***

There are generally significant differences between the religious aspects of church-related institutions of higher learning and parochial elementary and secondary schools. The "affirmative if not dominant policy" of the instruction in pre-college church schools is "to assure future adherents to a particular faith by having control of their total education at an early age." *Walz v. Tax Comm'n*, [397 U.S.], at 671. There is substance to the contention that college students are less impressionable and less susceptible to religious indoctrination. Common observation would seem to support that view, and Congress may well have entertained it. The skepticism of the college student is not an inconsiderable barrier to any attempt or tendency to subvert the congressional objectives and limitations. Furthermore, by their very nature, college and postgraduate courses tend to limit the opportunities for sectarian influence by virtue of their own internal disciplines. Many church-related colleges and universities are characterized by a high degree of academic freedom and seek to evoke free and critical responses from their students.

The record here would not support a conclusion that any of these four institutions departed from this general pattern. All four schools are governed by Catholic religious organizations, and the faculties and student bodies at each are predominantly Catholic. Nevertheless, the evidence shows that non-Catholics were admitted as students and given faculty appointments. Not one of these four institutions requires its students to attend religious services. Although all four schools require their students to take theology courses, the parties stipulated that these courses are taught according to the academic requirements of the subject matter and the teacher's concept of professional standards. The parties also stipulated that the courses covered a range of human religious experiences and are not limited to courses about the Roman Catholic religion. The schools introduced evidence that they made no attempt to indoctrinate students or to proselytize. Indeed, some of the required theology courses at Albertus Magnus and Sacred Heart are taught by rabbis. Finally, as we have noted, these four schools subscribe to a well-established set of principles of academic freedom, and nothing in this record shows that these principles are not in fact followed. In short, the evidence shows institutions with admittedly religious functions but whose predominant higher education mission is to provide their students with a secular education.

Since religious indoctrination is not a substantial purpose or activity of these church-related colleges and universities, there is less likelihood than in primary and secondary schools that religion will permeate the area of secular education. This reduces the risk that government aid will in fact serve to support religious activities. Correspondingly, the necessity for intensive government surveillance is diminished and the resulting entanglements between government and religion lessened. Such inspection as may be necessary to ascertain that the facilities are devoted to secular education is minimal and indeed hardly more than the inspections that States impose over all private schools within the reach of compulsory education laws.

The entanglement between church and state is also lessened here by the nonideological character of the aid that the Government provides. ***

Finally, government entanglements with religion are reduced by the circumstance that, unlike the direct and continuing payments under the Pennsylvania program, and all the incidents of regulation and surveillance, the Government aid here is a one-time, single-purpose construction grant. There are no continuing financial relationships or dependencies, no annual audits, and no government analysis of an institution's expenditures on secular as distinguished from religious activities. Inspection as to use is a minimal contact.

No one of these three factors standing alone is necessarily controlling; cumulatively all of them shape a narrow and limited relationship with government which involves fewer and less significant contacts than the two state schemes before us in *Lemon* and *DiCenso*. The relationship therefore has less potential for realizing the substantive evils against which the Religion Clauses were intended to protect. ***

MR. JUSTICE DOUGLAS, with whom MR. JUSTICE BLACK and MR. JUSTICE MARSHALL concur, dissenting in part.

The correct constitutional principle for this case was stated by President Kennedy in 1961 when questioned as to his policy respecting aid to private and parochial schools:

> "[T]he Constitution clearly prohibits aid to the school, to parochial schools. I don't think there is any doubt of that.
>
> "The Everson case, which is probably the most celebrated case, provided only by a 5 to 4 decision was it possible for a local community to provide bus rides to nonpublic school children. But all through the majority and minority statements on that particular question there was a very clear prohibition against aid to the school direct. The Supreme Court made its decision in the Everson case by determining that the aid was to the child, not to the school. Aid to the school is—there isn't any room for debate on that subject. It is prohibited by the Constitution, and the Supreme Court has made that very clear. And therefore there would be no possibility of our recommending it."

* * *

The public purpose in secular education is, to be sure, furthered by the program. Yet the sectarian purpose is aided by making the parochial school system viable. The purpose is to increase "student enrollment" and the students obviously aimed at are those of the particular faith now financed by taxpayers' money. Parochial schools are not beamed at agnostics, atheists, or those of a competing sect. The more sophisticated institutions may admit minorities; but the dominant religious character is not changed. ***

What I have said in *Lemon* and in the *DiCenso* cases decided today is relevant here. The facilities financed by taxpayers' funds are not to be used for "sectarian" purposes. Religious teaching and secular teaching are so enmeshed in parochial schools that only the strictest supervision and surveillance would insure compliance with the condition. Parochial schools may require religious exercises, even in the classroom. A parochial school operates on one budget. Money not spent for one purpose becomes available for other purposes. Thus the fact that there are no religious observances in federally financed facilities is not controlling because required religious observances will take place in other buildings. *** Once these schools become federally funded they become bound by federal standards and accordingly adherence to *Engel* would require an end to required religious exercises. ***

It is almost unbelievable that we have made the radical departure from Madison's Remonstrance memorialized in today's decision. I dissent not because of any lack of respect for parochial schools but out of a feeling of despair that the respect which through history has been accorded the First Amendment is this day lost.

It should be remembered that in this case we deal with federal grants and with the command that "Congress shall make no law respecting an establishment of religion, or prohibiting the free exercise thereof." The million-dollar grants sustained today put Madison's miserable "three pence" to shame. But he even thought, as I do, that even a small amount coming out of the pocket of taxpayers and going into the coffers of a church was not in keeping with our constitutional ideal.

I would reverse the judgment below.

WOLMAN v. WALTER*

433 U.S. 229 (1977)

MR. JUSTICE BLACKMUN delivered the opinion of the Court (Parts I, V, VI, VII, and VIII), together with an opinion (Parts II, III, and IV), in which THE CHIEF JUSTICE, MR. JUSTICE STEWART, and MR. JUSTICE POWELL joined.

This is still another case presenting the recurrent issue of the limitations imposed by the Establishment Clause of the First Amendment, made applicable to the States by the Fourteenth Amendment, on state aid to pupils in church-related elementary and secondary schools. Appellants are citizens and taxpayers of Ohio. They challenge all but one of the provisions of Ohio Rev. Code Ann. § 3317.06 (Supp. 1976) which authorize various forms of aid. A three judge court held the statute constitutional in all respects. We noted probable jurisdiction.

I

*** In broad outline, the statute authorizes the State to provide nonpublic school pupils with books, instructional materials and equipment, standardized testing and scoring, diagnostic services, therapeutic services, and field trip transportation.

The initial biennial appropriation by the Ohio Legislature for implementation of the statute was the sum of $88,800,000. Funds so appropriated are paid to the State's public school districts and are then expended by them. All disbursements made with respect to nonpublic schools have their equivalents in disbursements for public schools, and the amount expended per pupil in nonpublic schools may not exceed the amount expended per pupil in the public schools.

The parties stipulated that during the 1974-1975 school year there were 720 chartered nonpublic schools in Ohio. Of these, all but 29 were sectarian. More than 96% of the nonpublic enrollment attended sectarian schools, and more than 92% attended Catholic schools. ***

---

*. [**Ed. Note**. This case was subsequently overruled in part. *See* Mitchell v. Helms, 530 U.S. 793 (2000), *infra* at page 923.

II

The mode of analysis for Establishment Clause questions is defined by the three-part test that has emerged from the Court's decisions. In order to pass muster, a statute must have a secular legislative purpose, must have a principal or primary effect that neither advances nor inhibits religion, and must not foster an excessive government entanglement with religion. ***

In the present case we have no difficulty with the first prong of this three-part test. We are satisfied that the challenged statute reflects Ohio's legitimate interest in protecting the health of its youth and in providing a fertile educational environment for all the schoolchildren of the State. As is usual in our cases, the analytical difficulty has to do with the effect and entanglement criteria. ***

III

Textbooks

* * *

This system for the loan of textbooks to individual students bears a striking resemblance to the systems approved in Board of Education v. Allen, 392 U.S. 236 (1968). *** Accordingly, we conclude that § 3317.06 (A) is constitutional.

IV

Testing and Scoring

Section 3317.06 authorizes expenditure of funds:

> "(J) To supply for use by pupils attending nonpublic schools within the district such standardized tests and scoring services as are in use in the public schools of the state."

These tests "are used to measure the progress of students in secular subjects." Nonpublic school personnel are not involved in either the drafting or scoring of the tests. The statute does not authorize any payment to nonpublic school personnel for the costs of administering the tests. *** Under the section at issue, the State provides both the schools and the school district with the means of ensuring that the minimum standards are met. The nonpublic school does not control the content of the test or its result. *** Similarly, the inability of the school to control the test eliminates the need for the supervision that gives rise to excessive entanglement. We therefore agree with the District Court's conclusion that § 3317.06(J) is constitutional.

V

Diagnostic Services

Section 3317.06 authorizes expenditures of funds:

> "(D) To provide speech and hearing diagnostic services to pupils attending nonpublic schools within the district. Such service shall be provided in the nonpublic school attended by the pupil receiving the service. ***

> "(F) To provide diagnostic psychological services to pupils attending nonpublic schools within the district. Such services shall be provided in the school attended by the pupil receiving the service."

It will be observed that these speech and hearing and psychological diagnostic services are to be provided within the nonpublic school. It is stipulated, however, that the personnel (with the exception of physicians) who perform the services are employees of the local board of education; that physicians may be hired on a contract basis; that the purpose of these services is to determine the pupil's deficiency or need of assistance; and that treatment of any defect so found would take place off the nonpublic school premises.

[D]iagnostic services, unlike teaching or counseling, have little or no educational content and are not closely associated with the educational mission of the nonpublic school. The nature of the relationship between the diagnostician and the pupil does not provide the same opportunity for the transmission of sectarian views as attends the relationship between teacher and student or that between counselor and student.

We conclude that providing diagnostic services on the nonpublic school premises will not create an impermissible risk of the fostering of ideological views. It follows that there is no need for excessive surveillance, and there will not be impermissible entanglement. We therefore hold that §§ 3317.06 (D) and (F) are constitutional.
***

VI

Therapeutic Services

Sections 3317.06(G), (H), (I), and (K) authorize expenditures of funds for certain therapeutic, guidance, and remedial services for students who have been identified as having a need for specialized attention. Personnel providing the services must be employees of the local board of education or under contract with the State Department of Health. The services are to be performed only in public schools, in public centers, or in mobile units located off the nonpublic school premises.

Appellants concede that the provision of remedial, therapeutic, and guidance services in public schools, public centers , or mobile units is constitutional if both public and nonpublic school students are served simultaneously. Their challenge is limited to the situation where a facility is used to service only nonpublic school students.

The District Court construed the statute, as do we, to authorize services only on sites that are "neither physically nor educationally identified with the functions of the nonpublic schools." Thus, the services are to be offered under circumstances that reflect their religious neutrality.

We recognize that, unlike the diagnostician, the therapist may establish a relationship with the pupil in which there might be opportunities to transmit ideological views. But the influence on a therapist's behavior that is exerted by the fact that he serves a sectarian pupil is qualitatively different from the influence of the pervasive atmosphere of a religious institution.

Accordingly, we hold that providing therapeutic and remedial services at a neutral site off the premises of the nonpublic schools will not have the impermissible effect of advancing religion. Neither will there be any excessive entanglement arising from supervision of public employees to insure that they maintain a neutral stance.

VII

Instructional Materials and Equipment

Sections 3317.06(B) and (C) authorize expenditures of funds for the purchase and loan to pupils or their parents upon individual request of instructional materials and instructional equipment of the kind in use in the public schools within the district and which is "incapable of diversion to religious use." Section 3317.06 also provides that the materials and equipment may be stored on the premises of a nonpublic school and that publicly hired personnel who administer the lending program may perform their services upon the nonpublic school premises when necessary "for efficient implementation of the lending program."

Although the exact nature of the material and equipment is not clearly revealed, the parties have stipulated: "It is expected that materials and equipment loaned to pupils or parents under the new law will be similar to such former materials and equipment except that to the extent that the law requires that materials and equipment capable of diversion to religious issues will not be supplied." Equipment provided under the predecessor statute, included projectors, tape recorders, record players, maps and globes, science kits, weather forecasting charts, and the like. The District Court, found the statute, constitutional because the court could not distinguish the loan of material and equipment from the textbook provisions upheld in *Meek*, 421 U.S., at 359-362, and in *Allen*, 392 U.S., at 248.

In *Meek*, however, the Court considered the constitutional validity of a direct loan to nonpublic schools of instructional material and equipment, and, despite the apparent secular nature of the goods, held the loan impermissible. ***

Appellees seek to avoid *Meek* by emphasizing that it involved a program of direct loans to nonpublic schools. In contrast, the material and equipment at issue under the Ohio statute are loaned to the pupil or his parent. In our view, however, it would exalt form over substance if this distinction were found to justify a result different from that in *Meek*. Before *Meek* was decided by this Court, Ohio authorized the loan of material and equipment directly to the nonpublic schools. Then, in light of *Meek*, the state legislature decided to channel the goods through the parents and pupils. Despite the technical change in legal bailee, the program in substance is the same as before: The equipment is substantially the same; it will receive the same use by the students; and it may still be stored and distributed on the nonpublic school premises. In view of the impossibility of separating the secular education function from the sectarian, the state aid inevitably flows in part in support of the religious role of the schools. *** Accordingly, we hold §§ 3317.06(B) and (C) to be unconstitutional.

VIII
Field Trips

Section 3317.06 also authorizes expenditures of funds:

> "(L) To provide such field trip transportation and services to nonpublic school students as are provided to public school students in the district. School districts may contract with commercial transportation companies for such transportation service if school district busses are unavailable."

There is no restriction on the timing of field trips; the only restriction on number lies in the parallel the statute draws to field trips provided to public school students in the district. The parties have stipulated that the trips "would consist of visits to governmental, industrial, cultural, and scientific centers designed to enrich the secular studies of students." The choice of destination, however, will be made by the nonpublic school teacher from a wide range of locations.

The District Court held this feature to be constitutionally indistinguishable from that with which the Court was concerned in Everson v. Board of Education, 330 U.S. 1 (1947). We do not agree. In *Everson* the Court approved a system under which a New Jersey board of education reimbursed parents for the costs of sending their children to and from school, public or parochial, by public carrier. ***

The Ohio situation is in sharp contrast. First, the nonpublic school controls the timing of the trips and, within a certain range, their frequency and destinations. Thus, the schools, rather than the children, truly are the recipients of the service and, as this Court has recognized, this fact alone may be sufficient to invalidate the program as impermissible direct aid. Second, although a trip may be to a location that would be of interest to those in public schools, it is the individual teacher who makes a field trip meaningful. The experience begins with the study and discussion of the place to be visited; it continues on location with the teacher pointing out items of interest and stimulating the imagination; and it ends with a discussion of the experience. The field trips are an integral part of the educational experience, and where the teacher works within and for a sectarian institution, an unacceptable risk of fostering of religion is an inevitable byproduct. *** We hold § 3317.06(L) to be unconstitutional.

IX

In summary, we hold constitutional those portions of the Ohio statute authorizing the State to provide nonpublic school pupils with books, standardized testing and scoring, diagnostic services, and therapeutic and remedial services. We hold unconstitutional those portions relating to instructional materials and equipment and field trip services.

The judgment of the District Court is therefore affirmed in part and reversed in part.

THE CHIEF JUSTICE dissents from Parts VII and VIII of the Court's opinion. [Omitted.]

MR. JUSTICE BRENNAN, concurring in part and dissenting. [Omitted.]

MR. JUSTICE MARSHALL, concurring in part and dissenting in part.

* * *

The court upholds the textbook loan provision, § 3317.06(A), on the precedent of Board of Education v. Allen, 392 U.S. 236 (1968). *** It also recognizes, however, that there is "a tension" between *Allen* and the reasoning of the Court in Meek v. Pittenger, 421 U.S. 349 (1975). I would resolve that tension by overruling *Allen*. ***

MR. JUSTICE POWELL, concurring in part, concurring in the judgment in part, and dissenting in part. [Omitted.]

MR. JUSTICE STEVENS, concurring in part and dissenting in part.

The line drawn by the Establishment Clause of the First Amendment must also have a fundamental character. It should not differentiate between direct and indirect subsidies, or between instructional materials like globes and maps on the one hand and instructional materials like textbooks on the other. For that reason, rather than the three-part test described in Part II of the plurality's opinion, I would adhere to the test enunciated for the Court by Mr. Justice Black:

> "No tax in any amount, large or small, can be levied to support any religious activities or institutions, whatever they may be called, or whatever form they may adopt to teach or practice religion." Everson v. Board of Education, 330 U.S. 1, 16.

Under that test, a state subsidy of sectarian schools is invalid regardless of the form it takes. The financing of buildings, field trips, instructional materials, educational tests, and schoolbooks are all equally invalid. For all give aid to the school's educational mission, which at heart is religious. On the other hand, I am not prepared to exclude the possibility that some parts of the statute before us may be administered in a constitutional manner. The State can plainly provide public health services to children attending nonpublic schools. The diagnostic and therapeutic services described in Parts V and VI of the Court's opinion may fall into this category. Although I have some misgivings on this point, I am not prepared to hold this part of the statute invalid on its face. ***

C. THE GENERAL TEST MODIFIED AND IN RENEWED DISPUTE

MUELLER v. ALLEN
463 U.S. 388 (1983)

JUSTICE REHNQUIST delivered the opinion of the Court.

Minnesota allows taxpayers, in computing their state income tax, to deduct certain expenses incurred in providing for the education of their children.[1] ***

Minnesota, like every other State, provides its citizens with free elementary and secondary schooling. Minn. Stat. §§ 120.06, 120.72 (1982). It seems to be agreed that about 820,000 students attended this school system in the most recent school year. During the same year, approximately 91,000 elementary and secondary students attended some 500 privately supported schools located in Minnesota, and about 95% of these students attended schools considering themselves to be sectarian. ***

*** In this case we are asked to decide whether Minnesota's tax deduction bears greater resemblance to those types of assistance to parochial schools we have approved, or to those we have struck down. [I]n *Committee for Public Education v. Nyquist*, [413 U.S. 756], we held invalid a New York statute providing public funds for the maintenance and repair of the physical facilities of private schools and granting thinly disguised "tax benefits," actually amounting to tuition grants, to the parents of children attending private schools. As explained below, we conclude that § 290.09, subd. 22, bears less resemblance to the arrangement struck down in *Nyquist* than it does to assistance programs upheld in our prior decisions and those discussed with approval in *Nyquist*.

The general nature of our inquiry in this area has been guided, since the decision in *Lemon v. Kurtzman*, by the "three-part" test laid down in that case:

> "First, the statute must have a secular legislative purpose; second, its principal or primary effect must be one that neither advances nor inhibits religion ***;

---

1. Minnesota Stat. § 290.09, subd. 22 (1982), permits a taxpayer to deduct from his or her computation of gross income the following:

"Tuition and transportation expense. The amount he has paid to others, not to exceed $500 for each dependent in grades K to 6 and $700 for each dependent in grades 7 to 12, for tuition, textbooks and transportation of each dependent in attending an elementary or secondary school situated in Minnesota, North Dakota, South Dakota, Iowa, or Wisconsin, wherein a resident of this state may legally fulfill the state's compulsory attendance laws, which is not operated for profit, and which adheres to the provisions of the Civil Rights Act of 1964 and chapter 363. As used in this subdivision, 'textbooks' shall mean and include books and other instructional materials and equipment used in elementary and secondary schools in teaching only those subjects legally and commonly taught in public elementary and secondary schools in this state and shall not include instructional books and materials used in the teaching of religious tenets, doctrines or worship, the purpose of which is to inculcate such tenets, doctrines or worship, nor shall it include such books or materials for, or transportation to, extra-curricular activities including sporting events, musical or dramatic events, speech activities, driver's education, or programs of a similar nature."

finally, the statute must not foster 'an excessive government entanglement with religion.'"

* * *

Little time need be spent on the question of whether the Minnesota tax deduction has a secular purpose. Under our prior decisions, governmental assistance programs have consistently survived this inquiry even when they have run afoul of other aspects of the Lemon framework. See, e.g., *Lemon v. Kurtzman; Meek v. Pittenger*, [421 U.S.], at 363; *Wolman v. Walter*. This reflects, at least in part, our reluctance to attribute unconstitutional motives to the States, particularly when a plausible secular purpose for the State's program may be discerned from the face of the statute.

A State's decision to defray the cost of educational expenses incurred by parents —regardless of the type of schools their children attend—evidences a purpose that is both secular and understandable. An educated populace is essential to the political and economic health of any community, and a State's efforts to assist parents in meeting the rising cost of educational expenses plainly serves this secular purpose of ensuring that the State's citizenry is well educated. Similarly, Minnesota, like other States, could conclude that there is a strong public interest in assuring the continued financial health or private schools, both sectarian and nonsectarian. By educating a substantial number of students such schools relieve public schools of a correspondingly great burden—to the benefit of all taxpayers. In addition, private schools may serve as a benchmark for public schools, in a manner analogous to the "TVA yardstick" for private power companies. As JUSTICE POWELL has remarked:

> "Parochial schools, quite apart from their sectarian purpose, have provided an educational alternative for millions of young Americans; they often afford wholesome competition with our public schools; and in some States they relieve substantially the tax burden incident to the operation of public schools. The State has, moreover, a legitimate interest in facilitating education of the highest quality for all children within its boundaries, whatever school their parents have chosen for them." *Wolman v. Walter*, [433 U.S.], at 262 (concurring in part, concurring in judgment in part, and dissenting in part).

All these justifications are readily available to support § 290.09, subd. 22, and each is sufficient to satisfy the secular purpose inquiry of *Lemon*.

We turn therefore to the more difficult but related question whether the Minnesota statute has "the primary effect of advancing the sectarian aims of the nonpublic schools." In concluding that it does not, we find several features of the Minnesota tax deduction particularly significant. First, an essential feature of Minnesota's arrangement is the fact that § 290.09, subd. 22, is only one among many deductions —such as those for medical expenses, § 290.09, subd. 10, and charitable contributions, § 290.21, subd. 3—available under the Minnesota tax laws. Our decisions consistently have recognized that traditionally "[l]egislatures have especially broad latitude in creating classifications and distinctions in tax statutes." ***

Most importantly, the deduction is available for educational expenses incurred by all parents, including those whose children attend public schools and those whose children attend nonsectarian private schools or sectarian private schools. *** In this respect, as well as others, this case is vitally different from the scheme struck down in *Nyquist*. There, public assistance amounting to tuition grants, was provided only to parents of children in *nonpublic* schools. ***

We also agree with the Court of Appeals that, by channeling whatever assistance it may provide to parochial schools through individual parents, Minnesota has reduced the Establishment Clause objections to which its action is subject. It is true, of course, that financial assistance provided to parents ultimately has an economic effect comparable to that of aid given directly to the schools attended by their children. It is also true, however, that under Minnesota's arrangement public funds become available only as a result of numerous, private choices of individual parents of school-age children. For these reasons, we recognized in *Nyquist* that the means by which state assistance flows to private schools is of some importance: we said that "the fact that aid is disbursed to parents rather than to schools" is a material consideration in Establishment Clause analysis, albeit "only one among many factors to be considered." ***

Petitioners argue that, notwithstanding the facial neutrality of § 290.09, subd. 22, in application the statute primarily benefits religious institutions. Petitioners rely, as they did below, on a statistical analysis of the type of persons claiming the tax deduction. They contend that most parents of public school children incur no tuition expenses, and that other expenses deductible under § 290.09, subd. 22, are negligible in value; moreover, they claim that 96% of the children in private schools in 1978-1979 attended religiously affiliated institutions. Because of all this, they reason, the bulk of deductions taken under § 290.09, subd. 22, will be claimed by parents of children in sectarian schools. Respondents reply that petitioners have failed to consider the impact of deductions for items such as transportation, summer school tuition, tuition paid by parents whose children attended schools outside the school districts in which they resided, rental or purchase costs for a variety of equipment, and tuition for certain types of instruction not ordinarily provided in public schools.

We need not consider these contentions in detail. We would be loath to adopt a rule grounding the constitutionality of a facially neutral law on annual reports reciting the extent to which various classes of private citizens claimed benefits under the law. *** More fundamentally, whatever unequal effect may be attributed to the statutory classification can fairly be regarded as a rough return for the benefits, discussed above, provided to the State and all taxpayers by parents sending their children to parochial schools. In the light of all this, we believe it wiser to decline to engage in the type of empirical inquiry into those persons benefited by state law which petitioners urge.

Thus, we hold that the Minnesota tax deduction for educational expenses satisfies the primary effect inquiry of our Establishment Clause cases.

Turning to the third part of the *Lemon* inquiry, we have no difficulty in concluding that the Minnesota statute does not "excessively entangle" the State in religion. The only plausible source of the "comprehensive, discriminating, and continuing state surveillance," 403 U.S., at 619, necessary to run afoul of this standard would lie in the fact that state officials must determine whether particular textbooks qualify for a deduction. In making this decision, state officials must disallow deductions taken for "instructional books and materials used in the teaching of religious tenets, doctrines or worship, the purpose of which is to inculcate such tenets, doctrines or worship." Minn. Stat. § 290.09, subd. 22 (1982). Making decisions such as this does not differ substantially from making the types of decisions approved in earlier opinions of this Court. In Board of Education v. Allen, 392 U.S. 236 (1968), for example, the Court upheld the loan of secular textbooks to parents or children attending nonpublic schools; though state officials were required to determine whether particular books were or were not secular, the system was held not to violate the Establishment Clause. ***

For the foregoing reasons, the judgment of the Court of Appeals is [a]ffirmed.

JUSTICE MARSHALL, with whom JUSTICE BRENNAN, JUSTICE BLACKMUN, and JUSTICE STEVENS join, dissenting.

The Establishment Clause of the First Amendment prohibits a State from subsidizing religious education, whether it does so directly or indirectly. In my view, this principle of neutrality forbids not only the tax benefits struck down in Committee for Public Education v. Nyquist, 413 U.S. 756 (1973), but any tax benefit, including the tax deduction at issue here, which subsidizes tuition payments to sectarian schools. I also believe that the Establishment Clause prohibits the tax deductions that Minnesota authorizes for the cost of books and other instructional materials used for sectarian purposes.

I

The majority today does not question the continuing vitality of this Court's decision in *Nyquist*. That decision established that a State may not support religious education either through direct grants to parochial schools or through financial aid to parents of parochial school students. *** *Nyquist* also established that financial aid to parents of students attending parochial schools is no more permissible if it is provided in the form of a tax credit than if provided in the form of cash payments. ***

The majority attempts to distinguish *Nyquist* by pointing to two differences between the Minnesota tuition-assistance program and the program struck down in *Nyquist*. Neither of these distinctions can withstand scrutiny.

The majority first attempts to distinguish *Nyquist* on the ground that Minnesota makes all parents eligible to deduct up to $500 or $700 for each dependent, whereas the New York law allowed a deduction only for parents whose children attended nonpublic schools. Although Minnesota taxpayers who send their children to local public schools may not deduct tuition expenses because they incur none, they may deduct other expenses, such as the cost of gym clothes, pencils, and notebooks, which are shared by all parents of school-age children. This, in the majority's view, distinguishes the Minnesota scheme from the law at issue in*Nyquist*. *** It is simply undeniable that the single largest expense that may be deducted under the Minnesota statute is tuition. The statute is little more than a subsidy of tuition masquerading as a subsidy of general educational expenses. The other deductible expenses are *de minimis* in comparison to tuition expenses. *** The only factual inquiry necessary is the same as that employed in *Nyquist* and Sloan v. Lemon, 413 U.S. 825 (1973): whether the deduction permitted for tuition expenses primarily benefits those who send their children to religious schools. ***

The majority incorrectly asserts that Minnesota's tax deduction for tuition expenses "bears less resemblance to the arrangement struck down in *Nyquist* than it does to assistance programs upheld in our prior decisions and those discussed with approval in *Nyquist*." One might as well say that a tangerine bears less resemblance to an orange than to an apple. The two cases relied on by the majority, Board of Education v. Allen, 392 U.S. 236 (1968), and Everson v. Board of Education, 330 U.S. 1 (1947), are inapposite today for precisely the same reasons that they were inapposite in *Nyquist*. As previously noted, the Minnesota tuition tax deduction is not available to all parents, but only to parents whose children attend schools that charge tuition, which are comprised almost entirely of sectarian schools. More importantly, the assistance that flows to parochial schools as a result of the tax benefit is not restricted, and cannot be restricted, to the secular functions of those schools.

II-III

In my view, Minnesota's tax deduction for the cost of textbooks and other instructional materials is also constitutionally infirm. The majority is simply mistaken in concluding that a tax deduction, unlike a tax credit or a direct grant to parents, promotes religious education in a manner that is only "attenuated." *** A tax deduction has a primary effect that advances religion if it is provided to offset expenditures which are not restricted to the secular activities of parochial schools.

The instructional materials which are subsidized by the Minnesota tax deduction plainly may be used to inculcate religious values and belief. In Meek v. Pittenger, 421 U.S., at 366, we held that even the use of "wholly neutral, secular instructional material and equipment" by church-related schools contributes to religious instruction because "'[t]he secular education those schools provide goes hand in hand with the religious mission that is the only reason for the schools' existence.'" In Wolman v. Walter, 433 U.S., at 249-250, we concluded that precisely the same impermissible effect results when the instructional materials are loaned to the pupil or his parent, rather than directly to the schools. ***

There is no reason to treat Minnesota's tax deduction for textbooks any differently. Secular textbooks, like other secular instructional materials, contribute to the religious mission of the parochial schools that use those books. Although this

Court upheld the loan of secular textbooks to religious schools in *Board of Education v. Allen*, the Court believed at that time that it lacked sufficient experience to determine "based solely on judicial notice" that "the processes of secular and religious training are so intertwined that secular textbooks furnished to students by the public [will always be] instrumental in the teaching of religion." This basis for distinguishing secular instructional materials and secular textbooks is simply untenable, and is inconsistent with many of our more recent decisions concerning state aid to parochial schools. *** In any event, the Court's assumption in *Allen* that the textbooks at issue there might be used only for secular education was based on the fact that those very books had been chosen by the State for use in the public schools. In contrast, the Minnesota statute does not limit the tax deduction to those books which the State had approved for use in public schools. Rather, it permits a deduction for books that are chosen by the parochial schools themselves. Indeed, under the Minnesota statutory scheme, textbooks chosen by parochial schools but not used by public schools are likely to be precisely the ones purchased by parents for their children's use.

***

For the first time, the Court has upheld financial support for religious schools without any reason at all to assume that the support will be restricted to the secular functions of those schools and will not be used to support religious instruction. This result is flatly at odds with the fundamental principle that a State may provide no financial support whatsoever to promote religion. *** I dissent.

ZOBREST v. CATALINA FOOTHILLS SCHOOL DISTRICT
509 U.S. 1 (1993)

CHIEF JUSTICE REHNQUIST delivered the opinion of the Court.

Petitioner James Zobrest, who has been deaf since birth, asked respondent school district to provide a sign-language interpreter to accompany him to classes at a Roman Catholic high school in Tucson, Arizona, pursuant to the Individuals with Disabilities Education Act (IDEA). *** While he attended public school, respondent furnished him with a sign-language interpreter. For religious reasons, James' parents (also petitioners here) enrolled him for the ninth grade in Salpointe Catholic High School, a sectarian institution.[2] When petitioners requested that respondent supply James with an interpreter at Salpointe, respondent referred the matter to the County Attorney, who concluded that providing an interpreter on the school's premises would violate the United States Constitution.

---

2. The parties have stipulated: "The two functions of secular education and advancement of religious values or beliefs are inextricably intertwined throughout the operations of Salpointe."

Petitioners then instituted this action. [They] asserted that the IDEA and the Free Exercise Clause of the First Amendment require respondent to provide James with an interpreter at Salpointe, and that the Establishment Clause does not bar such relief. *** The court thereafter granted respondent summary judgment, on the ground that "[t]he interpreter would act as a conduit for the religious inculcation of James—thereby, promoting James' religious development at government expense."

*** The Court of Appeals affirmed by a divided vote, applying the three-part test announced in Lemon v. Kurtzman, 403 U.S. 602, 613 (1971). *** We granted certiorari and now reverse. ***

[W]e have consistently held that government programs that neutrally provide benefits to a broad class of citizens defined without reference to religion are not readily subject to an Establishment Clause challenge just because sectarian institutions may also receive an attenuated financial benefit. Nowhere have we stated this principle more clearly than in Mueller v. Allen, 463 U.S. 388 (1983), and Witters v. Washington Dept. of Services for Blind, 474 U.S. 481 (1986), two cases dealing specifically with government programs offering general educational assistance. ***

*** In [*Witters*] we upheld against an Establishment Clause challenge the State of Washington's extension of vocational assistance, as part of a general state program, to a blind person studying at a private Christian college to become a pastor, missionary, or youth director. Looking at the statute as a whole, we observed that "[a]ny aid provided under Washington's program that ultimately flows to religious institutions does so only as a result of the genuinely independent and private choices of aid recipients." In light of these factors, we held that Washington's program —even as applied to a student who sought state assistance so that he could become a pastor—would not advance religion in a manner inconsistent with the Establishment Clause.

That same reasoning applies with equal force here. The service at issue in this case is part of a general government program that distributes benefits neutrally to any child qualifying as "handicapped" under the IDEA, without regard to the "sectarian-nonsectarian, or public-nonpublic nature" of the school the child attends. ***

Respondent contends, however, that this case differs from *Mueller* and *Witters*, in that petitioners seek to have a public employee physically present in a sectarian school to assist in James' religious education. In light of this distinction, respondent argues that this case more closely resembles Meek v. Pittenger, 421 U.S. 349 (1975), and School Dist. of Grand Rapids v. Ball, 473 U.S. 373 (1985). In *Meek*, we struck down a statute that, provided "massive aid" to private schools—more than 75% of which were church related—through a direct loan of teaching material and equipment. The material and equipment covered by the statute included maps, charts, and tape recorders. According to respondent, if the government could not place a tape recorder in a sectarian school in *Meek*, then it surely cannot place an interpreter in Salpointe. The statute in *Meek* also authorized state-paid personnel to furnish "auxiliary services"—which included remedial and accelerated instruction and guidance counseling—on the premises of religious schools. We determined that this part of the statute offended the First Amendment as well. *Ball* similarly involved two public programs that provided services on private school premises; there, public employees taught classes to students in private school classrooms.[9] We found that those programs likewise violated the Constitution, relying largely on *Meek*. According to respondent, if the government could not provide educational services on the premises of sectarian schools in *Meek* and *Ball*, then it surely cannot provide James with an interpreter on the premises of Salpointe.

Respondent's reliance on *Meek* and *Ball* is misplaced for two reasons. First, the programs in *Meek* and *Ball*—through direct grants of government aid—relieved sectarian schools of costs they otherwise would have borne in educating their students. *** So, too, was the case in *Ball*: The programs challenged there, which provided teachers in addition to instructional equipment and material, "in effect subsidize[d] the religious functions of the parochial schools by taking over a substantial portion of their responsibility for teaching secular subjects." "This kind of direct aid," we determined, "is indistinguishable from the provision of a direct cash subsidy to the religious school." The extension of aid to petitioners, however, does not amount to "an impermissible 'direct subsidy'" of Salpointe. For Salpointe is not relieved of an expense that it otherwise would have assumed in educating its students. *** Handicapped children, not sectarian schools, are the primary beneficiaries of the IDEA; to the extent sectarian schools benefit at all from the IDEA, they are only incidental beneficiaries.

Second, the task of a sign-language interpreter seems to us quite different from that of a teacher or guidance counselor. Notwithstanding the Court of Appeals' intimations to the contrary, the Establishment Clause lays down no absolute bar to the placing of a public employee in a sectarian school.[10] Such a flat rule, smacking of antiquated notions of "taint," would indeed exalt form over substance.[11] Nothing in this record suggests that a sign-language interpreter would do more than accurately interpret whatever material is presented to the class as a whole. In fact, ethical guidelines require interpreters to "transmit everything that is said in exactly the same way it was intended." *** James' parents have chosen of their own free will to place him

9. Forty of the forty-one private schools involved in *Ball* were pervasively sectarian.

10. For instance, in Wolman v. Walter, 433 U.S. 229, 242 (1977), we made clear that "the provision of health services to all schoolchildren—public and nonpublic—does not have the primary effect of aiding religion," even when those services are provided within sectarian schools. We accordingly rejected a First Amendment challenge to the State's providing diagnostic speech and hearing services on sectarian school premises. ***

11. Indeed, respondent readily admits, as it must, that there would be no problem under the Establishment Clause if the IDEA funds instead went directly to James' parents, who, in turn, hired the interpreter themselves. Brief for Respondent 11 ("If such were the case, then the sign language interpreter would be the student's employee, not the School District's, and governmental involvement in the enterprise would end with the disbursement of funds").

in a pervasively sectarian environment. The sign-language interpreter they have requested will neither add to nor subtract from that environment, and hence the provision of such assistance is not barred by the Establishment Clause.

The IDEA creates a neutral government program dispensing aid not to schools but to individual handicapped children. If a handicapped child chooses to enroll in a sectarian school, we hold that the Establishment Clause does not prevent the school district from furnishing him with a sign-language interpreter there in order to facilitate his education. The judgment of the Court of Appeals is therefore [r]eversed.

JUSTICE BLACKMUN, with whom JUSTICE SOUTER joins, and with whom JUSTICE STEVENS and JUSTICE O'CONNOR join as to Part I, dissenting.

Today, the Court *** holds that placement in a parochial school classroom of a public employee whose duty consists of relaying religious messages does not violate the Establishment Clause of the First Amendment. I disagree [and] therefore dissent.

*** Until now, the Court never has authorized a public employee to participate directly in religious indoctrination. Yet that is the consequence of today's decision.

Let us be clear about exactly what is going on here. The parties have stipulated to the following facts. Petitioner requested the State to supply him with a sign-language interpreter at Salpointe High School, a private Roman Catholic school operated by the Carmelite Order of the Catholic Church. Salpointe is a "pervasively religious" institution where "[t]he two functions of secular education and advancement of religious values or beliefs are inextricably intertwined." Salpointe's overriding "objective" is to "instill a sense of Christian values." Its "distinguishing purpose" is "the inculcation in its students of the faith and morals of the Roman Catholic Church." ***

At Salpointe, where the secular and the sectarian are "inextricably intertwined," governmental assistance to the educational function of the school necessarily entails governmental participation in the school's inculcation of religion. A state-employed sign-language interpreter would be required to communicate the material covered in religion class, the nominally secular subjects that are taught from a religious perspective, and the daily Masses at which Salpointe encourages attendance for Catholic students. In an environment so pervaded by discussions of the divine, the interpreter's every gesture would be infused with religious significance. ***

The majority attempts to elude the impact of the record by offering three reasons why this sort of aid to petitioners survives Establishment Clause scrutiny. First, the majority observes that provision of a sign-language interpreter occurs as "part of a general government program that distributes benefits neutrally to any child qualifying as 'handicapped' under the IDEA, without regard to the 'sectarian-nonsectarian, or public-nonpublic' nature of the school the child attends." Second, the majority finds significant the fact that aid is provided to pupils and their parents, rather than directly to sectarian schools. And, finally, the majority opines that "the task of a sign-language interpreter seems to us quite different from that of a teacher or guidance counselor."

But the majority's arguments are unavailing. As to the first two, even a general welfare program may have specific applications that are constitutionally forbidden under the Establishment Clause. For example, a general program granting remedial assistance to disadvantaged schoolchildren attending public and private, secular and sectarian schools alike would clearly offend the Establishment Clause insofar as it authorized the provision of teachers. Such a program would not be saved simply because it supplied teachers to secular as well as sectarian schools. Nor would the fact that teachers were furnished to pupils and their parents, rather than directly to sectarian schools, immunize such a program from Establishment Clause scrutiny. See Wolman v. Walter, 433 U.S. 229, 250 (1977) (it would "exalt form over substance if this distinction [between equipment loaned to the pupil or his parent and equipment loaned directly to the school] were found to justify a *** different" result); *Grand Rapids*, 473 U.S., at 395 (rejecting "fiction that a *** program could be saved by masking it as aid to individual students"). The majority's decision must turn, then, upon the distinction between a teacher and a sign-language interpreter.

"Although Establishment Clause jurisprudence is characterized by few absolutes," at a minimum "the Clause does absolutely prohibit government-financed or government-sponsored indoctrination into the beliefs of a particular religious faith." *Grand Rapids*, 473 U.S., at 385. See Bowen v. Kendrick, 487 U.S., at 623 (O'Connor, J., concurring) ("[*A*]*ny* use of public funds to promote religious doctrines violates the Establishment Clause") (emphasis in original); *** Levitt v. Committee for Public Education and Religious Liberty, 413 U.S. 472, 480 (1973) ("[T]he State is constitutionally compelled to assure that the state-supported activity is not being used for religious indoctrination"). *** Although the Court generally has permitted the provision of "secular and nonideological services unrelated to the primary, religion-oriented educational function of the sectarian school," *Meek*, 421 U.S., at 364, it has always proscribed the provision of benefits that afford even "the opportunity for the transmission of sectarian views," *Wolman*, 433 U.S., at 244. ***

[O]ur cases make clear that government crosses the boundary when it furnishes the medium for communication of a religious message. If petitioners receive the relief they seek, it is beyond question that a state-employed sign-language interpreter would serve as the conduit for petitioner's religious education, thereby assisting Salpointe in its mission of religious indoctrination. ***

Witters, and Mueller v. Allen, 463 U.S. 388 (1983), are not to the contrary. Those cases dealt with the payment of cash or a tax deduction, where governmental involvement ended with the disbursement of funds or lessening of tax. This case, on the other hand, involves ongoing, daily, and intimate governmental participation in the teaching and propagation of religious doctrine. When government dispenses public funds to individuals who employ them to finance private choices, it is difficult to argue that government is actually endorsing religion. But the graphic symbol of the concert of church and state that results when a public employee or instrumentality mouths a religious message is likely to "enlis[t]—at least in the eyes of impressionable youngsters—the powers of government to the support of the religious denomination operating the school." *Grand Rapids*, 473 U.S., at 385. ***

JUSTICE O'CONNOR, with whom JUSTICE STEVENS joins, dissenting. [Omitted.]

ROSENBERGER v. RECTOR AND VISITORS OF THE UNIVERSITY OF VIRGINIA

515 U.S. 819 (1995)

Justice KENNEDY delivered the opinion of the Court.* ***

III

Before its brief on the merits in this Court, the University had argued at all stages of the litigation that inclusion of WAP's contractors in SAF funding authorization would violate the Establishment Clause.** ***

The governmental program here is neutral toward religion. There is no suggestion that the University created it to advance religion or adopted some ingenious device with the purpose of aiding a religious cause. The object of the SAF is to open a forum for speech and to support various student enterprises, including the publication of newspapers, in recognition of the diversity and creativity of student life. The University's SAF Guidelines have a separate classification for, and do not make third-party payments on behalf of, "religious organizations," which are those "whose purpose is to practice a devotion to an acknowledged ultimate reality or deity." The category of support here is for "student news, information, opinion, entertainment, or academic communications media groups," of which Wide Awake was 1 of 15 in the 1990 school year. WAP did not seek a subsidy because of its Christian editorial viewpoint; it sought funding as a student journal, which it was.

The neutrality of the program distinguishes the student fees from a tax levied for the direct support of a church or group of churches. A tax of that sort, of course, would run contrary to Establishment Clause concerns dating from the earliest days of the Republic. The apprehensions of our predecessors involved the levying of taxes upon the public for the sole and exclusive purpose of establishing and

---

*. **[Ed. Note**: For a reminder of the parties, facts, and issues addressed in Parts I and II of this case, *see* p.457 *supra*.]

. **[Ed. Note. In brief, the university sought to defend its refusal to use student fees to pay for publications sponsored by Wide Awake Productions (WAP) partly on the basis that it was constrained by the Establishment Clause not to do so — that any use it might make of mandatory student fees to subsidize religious organizations *by underwriting the costs of their religious publications*, was forbidden by the Establishment Clause — the university so understood the decisions of the Supreme Court.]

supporting specific sects. The exaction here, by contrast, is a student activity fee designed to reflect the reality that student life in its many dimensions includes the necessity of wide-ranging speech and inquiry and that student expression is an integral part of the University's educational mission. The fee is mandatory, and we do not have before us the question whether an objecting student has the First Amendment right to demand a pro rata return to the extent the fee is expended for speech to which he or she does not subscribe.[***] See *Keller v. State Bar of Cal.*, 496 U.S. 1, 15-16 (1990); *Abood v. Detroit Bd. of Ed.*, 431 U.S. 209, 235-236 (1977). We must treat it, then, as an exaction upon the students. But the $14 paid each semester by the students is not a general tax designed to raise revenue for the University. The SAF cannot be used for unlimited purposes, much less the illegitimate purpose of supporting one religion. Much like the arrangement in *Widmar*, the money goes to a special fund from which any group of students with CIO status can draw for purposes consistent with the University's educational mission; and to the extent the student is interested in speech, withdrawal is permitted to cover the whole spectrum of speech, whether it manifests a religious view, an antireligious view, or neither. Our decision, then, cannot be read as addressing an expenditure from a general tax fund. Here, the disbursements from the fund go to private contractors for the cost of printing that which is protected under the Speech Clause of the First Amendment. This is a far cry from a general public assessment designed and effected to provide financial support for a church.

Government neutrality is apparent in the State's overall scheme in a further meaningful respect. "*** [T]he government has not fostered or encouraged" any mistaken impression that the student newspapers speak for the University. *Capitol Square Review and Advisory Bd. v. Pinette*, 515 U.S. 753, 766. ***

The Court of Appeals (and the dissent) are correct to extract from our decisions the principle that we have recognized special Establishment Clause dangers where the government makes direct money payments to sectarian institutions. The error is not in identifying the principle, but in believing that it controls this case. Even assuming that WAP is no different from a church and that its speech is the same as the religious exercises conducted in *Widmar* (two points much in doubt), the Court of Appeals decided a case that was, in essence, not before it, and the dissent would have us do the same. We do not confront a case where, even under a neutral program that includes nonsectarian recipients, the government is making direct money payments to an institution or group that is engaged in religious activity. Neither the Court of Appeals nor the dissent, we believe, takes sufficient cognizance of the undisputed fact that no public funds flow directly to WAP's coffers.

It does not violate the Establishment Clause for a public university to grant access to its facilities on a religion-neutral basis to a wide spectrum of student

---

***. [**Ed. Note**. For the Court's response to this claim, *See* Board of Regents of the University of Wisconsin v. Southworth, 529 U.S. 217 (2000), this casebook *supra* at p. 568.

groups, including groups that use meeting rooms for sectarian activities, accompanied by some devotional exercises. This is so even where the upkeep, maintenance, and repair of the facilities attributed to those uses are paid from a student activities fund to which students are required to contribute. The government usually acts by spending money. Even the provision of a meeting room involve[s] governmental expenditure, if only in the form of electricity and heating or cooling costs. *** [I]t follows that a public university may maintain its own computer facility and give student groups access to that facility, including the use of the printers, on a religion neutral, say first-come-first-served, basis. If a religious student organization obtained access on that religion-neutral basis and used a computer to compose or a printer or copy machine to print speech with a religious content or viewpoint, the State's action in providing the group with access would no more violate the Establishment Clause than would giving those groups access to an assembly hall. There is no difference in logic or principle, and no difference of constitutional significance, between a school using its funds to operate a facility to which students have access, and a school paying a third-party contractor to operate the facility on its behalf. ***

By paying outside printers, the University in fact attains a further degree of separation from the student publication, for it avoids the duties of supervision, escapes the costs of upkeep, repair, and replacement attributable to student use, and has a clear record of costs. ***

Were the dissent's view to become law, it would require the University, in order to avoid a constitutional violation, to scrutinize the content of student speech, lest the expression in question — speech otherwise protected by the Constitution — contain too great a religious content. The dissent, in fact, anticipates such censorship as "crucial" in distinguishing between "works characterized by the evangelism of Wide Awake and writing that merely happens to express views that a given religion might approve." That eventuality raises the specter of governmental censorship, to ensure that all student writings and publications meet some baseline standard of secular orthodoxy. To impose that standard on student speech at a university is to imperil the very sources of free speech and expression. ***

To obey the Establishment Clause, it was not necessary for the University to deny eligibility to student publications because of their viewpoint. The neutrality commanded of the State by the separate Clauses of the First Amendment was compromised by the University's course of action. The viewpoint discrimination inherent in the University's regulation required public officials to scan and interpret student publications to discern their underlying philosophic assumptions respecting religious theory and belief. That course of action was a denial of the right of free speech and would risk fostering a pervasive bias or hostility to religion, which could undermine the very neutrality the Establishment Clause requires. There is no Establishment Clause violation in the University's honoring its duties under the Free Speech Clause.

The judgment of the Court of Appeals must be, and is, reversed.

Justice O'CONNOR, concurring. [omitted]

Justice THOMAS, concurring. [omitted]*

Justice SOUTER, with whom Justice STEVENS, Justice GINSBURG, and Justice BREYER join, dissenting.

*** The masthead of every issue bears St. Paul's exhortation, that "[t]he hour has come for you to awake from your slumber, because our salvation is nearer now than when we first believed. Romans 13:11." Each issue of Wide Awake contained in the record makes good on the editor's promise and echoes the Apostle's call to accept salvation:

> "The only way to salvation through Him is by confessing and repenting of sin. It is the Christian's duty to make sinners aware of their need for salvation. Thus, Christians must confront and condemn sin, or else they fail in their duty of love."

Using public funds for the direct subsidization of preaching the word is categorically forbidden under the Establishment Clause, and if the Clause was meant to accomplish nothing else, it was meant to bar this use of public money. *** Four years before the First Congress proposed the First Amendment, Madison gave his opinion on the legitimacy of using public funds for religious purposes, in the Memorial and Remonstrance Against Religious Assessments, which played the central role in ensuring the defeat of the Virginia tax assessment bill in 1786 and framed the debate upon which the Religion Clauses stand:

> "Who does not see that ... the same authority which can force a citizen to contribute three pence only of his property for the support of any one establishment, may force him to conform to any other establishment in all cases whatsoever?"

Madison wrote against a background in which nearly every Colony had exacted a tax for church support, *Everson*, at 10, n. 8, the practice having become "so commonplace as to shock the freedom-loving colonials into a feeling of abhorrence." Madison's Remonstrance captured the colonists' "conviction that individual religious liberty could be achieved best under a government which was stripped of all power to tax, to support, or otherwise to assist any or all religions, or to interfere with the

*. **[Ed. Note.** Justice Thomas expressly joins "the Court's Opinion," but goes further; he aggressively takes issue with the "no direct financial aid" to religious organizations and proposes that cash subsidies, inclusive of religious organizations as a subset of a larger class, should not be deemed forbidden by the Establishment clause...]

beliefs of any religious individual or group."[1]

The principle against direct funding with public money is patently violated by the contested use of today's student activity fee.[3] Like today's taxes generally, the fee is Madison's threepence. The University exercises the power of the State to compel a student to pay it, and the use of any part of it for the direct support of religious activity thus strikes at what we have repeatedlyheld to be the heart of the prohibition on establishment. *** The Court, accordingly, has never before upheld direct state funding of the sort of proselytizing published in WideAwake and, in fact, has categorically condemned state programs directly aiding religious activity. ***

II

There is no viewpoint discrimination in the University's application of its Guidelines to deny funding to Wide Awake. Under those Guidelines, a "religious activit[y]," which is not eligible for funding, is "an activity which primarily promotes or manifests a particular belief(s) in or about a deity or an ultimate reality." It is clear that this is the basis on which Wide Awake Productions was denied funding. *** If the Guidelines were written or applied so as to limit only such Christian advocacy and no other evangelical efforts that might compete with it, the discrimination would be based on viewpoint. But that is not what the regulation authorizes; it applies to Muslim and Jewish and Buddhist advocacy as well as to Christian. And since it limits funding to activities promoting or manifesting a particular belief not only "in" but "about" a deity or ultimate reality, it applies to agnostics and atheists as well as it does to deists and theists as the University maintained at oral argument, and as the Court recognizes. ***

The Guidelines are thus substantially different from the access restriction

---

1. Justice THOMAS suggests that Madison would have approved of the assessment bill if only it had satisfied the principle of evenhandedness. Nowhere in the Remonstrance, however, did Madison advance the view that Virginia should be able to provide financial support for religion as part of a generally available subsidy program. Indeed, while Justice THOMAS claims that the "funding provided by the Virginia assessment was to be extended only to Christian sects," it is clear that the bill was more general in scope than this. While the bill, ***, provided that each taxpayer could designate a religious society to which he wanted his levy paid, it would also have allowed a taxpayer to refuse to appropriate his levy to any religious society, in which case the legislature was to use these unappropriated sums to fund "seminaries of learning" (contrary to Justice THOMAS's unsupported assertion, this portion of the bill was no less obligatory than any other). While some of these seminaries undoubtedly would have been religious in character, others would not have been, as a seminary was generally understood at the time to be "any school, academy, college or university, in which young persons are instructed in the several branches of learning which may qualify them for their future employments." N. Webster, An American Dictionary of the English Language (1st ed. 1828); *see also* 14 The Oxford English Dictionary 956 (2d ed.1989). Not surprisingly, then, scholars have generally agreed that the bill would have provided funding for nonreligious schools. ***

3. In the District Court, the parties agreed to the following facts: "The University of Virginia has charged at all times relevant herein and currently charges each full-time student a compulsory student activity fee of $14.00 per semester. There is no procedural or other mechanism by which a student may decline to pay the fee."

considered in *Lamb's Chapel,* the case upon which the Court heavily relies in finding a viewpoint distinction here. *Lamb's Chapel* addressed a school board's regulation prohibiting the after-hours use of school premises "by any group for religious purposes," even though the forum otherwise was open for a variety of social, civic, and recreational purposes. "Religious" was understood to refer to the viewpoint of a believer, and the regulation did not purport to deny access to any speaker wishing to express a non-religious or expressly antireligious point of view on any subject. *** With this understanding, it was unremarkable that in *Lamb's Chapel* we unanimously determined that the access restriction, as applied to a speaker wishing to discuss family values from a Christian perspective, impermissibly distinguished between speakers on the basis of viewpoint. Equally obvious is the distinction between that case and this one, where the regulation is being applied, not to deny funding for those who discuss issues in general from a religious viewpoint, but to those engaged in promoting or opposing religious conversion and religious observances as such. If this amounts to viewpoint discrimination, the Court has all but eviscerated the line between viewpoint and content. *** I respectfully dissent.

BOARD OF EDUCATION OF KIRYAS JOEL VILLAGE SCHOOL DISTRICT v. GRUMET
512 U.S. 687 (1994)

JUSTICE SOUTER delivered the opinion of the Court.

The Village of Kiryas Joel in Orange County, New York, is a religious enclave of Satmar Hasidim, practitioners of a strict form of Judaism. *** 20 years ago, the Satmars purchased an approved but undeveloped subdivision in the town of Monroe and began assembling the community that has since become the Village of Kiryas Joel. When a zoning dispute arose in the course of settlement, the Satmars presented the Town Board of Monroe with a petition to form a new village within the town, a right that New York's Village Law gives almost any group of residents who satisfy certain procedural niceties. [A]fter arduous negotiations the proposed boundaries of the Village of Kiryas Joel were drawn to include just the 320 acres owned and inhabited entirely by Satmars. *** Rabbi Aaron Teitelbaum, eldest son of the current Grand Rebbe, serves as the village rov (chief rabbi) and rosh yeshivah (chief authority in the parochial schools).

The residents of Kiryas Joel are vigorously religious people who make few concessions to the modern world and go to great lengths to avoid assimilation into it. They interpret the Torah strictly; segregate the sexes outside the home; speak Yiddish as their primary language; eschew television, radio, and English-language publications; and dress in distinctive ways that include headcoverings and special garments for boys and modest dresses for girls. Children are educated in private religious schools, most boys at the United Talmudic Academy where they receive a thorough grounding in the Torah and limited exposure to secular subjects, and most girls at Bais Rochel, an affiliated school with a curriculum designed to prepare girls for their roles as wives and mothers.

These schools do not, however, offer any distinctive services to handicapped children, who are entitled under state and federal law to special education services even when enrolled in private schools. Starting in 1984 the Monroe-Woodbury Central School District provided such services for the children of Kiryas Joel at an annex to Bais Rochel, but a year later ended that arrangement in response to our decisions in Aguilar v. Felton, 473 U.S. 402 (1985), and School Dist. of Grand Rapids v. Ball, 473 U.S. 373 (1985). Children from Kiryas Joel who needed special education (including the deaf, the mentally retarded, and others suffering from a range of physical, mental, or emotional disorders) were then forced to attend public schools outside the village, which their families found highly unsatisfactory. Parents of most of these children withdrew them from the Monroe-Woodbury secular schools, citing "the panic, fear and trauma [the children] suffered in leaving their own community and being with people whose ways were so different," and some sought administrative review of the public-school placements. ***

By 1989, only one child from Kiryas Joel was attending Monroe-Woodbury's public schools; the village's other handicapped children received privately funded special services or went without. It was then that the New York Legislature passed the statute at issue in this litigation, which provided that the Village of Kiryas Joel "is constituted a separate school district, *** and shall have and enjoy all the powers and duties of a union free school district. ***" The statute thus empowered a locally elected board of education to take such action as opening schools and closing them, hiring teachers, prescribing textbooks, establishing disciplinary rules, and raising property taxes to fund operations. In signing the bill into law, Governor Cuomo recognized that the residents of the new school district were "all members of the same religious sect," but said that the bill was "a good faith effort to solve th[e] unique problem" associated with providing special education services to handicapped children in the village.

Although it enjoys plenary legal authority over the elementary and secondary education of all school-aged children in the village, the Kiryas Joel Village School District currently runs only a special education program for handicapped children. The other village children have stayed in their parochial schools, relying on the new school district only for transportation, remedial education, and health and welfare services. If any child without handicap in Kiryas Joel were to seek a public-school education, the district would pay tuition to send the child into Monroe-Woodbury or another school district nearby. Under like arrangements, several of the neighboring districts send their handicapped Hasidic children into Kiryas Joel, so that two thirds of the full-time students in the village's public school come from outside. In all, the new district serves just over 40 full-time students, and two or three times that many parochial school students on a part-time basis.

Several months before the new district began operations, the New York State School Boards Association and respondents Grumet and Hawk brought this action against the State Education Department and various state officials, challenging Chapter 748 under the national and state constitutions as an unconstitutional establishment of religion. *** On cross-motions for summary judgment, the trial court ruled for the plaintiffs (respondents here), finding that the statute failed all three prongs of the test in Lemon v. Kurtzman, 403 U.S. 602 (1971), and was thus unconstitutional under both the National and State Constitutions.

A divided Appellate Division affirmed on the ground that Chapter 748 had the primary effect of advancing religion, in violation of both constitutions, and the state Court of Appeals affirmed on the federal question, while expressly reserving the state constitutional issue. *** We stayed the mandate of the Court of Appeals, and granted certiorari.

II

"A proper respect for both the Free Exercise and the Establishment Clauses compels the State to pursue a course of 'neutrality' toward religion," Committee for Public Ed. & Religious Liberty v. Nyquist, 413 U.S. 756, 792-793 (1973), favoring neither one religion over others nor religious adherents collectively over nonadherents. Chapter 748, the statute creating the Kiryas Joel Village School District, departs from this constitutional command by delegating the State's discretionary authority over public schools to a group defined by its character as a religious community, in a legal and historical context that gives no assurance that governmental power has been or will be exercised neutrally. ***

It is undisputed that those who negotiated the village boundaries when applying the general village incorporation statute drew them so as to exclude all but Satmars, and that the New York Legislature was well aware that the village remained exclusively Satmar in 1989 when it adopted Chapter 748. The significance of this fact to the state legislature is indicated by the further fact that carving out the village school district ran counter to customary districting practices in the State. Indeed, the trend in New York is not toward dividing school districts but toward consolidating them. The Kiryas Joel Village School District, in contrast, has only 13 local, full-time students in all (even including out-of-area and part-time students leaves the number under 200), and in offering only special education and remedial programs it makes no pretense to be a full-service district.

Because the district's creation ran uniquely counter to state practice, following the lines of a religious community where the customary and neutral principles would not have dictated the same result, we have good reasons to treat this district as the reflection of a religious criterion for identifying the recipients of civil authority. Not even the special needs of the children in this community can explain the legislature's unusual Act, for the State could have responded to the concerns of the Satmar parents without implicating the Establishment Clause, as we explain in some detail further on. We therefore find the legislature's Act to be substantially equivalent to defining a political subdivision and hence the qualification for its franchise by a religious test, resulting in a purposeful and forbidden "fusion of governmental and religious functions."

***

Because the religious community of Kiryas Joel did not receive its new governmental authority simply as one of many communities eligible for equal treatment under a general law,[7] we have no assurance that the next similarly situated group seeking a school district of its own will receive one; unlike an administrative agency's denial of an exemption from a generally applicable law, a legislature's failure to enact a special law is itself unreviewable. Nor can the historical context in this case furnish us with any reason to suppose that the Satmars are merely one in a series of communities receiving the benefit of special school district laws. *** [W]hat petitioners seek is an adjustment to the Satmars' religiously grounded preferences[9] that our cases do not countenance. Prior decisions have allowed religious communities and institutions to pursue their own interests free from governmental interference, see Zorach v. Clauson, 343 U.S. 306 (1952) (government may allow public schools to release students during the school day to receive off-site religious education), but we have never hinted that an otherwise unconstitutional delegation of political power to a religious group could be saved as a religious accommodation. Petitioners' proposed accommodation singles out a particular religious sect for special treatment, and whatever the limits of permissible legislative accommodations may be, it is clear that neutrality as among religions must be honored.

This conclusion does not, however, bring the Satmar parents, the Monroe-Woodbury school district, or the State of New York to the end of the road in seeking ways to respond to the parents' concerns. Such services can perfectly well be offered to village children through the Monroe-Woodbury Central School District. Since the Satmars do not claim that separatism is religiously mandated, their children may receive bilingual and bicultural instruction at a public school already run by the Monroe-Woodbury district. Or if the educationally appropriate offering by Monroe-Woodbury should turn out to be a separate program of bilingual and bicultural education at a neutral site near one of the village's parochial schools, this Court has already made it clear that no Establishment Clause difficulty would inhere in such a scheme, administered in accordance with neutral principles that would not necessarily confine special treatment to Satmars. ***

In this case we are clearly constrained to conclude that the statute before us fails

---

7. This contrasts with the process by which the Village of Kiryas Joel itself was created, involving, as it did, the application of a neutral state law designed to give almost any group of residents the right to incorporate.

9. The Board of Education of the Kiryas Joel Village School District explains that the Satmars prefer to live together "to facilitate individual religious observance and maintain social, cultural and religious values," but that it is not "'against their religion' to interact with others."

the test of neutrality. It delegates a power this Court has said "ranks at the very apex of the function of a State," Wisconsin v. Yoder, 406 U.S. 205, 213 (1972), to an electorate defined by common religious belief and practice, in a manner that fails to foreclose religious favoritism. It therefore crosses the line from permissible accommodation to impermissible establishment. The judgment of the Court of Appeals of the State of New York is accordingly [a]ffirmed.

JUSTICE BLACKMUN, concurring.

For the reasons stated by Justice Souter and Justice Stevens, whose opinions I join, I agree that the New York statute under review violates the Establishment Clause of the First Amendment. I write separately only to note my disagreement with any suggestion that today's decision signals a departure from the principles described in Lemon v. Kurtzman, 403 U.S. 602 (1971). ***

JUSTICE STEVENS, with whom JUSTICE BLACKMUN and JUSTICE GINSBURG join, concurring.

New York created a special school district for the members of the Satmar religious sect in response to parental concern that children suffered "panic, fear and trauma" when "leaving their own community and being with people whose ways were so different." To meet those concerns, the State could have taken steps to alleviate the children's fear by teaching their schoolmates to be tolerant and respectful of Satmar customs. Action of that kind would raise no constitutional concerns and would further the strong public interest in promoting diversity and understanding in the public schools.

Instead, the State responded with a solution that affirmatively supports a religious sect's interest in segregating itself and preventing its children from associating with their neighbors. The isolation of these children, while it may protect them from "panic, fear and trauma," also unquestionably increased the likelihood that they would remain within the fold, faithful adherents of their parents' religious faith. By creating a school district that is specifically intended to shield children from contact with others who have "different ways," the State provided official support to cement the attachment of young adherents to a particular faith. ***

Affirmative state action in aid of segregation of this character is unlike the evenhanded distribution of a public benefit or service, a "release time" program for public school students involving no public premises or funds, or a decision to grant an exemption from a burdensome general rule. It is, I believe, fairly characterized as establishing, rather than merely accommodating, religion. For this reason, as well as the reasons set out in Justice Souter's opinion, I am persuaded that the New York law at issue in these cases violates the Establishment Clause of the First Amendment.

JUSTICE O'CONNOR, concurring in part and concurring in the judgment.

*** Religious needs can be accommodated through laws that are neutral with regard to religion. *** This emphasis on equal treatment is, I think, an eminently sound approach. I join *** the Court's opinion because I think this law, rather than being a general accommodation, singles out a particular religious group for favorable treatment. *** Our invalidation of this statute in no way means that the Satmars' needs cannot be accommodated. There is nothing improper about a legislative intention to accommodate a religious group, so long as it is implemented through generally applicable legislation. New York may, for instance, allow all villages to operate their own school districts. If it does not want to act so broadly, it may set forth neutral criteria that a village must meet to have a school district of its own; these criteria can then be applied by a state agency, and the decision would then be reviewable by the judiciary. A district created under a generally applicable scheme would be acceptable even though it coincides with a village which was consciously created by its voters as an enclave for their religious group. I do not think the Court's opinion holds the contrary. ***

JUSTICE KENNEDY, concurring in the judgment.

The Court's ruling that the Kiryas Joel Village School District violates the Establishment Clause is in my view correct, but my reservations about what the Court's reasoning implies for religious accommodations in general are sufficient to require a separate writing. As the Court recognizes, a legislative accommodation that discriminates among religions may become an establishment of religion. But the Court's opinion can be interpreted to say that an accommodation for a particular religious group is invalid because of the risk that the legislature will not grant the same accommodation to another religious group suffering some similar burden. This rationale seems to me without grounding in our precedents and a needless restriction upon the legislature's ability to respond to the unique problems of a particular religious group. The real vice of the school district, in my estimation, is that New York created it by drawing political boundaries on the basis of religion. I would decide the issue we confront upon this narrower theory, though in accord with many of the Court's general observations about the State's actions in this case. ***

JUSTICE SCALIA, with whom THE CHIEF JUSTICE and JUSTICE THOMAS join, dissenting.

I

Unlike most of our Establishment Clause cases involving education, th[is] case involve[s] no public funding, however slight or indirect, to private religious schools. The school under scrutiny is a public school specifically designed to provide a public secular education to handicapped students. The superintendent of the school, who is not Hasidic, is a 20-year veteran of the New York City public school system, with expertise in the area of bilingual, bicultural, special education. The teachers and therapists at the school all live outside the village of Kiryas Joel. While the village's private schools are profoundly religious and strictly segregated by sex, classes at the public school are co-ed and the curriculum secular. The school building has the bland appearance of a public school, unadorned by religious symbols or markings;

and the school complies with the laws and regulations governing all other New York State public schools. In sum, these cases involve only public aid to a school that is public as can be. The only thing distinctive about the school is that all the students share the same religion. ***

For these very good reasons, JUSTICE SOUTER's opinion does not focus upon the school, but rather upon the school district and the New York Legislature that created it. His arguments, though sometimes intermingled, are two: that reposing governmental power in the Kiryas Joel School District is the same as reposing governmental power in a religious group; and that in enacting the statute creating the district, the New York State Legislature was discriminating on the basis of religion, *i.e.*, favoring the Satmar Hasidim over others. I shall discuss these arguments in turn.

II

For his thesis that New York has unconstitutionally conferred governmental authority upon the Satmar sect, JUSTICE SOUTER relies extensively, and virtually exclusively, upon Larkin v. Grendel's Den, Inc., 459 U.S. 116 (1982). *** The statute at issue there gave churches veto power over the State's authority to grant a liquor license to establishments in the vicinity of the church. *** The uniqueness of the case stemmed from the grant of governmental power directly to a religious institution, and the Court's opinion focused on that fact, remarking that the transfer of authority was to "churches" (10 times), the "governing body of churches" (twice), "religious institutions" (twice) and "religious bodies" (once).

JUSTICE SOUTER's steamrolling of the difference between civil authority held by a church, and civil authority held by members of a church, is breathtaking. To accept it, one must believe that large portions of the civil authority exercised during most of our history were unconstitutional, and that much more of it than merely the Kiryas Joel School District is unconstitutional today. *** If the conferral of governmental power upon a religious institution *as such* (rather than upon American citizens who belong to the religious institution) is not the test of *Grendel's Den* invalidity, there is no reason why giving power to a body that is overwhelmingly dominated by the members of one sect would not suffice to invoke the Establishment Clause. That might have made the entire States of Utah and New Mexico unconstitutional at the time of their admission to the Union,[1] and would undoubtedly make many units of local government unconstitutional today.[2] ***

---

1. A census taken in 1906, 10 years after statehood was granted to Utah, and 6 years before it was granted to New Mexico, showed that in Utah 87.7% of all church members were Mormon, and in New Mexico 88.7% of all church members were Roman Catholic. See Bureau of the Census, Special Reports, Religious Bodies, Part I, p. 55 (1910).

2. At the county level, the smallest unit for which comprehensive data is available, there are a number of counties in which the overwhelming majority of churchgoers are of a single religion: Rich County, Utah (100% Mormon); Kennedy County, Texas (100% Roman Catholic); Emery County, Utah (99.2% Mormon); Franklin and Madison Counties, Idaho (99% or more Mormon); Graham County, North Carolina (93.7% Southern Baptist); Mora County, New Mexico (92.6% Roman Catholic). ***

III

I turn, next, to JUSTICE SOUTER's second justification for finding an establishment of religion: his facile conclusion that the New York Legislature's creation of the Kiryas Joel School District was religiously motivated. But in the Land of the Free, democratically adopted laws are not so easily impeached by unelected judges. To establish the unconstitutionality of a facially neutral law on the mere basis of its asserted religiously preferential (or discriminatory) effects—or at least to establish it in conformity with our precedents—JUSTICE SOUTER "must be able to show the absence of a neutral, secular basis" for the law.

There is of course no possible doubt of a secular basis here. The New York Legislature faced a unique problem in Kiryas Joel: a community in which all the non-handicapped children attend private schools, and the physically and mentally disabled children who attend public school suffer the additional handicap of cultural distinctiveness. *** The handicapped children suffered sufficient emotional trauma from their predicament that their parents kept them home from school. Surely the legislature could target this problem, and provide a public education for these students, in the same way it addressed, *by a similar law*, the unique needs of children institutionalized in a hospital. See *e.g.*, 1970 N.Y. Laws, ch. 843 (authorizing a union free school district for the area owned by Blythedale Children's Hospital). *** There was really nothing so "special" about the formation of a school district by an Act of the New York Legislature. The State has created both large school districts, see *e.g.*, 1972 N.Y. Laws, ch. 928 (creating the Gananda School District out of land previously in two other districts), and small specialized school districts for institutionalized children, see *e.g.*, 1972 N.Y. Laws, ch. 559 (creating a union free school district for the area owned by Abbott House), through these special Acts. *** To be sure, when there is no special treatment there is no possibility of religious favoritism; but it is not logical to suggest that when there *is* special treatment there is *proof* of religious favoritism.

***

I have little doubt that JUSTICE SOUTER would laud this humanitarian legislation if all of the distinctiveness of the students of Kiryas Joel were attributable to the fact that their parents were nonreligious commune-dwellers, or American Indians, or gypsies. The creation of a special, one-culture school district for the benefit of those children would pose no problem. The neutrality demanded by the Religion Clauses requires the same indulgence towards cultural characteristics that are accompanied by religious belief. ***

The Court's decision today is astounding. Chapter 748 involves no public aid to private schools and does not mention religion. In order to invalidate it, the Court casts aside, on the flimsiest of evidence, the strong presumption of validity that attaches to facially neutral laws, and invalidates the present accommodation because it does not trust New York to be as accommodating toward other religions (presumably those less powerful than the Satmar Hasidim) in the future. This is unprece dented-except that it continues, and takes to new extremes, a recent tendency in the opinions of this Court to turn the Establishment Clause into a repealer of our Nation's tradition of religious toleration. I dissent.

NOTES AND SUBSEQUENT DEVELOPMENTS

In *Kiryas Joel*, as the Court noted in its Opinion, special education services were required by a federal spending measure designating how certain federal funds were to be spent in aid of certain "at-risk" elementary and secondary school children (Title I of the Elementary and Secondary Education Act of 1965, 20 U.S.C. § 6301 et seq). The act required special (remedial) services to be provided through the state to eligible students identified as students: (a) residing in a low-income area; and (b) disadvantaged in being at risk of failing, educationally, because of impaired hearing, mental retardation, or other physical, mental, or emotional disorders, whether attending a private school or a public school.

As noted in *Kiryas Joel*, these required services were first provided by the Monroe-Woodbury Central School District *on site* of the Satmar religious school, integrated in the daily operation of the school. As also noted, however, that arrangement had been discontinued because the Supreme Court had held that the direct, ongoing engagement of public school personnel in furnishing tax-supported educational services *administratively integrated* on parochial school premises was not permissible under the first or fourteenth amendments. Specifically, in *Aguilar v. Felton*, 473 U.S. 402 (1985), and *School Dist. of Grand Rapids v. Ball*, 473 U.S. 383 (1984) (a case involving "enrichment" programs rather than merely "remedial" programs as in *Aguilar*), the Court had held that such arrangements were inconsistent with the "primary effect" and "no entanglement" requirements of the three-part *Lemon* test.

After *Aguilar*, as also noted by the Court, the public school district had sought to supply such services by making arrangements for eligible children in the Satmar religious schools to receive the same services in nearby public schools of the Monroe-Woodbury Central School District.[1] This provision was satisfactory under the federal statute, but not satisfactory to the parents of the handicapped Hasidic children who, held out from the public school, now only "received privately funded special services or went without," until the New York legislature adopted the special legislation facilitating the "public school district" precisely tailored to the exact 320 acres "owned and inhabited entirely by Satmars." The New York law, in turn, was

---

1. In other instances, in New York and elsewhere, immediately following the Court's decisions in *Aguilar* and in *Ball*, suitably equipped mobile vans were utilized, parking nearby parochial schools, with arrangements made with the parochial schools to schedule eligible students to receive the special education services immediately adjacent to the parochial school.

held invalid (albeit by a sharply divided Court), as we have just seen, as a religious gerrymander — an impermissible act in aid of a religious establishment in *Kiryas Joel.*[2]

In *Kiryas Joel* itself, however, the Court also noted the case had come to the Court only one year after the Court's then-recent (5/4) decision in *Zobrest v. Catalina Foothills School Dist.*, 509 U.S. 1 (1993) (the case sustaining the use of an assigned public employee to serve as sign-language interpreter to a hearing impaired student in all of his classes inside a Catholic school. And in light of the Court's decision in *Zobrest,* several Justices openly expressed doubts in the *Kiryas Joel* case as to whether the Court's own prior decisions in *Aguilar* and *Ball* were reconcilable with the Court's (new?) view as reflected in *Zobrest.* And nearly at once, proceedings were reopened in federal district court in New York by those who had lost in *Aguilar*, seeking lifting of the injunction that had previously issued in *Aguilar.*

The case proceeded through the two lower federal courts both of which refused the request to lift the injunction, essentially on the ground that until the Supreme Court expressly addressed the issue and declared otherwise, they were bound by the decision in *Aguilar* as the "law of the case." Following grant of certiorari by the Supreme Court, however, on May 23, 1997, the Court did overrule both *Aguilar* and a portion of *Ball.* Excerpts from the principal Opinions by O'Connor, J., for the Court and in dissent by Souter, J. (joined by Stevens and Ginsburg, J.J., and by Breyer, J., as to Part II), immediately follow.

---

2. In an editor's note to Justice O'Connor's concurring opinion in *Kiryas Joel,* the question was raised whether a less targeted (i.e. "less targeted" solely to the village of Kiryas Joel) act of the New York legislature could be adopted, and whether, were such legislation to be adopted, pursuant to which the village were once again to form the same de facto wholly Satmar separate school district, it might now be sustained (i.e. as not void under the Establishment Clause). In fact the New York legislature did adopt such a law within two weeks. The "neutral criteria" were framed to ensure that the village of Kiryas Joel would qualify, and the village once again opted out of the Monroe-Woodbury school district. In the end, however, the New York Court of Appeals held the new state law invalid. The "neutral criteria" were such that few (if any) other municipalities within an existing school district could qualify; and the defendants in litigation acknowledged the law was enacted in direct response to the Supreme Court's decision in *Kiryas Joel,* and was designed explicitly to provide the Satmar village with a mechanism to secure their own school district. The New York Court of Appeals reasoned that chapter 241 was not a "religion-neutral law of general applicability" that Kiryas Joel happened to have invoked just as others might have. Chapter 241, the court concluded, simply replicated the prior unconstitutional law. See 90 N.Y.2d 57 (1997). The New York legislature did attempt a third time, using "neutral" criteria such that two municipalities (Kiryas Joel and one other) qualified, but the New York Court of Appeals again found the scheme unconstitutional. See *Grumet v. Pataki,* 93 N.Y. 2d 677,720 N.E. 2d 66 (N.Y. 1999), *cert. pending.* The Court's subsequent decision in *Agostini* 93 N.Y 2d 677, *cert. denied,* 528 U.S. 546 (1999) may offer the Satmar Hasidim in question another alternative.

AGOSTINI v. FELTON

117 U.S. 771 (1997)

JUSTICE O'CONNOR delivered the opinion of the Court. ***

III (A)

In order to evaluate whether *Aguilar* has been eroded by our subsequent Establishment Clause cases, it is necessary to understand the rationale upon which *Aguilar*, as well as its companion case, *School Dist. of Grand Rapids v. Ball*, 473 U.S. 373 (1985), rested.

In *Ball*, the Court evaluated two programs implemented by the School District of Grand Rapids, Michigan. The district's Shared Time program, the one most analogous to Title I, provided remedial and "enrichment" classes, at public expense, to students attending nonpublic schools. The classes were taught during regular school hours by publicly employed teachers, using materials purchased with public funds, on the premises of nonpublic schools. *** Our cases subsequent to *Aguilar* [and *Ball*]have *** abandoned the presumption *** that the placement of public employees on parochial school grounds inevitably results in the impermissible effect of state-sponsored indoctrination or constitutes a symbolic union between government and religion. In *Zobrest v. Catalina Foothills School Dist.*, we examined whether the IDEA, 20 U.S.C. § 1400 et seq., was constitutional as applied to a deaf student who sought to bring his state-employed sign-language interpreter with him to his Roman Catholic high school. *** Because the only government aid in *Zobrest* was the interpreter, who was herself not inculcating any religious messages, no government indoctrination took place and we were able to conclude that "the provision of such assistance [was] not barred by the Establishment Clause." *Zobrest* therefore expressly rejected the notion — relied on in *Ball* and *Aguilar* — that, solely because of her presence on private school property, a public employee will be presumed to inculcate religion in the students. *Zobrest* also implicitly repudiated another assumption on which *Ball* and *Aguilar* turned: that the presence of a public employee on private school property creates an impermissible "symbolic link" between government and religion. ***

Second, we have departed from the rule relied on in *Ball* that all government aid that directly aids the educational function of religious schools is invalid. In *Witters v. Washington Dept. of Servs. for Blind*, 474 U.S. 481 (1986), we held that the Establishment Clause did not bar a State from issuing a vocational tuition grant to a blind person who wished to use the grant to attend a Christian college and become a pastor, missionary, or youth director. *** The grants were disbursed directly to students, who then used the money to pay for tuition at the educational institution of their choice. ***

Zobrest and *Witters* make clear that, under current law, the Shared Time program in *Ball* and New York City's Title I program in *Aguilar* will not, as a matter of law, be deemed to have the effect of advancing religion through indoctrination. ***

In all relevant respects, the provision of instructional services under Title I is indistinguishable from the provision of sign-language interpreters under the IDEA. Both programs make aid available only to eligible recipients. That aid is provided to students at whatever school they choose to attend. Although Title I instruction is provided to several students at once, whereas an interpreter provides translation to a single student, this distinction is not constitutionally significant. Moreover, as in *Zobrest*, Title I services are by law supplemental to the regular curricula. These services do not, therefore, "reliev[e] sectarian schools of costs they otherwise would have borne in educating their students." *** No Title I funds ever reach the coffers of religious schools, compare *Committee for Public Ed. & Religious Liberty v. Regan*, (involving a program giving "direct cash reimbursement" to religious schools for performing certain state- mandated tasks), and Title I services may not be provided to religious schools on a school-wide basis, 34 CFR § 200.12(b) (1996). Title I funds are instead distributed to a public agency (an LEA) that dispenses services directly to the eligible students within its boundaries, no matter where they choose to attend school. ***

What is most fatal to the argument that New York City's Title I program directly subsidizes religion is that it applies with equal force when those services are provided off-campus, and *Aguilar* implied that providing the services off-campus is entirely consistent with the Establishment Clause. JUSTICE SOUTER resists the impulse to upset this implication, contending that it can be justified on the ground that Title I services are "less likely to supplant some of what would otherwise go on inside [the sectarian schools] and to subsidize what remains" when those services are offered off-campus. But JUSTICE SOUTER does not explain why a sectarian school would not have the same incentive to "make patently significant cut-backs" in its curriculum no matter where Title I services are offered, since the school would ostensibly be excused from having to provide the Title I-type services itself. Because the incentive is the same either way, we find no logical basis upon which to conclude that Title I services are an impermissible subsidy of religion when offered on-campus, but not when offered off-campus. ***

***

We turn now to *Aguilar*'s conclusion that New York City's Title I program resulted in an excessive entanglement between church and state. Whether a government aid program results in such an entanglement has consistently been an aspect of our Establishment Clause analysis. *** [T]he Court's finding of "excessive" entanglement in *Aguilar* rested on three grounds: (I) the program would require "pervasive monitoring by public authorities" to ensure that Title I employees did not inculcate religion; (ii) the program required "administrative cooperation" between the Board and parochial schools; and (iii) the program might increase the dangers of "political divisiveness." Under our current understanding of the Establishment Clause, the last two considerations are insufficient by themselves to create an "excessive" entanglement. They are present no matter where Title I services are offered, and no court has held that Title I services cannot be offered off-campus. Further, the assumption underlying the first consideration has been undermined. *** [A]fter *Zobrest* we no longer presume that public employees will inculcate religion simply because they happen to be in a sectarian environment. ***

To summarize, New York City's Title I program does not run afoul of any of three primary criteria we currently use to evaluate whether government aid has the effect of advancing religion: it does not result in governmental indoctrination; define its recipients by reference to religion; or create an excessive entanglement. *** Accordingly, we must acknowledge that *Aguilar*, as well as the portion of *Ball* addressing Grand Rapids' Shared Time program, are no longer good law. ***

JUSTICE SOUTER, with whom JUSTICE STEVENS and JUSTICE GINSBURG join, and with whom JUSTICE BREYER joins as to Part II, dissenting.

I believe *Aguilar* was a correct and sensible decision, and my only reservation about its opinion is that the emphasis on the excessive entanglement produced by monitoring religious instructional content obscured those facts that independently called for the application of two central tenets of Establishment Clause jurisprudence. The State is forbidden to subsidize religion directly and is just as surely forbidden to act in any way that could reasonably be viewed as religious endorsement. ***

These principles were violated by the programs at issue in *Aguilar* and *Ball*, as a consequence of several significant features common to both Title I, as implemented in New York City before *Aguilar*, and the Grand Rapids Shared Time program: each provided classes on the premises of the religious schools, covering a wide range of subjects including some at the core of primary and secondary education, like reading and mathematics; while their services were termed "supplemental," the programs and their instructors necessarily assumed responsibility for teaching subjects that the religious schools would otherwise have been obligated to provide, *** Calling some classes remedial does not distinguish their subjects from the schools' basic subjects, however inadequately the schools may have been addressing them. ***

It may be objected that there is some subsidy in remedial education even when it takes place off the religious premises, some subsidy, that is, even in the way New York City has administered the Title I program after *Aguilar*. In these circumstances, too, what the State does, the religious school need not do; the schools save money and the program makes it easier for them to survive and concentrate their resources on their religious objectives. This argument may, of course, prove too much, but if it is not thought strong enough to bar even off-premises aid in teaching the basics to religious school pupils (an issue not before the Court in *Aguilar* or today), it does nothing to undermine the sense of drawing a line between remedial teaching on and off-premises. The off-premises teaching is arguably less likely to open the door to relieving religious schools of their responsibilities for secular subjects ***. On top of that, the difference in the degree of reasonably perceptible endorsement is substantial. Sharing the teaching responsibilities within a school having religious objectives is far more likely to telegraph approval of the school's mission than keeping the State's distance would do. *** As the Court observed in *Ball*, "[t]he symbolism of a union between church and state [effected by placing the public school teachers into the religious schools] is most likely to influence children of tender years, whose experience is limited and whose beliefs consequently are the function of environment as much as of free and voluntary choice." *** In sum, if a line is to be drawn short of barring all state aid to religious schools for teaching standard subjects, the *Aguilar-Ball* line was a sensible one capable of principled adherence. ***

II

Zobrest held that the Establishment Clause does not prevent a school district from providing a sign-language interpreter to a deaf student enrolled in a sectarian school. *** [T]he Court did indeed recognize that the Establishment Clause lays down no absolute bar to placing public employees in a sectarian school, but the rejection of such a per se rule was hinged expressly on the nature of the employee's job, sign- language interpretation (or signing) and the circumscribed role of the signer. *** The signer could thus be seen as more like a hearing aid than a teacher, and the signing could not be understood as an opportunity to inject religious content in what was supposed to be secular instruction. *** *Zobrest* did not, implicitly or otherwise, repudiate the view that the involvement of public teachers in the instruction provided within sectarian schools looks like a partnership or union and implies approval of the sectarian aim. On the subject of symbolic unions and the strength of their implications, the lesson of *Zobrest* is merely that less is less. *** *Witters* and *Zobrest* did nothing to repudiate the principle, emphasizing rather the limited nature of the aid at issue in each case as well as the fact that religious institutions did not receive it directly from the State.

It is accordingly puzzling to find the Court insisting that the aid scheme administered under Title I and considered in *Aguilar* was comparable to the programs in *Witters* and *Zobrest*. Instead of aiding isolated individuals within a school system, New York City's Title I program before *Aguilar* served about 22,000 private school students, all but 52 of whom attended religious schools. Instead of serving individual blind or deaf students, as such, Title I as administered in New York City before *Aguilar* (and as now to be revived) funded instruction in core subjects (remedial reading, reading skills, remedial mathematics, English as a second language) and provided guidance services. Instead of providing a service the school would not otherwise furnish, the Title I services necessarily relieved a religious school of "an expense that it otherwise would have assumed," and freed its funds for other, and sectarian uses.

Finally, instead of aid that comes to the religious school indirectly in the sense that its distribution results from private decisionmaking, a public educational agency distributes Title I aid in the form of programs and services directly to the religious schools. In sum, nothing since *Ball* and *Aguilar* and before this case has eroded the distinction between "direct and substantial" and "indirect and incidental." That principled line is being breached only here and now. ***

JUSTICE GINSBURG, with whom JUSTICE STEVENS, JUSTICE SOUTER, and JUSTICE BREYER join, dissenting. [Omitted.]

GUY MITCHELL ET AL., v. MARY L. HELMS ET AL.
530 U.S. 793 (2000)

Justice THOMAS announced the judgment of the Court and delivered an opinion, in which The Chief Justice, Justice SCALIA, and Justice KENNEDY join.

As part of a longstanding school aid program known as Chapter 2, the Federal Government distributes funds to state and local governmental agencies, which in turn lend educational materials and equipment to public and private schools, with the enrollment of each participating school determining the amount of aid that it receives. The question is whether Chapter 2, as applied in Jefferson Parish, Louisiana, is a law respecting an establishment of religion, because many of the private schools receiving Chapter 2 aid in that parish are religiously affiliated. We hold that Chapter 2 is not such a law.

Chapter 2 of the Education Consolidation and Improvement Act of 1981,—is a close cousin of the provision of the ESEA that we recently considered in *Agostini* v. *Felton*. Like the provision at issue in *Agostini*, Chapter 2 channels federal funds to local educational agencies (LEAs), which are usually public school districts, via state educational agencies (SEAs), to implement programs to assist children in elementary and secondary schools. Among other things, Chapter 2 provides aid

> "for the acquisition and use of instructional and educational materials, including library services and materials (including media materials), assessments, reference materials, computer software and hardware for instructional use, and other curricular materials."

LEAs and SEAs must offer assistance to both public and private schools (although any private school must be nonprofit). Participating private schools receive Chapter 2 aid based on the number of children enrolled in each school

Several restrictions apply to aid to private schools. Most significantly, the "services, materials, and equipment" provided to private schools must be "secular, neutral, and nonideological." In addition, private schools may not acquire control of Chapter 2 funds or title to Chapter 2 materials, equipment, or property. A private school receives the materials and equipment by submitting to the LEA an application detailing which items the school seeks and how it will use them; the LEA, if it approves the application, purchases those items from the school's allocation of funds, and then lends them to that school.

In the 1986–1987 fiscal year, 44% of the money budgeted for private schools in Jefferson Parish was spent by LEAs for acquiring library and media materials, and 48% for instructional equipment. Among the materials and equipment provided have been library books, computers, and computer software, and also slide and movie projectors, overhead projectors, television sets, tape recorders, VCR's, projection screens, laboratory equipment, maps, globes, filmstrips, slides, and cassette recordings.

About 30% of Chapter 2 funds spent in Jefferson Parish are allocated for private schools. For 1987, 46 participated, and the participation level has remained relatively constant since then. Of these 46, 34 were Roman Catholic; 7 were otherwise religiously affiliated; and 5 were not religiously affiliated.

***

II

The Establishment Clause of the First Amendment dictates that "Congress shall make no law respecting an establishment of religion." In the over 50 years since *Everson*, we have consistently struggled to apply these simple words in the context of governmental aid to religious schools. *** In *Agostini*, we brought some clarity to our case law, by overruling two anomalous precedents (one in whole, the other in part) and by consolidating some of our previously disparate considerations under a revised test. Whereas in *Lemon* we had considered whether a statute (1) has a secular purpose, (2) has a primary effect of advancing or inhibiting religion, or (3) creates an excessive entanglement between government and religion, in *Agostini* we modified *Lemon* for purposes of evaluating aid to schools and examined only the first and second factors. *** We then set out revised criteria for determining the effect of a statute:

> "To summarize, New York City's Title I program does not run afoul of any of three primary criteria we currently use to evaluate whether government aid has the effect of advancing religion: It does not result in governmental indoctrination; define its recipients by reference to religion; or create an excessive entanglement."

In this case, our inquiry under *Agostini*'s purpose and effect test is a narrow one. Because respondents do not challenge the District Court's holding that Chapter 2 has a secular purpose, and because the Fifth Circuit also did not question that holding, we will consider only Chapter 2's effect. Further, in determining that effect, we will consider only the first two *Agostini* criteria, since neither respondents nor the Fifth Circuit has questioned the District Court's holding, that Chapter 2 does not create an excessive entanglement. Considering Chapter 2 in light of our more recent case law, we conclude that it neither results in religious indoctrination by the government nor defines its recipients by reference to religion. We therefore hold that Chapter 2 is not a "law respecting an establishment of religion." In so holding, we acknowledge — *Meek* and *Wolman* are anomalies in our case law. We therefore conclude that they are no longer good law.

A

***

In distinguishing between indoctrination that is attributable to the State and indoctrination that is not, we have consistently turned to the principle of neutrality, upholding aid that is offered to a broad range of groups or persons without regard to their religion. If the religious, irreligious, and areligious are all alike eligible for governmental aid, no one would conclude that any indoctrination that any particular recipient conducts has been done at the behest of the government. For attribution of indoctrination is a relative question. If the government is offering assistance to recipients who provide, so to speak, a broad range of indoctrination, the government itself is not thought responsible for any particular indoctrination. To put the point differently, if the government, seeking to further some legitimate secular purpose, offers aid on the same terms, without regard to religion, to all who adequately further that purpose, — then it is fair to say that any aid going to a religious recipient only has the effect of furthering that secular purpose. *** As a way of assuring neutrality, we have repeatedly considered whether any governmental aid that goes to a religious institution does so "only as a result of the genuinely independent and private choices of individuals." ***

The principles of neutrality and private choice, and their relationship to each other, were prominent not only in *Agostini*, but also in *Zobrest*, *Witters*, and *Mueller*. The heart of our reasoning in *Zobrest*, upholding governmental provision of a sign language interpreter to a deaf student at his Catholic high school, was as follows:

> ***[that] because the [statute] creates no financial incentive for parents to choose a sectarian school, an interpreter's presence there cannot be attributed to state decisionmaking."

As this passage indicates, the private choices helped to ensure neutrality, and neutrality and private choices together eliminated any possible attribution to the government even when the interpreter translated classes on Catholic doctrine. ***

The second criterion requires a court to consider whether an aid program "define[s] its recipients by reference to religion." As we briefly explained in *Agostini*, this second criterion looks to the same set of facts as does our focus, under the first criterion, on neutrality, but the second criterion uses those facts to answer a somewhat different question—whether the criteria for allocating the aid "creat[e] a financial incentive to undertake religious indoctrination." In *Agostini* we set out the following rule for answering this question:

> "This incentive is not present where the aid is allocated on the basis of neutral, secular criteria that neither favor nor disfavor religion, and is made available to both religious and secular beneficiaries on a nondiscriminatory basis.***

We hasten to add, what should be obvious from the rule itself, that simply because an aid program offers private schools, and thus religious schools, a benefit that they did not previously receive does not mean that the program, by reducing the cost of securing a religious education, creates, under *Agostini*'s second criterion, an "incentive" for parents to choose such an education for their children. For *any* aid will have some such effect.

B

Respondents *** argue first, and chiefly, that "direct, nonincidental" aid to the primary educational mission of religious is always impermissible. Second, they argue that provision to religious schools of aid that is divertible to religious use is similarly impermissible.[7] Respondents' arguments are inconsistent with our more recent case law, in particular *Agostini* and *Zobrest*, and we therefore reject them.

1

If aid to schools, even "direct aid," is neutrally available and, before reaching or benefiting any religious school, first passes through the hands (literally or figuratively) of numerous private citizens who are free to direct the aid elsewhere, the government has not provided any "support of religion." Although the presence of private choice is easier to see when aid literally passes through the hands of individuals—which is why we have mentioned directness in the same breath with private choice,— there is no reason why the Establishment Clause requires such a form.

***

[R]espondents' formalistic line breaks down in the application to real-world programs. In *Allen*, for example, although we did recognize that students themselves received and owned the textbooks, we also noted that the books provided were those that the private schools required for courses, that the schools could collect students' requests for books and submit them to the board of education, that the schools could store the textbooks, and that the textbooks were essential to the schools' teaching of secular subjects. Whether one chooses to label this program "direct" or "indirect" is a rather arbitrary choice, one that does not further the constitutional analysis.

Of course, we have seen "special Establishment Clause dangers," when *money* is given to religious schools or entities directly rather than, as in *Witters* and *Mueller*, indirectly.[8] But direct payments of money are not at issue in this case, and we refuse to allow a "special" case to create a rule for all cases.

2

Respondents also contend that the Establishment Clause requires that aid to religious schools not be impermissibly religious in nature or be divertible to religious

---

7. Respondents also contend that Chapter 2 aid supplants, rather than supplements, the core educational function of parochial schools and therefore has the effect of furthering religion. Our case law does provide some indication that this distinction may be relevant to determining whether aid results in governmental indoctrination, but we have never delineated the distinction's contours or held that it is constitutionally required.

8. The reason for such concern is not that the form *per se* is bad, but that such a form creates special risks that governmental aid will have the effect of advancing religion (or, even more, a purpose of doing so). An indirect form of payment reduces these risks. It is arguable, however, at least after *Witters*, that the principles of neutrality and private choice would be adequate to address those special risks, for it is hard to see the basis for deciding *Witters* differently simply if the State had sent the tuition check directly to whichever school Witters chose to attend.

use. We agree with the first part of this argument but not the second. Respondents' "no divertibility" rule is inconsistent with our more recent case law and is unworkable. So long as the governmental aid is not itself "unsuitable for use in the public schools because of religious content," and eligibility for aid is determined in a constitutionally permissible manner, any use of that aid to indoctrinate cannot be attributed to the government and is thus not of constitutional concern. *** The issue is not divertibility of aid but rather whether the aid itself has an impermissible content. Where the aid would be suitable for use in a public school, it is also suitable for use in any private school.

A concern for divertibility, as opposed to improper content, is misplaced not only because it fails to explain why the sort of aid that we have allowed is permissible, but also because it is boundless—enveloping all aid, no matter how trivial—and thus has only the most attenuated (if any) link to any realistic concern for preventing an "establishment of religion." Presumably, for example, government-provided lecterns, chalk, crayons, pens, paper, and paintbrushes would have to be excluded from religious schools under respondents' proposed rule.***

C

*** One of the dissent's factors deserves special mention: whether a school that receives aid (or whose students receive aid) is pervasively sectarian. The dissent is correct that there was a period when this factor mattered, particularly if the pervasively sectarian school was a primary or secondary school. But that period is one that the Court should regret, and it is thankfully long past.

There are numerous reasons to formally dispense with this factor. First, its relevance in our precedents is in sharp decline. Although our case law has consistently mentioned it even in recent years, we have not struck down an aid program in reliance on this factor since 1985.***

Hostility to aid to pervasively sectarian schools has a shameful pedigree that we do not hesitate to disavow. ***Opposition to aid to "sectarian" schools acquired prominence in the 1870' s with Congress's consideration (and near passage) of the Blaine Amendment, which would have amended the Constitution to bar any aid to sectarian institutions. Consideration of the amendment arose at a time of pervasive hostility to the Catholic Church and to Catholics in general, and it was an open secret that "sectarian" was code for "Catholic."***

In short, nothing in the Establishment Clause requires the exclusion of pervasively sectarian schools from otherwise permissible aid programs, and other doctrines of this Court bar it. This doctrine, born of bigotry, should be buried now.

III

Applying the two relevant *Agostini* criteria, we see no basis for concluding that Jefferson Parish's Chapter 2 program "has the effect of advancing religion." Chapter 2 does not result in governmental indoctrination, because it determines eligibility for aid neutrally, allocates that aid based on the private choices of the parents of schoolchildren, and does not provide aid that has an impermissible content. Nor does Chapter 2 define its recipients by reference to religion.

Chapter 2 also satisfies the first *Agostini* criterion. The program makes a broad array of schools eligible for aid without regard to their religious affiliations or lack thereof. We therefore have no difficulty concluding that Chapter 2 is neutral with regard to religion. Chapter 2 aid also, like the aid in *Agostini*, *Zobrest*, and *Witters*, reaches participating schools only "as a consequence of private decisionmaking."***

Because Chapter 2 aid is provided pursuant to private choices, it is not problematic that one could fairly describe Chapter 2 as providing "direct" aid. The ultimate beneficiaries of Chapter 2 aid are the students who attend the schools that receive that aid, and this is so regardless of whether individual students lug computers to school each day or, as Jefferson Parish has more sensibly provided, the schools receive the computers.

***

There is evidence that equipment has been, or at least easily could be, diverted for use in religious classes. *** [W]e agree with the dissent that there is evidence of actual diversion and that, were the safeguards anything other than anemic, there would almost certainly be more such evidence. [F]or reasons we discussed in Part II–B–2, *supra*, the evidence of actual diversion and the weakness of the safeguards against actual diversion are not relevant to the constitutional inquiry, whatever relevance they may have under the statute and regulations.

***

The judgment of the Fifth Circuit is reversed.

JUSTICE O' CONNOR, with whom JUSTICE BREYER joins, concurring in the judgment.

To the extent our decisions in *Meek* v. *Pittenger*, and *Wolman* v. *Walter*, are inconsistent with the Court's judgment today, I agree that those decisions should be overruled....

[T]wo specific aspects of the opinion compel me to write separately. First, the plurality's treatment of neutrality comes close to assigning that factor singular importance in the future adjudication of Establishment Clause challenges to government school-aid programs. Second, the plurality's approval of actual diversion of government aid to religious indoctrination is in tension with our precedents and, in any event, unnecessary to decide the instant case.***

I

[W]e have never held that a government-aid program passes constitutional muster *solely* because of the neutral criteria it employs as a basis for distributing aid. For example, in *Agostini*, neutrality was only one of several factors we considered in determining that New York City's Title I program did not have the impermissible effect of advancing religion. See *Agostini* at 226–228 (noting lack of evidence of inculcation of religion by Title I instructors, legal requirement that Title I services be supplemental to regular curricula, and that no Title I funds reached religious schools' coffers). ***

I also disagree with the plurality's conclusion that actual diversion of government aid to religious indoctrination is consistent with the Establishment Clause. In both *Agostini*, and *Allen*, we rested our approval of the relevant programs in part on the fact that the aid had not been used to advance the religious missions of the recipient schools.***

The plurality bases its holding that actual diversion is permissible on *Witters* and *Zobrest*. *Ante*, at 21–22. Those decisions, however, rested on a significant factual premise missing from this case, as well as from the majority of cases thus far considered by the Court involving Establishment Clause challenges to school-aid programs. Specifically, we decided *Witters* and *Zobrest* on the understanding that the aid was provided directly to the individual student who, in turn, made the choice of where to put that aid to use. ***Like JUSTICE SOUTER, I do not believe that we should treat a per-capita-aid program the same as the true private-choice programs considered in *Witters* and *Zobrest*.

First, when the government provides aid directly to the student beneficiary, that student can attend a religious school and yet retain control over whether the secular government aid will be applied toward the religious education. The fact that aid flows to the religious school and is used for the advancement of religion is therefore *wholly* dependent on the student's private decision. ***

Second, I believe the distinction between a per-capita school-aid program and a true private-choice program is significant for purposes of endorsement. ***Because the religious indoctrination is supported by government assistance, the reasonable observer would naturally perceive the aid program as *government* support for the advancement of religion. ***

Finally, the distinction between a per-capita-aid program and a true private-choice program is important when considering aid that consists of direct monetary subsidies. ***To be sure, the plurality does not actually hold that its theory extends to direct money payments.... That omission, however, is of little comfort. In its logic as well as its specific advisory language,...the plurality opinion foreshadows the approval of direct monetary subsidies to religious organizations, even when they use the money to advance their religious objectives. ***For these reasons, as well as my disagreement with the plurality's approach, I would decide today's case by applying the criteria set forth in *Agostini*.

II

Like the Title I program considered in *Agostini*, all Chapter 2 funds are controlled by public agencies—the SEAs and LEAs. The LEAs purchase instructional and educational materials and then lend those materials to public and private schools. [T]he statute provides that all Chapter 2 materials and equipment must be "secular, neutral, and nonideological." That restriction is reinforced by a further statutory prohibition on "the making of any payment...for religious worship or instruction." Although respondents claim that Chapter 2 aid has been diverted to religious instruction, that evidence is *de minimis*....

*** Because I believe that the Court should abandon the presumption adopted in *Meek* and *Wolman* respecting the use of instructional materials and equipment by religious-school teachers, I see no constitutional need for*pervasive* monitoring under the Chapter 2 program.

[A]t the state level, the Louisiana Department of Education (the relevant SEA for Louisiana) requires all nonpublic schools to submit signed assurances that they will use Chapter 2 aid only to supplement and not to supplant non-Federal funds, and that the instructional materials and equipment "will only be used for secular, neutral and nonideological purposes."*** Regardless of whether these factors are constitutional requirements, they are surely sufficient to find that the program at issue here does not have the impermissible effect of advancing religion. For the same reasons, "this carefully constrained program also cannot reasonably be viewed as an endorsement of religion."

Accordingly, I concur in the judgment.

JUSTICE SOUTER, with whom JUSTICE STEVENS and JUSTICE GINSBURG join, dissenting. *

[Justice Souter begins the dissent by reasserting a bedrock principle to which, he says, all nine Justices subscribed, in *Everson v. Board of Education*.[2] All agreed, in *Everson*, that the establishment clause forbids the state to use public funds to subsidize or to support religious establishments as such,[3] consistent with the principle putting every religion on an independent foundation of voluntarism (rather than "state support").

It follows, and so the Court had consistently held (and indeed could not hold otherwise), that insofar as a religious school is itself established by a church or

---

*. **[Ed. Note**: The dissent by Justice Souter, joined by Justice Stevens and Justice Ginsburg, is both elaborate and complex. It reviews virtually all of the Court's establishment clause doctrinal history and case law, and fills a full fifty pages in the U.S. Reports. The following edited summary is, unavoidably, a very severe abridgment. (So, for example, it entirely omits his elaborate review of previous cases–to explain, reconcile, defend, and account for the critical distinctions students have struggled to understand up to now, many of which are now abandoned in the opinion by Justice Thomas, writing for a plurality of the Court.) The reader may well want to see the full opinion; as it may likewise be helpful to see also the more complete opinion of Justice O'Connor (especially, as, for the moment, it may represent the critical "voice" on the Court).]

2. 330 U.S. 1 (1947) (casebook at p. 833).

3. (That is, *all* agreed that this was so, in *Everson*; rather, the only difference in the case was that five of the Justices simply did not see that there was any departure from, or inconsistency with, this understanding simply because parents of school-age children (not excluding those of parochial school students) were eligible to be reimbursed for ordinary bus fare, on *ordinary public buses moving along their regular routes*, in securing to their children a common means of safe travel (though, even then, four Justices disagreed and thought the mere bus-fare reimbursement plan as such was not permissible).

congregation, and so established and conducted under religious auspices as a means of propagating the faith of its sponsoring religion, the state may no more use public funds to relieve it of depending upon the support of those who share its faith and mission, to advance its religious mission, any more than in respect to a church. The one is equally a breach of the establishment clause as is the other. And, he says, there has never been any departure from *this* understanding of basic establishment clause doctrine at any time during the half-century since the Court first addressed the meaning of the establishment clause, in 1947.

Coming, then, to this case, it is plain to Justice Souter that *that* line of separation was clearly crossed by the forms of religious assistance provided by the state in this case: (a) in the *nature* of the *direct* aid furnished *to* the religious schools themselves; (b) in the *manner* and *amount* of that aid; (c) in the *inextricability* of its use in the religious school setting in directly and substantially advancing the religious inculcative functions of the recipient religious schools; and (d) *in the actual uses* made of the materials supplied by state, even as the plurality opinion itself acknowledged had taken place. Under *all* previous precedent, he says, this would clearly require the court to sustain the original complaint--even as the lower court agreed--and require it to hold in favor of the complaining parties and enjoin the state's continuing disbursements of its various forms of substantial assistance. In short, the decision by the court of appeals was inevitable and correct.

Justice Souter then contrasts "the plurality's approach" (i.e., the opinion for four members of the Court by Justice Thomas *supra*). He declares it is "an utter departure" and "would break with the law." To be sure, he notes, because of the view taken of the case in the concurring opinion--by Justice O'Connor in which Justice Breyer joined--the plurality view is not yet the view of the Court.[4] Turning directly to the plurality opinion, however, he says (emphasis added): "[T]here is no mistaking the abandonment of doctrine that would occur if the plurality were to become a majority.****The plurality is candid in pointing out the extent of actual diversion of Chapter 2 aid to religious use in the case before us, and equally candid in saying it does not matter*."

But, he asks, why doesn't it matter, when heretofore (he says), it has always not merely mattered but been decisive?

--The reason it "does not matter" to the plurality of the four Justices, when previously it always had, Justice Souter declares, is evidently this: "To the plurality there is nothing wrong[5] with [using taxpayer public funds even in direct aid of] a [church-related] school's religious mission," when accomplished through a plan merely "also providing assistance to the public schools." This is the "doctrinal coup," he says, and, indeed, "it is a break with consistent doctrine...unequaled in the history of Establishment Clause interpretation."

---

4. (Thus, he says, this case does not itself "stage a doctrinal coup.")

5. (I.e., nothing inconsistent with the establishment clause.)

How? In what way? In just this way: "***[I]n rejecting the principle of no [taxpayer funded] aid to a school's religious mission the plurality is attacking the most fundamental assumption underlying the Establishment Clause." "Religious missions" are not the business of government, either to subsidize or to subvert, under *Everson*, Souter says, but (in his view) the view now taken by four members of the Court represent the clearest evidence yet that this understanding is increasingly fragile and at risk.]

NOTE ON SCHOOL VOUCHERS

Increasingly in the last decade, states have enacted so-called "school voucher programs" which — although they vary in their precise features from state to state — at bottom provide state (taxpayer) funds to pay (at least a portion of) private and parochial school tuition for children in low income families. The Ohio program, for instance, which was recently sustained by the Ohio Supreme Court, *Simmons-Harris v. Goff*, 711 N.E.2d 203 (Ohio, May 27, 1999), but held to be in violation of the establishment clause by the sixth circuit Federal Court, *Simmons-Harris v. Zelman*, 234 F.3d 945 (6th Cir. 2000) required the state superintendent to give scholarships to Cleveland students to attend a "registered" private school; scholarships are for 75 to 90 percent of actual tuition (depending on the family income) or up to $2500; and the tuition checks are made payable to the parents, but sent to the schools where the parents would then endorse the check over to the schools. *See also Kotterman v. Killian*, 972 P.2d 606 (Ariz. 1999) (sustaining voucher scheme); *Jackson v. Bensen*, 578 N.W.2d 602 (Wisc. 1998) (sustaining voucher scheme), *cert. denied*, 119 S. Ct. 466 (1999); *but see Chittenden Town School District v. Vermont Department of Education*, 738 A.2d 539 (Vt., June 11, 1999) (finding voucher program violates Compelled Support Clause of Vermont constitution).

The constitutionality of these schemes has been intensely debated, and although the Court denied certiorari in the Wisconsin case in 1999, it is expected one of these arrangements will wend its way to the Court in due time. Would these arrangements fail under *Everson* ("No tax in any amount, large or small, can be levied to support any religious activities or institutions . . .") or might some fall within the cases in this section (e.g., *Mueller v. Allen*, and *Agostini*, and *Mitchell v. Helms*)? *See* Eugene Volokh, Equal Treatment is Not Establishment, 13 Notre Dame J.L. Ethics & Pub. Pol'y 341 (1999); Laura Underkuffler, Voucher and Beyond: The Individual as Causative Agent in Establishment Clause Jurisprudence, 75 Indiana L.J. 167 (2000).

D. THE ESTABLISHMENT CLAUSE AND "THEOCRACY"[6]

1. Enforcing God's laws as the law of the civil state

The cases thus far reviewed show the extent to which the establishment clause has been construed to draw lines between laws "accommodating" religious needs[7] and those "aiding" or "advancing" religion, i.e. laws "establishing" religion through some kind of government support.[8] A different form of the same problem may arise when civil government enacts positive law the very predicate of which is that "the law of God should also be the law of the state"—to be enforced against believers and nonbelievers alike. Government by such rule is usually identified to theocratic states.[9]

The establishment clause, plus the Article VI clause forbidding any religious test as a qualification of office or trust under the authority of the United States, plus the "support and defend" oath requirement of Article VI—the oath to support and defend the Constitution (including the establishment clause as part of the Constitution one is pledged to support and defend)—are the principal clauses directed to concerns of this kind. In some measure, of course, the free exercise clause may also be relevant as well.

In some states, particular state constitutional provisions may also be pertinent—i.e. we have already noted that state constitutional clauses antedating or modeled on the Blaine amendment have sometimes been given a wider scope than the establishment clause itself.[10] In some states there have been explicit state constitutional limitations on office holding by members of the clergy. [T]he majority of these provisions have reflected a strong view that members of the clergy ought not share power in legislative bodies while simultaneously holding office as ministers or as

---

6. "Theocracy: 1. Government by a god regarded as the ruling power or by priests or officials claiming divine sanction. 2. A state so governed. [Greek *theokratia*]" American Heritage Dictionary 1334 (1971 ed.)

7. E.g., *Pierce, Zorach, Allen, Walz, Mueller, Tilton.*

8. E.g., *McCollum, Engel, Schempp, Wolman, Lemon, Nyquist.*

9. See Kent Greenawalt, Religious Convictions and Political Choices (1988); Kent Greenawalt, Religious Convictions and Lawmaking, 84 Mich.L.Rev. 352, 401 (1985) ("[T]o demand that other people act in accord with dominant religious beliefs is to promote or impose those beliefs in an impermissible way."). Cf. John Thomas Noonan, The Believer and the Powers That Are (1987); Berman, The Challenge of the Modern State, in Articles of Faith, Articles of Peace 47 (James Davison Hunter & Os Guinness eds. 1990) ("[I]n 1787 religion played a guiding role, and government an implementing role, in family law and criminal law.")

10. In a number of states, arrangements of the sort narrowly sustained in *Everson* have been held invalid under such state constitutional clauses. See, *e.g.*, Judd v. Board of Educ. of Union Free Sch. Dist., 15 N.E.2d 576 (N.Y. Ct. App. 1938). (*Everson*-type appropriation of local tax funds to furnish bus transport to private and parochial schools, additional to public schools, held invalid pursuant to state constitutional provision providing: "Neither the State nor any subdivision thereof, shall use its property or credit or any public money *** directly or indirectly, in aid *** of any school *** wholly or in part under the control or direction of any religious denomination ***.")

priests bound by vows as keepers of a sectarian faith.

In 1978, in *McDaniel v. Paty*,[11] however, the Supreme Court held that a state constitutional provision disqualifying "ministers of the gospel" from eligibility for election to the state legislature was unconstitutional under the fourteenth amendment.[12] The state constitutional provision involved in the case was very old, established in the Tennessee Constitution in 1796. It was of a kind fairly common to a number of states during the nineteenth century. The general purpose of such elective office restrictions "was primarily to assure the success of a new political experiment, the separation of church and state."[13] Provisions of this kind had in fact been supported by John Locke and Thomas Jefferson, and originally by James Madison as well.

In *McDaniel v. Paty*, the Court held that even assuming the state had a substantial interest in adopting office holding eligibility standards to provide some assurance that such acts as its General Assembly might adopt would not seek to enact sectarian religious interests (but would, rather, be guided by the separation principles of the establishment clause), the state's categorical presumption that ordained ministers would be unable to abide by the civil oath required of them—to support and defend the Constitution—was unwarranted. So the flat ban on legislative eligibility was struck down.[14] The Court acknowledged that such notables as John Locke and

---

11. 435 U.S. 618 (1978).

12. The immediate issue before the Court involved a state statutory restriction on candidate eligibility to serve as a delegate to the state's limited constitutional convention, rather than eligibility to serve in the state legislature. The constitutional convention delegate eligibility standard, however, was set by reference to the state constitutional provision regarding eligibility for election to the House of Representatives of the Tennessee General Assembly, and the Court therefore directly addressed the latter provision as well. The state supreme court had held that the restriction on ordained ministers from holding legislative office did not violate the fourteenth amendment, insofar as the disqualification was not based on religious belief but more narrowly, on vocational status as an ordained minister; it upheld the limitation in light of the constitutional interest to separate legislative action from religious action in "the lawmaking process of government—*where religious action is absolutely prohibited by the establishment clause* ***." 547 S.W.2d 897, 903 (Tenn. 1977) (emphasis added).

13. 435 U.S. at 622.

14. The plurality opinion was written by Chief Justice Burger for himself, Powell, Rehnquist, and Stevens. A concurring opinion by Brennan (for himself and Marshall) treated the state constitutional provision as a form of unconstitutional condition, i.e. requiring one who is an ordained minister (one form of exercising one's freedom of religion) either to give up his office as a minister or to be deemed ineligible for elective offices open to others. Justice Brennan, 435 U.S. at 642, relied on "judicial enforcement of the Establishment Clause" to provide the necessary safeguard against such sectarian actions ministers-as-legislators might be tempted to take, to the extent that they might not themselves live up to the oath of office otherwise required of them—to support and defend the Constitution (including the establishment clause). Stewart concurred separately on the basis that disqualification from office because of one's religious vocation (as a minister) was indistinguishable from disqualification on grounds of religious belief or lack of religious belief, a kind of disqualification the Court had earlier held to be unconstitutional in Torcaso v. Watkins, 367 U.S. 488 (1961). White concurred separately on the basis of the fourteenth amendment equal protection clause, opining that the

Thomas Jefferson had supported such limitations. It also noted that James Madison originally agreed with that view but that Madison came to believe otherwise (i.e. that such restrictions were not really necessary and were, moreover, quite unfair)—and eventually, so had every state except Tennessee, the last state still to retain such a limitation on ordained ministers or priests and eligibility for legislative election.

The Court's decision in *McDaniel v. Paty* serves as a reminder that priests, ministers, mullahs, rabbis, etc. may not be deemed ineligible for elective office.[15] And of course each person is free to support whomever he or she wishes for elective office, according to one's own preference for such legislation one desires to see enacted—including that based on a strongly-held religious conviction that the civil law *ought* to report what scripture and/or religious teaching prescribes—including laws characteristic of theocratic states.

The principal safeguards against tendencies of a theocratic state, therefore, are *not* safeguards limiting office-holding eligibility to nonclergy, or limitations on first amendment rights to form parties committed to certain religious aims, or limitations on how people choose to vote. Rather, such as they are, they arise merely from the Article VI requirement nominally binding federal and state officials to support and defend the Constitution in their role as civil legislators, executives, and judges, and from the judicial enforcement of the establishment clause itself—directly as to Congress and indirectly (i.e. via the fourteenth amendment) as to the states. But how is this latter "safeguard" expected to work? This is the topic we now explore.

As a hypothetical example, suppose it is contrary to the tenets of a particular religion to eat pork. And suppose, moreover, that the eating of pork is deemed by the scriptures of that religion to be a sin generally, condemned in the sight of God. Suppose the religion is or becomes of controlling influence within a given state legislature such that a general law is enacted which forbids the sale of pork for human consumption, punishing those who do eat it as criminal misdemeanants, by criminal fines up to $500 or jail up to thirty days.

Insofar as the predicate for this legislation is that "the human consumption of pork is an abomination in the sight of God, and therefore on that account is to be forbidden in a community founded on God's will," it would seem to be vulnerable pursuant to the establishment clause of the first amendment. Accordingly, one might expect that a person prosecuted for violating such a law would have a valid constitutional defense. The defense would *not* be that the law abridges the defendant's freedom of religion (the defendant's religion, if he or she has one, may

---

disqualification swept too broadly (and thus was over inclusive) since it disqualified ministers whose religious beliefs would not necessarily prevent them from properly discharging their obligations in office.

15. Neither may any restriction of eligibility for election to the House, the Senate, presidency, or vice presidency disqualify religious leaders, heads of churches, clergy, ministers, etc. for such offices. See, e.g., Powell v. McCormack, 395 U.S. 486 (1969) (the criteria of eligibility for election to the House provided in the Constitution are exclusive, i.e. no other criteria may constitutionally be required).

say nothing one way or the other about eating pork). Rather, it would be that the law violates the establishment clause's separation of the civil from the theocratic state.

Perhaps the following is another suitable example. In the Book of Exodus, chapt. 20, the following Commandment appears:

> Remember the sabbath day, to keep it holy. Six days you shall labor, and do all your work; but the seventh day is a sabbath to the Lord your god; in it you shall not do any work ***

Consistent with the establishment clause, may the civil state require all to conform according to the dictates of this religious text on pain of fine or jail? And more generally, to whatever extent the state attempts to carry into positive law "God's will" in prescribing (and proscribing) what may (and may not) be done,[16] is this not a manifestation of a "theocratic," rather than of a "civil," state?[17] Isn't the legislative predicate of a theocratic state at odds with the establishment clause of the first amendment?[18] Consider the following reported case. How does one disentangle a "religious" from a "civil" or "secular" predicate for legislative action? How will the three-part *Lemon* establishment clause test apply?[19]

---

16. Does it matter whether the legislators are themselves ministers, priests, or ayatollahs or (if not) whether they nonetheless legislate according to the dictates of the politically dominate religion either because they agree with its tenets, or because they seek to avoid losing elections?

17. If sodomy is criminalized "because it is an abomination in the sight of God" (according to the tenets of the religion dominantly of influence with the particular legislature), does its criminalization thereby enact the compulsory observance of the religious tenets of the dominant faith? Is this to establish a religion (i.e. its tenets) under secular auspices, enacting a theocracy on the installment plan? Cf. Bowers v. Hardwick, 478 U.S. 186 (1986). If the reading or willing viewing of obscenity is condemned as a "sin" —and for that reason made criminal, how does one describe the foundation of the law in nontheocratic terms? See Henkin, Morals and the Constitution: The Sin of Obscenity, 63 Colum.L.Rev. 391 (1963). See also Webster v. Reproductive Health Services, 492 U.S. 490 (1989) (Stevens, J., dissenting) (finding no non-religious legislative basis to distinguish a gamete and a zygote, for purposes of drawing any constitutional distinction for an anti-abortion act applicable at the moment of conception as distinct from a later time in the gestation of the fetus).

18. But see Douglas, J., in Zorach v. Clauson, 343 U.S. 306 (1952) ("We are a religious people *whose institutions presuppose a Supreme Being.*") (emphasis added).

19. Cf. Stone v. Graham, 449 U.S. 39 (1980) (posting of the Ten Commandments on public classroom walls, held unconstitutional as serving solely a religious purpose, despite required notation printed at the bottom of each posted copy declaring: "The secular application of the Ten Commandments is clearly seen in its adoption as the fundamental legal code of Western Civilization and the Common Law of the United States"). See also Epperson v. Arkansas, 393 U.S. 97 (1968) (legislative ban on public school instruction on evolution held invalid as applied to high school biology teacher, for failure to satisfy the "secular purpose" prong of the *Lemon* test).

MCGOWAN v. MARYLAND
366 U.S. 420 (1961)

MR. CHIEF JUSTICE WARREN delivered the opinion of the Court.

The issues in this case concern the constitutional validity of Maryland criminal statutes, commonly known as Sunday Closing Laws or Sunday Blue Laws. ***

Appellants are seven employees of a large discount department store located on a highway in Anne Arundel County, Maryland. They were indicted for the Sunday sale of a three-ring loose-leaf binder, a can of floor wax, a stapler and staples, and a toy submarine in violation of Md. Ann. Code, Art. 27, § 521. Generally, this section prohibited, throughout the State, the Sunday sale of all merchandise except the retail sale of tobacco products, confectioneries, milk, bread, fruits, gasoline, oils, greases, drugs and medicines, and newspapers and periodicals. Recently amended, this section also now excepts from the general prohibition the retail sale in Anne Arundel County of all foodstuffs, automobile and boating accessories, flowers, toilet goods, hospital supplies and souvenirs. Appellants were convicted and each was fined five dollars and costs. The Maryland Court of Appeals affirmed, [and] we noted probable jurisdiction.

I

* * *

[A]ppellants contend here that the statutes applicable to Anne Arundel County violate the constitutional guarantee of freedom of religion in that the statutes' effect is to prohibit the free exercise of religion in contravention of the First Amendment, made applicable to the States by the Fourteenth Amendment. But appellants allege only economic injury to themselves; they do not allege any infringement of their own religious freedoms due to Sunday closing. In fact, the record is silent as to what appellants' religious beliefs are.

Secondly, appellants contend that the statutes violate the guarantee of separation of church and state in that the statutes are laws respecting an establishment of religion contrary to the First Amendment, made applicable to the States by the Fourteenth Amendment. If the purpose of the "establishment" clause was only to insure protection for the "free exercise" of religion, then what we have said above concerning appellants' standing to raise the "free exercise" contention would appear to be true here. However, the writings of Madison, who was the First Amendment's architect, demonstrate that the establishment of a religion was equally feared because of its tendencies to political tyranny and subversion of civil authority. Thus, in *Everson v. Board of Education*, the Court permitted a district taxpayer to challenge, on "establishment" grounds, a state statute which authorized district boards of education to reimburse parents for fares paid for the transportation of their children to both public and Catholic schools. Appellants here concededly have suffered direct economic injury, allegedly due to the imposition on them of the tenets of the Christian religion.

The essence of appellants' "establishment" argument is that Sunday is the Sabbath day of the predominant Christian sects; that the purpose of the enforced stoppage of labor on that day is to facilitate and encourage church attendance; that the purpose of setting Sunday as a day of universal rest is to induce people with no religion or people with marginal religious beliefs to join the predominant Christian sects; that the purpose of the atmosphere of tranquility created by Sunday closing is to aid the conduct of church services and religious observance of the sacred day. In substantiating their "establishment" argument, appellants rely on the wording of the present Maryland statutes, on earlier versions of the current Sunday laws and on prior judicial characterizations of these laws by the Maryland Court of Appeals. Although only the constitutionality of § 521, the section under which appellants have been convicted, is immediately before us in this litigation, inquiry into the history of Sunday Closing Laws in our country, in addition to an examination of the Maryland Sunday closing statutes in their entirety and of their history, is relevant to the decision of whether the Maryland Sunday law in question is one respecting an establishment of religion. There is no dispute that the original laws which dealt with Sunday labor were motivated by religious forces. But what we must decide is whether present Sunday legislation, having undergone extensive changes from the earliest forms, still retains its religious character.

Sunday Closing Laws go far back into American history, having been brought to the colonies with a background of English legislation dating to the thirteenth century. In 1237, Henry III forbade the frequenting of markets on Sunday; the Sunday showing of wools at the staple was banned by Edward III in 1354; in 1409, Henry IV prohibited the playing of unlawful games on Sunday; Henry VI proscribed Sunday fairs in churchyards in 1444 and, four years later, made unlawful all fairs and markets and all showings of any goods or merchandise; Edward VI disallowed Sunday bodily labor by several injunctions in the mid-sixteenth century; various Sunday sports and amusements were restricted in 1625 by Charles I. *** Observation of the above language, and of that of the prior mandates, reveals clearly that the English Sunday legislation was in aid of the established church.

The American colonial Sunday restrictions arose soon after settlement. Starting in 1650, the Plymouth Colony proscribed servile work, unnecessary traveling, sports, and the sale of alcoholic beverages on the Lord's day and enacted laws concerning church attendance. The Massachusetts Bay Colony and the Connecticut and New Haven Colonies enacted similar prohibitions, some even earlier in the seventeenth century. The religious orientation of the colonial statutes was equally apparent. For example, a 1629 Massachusetts Bay instruction began, "And to the end the Sabbath may be celebrated in a religious manner. ***" A 1653 enactment spoke of Sunday activities "which things tend much to the dishonor of God, the reproach of religion, and the profanation of his holy Sabbath, the sanctification whereof is sometimes put for all duties immediately respecting the service of God. ***" ***

But, despite the strongly religious origin of these laws, beginning before the eighteenth century, nonreligious arguments for Sunday closing began to be heard more distinctly and the statutes began to lose some of their totally religious flavor. In the middle 1700's Blackstone wrote, "[T]he keeping one day in the seven holy, as a time of relaxation and refreshment as well as for public worship, is of admirable service to a state considered merely as a civil institution. It humanizes, by the help of conversation and society, the manners of the lower classes; which would otherwise degenerate into a sordid ferocity and savage selfishness of spirit; it enables the industrious workman to pursue his occupation in the ensuing week with health and cheerfulness." 4 Bl. Comm. 63. ***

The proponents of Sunday closing legislation are no longer exclusively representatives of religious interests. *** Some of our States now enforce their Sunday legislation through Departments of Labor, *e.g.*, 6 S.C. Code Ann. (1952), § 64-5. Thus have Sunday laws evolved from the wholly religious sanctions that originally were enacted.

Moreover, litigation over Sunday closing laws is not novel. Scores of cases may be found in the state appellate courts relating to sundry phases of Sunday enactments. Religious objections have been raised there on numerous occasions but sustained only once, in *Ex parte* Newman, 9 Cal. 502 (1858); and that decision was overruled three years later, in *Ex parte* Andrews, 18 Cal. 678. ***

[T]he "Establishment" Clause does not ban federal or state regulation of conduct whose reason or effect merely happens to coincide or harmonize with the tenets of some or all religions. In many instances, the Congress or state legislatures conclude that the general welfare of society, wholly apart from any religious considerations, demands such regulation. Thus, for temporal purposes, murder is illegal. And the fact that this agrees with the dictates of the Judaeo- Christian religions while it may disagree with others does not invalidate the regulation. So too with the questions of adultery and polygamy. The same could be said of theft, fraud, etc., because those offenses were also proscribed in the Decalogue. ***

In light of the evolution of our Sunday Closing Laws through the centuries, and of their more or less recent emphasis upon secular considerations, it is not difficult to discern that as presently written and administered, most of them, at least, are of a secular rather than of a religious character, and that presently they bear no relationship to establishment of religion as those words are used in the Constitution of the United States.

Throughout this century and longer, both the federal and state governments have oriented their activities very largely toward improvement of the health, safety, recreation and general well-being of our citizens. Numerous laws affecting public health, safety factors in industry, laws affecting hours and conditions of labor of women and children, week-end diversion at parks and beaches, and cultural activities of various kinds, now point the way toward the good life for all. Sunday Closing Laws, like those before us, have become part and parcel of this great governmental concern wholly apart from their original purposes or connotations. The present purpose and effect of most of them is to provide a uniform day of rest for all citizens; the fact that this day is Sunday, a day of particular significance for the dominant Christian sects, does not bar the State from achieving its secular goals. To say that the States cannot prescribe Sunday as a day of rest for these purposes solely because centuries ago such laws had their genesis in religion would give a constitutional interpretation of hostility to the public welfare rather than one of mere separation of church and State.

We now reach the Maryland statutes under review. The title of the major series of sections of the Maryland Code dealing with Sunday closing—Art. 27, §§ 492-534C—is "Sabbath Breaking"; § 492 proscribes work or bodily labor on the "Lord's day," and forbids persons to "profane the Lord's day" by gaming, fishing et cetera; § 522 refers to Sunday as the "Sabbath day." *** The predecessors of the existing Maryland Sunday laws are undeniably religious in origin. ***

Considering the language and operative effect of the current statutes, we no longer find the blanket prohibition against Sunday work or bodily labor. To the contrary, we find that § 521 of Art. 27, the section which appellants violated, permits the Sunday sale of tobaccos and sweets and a long list of sundry articles which we have enumerated above; we find that § 509 of Art. 27 permits the Sunday operation of bathing beaches, amusement parks and similar facilities; we find that Art. 2B, § 28, permits the Sunday sale of alcoholic beverages, products strictly forbidden by predecessor statutes; we are told that Anne Arundel County allows Sunday bingo and the Sunday playing of pinball machines and slot machines, activities generally condemned by prior Maryland Sunday legislation. Certainly, these are not works of charity or necessity. Section 521's current stipulation that shops with only one employee may remain open on Sunday does not coincide with a religious purpose. These provisions, along with those which permit various sports and entertainments on Sunday, seem clearly to be fashioned for the purpose of providing a Sunday atmosphere of recreation, cheerfulness, repose and enjoyment. Coupled with the general proscription against other types of work, we believe that the air of the day is one of relaxation rather than one of religion.

The existing Maryland Sunday laws are not simply verbatim re-enactments of their religiously oriented antecedents. Only § 492 retains the appellation of "Lord's day" and even that section no longer makes recitation of religious purpose. It does talk in terms of "[profaning] the Lord's day," but other sections permit the activities previously thought to be profane. Prior denunciation of Sunday drunkenness is now gone. Contemporary concern with these statutes is evidenced by the dozen changes made in 1959 and by the recent enactment of a majority of the exceptions. *** After engaging in the close scrutiny demanded of us when First Amendment liberties are at issue, we accept the State Supreme Court's determination that the statutes' present purpose and effect is not to aid religion but to set aside a day of rest and recreation.

But this does not answer all of appellants' contentions. We are told that the State has other means at its disposal to accomplish its secular purpose, other courses that would not even remotely or incidentally give state aid to religion. On this basis, we are asked to hold these statutes invalid on the ground that the State's power to regulate conduct in the public interest may only be executed in a way that does not unduly or unnecessarily infringe upon the religious provisions of the First Amendment. ***

However, the State's purpose is not merely to provide a one-day-in-seven work stoppage. In addition to this, the State seeks to set one day apart from all others as a day of rest, repose, recreation and tranquility—a day which all members of the family and community have the opportunity to spend and enjoy together, a day on which there exists relative quiet and disassociation from the everyday intensity of commercial activities, a day on which people may visit friends and relatives who are not available during working days.

Obviously, a State is empowered to determine that a rest-one-day-in-seven statute would not accomplish this purpose; that it would not provide for a general cessation of activity, a special atmosphere of tranquility, a day which all members of the family or friends and relatives might spend together. Furthermore, it seems plain that the problems involved in enforcing such a provision would be exceedingly more difficult than those in enforcing a common-day-of-rest provision.

Moreover, it is common knowledge that the first day of the week has come to have special significance as a rest day in this country. People of all religions and people with no religion regard Sunday as a time for family activity, for visiting friends and relatives, for late sleeping, for passive and active entertainments, for dining out, and the like. *** It would seem unrealistic for enforcement purposes and perhaps detrimental to the general welfare to require a State to choose a common day of rest other than that which most persons would select of their own accord. For these reasons, we hold that the Maryland statutes are not laws respecting an establishment of religion. ***

Separate opinion of MR. JUSTICE FRANKFURTER, whom MR. JUSTICE HARLAN joins.

[T]he Establishment Clause withdrew from the sphere of legitimate legislative concern and competence a specific, but comprehensive, area of human conduct: man's belief or disbelief in the verity of some transcendental idea and man's expression in action of that belief or disbelief. Congress may not make these matters, as such, the subject of legislation, nor, now, may any legislature in this country. Neither the National Government nor, under the Due Process Clause of the Fourteenth Amendment, a State may, by any device, support belief or the expression of belief for its own sake, whether from conviction of the truth of that belief, or from conviction that by the propagation of that belief the civil welfare of the State is served, or because a majority of its citizens, holding that belief, are offended when all do not hold it.

With regulations which have other objectives the Establishment Clause, and the fundamental separationist concept which it expresses, are not concerned. These regulations may fall afoul of the constitutional guarantee against infringement of the free exercise or observance of religion. Where they do, they must be set aside at the instance of those whose faith they prejudice. But once it is determined that a challenged statute is supportable as implementing other substantial interests than the promotion of belief, the guarantee prohibiting religious "establishment" is satisfied.

To ask what interest, what objective, legislation serves, of course, is not to psychoanalyze its legislators, but to examine the necessary effects of what they have enacted. If the primary end achieved by a form of regulation is the affirmation or promotion of religious doctrine—primary, in the sense that all secular ends which it purportedly serves are derivative from, not wholly independent of, the advancement of religion—the regulation is beyond the power of the state. *** Or if a statute furthers both secular and religious ends by means unnecessary to the effectuation of the secular ends alone—where the same secular ends could equally be attained by means which do not have consequences for promotion of religion—the statute cannot stand.

In the present cases the Sunday retail sellers and their employees and customers, in attacking statutes banning various activities on a day which most Christian creeds consecrate, do assert that these statutes have no other purpose. ***

To be sure, the Massachusetts statute now before the Court, and statutes in Pennsylvania and Maryland, still call Sunday the "Lord's day" or the "Sabbath." So do the Sunday laws in many other States. But the continuation of seventeenth century language does not of itself prove the continuation of the purposes for which the colonial governments enacted these laws, or that these are the purposes for which their successors of the twentieth have retained them and modified them. We know, for example, that Committees of the New York Legislature, considering that State's Sabbath Laws on two occasions more than a century apart, twice recommended no repeal of those laws, both times on the ground that the laws did not involve "any partisan religious issue, but rather economic and health regulation of the activities of the people on a universal day of rest," and that a Massachusetts legislative committee rested on the same views. Sunday legislation has been supported not only by such clerical organizations as the Lord's Day Alliance, but also by labor and trade groups. ***

Appellees in the *Gallagher* case and appellants in the *Braunfeld* case contend that, as applied to them, Orthodox Jewish retailers and their Orthodox Jewish customers, the Massachusetts Lord's day statute and the Pennsylvania Sunday retail sales act violate the Due Process Clause of the Fourteenth Amendment because, in effect, the statutes deter the exercise and observance of their religion. The argument runs that by compelling the Sunday closing of retail stores and thus making unavailable for business and shopping uses one-seventh part of the week, these statutes force them either to give up the Sabbath observance—an essential part of their faith —or to forego advantages enjoyed by the non-Sabbatarian majority of the community.

The claim which these litigants urge assumes a number of aspects. First, they argue that any one-common-day-of-closing regulation which selected a day other than their Sabbath would be *ipso facto* unconstitutional in its application to them because of its effect in preferring persons who observe no Sabbath, therefore creating economic pressures which urge Sabbatarians to give up their usage The creation of this pressure by the Sunday statutes, it is said, is not so necessary a means to the achievement of the ends of day-of-rest legislation as to justify its employment when weighed against the injury to Sabbatarian religion which it entails. Six-day- week regulation, with the closing day left to individual choice, is urged as a more reasonable alternative.

Second, they argue that even if legitimate state interests justify the enforcement against persons generally of a single common day of rest, the choice of Sunday as that day violates the rights of religious freedom of the Sabbatarian minority. By choosing a day upon which Sunday-observing Christians worship and abstain from labor, the statutes are said to discriminate between religions. ***

In urging that an exception in favor of those who observe some other day as sacred would not defeat the ends of Sunday legislation, and therefore that failure to provide such an exception is an unnecessary—hence an unconstitutional—burden on Sabbatarians, the *Gallagher* appellees and *Braunfeld* appellants point to such exceptions in twenty-one of the thirty-four jurisdictions which have statutes banning labor or employment or the selling of goods on Sunday. Actually, in less than half of these twenty-one States does the exemption extend to sales activity as well as to labor. There are tenable reasons why a legislature might choose not to make such an exception. To whatever extent persons who come within the exception are present in a community, their activity would disturb the atmosphere of general repose and reintroduce into Sunday the business tempos of the week. Administration would be more difficult, with violations less evident and, in effect, two or more days to police instead of one. If it is assumed that the retail demand for consumer items is approximately equivalent on Saturday and on Sunday, the Sabbatarian, in proportion as he is less numerous, and hence the competition less severe, might incur through the exception a competitive advantage over the non-Sabbatarian, who would then be in a position, presumably, to complain of discrimination against his religion. Employers who wished to avail themselves of the exception would have to employ only their coreligionists, and there might be introduced into private employment practices an element of religious differentiation which a legislature could regard as undesirable.[106]

Finally, a relevant consideration which might cause a State's lawmakers to reject exception for observers of another day than Sunday is that administration of such a provision may require judicial inquiry into religious belief.

Surely, in light of the delicate enforcement problems to which these provisions bear witness, the legislative choice of a blanket Sunday ban applicable to observers of all faiths cannot be held unreasonable. A legislature might in reason find that the

---

106. Both Pennsylvania and Massachusetts have fair employment practices acts prohibiting religious discrimination in hiring. ***

alternative of exempting Sabbatarians would impede the effective operation of the Sunday statutes, produce harmful collateral effects, and entail, itself, a not inconsiderable intrusion into matters of religious faith. However preferable, personally, one might deem such an exception, I cannot find that the Constitution compels it. ***

MR. JUSTICE DOUGLAS, dissenting.

* * *

The Court picks and chooses language from various decisions to bolster its conclusion that these Sunday laws in the modern setting are "civil regulations." No matter how much is written, no matter what is said, the parentage of these laws is the Fourth Commandment; and they serve and satisfy the religious predispositions of our Christian communities. ***

It seems to me plain that by these laws the States compel one, under sanction of law, to refrain from work or recreation on Sunday because of the majority's religious views about that day. The State by law makes Sunday a symbol of respect or adherence. Refraining from work or recreation in deference to the majority's religious feelings about Sunday is within every person's choice. By what authority can government compel it?

Cases are put where acts that are immoral by our standards but not by the standards of other religious groups are made criminal. That category of cases, until today, has been a very restricted one confined to polygamy (Reynolds v. United States, 98 U.S. 145) and other extreme situations. The latest example is Prince v. Massachusetts, 321 U.S. 158, which upheld a statute making it criminal for a child under twelve to sell papers, periodicals, or merchandise on a street or in any public place. It was sustained in spite of the finding that the child thought it was her religious duty to perform the act. *** None of the acts involved here implicates minors. None of the actions made constitutionally criminal today involves the doing of any act that any society has deemed to be immoral.

The State can, of course, require one day of rest a week: one day when every shop or factory is closed. Quite a few States make that requirement. Then the "day of rest" becomes purely and simply a health measure. But the Sunday laws operate differently. They force minorities to obey the majority's religious feelings of what is due and proper for a Christian community; they provide a coercive spur to the "weaker brethren," to those who are indifferent to the claims of a Sabbath through apathy or scruple. Can there be any doubt that Christians, now aligned vigorously in favor of these laws, would be as strongly opposed if they were prosecuted under a Moslem law that forbade them from engaging in secular activities on days that violated Moslem scruples?

There is an "establishment" of religion in the constitutional sense if any practice of any religious group has the sanction of law behind it. There is an interference with the "free exercise" of religion if what in conscience one can do or omit doing is required because of the religious scruples of the community. Hence I would declare each of those laws unconstitutional as applied to the complaining parties, whether or not they are members of a sect which observes as its Sabbath a day other than Sunday. When these laws are applied to Orthodox Jews, or to Sabbatarians their vice is accentuated. *** When, however, the State uses its coercive powers— here the criminal law—to compel minorities to observe a second Sabbath, not their own, the State undertakes to aid and "prefer one religion over another"—contrary to the command of the Constitution.

NOTE

1. In light of *McGowan v. Maryland, Stone v. Graham,*[20] and *Epperson v. Arkansas,*[21] consider the following case reported in the New York Times.[22]

SUPREME COURT LETS STAND A MISSOURI TOWN'S BAN ON SCHOOL DANCES

Washington, April 16 [1990]: — A ban on school dances in a small Missouri town survived Supreme Court review today.

Without comment, the Court refused to hear a challenge by a group of students and their parents in Purdy, Mo., to the ban. They argued that the policy, reflecting the Christian fundamentalist view that social dancing is sinful, violated the constitutionally required separation of church and state.

Fundamentalist Christians make up a majority of Purdy's residents, and a group of ministers took the leading role in preserving the century old ban when school officials considered modifying it in 1986. A school board officials, asked at one community meeting whether he thought the ban might violate the separation of church and state, replied, "You better hope there's never a separation of God and school."

A Federal District Judge in Missouri, Russell G. Clark, ruled in 1988 that the ban amounted to an unconstitutional "establishment" of religion. But a three-judge panel of the United States Court of Appeals for the Eight Circuit overturned the decision.

The appeals court said that dancing was a "secular" activity and that a prohibition against school dances could be defended as an appropriately "neutral" policy, whatever the motivation behind it.

"We simply do not believe elected government officials are required to check at the door whatever religious background they carry with them before they act on rules that are otherwise [un]objectionable," the appellate panel said.

---

20. 449 U.S. 39 (1980).

21. 393 U.S. 97 (1968). (For brief descriptions of *Stone* and *Epperson*, see note 19, p. 935 *supra.*

22. For additional facts and discussion, see Clayton v. Place, 690 F.Supp. 850 (W.D. Mo. 1988), *rev'd*, 884 F.2d 376 (8th Cir. 1989), *reh'g denied*, 889 F.2d 192 (8th Cir. 1989).

The full Eight Circuit voted 5 to 4 against rehearing the case. The dissenting judges declared that "this is a case about religious tyranny."

In their Supreme Court appeal, Clayton v. Place, No. 89-1348, the students argued that the appeals court had failed to give proper consideration to the religious motivation behind the ban. They said the decision indicated that "public school boards may endorse and promote the religious beliefs of a locally dominant religious sect as official school policy, so long as the school policy is 'facially neutral.'"

But the school board, in turn, warned the Justices that to strike down the dancing ban on church-state ground would call into question a number of other "public school rules and decisions which have their basis in traditional morality," like dress codes and rules against swearing.

The school board's brief continued: "All citizens are allowed to participate equally in public policy formulation. To exclude those who are informed in their moral vision by an underlying religious faith would deny them freedom of speech and their right to engage in the political process."

2. As observed in a recent student Note,[23] "[E]ach year on a Friday in late March or early April — two days before Easter — Christians commemorate the crucifixion of their savior Jesus Christ. They call that day Good Friday. Many states have given Good Friday the status for a legal holiday, closing government offices and schools." The public employees (e.g., public school teachers, employees at closed state departments of motor vehicles offices, etc.) are paid their usual salaries, though no work is being done. Most of these state laws are of fairly recent origin. Several have been challenged under the establishment clause, though none has reached the Supreme Court. Would the rationale of *McGowan* apply to sustain these laws? Would the rationale of the next principal case (*Marsh*)?

2. Religion in government

A different aspect of the theocratic state might be the installation of theology *within* government. For example, a government might formally incorporate a clear theocratic commitment in its official self-description—e.g., "One Nation, Under Allah." Such a government might thereby proclaim itself to be subordinate to and faithful to Allah, and thereby suggest it would reflect the will of Allah in its proceedings as well as arrange its laws according to what the Qu'ran allegedly requires. For example, it might forbid the charging of interest on loans, reasoning that this practice is wrong in the sight of Allah.

Another example might be a nation proclaiming itself "One Nation, Under God,"—a nation wherein the legislative assemblies are even called to order by ministers offering prayers (ministers appointed under government auspices and paid

23. *See* Justin Brookman, Note, *The Constitutionality of The Good Friday Holiday, 73 N.Y.U.L.* Rev. 193 (1998).

from tax monies)—a nation also proclaiming "In God We Trust" as its national motto,—a nation administering theistic oaths as an incident of its elected officials taking public office—a nation administering the same theistic oath even to private citizens appearing as witnesses before its formal legislative committees or before its official courts.

How does one reconcile the "no establishment" clause with installed government practices such as these?[24]

MARSH v. CHAMBERS
463 U.S. 783 (1983)

CHIEF JUSTICE BURGER delivered the opinion of the Court.

The question presented is whether the Nebraska Legislature's practice of opening each legislative day with a prayer by a chaplain paid by the State violates the Establishment Clause of the First Amendment.

I

The Nebraska Legislature begins each of its sessions with a prayer offered by a chaplain who is chosen biennially by the Executive Board of the Legislative Council and paid out of public funds.[1] Robert E. Palmer, a Presbyterian minister, has served as chaplain since 1965 at a salary of $319.75 per month for each month the legislature is in session.

Ernest Chambers is a member of the Nebraska Legislature and a taxpayer of Nebraska. Claiming that the Nebraska Legislature's chaplaincy practice violates the Establishment Clause of the First Amendment, he brought this action under 42 U.S.C. § 1983, seeking to enjoin enforcement of the practice.[2] After denying a motion to dismiss on the ground of legislative immunity, the District Court held that the Establishment Clause was not breached by the prayers, but was violated by paying the chaplain from public funds. It therefore enjoined the legislature from using public funds to pay the chaplain; it declined to enjoin the policy of beginning

---

24. For additional discussion of these and similar practices, see Steven B. Epstein, *Rethinking the Constitutionality of Ceremonial Deism*, 96 Colum. L. Rev. 2083 (1996). See also ACLU of Ohio v. Capitol Square Review and Advisory Bd., 243 F. 3d 289 (6th Cir. 2001).

1. Rules of the Nebraska Unicameral, Rules 1, 2, and 21. These prayers are recorded in the Legislative Journal and, upon the vote of the legislature, collected from time to time into prayerbooks, which are published at public expense. In 1975, 200 copies were printed; prayerbooks were also published in 1978 (200 copies), and 1979 (100 copies). In total, publication costs amounted to $458.56.

2. Respondent named as defendants State Treasurer Frank Marsh, Chaplain Palmer, and the members of the Executive Board of the Legislative Council in their official capacity. All appear as petitioners before us.

sessions with prayers. Cross-appeals were taken.[3]

The Court of Appeals for the Eighth Circuit rejected arguments that the case should be dismissed on Tenth Amendment, legislative immunity, standing, or federalism grounds. ***

Applying the three-part test of Lemon v. Kurtzman, 403 U.S. 602, 612-613 (1971), as set out in Committee for Public Education & Religious Liberty v. Nyquist, 413 U.S. 756, 773 (1973), the court held that the chaplaincy practice violated all three elements of the test: the purpose and primary effect of selecting the same minister for 16 years and publishing his prayers was to promote a particular religious expression; use of state money for compensation and publication led to entanglement Accordingly, the Court of Appeals modified the District Court's injunction and prohibited the State from engaging in any aspect of its established chaplaincy practice.

We granted certiorari limited to the challenge to the practice of opening sessions with prayers by a state-employed clergyman, and we reverse.

II

The opening of sessions of legislative and other deliberative public bodies with prayer is deeply embedded in the history and tradition of this country. From colonial times through the founding of the Republic and ever since, the practice of legislative prayer has coexisted with the principles of disestablishment and religious freedom. In the very courtrooms in which the United States District Judge and later three Circuit Judges heard and decided this case, the proceedings opened with an announcement that concluded, "God save the United States and this Honorable Court." The same invocation occurs at all sessions of this Court.

The tradition in many of the Colonies was, of course, linked to an established church, but the Continental Congress, beginning in 1774, adopted the traditional procedure of opening its sessions with a prayer offered by a paid chaplain. Although prayers were not offered during the Constitutional Convention, the First Congress, as one of its early items of business, adopted the policy of selecting a chaplain to open each session with prayer. A statute providing for the payment of these chaplains was enacted into law on September 22, 1789.

On September 25, 1789, three days after Congress authorized the appointment of paid chaplains, final agreement was reached on the language of the Bill of Rights, Clearly the men who wrote the First Amendment Religion Clause did not view paid legislative chaplains and opening prayers as a violation of that Amendment, for the practice of opening sessions with prayer has continued without interruption ever since that early session of Congress. It has also been followed consistently in most

---

3. The District Court also enjoined the State from using public funds to publish the prayers holding that this practice violated the Establishment Clause. Petitioners have represented to us that they did not challenge this facet of the District Court's decision, Tr. of Oral Arg. 19-20. Accordingly, no issue as to publishing these prayers is before us.

of the states, including Nebraska, where the institution of opening legislative sessions with prayer was adopted even before the State attained statehood. ***

In Walz v. Tax Comm'n, 397 U.S. 664, 678 (1970), we considered the weight to be accorded to history:

> "It is obviously correct that no one acquires a vested or protected right in violation of the Constitution by long use, even when that span of time covers our entire national existence and indeed predates it. Yet an unbroken practice *** is not something to be lightly cast aside."

No more is Nebraska's practice of over a century, consistent with two centuries of national practice, to be cast aside. It can hardly be thought that in the same week Members of the First Congress voted to appoint and to pay a chaplain for each House and also voted to approve the draft of the First Amendment for submission to the states, they intended the Establishment Clause of the Amendment to forbid what they had just declared acceptable. In applying the First Amendment to the states through the Fourteenth Amendment, Cantwell v. Connecticut, 310 U.S. 296 (1940), it would be incongruous to interpret that Clause as imposing more stringent First Amendment limits on the states than the draftsmen imposed on the Federal Government.

This unique history leads us to accept the interpretation of the First Amendment draftsmen who saw no real threat to the Establishment Clause arising from a practice of prayer similar to that now challenged. We conclude that legislative prayer presents no more potential for establishment than the provision of school transportation, Everson v. Board of Education, 330 U.S. 1 (1947), beneficial grants for higher education, Tilton v. Richardson, 403 U.S. 672 (1971), or tax exemptions for religious organizations, *Walz, supra.* ***

III

We turn then to the question of whether any features of the Nebraska practice violate the Establishment Clause. Beyond the bare fact that a prayer is offered, three points have been made: first, that a clergyman of only one denomination— Presbyterian—has been selected for 16 years; second, that the chaplain is paid at public expense; and third, that the prayers are in the Judeo- Christian tradition. Weighed against the historical background, these factors do not serve to invalidate Nebraska's practice.

The Court of Appeals was concerned that Palmer's long tenure has the effect of giving preference to his religious views. We cannot, any more than Members of the Congresses of this century, perceive any suggestion that choosing a clergyman of one denomination advances the beliefs of a particular church. To the contrary, the evidence indicates that Palmer was reappointed because his performance and personal qualities were acceptable to the body appointing him.

Nor is the compensation of the chaplain from public funds a reason to invalidate the Nebraska Legislature's chaplaincy; remuneration is grounded in historic practice initiated, as we noted earlier, by the same Congress that drafted the Establishment

Clause of the First Amendment. The content of the prayer is not of concern to judges where, as here, there is no indication that the prayer opportunity has been exploited to proselytize or advance any one, or to disparage any other, faith or belief. That being so, it is not for us to embark on a sensitive evaluation or to parse the content of a particular prayer. ***

The judgment of the Court of Appeals is [r]eversed.

JUSTICE BRENNAN, with whom JUSTICE MARSHALL joins, dissenting.

* * *

The Court makes no pretense of subjecting Nebraska's practice of legislative prayer to any of the formal "tests" that have traditionally structured our inquiry under the Establishment Clause. That it fails to do so is, in a sense, a good thing, for it simply confirms that the Court is carving out an exception to the Establishment Clause rather than reshaping Establishment Clause doctrine to accommodate legislative prayer. [I]f the Court were to judge legislative prayer through the unsentimental eye of our settled doctrine, it would have to strike it down as a clear violation of the Establishment Clause.

The most commonly cited formulation of prevailing Establishment Clause doctrine is found in Lemon v. Kurtzman, 403 U.S. 602 (1971):

> Every analysis in this area must begin with consideration of the cumulative criteria developed by the Court over many years. Three such tests may be gleaned from our cases. First, the statute [at issue] must have a secular legislative purpose; second, its principal or primary effect must be one that neither advances nor inhibits religion; finally, the statute must not foster 'an excessive government entanglement with religion.

That the "purpose" of legislative prayer is pre-eminently religious rather than secular seems to me to be self-evident. "To invoke Divine guidance on a public body entrusted with making the laws," is nothing but a religious act. Moreover, whatever secular functions legislative prayer might play—formally opening the legislative session, getting the members of the body to quiet down, and imbuing them with a sense of seriousness and high purpose—could so plainly be performed in a purely nonreligious fashion that to claim a secular purpose for the prayer is an insult to the perfectly honorable individuals who instituted and continue the practice. ***

Finally, there can be no doubt that the practice of legislative prayer leads to excessive "entanglement" between the State and religion. *Lemon* pointed out that "entanglement" can take two forms: First, a state statute or program might involve the state impermissibly in monitoring and overseeing religious affairs. In the case of legislative prayer, the process of choosing a "suitable" chaplain, whether on a permanent or rotating basis, and insuring that the chaplain limits himself or herself to "suitable" prayers, involves precisely the sort of supervision that agencies of government should if at all possible avoid.

Second, excessive "entanglement" might arise out of "the divisive political potential" of a state statute or program. *** In this case, this second aspect of entanglement is also clear. The controversy between Senator Chambers and his colleagues, which had reached the stage of difficulty and rancor long before this lawsuit was brought, has split the Nebraska Legislature precisely on issues of religion and religious conformity. The record in this case also reports a series of instances, involving legislators other than Senator Chambers, in which invocations by Reverend Palmer and others led to controversy along religious lines. And in general, the history of legislative prayer has been far more eventful—and divisive—than a hasty reading of the Court's opinion might indicate.[10]

In sum, I have no doubt that, if any group of law students were asked to apply the principles of *Lemon* to the question of legislative prayer, they would nearly unanimously find the practice to be unconstitutional. ***

Nor should it be thought that this view of the Establishment Clause is a recent concoction of an overreaching judiciary. Even before the First Amendment was written, the Framers of the Constitution broke with the practice of the Articles of Confederation and many state constitutions, and did not invoke the name of God in the document. This "omission of a reference to the Deity was not inadvertent; nor did it remain unnoticed."[18] Moreover, Thomas Jefferson and Andrew Jackson, during their respective terms as President, both refused on Establishment Clause grounds to declare national days of thanksgiving or fasting.[19] And James Madison, writing subsequent to his own Presidency on essentially the very issue we face today, stated:

> "Is the appointment of Chaplains to the two Houses of Congress consistent with the Constitution, and with the pure principle of religious freedom?

---

10. *** In more recent years, particular prayers and particular chaplains in the state legislatures have periodically led to serious political divisiveness along religious lines. See, e.g., The Oregonian, Apr. 1, 1983, p. C8 ("Despite protests from at least one representative, a follower of an Indian guru was allowed to give the prayer at the start of Thursday's [Oregon] House [of Representatives] session. Shortly before Ma Anand Sheela began the invocation, about a half-dozen representatives walked off the House floor in apparent protest of the prayer"); Cal. Senate Jour., 37th Sess., 171-173, 307-308 (1907) (discussing request by a State Senator that State Senate Chaplain not use the name of Christ in legislative prayer, and response by one local clergyman claiming that the legislator who made the request had committed a "crowning infamy" and that his "words were those of an irreverent and godless man").***

18. Pfeffer, The Deity in American Constitutional History, 23 J. Church & State 215, 217 (1981). See also 1 Stokes 523.

19. See L. Pfeffer, Church, State, and Freedom 266 (rev. ed. 1967). Jefferson expressed his views as follows: "'I consider the government of the United States as interdicted by the Constitution from intermeddling with religious institutions, their doctrines, discipline, or exercises. [I]t is only proposed that I should recommend not prescribe a day of fasting and prayer. [But] I do not believe it is for interest of religion to invite the civil magistrate to direct its exercises, its discipline, or its doctrine. *** Fasting and prayer are religious exercises; the enjoining of them an act of discipline. Every religious society has a right to determine for itself the times for these exercises, and the objects proper for them, according to their own particular tenets; and the right can never be safer than in their hands, where the Constitution has deposited it.'" *Ibid.*, quoting 11 Jefferson's Writings 428-430 (Monticello ed. 1905).

"In strictness, the answer on both points must be in the negative. The Constitution of the U.S. forbids everything like an establishment of a national religion. The law appointing Chaplains establishes a religious worship for the national representatives, to be performed by Ministers of religion, elected by a majority of them; and these are to be paid out of the national taxes. Does not this involve the principle of a national establishment, applicable to a provision for a religious worship for the Constituent as well as of the representative Body, approved by the majority, and conducted by Ministers of religion paid by the entire nation." Fleet, Madison's "Detached Memoranda," 3 Wm. & Mary Quarterly 534, 558 (1946).

Legislative prayer clearly violates the principles of neutrality and separation that are embedded within the Establishment Clause. It is contrary to the fundamental message of *Engel* and *Schempp*. It intrudes on the right to conscience by forcing some legislators either to participate in a "prayer opportunity," with which they are in basic disagreement, or to make their disagreement a matter of public comment by declining to participate. It forces all residents of the State to support a religious exercise that may be contrary to their own beliefs. It requires the State to commit itself on fundamental theological issues. It has the potential for degrading religion by allowing a religious call to worship to be intermeshed with a secular call to order. And it injects religion into the political sphere by creating the potential that each and every selection of a chaplain, or consideration of a particular prayer, or even reconsideration of the practice itself, will provoke a political battle along religious lines and ultimately alienate some religiously identified group of citizens. ***

The Court's main argument for carving out an exception sustaining legislative prayer is historical. This is a case, however, in which—absent the Court's invocation of history—there would be no question that the practice at issue was unconstitutional. And despite the surface appeal of the Court's argument, there are at least three reasons why specific historical practice should not in this case override that clear constitutional imperative.[30]

First, it is significant that the Court's historical argument does not rely on the legislative history of the Establishment Clause itself. Indeed, that formal history is profoundly unilluminating on this and most other subjects. Rather, the Court assumes that the Framers of the Establishment Clause would not have themselves authorized a practice that they thought violated the guarantees contained in the Clause. This assumption, however, is questionable. Legislators, influenced by the

---

30. Indeed, the sort of historical argument made by the Court should be advanced with some hesitation in light of certain other skeletons in the congressional closet. See, e.g., An Act for the Punishment of certain Crimes against the United States, § 16, 1 Stat. 116 (1790) (enacted by the First Congress and requiring that persons convicted of certain theft offenses "be publicly whipped, not exceeding thirty-nine stripes"); Act of July 23, 1866, 14 Stat. 216 (reaffirming the racial segregation of the public schools in the District of Columbia; enacted exactly one week after Congress proposed Fourteenth Amendment to the States).

passions and exigencies of the moment, the pressure of constituents and colleagues, and the press of business, do not always pass sober constitutional judgment on every piece of legislation they enact, and this must be assumed to be as true of the Members of the First Congress as any other. Indeed, the fact that James Madison, who voted for the bill authorizing the payment of the first congressional chaplains, later expressed the view that the practice was unconstitutional, is instructive on precisely this point. ***

Finally, and most importantly, the argument tendered by the Court is misguided because the Constitution is not a static document whose meaning on every detail is fixed for all time by the life experience of the Framers. *** "[O]ur religious composition makes us a vastly more diverse people than were our forefathers. *** In the face of such profound changes, practices which may have been objectionable to no one in the time of Jefferson and Madison may today be highly offensive to many persons, the deeply devout and the nonbelievers alike." *Schempp, supra,* at 240-241 (BRENNAN, J., concurring). *** Indeed, a proper respect for the Framers themselves forbids us to give so static and lifeless a meaning to their work. To my mind, the Court's focus here on a narrow piece of history is, in a fundamental sense, a betrayal of the lessons of history. ***

JUSTICE STEVENS, dissenting. [Omitted.]

LYNCH, MAYOR OF PAWTUCKET v. DONNELLY

465 U.S. 668 (1984)

CHIEF JUSTICE BURGER delivered the opinion of the Court.

We granted certiorari to decide whether the Establishment Clause of the First Amendment prohibits a municipality from including a crèche, or Nativity scene, in its annual Christmas display.

***

Each year, in cooperation with the downtown retail merchants' association, the city of Pawtucket, R.I., erects a Christmas display as part of its observance of the Christmas holiday season. The display is situated in a park owned by a nonprofit organization and located in the heart of the shopping district. The display is essentially like those to be found in hundreds of towns or cities across the Nation—often on public grounds—during the Christmas season. The Pawtucket display comprises many of the figures and decorations traditionally associated with Christmas, including, among other things, a Santa Claus house, reindeer pulling Santa's sleigh, candy-striped poles, a Christmas tree, carolers, cutout figures representing such characters as a clown, an elephant, and a teddy bear, hundreds of colored lights, a large banner that reads "SEASONS GREETINGS," and the crèche at issue here. All components of this display are owned by the city.

The crèche, which has been included in the display for 40 or more years, consists of the traditional figures, including the Infant Jesus, Mary and Joseph, angels, shepherds, kings, and animals, all ranging in height from 5" to 5'. In 1973, when the present crèche was acquired, it cost the city $1,365; it now is valued at $200. The erection and dismantling of the crèche costs the city about $20 per year; nominal expenses are incurred in lighting the crèche. No money has been expended on its maintenance for the past 10 years.

Respondents, Pawtucket residents and individual members of the Rhode Island affiliate of the American Civil Liberties Union, and the affiliate itself, brought this action in the United States District Court for Rhode Island, challenging the city's inclusion of the crèche in the annual display. The District Court held that the city's inclusion of the crèche in the display violates the Establishment Clause, which is binding on the states through the Fourteenth Amendment. The District Court found that, by including the crèche in the Christmas display, the city has "tried to endorse and promulgate religious beliefs," and that "erection of the crèche has the real and substantial effect of affiliating the City with the Christian beliefs that the crèche represents."

A divided panel of the Court of Appeals for the First Circuit affirmed. We granted certiorari, and we reverse.

II

***

The Court has sometimes described the Religion Clauses as erecting a "wall" between church and state, see, e.g., Everson v. Board of Education, 330 U.S. 1, 18 (1947). The concept of a "wall" of separation is a useful figure of speech probably deriving from views of Thomas Jefferson. The metaphor has served as a reminder that the Establishment Clause forbids an established church or anything approaching it. But the metaphor itself is not a wholly accurate description of the practical aspects of the relationship that in fact exists between church and state. *** Nor does the Constitution require complete separation of church and state; it affirmatively mandates accommodation, not merely tolerance, of all religions, and forbids hostility toward any.

*** In Marsh v. Chambers, 463 U.S. 783 (1983), we noted that 17 Members of that First Congress had been Delegates to the Constitutional Convention where freedom of speech, press, and religion and antagonism toward an established church were subjects of frequent discussion. *** It is clear that neither the 17 draftsmen of the Constitution who were Members of the First Congress, nor the Congress of 1789, saw any establishment problem in the employment of congressional Chaplains to offer daily prayers in the Congress, a practice that has continued for nearly two centuries. It would be difficult to identify a more striking example of the accommodation of religious belief intended by the Framers.

There is an unbroken history of official acknowledgment by all three branches of government of the role of religion in American life from at least 1789. Seldom in our opinions was this more affirmatively expressed than in Justice Douglas' opinion for the Court validating a program allowing release of public school students from classes to attend off-campus religious exercise. Rejecting a claim that the program violated the Establishment Clause, the Court asserted pointedly:

> "We are a religious people whose institutions presuppose a Supreme Being." *Zorach v. Clauson*, [343 U.S.], at 313.

Our history is replete with official references to the value and invocation of Divine guidance in deliberations and pronouncements of the Founding Fathers and contemporary leaders. Beginning in the early colonial period long before Independence, a day of Thanksgiving was celebrated as a religious holiday to give thanks for the bounties of Nature as gifts from God. President Washington and his successors proclaimed Thanksgiving, with all its religious overtones, a day of national celebration and Congress made it a National Holiday more than a century ago. That holiday has not lost its theme of expressing thanks for Divine aid any more than has Christmas lost its religious significance.

Executive Orders and other official announcements of Presidents and of the Congress have proclaimed both Christmas and Thanksgiving National Holidays in religious terms. And, by Acts of Congress, it has long been the practice that federal employees are released from duties on these National Holidays, while being paid from the same public revenues that provide the compensation of the Chaplains of the Senate and the House and the military services. Thus, it is clear that Government has long recognized—indeed it has subsidized—holidays with religious significance.

Other examples of reference to our religious heritage are found in the statutorily prescribed national motto "In God We Trust," 36 U.S.C. § 186, which Congress and the President mandated for our currency, see 31 U.S.C. § 5112(d)(1) (1982 ed.), and in the language "One nation under God," as part of the Pledge of Allegiance to the American flag. That pledge is recited by many thousands of public school children —and adults—every year.

Art galleries supported by public revenues display religious paintings of the 15th and 16th centuries, predominantly inspired by one religious faith. *** The very chamber in which oral arguments on this case were heard is decorated with a notable and permanent—not seasonal—symbol of religion: Moses with the Ten Commandments. Congress has long provided chapels in the Capitol for religious worship and meditation. ***

III

* * *

In this case, the focus of our inquiry must be on the crèche in the context of the Christmas season. See, e.g., Stone v. Graham, 449 U.S. 39 (1980) (*per curiam*); Abington School District v. Schempp, 374 U.S. 203 (1963). In *Stone*, for example, we invalidated a state statute requiring the posting of a copy of the Ten Commandments on public classroom walls. But the Court carefully pointed out that the Commandments were posted purely as a religious admonition, not "integrated into the school curriculum, where the Bible may constitutionally be used in an appropriate study of history, civilization, ethics, comparative religion, or the like." Similarly, in

Abington, although the Court struck down the practices in two States requiring daily Bible readings in public schools, it specifically noted that nothing in the Court's holding was intended to "indicat[e] that such study of the Bible or of religion, when presented objectively as part of a secular program of education, may not be effected consistently with the First Amendment." Focus exclusively on the religious component of any activity would inevitably lead to its invalidation under the Establishment Clause.

The District Court inferred from the religious nature of the crèche that the city has no secular purpose for the display. In so doing, it rejected the city's claim that its reasons for including the crèche are essentially the same as its reasons for sponsoring the display as a whole. The District Court plainly erred by focusing almost exclusively on the crèche. When viewed in the proper context of the Christmas Holiday season, it is apparent that, on this record, there is insufficient evidence to establish that the inclusion of the crèche is a purposeful or surreptitious effort to express some kind of subtle governmental advocacy of a particular religious message. In a pluralistic society a variety of motives and purposes are implicated. The city, like the Congresses and Presidents, however, has principally taken note of a significant historical religious event long celebrated in the Western World. The crèche in the display depicts the historical origins of this traditional event long recognized as a National Holiday. ***

The narrow question is whether there is a secular purpose for Pawtucket's display of the crèche. The display is sponsored by the city to celebrate the Holiday and to depict the origins of that Holiday. These are legitimate secular purposes.[6] The District Court's inference, drawn from the religious nature of the crèche, that the city has no secular purpose was, on this record, clearly erroneous.[7]

The District Court found that the primary effect of including the crèche is to confer a substantial and impermissible benefit on religion in general and on the Christian faith in particular. Comparisons of the relative benefits to religion of different forms of governmental support are elusive and difficult to make. But to conclude that the primary effect of including the crèche is to advance religion in violation of the Establishment Clause would require that we view it as more beneficial to and more an endorsement of religion, for example, than expenditure of large sums of public money for textbooks supplied throughout the country to students attending church-sponsored schools, *Board of Education v. Allen*; expenditure of public funds for transportation of students to church-sponsored schools, *Everson v. Board of Edu-*

---

6. The city contends that the purposes of the display are "exclusively secular." We hold only that Pawtucket has a secular purpose for its display, which is all that Lemon v. Kurtzman, 403 U.S. 602 (1971), requires. Were the test that the government must have "exclusively secular" objectives, much of the conduct and legislation this Court has approved in the past would have been invalidated.

7. Justice Brennan argues that the city's objectives could have been achieved without including the crèche in the display ***. True or not, that is irrelevant. The question is whether the display of the crèche violates the Establishment Clause.

cation; [and] the tax exemptions for church properties sanctioned in Walz v. Tax Comm'n, 397 U.S. 664 (1970). It would also require that we view it as more of an endorsement of religion than the Sunday Closing Laws upheld in McGowan v. Maryland, 366 U.S. 420 (1961); the release time program for religious training in Zorach v. Clauson, 343 U.S. 306 (1952); and the legislative prayers upheld in Marsh v. Chambers, 463 U.S. 783 (1983).

We are unable to discern a greater aid to religion deriving from inclusion of the crèche than from these benefits and endorsements previously held not violative of the Establishment Clause. ***

We can assume, *arguendo*, that the display advances religion in a sense; but our precedents plainly contemplate that on occasion some advancement of religion will result from governmental action. *** Here, whatever benefit there is to one faith or religion or to all religions, is indirect, remote, and incidental; display of the crèche is no more an advancement or endorsement of religion than the Congressional and Executive recognition of the origins of the Holiday itself as "Christ's Mass," or the exhibition of literally hundreds of religions paintings in governmentally supported museums. ***

The Court of Appeals correctly observed that this Court has not held that political divisiveness alone can serve to invalidate otherwise permissible conduct. And we decline to so hold today. This case does not involve a direct subsidy to church-sponsored schools or colleges, or other religious institutions, and hence no inquiry into potential political divisiveness is even called for, Mueller v. Allen, 463 U.S. 388, 403- 404, n. 11 (1983). ***

We are satisfied that the city has a secular purpose for including the crèche, that the city has not impermissibly advanced religion, and that including the crèche does not create excessive entanglement between religion and government.

IV

Of course the crèche is identified with one religious faith but no more so than the examples we have set out from prior cases in which we found no conflict with the Establishment Clause. See, e.g., McGowan v. Maryland, 366 U.S. 420 (1961); Marsh v. Chambers, 463 U.S. 783 (1983). It would be ironic, however, if the inclusion of a single symbol of a particular historic religious event, as part of a celebration acknowledged in the Western World for 20 centuries, and in this country by the people, by the Executive Branch, by the Congress, and the courts for 2 centuries, would so "taint" the city's exhibit as to render it violative of the Establishment Clause. To forbid the use of this one passive symbol—the crèche—at the very time people are taking note of the season with Christmas hymns and carols in public schools and other public places, and while the Congress and legislatures open sessions with prayers by paid chaplains would be a stilted overreaction contrary to our history and to our holdings. If the presence of the crèche in this display violates the Establishment Clause, a host of other forms of taking official note of Christmas, and of our religious heritage, are equally offensive to the Constitution. *** Any notion that these symbols pose a real danger of establishment of a state church is farfetched indeed. ***

JUSTICE O'CONNOR, concurring.

I concur in the opinion of the Court. I write separately to suggest a clarification of our Establishment Clause doctrine. The suggested approach leads to the same result in this case as that taken by the Court, and the Court's opinion, as I read it, is consistent with my analysis.

I

The Establishment Clause prohibits government from making adherence to a religion relevant in any way to a person's standing in the political community. Government can run afoul of that prohibition in two principal ways. One is excessive entanglement with religious institutions, which may interfere with the independence of the institutions, give the institutions access to government or governmental powers not fully shared by nonadherents of the religion, and foster the creation of political constituencies defined along religious lines. E.g., Larkin v. Grendel's Den, Inc., 459 U.S. 116 (1982). The second and more direct infringement is government endorsement or disapproval of religion. Endorsement sends a message to nonadherents that they are outsiders, not full members of the political community, and an accompanying message to adherents that they are insiders, favored members of the political community. Disapproval sends the opposite message. See generally Abington School District v. Schempp, 374 U.S. 203 (1963).

Our prior cases have used the three-part test articulated in Lemon v. Kurtzman, 403 U.S. 602, 612-613 (1971), as a guide to detecting these two forms of unconstitutional government action. It has never been entirely clear, however, how the three parts of the test relate to the principles enshrined in the Establishment Clause. Focusing on institutional entanglement and on endorsement or disapproval of religion clarifies the *Lemon* test as an analytical device.

II

***

Although several of our cases have discussed political divisiveness under the entanglement prong of *Lemon*, see, *e.g.*, Committee for Public Education & Religious Liberty v. Nyquist, 413 U.S. 756, 796 (1973); *Lemon v. Kurtzman, supra*, at 623, we have never relied on divisiveness as an independent ground for holding a government practice unconstitutional. Guessing the potential for political divisiveness inherent in a government practice is simply too speculative an enterprise, in part because the existence of the litigation, as this case illustrates, itself may affect the political response to the government practice. Political divisiveness is admittedly an evil addressed by the Establishment Clause. Its existence may be evidence that institutional entanglement is excessive or that a government practice is perceived as an endorsement of religion. But the constitutional inquiry should focus ultimately on the character of the government activity that might cause such divisiveness, not on the divisiveness itself. The entanglement prong of the *Lemon* test is properly limited to institutional entanglement.

III

The central issue in this case is whether Pawtucket has endorsed Christianity by its display of the crèche. To answer that question, we must examine both what Pawtucket intended to communicate in displaying the crèche and what message the city's display actually conveyed. The purpose and effect prongs of the *Lemon* test represent these two aspects of the meaning of the city's action.

The meaning of a statement to its audience depends both on the intention of the speaker and on the "objective" meaning of the statement in the community. Some listeners need not rely solely on the words themselves in discerning the speaker's intent: they can judge the intent by, for example, examining the context of the statement or asking questions of the speaker. Other listeners do not have or will not seek access to such evidence of intent. They will rely instead on the words themselves; for them the message actually conveyed may be something not actually intended. If the audience is large, as it always is when government "speaks" by word or deed, some portion of the audience will inevitably receive a message determined by the "objective" content of the statement, and some portion will inevitably receive the intended message. Examination of both the subjective and the objective components of the message communicated by a government action is therefore necessary to determine whether the action carries a forbidden meaning.

The purpose prong of the *Lemon* test asks whether government's actual purpose is to endorse or disapprove of religion. The effect prong asks whether, irrespective of government's actual purpose, the practice under review in fact conveys a message of endorsement or disapproval. An affirmative answer to either question should render the challenged practice invalid.

A

The purpose prong of the *Lemon* test requires that a government activity have a secular purpose. That requirement is not satisfied, however, by the mere existence of some secular purpose, however dominated by religious purposes. *** The proper inquiry under the purpose prong of *Lemon*, I submit, is whether the government intends to convey a message of endorsement or disapproval of religion.

Applying that formulation to this case, I would find that Pawtucket did not intend to convey any message of endorsement of Christianity or disapproval of non-Christian religions. The evident purpose of including the crèche in the larger display was not promotion of the religious content of the crèche but celebration of the public holiday through its traditional symbols. Celebration of public holidays, which have cultural significance even if they also have religious aspects, is a legitimate secular purpose.

The District Court's finding that the display of the crèche had no secular purpose was based on erroneous reasoning. The District Court believed that it should ascertain the city's purpose in displaying the crèche separate and apart from the general purpose in setting up the display. It also found that, because the tradition-celebrating purpose was suspect in the court's eyes, the city's use of an unarguably religious symbol "raises an inference" of intent to endorse. When viewed in light of correct legal principles, the District Court's finding of unlawful purpose was clearly erroneous.

B

Focusing on the evil of government endorsement or disapproval of religion makes clear that the effect prong of the *Lemon* test is properly interpreted not to require invalidation of a government practice merely because it in fact causes, even as a primary effect, advancement or inhibition of religion. *** What is crucial is that a government practice not have the effect of communicating a message of government endorsement or disapproval of religion. It is only practices having that effect, whether intentionally or unintentionally, that make religion relevant, in reality or public perception, to status in the political community.

Pawtucket's display of its crèche, I believe, does not communicate a message that the government intends to endorse the Christian beliefs represented by the crèche. Although the religious and indeed sectarian significance of the crèche, as the District Court found, is not neutralized by the setting, the overall holiday setting changes what viewers may fairly understand to be the purpose of the display—as a typical museum setting, though not neutralizing the religious content of a religious painting, negates any message of endorsement of that content. The display celebrates a public holiday, and no one contends that declaration of that holiday is understood to be an endorsement of religion. The holiday itself has very strong secular components and traditions. Government celebration of the holiday, which is extremely common, generally is not understood to endorse the religious content of the holiday, just as government celebration of Thanksgiving is not so understood. The crèche is a traditional symbol of the holiday that is very commonly displayed along with purely secular symbols, as it was in Pawtucket. ***

The city of Pawtucket is alleged to have violated the Establishment Clause by endorsing the Christian beliefs represented by the crèche included in its Christmas display. Giving the challenged practice the careful scrutiny it deserves, I cannot say that the particular crèche display at issue in this case was intended to endorse or had the effect of endorsing Christianity. I agree with the Court that the judgment below must be reversed.

JUSTICE BRENNAN, with whom JUSTICE MARSHALL, JUSTICE BLACKMUN, and JUSTICE STEVENS join, dissenting.

The principles announced in the compact phrases of the Religion Clauses have, as the Court today reminds us, *** proved difficult to apply. Faced with that uncertainty, the Court properly looks for guidance to the settled test announced in Lemon v. Kurtzman, 403 U.S. 602 (1971), for assessing whether a challenged governmental practice involves an impermissible step toward the establishment of religion. *** Applying that test to this case, the Court reaches an essentially narrow result which turns largely upon the particular holiday context in which the city of Pawtucket's nativity scene appeared. The Court's decision implicitly leaves open questions concerning the constitutionality of the public display on public property of a crèche standing alone, or the public display of other distinctively religious symbols such as a cross. Despite the narrow contours of the Court's opinion, our precedents in my view compel the holding that Pawtucket's inclusion of a life- sized display depicting the biblical description of the birth of Christ as part of its annual Christmas celebration is unconstitutional. Nothing in the history of such practices or the setting in which the city's crèche is presented obscures or diminishes the plain fact that Pawtucket's action amounts to an impermissible governmental endorsement of a particular faith.

Last Term, I expressed the hope that the Court's decision in Marsh v. Chambers, 463 U.S. 783 (1983), would prove to be only a single, aberrant departure from our settled method of analyzing Establishment Clause cases. *Id.*, at 796 (BRENNAN, J., dissenting). That the Court today returns to the settled analysis of our prior cases gratifies that hope. At the same time, the Court's less-than-vigorous application of the *Lemon* test suggests that its commitment to those standards may only be superficial. After reviewing the Court's opinion, I am convinced that this case appears hard not because the principles of decision are obscure, but because the Christmas holiday seems so familiar and agreeable. Although the Court's reluctance to disturb a community's chosen method of celebrating such an agreeable holiday is understandable, that cannot justify the Court's departure from controlling precedent. ***

*** To be found constitutional, Pawtucket's seasonal celebration must at least be nondenominational and not serve to promote religion. The inclusion of a distinctively religious element like the crèche, however, demonstrates that a narrower sectarian purpose lay behind the decision to include a nativity scene. That the crèche retained this religious character for the people and municipal government of Pawtucket is suggested by the Mayor's testimony at trial in which he stated that for him, as well as others in the city, the effort to eliminate the nativity scene from Pawtucket's Christmas celebration "is a step towards establishing another religion, non-religion that it may be." *** Plainly, the city and its leaders understood that the inclusion of the crèche in its display would serve the wholly religious purpose of "keep[ing] 'Christ in Christmas.'" 525 F. Supp. 1150, 1173 (RI 1981). From this record, therefore, it is impossible to say with the kind of confidence that was possible in McGowan v. Maryland, 366 U.S. 420, 445 (1961), that a wholly secular goal predominates.

The "primary effect" of including a nativity scene in the city's display is, as the District Court found, to place the government's imprimatur of approval on the particular religious beliefs exemplified by the crèche. The effect on minority religious groups, as well as on those who may reject all religion, is to convey the message that their views are not similarly worthy of public recognition nor entitled to public support. ***

The American historical experience concerning the public celebration of Christmas, if carefully examined, provides no support for the Court's decision. *** Two features of this history are worth noting. First, at the time of the adoption of the Constitution and the Bill of Rights, there was no settled pattern of celebrating Christmas, either as a purely religious holiday or as a public event. Second, the historical evidence, such as it is, offers no uniform pattern of widespread acceptance of the holiday and indeed suggests that the development of Christmas as a public holiday is a comparatively recent phenomenon.[25] ***

Many of the same religious sects that were devotedly opposed to the celebration of Christmas on purely religious grounds, were also some of the most vocal and dedicated foes of established religions in the period just prior to the Revolutionary War. In the eyes of these dissenting religious sects, therefore, the groups most closely associated with established religion—the Churches of England and of Rome—were also most closely linked to the profane practice of publicly celebrating Christmas.

In sum, there is no evidence whatsoever that the Framers would have expressly approved a federal celebration of the Christmas holiday including public displays of a nativity scene; accordingly, the Court's repeated invocation of the decision in is not only baffling, it is utterly irrelevant. Nor is there any suggestion that publicly financed and supported displays of Christmas crèches are supported by a record of widespread, undeviating acceptance that extends throughout our history. Therefore, our prior decisions which relied upon concrete, specific historical evidence to support a particular practice simply have no bearing on the question presented in this case. Contrary to today's careless decision, those prior cases have all recognized that the "illumination" provided by history must always be focused on the particular practice at issue in a given case. Without that guiding principle and the intellectual discipline it imposes, the Court is at sea, free to select random elements of America's varied history solely to suit the views of five members of this Court. ***

JUSTICE BLACKMUN, with whom JUSTICE STEVENS joins, dissenting. [Omitted.]

---

25. The Court's insistence upon pursuing this vague historical analysis is especially baffling since even the petitioners and their supporting *amici* concede that no historical evidence equivalent to that relied upon in *Marsh, McGowan*, or *Walz* supports publicly sponsored Christmas displays. At oral argument, counsel for petitioners was asked whether there is "anything we can refer to to let us know how long it has been the practice in this country for public bodies to have nativity scenes displayed?" Counsel responded: "Specifically, I cannot. *** The recognition of Christmas [as a public holiday] began in the middle part of the last century *** but specifically with respect to the use of the nativity scene, we have been unable to locate that data."

COUNTY OF ALLEGHENY v. AMERICAN CIVIL LIBERTIES UNION

492 U.S. 573 (1989)

MR. JUSTICE BLACKMUN announced the judgment of the Court[.]

* * *

This litigation concerns the constitutionality of two recurring holiday displays located on public property in downtown Pittsburgh. The first is a crèche placed on the Grand Staircase of the Allegheny County Courthouse. The second is a Chanukah menorah placed just outside the City- County Building, next to a Christmas tree and a sign saluting liberty. The Court of Appeals for the Third Circuit ruled that each display violates the Establishment Clause of the First Amendment because each has the impermissible effect of endorsing religion. We agree that the crèche display has that unconstitutional effect but reverse the Court of Appeals' judgment regarding the menorah display.

I-II

* * *

The crèche in the County Courthouse, like other crèches, is a visual representation of the scene in the manger in Bethlehem shortly after the birth of Jesus, as described in the Gospels of Luke and Matthew. The crèche includes figures of the infant Jesus, Mary, Joseph, farm animals, shepherds, and wise men, all placed in or before a wooden representation of a manger, which has at its crest an angel bearing a banner that proclaims "Gloria in Excelsis Deo!"

During the 1986-87 holiday season, the crèche was on display on the Grand Staircase from November 26 to January 9. It had a wooden fence on three sides and bore a plaque stating: "This Display Donated by the Holy Name Society." Sometime during the week of December 2, the county placed red and white poinsettia plants around the fence. The angel was at the apex of the crèche display. Altogether, the crèche, the fence, the poinsettias, and the trees occupied a substantial amount of space on the Grand Staircase. No figures of Santa Claus or other decorations appeared on the Grand Staircase.

The City-County Building is separate and a block removed from the county courthouse and, as the name implies, is jointly owned by the city of Pittsburgh and Allegheny County. For a number of years, the city has had a large Christmas tree under the middle arch outside the Grant Street entrance. Following this practice, city employees on November 17, 1986, erected a 45-foot tree under the middle arch and decorated it with lights and ornaments. A few days later, the city placed at the foot of the tree a sign bearing the Mayor's name and entitled "Salute to Liberty." Beneath the title, the sign stated:

> During this holiday season, the City of Pittsburgh salutes liberty. Let these festive lights remind us that we are the keepers of the flame of liberty and our legacy of freedom." ***

At least since 1982, the city has expanded its Grant Street holiday display to include a symbolic representation of Chanukah, an 8-day Jewish holiday that begins on the 25th day of the Jewish lunar month of Kislev. [T]he city placed at the Grant Street entrance to the City-County Building an 18-foot Chanukah menorah of an abstract tree-and-branch design. The menorah was placed next to the city's 45-foot Christmas tree, against one of the columns that supports the arch into which the tree was set. The menorah is owned by Chabad, a Jewish group,[35] but is stored, erected, and removed each year by the city. The tree, the sign, and the menorah were all removed on January 13. ***

This litigation began on December 10, 1986, when respondents, the Greater Pittsburgh Chapter of the American Civil Liberties Union and seven local residents, filed suit against the county and the city, seeking permanently to enjoin the county from displaying the crèche in the county courthouse and the city from displaying the menorah in front of the City-County Building. Respondents claim that the displays of the crèche and the menorah each violate the Establishment Clause of the First Amendment, made applicable to state governments by the Fourteenth Amendment. ***

III

* * *

In the course of adjudicating specific cases, this Court has come to understand the Establishment Clause to mean that government may not promote or affiliate itself with any religious doctrine or organization, may not discriminate among persons on the basis of their religious beliefs and practices, may not delegate a governmental power to a religious institution, and may not involve itself too deeply in such an institution's affairs. ***

In *Lemon v. Kurtzman*, the Court sought to refine these principles by focusing on three "tests" for determining whether a government practice violates the Establishment Clause. Under the *Lemon* analysis, a statute or practice which touches upon religion, if it is to be permissible under the Establishment Clause, must have a secular purpose; it must neither advance nor inhibit religion in its principal or primary effect; and it must not foster an excessive entanglement with religion. This trilogy of tests has been applied regularly in the Court's later Establishment Clause cases.

Our subsequent decisions further have refined the definition of governmental action that unconstitutionally advances religion. In recent years, we have paid particularly close attention to whether the challenged governmental practice either has the purpose or effect of "endorsing" religion, a concern that has long had a place in our Establishment Clause jurisprudence. ***

Under the Court's holding in *Lynch*, the effect of a crèche display turns on its setting. Here, unlike in *Lynch*, nothing in the context of the display detracts from the

---

35. Chabad, also known as Lubavitch, is an organization of Hasidic Jews who follow the teachings of a particular Jewish leader, the Lubavitch Rebbe. *** The Lubavitch movement is a branch of Hasidism, which itself is a branch of orthodox Judaism. *** Pittsburgh has a total population of 45,000 Jews; of these, 100 to 150 families attend synagogue at Pittsburgh's Lubavitch Center. ***

crèche's religious message. The *Lynch* display comprised a series of figures and objects, each group of which had its own focal point. Santa's house and his reindeer were objects of attention separate from the crèche, and had their specific visual story to tell. Similarly, whatever a "talking" wishing well may be, it obviously was a center of attention separate from the crèche. Here, in contrast, the crèche stands alone: it is the single element of the display on the Grand Staircase.

The floral decoration surrounding the crèche cannot be viewed as somehow equivalent to the secular symbols in the overall *Lynch* display. The floral frame, like all good frames, serves only to draw one's attention to the message inside the frame. The floral decoration surrounding the crèche contributes to, rather than detracts from, the endorsement of religion conveyed by the crèche. It is as if the county had allowed the Holy Name Society to display a cross on the Grand Staircase at Easter, and the county had surrounded the cross with Easter lilies.

Furthermore, the crèche sits on the Grand Staircase, the "main" and "most beautiful part" of the building that is the seat of county government. No viewer could reasonably think that it occupies this location without the support and approval of the government. Thus, by permitting the "display of the crèche in this particular physical setting." *Lynch*, 465 U. S., at 692, (O'CONNOR, J., concurring), the county sends an unmistakable message that it supports and promotes the Christian praise to God that is the crèche's religious message.

The fact that the crèche bears a sign disclosing its ownership by a Roman Catholic organization does not alter this conclusion. On the contrary, the sign simply demonstrates that the government is endorsing the religious message of that organization, rather than communicating a message of its own.

In sum, *Lynch* teaches that government may celebrate Christmas in some manner and form, but not in a way that endorses Christian doctrine. Here, Allegheny County has transgressed this line. It has chosen to celebrate Christmas in a way that has the effect of endorsing a patently Christian message: Glory to God for the birth of Jesus Christ. Under *Lynch*, and the rest of our cases, nothing more is required to demonstrate a violation of the Establishment Clause. The display of the crèche in this context, therefore, must be permanently enjoined. ***

V

*** JUSTICE KENNEDY, however, argues that *Marsh* legitimates all "practices with no greater potential for an establishment of religion" than those "accepted traditions dating back to the Founding." ***

Our previous opinions have considered in dicta the motto and the pledge, characterizing them as consistent with the proposition that government may not communicate an endorsement of religious belief. *Lynch*, 465 U. S., at 693 (O'CONNOR, J., concurring); *id.*, at 716-717 (BRENNAN, J., dissenting). We need not return to the subject of "ceremonial deism," *** because there is an obvious distinction between crèche displays and references to God in the motto and the pledge. However history may affect the constitutionality of nonsectarian references to religion by the government,[52] history cannot legitimate practices that demonstrate the government's allegiance to a particular sect or creed.

Indeed, in *Marsh* itself, the Court recognized that not even the "unique history" of legislative prayer, can justify contemporary legislative prayers that have the effect of affiliating the government with any one specific faith or belief. The legislative prayers involved in *Marsh* did not violate this principle because the particular chaplain had "removed all references to Christ." ***

VI

The display of the Chanukah menorah in front of the City-County Building may well present a closer constitutional question. The menorah, one must recognize, is a religious symbol: it serves to commemorate the miracle of the oil as described in the Talmud. But the menorah's message is not exclusively religious. The menorah is the primary visual symbol for a holiday that, like Christmas, has both religious and secular dimensions.

Moreover, the menorah here stands next to a Christmas tree and a sign saluting liberty. While no challenge has been made here to the display of the tree and the sign, their presence is obviously relevant in determining the effect of the menorah's display. *** The conclusion here that, in this particular context, the menorah's display does not have an effect of endorsing religious faith does not foreclose the possibility that the display of the menorah might violate either the "purpose" or "entanglement" prong of the *Lemon* analysis. These issues were not addressed by the Court of Appeals and may be considered by that court on remand. ***

JUSTICE O'CONNOR, with whom JUSTICE BRENNAN and JUSTICE STEVENS join as to Part II, concurring in part and concurring in the judgment.

* * *

In my concurrence in *Lynch*, I suggest a clarification of our Establishment Clause doctrine to reinforce the concept that the Establishment Clause "prohibits government from making adherence to a religion relevant in any way to a person's standing in the political community." ***

I agree that the crèche displayed on the Grand Staircase of the Allegheny County Courthouse, the seat of county government, conveys a message to nonadherents of Christianity that they are not full members of the political community, and a corresponding message to Christians that they are favored members of the political community. In contrast to the crèche in *Lynch*, which was displayed in a private park in the city's commercial district as part of a broader display of traditional secular

52. It is worth noting that just because *Marsh* sustained the validity of legislative prayer, it does not necessarily follow that practices like proclaiming a National Day of Prayer are constitutional. Legislative prayer does not urge citizens to engage in religious practices, and on that basis could well be distinguishable from an exhortation from government to the people that they engage in religious conduct. But, as this practice is not before us, we express no judgment about its constitutionality.

symbols of the holiday season, this crèche stands alone in the county courthouse. The display of religious symbols in public areas of core government buildings runs a special risk of "mak[ing] religion relevant, in reality or public perception, to status in the political community." The Court correctly concludes that placement of the central religious symbol of the Christmas holiday season at the Allegheny County Courthouse has the unconstitutional effect of conveying a government endorsement of Christianity.

For reasons which differ somewhat from those set forth in JUSTICE BLACKMUN's opinion, I also conclude that the city of Pittsburgh's combined holiday display of a Chanukah menorah, a Christmas tree, and a sign saluting liberty does not have the effect of conveying an endorsement of religion. *** In my view, the relevant question for Establishment Clause purposes is whether the city of Pittsburgh's display of the menorah, the religious symbol of a religious holiday, next to a Christmas tree and a sign saluting liberty sends a message of government endorsement of Judaism or whether it sends a message of pluralism and freedom to choose one's own beliefs. ***

JUSTICE BRENNAN, with whom JUSTICE MARSHALL and JUSTICE STEVENS join, concurring in part and dissenting in part. [Omitted.]

JUSTICE STEVENS, with whom JUSTICE BRENNAN and JUSTICE MARSHALL join, concurring in part and dissenting in part.

* * *

In my opinion the Establishment Clause should be construed to create a strong presumption against the display of religious symbols on public property. There is always a risk that such symbols will offend nonmembers of the faith being advertised as well as adherents who consider the particular advertisement disrespectful. Some devout Christians believe that the crèche should be placed only in reverential settings, such as a church or perhaps a private home; they do not countenance its use as an aid to commercialization of Christ's birthday. Cf. *Lynch*, 465 U.S., at 726-727 (BLACKMUN, J., dissenting).[8] In this very suit, members of the Jewish faith firmly opposed the use of which the menorah was put by the particular sect that sponsored the display at Pittsburgh's City-County Building.[9] Even though "[p]assersby who disagree with the message conveyed by these displays are free to ignore them, or even turn their backs," (KENNEDY, J., concurring in judgment in part and dissenting in part), displays of this kind inevitably have a greater tendency to emphasize sincere

---

8. The point is reiterated here by *amicus* the Governing Board of the National Counsel of Churches of Christ in the U.S.A., which argues that "government acceptance of a crèche on public property *** secularizes and degrades a sacred symbol of Christianity." See also *Engel*, 370 U.S., at 431. Indeed two Roman Catholics testified before the District Court in this case that the creche display offended them.

9. See Brief for American Jewish Committee et al. as *Amici Curiae* i-ii; Brief for American Jewish Congress et al. as *Amici Curiae* 1-2; Tr. of Oral Arg. 44.

and deeply felt differences among individuals than to achieve an ecumenical goal. The Establishment Clause does not allow public bodies to foment such disagreement.[10] ***

I cannot agree with the Court's conclusion that the display at Pittsburgh's City-County Building was constitutional. Standing alone in front of a governmental headquarters, a lighted, 45-foot evergreen tree might convey holiday greetings linked too tenuously to Christianity to have constitutional moment. Juxtaposition of this tree with an 18-foot menorah does not make the latter secular, as JUSTICE BLACKMUN contends, Rather, the presence of the Chanukah menorah, unquestionably a religious symbol, gives religious significance to the Christmas tree. The overall display thus manifests governmental approval of the Jewish and Christian religions. ***

JUSTICE KENNEDY, with whom THE CHIEF JUSTICE, JUSTICE WHITE, and JUSTICE SCALIA join, concurring in the judgment in part and dissenting in part.

I

In keeping with the usual fashion of recent years, the majority applies the *Lemon* test to judge the constitutionality of the holiday displays here in question. I am content for present purposes to remain within the *Lemon* framework, but do not wish to be seen as advocating, let alone adopting, that test as our primary guide in this difficult area. ***

The only *Lemon* factor implicated in this case directs us to inquire whether the "principal or primary effect" of the challenged government practice is "one that neither advances nor inhibits religion." The requirement of neutrality inherent in that formulation has sometimes been stated in categorical terms. For example, in Everson v. Board of Education, 330 U.S. 1 (1947), the first case in our modern Establishment Clause jurisprudence, Justice Black wrote that the Clause forbids laws "which aid one religion, aid all religions, or prefer one religion over another." *Id.*, at 15-16.

These statements must not give the impression of a formalism that does not exist. Taken to its logical extreme, some of the language quoted above would require a relentless extirpation of all contact between government and religion. But that is not the history or the purpose of the Establishment Clause. Government policies of accommodation, acknowledgment, and support for religion are an accepted part of our political and cultural heritage. ***

Our cases disclose two limiting principles: government may not coerce anyone to support or participate in any religion or its exercise; and it may not, in the guise

---

10. This case illustrates the danger that governmental displays of religious symbols may give rise to unintended divisiveness, for the net result of the Court's disposition is to disallow the display of the crèche but to allow the display of the menorah. Laypersons unfamiliar with the intricacies of Establishment Clause jurisprudence may reach the wholly unjustified conclusion that the Court itself is preferring one faith over another. ***

of avoiding hostility or callous indifference, give direct benefits to religion in such a degree that it in fact "establishes a [state] religion or religious faith, or tends to do so." *Lynch v. Donnelly, supra*, at 678. These two principles, while distinct, are not unrelated, for it would be difficult indeed to establish a religion without some measure of more or less subtle coercion, be it in the form of taxation to supply the substantial benefits that would sustain a state-established faith, direct compulsion to observance, or governmental exhortation to religiousity that amounts in fact to proselytizing. ***

Symbolic recognition or accommodation of religious faith may violate the Clause in an extreme case. I doubt not, for example, that the Clause forbids a city to permit the permanent erection of a large Latin cross on the roof of city hall. This is not because government speech about religion is *per se* suspect, as the majority would have it, but because such an obtrusive year-round religious display would place the government's weight behind an obvious effort to proseltyze on behalf of a particular religion. *** Non-coercive government action within the realm of flexible accommodation or passive acknowledgment of existing symbols does not violate the Establishment Clause unless it benefits religion in a way more direct and more substantial than practices that are accepted in our national heritage.

II

* * *

There is no suggestion here that the government's power to coerce has been used to further the interests of Christianity or Judaism in any way. No one was compelled to observe or participate in any religious ceremony or activity. Neither the city nor the county contributed significant amounts of tax money to serve the cause of one religious faith. The crèche and the menorah are purely passive symbols of religious holidays. Passersby who disagree with the message conveyed by these displays are free to ignore them, or even to turn their backs, just as they are free to do when they disagree with any other form of government speech.

There is no realistic risk that the crèche or the menorah represent an effort to proselytize or are otherwise the first step down the road to an establishment of religion. *Lynch* is dispositive of this claim with respect to the crèche, and I find no reason for reaching a different result with respect to the menorah. Both are the traditional symbols of religious holidays that over time have acquired a secular component. ***

Nor can I comprehend why it should be that placement of a government-owned crèche on private land is lawful while placement of a privately owned crèche on public land is not.[5] If anything, I should have thought government ownership of a religious symbol presented the more difficult question under the Establishment Clause, but as *Lynch* resolved that question to sustain the government action, the sponsorship here ought to be all the easier to sustain. In short, nothing about the religious dis-

---

5. The crèche in *Lynch* was owned by Pawtucket. Neither the crèche nor the menorah at issue in this case is owned by a governmental entity.

plays here distinguishes them in any meaningful way from the crèche we permitted in *Lynch*. ***

III-IV

Even if *Lynch* did not control, I would not commit this Court to the test applied by the majority today. The notion that cases arising under the Establishment Clause should be decided by an inquiry into whether a "'reasonable observer'" may "'fairly understand'" government action to "'sen[d] a message to nonadherents that they are outsiders, not full members of the political community,'" is a recent, and in my view most unwelcome, addition to our tangled Establishment Clause jurisprudence. ***

If the endorsement test, applied without artificial exceptions for historical practice, reached results consistent with history, my objections to it would have less force. But, as I understand that test, the touchstone of an Establishment Clause violation is whether nonadherents would be made to feel like "outsiders" by government recognition or accommodation of religion. Few of our traditional practices recognizing the part religion plays in our society can withstand scrutiny under a faithful application of this formula. ***

The approach adopted by the majority contradicts important values embodied in the Clause. Obsessive, implacable resistance to all but the most carefully scripted and secularized forms of accommodation requires this Court to act as a censor, issuing national decrees as to what is orthodox and what is not. What is orthodox, in this context, means what is secular; the only Christmas the State can acknowledge is one in which references to religion have been held to a minimum. The Court thus lends its assistant to an Orwellian rewriting of history as many understand it. I can conceive of no judicial function more antithetical to the First Amendment.

A further contradiction arises from the majority's approach, for the Court also assumes the difficult and inappropriate task of saying what every religious symbol means. Before studying this case, I had not known the full history of the menorah, and I suspect the same was true of my colleagues. More important, this history was, and is, likely unknown to the vast majority of people of all faiths who saw the symbol displayed in Pittsburgh. Even if the majority is quite right about the history of the menorah, it hardly follows that this same history informed the observers' view of the symbol and the reason for its presence. This Court is ill-equipped to sit as a national theology board, and I question both the wisdom and the constitutionality of its doing so. Indeed, were I required to choose between the approach taken by the majority and a strict separationist view, I would have to respect the consistency of the latter.

The suit before us is admittedly a troubling one. It must be conceded that, however neutral the purpose of the city and county, the eager proselytizer may seek to use these symbols for his own ends. The urge to use them to teach or to taunt is always present. It is also true that some devout adherents of Judaism or Christianity may be as offended by the holiday display as are nonbelievers, if not more so. To place these religious symbols in a common hallway or sidewalk, where they may be ignored or even insulted, must be distasteful to many who cherish their meaning.

For these reasons, I might have voted against installation of these particular displays were I a local legislative official. But we have no jurisdiction over matters of taste within the realm of constitutionally permissible discretion. *** In my view, the principles of the Establishment Clause and our Nation's historic traditions of diversity and pluralism allow communities to make reasonable judgments respecting the accommodation or acknowledgment of holidays with both cultural and religious aspects. No constitutional violation occurs when they do so by displaying a symbol of the holiday's religious origins.

LEE v. WEISMAN

505 U.S. 577 (1992)

JUSTICE KENNEDY delivered the opinion of the Court.

School principals in the public school system of the city of Providence, Rhode Island, are permitted to invite members of the clergy to offer invocation and benediction prayers as part of the formal graduation ceremonies for middle schools and for high schools. *** Many, but not all, of the principals elected to include prayers as part of the graduation ceremonies. Acting for himself and his daughter, Deborah's father, Daniel Weisman, objected to any prayers at Deborah's middle school graduation, but to no avail. The school principal, petitioner Robert E. Lee, invited a rabbi to deliver prayers at the graduation exercises for Deborah's class. Rabbi Leslie Gutterman, of the Temple Beth El in Providence, accepted.

It has been the custom of Providence school officials to provide invited clergy with a pamphlet entitled "Guidelines for Civic Occasions," prepared by the National Conference of Christians and Jews. *** Rabbi Gutterman's prayers were as follows:

INVOCATION

God of the Free, Hope of the Brave:

For the legacy of America where diversity is celebrated and the rights of minorities are protected, we thank You. May these young men and women grow up to enrich it.

For the liberty of America, we thank You. May these new graduates grow up to guard it.

For the political process of America in which all its citizens may participate, for its court system where all may seek justice we thank You. May those we honor this morning always turn to it in trust.

For the destiny of America we thank You. May the graduates of Nathan Bishop Middle School so live that they might help to share it.

May our aspirations for our country and for these young people, who are our hope for the future, be richly fulfilled. AMEN.

BENEDICTION

O God, we are grateful to You for having endowed us with the capacity for learning which we have celebrated on this joyous commencement.

> Happy families give thanks for seeing their children achieve an important milestone. Send Your blessings upon the teachers and administrators who helped prepare them.
> The graduates now need strength and guidance for the future, help them to understand that we are not complete with academic knowledge alone. We must each strive to fulfill what You require of us all: To do justly, to love mercy, to walk humbly.
> We give thanks to You, Lord, for keeping us alive, sustaining us and allowing us to reach this special, happy occasion. AMEN. ***

The District Court held that petitioners' practice of including invocations and benedictions in public school graduations violated the Establishment Clause of the First Amendment, and it enjoined petitioners from continuing the practice. *** We granted certiorari, and now affirm.

These dominant facts mark and control the confines of our decision: State officials direct the performance of a formal religious exercise at promotional and graduation ceremonies for secondary schools. Even for those students who object to the religious exercise, their attendance and participation in the state-sponsored religious activity are in a fair and real sense obligatory, though the school district does not require attendance as a condition for receipt of the diploma.

This case does not require us to revisit the difficult questions dividing us in recent cases, questions of the definition and full scope of the principles governing the extent of permitted accommodation by the State for the religious beliefs and practices of many of its citizens. *** [W]ithout reference to those principles in other contexts, the controlling precedents as they relate to prayer and religious exercise in primary and secondary public schools compel the holding here that the policy of the city of Providence is an unconstitutional one. We can decide the case without reconsidering the general constitutional framework by which public schools' efforts to accommodate religion are measured. Thus we do not accept the invitation of petitioners and amicus the United States to reconsider our decision in *Lemon v. Kurtzman*. The government involvement with religious activity in this case is pervasive, to the point of creating a state-sponsored and state-directed religious exercise in a public school. Conducting this formal religious observance conflicts with settled rules pertaining to prayer exercises for students, and that suffices to determine the question before us.

The principle that government may accommodate the free exercise of religion does not supersede the fundamental limitations imposed by the Establishment Clause. It is beyond dispute that, at a minimum, the Constitution guarantees that government may not coerce anyone to support or participate in religion or its exercise, or otherwise act in a way which "establishes a [state] religion or religious faith, or tends to do so." *Lynch*, [492 U.S.], at 678; see also *Allegheny County*, [465 U.S.], at 591 quoting Everson v. Board of Education of Ewing, 330 U.S. 1, 15-16 (1947). The State's involvement in the school prayers challenged today violates these central principles.

That involvement is as troubling as it is undenied. A school official, the principal, decided that an invocation and a benediction should be given; this is a choice attributable to the State, and from a constitutional perspective it is as if a state statute decreed that the prayers must occur. The principal chose the religious participant, here a rabbi, and that choice is also attributable to the State. The reason for the choice of a rabbi is not disclosed by the record, but the potential for divisiveness over the choice of a particular member of the clergy to conduct the ceremony is apparent.

Divisiveness, of course, can attend any state decision respecting religions, and neither its existence nor its potential necessarily invalidates the State's attempts to accommodate religion in all cases. The potential for divisiveness is of particular relevance here though, because it centers around an overt religious exercise in a secondary school environment where *** subtle coercive pressures exist and where the student had no real alternative which would have allowed her to avoid the fact or appearance of participation.

The State's role did not end with the decision to include a prayer and with the choice of clergyman. Principal Lee provided Rabbi Gutterman with a copy of the "Guidelines for Civic Occasions," and advised him that his prayers should be nonsectarian. Through these means the principal directed and controlled the content of the prayer. Even if the only sanction for ignoring the instructions were that the rabbi would not be invited back, we think no religious representative who valued his or her continued reputation and effectiveness in the community would incur the State's displeasure in this regard. It is a cornerstone principle of our Establishment Clause jurisprudence that "it is no part of the business of government to compose official prayers for any group of the American people to recite as a part of a religious program carried on by government," Engel v. Vitale, 370 U.S. 421, 425 (1962), and that is what the school officials attempted to do.

Petitioners argue, and we find nothing in the case to refute it, that the directions for the content of the prayers were a good-faith attempt by the school to ensure that the sectarianism which is so often the flashpoint for religious animosity be removed from the graduation ceremony. The concern is understandable, as a prayer which uses ideas or images identified with a particular religion may foster a different sort of sectarian rivalry than an invocation or benediction in terms more neutral. The school's explanation, however, does not resolve the dilemma caused by its participation. The question is not the good faith of the school in attempting to make the prayer acceptable to most persons, but the legitimacy of its undertaking that enterprise at all when the object is to produce a prayer to be used in a formal religious exercise which students, for all practical purposes, are obliged to attend. ***

*** By the time they are seniors, high school students no doubt have been required to attend classes and assemblies and to complete assignments exposing them to ideas they find distasteful or immoral or absurd or all of these. Against this background, students may consider it an odd measure of justice to be subjected during the course of their educations to ideas deemed offensive and irreligious, but to be denied a brief, formal prayer ceremony that the school offers in return. This argument cannot prevail, however. It overlooks a fundamental dynamic of the Constitution.

The explanation lies in the lesson of history that was and is the inspiration for the Establishment Clause, the lesson that in the hands of government what might begin as a tolerant expression of religious views may end in a policy to indoctrinate and coerce. A state-created orthodoxy puts at grave risk that freedom of belief and conscience which are the sole assurance that religious faith is real, not imposed.

As we have observed before, there are heightened concerns with protecting freedom of conscience from subtle coercive pressure in the elementary and secondary public schools. Our decisions in Engel v. Vitale, 370 U.S. 421 (1962), and *Abington School District* recognize, among other things, that prayer exercises in public schools carry a particular risk of indirect coercion. The concern may not be limited to the context of schools, but it is most pronounced there. *** Finding no violation under these circumstances would place objectors in the dilemma of participating, with all that implies, or protesting. We do not address whether that choice is acceptable if the affected citizens are mature adults, but we think the State may not, consistent with the Clause, place primary and secondary school children in this position. Research in psychology supports the common assumption that adolescents are often susceptible to pressure from their peers towards conformity, and that the influence is strongest in matters of social convention. [Citations omitted.] To recognize that the choice imposed by the State constitutes an unacceptable constraint only acknowledges that the government may no more use social pressure to enforce orthodoxy than it may use more direct means.

There was a stipulation in the District Court that attendance at graduation and promotional ceremonies is voluntary. Petitioners and the United States, as *amicus*, made this a center point of the case, arguing that the option of not attending the graduation excuses any inducement or coercion in the ceremony itself. The argument lacks all persuasion. Law reaches past formalism. And to say a teenage student has a real choice not to attend her high school graduation is formalistic in the extreme. True, Deborah could elect not to attend commencement without renouncing her diploma; but we shall not allow the case to turn on this point. *** The Constitution forbids the State to exact religious conformity from a student as the price of attending her own high school graduation. This is the calculus the Constitution commands.***

No holding by this Court suggests that a school can persuade or compel a student to participate in a religious exercise. That is being done here, and it is forbidden by the Establishment Clause of the First Amendment.

For the reasons we have stated, the judgment of the Court of Appeals is [a]ffirmed.

JUSTICE BLACKMUN, with whom JUSTICE STEVENS and JUSTICE O'CONNOR join, concurring. ***

I join the Court's opinion today because I find nothing in it inconsistent with the essential precepts of the Establishment Clause developed in our precedents. The Court holds that the graduation prayer is unconstitutional because the State "in effect required participation in a religious exercise." Although our precedents make clear that proof of government coercion is not necessary to prove an Establishment Clause violation, it is sufficient. Government pressure to participate in a religious activity is an obvious indication that the government is endorsing or promoting religion.

But it is not enough that the government restrain from compelling religious practices: It must not engage in them either. ***

When the government arrogates to itself a role in religious affairs, it abandons its obligation as guarantor of democracy. *** Madison warned that government officials who would use religious authority to pursue secular ends "exceed the commission from which they derive their authority and are Tyrants. The People who submit to it are governed by laws made neither by themselves, nor by an authority derived from them, and are slaves." Memorial and Remonstrance against Religious Assessments (1785) in The Complete Madison 300 (S. Padover, ed. 1953). Democratic government will not last long when proclamation replaces persuasion as the medium of political exchange. ***

I remain convinced that our jurisprudence is not misguided, and that it requires the decision reached by the Court today. Accordingly, I join the Court in affirming the judgment of the Court of Appeals.

JUSTICE SOUTER, with whom JUSTICE STEVENS and JUSTICE O'CONNOR join, concurring.

I join the whole of the Court's opinion, and fully agree that prayers at public school graduation ceremonies indirectly coerce religious observance. I write separately nonetheless on two issues of Establishment Clause analysis that underlie my independent resolution of this case: whether the Clause applies to governmental practices that do not favor one religion or denomination over others, and whether state coercion of religious conformity, over and above state endorsement of religious exercise or belief, is a necessary element of an Establishment Clause violation.

I

Forty-five years ago, this Court announced a basic principle of constitutional law from which it has not strayed: the Establishment Clause forbids not only state practices that "aid one religion *** or prefer one religion over another," but also those that "aid all religions." Everson v. Board of Education of Ewing, 330 U.S. 1, 15 (1947). Today we reaffirm that principle, holding that the Establishment Clause forbids state-sponsored prayers in public school settings no matter how nondenominational the prayers may be. In barring the State from sponsoring generically Theistic prayers where it could not sponsor sectarian ones, we hold true to a line of precedent from which there is no adequate historical case to depart. ***

Some have challenged this precedent by reading the Establishment Clause to permit "nonpreferential" state promotion of religion. The challengers argue that, as originally understood by the Framers, "[t]he Establishment Clause did not require government neutrality between religion and irreligion nor did it prohibit the Federal Government from providing nondiscriminatory aid to religion." *Wallace*, [472 U.S.], at 106 (REHNQUIST, J., dissenting); see also R. Cord, Separation of Church and State: Historical Fact and Current Fiction (1988). While a case has been made for this position, it is not so convincing as to warrant reconsideration of our settled law; indeed, I find in the history of the Clause's textual development a more powerful argument supporting the Court's jurisprudence following *Everson*.

When James Madison arrived at the First Congress with a series of proposals to amend the National Constitution, one of the provisions read that "[t]he civil rights of none shall be abridged on account of religious belief or worship, nor shall any national religion be established, nor shall the full and equal rights of conscience be in any manner, or on any pretext, infringed." *** Madison's language did not last long. It was sent to a Select Committee of the House, which, without explanation, changed it to read that "no religion shall be established by law, nor shall the equal rights of conscience be infringed." *** Thence the proposal went to the Committee of the Whole, which was in turn dissatisfied with the Select Committee's language and adopted an alternative proposed by Samuel Livermore of New Hampshire: "Congress shall make no laws touching religion, or infringing the rights of conscience." *** Livermore's proposal would have forbidden laws having anything to do with religion and was thus not only far broader than Madison's version, but broader even than the scope of the Establishment Clause as we now understand it. ***

The House rewrote the amendment once more before sending it to the Senate, this time adopting, without recorded debate, language derived from a proposal by Fisher Ames of Massachusetts: "Congress shall make no law establishing Religion, or prohibiting the free exercise thereof, nor shall the rights of conscience be infringed." [T]he House rejected the Select Committee's version, which arguably ensured only that "no religion" enjoyed an official preference over others, and deliberately chose instead a prohibition extending to laws establishing "religion" in general *** an establishment of "a religion," "a national religion," "one religious sect," or specific "articles of faith." The Framers repeatedly considered and deliberately rejected such narrow language and instead extended their prohibition to state support for "religion" in general. ***

What we thus know of the Framers' experience underscores the observation of one prominent commentator, that confining the Establishment Clause to a prohibition on preferential aid "requires a premise that the Framers were extraordinarily bad drafters—that they believed one thing but adopted language that said something substantially different, and that they did so after repeatedly attending to the choice of language." Laycock, "Nonpreferential" Aid 882-883; see also Allegheny County v. American Civil Liberties Union, Greater Pittsburgh Chapter, 492 U.S. 573, 647-648 (1989) (opinion of STEVENS, J.). We must presume, since there is no conclusive evidence to the contrary, that the Framers embraced the significance of their textual judgment.[3] Thus, on balance, history neither contradicts nor warrants reconsideration of the settled principle that the Establishment Clause forbids support for religion in general no less than support for one religion or some.

While these considerations are, for me, sufficient to reject the non-preferentialist position, one further concern animates my judgment. In many contexts, including this one, nonpreferentialism requires some distinction between "sectarian" religious practices and those that would be, by some measure, ecumenical enough to pass Establishment Clause muster. Simply by requiring the enquiry, nonpreferentialists invite the courts to engage in comparative theology. I can hardly imagine a subject less amenable to the competence of the federal judiciary, or more deliberately to be avoided where possible.

This case is nicely in point. Since the nonpreferentiality of a prayer must be judged by its text, JUSTICE BLACKMUN pertinently observes *** that Rabbi Gutterman drew his exhortation "[t]o do justly, to love mercy, to walk humbly" straight from the King James version of Micah, Ch. 9, v. 8. At some undefinable point, the similarities between a state-sponsored prayer and the sacred text of a specific religion would so closely identify the former with the latter that even a nonpreferentialist would have to concede a breach of the Establishment Clause. And even if Micah's thought is sufficiently generic for most believers, it still embodies a straightforwardly Theistic premise, and so does the Rabbi's prayer. Many Americans who consider themselves religious are not Theistic; some, like several of the Framers, are Deists who would question Rabbi Gutterman's plea for divine advancement of the country's political and moral good. ***

Nor does it solve the problem to say that the State should promote a "diversity" of religious views; that position would necessarily compel the government and, inevitably, the courts to make wholly inappropriate judgments about the number of religions the State should sponsor and the relative frequency with which it should sponsor each. In fact, the prospect would be even worse than that. As Madison observed in criticizing religious presidential proclamations, the practice of sponsoring religious messages tends, over time, "to narrow the recommendation to the standard

---

3. In his dissent in Wallace v. Jaffree, 472 U.S. 38 (1985), THE CHIEF JUSTICE rested his nonpreferentialist interpretation partly on the post-ratification actions of the early national government. Aside from the willingness of some (but not all) early Presidents to issue ceremonial religious proclamations, which were at worst trivial breaches of the Establishment Clause, *** he cited such seemingly preferential aid as a treaty provision, signed by Jefferson, authorizing federal subsidization of a Roman Catholic priest and church for the Kaskaskia Indians. But this proves too much, for if the Establishment Clause permits a special appropriation of tax money for the religious activities of a particular sect, it forbids virtually nothing. Although evidence of historical practice can indeed furnish valuable aid in the interpretation of contemporary language, acts like the one in question prove only that public officials, no matter when they serve, can turn a blind eye to constitutional principle. ***

of the predominant sect." Madison's "Detached Memoranda," 3 Wm. & Mary Q. 534, 561 (E. Fleet ed. 1946) (hereinafter Madison's "Detached Memoranda"). ***

II-III

* * *

Petitioners contend that because the early Presidents included religious messages in their inaugural and Thanksgiving Day addresses, the Framers could not have meant the Establishment Clause to forbid noncoercive state endorsement of religion. The argument ignores the fact, however, that Americans today find such proclamations less controversial than did the founding generation, whose published thoughts on the matter belie petitioners' claim. President Jefferson, for example, steadfastly refused to issue Thanksgiving proclamations of any kind, in part because he thought they violated the Religion Clauses. Letter from Thomas Jefferson to Rev. S. Miller (Jan. 23, 1808), in 5 The Founders' Constitution, at 98. ***

During his first three years in office, James Madison also refused to call for days of thanksgiving and prayer, though later, amid the political turmoil of the War of 1812, he did so on four separate occasions. See Madison's "Detached Memoranda," 562, and n.54. Upon retirement, in an essay condemning as an unconstitutional "establishment" the use of public money to support congressional and military chaplains, *id.*, at 558-560, he concluded that "[r]eligious proclamations by the Executive recommending thanksgivings & fasts are shoots from the same root with the legislative acts reviewed. ***"

Madison's failure to keep pace with his principles in the face of congressional pressure cannot erase the principles. He admitted to backsliding, and explained that he had made the content of his wartime proclamations inconsequential enough to mitigate much of their impropriety. See *ibid.*; see also Letter from J. Madison to E. Livingston (July 10, 1822), in 5 The Founders' Constitution, at 105. While his writings suggest mild variations in his interpretation of the Establishment Clause, Madison was no different in that respect from the rest of his political generation. That he expressed so much doubt about the constitutionality of religious proclamations, however, suggests a brand of separationism stronger even than that embodied in our traditional jurisprudence. So too does his characterization of public subsidies for legislative and military chaplains as unconstitutional "establishments," *** for the federal courts, however expansive their general view of the Establishment Clause, have upheld both practices. See Marsh v. Chambers, 463 U.S. 783 (1983) (legislative chaplains); Katcoff v. Marsh, 755 F.2d 223 (CA2 1985) (military chaplains).

To be sure, the leaders of the young Republic engaged in some of the practices that separationists like Jefferson and Madison criticized. The First Congress did hire institutional chaplains, and Presidents Washington and Adams unapologetically marked days of "public thanksgiving and prayer." Yet in the face of the separationist dissent, those practices prove, at best, that the Framers simply did not share a common understanding of the Establishment Clause, and, at worst, that they, like other politicians, could raise constitutional ideals one day and turn their backs on them the next. *** Ten years after proposing the First Amendment, Congress passed the Alien and Sedition Acts, measures patently unconstitutional by modern standards. If the early Congress's political actions were determinative, and not merely relevant, evidence of constitutional meaning, we would have to gut our current First Amendment doctrine to make room for political censorship. ***

Religious students cannot complain that omitting prayers from their graduation ceremony would, in any realistic sense, "burden" their spiritual callings. To be sure, many of them invest this rite of passage with spiritual significance, but they may express their religious feelings about it before and after the ceremony. They may even organize a privately sponsored baccalaureate if they desire the company of likeminded students. Because they accordingly have no need for the machinery of the State to affirm their beliefs, the government's sponsorship of prayer at the graduation ceremony is most reasonably understood as an official endorsement of religion and, in this instance, of Theistic religion. One may fairly say, as one commentator has suggested, that the government brought prayer into the ceremony "precisely because some people want a symbolic affirmation that government approves and endorses their religion, and because many of the people who want this affirmation place little or no value on the costs to religious minorities." Laycock, Summary and Synthesis: The Crisis in Religious Liberty, 60 Geo. Wash. L. Rev. 841, 844 (1992).

Petitioners would deflect this conclusion by arguing that graduation prayers are no different from presidential religious proclamations and similar official "acknowledgments" of religion in public life. But religious invocations in Thanksgiving Day addresses and the like, rarely noticed, ignored without effort, conveyed over an impersonal medium, and directed at no one in particular, inhabit a pallid zone worlds apart from official prayers delivered to a captive audience of public school students and their families. Madison himself respected the difference between the trivial and the serious in constitutional practice. Realizing that his contemporaries were unlikely to take the Establishment Clause seriously enough to forgo a legislative chaplainship, he suggested that "[r]ather than let this step beyond the landmarks of power have the effect of a legitimate precedent, it will be better to apply to it the legal aphorism de minimis non curat lex. ***" Madison's "Detached Memoranda" 559; see also Letter from J. Madison to E. Livingston, 10 July 1822, in 5 The Founders' Constitution, at 105. But that logic permits no winking at the practice in question here. When public school officials, armed with the State's authority, convey an endorsement of religion to their students, they strike near the core of the Establishment Clause. However "ceremonial" their messages may be, they are flatly unconstitutional.

JUSTICE SCALIA, with whom THE CHIEF JUSTICE, JUSTICE WHITE, and JUSTICE THOMAS join, dissenting.

* * *

I

Justice Holmes' aphorism that "a page of history is worth a volume of logic," New York Trust Co. v. Eisner, 256 U.S. 345, 349 (1921), applies with particular force to our Establishment Clause jurisprudence. ***

From our Nation's origin, prayer has been a prominent part of governmental ceremonies and proclamations. The Declaration of Independence, the document marking our birth as a separate people, "appeal[ed] to the Supreme Judge of the world for the rectitude of our intentions" and avowed "a firm reliance on the protection of divine Providence." In his first inaugural address, after swearing his oath of office on a Bible, George Washington deliberately made a prayer a part of his first official act as President:

> "it would be peculiarly improper to omit in this first official act my fervent supplications to that Almighty Being who rules over the universe, who presides in the councils of nations, and whose providential aids can supply every human defect, that His benediction may consecrate to the liberties and happiness of the people of the United States a Government instituted by themselves for these essential purposes." Inaugural Addresses of the Presidents of the United States 2 (1989).

Such supplications have been a characteristic feature of inaugural addresses ever since. Thomas Jefferson, for example, prayed in his first inaugural address: "may that Infinite Power which rules the destinies of the universe lead our councils to what is best, and give them a favorable issue for your peace and prosperity." Similarly, James Madison, in his first inaugural address, placed his confidence

> "in the guardianship and guidance of that Almighty Being whose power regulates the destiny of nations, whose blessings have been so conspicuously dispensed to this rising Republic, and to whom we are bound to address our devout gratitude for the past, as well as our fervent supplications and best hopes for the future." ***

Most recently, President Bush, continuing the tradition established by President Washington, asked those attending his inauguration to bow their heads, and made a prayer his first official act as President. ***

The other two branches of the Federal Government also have a long-established practice of prayer at public events. As we detailed in *Marsh*, Congressional sessions have opened with a chaplain's prayer ever since the First Congress. And this Court's own sessions have opened with the invocation "God save the United States and this Honorable Court" since the days of Chief Justice Marshall. 1 C. Warren, The Supreme Court in United States History 469 (1922).

In addition to this general tradition of prayer at public ceremonies, there exists a more specific tradition of invocations and benedictions at public-school graduation exercises. By one account, the first public-high-school graduation ceremony took place in Connecticut in July 1868—the very month, as it happens, that the Fourteenth

Amendment (the vehicle by which the Establishment Clause has been applied against the States) was ratified—when "15 seniors from the Norwich Free Academy marched in their best Sunday suits and dresses into a church hall and waited through majestic music and long prayers." ***

II-III

The Court presumably would separate graduation invocations and benedictions from other instances of public "preservation and transmission of religious beliefs" on the ground that they involve "psychological coercion." ***

The opinion manifests that the Court itself has not given careful consideration to its test of psychological coercion. For if it had, how could it observe, with no hint of concern or disapproval, that students stood for the Pledge of Allegiance, which immediately preceded Rabbi Gutterman's invocation? *** The government can, of course, no more coerce political orthodoxy than religious orthodoxy. West Virginia Board of Education v. Barnette, 319 U.S. 624, 642 (1943). Moreover, since the Pledge of Allegiance has been revised since *Barnette* to include the phrase "under God," recital of the Pledge would appear to raise the same Establishment Clause issue as the invocation and benediction. If students were psychologically coerced to remain standing during the invocation, they must also have been psychologically coerced, moments before, to stand for (and thereby, in the Court's view, take part in or appear to take part in) the Pledge. Must the Pledge therefore be barred from the public schools (both from graduation ceremonies and from the classroom)? ***

To characterize the "subtle coercive pressures," allegedly present here as the "practical" equivalent of the legal sanctions in *Barnette* is *** well, let me just say it is not a "delicate and fact-sensitive" analysis.

The Court relies on our "school prayer" cases, Engel v. Vitale, 370 U.S. 421 (1962), and Abington School District v. Schempp, 374 U.S. 203 (1963). But whatever the merit of those cases, they do not support, much less compel, the Court's psycho-journey. *Engel* and *Schempp* do not constitute an exception to the rule, distilled from historical practice, that public ceremonies may include prayer. [R]ather, they simply do not fall within the scope of the rule (for the obvious reason that school instruction is not a public ceremony). ***

IV

Our religion-clause jurisprudence has become bedeviled (so to speak) by reliance on formulaic abstractions that are not derived from, but positively conflict with, our long-accepted constitutional traditions. Foremost among these has been the so-called *Lemon* test, which has received well-earned criticism from many members of this Court. The Court today demonstrates the irrelevance of*Lemon* by essentially ignoring it, and the interment of that case may be the one happy byproduct of the Court's otherwise lamentable decision. ***

Another happy aspect of the case is that it is only a jurisprudential disaster and not a practical one. Given the odd basis for the Court's decision, invocations and benedictions will be able to be given at public-school graduations next June, as they have for the past century and a half, so long as school authorities make clear that anyone who abstains from screaming in protest does not necessarily participate in the prayers. All that is seemingly needed is an announcement, or perhaps a written insertion at the beginning of the graduation Program, to the effect that, while all are asked to rise for the invocation and benediction, none is compelled to join in them, nor will be assumed, by rising, to have done so. That obvious fact recited, the graduates and their parents may proceed to thank God, as Americans have always done, for the blessings He has generously bestowed on them and on their country. *** For the foregoing reasons, I dissent.

SANTA FE INDEPENDENT SCHOOL DISTRICT v. JANE DOE, ET AL.

530 U.S. 271 [2000]

JUSTICE STEVENS delivered the opinion of the Court.

I

The Santa Fe Independent School District is responsible for the education of more than 4,000 students in a small community in the southern part of the State of Texas.***In their complaint the Does alleged that the District had engaged in several proselytizing practices, such as promoting attendance at a Baptist revival meeting, encouraging membership in religious clubs, chastising children who held minority religious beliefs, and distributing Gideon Bibles on school premises. They also alleged that the District allowed students to read Christian invocations and benedictions from the stage at graduation ceremonies, and to deliver overtly Christian prayers over the public address system at home football games.

On May 10, 1995, the District Court entered an interim order addressing a number of different issues. In response, the District adopted a series of policies over several months dealing with prayer at school functions. The policies enacted in May and July for graduation ceremonies provided the format for the August and October policies for football games. The August policy, which was titled "Prayer at Football Games," authorized two student elections, the first to determine whether "invocations" should be delivered, and the second to select the spokesperson to deliver them. The final policy (October policy) is essentially the same as the August policy, though it omits the word "prayer" from its title, and refers to "messages" and "statements" as well as "invocations." It is the validity of that policy that is before us.[6] We granted the District's petition for certiorari, limited to th[is] question:

---

6. "STUDENT ACTIVITIES: PRE-GAME CEREMONIES AT FOOTBALL GAMES. The board has chosen to permit students to deliver a brief invocation and/or message to be delivered during the pre-game ceremonies of home varsity football games to solemnize the event, to promote good sportsmanship and

"Whether petitioner's policy permitting student-led, student-initiated prayer at football games violates the Establishment Clause." We conclude, as did the Court of Appeals, that it does.

II

Although this case involves student prayer at a different type of school function, our analysis is properly guided by the principles that we endorsed in *Lee v. Weisman*: "It is beyond dispute that, at a minimum, the Constitution guarantees that government may not coerce anyone to support or participate in religion or its exercise, or otherwise act in a way which 'establishes a [state] religion or religious faith, or tends to do so.'"

[T]he District first argues that this principle is inapplicable to its October policy because the messages are private student speech, not public speech. It reminds us that "there is a crucial difference between government speech endorsing religion, which the Establishment Clause forbids, and private speech endorsing religion, which the Free Speech and Free Exercise Clauses protect." We certainly agree with that distinction, but we are not persuaded that the pregame invocations should be regarded as "private speech."

These invocations are authorized by a government policy and take place on government property at government-sponsored school-related events. Of course, not every message delivered under such circumstances is the government's own. We have held, for example, that an individual's contribution to a government-created forum was not government speech. See *Rosenberger v. Rector and Visitors of Univ. of Virginia* (1995). Although the District relies heavily on *Rosenberger* and similar cases involving such forums, it is clear that the pregame ceremony is not the type of forum discussed in those cases. *** Rather, the school allows only one student, the same student for the entire season, to give the invocation. The statement or invocation, moreover, is subject to particular regulations that confine the content and topic of the student's message.***Granting only one student access to the stage at a time does not, of course, necessarily preclude a finding that a school has created a limited public forum. Here, however, Santa Fe's student election system ensures that only those messages deemed "appropriate" under the District's policy may be delivered. That is, the majoritarian process implemented by the District guarantees, by definition, that minority candidates will never prevail and that their views will be effectively silenced.

---

student safety, and to establish the appropriate environment for the competition.

Upon advice and direction of the high school principal, each spring, the high school student council shall conduct an election, by the high school student body, by secret ballot, to determine whether such a statement or invocation will be a part of the pre-game ceremonies and if so, shall elect a student, from a list of student volunteers, to deliver the statement or invocation. The student volunteer who is selected by his or her classmates may decide what message and/or invocation to deliver, consistent with the goals and purposes of this policy."

Recently, in *Board of Regents of Univ. of Wis. System v. Southworth*, we explained why student elections that determine, by majority vote, which expressive activities shall receive or not receive school benefits are constitutionally problematic: "To the extent the referendum substitutes majority determinations for viewpoint neutrality it would undermine the constitutional protection the program requires." Like the student referendum for funding in *Southworth*, this student election does nothing to protect minority views but rather places the students who hold such views at the mercy of the majority.[15]
***

Moreover, the District has failed to divorce itself from the religious content in the invocations. It has not succeeded in doing so, either by claiming that its policy is "one of neutrality rather than endorsement"or by characterizing the individual student as the "circuit-breaker" in the process.***In addition to involving the school in the selection of the speaker, the policy, by its terms, invites and encourages religious messages. The policy itself states that the purpose of the message is "to solemnize the event." Moreover, the requirements that the message "promote good citizenship" and "establish the appropriate environment for competition" further narrow the types of message deemed appropriate, suggesting that a solemn, yet nonreligious, message, such as commentary on United States foreign policy, would be prohibited. Indeed, the only type of message that is expressly endorsed in the text is an "invocation"—a term that primarily describes an appeal for divine assistance. In fact, as used in the past at Santa Fe High School, an "invocation" has always entailed a focused religious message.[21]

The actual or perceived endorsement of the message, moreover, is established by factors beyond just the text of the policy. Once the student speaker is selected and the message composed, the invocation is then delivered to a large audience assembled as part of a regularly scheduled, school-sponsored function conducted on school property. The message is broadcast over the school's public address system, which remains subject to the control of school officials.

Most striking to us is the evolution of the current policy from the long-sanctioned office of "Student Chaplain" to the candidly titled "Prayer at Football Games" regulation. This history indicates that the District intended to preserve the practice of prayer before football games. The conclusion that the District viewed the October policy simply as a continuation of the previous policies is dramatically

---

15. If instead of a choice between an invocation and no pregame message, the first election determined whether a political speech should be made, and the second election determined whether the speaker should be a Democrat or a Republican, it would be rather clear that the public address system was being used to deliver a partisan message reflecting the viewpoint of the majority rather than a random statement by a private individual.

21. Even if the plain language of the October policy were facially neutral, the Establishment Clause forbids a State to hide behind the application of formally neutral criteria and remain studiously oblivious to the effects of its actions.

illustrated by the fact that the school did not conduct a new election, pursuant to the current policy, to replace the results of the previous election, which occurred under the former policy.

School sponsorship of a religious message is impermissible because it sends the ancillary message to members of the audience who are nonadherants "that they are outsiders, not full members of the political community, and an accompanying message to adherants that they are insiders, favored members of the political community." *Lynch v. Donnelly*, 465 U.S. at 688 (1984) (O'Connor, J., concurring). The delivery of such a message—over the school's public address system, by a speaker representing the student body, under the supervision of school faculty, and pursuant to a school policy that explicitly and implicitly encourages public prayer—is not properly characterized as "private" speech.

III

***

One of the purposes served by the Establishment Clause is to remove debate over this kind of issue from governmental supervision or control. The two student elections authorized by the policy, coupled with the debates that presumably must precede each, impermissibly invade that private sphere. The election mechanism, when considered in light of the history in which the policy in question evolved, reflects a device the District put in place that determines whether religious messages will be delivered at home football games. The mechanism encourages divisiveness along religious lines in a public school setting, a result at odds with the Establishment Clause. Although it is true that the ultimate choice of student speaker is attributable to the students, the District's decision to hold the constitutionally problematic election is clearly a choice attributable to the State.

The District further argues that attendance at the commencement ceremonies at issue in *Lee* "differs dramatically" from attendance at high school football games. Attendance at a high school football game, unlike showing up for class, is certainly not required in order to receive a diploma. Moreover, we may assume that the District is correct in arguing that the informal pressure to attend an athletic event is not as strong as a senior's desire to attend her own graduation ceremony.

There are some students, however, such as cheerleaders, members of the band, and, of course, the team members themselves, for whom seasonal commitments mandate their attendance, sometimes for class credit. The District also minimizes the importance to many students of attending and participating in extracurricular activities as part of a complete educational experience. ***

Even if we regard every high school student's decision to attend a home football game as purely voluntary, we are nevertheless persuaded that the delivery of a pregame prayer has the improper effect of coercing those present to participate in an act of religious worship. "[T]he government may no more use social pressure to enforce orthodoxy than it may use more direct means." *Lee* at 594. As in *Lee*, "what to most believers may seem nothing more than a reasonable request that the nonbeliever respect their religious practices, in a school context may appear to the nonbeliever or dissenter to be an attempt to employ the machinery of the State to enforce a religious orthodoxy." The constitutional command will not permit the District "to exact religious conformity from a student as the price" of joining her classmates at a varsity football game.

IV

Finally, the District argues repeatedly that the Does have made a premature facial challenge to the October policy that necessarily must fail. The District emphasizes that until a student actually delivers a solemnizing message under the latest version of the policy, there can be no certainty that any of the statements or invocations will be religious.

This argument, however, assumes that we are concerned only with the serious constitutional injury that occurs when a student is forced to participate in an act of religious worship because she chooses to attend a school event. But the Constitution also requires that we keep in mind "the myriad, subtle ways in which Establishment Clause values can be eroded," *Lynch* (O'Connor, J., concurring). One is the mere passage by the District of a policy that has the purpose and perception of government establishment of religion. Another is the implementation of a governmental electoral process that subjects the issue of prayer to a majoritarian vote. Under the *Lemon* standard, a court must invalidate a statute if it lacks "a secular legislative purpose." It is therefore proper, as part of this facial challenge, for us to examine the purpose of the October policy.

As [we have already noted], the text of the October policy alone reveals that it has an unconstitutional purpose. The plain language of the policy clearly spells out the extent of school involvement in both the election of the speaker and the content of the message. Additionally, the text of the October policy specifies only one, clearly preferred message—that of Santa Fe's traditional religious "invocation." Our examination, however, need not stop at an analysis of the text of the policy.

This case comes to us as the latest step in developing litigation brought as a challenge to institutional practices that unquestionably violated the Establishment Clause. One of those practices was the District's long-established tradition of sanctioning student-led prayer at varsity football games. The District asks us to pretend that we do not recognize what every Santa Fe High School student understands clearly—that this policy is about prayer. The District further asks us to accept what is obviously untrue: that these messages are necessary to "solemnize" a football game and that this single-student, year-long position is essential to the protection of student speech. We refuse to turn a blind eye to the context in which this policy arose, and that context quells any doubt that this policy was implemented with the purpose of endorsing school prayer. Therefore, the simple enactment of this policy, with the purpose and perception of school endorsement of student prayer, was a constitutional violation.

This policy likewise does not survive a facial challenge because it impermissibly imposes upon the student body a majoritarian election on the issue of prayer. Through its election scheme, the District has established a governmental electoral mechanism that turns the school into a forum for religious debate. It further empowers the student body majority with the authority to subject students of minority views to constitutionally improper messages. The award of that power alone, regardless of the students' ultimate use of it, is not acceptable.[23] No further injury is required for the policy to fail a facial challenge. The policy is invalid on its face because it establishes an improper majoritarian election on religion, and unquestionably has the purpose and creates the perception of encouraging the delivery of prayer at a series of important school events.

CHIEF JUSTICE REHNQUIST, with whom JUSTICE SCALIA and JUSTICE THOMAS join, dissenting.

The Court, venturing into the realm of prophesy, decides that it "need not wait for the inevitable" and invalidates the district's policy on its face. To do so, it applies the most rigid version of the oft-criticized test of*Lemon v. Kurtzman*. *Lemon* has had a checkered career in the decisional law of this Court. In two cases, the Court did not even apply the *Lemon* 'test.' Indeed, in *Lee v. Weisman,* an opinion upon which the Court relies heavily today, we mentioned but did not feel compelled to apply the *Lemon* test. Even if it were appropriate to apply the *Lemon* test here, the district's student-message policy should not be invalidated on its face.

First, the Court misconstrues the nature of the "majoritarian election" permitted by the policy as being an election on "prayer" and "religion." To the contrary, the election permitted by the policy is a two-fold process whereby students vote first on whether to have a student speaker before football games at all, and second, if the students vote to have such a speaker, on who that speaker will be. It is conceivable that the election could become one in which student candidates campaign on platforms that focus on whether or not they will pray if elected. It is also conceivable that the election could lead to a Christian prayer before 90 percent of the football games. If, upon implementation, the policy operated in this fashion, we would have a record before us to review whether the policy, as applied, violated the Establishment Clause or unduly suppressed minority viewpoints. But it is possible that the students might vote not to have a pregame speaker, in which case there would be no threat of a constitutional violation. It is also possible that the election would not focus on prayer, but on public speaking ability or social popularity.

But the Court ignores these possibilities by holding that merely granting the student body the power to elect a speaker that may choose to pray, regardless of the

23. The Chief Justice accuses us of "essentially invalidating all student elections." This is obvious hyperbole. We have concluded that the resulting religious message under this policy would be attributable to the school, not just the student. For this reason, we now hold only that the District's decision to allow the student majority to control whether students of minority views are subjected to a school-sponsored prayer violates the Establishment Clause.

students ultimate use of it, is not acceptable. The Court so holds despite that any speech that may occur as a result of the election process here would be private, not government, speech. The elected student, not the government, would choose what to say. Support for the Court's holding cannot be found in any of our cases. And it essentially invalidates all student elections. A newly elected student body president, or even a newly elected prom king or queen, could use opportunities for public speaking to say prayers. Under the Court's view, the mere grant of power to the students to vote for such offices, in light of the fear that those elected might publicly pray, violates the Establishment Clause.

Second, with respect to the policy's purpose, the Court holds that "the simple enactment of this policy, with the purpose and perception of school endorsement of student prayer, was a constitutional violation." But the policy itself has plausible secular purposes: "To solemnize the event, to promote good sportsmanship and student safety, and to establish the appropriate environment for the competition." Where a governmental body expresses a plausible secular purpose for an enactment, courts should generally defer to that stated intent. The Court grants no deference to—and appears openly hostile toward—the policy's stated purposes, and wastes no time in concluding that they are a sham.

The Court bases its conclusion that the true purpose of the policy is to endorse student prayer on its view of the school district's history of Establishment Clause violations and the context in which the policy was written. *** But the context—attempted compliance with a District Court order—actually demonstrates that the school district was acting diligently to come within the governing constitutional law.

The Court also relies on our decision in *Lee v. Weisman*, to support its conclusion. In *Lee*, we concluded that the content of the speech at issue, a graduation prayer given by a rabbi, was "directed and controlled" by a school official. In other words, at issue in *Lee* was government speech. Here, by contrast, the potential speech at issue, if the policy had been allowed to proceed, would be a message or invocation selected or created by a student. Had the policy been put into practice, the students may have chosen a speaker according to wholly secular criteria—like good public speaking skills or social popularity—and the student speaker may have chosen, on her own accord, to deliver a religious message. Such an application of the policy would likely pass constitutional muster. See *Lee* (Souter, J., concurring) ("If the State had chosen its graduation day speakers according to wholly secular criteria, and if one of those speakers (not a state actor) had individually chosen to deliver a religious message, it would be harder to attribute an endorsement of religion to the State"). The policy at issue here may be applied in an unconstitutional manner, but it will be time enough to invalidate it if that is found to be the case. I would reverse the judgment of the Court of Appeals.

———

NOTE

Against the background of these cases, reporting the judicial effort to reconcile tradition and historical practices in the United States with some sensitivity to the first amendment,[23] consider the following hypothetical case:

> In Collander County, Idaho, during the past thirty years a major population change has occurred. The earlier residents, discouraged by farm conditions, have tended to move away. New, darker skinned residents, with customs of their own, principally from different parts of Southeast Asia, Indonesia, and Pakistan have tended to move in. By 1995, they had become a majority of the voting age population in Collander County. By 1998, a majority of the elected county commissioners reflected the new political success of the newer residents of Collander county.
>
> Thinking it appropriate to have the county reflect the recent changes, in 2000 the county commissioners voted in favor of reflecting the different traditions of the newer, rather than of the older, residents. Formerly, the county commission had opened with a prayer provided by a local Presbyterian minister, paid an annual $500 fee for his service, from the county fund. In 2000, the county commission let the local minister's contract lapse, in favor of extending the same arrangement instead to a resident mullah (a Moslem teacher or religious leader) to lead the commission, when meeting in public session, in Islamic prayer.
>
> Concurrently, the county commission meeting chamber was redone. Where formerly there had been several painted pictures and scenes on the walls, mosaic patterns were substituted (pictures being regarded as inappropriate to the tradition of Islam). Where formerly the motif up behind the semi-circular dais in the commission public chamber reported the motto "In God We Trust," it was replaced with letters merely of the same size reporting "Allah Akbar" ("God Is Great").
>
> The majority of the residents being Moslem, moreover, the day previously established by county ordinance as a day requiring most businesses to close (Sunday) was determined to be less convenient than once it was. This, because Sunday was a relatively indifferent day for most of the current residents, many of whom spent much of Friday as the Moslem day for prayer, and accordingly, for whom missing work also on Sunday was an unwelcome loss. Consistent still with providing one uniform day free from required employment by

---

23. See William Lee Miller, The Moral Project of the American Founders, in Articles of Faith, Articles of Peace 36 (James Davison Hunter & Os Guinness eds. 1990). ("Whereas later believers look back at the founding through the screen of the evangelical revivals and of their own sympathies to find more piety than there was in early America, the cultured among the despisers look back through the screen of their unbelief to find only Thomas Jefferson and Tom Paine and more unabashed secularism than there really was.") See also Jesse H. Choper, Securing Religious Liberty: Principles for Judicial Interpretation of the Religion Clauses 154-55 (1995).

businesses for more than six consecutive days, the county commissioners voted affirmatively to repeal the Sunday closing law and enact a uniform Friday closing day.

By state law, in Idaho, the consumption and sale of alcoholic beverages has always been subject to local option, i.e. determined by county commission choice. Collander County has generally been a "dry" county; possession, sale, or consumption of alcoholic beverages except for medicinal uses (on a doctor's written prescription) is generally forbidden, though the ordinance, while not actually providing any other express exception, had not been enforced in respect to the mere use of sacramental wine as part of holy communion, at the local Catholic church.

The new county commission, however, took the county ordinance somewhat more seriously than had their predecessors. They fully agreed with Collander County being a dry county (Islam is as much opposed to the use of alcohol as the more fundamentalist Christian groups have traditionally been), so they fully endorsed the current ordinance. They saw no reason for continuing the *de facto* exemption of wine use inconsistent with the ordinance, however, and directed the county sheriff to give notice that hereafter the ordinance would be uniformly enforced.

These changes in Collander County have not been free of controversy. Indeed, a number of residents previously satisfied with things as they were, are now angry and in a serious litigative mood. Accordingly, the following actions have been filed in state court. Your task is to assess their likelihood of success or failure, and briefly to indicate on what basis each might have been brought in first amendment terms, and the grounds on which they may fail or succeed:

1. An action by the priest of the local Catholic church, on his own behalf and on behalf of resident Catholic communicants, naming the county prosecutor as defendant, for declaratory relief against threatened criminal enforcement of the alcohol prohibition ordinance;

2. An action by a local businessman, a practicing Protestant, on his own behalf and on behalf of his employees and customers, naming the County Commission as defendant, for declaratory judgment voiding the Friday closing law;

3. An action by a local resident for declaratory judgment and mandatory injunction, naming the County Commission as defendant, to direct the Commission to remove the new motto from the rear wall of the public county commission chamber, to modify the mosaic motif, to desist from paying or permitting the mullah (also named as defendant) to commence public commission sessions with Islamic prayer;

4. An action by the nonrenewed Presbyterian minister for mandatory injunction against the County Commission as defendant to reinstate the previous arrangement he had with the county; in the alternative, an injunction requiring

that he be paid and treated in rotation of service on equal terms as the commission provides to the mullah.

Chapter 10

"*** OR PROHIBITING THE FREE EXERCISE THEREOF."

A. THE GENERAL TEST

REYNOLDS v. UNITED STATES
98 U.S. 145 (1878)

MR. CHIEF JUSTICE WAITE delivered the opinion of the court.

* * *

On the trial, the plaintiff in error, proved that at the time of his alleged second marriage he was, and for many years before had been, a member of the Church of Jesus Christ of Latter-Day Saints, commonly called the Mormon Church, and a believer in its doctrines; that it was an accepted doctrine of that church "that it was the duty of male members of said church, circumstances permitting, to practise polygamy; that this duty was enjoined by different books which the members of said church believed to be of divine origin, and among others the Holy Bible, and also that the members of the church believed that the practice of polygamy was directly enjoined upon the male members thereof by the Almighty God, in a revelation to Joseph Smith, the founder and prophet of said church; that the failing or refusing to practise polygamy by such male members of said church, when circumstances would admit, would be punished, and that the penalty for such failure and refusal would be damnation in the life to come." He also proved "that he had received permission from the recognized authorities in said church to enter into polygamous marriage; that Daniel H. Wells, one having authority in said church to perform the marriage ceremony, married the said defendant on or about the time the crime is alleged to have been committed, to some woman by the name of Schofield, and that such marriage ceremony was performed under and pursuant to the doctrines of said church."

Upon this proof he asked the court to instruct the jury that if they found from the evidence that he "was married as charged—if he was married—in pursuance of and in conformity with what he believed at the time to be a religious duty, that the verdict must be 'not guilty.'" This request was refused, and the court did charge "that there must have been a criminal intent, but that if the defendant, under the influence of a religious belief that it was right,—under an inspiration, if you please, that it was right,—deliberately married a second time, having a first wife living, the want of consciousness of evil intent—the want of understanding on his part that he was committing a crime—did not excuse him; but the law inexorably in such case implies the criminal intent."

Upon this charge and refusal to charge the question is raised, whether religious belief can be accepted as a justification of an overt act made criminal by the law of the land. The inquiry is not as to the power of Congress to prescribe criminal laws for the Territories, but as to the guilt of one who knowingly violates a law which has been properly enacted, if he entertains a religious belief that the law is wrong.

Congress cannot pass a law for the government of the Territories which shall prohibit the free exercise of religion. The first amendment to the Constitution expressly forbids such legislation. Religious freedom is guaranteed everywhere throughout the United States, so far as congressional interference is concerned. The question to be determined is, whether the law now under consideration comes within this prohibition.

The word "religion" is not defined in the Constitution. We must go elsewhere, therefore, to ascertain its meaning, and nowhere more appropriately, we think, than to the history of the times in the midst of which the provision was adopted. The precise point of the inquiry is, what is the religious freedom which has been guaranteed.

Before the adoption of the Constitution, attempts were made in some of the colonies and States to legislate not only in respect to the establishment of religion, but in respect to its doctrines and precepts as well. The people were taxed, against their will, for the support of religion, and sometimes for the support of particular sects to whose tenets they could not and did not subscribe. Punishments were prescribed for a failure to attend upon public worship, and sometimes for entertaining heretical opinions. The controversy upon this general subject was animated in many of the States, but seemed at last to culminate in Virginia. In 1784, the House of Delegates of that State having under consideration "a bill establishing provision for teachers of the Christian religion," postponed it until the next session, and directed that the bill should be published and distributed, and that the people be requested "to signify their opinion respecting the adoption of such a bill at the next session of assembly."

This brought out a determined opposition. Amongst others, Mr. Madison prepared a "Memorial and Remonstrance," which was widely circulated and signed, and in which he demonstrated "that religion, or the duty we owe the Creator," was not within the cognizance of civil government. *** At the next session the proposed bill was not only defeated, but another, "for establishing religious freedom," drafted by Mr. Jefferson, was passed. In the preamble of this act (12 Hening's Stat. 84) religious freedom is defined; and after a recital "that to suffer the civil magistrate to intrude his powers into the field of opinion, and to restrain the profession or propagation of principles on supposition of their ill tendency, is a dangerous fallacy which at once destroys all religious liberty," it is declared "that it is time enough for the rightful purposes of civil government for its officers to interfere when principles break out into overt acts against peace and good order." In these two sentences is found the true distinction between what properly belongs to the church and what to the State.

In a little more than a year after the passage of this statute the convention met which prepared the "Constitution of the United States." Of this convention Mr. Jefferson was not a member, he being then absent as minister to France. As soon as he saw the draft of the Constitution proposed for adoption, he, in a letter to a friend, expressed his disappointment at the absence of an express declaration insuring the freedom of religion, but was willing to accept it as it was, trusting that the good sense and honest intentions of the people would bring about the necessary alterations. Five of the States, while adopting the Constitution, proposed amendments. Three—New Hampshire, New York, and Virginia—included in one form or another a declaration of religious freedom in the changes they desired to have made, as did also North Carolina, where the convention at first declined to ratify the Constitution until the proposed amendments were acted upon. Accordingly, at the first session of the first Congress the amendment now under consideration was proposed with others by Mr. Madison. It met the views of the advocates of religious freedom, and was adopted. Mr. Jefferson afterwards, in reply to an address to him by a committee of the Danbury Baptist Association, took occasion to say: "Believing with you that religion is a matter which lies solely between man and his God; that he owes account to none other for his faith or his worship; that the legislative powers of the government reach actions only, and not opinions,—I contemplate with sovereign reverence that act of the whole American people which declared that their legislature should 'make no law respecting an establishment of religion or prohibiting the free exercise thereof,' thus building a wall of separation between church and State. Adhering to this expression of the supreme will of the nation in behalf of the rights of conscience, I shall see with sincere satisfaction the progress of those sentiments which tend to restore man to all his natural rights, convinced he has no natural right in opposition to his social duties." Coming as this does from an acknowledged leader of the advocates of the measure, it may be accepted almost as an authoritative declaration of the scope and effect of the amendment thus secured. Congress was deprived of all legislative power over mere opinion, but was left free to reach actions which were in violation of social duties or subversive of good order.

Polygamy has always been odious among the northern and western nations of Europe, and, until the establishment of the Mormon Church, was almost exclusively a feature of the life of Asiatic and of African people. ***

By the statute of 1 James I. (c. 11), the offence, if committed in England or Wales, was made punishable in the civil courts, and the penalty was death. As this statute was limited in its operation to England and Wales, it was at a very early period re-enacted, generally with some modifications, in all the colonies. In connection with the case we are now considering, it is a significant fact that on the 8th of December, 1788, after the passage of the act establishing religious freedom, and after the convention of Virginia had recommended as an amendment to the Constitution of the United States the declaration in a bill of rights that "all men have an equal, natural, and unalienable right to the free exercise of religion, according to the dictates of conscience," the legislature of that State substantially enacted the statute of James I., death penalty included, because, as recited in the preamble, "it hath been doubted whether bigamy or poligamy be punishable by the laws of this Commonwealth." 12 Hening's Stat. 691. From that day to this we think it may safely be said there never has been a time in any State of the Union when polygamy has not been an offence against society, cognizable by the civil courts and punishable with more or less severity. In the face of all this evidence, it is impossible to believe that the constitutional guaranty of religious freedom was intended to prohibit legislation in respect to this most important feature of social life. Marriage, while from its very nature a sacred obligation, is nevertheless, in most civilized nations, a civil contract, and usually regulated by law. Upon it society may be said to be built, and out of its fruits spring social relations and social obligations and duties, with which government is necessarily required to deal. In fact, according as monogamous or polygamous marriages are allowed, do we find the principles on which the government of the people, to a greater or less extent, rests. Professor Lieber says, polygamy leads to the patriarchal principle, and which, when applied to large communities, fetters the people in stationary despotism, while that principle cannot long exist in connection with monogamy. ***

In our opinion, the statute immediately under consideration is within the legislative power of Congress. It is constitutional and valid as prescribing a rule of action for all those residing in the Territories, and in places over which the United States have exclusive control. This being so, the only question which remains is, whether those who make polygamy a part of their religion are excepted from the operation of the statute. If they are, then those who do not make polygamy a part of their religious belief may be found guilty and punished, while those who do, must be acquitted and go free. This would be introducing a new element into criminal law. Laws are made for the government of actions, and while they cannot interfere with mere religious belief and opinions, they may with practices. Suppose one believed that human sacrifices were a necessary part of religious worship, would it be seriously contended that the civil government under which he lived could not interfere to prevent a sacrifice? Or if a wife religiously believed it was her duty to burn herself upon the funeral pile of her dead husband, would it be beyond the power of the civil government to prevent her carrying her belief into practice?

So here, as a law of the organization of society under the exclusive dominion of the United States, it is provided that plural marriages shall not be allowed. Can a man excuse his practices to the contrary because of his religious belief? To permit this would be to make the professed doctrines of religious belief superior to the law of the land, and in effect to permit every citizen to become a law unto himself. Government could exist only in name under such circumstances.

A criminal intent is generally an element of crime, but every man is presumed to intend the necessary and legitimate consequences of what he knowingly does. Here the accused knew he had been once married, and that his first wife was living. He also knew that his second marriage was forbidden by law. When, therefore, he married the second time, he is presumed to have intended to break the law. And the breaking of the law is the crime. Every act necessary to constitute the crime was knowingly done, and the crime was therefore knowingly committed. Ignorance of a fact may sometimes be taken as evidence of a want of criminal intent, but not ignorance of the law. The only defence of the accused in this case is his belief that the law ought not to have been enacted. It matters not that his belief was a part of his professed religion: it was still belief, and belief only.

In Regina v. Wagstaff (10 Cox Crim. Cases, 531), the parents of a sick child, who omitted to call in medical attendance because of their religious belief that what they did for its cure would be effective, were held not to be guilty of manslaughter, while it was said the contrary would have been the result if the child had actually been starved to death by the parents, under the notion that it was their religious duty to abstain from giving it food. But when the offence consists of a positive act which is knowingly done, it would be dangerous to hold that the offender might escape punishment because he religiously believed the law which he had broken ought never to have been made. No case, we believe, can be found that has gone so far. ***

Upon a careful consideration of the whole case, we are satisfied that no error was committed by the court below.

Judgment affirmed.

CANTWELL v. CONNECTICUT
310 U.S. 296 (1940)

MR. JUSTICE ROBERTS delivered the opinion of the Court.

Newton Cantwell and his two sons, Jesse and Russell, members of a group known as Jehovah's Witnesses, and claiming to be ordained ministers, were arrested in New Haven, Connecticut, and each was charged by information in five counts, with statutory and common law offenses. After trial in the Court of Common Pleas of New Haven County each of them was convicted on the third count, which charged a violation of § 6294 of the General Statutes of Connecticut, and on the fifth count, which charged commission of the common law offense of inciting a breach of the peace. On appeal to the Supreme Court the conviction of all three on the third count was affirmed. The conviction of Jesse Cantwell, on the fifth count, was also affirmed. ***

The facts adduced to sustain the convictions on the third count follow. On the day of their arrest the appellants were engaged in going singly from house to house on Cassius Street in New Haven. They were individually equipped with a bag containing books and pamphlets on religious subjects, a portable phonograph and a set of records, each of which, when played, introduced, and was a description of, one of the books. Each appellant asked the person who responded to his call for permission to play one of the records. If permission was granted he asked the person to buy the book described and, upon refusal, he solicited such contribution towards the publication of the pamphlets as the listener was willing to make. If a contribution was received a pamphlet was delivered upon condition that it would be read.

Cassius Street is in a thickly populated neighborhood, where about ninety per cent of the residents are Roman Catholics. A phonograph record, describing a book entitled "Enemies," included an attack on the Catholic religion. None of the persons interviewed were members of Jehovah's Witnesses.

The statute under which the appellants were charged provides:

> No person shall solicit money, services, subscriptions or any valuable thing for any alleged religious, charitable or philanthropic cause, from other than a member of the organization for whose benefit such person is soliciting or within the county in which such person or organization is located unless such cause shall have been approved by the secretary of the public welfare council. Upon application of any person in behalf of such cause, the secretary shall determine whether such cause is a religious one or is a bona fide object of charity or philanthropy and conforms to reasonable standards of efficiency and integrity, and, if he shall so find, shall approve the same and issue to the authority in charge a certificate to that effect. Such certificate may be revoked at any time. Any person violating any provision of this section shall be fined not more than one hundred dollars or imprisoned not more than thirty days or both.

The appellants claimed that their activities were not within the statute but consisted only of distribution of books, pamphlets, and periodicals. The State Supreme Court construed the finding of the trial court to be that "in addition to the sale of the books and the distribution of the pamphlets the defendants were also soliciting contributions or donations of money for an alleged religious cause, and thereby came within the purview of the statute." It overruled the contention that the Act, as applied to the appellants, offends the due process clause of the Fourteenth Amendment, because it abridges or denies religious freedom and liberty of speech and press. The court stated that it was the solicitation that brought the appellants within the sweep of the Act and not their other activities in the dissemination of literature. It declared the legislation constitutional as an effort by the State to protect the public against fraud and imposition in the solicitation of funds for what purported to be religious, charitable, or philanthropic causes.

The facts which were held to support the conviction of Jesse Cantwell on the fifth count were that he stopped two men in the street, asked, and received, permission to play a phonograph record, and played the record "Enemies," which attacked the religion and church of the two men, who were Catholics. Both were incensed by the contents of the record and were tempted to strike Cantwell unless he went away. On being told to be on his way he left their presence. There was no evidence that he was personally offensive or entered into any argument with those he interviewed.

The court held that the charge was not assault or breach of the peace or threats on Cantwell's part, but invoking or inciting others to breach of the peace, and that the facts supported the conviction of that offense.

First. We hold that the statute, as construed and applied to the appellants, deprives them of their liberty without due process of law in contravention of the Fourteenth Amendment. The fundamental concept of liberty embodied in that Amendment embraces the liberties guaranteed by the First Amendment. The First Amendment declares that Congress shall make no law respecting an establishment of religion or prohibiting the free exercise thereof. The Fourteenth Amendment has rendered the legislatures of the states as incompetent as Congress to enact such laws. The constitutional inhibition of legislation on the subject of religion has a double aspect. On the one hand, it forestalls compulsion by law of the acceptance of any creed or the practice of any form of worship. Freedom of conscience and freedom to adhere to such religious organization or form of worship as the individual may choose cannot be restricted by law. On the other hand, it safeguards the free exercise of the chosen form of religion. Thus the Amendment embraces two concepts, —freedom to believe and freedom to act. The first is absolute but, in the nature of things, the second cannot be. Conduct remains subject to regulation for the protection of society.[4] The freedom to act must have appropriate definition to preserve the enforcement of that protection. In every case the power to regulate must be so exercised as not, in attaining a permissible end, unduly to infringe the protected freedom. No one would contest the proposition that a State may not, by statute, wholly deny the right to preach or to disseminate religious views. Plainly such a previous and absolute restraint would violate the terms of the guarantee. It is equally clear that a State may by general and non-discriminatory legislation regulate the times, the places, and the manner of soliciting upon its streets, and of holding meetings thereon; and may in other respects safeguard the peace, good order and comfort of the community, without unconstitutionally invading the liberties protected by the Fourteenth Amendment. The appellants are right in their insistence that the Act in question is not such a regulation. If a certificate is procured, solicitation is permitted without restraint but, in the absence of a certificate, solicitation is altogether prohibited.

The appellants urge that to require them to obtain a certificate as a condition of soliciting support for their views amounts to a prior restraint on the exercise of their religion within the meaning of the Constitution. The State insists that the Act, as construed by the Supreme Court of Connecticut, imposes no previous restraint upon the dissemination of religious views or teaching but merely safeguards against the perpetration of frauds under the cloak of religion. Conceding that this is so, the question remains whether the method adopted by Connecticut to that end transgresses the liberty safeguarded by the Constitution.

---

4. Reynolds v. United States, 98 U.S. 145; Davis v. Beason, 133 U.S. 333.

The general regulation, in the public interest, of solicitation, which does not involve any religious test and does not unreasonably obstruct or delay the collection of funds, is not open to any constitutional objection, even though the collection be for a religious purpose. Such regulation would not constitute a prohibited previous restraint on the free exercise of religion or interpose an inadmissible obstacle to its exercise.

It will be noted, however, that the Act requires an application to the secretary of the public welfare council of the State; that he is empowered to determine whether the cause is a religious one, and that the issue of a certificate depends upon his affirmative action. If he finds that the cause is not that of religion, to solicit for it becomes a crime. He is not to issue a certificate as a matter of course. His decision to issue or refuse it involves appraisal of facts, the exercise of judgment, and the formation of an opinion. He is authorized to withhold his approval if he determines that the cause is not a religious one. Such a censorship of religion as the means of determining its right to survive is a denial of liberty protected by the First Amendment and included in the liberty which is within the protection of the Fourteenth.

The State asserts that if the licensing officer acts arbitrarily, capriciously, or corruptly, his action is subject to judicial correction. *** It is suggested that the statute is to be read as requiring the officer to issue a certificate unless the cause in question is clearly not a religious one; and that if he violates his duty his action will be corrected by a court.

To this suggestion there are several sufficient answers. The line between a discretionary and a ministerial act is not always easy to mark and the statute has not been construed by the state court to impose a mere ministerial duty on the secretary of the welfare council. Upon his decision as to the nature of the cause, the right to solicit depends. Moreover, the availability of a judicial remedy for abuses in the system of licensing still leaves that system one of previous restraint which, in the field of free speech and press, we have held inadmissible. A statute authorizing previous restraint upon the exercise of the guaranteed freedom by judicial decision after trial is as obnoxious to the Constitution as one providing for like restraint by administrative action.[7]

Nothing we have said is intended even remotely to imply that, under the cloak of religion, persons may, with impunity, commit frauds upon the public. Certainly penal laws are available to punish such conduct. Even the exercise of religion may be at some slight inconvenience in order that the State may protect its citizens from injury. Without doubt a State may protect its citizens from fraudulent solicitation by requiring a stranger in the community, before permitting him publicly to solicit funds for any purpose, to establish his identity and his authority to act for the cause which he purports to represent. The State is likewise free to regulate the time and manner

---

7. Near v. Minnesota, 283 U.S. 697.

of solicitation generally, in the interest of public safety, peace, comfort or convenience. But to condition the solicitation of aid for the perpetuation of religious views or systems upon a license, the grant of which rests in the exercise of a determination by state authority as to what is a religious cause, is to lay a forbidden burden upon the exercise of liberty protected by the Constitution.

Second. We hold that, in the circumstances disclosed, the conviction of Jesse Cantwell on the fifth count must be set aside. Decision as to the lawfulness of the conviction demands the weighing of two conflicting interests. The fundamental law declares the interest of the United States that the free exercise of religion be not prohibited and that freedom to communicate information and opinion be not abridged. The State of Connecticut has an obvious interest in the preservation and protection of peace and good order within her borders. We must determine whether the alleged protection of the State's interest, means to which end would, in the absence of limitation by the Federal Constitution, lie wholly within the State's discretion, has been pressed, in this instance, to a point where it has come into fatal collision with the overriding interest protected by the federal compact. ***

The offense known as breach of the peace embraces a great variety of conduct destroying or menacing public order and tranquility. It includes not only violent acts but acts and words likely to produce violence in others. No one would have the hardihood to suggest that the principle of freedom of speech sanctions incitement to riot or that religious liberty connotes the privilege to exhort others to physical attack upon those belonging to another sect. When clear and present danger of riot, disorder, interference with traffic upon the public streets, or other immediate threat to public safety, peace, or order, appears, the power of the State to prevent or punish is obvious. Equally obvious is it that a State may not unduly suppress free communication of views, religious or other, under the guise of conserving desirable conditions. Here we have a situation analogous to a conviction under a statute sweeping in a great variety of conduct under a general and indefinite characterization, and leaving to the executive and Judicial branches too wide a discretion in its application.

Having these considerations in mind, we note that Jesse Cantwell, on April 26, 1938, was upon a public street, where he had a right to be, and where he had a right peacefully to impart his views to others. There is no showing that his deportment was noisy, truculent, overbearing or offensive. He requested of two pedestrians permission to play to them a phonograph record. The permission was granted. It is not claimed that he intended to insult or affront the hearers by playing the record. It is plain that he wished only to interest them in his propaganda. The sound of the phonograph is not shown to have disturbed residents of the street, to have drawn a crowd, or to have impeded traffic. Thus far he had invaded no right or interest of the public or of the men accosted.

The record played by Cantwell embodies a general attack on all organized religious systems as instruments of Satan and injurious to man; it then singles out the Roman Catholic Church for strictures couched in terms which naturally would offend not only persons of that persuasion, but all others who respect the honestly held religious faith of their fellows. The hearers were in fact highly offended. One of them said he felt like hitting Cantwell and the other that he was tempted to throw Cantwell off the street. The one who testified he felt like hitting Cantwell said, in answer to the question "Did you do anything else or have any other reaction?" "No, sir, because he said he would take the victrola and he went." The other witness testified that he told Cantwell he had better get off the street before something happened to him and that was the end of the matter as Cantwell picked up his books and walked up the street. ***

We find in the instant case no assault or threatening of bodily harm, no truculent bearing, no intentional discourtesy, no personal abuse. On the contrary, we find only an effort to persuade a willing listener to buy a book or to contribute money in the interest of what Cantwell, however misguided others may think him, conceived to be true religion.

In the realm of religious faith, and in that of political belief, sharp differences arise. In both fields the tenets of one man may seem the rankest error to his neighbor. To persuade others to his own point of view, the pleader, as we know, at times, resorts to exaggeration, to vilification of men who have been, or are, prominent in church or state, and even to false statement. But the people of this nation have ordained in the light of history, that, in spite of the probability of excesses and abuses, these liberties are, in the long view, essential to enlightened opinion and right conduct on the part of the citizens of a democracy.

The essential characteristic of these liberties is, that under their shield many types of life, character, opinion and belief can develop unmolested and unobstructed. Nowhere is this shield more necessary than in our own country for a people composed of many races and of many creeds. There are limits to the exercise of these liberties. The danger in these times from the coercive activities of those who in the delusion of racial or religious conceit would incite violence and breaches of the peace in order to deprive others of their equal right to the exercise of their liberties, is emphasized by events familiar to all. These and other transgressions of those limits the States appropriately may punish.

Although the contents of the record not unnaturally aroused animosity, we think that, in the absence of a statute narrowly drawn to define and punish specific conduct as constituting a clear and present danger to a substantial interest of the State, the petitioner's communication, considered in the light of the constitutional guarantees, raised no such clear and present menace to public peace and order as to render him liable to conviction of the common law offense in question.[10]

The judgment affirming the convictions on the third and fifth counts is reversed and the cause is remanded for further proceedings not inconsistent with this opinion.

---

10. Compare Schenck v. United States, 249 U. S. 47, 52; Herndon v. Lowry, 301 U. S. 242, 256.

PRINCE v. MASSACHUSETTS
321 U.S. 158 (1944)

MR. JUSTICE RUTLEDGE delivered the opinion of the court.

The case brings for review another episode in the conflict between Jehovah's Witnesses and state authority. This time Sarah Prince appeals from convictions for violating Massachusetts' child labor laws, by acts said to be a rightful exercise of her religious convictions.

When the offenses were committed she was the aunt and custodian of Betty M. Simmons, a girl nine years of age. Originally there were three separate complaints. They were, shortly, for (1) refusal to disclose Betty's identity and age to a public officer whose duty was to enforce the statutes; (2) furnishing her with magazines, knowing she was to sell them unlawfully, that is, on the street; and (3) as Betty's custodian, permitting her to work contrary to law. The complaints were made, respectively, pursuant to §§ 79, 80 and 81 of Chapter 149, Gen.Laws of Mass. (Ter. Ed.). The Supreme Judicial Court reversed the conviction under the first complaint on state grounds; but sustained the judgments founded on the other two. They present the only questions for our decision. These are whether §§ 80 and 81, as applied, contravene the Fourteenth Amendment by denying or abridging appellant's freedom of religion and by denying to her the equal protection of the laws.

Sections 80 and 81 form parts of Massachusetts' comprehensive child labor law. They provide methods for enforcing the prohibitions of § 69, which is as follows:

> No boy under twelve and no girl under eighteen shall sell, expose or offer for sale any newspapers, magazines, periodicals or any other articles of merchandise of any description, or exercise the trade of bootblack or scavenger, or any other trade, in any street or public place.

Section 80 and 81, so far as pertinent, read:

> Whoever furnishes or sells to any minor any article of any description with the knowledge that the minor intends to sell such article in violation of any provision of sections sixty-nine to seventy-three, inclusive, or after having received written notice to this effect from any officer charged with the enforcement thereof, or knowingly procures or encourages any minor to violate any provisions of said sections, shall be punished by a fine of not less than ten nor more than two hundred dollars or by imprisonment for not more than two months, or both. § 80.
>
> Any parent, guardian or custodian having a minor under his control who compels or permits such minor to work in violation of any provision of sections sixty to seventy-four, inclusive, *** shall for a first offence be punished by a fine of not less than two nor more than ten dollars or by imprisonment for not more than five days, or both ***. § 81.

The story told by the evidence has become familiar. It hardly needs repeating, except to give setting to the variations introduced through the part played by a child of tender years. Mrs. Prince, living in Brockton, is the mother of two young sons. She also has legal custody of Betty Simmons who lives with them. The children too are Jehovah's Witnesses and both Mrs. Prince and Betty testified they were ordained ministers. The former was accustomed to go each week on the streets of Brockton to distribute "Watchtower" and "Consolation," according to the usual plan.[4] She had permitted the children to engage in this activity previously, and had been warned against doing so by the school attendance officer, Mr. Perkins. But, until December 18, 1941, she generally did not take them with her at night.

That evening, as Mrs. Prince was preparing to leave her home, the children asked to go. She at first refused. Childlike, they resorted to tears; and, motherlike, she yielded. Arriving downtown, Mrs. Prince permitted the children "to engage in the preaching work with her upon the sidewalks." That is, with specific reference to Betty, she and Mrs. Prince took positions about twenty feet apart near a street intersection. Betty held up in her hand, for passersby to see, copies of "Watch Tower" and "Consolation." From her shoulder hung the usual canvas magazine bag, on which was printed "Watchtower and Consolation 5¢ per copy." No one accepted a copy from Betty that evening and she received no money. Nor did her aunt. But on other occasions, Betty had received funds and given out copies.

Mrs. Prince and Betty remained until 8:45 p.m. A few minutes before this Mr. Perkins approached Mrs. Prince. A discussion ensued. He inquired and she refused to give Betty's name. However, she stated the child attended the Shaw School. Mr. Perkins referred to his previous warnings and said he would allow five minutes for them to get off the street. Mrs. Prince admitted she supplied Betty with the magazines and said, "[N]either you nor anybody else can stop me ***. This child is exercising her God-given right and her constitutional right to preach the gospel, and no creature has a right to interfere with God's commands." However, Mrs. Prince and Betty departed. She remarked as she went, "I'm not going through this any more. We've been through it time and time again. I'm going home and put the little girl to bed." It may be added that testimony, by Betty, her aunt and others, was offered at the trials, and was excluded, to show that Betty believed it was her religious duty to perform this work and failure would bring condemnation "to everlasting destruction at Armageddon." ***

Appellant does not stand on freedom of the press. Regarding it as secular, she concedes it may be restricted as Massachusetts has done. Hence, she rests squarely on freedom of religion under the First Amendment, applied by the Fourteenth to the states. She buttresses this foundation, however, with a claim of parental right as

4. Cf. the facts as set forth in Jamison v. Texas, 318 U.S. 413; Largent v. Texas, 318 U.S. 418; Murdock v. Pennsylvania, 319 U.S. 105; Busey v. District of Columbia, 75 U.S.App.D.C. 352, 129 F.2d 24. A common feature is that specified small sums are generally asked and received but the publications may be had without the payment if so desired.

secured by the due process clause of the latter Amendment. Cf. Meyer v. Nebraska, 262 U.S. 390. These guaranties, she thinks, guard alike herself and the child in what they have done. Thus, two claimed liberties are at stake. One is the parent's, to bring up the child in the way he should go, which for appellant means to teach him the tenets and the practices of their faith. The other freedom is the child's, to observe these; and among them is "to preach the gospel *** by public distribution" of "Watchtower" and "Consolation," in conformity with the scripture: "A little child shall lead them."

If by this position appellant seeks for freedom of conscience a broader protection than for freedom of the mind, it may be doubted that any of the great liberties insured by the First Article can be given higher place than the others. All have preferred position in our basic scheme. ***

To make accommodation between these freedoms and an exercise of state authority always is delicate. It hardly could be more so than in such a clash as this case presents. On one side is the obviously earnest claim for freedom of conscience and religious practice. With it is allied the parent's claim to authority in her own household and in the rearing of her children. The parent's conflict with the state over control of the child and his training is serious enough when only secular matters are concerned. It becomes the more so when an element of religious conviction enters. Against these sacred private interests, basic in a democracy, stand the interests of society to protect the welfare of children, and the state's assertion of authority to that end, made here in a manner conceded valid if only secular things were involved. ***

The rights of children to exercise their religion, and of parents to give them religious training and to encourage them in the practice of religious belief, as against preponderant sentiment and assertion of state power voicing it, have had recognition here, most recently in West Virginia State Board of Education v. Barnette, 319 U.S. 624. Previously in Pierce v. Society of Sisters, 268 U.S. 510, this Court had sustained the parent's authority to provide religious with secular schooling, and the child's right to receive it, as against the state's requirement of attendance at public schools. And in Meyer v. Nebraska, 262 U.S. 390, children's rights to receive teaching in languages other than the nation's common tongue were guarded against the state's encroachment. It is cardinal with us that the custody, care and nurture of the child reside first in the parents, whose primary function and freedom include preparation for obligations the state can neither supply nor hinder. *Pierce v. Society of Sisters*. And it is in recognition of this that these decisions have respected the private realm of family life which the state cannot enter.

But the family itself is not beyond regulation in the public interest, as against a claim of religious liberty. Reynolds v. United States, 98 U.S. 145 ***. Thus, he cannot claim freedom from compulsory vaccination for the child more than for himself on religious grounds.[12] The right to practice religion freely does not include liberty to expose the community or the child to communicable disease or the latter to ill health or death. *** The catalogue need not be lengthened. It is sufficient to show what indeed appellant hardly disputes, that the state has a wide range of power for limiting parental freedom and authority in things affecting the child's welfare; and that this includes, to some extent, matters of conscience and religious conviction.

But it is said the state cannot do so here. This, first, because when state action impinges upon a claimed religious freedom, it must fall unless shown to be necessary for or conducive to the child's protection against some clear and present danger, cf. Schenck v. United States, 249 U.S. 47; and, it is added, there was no such showing here. The child's presence on the street, with her guardian, distributing or offering to distribute the magazines, it is urged, was in no way harmful to her, nor in any event more so than the presence of many other children at the same time and place, engaged in shopping and other activities not prohibited. Accordingly, in view of the preferred position the freedoms of the First Article occupy, the statute in its present application must fall. It cannot be sustained by any presumption of validity. Cf. Schneider v. State, 308 U.S. 147. And, finally, it is said, the statute is, as to children, an absolute prohibition, not merely a reasonable regulation, of the denounced activity.

Concededly a statute or ordinance identical in terms with § 69, except that it is applicable to adults or all persons generally, would be invalid. *** But the mere fact a state could not wholly prohibit this form of adult activity, whether characterized locally as a "sale" or otherwise, does not mean it cannot do so for children. Such a conclusion granted would mean that a state could impose no greater limitation upon child labor than upon adult labor. ***

The state's authority over children's activities is broader than over like actions of adults. This is peculiarly true of public activities and matters of employment. A democratic society rests, for its continuance, upon the healthy, well-rounded growth of young people into full maturity as citizens, with all that implies. It may secure this against impeding restraints and dangers, within a broad range of selection. Among evils most appropriate for such action are the crippling effects of child employment, more especially in public places, and the possible harms arising from other activities subject to all the diverse influences of the street. It is too late now to doubt that legislation appropriately designed to reach such evils is within the state's police power, whether against the parents claim to control of the child or one that religious scruples dictate contrary action. ***

Street preaching, whether oral or by handing out literature, is not the primary use of the highway, even for adults. While for them it cannot be wholly prohibited, it can be regulated within reasonable limits in accommodation to the primary and

---

12. Jacobson v. Massachusetts, 197 U.S. 11.

other incidental uses.[17] But, for obvious reasons, notwithstanding appellant's contrary view,[18] the validity of such a prohibition applied to children not accompanied by an older person hardly would seem open to question. The case reduces itself therefore to the question whether the presence of the child's guardian puts a limit to the state's power. That fact may lessen the likelihood that some evils the legislation seeks to avert will occur. But it cannot forestall all of them. The zealous though lawful exercise of the right to engage in propagandizing the community, whether in religious, political or other matters, may and at times does create situations difficult enough for adults to cope with and wholly inappropriate for children, especially of tender years, to face. Other harmful possibilities could be stated, of emotional excitement and psychological or physical injury. Parents may be free to become martyrs themselves. But it does not follow they are free, in identical circumstances, to make martyrs of their children before they have reached the age of full and legal discretion when they can make that choice for themselves. Massachusetts has determined that an absolute prohibition, though one limited to streets and public places and to the incidental uses proscribed, is necessary to accomplish its legitimate objectives. Its power to attain them is broad enough to reach these peripheral instances in which the parent's supervision may reduce but cannot eliminate entirely the ill effects of the prohibited conduct. We think that with reference to the public proclaiming of religion, upon the streets and in other similar public places, the power of the state to control the conduct of children reaches beyond the scope of its authority over adults, as is true in the case of other freedoms, and the rightful boundary of its power has not been crossed in this case.
***

Our ruling does not extend beyond the facts the case presents. We neither lay the foundation "for any [that is, every] state intervention in the indoctrination and participation of children in religion" which may be done "in the name of their health and welfare" nor give warrant for "every limitation on their religious training and activities." The religious training and indoctrination of children may be accomplished in many ways, some of which, as we have noted, have received constitutional protection through decisions of this Court. These and all others except the public proclaiming of religion on the streets, if this may be taken as either training or indoctrination of the proclaimer, remain unaffected by the decision.

The judgment is affirmed.

MR. JUSTICE MURPHY, dissenting.

* * *

17. Cox v. New Hampshire, 312 U.S. 569; Chaplinsky v. New Hampshire, 315 U.S. 568.

18. Although the argument points to the guardian's presence as showing the child's activities here were not harmful, it is nowhere conceded in the briefs that the statute could be applied, consistently with the guaranty of religious freedom, if the facts had been altered only by the guardian's absence.

In dealing with the validity of statutes which directly or indirectly infringe religious freedom and the right of parents to encourage their children in the practice of a religious belief, we are not aided by any strong presumption of the constitutionality of such legislation. United States v. Carolene Products Co., 304 U.S. 144, 152, note 4. On the contrary, the human freedoms enumerated in the First Amendment and carried over into the Fourteenth Amendment are to be presumed to be invulnerable and any attempt to sweep away those freedoms is prima facie invalid. It follows that any restriction or prohibition must be justified by those who deny that the freedoms have been unlawfully invaded. The burden was therefore on the state of Massachusetts to prove the reasonableness and necessity of prohibiting children from engaging in religious activity of the type involved in this case. ***

The state, in my opinion, has completely failed to sustain its burden of proving the existence of any grave or immediate danger to any interest which it may lawfully protect. There is no proof that Betty Simmons' mode of worship constituted a serious menace to the public. It was carried on in an orderly, lawful manner at a public street corner. And "one who is rightfully on a street which the state has left open to the public carries with him there as elsewhere the constitutional right to express his views in an orderly fashion. This right extends to the communication of ideas by handbills and literature as well as by the spoken word." Jamison v. Texas, 318 U.S. 413, 416. The sidewalk, no less than the cathedral or the evangelist's tent, is a proper place, under the Constitution, for the orderly worship of God. Such use of the streets is as necessary to the Jehovah's Witnesses, the Salvation Army and others who practice religion without benefit of conventional shelters as is the use of the streets for purposes of passage.

It is claimed, however, that such activity was likely to affect adversely the health, morals and welfare of the child. Reference is made in the majority opinion to "the crippling effects of child employment, more especially in public places, and the possible harms arising from other activities subject to all the diverse influences of the street." To the extent that they flow from participation in ordinary commercial activities, these harms are irrelevant to this case. And the bare possibility that such harms might emanate from distribution of religious literature is not, standing alone, sufficient justification for restricting freedom of conscience and religion. Nor can parents or guardians be subjected to criminal liability because of vague possibilities that their teachings might cause injury to the child. The evils must be grave, immediate, substantial. Cf. Bridges v. California, 314 U.S. 252, 262. ***

UNITED STATES v. BALLARD
322 U.S. 78 (1944)

MR. JUSTICE DOUGLAS delivered the opinion of the court.

Respondents were indicted and convicted for using, and conspiring to use, the mails to defraud. *** The indictment was in twelve counts. It charged a scheme to defraud by organizing and promoting the I Am movement through the use of the mails. The charge was that certain designated corporations were formed, literature distributed and sold, funds solicited, and memberships in the I Am movement sought "by means of false and fraudulent representations, pretenses and promises." The false representations charged were eighteen in number. It is sufficient at this point to say that they covered respondents' alleged religious doctrines or beliefs. They were all set forth in the first count. The following are representative:

> that Guy W. Ballard, now deceased, alias Saint Germain, Jesus, George Washington, and Godfre Ray King, had been selected and thereby designated by the alleged "ascertained masters," Saint Germain, as a divine messenger; and that the words of 'ascended masters' and the words of the alleged divine entity, Saint Germain, would be transmitted to mankind through the medium of the said Guy W. Ballard;
>
> * * *
>
> that Guy W. Ballard, during his lifetime, and Edna W. Ballard and Donald Ballard had, by reason of supernatural attainments, the power to heal persons of ailments and diseases and to make well persons afflicted with any diseases, injuries, or ailments, and did falsely represent to persons intended to be defrauded that the three designated persons had the ability and power to cure persons of those diseases normally classified as curable and also of diseases which are ordinarily classified by the medical profession as being incurable diseases; and did further represent that the three designated persons had in fact cured either by the activity of one, either, or all of said persons, hundreds of persons afflicted with diseases and ailments;

Each of the representations enumerated in the indictment was followed by the charge that respondents "well knew" ***

> *** all of said aforementioned representations were false and untrue and were made with the intention on the part of the defendants, and each of them, to cheat, wrong, and defraud persons intended to be defrauded, and to obtain from persons intended to be defrauded by the defendants, money, property, and other things of value and to convert the same to the use and the benefit of the defendants, and each of them;

Early in the trial objections were raised to the admission of certain evidence concerning respondents' religious beliefs. The court conferred with counsel in absence of the jury and with the acquiescence of counsel for the United States and for respondents confined the issues on this phase of the case to the question of the good faith of respondents. At the request of counsel for both sides the court advised the jury of that action in the following language:

> First, the defendants in this case made certain representations of belief in a divinity and in a supernatural power. Some of the teachings of the defendants, representations, might seem extremely improbable to a great many people. For instance, the appearance of Jesus to dictate some of the works that we have had introduced in evidence, as testified to here at the opening transcription, or shaking hands with Jesus, to some people that might seem highly improbable. I point that out as one of the many statements.
>
> Whether that is true or not is not the concern of this Court and is not the concern of the jury. *** They are not going to be permitted to speculate on the actuality of the happening of those incidents. Now, I think I have made that as clear as I can. Therefore, the religious beliefs of these defendants cannot be an issue in this court.
>
> The issue is: Did these defendants honestly and in good faith believe those things? If they did, they should be acquitted. I cannot make it any clearer than that.

As we have said, counsel for the defense acquiesced in this treatment of the matter, made no objection to it during the trial, and indeed treated it without protest as the law of the case throughout the proceedings prior to the verdict. Respondents did not change their position before the District Court after verdict and contend that the truth or verity of their religious doctrines or beliefs should have been submitted to the jury. In their motion for new trial they did contend, however, that the withdrawal of these issues from the jury was error because it was in effect an amendment of the indictment. That was also one of their specifications of errors on appeal.

The Circuit Court of Appeals reversed the judgment of conviction and granted a new trial, one judge dissenting. Its reason was that the scheme to defraud alleged in the indictment was that respondents made the eighteen alleged false representations; and that to prove that defendants devised the scheme described in the indictment "it was necessary to prove that they schemed to make some, at least, of the (eighteen) representations and that some, at least, of the representations which they schemed to make were false."

A careful reading of the whole charge leads us to agree with the Circuit Court of Appeals on this phase of the case that the only issue submitted to the jury was the question as stated by the District Court, of respondents' "belief in their representations and promises."

The United States contends that respondents acquiesced in the withdrawal from the jury of the truth of their religious doctrines or beliefs and that their consent bars them from insisting on a different course once that one turned out to be unsuccessful. In fairness to respondents that principle cannot be applied here. The real objection of respondents is not that the truth of their religious doctrines or beliefs should have been submitted to the jury. Their demurrer and motion to quash made clear their position that that issue should be withheld from the jury on the basis of the First Amendment. Moreover, their position at all times was and still is that the court should have gone the whole way and withheld from the jury both that issue and the issue of their good faith. Their demurrer and motion to quash asked for dismissal of the entire indictment. Their argument that the truth of their religious doctrines or beliefs should have gone to the jury when the question of their good faith was submitted was and is merely an alternative argument. ***

As we have noted, the Circuit Court of Appeals held that the question of the truth of the representations concerning respondent's religious doctrines or beliefs should have been submitted to the jury. And it remanded the case for a new trial. It may be that the Circuit Court of Appeals took that action because it did not think that the indictment could be properly construed as charging a scheme to defraud by means other than misrepresentations of respondents' religious doctrines or beliefs. Or that court may have concluded that the withdrawal of the issue of the truth of those religious doctrines or beliefs was unwarranted because it resulted in a substantial change in the character of the crime charged. But on whichever basis that court rested its action, we do not agree that the truth or verity of respondents' religious doctrines or beliefs should have been submitted to the jury. Whatever this particular indictment might require, the First Amendment precludes such a course, as the United States seems to concede. *** Heresy trials are foreign to our Constitution. Men may believe what they cannot prove. They may not be put to the proof of their religious doctrines or beliefs. Religious experiences which are as real as life to some may be incomprehensible to others. Yet the fact that they may be beyond the ken of mortals does not mean that they can be made suspect before the law. Many take their gospel from the New Testament. But it would hardly be supposed that they could be tried before a jury charged with the duty of determining whether those teachings contained false representations. The miracles of the New Testament, the Divinity of Christ, life after death, the power of prayer are deep in the religious convictions of many. If one could be sent to jail because a jury in a hostile environment found those teachings false, little indeed would be left of religious freedom. *** The religious views espoused by respondents might seem incredible, if not preposterous, to most people. But if those doctrines are subject to trial before a jury charged with finding their truth or falsity, then the same can be done with the religious beliefs of any sect. When the triers of fact undertake that task, they enter a forbidden domain. The First Amendment does not select any one group or any one type of religion for preferred treatment. It puts them all in that position. *** So we conclude that the District Court ruled properly when it withheld from the jury all questions concerning the truth or falsity of the religious beliefs or doctrines of respondents. ***

The judgment is reversed and the cause is remanded to the Circuit Court of Appeals for further proceedings in conformity to this opinion.

MR. CHIEF JUSTICE STONE, dissenting [joined by ROBERTS and FRANKFURTER, JJ.]

* * *

The indictment charges respondents' use of the mails to defraud and a conspiracy to commit that offense by false statements of their religious experiences which had not in fact occurred. But it also charged that the representations were "falsely and fraudulently" made, that respondents "well knew" that these representations were untrue, and that they were made by respondents with the intent to cheat and defraud those to whom they were made. With the assent of the prosecution and the defense the trial judge withdrew from the consideration of the jury the question whether the alleged religious experiences had in fact occurred, but submitted to the jury the single issue whether petitioners honestly believed that they had occurred, with the instruction that if the jury did not so find, then it should return a verdict of guilty. On this issue the jury, on ample evidence that respondents were without belief in the statements which they had made to their victims, found a verdict of guilty. *** Certainly none of respondents' constitutional rights are violated if they are prosecuted for the fraudulent procurement of money by false representations as to their beliefs, religious or otherwise.

Obviously if the question whether the religious experiences in fact occurred could not constitutionally have been submitted to the jury the court rightly withdrew it. If it could have been submitted I know of no reason why the parties could not, with the advice of counsel, assent to its withdrawal from the jury. And where, as here, the indictment charges two sets of false statements, each independently sufficient to sustain the conviction, I cannot accept respondents' contention that the withdrawal of one set and the submission of the other to the jury amounted to an amendment of the indictment. ***

On the issue submitted to the jury in this case it properly rendered a verdict of guilty. As no legally sufficient reason for disturbing it appears, I think the judgment below should be reversed and that of the District Court reinstated.

MR. JUSTICE JACKSON, dissenting.

I should say the defendants have done just that for which they are indicted. If I might agree to their conviction without creating a precedent, I cheerfully would do so. I can see in their teachings nothing but humbug, untainted by any trace of truth. But that does not dispose of the constitutional question whether misrepresentation of religious experience or belief is prosecutable; it rather emphasizes the danger of such prosecutions. ***

In the first place, as a matter of either practice or philosophy I do not see how we can separate an issue as to what is believed from considerations as to what is believable. The most convincing proof that one believes his statements is to show that they have been true in his experience. Likewise, that one knowingly falsified is best proved by showing that what he said happened never did happen. How can the Government prove these persons knew something to be false which it cannot prove to be false? If we try religious sincerity severed from religious verity, we isolate the dispute from the very considerations which in common experience provide its most reliable answer. *** When one comes to trial which turns on any aspect of religious belief or representation, unbelievers among his judges are likely not to understand and are almost certain not to believe him.

And then I do not know what degree of skepticism or disbelief in a religious representation amounts to actionable fraud. James points out that "Faith means belief in something concerning which doubt is theoretically possible."[2] Belief in what one may demonstrate to the senses is not faith. All schools of religious thought make enormous assumptions, generally on the basis of revelations authenticated by some sign or miracle. The appeal in such matters is to a very different plane of credulity than is invoked by representations of secular fact in commerce. ***

There appear to be persons—let us hope not many—who find refreshment and courage in the teachings of the "I Am" cult. If the members of the sect get comfort from the celestial guidance of their "Saint Germain," however doubtful it seems to me, it is hard to say that they do not get what they pay for. Scores of sects flourish in this country by teaching what to me are queer notions. It is plain that there is wide variety in American religious taste. The Ballards are not alone in catering to it with a pretty dubious product.

The chief wrong which false prophets do to their following is not financial. The collections aggregate a tempting total, but individual payments are not ruinous. I doubt if the vigilance of the law is equal to making money stick by over-credulous people. But the real harm is on the mental and spiritual plane. There are those who hunger and thirst after higher values which they feel wanting in their humdrum lives. They live in mental confusion or moral anarchy and seek vaguely for truth and beauty and moral support. When they are deluded and then disillusioned, cynicism and confusion follow. The wrong of these things, as I see it, is not in the money the victims part with half so much as in the mental and spiritual poison they get. But that is precisely the thing the Constitution put beyond the reach of the prosecutor, for the price of freedom of religion or of speech or of the press is that we must put up with, and even pay for, a good deal of rubbish.

Prosecutions of this character easily could degenerate into religious persecution. I do not doubt that religious leaders may be convicted of fraud for making false representations on matters other than faith or experience, as for example if one represents that funds are being used to construct a church when in fact they are being used for personal purposes. But that is not this case, which reaches into wholly

2. William James, The Will to Believe, p. 90.

dangerous ground. When does less than full belief in a professed credo become actionable fraud if one is soliciting gifts or legacies? Such inquiries may discomfort orthodox as well as unconventional religious teachers, for even the most regular of them are sometimes accused of taking their orthodoxy with a grain of salt.

I would dismiss the indictment and have done with this business of judicially examining other people's faiths.

B. THE GENERAL TEST REFINED, MODIFIED, AND IN DISPUTE

From *Wisconsin v. Yoder* and *Sherbert v. Verner*, through *Employment Division v. Smith* and the Religious Freedom Restoration Act.

WISCONSIN v. YODER
406 U.S. 205 (1972)

MR. CHIEF JUSTICE BURGER delivered the opinion of the Court.

Respondents Jonas Yoder and Wallace Miller are members of the Old Order Amish religion, and respondent Adin Yutzy is a member of the Conservative Amish Mennonite Church. They and their families are residents of Green County, Wisconsin. Wisconsin's compulsory school-attendance law required them to cause their children to attend public or private school until reaching age 16 but the respondents declined to send their children, ages 14 and 15, to public school after they complete the eighth grade. The children were not enrolled in any private school, or within any recognized exception to the compulsory-attendance law, and they are conceded to be subject to the Wisconsin statute.

On complaint of the school district administrator for the public schools, respondents were charged, tried, and convicted of violating the compulsory-attendance law in Green County Court and were fined the sum of $5 each. *** The trial testimony showed that respondents believed, in accordance with the tenets of Old Order Amish communities generally, that their children's attendance at high school, public or private, was contrary to the Amish religion and way of life. They believed that by sending their children to high school, they would not only expose themselves to the danger of the censure of the church community, but, as found by the county court, also endanger their own salvation and that of their children. The State stipulated that respondents' religious beliefs were sincere.

In support of their position, respondents presented as expert witnesses scholars on religion and education whose testimony is uncontradicted. *** As a result of their common heritage, Old Order Amish communities today are characterized by a fundamental belief that salvation requires life in a church community separate and apart from the world and worldly influence. *** Amish beliefs require members of the community to make their living by farming or closely related activities.

Amish objection to formal education beyond the eighth grade is firmly grounded in these central religious concepts. They object to the high school, and higher education generally, because the values they teach are in marked variance with Amish values and the Amish way of life; they view secondary school education as an impermissible exposure of their children to a "worldly" influence in conflict with their beliefs. The high school tends to emphasize intellectual and scientific accomplishments, self-distinction, competitiveness, worldly success, and social life with other students. Amish society emphasizes informal learning-through-doing; a life of "goodness," rather than a life of intellect; wisdom, rather than technical knowledge, community welfare, rather than competition; and separation from, rather than integration with, contemporary worldly society. *** In the Amish belief higher learning tends to develop values they reject as influences that alienate man from God.

The testimony of Dr. Donald A. Erickson, an expert witness on education, also showed that the Amish succeed in preparing their high school age children to be productive members of the Amish community. He described their system of learning through doing the skills directly relevant to their adult roles in the Amish community as "ideal" and perhaps superior to ordinary high school education. The evidence also showed that the Amish have an excellent record as law-abiding and generally self-sufficient members of society.

Although the trial court in its careful findings determined that the Wisconsin compulsory school-attendance law "does interfere with the freedom of the Defendants to act in accordance with their sincere religious belief" it also concluded that the requirement of high school attendance until age 16 was a "reasonable and constitutional" exercise of governmental power, and therefore denied the motion to dismiss the charges. The Wisconsin Circuit Court affirmed the convictions. The Wisconsin Supreme Court, however, sustained respondents' claim under the Free Exercise Clause of the First Amendment and reversed the convictions. ***

I

There is no doubt as to the power of a State, having a high responsibility for education of its citizens, to impose reasonable regulations for the control and duration of basic education. See, e.g., Pierce v. Society of Sisters, 268 U.S. 510, 534 (1925). Providing public schools ranks at the very apex of the function of a State. Yet even this paramount responsibility was, in *Pierce*, made to yield to the right of parents to provide an equivalent education in a privately operated system. There the Court held that Oregon's statute compelling attendance in a public school from age eight to age 16 unreasonably interfered with the interest of parents in directing the rearing of their off-spring, including their education in church-operated schools. As that case suggests, the values of parental direction of the religious upbringing and education of their children in their early and formative years have a high place in our society. Thus, a State's interest in universal education, however highly we rank it, is not totally free from a balancing process when it impinges on fundamental rights and interests, such as those specifically protected by the Free Exercise Clause of the First Amendment, and the traditional interest of parents with respect to the religious upbringing of their children so long as they, in the words of *Pierce*, "prepare [them] for additional obligations."

It follows that in order for Wisconsin to compel school attendance beyond the eighth grade against a claim that such attendance interferes with the practice of a legitimate religious belief, it must appear either that the State does not deny the free exercise of religious belief by its requirement, or that there is a state interest of sufficient magnitude to override the interest claiming protection under the Free Exercise Clause. ***

The essence of all that has been said and written on the subject is that only those interests of the highest order and those not otherwise served can overbalance legitimate claims to the free exercise of religion.

II

We come then to the quality of the claims of the respondents concerning the alleged encroachment of Wisconsin's compulsory school-attendance statute on their rights and the rights of their children to the free exercise of the religious beliefs they and their forbears have adhered to for almost three centuries. In evaluating those claims we must be careful to determine whether the Amish religious faith and their mode of life are, as they claim, inseparable and interdependent. A way of life, however virtuous and admirable, may not be interposed as a barrier to reasonable state regulation of education if it is based on purely secular considerations; to have the protection of the Religion Clauses, the claims must be rooted in religious belief. Thus, if the Amish asserted their claims because of their subjective evaluation and rejection of the contemporary secular values accepted by the majority, much as Thoreau rejected the social values of his time and isolated himself at Walden Pond, their claims would not rest on a religious basis. Thoreau's choice was philosophical and personal rather than religious, and such belief does not rise to the demands of the Religion Clauses.

Giving no weight to such secular considerations, however, we see that the record in this case abundantly supports the claim that the traditional way of life of the Amish is not merely a matter of personal preference, but one of deep religious conviction, shared by an organized group, and intimately related to daily living. That the Old Order Amish daily life and religious practice stem from their faith is shown by the fact that it is in response to their literal interpretation of the Biblical injunction from the Epistle of Paul to the Romans, "be not conformed to this world." This command is fundamental to the Amish faith. Moreover, for the Old Order Amish, religion is not simply a matter of theocratic belief. As the expert witnesses explained, the Old Order Amish religion pervades and determines virtually their entire way of life, regulating it with the detail of the Talmudic diet through the strictly enforced rules of the church community. ***

So long as compulsory education laws were confined to eight grades of elementary basic education imparted in a nearby rural schoolhouse, with a large proportion of students of the Amish faith, the Old Order Amish had little basis to fear that school attendance would expose their children to the worldly influence they reject. But modern compulsory secondary education in rural areas is now largely carried on in a consolidated school, often remote from the student's home and alien to his daily home life. As the record so strongly shows, the values and programs of the modern secondary school are in sharp conflict with the fundamental mode of life mandated by the Amish religion. The conclusion is inescapable that secondary schooling, by exposing Amish children to worldly influences in terms of attitudes, goals, and values contrary to beliefs, and by substantially interfering with the religious development of the Amish child and his integration into the way of life of the Amish faith community at the crucial adolescent stage of development, contravenes the basic religious tenets and practice of the Amish faith, both as to the parent and the child.

In sum, the unchallenged testimony of acknowledged experts in education and religious history, almost 300 years of consistent practice, and strong evidence of a sustained faith pervading and regulating respondents' entire mode of life support the claim that enforcement of the State's requirement of compulsory formal education after the eighth grade would gravely endanger if not destroy the free exercise of respondents' religious beliefs.

III

* * *

Wisconsin concedes that under the Religion Clauses religious beliefs are absolutely free from the State's control, but it argues that "actions," even though religiously grounded, are outside the protection of the First Amendment. But our decisions have rejected the idea that religiously grounded conduct is always outside the protection of the Free Exercise Clause. It is true that activities of individuals, even when religiously based, are often subject to regulation by the States in the exercise of their undoubted power to promote the health, safety, and general welfare, or the Federal Government in the exercise of its delegated powers. But to agree that religiously grounded conduct must often be subject to the broad police power of the State is not to deny that there are areas of conduct protected by the Free Exercise Clause of the First Amendment and thus beyond the power of the State to control, even under regulations of general applicability. *** Nor can this case be disposed of on the grounds that Wisconsin's requirement for school attendance to age 16 applies uniformly to all citizens of the State and does not, on its face, discriminate against religions or a particular religion, or that it is motivated by legitimate secular concerns. A regulation neutral on its face may, in its application, nonetheless offend the constitutional requirement for governmental neutrality if it unduly burdens the free exercise of religion. The Court must not ignore the danger that an exception from a general obligation of citizenship on religious grounds may run afoul of the Establishment Clause, but that danger cannot be allowed to prevent any exception no matter how vital it may be to the protection of values promoted by the right of free exercise. ***

The State advances two primary arguments in support of its system of compulsory education. It notes, as Thomas Jefferson pointed out early in our history, that some degree of education is necessary to prepare citizens to participate effectively and intelligently in our open political system if we are to preserve freedom and independence. Further, education prepares individuals to be self-reliant and self-sufficient participants in society. We accept these propositions.

However, the evidence adduced by the Amish in this case is persuasively to the effect that an additional one or two years of formal high school for Amish children in place of their long-established program of informal vocational education would do little to serve those interests. Respondents' experts testified at trial, without challenge, that the value of all education must be assessed in terms of its capacity to prepare the child for life. It is one thing to say that compulsory education for a year or two beyond the eighth grade may be necessary when its goal is the preparation of the child for life in modern society as the majority live, but it is quite another if the goal of education be viewed as the preparation of the child for life in the separated agrarian community that is the keystone of the Amish faith.

The State attacks respondents' position as one fostering "ignorance" from which the child must be protected by the State. No one can question the State's duty to protect children from ignorance but this argument does not square with the facts disclosed in the record. Whatever their idiosyncrasies as seen by the majority, this record strongly shows that the Amish community has been a highly successful social unit within our society, even if apart from the conventional "mainstream." Its members are productive and very law-abiding members of society; they reject public welfare in any of its usual modern forms.

It is neither fair nor correct to suggests that the Amish are opposed to education beyond the eighth grade level. What this record shows is that they are opposed to conventional formal education of the type provided by a certified high school because it comes at the child's crucial adolescent period of religious development.

The State, however, supports its interest in providing an additional one or two years of compulsory high school education to Amish children because of the possibility that some such children will choose to leave the Amish community, and that if this occurs they will be ill-equipped for life. The State argues that if Amish children leave their church they should not be in the position of making their way in the world without the education available in the one or two additional years the State requires. However, on this record, that argument is highly speculative.

There is nothing in this record to suggest that the Amish qualities of reliability, self-reliance, and dedication to work would fail to find ready markets in today's society. Absent some contrary evidence supporting the State's position, we are unwilling to assume that persons possessing such valuable vocational skills and habits are doomed to become burdens on society should they determine to leave the Amish faith, nor is there any basis in the record to warrant a finding that an additional one or two years of formal school education beyond the eighth grade would serve to eliminate any such problem that might exist.

Insofar as the State's claim rests on the view that a brief additional period of formal education is imperative to enable the Amish to participate effectively and intelligently in our democratic process, it must fall. The Amish alternative to formal secondary school education has enabled them to function effectively in their day-to-day life under self-imposed limitations on relations with the world, and to survive and prosper in contemporary society as a separate, sharply identifiable and highly self-sufficient community for more than 200 years in this country. In itself this is strong evidence that they are capable of fulfilling the social and political responsibilities of citizenship without compelled attendance beyond the eighth grade at the price of jeopardizing their free exercise of religious belief.[13] ***

The requirement for compulsory education beyond the eighth grade is a relatively recent development in our history. ***

The requirement of compulsory schooling to age 16 must *** be viewed as aimed not merely at providing educational opportunities for children, but as an alternative to the equally undesirable consequence of unhealthful child labor displacing adult workers, or, on the other hand, forced idleness. The two kinds of statutes—compulsory school attendance and child labor laws—tend to keep children of certain ages off the labor market and in school; this regimen in turn provides opportunity to prepare for a livelihood of a higher order than that which children could pursue without education and protects their health in adolescence.

In these terms, Wisconsin's interest in compelling the school attendance of Amish children to age 16 emerges as somewhat less substantial than requiring such attendance for children generally. For, while agricultural employment is not totally outside the legitimate concerns of the child labor laws, employment of children under parental guidance and on the family farm from age 14 to age 16 is an ancient tradition that lies at the periphery of the objectives of such laws. There is no intimation that the Amish employment of their children on family farms is in any way deleterious to their health or that Amish parents exploit children at tender years. Any such inference would be contrary to the record before us. Moreover, employment of Amish children on the family farm does not present the undesirable economic aspects of eliminating jobs that might otherwise be held by adults.

IV

Finally, the State, on authority of *Prince v. Massachusetts*, argues that a decision exempting Amish children from the State's requirement fails to recognize the substantive right of the Amish child to a secondary education, and fails to give due regard to the power of the State as *parens patriae* to extend the benefit of secondary

---

13. All of the children involved in this case are graduates of the eighth grade. In the county court, the defense introduced a study by Dr. Hostetler indicating that Amish children in the eighth grade achieved comparably to non-Amish children in the basic skills. ***

education to children regardless of the wishes of their parents. Taken at its broadest sweep, the Court's language in *Prince*, might be read to give support to the State's position. However, the Court was not confronted in *Prince* with a situation comparable to that of the Amish as revealed in this record; this is shown by the Court's severe characterization of the evils that it thought the legislature could legitimately associate with child labor, even when performed in the company of an adult. *** This case, of course, is not one in which any harm to the physical or mental health of the child or to the public safety, peace, order, or welfare has been demonstrated or may be properly inferred. The record is to the contrary, and any reliance on that theory would find no support in the evidence.

Contrary to the suggestion of the dissenting opinion of MR. JUSTICE DOUGLAS, our holding today in no degree depends on the assertion of the religious interest of the child as contrasted with that of the parents. *** The State has at no point tried this case on the theory that respondents were preventing their children from attending school against their expressed desires, and indeed the record is to the contrary.[21] The State's position from the outset has been that it is empowered to apply its compulsory-attendance law to Amish parents in the same manner as to other parents—that is, without regard to the wishes of the child. That is the claim we reject today.

Our holding in no way determines the proper resolution of possible competing interests of parents, children, and the State in an appropriate state court proceeding in which the power of the State is asserted on the theory that Amish parents are preventing their minor children from attending high school despite their expressed desires to the contrary. *** It is clear that such an intrusion by a State into family decisions in the area of religious training would give rise to grave questions of religious freedom comparable to those raised here and those presented in Pierce v. Society of Sisters, 268 U.S. 510, (1925). On this record we neither reach nor decide those issues. ***

However read, the Court's holding in *Pierce* stands as a charter of the rights of parents to direct the religious upbringing of their children. And, when the interests of parenthood are combined with a free exercise claim of the nature revealed by this record, more than merely a "reasonable relation to some purpose within the competency of the State" is required to sustain the validity of the State's requirement under the First Amendment. To be sure, the power of the parent, even when linked to a free exercise claim, may be subject to limitation under *Prince* if it appears that parental decisions will jeopardize the health or safety of the child, or have a potential for significant social burdens. But in this case, the Amish have introduced

21. The only relevant testimony in the record is to the effect that the wishes of the one child who testified corresponded with those of her parents. Testimony of Frieda Yoder to the effect that her personal religious beliefs guided her decision to discontinue school attendance after the eighth grade. The other children were not called by either side.

persuasive evidence undermining the arguments the State has advanced to support its claims in terms of the welfare of the child and society as a whole. ***

V

For the reasons stated we hold, with the Supreme Court of Wisconsin, that the First and Fourteenth Amendments prevent the State from compelling respondents to cause their children to attend formal high school to age 16. Our disposition of this case, however, in no way alters our recognition of the obvious fact that courts are not school boards or legislatures, and are ill-equipped to determine the "necessity" of discrete aspects of a State's program of compulsory education. This should suggest that courts must move with great circumspection in performing the sensitive and delicate task of weighing a State's legitimate social concern when faced with religious claims for exemption from generally applicable educational requirements. It cannot be overemphasized that we are not dealing with a way of life and mode of education by a group claiming to have recently discovered some "progressive" or more enlightened process for rearing children for modern life. ***

Affirmed.

MR. JUSTICE POWELL and MR. JUSTICE REHNQUIST took no part in the consideration or decision of this case.

MR. JUSTICE STEWART, with whom MR. JUSTICE BRENNAN joins, concurring.

[T]his record simply does not present the interesting and important issue discussed in Part II of the dissenting opinion of MR. JUSTICE DOUGLAS. With this observation, I join the opinion and the judgment of the Court.

MR. JUSTICE WHITE, with whom MR. JUSTICE BRENNAN and MR. JUSTICE STEWART join, concurring.

I join the opinion and judgment of the Court because I cannot say that the State's interest in requiring two more years of compulsory education in the ninth and tenth grades outweighs the importance of the concededly sincere Amish religious practice to the survival of that sect. ***

MR. JUSTICE DOUGLAS, dissenting in part.

I-II

*** If the parents in this case are allowed a religious exemption, the inevitable effect is to impose the parents' notions of religious duty upon their children. Where the child is mature enough to express potentially conflicting desires, it would be an invasion of the child's rights to permit such an imposition without canvassing his views. As in Prince v. Massachusetts, 321 U.S. 158, it is an imposition resulting from this very litigation. As the child has no other effective forum, it is in this litigation that his rights should be considered. And, if an Amish child desires to attend high school, and is mature enough to have that desire respected, the State may well be able to override the parents' religiously motivated objections.

Religion is an individual experience. It is not necessary, nor even appropriate, for every Amish child to express his views on the subject in a prosecution of a single adult. Crucial, however, are the views of the child whose parent is the subject of the suit. Frieda Yoder has in fact testified that her own religious views are opposed to high-school education. I therefore join the judgment of the Court as to respondent Jonas Yoder. But Frieda Yoder's views may not be those of Vernon Yutzy or Barbara Miller. I must dissent, therefore, as to respondents Adin Yutzy and Wallace Miller as their motion to dismiss also raised the question of their children's religious liberty.

The views of the two children in question were not canvassed by the Wisconsin courts. The matter should be explicitly reserved so that new hearings can be held on remand of the case.

III

* * *

The Court rightly rejects the notion that actions, even though religiously grounded, are always outside the protection of the Free Exercise Clause of the First Amendment. In so ruling, the Court departs from the teaching of Reynolds v. United States, 98 U.S. 145, 164, where it was said concerning the reach of the Free Exercise Clause of the First Amendment, "Congress was deprived of all legislative power over mere opinion, but was left free to reach actions which were in violation of social duties or subversive of good order." In that case it was conceded that polygamy was a part of the religion of the Mormons. Yet the Court said, "It matters not that his belief [in polygamy] was a part of his professed religion: it was still belief and belief only." *Id.*, at 167.

Action, which the Court deemed to be antisocial, could be punished even though it was grounded on deeply held and sincere religious convictions. What we do today, at least in this respect, opens the way to give organized religion a broader base than it has ever enjoyed; and it even promises that in time *Reynolds* will be overruled.

SHERBERT v. VERNER
374 U.S. 398 (1963)

MR. JUSTICE BRENNAN delivered the opinion of the Court.

Appellant, a member of the Seventh-day Adventist Church was discharged by her South Carolina employer because she would not work on Saturday, the Sabbath Day of her faith.[1] When she was unable to obtain other employment because from

---

1. Appellant became a member of the Seventh-day Adventist Church in 1957, at a time when her employer, a textile-mill operator, permitted her to work a five-day week. It was not until 1959 that the work week was changed to six days, including Saturday, for all three shifts in the employer's mill. No

conscientious scruples she would not take Saturday work,[2] she filed a claim for unemployment compensation benefits under the South Carolina Unemployment Compensation Act. That law provides that, to be eligible for benefits, a claimant must be "able to work and available for work"; and, further, that a claimant is ineligible for benefits "[i]f he has failed, without good cause to accept available suitable work when offered him by the employment office or the employer." The appellee Employment Security Commission, in administrative proceedings under the statute, found that appellant's restriction upon her availability for Saturday work brought her within the provision disqualifying for benefits insured workers who fail, without good cause, to accept "suitable work when offered by the employment office or the employer." The Commission's finding was sustained by the Court of Common Pleas for Spartanburg County. That court's judgment was in turn affirmed by the South Carolina Supreme Court, which rejected appellant's contention that, as applied to her, the disqualifying provisions of the South Carolina statute abridged her right to the free exercise of her religion secured under the Free Exercise Clause of the First Amendment through the Fourteenth Amendment. The State Supreme Court held specifically that appellant's ineligibility infringed no constitutional liberties because such a construction of the statute "places no restriction upon the appellant's freedom of religion nor does it in any way prevent her in the exercise of her right and freedom to observe her religious beliefs in accordance with the dictates of her conscience."[4] *** We reverse the judgment of the South Carolina Supreme Court and remand for further proceedings not inconsistent with this opinion.

I-II

We turn first to the question whether the disqualification for benefits imposes any burden on the free exercise of appellant's religion. We think it is clear that it does. In a sense the consequences of such a disqualification to religious principles and practices may be only an indirect result of welfare legislation within the State's general competence to enact; it is true that no criminal sanctions directly compel

---

question has been raised in this case concerning the sincerity of appellant's religious beliefs. Nor is there any doubt that the prohibition against Saturday labor is a basic tenet of the Seventh-day Adventist creed, based upon that religion's interpretation of the Holy Bible.

2. After her discharge, appellant sought employment with three other mills in the Spartanburg area, but found no suitable five-day work available at any of the mills. In filing her claim with the Commission, she expressed a willingness to accept employment at other mills, or even in another industry, so long as Saturday work was not required. The record indicates that of the 150 or more Seventh-day Adventists in the Spartanburg area, only appellant and one other have been unable to find suitable non-Saturday employment.

4. It has been suggested that appellant is not within the class entitled to benefits under the South Carolina statute because her unemployment did not result from discharge or layoff due to lack of work. It is true that unavailability for work for some personal reasons not having to do with matters of conscience or religion has been held to be a basis of disqualification for benefits. But appellant claims that the Free Exercise Clause prevents the State from basing the denial of benefits upon the "personal reason" she gives for not working on Saturday. ***

appellant to work a six-day week. But this is only the beginning, not the end, of our inquiry.[5] For "[i]f the purpose or effect of a law is to impede the observance of one or all religions or is to discriminate invidiously between religions, that law is constitutionally invalid even though the burden may be characterized as being only indirect." *Braunfeld v. Brown*, 366 U.S., at 607. Here not only is it apparent that appellant's declared ineligibility for benefits derives solely from the practice of her religion, but the pressure upon her to forego that practice is unmistakable. The ruling forces her to choose between following the precepts of her religion and forfeiting benefits, on the one hand, and abandoning one of the precepts of her religion in order to accept work, on the other hand. Governmental imposition of such a choice puts the same kind of burden upon the free exercise of religion as would a fine imposed against appellant for her Saturday worship.

Nor may the South Carolina court's construction of the statute be saved from constitutional infirmity on the ground that unemployment compensation benefits are not appellant's "right" but merely a "privilege." It is too late in the day to doubt that the liberties of religion and expression may be infringed by the denial of or placing of conditions upon a benefit or privilege. ***

Significantly South Carolina expressly saves the Sunday worshipper from having to make the kind of choice which we here hold infringes the Sabbatarian's religious liberty. When in times of "national emergency" the textile plants are authorized by the State Commissioner of Labor to operate on Sunday, "no employee shall be required to work on Sunday who is conscientiously opposed to Sunday work; and if any employee should refuse to work on Sunday on account of conscientious objections he or she shall not jeopardize his or her seniority by such refusal or be discriminated against in any other manner." S.C.Code, § 64—4. No question of the disqualification of a Sunday worshipper for benefits is likely to arise, since we cannot suppose that an employer will discharge him in violation of this statute. The unconstitutionality of the disqualification of the Sabbatarian is thus compounded by the religious discrimination which South Carolina's general statutory scheme necessarily effects.

III

We must next consider whether some compelling state interest enforced in the eligibility provisions of the South Carolina statute justifies the substantial infringement of appellant's First Amendment right. It is basic that no showing merely of a rational relationship to some colorable state interest would suffice; in this highly sensitive constitutional area, "[o]nly the gravest abuses, endangering

---

5. In a closely analogous context, this Court said:

"*** the fact that no direct restraint or punishment is imposed upon speech or assembly does not determine the free speech question. Under some circumstances, indirect 'discouragements' undoubtedly have the same coercive effect upon the exercise of First Amendment rights as imprisonment, fines, injunctions or taxes. A requirement that adherents of particular religious faiths or political parties wear identifying arm-bands, for example, is obviously of this nature."

paramount interest, give occasion for permissible limitation," Thomas v. Collins, 323 U.S. 516, 530. No such abuse or danger has been advanced in the present case. The appellees suggest no more than a possibility that the filing of fraudulent claims by unscrupulous claimants feigning religious objections to Saturday work might not only dilute the unemployment compensation fund but also hinder the scheduling by employers of necessary Saturday work. But that possibility is not apposite here because no such objection appears to have been made before the South Carolina Supreme Court, and we are unwilling to assess the importance of an asserted state interest without the views of the state court. [E]ven if the possibility of spurious claims did threaten to dilute the fund and disrupt the scheduling of work, it would plainly be incumbent upon the appellees to demonstrate that no alternative forms of regulation would combat such abuses without infringing First Amendment rights.[7] ***

In these respects, then, the state interest asserted in the present case is wholly dissimilar to the interests which were found to justify the less direct burden upon religious practices in *Braunfeld v. Brown.* The Court recognized that the Sunday closing law which that decision sustained undoubtedly served "to make the practice of [the Orthodox Jewish merchants'] religious beliefs more expensive." But the statute was nevertheless saved by a countervailing factor which finds no equivalent in the instant case—a strong state interest in providing one uniform day of rest for all workers. That secular objective could be achieved, the Court found, only by declaring Sunday to be that day of rest. Requiring exemptions for Sabbatarians, while theoretically possible, appeared to present an administrative problem of such magnitude, or to afford the exempted class so great a competitive advantage, that such a requirement would have rendered the entire statutory scheme unworkable. In the present case no such justifications underlie the determination of the state court that appellant's religion makes her ineligible to receive benefits.

IV

In holding as we do, plainly we are not fostering the "establishment" of the Seventh-day Adventist religion in South Carolina, for the extension of unemployment benefits to Sabbatarians in common with Sunday worshippers reflects nothing more than the governmental obligation of neutrality in the face of religious differences, and does not represent that involvement of religious with secular institutions which it is the object of the Establishment Clause to forestall. See

---

7. We note that before the instant decision, state supreme courts had, without exception, granted benefits to persons who were physically available for work but unable to find suitable employment solely because of a religious prohibition against Saturday work. *** Of the 47 States which have eligibility provisions similar to those of the South Carolina statute, only 28 appear to have given administrative rulings concerning the eligibility of persons whose religious convictions prevented them from accepting available work. Twenty-two of those States have held such persons entitled to benefits, although apparently only one such decision rests exclusively upon the federal constitutional ground which constitutes the basis of our decision. ***

School District of Abington Township v. Schempp, [374 U.S.] 203. Nor does the recognition of the appellant's right to unemployment benefits under the state statute serve to abridge any other person's religious liberties. Nor do we, by our decision today, declare the existence of a constitutional right to unemployment benefits on the part of all persons whose religious convictions are the cause of their unemployment. This is not a case in which an employee's religious convictions serve to make him a nonproductive member of society. See note 2, *supra.* Finally, nothing we say today constrains the States to adopt any particular form or scheme of unemployment compensation. Our holding today is only that South Carolina may not constitutionally apply the eligibility provisions so as to constrain a worker to abandon his religious convictions respecting the day of rest. *** The judgment of the South Carolina Supreme Court is reversed and the case is remanded for further proceedings not inconsistent with this opinion.

MR. JUSTICE DOUGLAS, concurring.

* * *

This case is resolvable not in terms of what an individual can demand of government, but solely in terms of what government may not do to an individual in violation of his religious scruples. The fact that government cannot exact from me a surrender of one iota of my religious scruples does not, of course, mean that I can demand of government a sum of money, the better to exercise them. For the Free Exercise Clause is written in terms of what the government cannot do to the individual, not in terms of what the individual can exact from the government.

Those considerations, however, are not relevant here. If appellant is otherwise qualified for unemployment benefits, payments will be made to her not as a Seventh-day Adventist, but as an unemployed worker. Conceivably these payments will indirectly benefit her church, but no more so than does the salary of any public employee. Thus, this case does not involve the problems of direct or indirect state assistance to a religious organization—matters relevant to the Establishment Clause, not in issue here.

MR. JUSTICE STEWART, concurring in the result.

Although fully agreeing with the result which the Court reaches in this case, I cannot join the Court's opinion. This case presents a double-barreled dilemma, which in all candor I think the Court's opinion has not succeeded in papering over. The dilemma ought to be resolved. ***

South Carolina would deny unemployment benefits to a mother unavailable for work on Saturdays because she was unable to get a babysitter.[3] Thus, we do not have before us a situation where a State provides unemployment compensation generally, and singles out for disqualification only those persons who are unavailable for work

---

3. See Judson Mills v. South Carolina Unemployment Compensation Comm., 28 S.E.2d 535; Hartsville Cotton Mill v. South Carolina Employment Security Comm., 79 S.E.2d 381.

on religious grounds. This is not, in short, a scheme which operates so as to discriminate against religion as such. But the Court nevertheless holds that the State must prefer a religious over a secular ground for being unavailable for work—that state financial support of the appellant's religion is constitutionally required to carry out "the governmental obligation of neutrality in the face of religious differences. ***"

Yet in cases decided under the Establishment Clause the Court has decreed otherwise. It has decreed that government must blind itself to the differing religious beliefs and traditions of the people. With all respect, I think it is the Courts duty to face up to the dilemma posed by the conflict between the Free Exercise Clause of the Constitution and the Establishment Clause as interpreted by the Court. It is a duty, I submit, which we owe to the people, the States, and the Nation, and a duty which we owe to ourselves. ***

My second difference with the Court's opinion is that I cannot agree that today's decision can stand consistently with *Braunfeld v. Brown.* The Court says that there was a "less direct burden upon religious practices" in that case than in this. With all respect, I think the Court is mistaken, simply as a matter of fact. The *Braunfeld* case involved a state *criminal* statute. The undisputed effect of that statute, as pointed out by MR. JUSTICE BRENNAN in his dissenting opinion in that case, was that "'Plaintiff, Abraham Braunfeld, will be unable to continue in his business if he may not stay open on Sunday and he will thereby lose his capital investment.' In other words, the issue in this case—and we do not understand either appellees or the Court to contend otherwise—is whether a State may put an individual to a choice between his business and his religion." The impact upon the appellant's religious freedom in the present case is considerably less onerous. We deal here not with a criminal statute, but with the particularized administration of South Carolina's Unemployment Compensation Act. Even upon the unlikely assumption that the appellant could not find suitable non-Saturday employment,[4] the appellant at the worst would be denied a maximum of 22 weeks of compensation payments. I agree with the Court that the possibility of that denial is enough to infringe upon the appellant's constitutional right to the free exercise of her religion. But it is clear to me that in order to reach this conclusion the court must explicitly reject the reasoning of *Braunfeld v. Brown.* I think the *Braunfeld* case was wrongly decided and should be overruled, and accordingly I concur in the result reached by the Court in the case before us.

MR. JUSTICE HARLAN, whom MR. JUSTICE WHITE joins, dissenting.

Today's decision is disturbing both in its rejection of existing precedent and in its implications for the future. The significance of the decision can best be understood after an examination of the state law applied in this case.

---

4. As noted by the Court, "The record indicates that of the 150 or more Seventh-day Adventists in the Spartanburg area, only appellant and one other have been unable to find suitable non-Saturday employment."

South Carolina's Unemployment Compensation Law was enacted in 1936 in response to the grave social and economic problems that arose during the depression of that period. As stated in the statute itself:

> "Economic insecurity due to unemployment is a serious menace to health, morals and welfare of the people of this State; *involuntary unemployment* is therefore a subject of general interest and concern ***; the achievement of social security requires protection against this greatest hazard of our economic life; this can be provided by encouraging the employers *to provide more stable employment and by the systematic accumulation of funds during periods of employment to provide benefits for periods of unemployment*, thus maintaining purchasing power and limiting the serious social consequences of poor relief assistance." § 68— 38. (Emphasis added.)

Thus the purpose of the legislature was to tide people over, and to avoid social and economic chaos, during periods when *work was unavailable*. But at the same time there was clearly no intent to provide relief for those who for purely personal reasons were or became *unavailable for work*. In accordance with this design, the legislature provided, in § 68—113, that "[a]n unemployed insured worker shall be eligible to receive benefits with respect to any week *only* if the Commission finds that [h]e is able to work and is available for work." (Emphasis added.)

The South Carolina Supreme Court has uniformly applied this law in conformity with its clearly expressed purpose. It has consistently held that one is not "available for work" if his unemployment has resulted not from the inability of industry to provide a job but rather from personal circumstances, no matter how compelling. The reference to "involuntary unemployment" in the legislative statement of policy, whatever a sociologist, philosopher, or theologian might say, has been interpreted not to embrace such personal circumstances.

In the present case all that the state court has done is to apply these accepted principles. Since virtually all of the mills in the Spartanburg area were operating on a six-day week, the appellant was "unavailable for work," and thus ineligible for benefits, when personal considerations prevented her from accepting employment on a full-time basis in the industry and locality in which she had worked. The fact that these personal considerations sprang from her religious convictions was wholly without relevance to the state court's application of the law. Thus in no proper sense can it be said that the State discriminated against the appellant on the basis of her religious beliefs or that she was denied benefits *because* she was a Seventh-day Adventist. She was denied benefits just as any other claimant would be denied benefits who was not "available for work" for personal reasons.[1]

---

1. I am completely at a loss to understand note 4 of the Court's opinion. Certainly the Court is not basing today's decision on the unsupported supposition that *some* day, the South Carolina Supreme Court may conclude that there is *some* personal reason for unemployment that may not disqualify a claimant for relief. In any event, I submit it is perfectly clear that South Carolina would not compensate

With this background, this Court's decision comes into clearer focus. What the Court is holding is that if the State chooses to condition unemployment compensation on the applicant's availability for work, it is constitutionally compelled *to carve out an exception*—and to provide benefits—for those whose unavailability is due to their religious convictions.[2] Such a holding has particular significance in two respects.

First, despite the Court's protestations to the contrary, the decision necessarily overrules Braunfeld v. Brown. *** *Second*, the implications of the present decision are far more troublesome than its apparently narrow dimensions would indicate at first glance. The meaning of today's holding, as already noted, is that the State must furnish unemployment benefits to one who is unavailable for work if the unavailability stems from the exercise of religious convictions. The State, in other words, must *single out* for financial assistance those whose behavior is religiously motivated, even though it denies such assistance to others whose identical behavior (in this case, inability to work no Saturdays) is not religiously motivated.

It has been suggested that such singling out of religious conduct for special treatment may violate the constitutional limitations on state action. See Kurland, Of Church and State and the Supreme Court, 29 U. of Chi.L.Rev. 1. My own view, however, is that at least under the circumstances of this case it would be a permissible accommodation of religion for the State, if it *chose* to do so, to create an exception to its eligibility requirements for persons like the appellant. *** There are too*** many areas in which the pervasive activities of the State [may] justify some special provision for religion to prevent it from being submerged by an all-embracing secularism. ***

For very much the same reasons, however, I cannot subscribe to the conclusion that the State is constitutionally *compelled* to carve out an exception to its general rule of eligibility in the present case. Those situations in which the Constitution may require special treatment on account of religion are, in my view, few and far between, and this view is amply supported by the course of constitutional litigation in this area. *** Such compulsion in the present case is particularly inappropriate in light of the indirect, remote, and insubstantial effect of the decision below on the

---

persons who became unemployed for *any* personal reason, as distinguished from layoffs or lack of work, since the State Supreme Court's decisions make it plain that such persons would not be regarded as "available for work" within the manifest meaning of the eligibility requirements. ***

2. The Court does suggest, in a rather startling disclaimer, that its holding is limited in applicability to those whose religious convictions do not make them "nonproductive" members of society, noting that most of the Seventh-day Adventists in the Spartanburg area are employed. But surely this disclaimer cannot be taken seriously, for the Court cannot mean that the case would have come out differently if none of the Seventh-day Adventists in Spartanburg had been gainfully employed, or if the appellant's religion had prevented her from working on Tuesdays instead of Saturdays. Nor can the Court be suggesting that it will make a value judgment in each case as to whether a particular individual's religious convictions prevent him from being "productive." I can think of no more inappropriate function for this Court to perform.

exercise of appellant's religion and in light of the direct financial assistance to religion that today's decision requires.

For these reasons I respectfully dissent from the opinion and judgment of the Court.[4]

AN EXTENDED NOTE ON *SHERBERT V. VERNER*

I. Note that *Sherbert v. Verner* presents no *direct* conflict between the plaintiff's religiously-felt obligation and the state law. It does not involve a free exercise clause claim frustrated by a law that commands one to do that which is forbidden by one's religion; neither does it involve a law forbidding one to do that which one's religion commands. As the Court acknowledges, Ms. Sherbert was not confronted with the kind of dilemma presented by *Prince v. Massachusetts*, of *either* obeying God *or* obeying the law of the civil state, there being no possibility of obeying both. Either of these arrangements, characteristic of the cases thus far examined[1] and of most others one will encounter, describes a direct conflict between the free exercise of religion and the civil state. Ms. Sherbert, however, was not required by state law to work on Saturday or, for that matter, on any other day. She broke no law of the state by abstaining from work on Saturday, as she was free to do as she saw fit. Her dilemma, rather, was more like that of the Jewish merchant in *McGowan* or in *Braunfield*. Moreover, the legal and financial consequences of exercising her religious choice seem no different from the legal and financial consequences of any nonreligious person exercising a like choice. Why, then, is the case treated as it is?

II. Is it the case, rather, that the statute operates in the mode of an "unconstitutional condition," as Justice Brennan's opinion suggests? That if Ms. Sherbert adheres to her religion she will be made to forfeit an advantage provided to others, and while something similar was present for the observant Jewish merchant in *Braunfield*, that was a very different case in that the resulting disadvantage was the consequence of the merchant's religion, but not a consequence of the law? Whereas in this instance the law itself subjected her to a "forfeiture" (of unemployment compensation benefits) for what her religion required her to do?[2]

---

4. Since the Court states, that it does not reach the appellant's "equal protection" argument, based upon South Carolina's emergency Sunday-work provisions, §§ 64-4, 64-6, I do not consider it appropriate for me to do so.

1. See, e.g., *West Virginia Bd. of Education v. Barnette* (if one salutes the flag, one thereby directly breaks God's commandment not to do so; but if one fails to salute the flag, one will be suspended from school, be taken from one's home, and be placed in a place of detention for delinquent children under superintendence of the state). See also *Reynolds v. United States* and *Wisconsin v. Yoder* (each presenting an equivalent direct conflict under the law).

2. But this effort to distinguish *Braunfield* is not correct, is it? The law to which Braunfield objected was the Sunday closing law which was, itself, the cause of his hardship. That is, insofar as he obeyed his religious obligation not to do business on Saturday, the Sunday closing law would force him

But note that insofar as Ms. Sherbert declined to accept work on Saturday because it conflicted with her religion, she evidently was not treated differently than any other person declining such work for reasons that would be equally compelling to them albeit without reference to any particular religion or religious belief. How, then, is it appropriate to describe the case as one imposing a special cost or penalty or forfeiture, on the exercise of one's religious belief?

Justice Stewart, while concurring in the Court's judgment, noted that unemployment benefits would also be unavailable under the South Carolina act "to a mother unavailable for work on Saturdays because she was unable to get a babysitter." Justice Harlan, in dissent, was similarly emphatic— that Ms. Sherbert was denied benefits "just as any other claimant would be denied benefits who was not 'available for work' for personal reasons,"[3] adding by way of footnote: "I submit it is perfectly clear that South Carolina would not compensate persons who became unemployed for any personal reason, as distinguished from layoffs or lack of work * * *."[4]

Insofar as this was the actual case, how then can the issue be described as one involving the doctrine of unconstitutional conditions in the usual sense of that doctrine's application, i.e. a case in which certain valuable benefits controlled by the state (here, rights to the unemployment compensation fund) will be withheld by a classificatory trait of ineligibility deemed specially protected by the Constitution—such as what political party one affiliates with, what social or political

---

to miss two days of business—while others would miss only one. Consistent with the Court's free exercise clause decision in *Sherbert v. Verner*, may it now be the case that *Braunfield* is no longer valid? How, if at all, is the case to be distinguished? In *Everson*, all nine Justices of the Supreme Court assumed it would be valid to subsidize the bus transport of public school students only (indeed, the Court divided five-to-four whether it was even allowable to include parochial school parents in the reimbursement plan). After *Sherbert*, would it be *unconstitutional* to limit bus fare reimbursement *solely* to parents of public school children? (Would such a law operate as an "unconstitutional condition" upon the free exercise of religion of those placing their children in parochial schools, working a forfeiture of bus transportation reimbursement eligibility insofar as they opt out of the public schools, albeit on religious grounds?)

3. See also the three cases, following *Sherbert*, cited in note 11 p. 1034 *infra*. In these cases, also, the statute made no distinction between religious and nonreligious reasons; the criterion of ineligibility was not tied to the exercise of any constitutional right.

4. The point was stressed both in the state's brief (at p. 21) and in the state's oral argument in the Supreme Court. At oral argument the state attorney general drew the distinction and gave as an additional example:

> "For instance, a workman, a worker having to care for children, having to care for a sick husband—a very laudable purpose that would require that she not be at her job. But nevertheless, in circumstances such as that, compensation is denied. *** Cases involving the cessation of work by a wife when her husband has been transferred away from the site of her employment. She may from religious or other reasons feel compelled to be by the side of her husband, but nevertheless that is not held to be a suitable ground for ceasing work and in that case unemployment benefits are [also] withheld."

Oral Argument of Appellee, at 9, *reprinted in* 57 Landmark Briefs and Arguments of the Supreme Court of the United States: Constitutional Law 1282 (Philip B. Kurland & Gerhard Casper eds. 1975).

causes one supports, or what religion one may or may not profess—when no such classificatory standard was involved in this law? Is this not, rather, an instance where one seeks an advantage of eligibility that others who are otherwise similarly situated *will be denied*?

It was not the case that Ms. Sherbert was deemed ineligible "because" she was a Seventh Day Adventist, or "because" of any religious practice or belief, was it? Rather, she was deemed ineligible "because" she was unavailable for work in the same sense as would characterize another who stayed at home to care for a dying relative, or another who moved away in order not to be separated from a spouse who found work somewhere else.[5] And insofar as this appears to have been the case,[6] *Sherbert v. Verner* may not fit comfortably within the usual profile of unconstitutional conditions kinds of cases, whatever the scope of the doctrine may be.

In brief, there appears to have been no singling out of religiously-actuated conduct as the trigger for the disqualification at stake.[7] Applying the doctrine of unconstitutional conditions in this setting seems therefore to require something special *just on account of* the free exercise clause, namely, the special *affirmative* favoring of persons identified by their religious practice, in a manner and in a form *denied* to others who are otherwise like themselves. Moreover, it requires an affirmative payment of *money* to them and not merely an exemption from an otherwise valid regulation (as was sought in *Braunfield, Reynolds*, or *Prince*), though others who are otherwise similarly situated will not be eligible for the same financial payments.

The apparent tension with the Court's own establishment clause cases is noted in the Stewart concurrence and in the Harlan dissent. How does one reconcile the apparent contradiction of the Court's own previous views of what it is that the establishment clause forbids, on the one hand, and what the free exercise clause—according to *Sherbert*—requires?

---

5. See Wimberly v. Labor & Indus. Rel. Comm'n, 479 U.S. 511 (1987). Following *Sherbert*, compare these two cases: (a) Mrs. Smith stays away from work because her child is very young and she feels strongly the duty to be with and to nurture her child; (b) Mrs. Smith stays away from work because her child is very young *and* according to her religion it would be contrary to God's law were she not to be with and to nurture her child. Is it the case that in case (a) the state need not pay unemployment compensation benefits, but that in case (b) the free exercise clause *requires* such benefits to be paid? (Insofar as no benefits are paid in case (a), how is the failure to pay benefits in case (b) an unconstitutional condition attached to the unemployment compensation law?)

6. It was not in fact quite the case (e.g., in oral argument the state attorney general suggested that leaving work on account of pregnancy might not have disqualified the employee from eligibility for unemployment compensation), but overall the case was approximately this.

7. Compare Rosenberger v. Rector and Visitors of the University of Virginia, 515 U.S. 819 (1995) (university subsidy generally available for covering printing cost of publications sponsored by recognized student organizations, not available if publication reflected the student group's religious perspective). (In *Rosenberger*, unlike *Sherbert*, it is the religious identity of the activity that triggered the ineligibility for assistance that would be received but for that fact—so it is plausible to regard the specified ground of ineligibility as a "penalty" for engaging in religious speech.)

Even assuming that it might not be inconsistent with those establishment clause decisions for the state to make an exception so to merely *permit* payments to be made to those unavailable for work due to religious dictates, even while withholding them from others who are unavailable for any other reason, what is the basis for the holding that in fact the free exercise clause not only affords a suitable public purpose sufficient to permit such payments, but indeed *requires* the state to treat religious absentees better than others whom it will continue to regard as unavailable for work? (How is this different from a tax on some, to be paid to others, to enable them to practice their religious faith?[8]

III

Sherbert v. Verner has sometimes been thought to turn on the fact that South Carolina's unemployment compensation statute did not exist in a vacuum. The point is not that the preceding critical review misrepresents the unemployment compensation statute, but that it nonetheless leaves several other matters out of account. The point is to see whether these other matters properly affected the case (and to see also whether they may therefore limit it such that the tension with the establishment clause is not, after all, nearly so severe as the foregoing review makes it appear to be).

Specifically, South Carolina also:

(a) Already maintained a general Sunday closing law such that, if merely as a consequence of that law, those bound by religious belief to do no work *on Sunday* would themselves *not* confront the need to choose between having to work on the day set aside by their religion, in violation of their religion, and being without work with no unemployment compensation; and South Carolina –

(b) Further provided that even when textile mills could lawfully operate on Sunday (namely in times of designated national emergency), no mill could discharge any employee for refusal to work on Sunday insofar as that particular employee was "conscientiously opposed to Sunday work."[9] So Sunday observant religionists were already protected in a way Ms. Sherbert was not.

---

8. See Jesse Choper, The Religion Clauses of the First Amendment: Reconciling the Conflict, 41 U.Pitt.L.Rev. 673, 698 (1980) (*Sherbert* irreconcilable insofar as it involves forced tax subsidy of religious practice); Michael W. McConnell & Richard A. Posner, An Economic Approach to Issues of Religious Freedom, 56 U.Chi.L.Rev. 1, 38-41 (1989). ("Under *Sherbert*, religious workers are insured [without additional charge] against an additional risk, not borne by nonreligious workers: the risk that their work may become unsuitable for religious reasons.")

9. The quoted language is taken from the pertinent South Carolina statute. (Cf. Estate of Thorton v. Caldor, 472 U.S. 703 (1985) (state statute granting absolute protection from dismissal to any employee declining work on a day forbidden by their religion as a work day; *held*, unconstitutional under the establishment clause), distinguishing Trans World Airlines, Inc. v. Hardison, 432 U.S. 63 (1977) (sustaining Act of Congress forbidding religious as well as sex, race, and national origin employment discrimination, and requiring "reasonable" accommodation of employee religiously-based concerns; *held*, not invalid under the establishment clause).)

The majority in *Sherbert* noted that the state's Sunday closing law had the effect (if not the purpose) of benefitting some religious persons, notably mainline Protestants and Catholics: losing *their* job, without benefit of unemployment compensation, triggered by a conflict between a particular kind of religious duty and an employer's needs, was not a real possibility as to them in most circumstances. The effect of the two laws combined, moreover, virtually eliminated one kind of unemployment risk (the risk of unemployment due to one kind of religious conflict, i.e. a conflict affecting the day one might be unable to work), for all workers save only those like Ms. Sherbert. Restoring Ms. Sherbert to a position of compensation eligibility in *these* circumstances might thus be seen as warranted by the need to have her treated merely on approximately equal—not better—terms with them, as to the particular kind of unemployment risk only those in her position effectively incurred.

IV

Influential as these considerations may or might have been in *Sherbert* itself, however, the case does not appear to have been reasoned in this way.[10] At least it is no longer so regarded by the Court as limiting the application of the decision itself. In three subsequent cases otherwise much like *Sherbert*, no use is made of these observations to limit the Court's holding in *Sherbert*. (Indeed no equivalent form of "equality-among-religions" rationale was available to help explain two of these three subsequent cases, or relied upon in any of the cases decided so to require the payment of unemployment benefits.[11])

How then shall one describe the free exercise "test" as modified and applied in *Sherbert v. Verner*? In what other environments may it apply, and especially its in-

---

10. Nor of course is this analysis of the case necessarily a proper one, is it? (E.g., if the unemployment compensation law is otherwise valid, then even granted that the Sunday closing law has the effect of reducing the hazard of one possible kind of hardship for some religionists which is not equally reduced for all other religionists, namely those in Ms. Sherbert's position, that may simply be an implicit consequence of the closing law as such—a consequence already sustained in the Court's own decisions in *McGowan* and in *Braunfield*; by itself it establishes no objection to the unemployment compensation law either on its face or as applied.) *Sherbert* may in fact represent an unusual extension of the free exercise clause in requiring payments facilitating religiously-motivated acts.

11. See Frazee v. Illinois Dept. of Employment Security, 489 U.S. 829 (1989) (*Sunday* observer refused retail clerk position because it required Sunday work, *Sherbert* applied to require the state to treat the claimant as eligible for unemployment compensation); Hobbie v. Unemployment Comm'n of Florida, 480 U.S. 136 (1987) (convert to Seventh Day Adventist discharged after refusing to work on Saturdays, *Sherbert* applied to require state payment of unemployment compensation) (Rehnquist, J., dissenting); Thomas v. Review Bd. of Ind. Employment Sec. Div., 450 U.S. 707 (1981) (*Sherbert* applied to require unemployment compensation payments to religious person who quit for religious reasons not involving the day, but rather when he learned the steel production in which he was engaged was for armaments, Court held that unemployment compensation must nonetheless be paid, Rehnquist dissenting—and noting evident inconsistency with prior establishment clause cases which would, absent the *Sherbert* decision, forbid a state from doing that which the Court says the free exercise clause requires).

volvement of the affirmative payment of tax funds, in order that one's free exercise of religion not be accompanied by personal financial loss?[12] Is *Everson* itself such a case? (If not, why not?)

GOLDMAN v. WEINBERGER

475 U.S. 503 (1986)

JUSTICE REHNQUIST delivered the opinion of the Court.

Petitioner S. Simcha Goldman contends that the Free Exercise Clause of the First Amendment to the United States Constitution permits him to wear a yarmulke while in uniform, notwithstanding an Air Force regulation mandating uniform dress for Air Force personnel. The District Court for the District of Columbia permanently enjoined the Air Force from enforcing its regulation against petitioner and from penalizing him for wearing his yarmulke. The Court of Appeals for the District of Columbia Circuit reversed on the ground that the Air Force's strong interest in discipline justified the strict enforcement of its uniform dress requirements. We granted certiorari because of the importance of the question, and now affirm.

Petitioner Goldman is an Orthodox Jew and ordained rabbi. In 1973, he was accepted into the Armed Forces Health Professions Scholarship Program and placed on inactive reserve status in the Air Force while he studied clinical psychology at Loyola University of Chicago. During his three years in the scholarship program, he received a monthly stipend and an allowance for tuition, books, and fees. After completing his Ph.D. in psychology, petitioner entered active service in the United States Air Force as a commissioned officer, in accordance with a requirement that participants in the scholarship program serve one year of active duty for each year of subsidized education. Petitioner was stationed at March Air Force Base in Riverside, California, and served as a clinical psychologist at the mental health clinic on the base.

Until 1981, petitioner was not prevented from wearing his yarmulke on the base. He avoided controversy by remaining close to his duty station in the health clinic and by wearing his service cap over the yarmulke when out of doors. But in April 1981, after he testified as a defense witness at a court-martial wearing his yarmulke but not his service cap, opposing counsel lodged a complaint with Colonel Joseph Gregory, the Hospital Commander, arguing that petitioner's practice of wearing his yarmulke

---

12. The Court subsequently rejected most free exercise claims premised on the *Sherbert* "test" outside the immediate subject area of unemployment compensation—either by finding the "burden" on religion insufficient to trigger the *Sherbert* "test," or by finding the government interests sufficiently compelling to pass the test. See Kenneth Karst, Religious Freedom and Equal Citizenship: Reflections on *Lukumi*, 69 Tulane L.Rev. 335, 337 (1994); and see Justice Scalia's opinion in *Employment Division v. Smith*, 494 U.S. 872 (1990) ("In recent years we have abstained from applying the *Sherbert* test outside the employment compensation field at all.").

was a violation of Air Force Regulation (AFR) 35-10. This regulation states in pertinent part that "[h]eadgear will not be worn [w]hile indoors except by armed security police in the performance of their duties." Petitioner argues that AFR 35-10, as applied to him, prohibits religiously motivated conduct and should therefore be analyzed under the standard enunciated in Sherbert v. Verner, 374 U.S. 398 (1963).

Our review of military regulations challenged on First Amendment grounds is far more deferential than constitutional review of similar laws or regulations designed for civilian society. The military need not encourage debate or tolerate protest to the extent that such tolerance is required of the civilian state by the First Amendment; to accomplish its mission the military must foster instinctive obedience, unity, commitment, and esprit de corps.

The considered professional judgment of the Air Force is that the traditional outfitting of personnel in standardized uniforms encourages the subordination of personal preferences and identities in favor of the overall group mission. Uniforms encourage a sense of hierarchical unity by tending to eliminate outward individual distinctions except for those of rank. The Air Force considers them as vital during peacetime as during war because its personnel must be ready to provide an effective defense on a moment's notice; the necessary habits of discipline and unity must be developed in advance of trouble. We have acknowledged that "[t]he inescapable demands of military discipline and obedience to orders cannot be taught on battlefields; the habit of immediate compliance with military procedures and orders must be virtually reflex with no time for debate or reflection." ***

Petitioner Goldman contends that the Free Exercise Clause of the First Amendment requires the Air Force to make an exception to its uniform dress requirements for religious apparel unless the accoutrements create a "clear danger" of undermining discipline and esprit de corps. He asserts that in general, visible but "unobtrusive" apparel will not create such a danger and must therefore be accommodated. He argues that the Air Force failed to prove that a specific exception for his practice of wearing an unobtrusive yarmulke would threaten discipline. He contends that the Air Force's assertion to the contrary is mere *ipse dixit*, with no support from actual experience or a scientific study in the record, and is contradicted by expert testimony that religious exceptions to AFR 35-10 are in fact desirable and will increase morale by making the Air Force a more humane place.

But whether or not expert witnesses may feel that religious exceptions to AFR 35-10 are desirable is quite beside the point. The desirability of dress regulations in the military is decided by the appropriate military officials, and they are under no constitutional mandate to abandon their considered professional judgment. Quite obviously, to the extent the regulations do not permit the wearing of religious apparel such as a yarmulke, a practice described by petitioner as silent devotion akin to prayer, military life may be more objectionable for petitioner and probably others. But the First Amendment does not require the military to accommodate such practices in the face of its view that they would detract from the uniformity sought by the dress regulations. The Air Force has drawn the line essentially between religious apparel which is visible and that which is not, and we hold that those portions of the regulations challenged here reasonably and evenhandedly regulate dress in the interest of the military's perceived need for uniformity. The First Amendment therefore does not prohibit them from being applied to petitioner even though their effect is to restrict the wearing of the headgear required by his religious beliefs.

The judgment of the Court of Appeals is [a]ffirmed.

JUSTICE STEVENS, with whom JUSTICE WHITE and JUSTICE POWELL join, concurring.

Captain Goldman presents an especially attractive case for an exception from the uniform regulations that are applicable to all other Air Force personnel. His devotion to his faith is readily apparent. The yarmulke is a familiar and accepted sight. In addition to its religious significance for the wearer, the yarmulke may evoke the deepest respect and admiration—the symbol of a distinguished tradition and an eloquent rebuke to the ugliness of anti-Semitism.[3] Captain Goldman's military duties are performed in a setting in which a modest departure from the uniform regulation creates almost no danger of impairment of the Air Force's military mission. Moreover, on the record before us, there is reason to believe that the policy of strict enforcement against Captain Goldman had a retaliatory motive—he had worn his yarmulke while testifying on behalf of a defendant in a court-martial proceeding. Nevertheless, as the case has been argued,[5] I believe we must test the validity of the Air Force's rule not merely as it applies to Captain Goldman but also as it applies to all service personnel who have sincere religious beliefs that may conflict with one or more military commands.

JUSTICE BRENNAN is unmoved by the Government's concern "that while a yarmulke might not seem obtrusive to a Jew, neither does a turban to a Sikh, a saffron robe to a Satchidananda Ashram-Integral Yogi, nor do dreadlocks to a Rastafarian." He correctly points out that "turbans, saffron robes, and dreadlocks are not before us in this case," and then suggests that other cases may be fairly decided by reference to a reasonable standard based on "functional utility, health and safety considerations, and the goal of a polished, professional appearance." As the Court

---

3. Cf. N. Belth, A Promise to Keep (1979) (recounting history of anti-Semitism in the United States). The history of intolerance in our own country can be glimpsed by reviewing Justice Story's observation that the purpose of the First Amendment was "not to countenance, much less to advance Mahometanism, or Judaism, or infidelity, by prostrating Christianity; but to exclude all rivalry among Christian sects," 2 J. Story, Commentaries on the Constitution of the United States § 1877, p. 594 (1851)—a view that the Court has, of course, explicitly rejected. See Wallace v. Jaffree, 472 U.S. 38, 52-55 (1985).

5. Captain Goldman has mounted a broad challenge to the prohibition on visible religious wear as it applies to yarmulkes. He has not argued the far narrower ground that, even if the general prohibition is valid, its application in his case was retaliatory and impermissible. ***

has explained, this approach attaches no weight to the separate interest in uniformity itself. Because professionals in the military service attach great importance to that plausible interest, it is one that we must recognize as legitimate and rational even though personal experience or admiration for the performance of the "rag-tag band of soldiers" that won us our freedom in the revolutionary war might persuade us that the Government has exaggerated the importance of that interest.

The interest in uniformity, however, has a dimension that is of still greater importance for me. It is the interest in uniform treatment for the members of all religious faiths. The very strength of Captain Goldman's claim creates the danger that a similar claim on behalf of a Sikh or a Rastafarian might readily be dismissed as "so extreme, so unusual, or so faddish an image that public confidence in his ability to perform his duties will be destroyed." If exceptions from dress code regulations are to be granted on the basis of a multifactored test such as that proposed by JUSTICE BRENNAN, inevitably the decisionmaker's evaluation of the character and the sincerity of the requestor's faith—as well as the probable reaction of the majority to the favored treatment of a member of that faith—will play a critical part in the decision. For the difference between a turban or a dreadlock on the one hand, and a yarmulke on the other, is not merely a difference in "appearance"—it is also the difference between a Sikh or a Rastafarian, on the one hand, and an Orthodox Jew on the other.

As the Court demonstrates, the rule that is challenged in this case is based on a neutral, completely objective standard—visibility. It was not motivated by hostility against, or any special respect for, any religious faith. An exception for yarmulkes would represent a fundamental departure from the true principle of uniformity that supports that rule. For that reason, I join the Court's opinion and its judgment.

JUSTICE BRENNAN, with whom JUSTICE MARSHALL joins, dissenting.

Simcha Goldman invokes this Court's protection of his First Amendment right to fulfill one of the traditional religious obligations of a male Orthodox Jew—to cover his head before an omnipresent God. *** If Dr. Goldman wanted to wear a hat to keep his head warm or to cover a bald spot I would join the majority. Mere personal preferences in dress are not constitutionally protected. The First Amendment, however, restrains the Government's ability to prevent an Orthodox Jewish serviceman from, or punish him for, wearing a yarmulke. *** When a military service burdens the free exercise rights of its members in the name of necessity, it must provide, as an initial matter and at a minimum, a credible explanation of how the contested practice is likely to interfere with the proffered military interest.[2] Unabashed *ipse dixit* cannot outweigh a constitutional right. ***

---

2. I continue to believe that Government restraints on First Amendment rights, including limitations placed on military personnel, may be justified only upon showing a compelling state interest which is precisely furthered by a narrowly tailored regulation. See, e.g., Brown v. Glines, 444 U.S. 348, 367 (1980) (BRENNAN, J., dissenting). I think that any special needs of the military can be accommodated

The contention that the discipline of the armed forces will be subverted if Orthodox Jews are allowed to wear yarmulkes with their uniforms surpasses belief. It lacks support in the record of this case and the Air Force offers no basis for it as a general proposition. While the perilous slope permits the services arbitrarily to refuse exceptions requested to satisfy mere personal preferences, before the Air Force may burden free exercise rights it must advance, at the *very least*, a rational reason for doing so. Furthermore, the Air Force cannot logically defend the content of its rule by insisting that discipline depends upon absolute adherence to whatever rule is established. If, as General Usher admitted at trial, the dress code codified religious exemptions from the "no-headgear-indoors" regulation, then the wearing of a yarmulke would be sanctioned by the code and could not be considered an unauthorized deviation from the rules.

The Government also argues that the services have an important interest in uniform dress, because such dress establishes the preeminence of group identity, thus fostering esprit de corps and loyalty to the service that transcends individual bonds. In its brief, the Government characterizes the yarmulke as an assertion of individuality and as a badge of religious and ethnic identity, strongly suggesting that, as such, it could drive a wedge of divisiveness between members of the services.

I find totally implausible the suggestion that the overarching group identity of the Air Force would be threatened if Orthodox Jews were allowed to wear yarmulkes with their uniforms. To the contrary, a yarmulke worn with a United States military uniform is an eloquent reminder that the shared and proud identity of United States serviceman embraces and unites religious and ethnic pluralism.

The Government dangles before the Court a classic parade of horribles, the specter of a brightly-colored, "rag-tag band of soldiers." Although turbans, saffron robes, and dreadlocks are not before us in this case and must each be evaluated against the reasons a service branch offers for prohibiting personnel from wearing them while in uniform, a reviewing court could legitimately give deference to dress and grooming rules that have a *reasoned* basis in, for example, functional utility, health and safety considerations, and the goal of a polished, professional appearance.[4]

Furthermore, contrary to its intimations, the Air Force has available to it a familiar standard for determining whether a particular style of yarmulke is consistent with a polished, professional military appearance—the "neat and conservative" standard by which the service judges jewelry. No rational reason exists why yarmulkes cannot be judged by the same criterion. Indeed, at argument Dr. Goldman declared

---

in the compelling interest prong of the test. My point here is simply that even under a more deferential test Dr. Goldman should prevail. ***

4. For example, the Air Force could no doubt justify regulations ordering troops to wear uniforms, prohibiting garments that could become entangled in machinery, and requiring hair to be worn short so that it may not be grabbed in combat and may be kept louse-free in field conditions.

himself willing to wear whatever style and color yarmulke the Air Force believes best comports with its uniform. ***

Department of Defense Directive 1300.17 (June 18, 1985) grants commanding officers the discretion to permit service personnel to wear religious items and apparel that are not visible with the uniform, such as crosses, temple garments, and scapulars. JUSTICE STEVENS favors this "visibility test" because he believes that it does not involve the Air Force in drawing distinctions among faiths. He rejects functional utility, health, and safety considerations, and similar grounds as criteria for religious exceptions to the dress code, because he fears that these standards will allow some servicepersons to satisfy their religious dress and grooming obligations, while preventing others from fulfilling theirs. But, the visible/not visible standard has that same effect. Furthermore, it restricts the free exercise rights of a larger number of service persons. The visibility test permits only individuals whose outer garments and grooming are indistinguishable from those of mainstream Christians to fulfill their religious duties. In my view, the Constitution requires the selection of criteria that permit the greatest possible number of persons to practice their faiths freely.

The Court and the military services have presented patriotic Orthodox Jews with a painful dilemma—the choice between fulfilling a religious obligation and serving their country. Should the draft be reinstated, compulsion will replace choice. Although the pain the services inflict on Orthodox Jewish servicemen is clearly the result of insensitivity rather than design, it is unworthy of our military because it is unnecessary. The Court and the military have refused these servicemen their constitutional rights; we must hope that Congress will correct this wrong.

JUSTICE BLACKMUN, dissenting. [Omitted.]

JUSTICE O'CONNOR, with whom JUSTICE MARSHALL joins, dissenting.

* * *

Like the Court today in this case involving the military, the Court in the past has had some difficulty, even in the civilian context, in articulating a clear standard for evaluating free exercise claims that result from the application of general state laws burdening religious conduct. In Sherbert v. Verner, 374 U.S. 398 (1963), and Thomas v. Review Board, 450 U.S. 707 (1981), the Court required the States to demonstrate that their challenged policies were "the least restrictive means of achieving some compelling state interest" in order to deprive claimants of unemployment benefits when the refusal to work was based on sincere religious beliefs. In Wisconsin v. Yoder, 406 U.S. 205, 215, (1972), the Court noted that "only those interests of the highest order and those not otherwise served can overbalance legitimate claims to the free exercise of religion" in deciding that the Amish were exempt from a State's requirement that children attend school through the age of 16. ***

These tests, though similar, are not identical. One can, however, glean at least two consistent themes from this Court's precedents. First, when the government attempts to deny a Free Exercise claim, it must show that an unusually important interest is at stake, whether that interest is denominated "compelling," "of the highest order," or "overriding." Second, the government must show that granting the requested exemption will do substantial harm to that interest, whether by showing that the means adopted is the "least restrictive" or "essential," or that the interest will not "otherwise be served." These two requirements are entirely sensible in the context of the assertion of a free exercise claim. *** There is no reason why these general principles should not apply in the military, as well as the civilian, context.

The first question that the Court should face here, therefore, is whether the interest that the Government asserts against the religiously based claim of the individual is of unusual importance. It is perfectly appropriate at this of the analysis to take account of the special role of the military. The mission of our armed services is to protect our Nation from those who would destroy all our freedoms. The need for military discipline and esprit de corps is unquestionably an especially important governmental interest. *** Nonetheless, as JUSTICE BRENNAN persuasively argues, the Government can present no sufficiently convincing proof in this case to support an assertion that granting an exemption of the type requested here would do substantial harm to military discipline and esprit de corps.

First, the Government's asserted need for absolute uniformity is contradicted by the Government's own exceptions to its rule. As JUSTICE BRENNAN notes, an Air Force dress code in force at the time of Captain Goldman's service states:

> "Neither the Air Force nor the public expects absolute uniformity of appearance. Each member has the right, within limits, to express individuality through his or her appearance. However, the image of a disciplined service member who can be relied on to do his or her job excludes the extreme, the unusual, and the fad." AFR 35-10, P 1-12.a.(2) (1978).

Furthermore, the Government does not assert, and could not plausibly argue, that petitioner's decision to wear his yarmulke while indoors at the hospital presents a threat to health or safety. And finally, the District Court found as fact that in this particular case, far from creating discontent or indiscipline in the hospital where Captain Goldman worked, "[f]rom September 1977 to May 7, 1981, *no objection* was raised to Goldman's wearing of his yarmulke while in uniform."

In the rare instances where the military has not consistently or plausibly justified its asserted need for rigidity of enforcement, and where the individual seeking the exemption establishes that the assertion by the military of a threat to discipline or esprit de corps is in his or her case completely unfounded, I would hold that the Government's policy of uniformity must yield to the individual's assertion of the right of free exercise of religion. *** Napoleon may have been correct to assert that, in the military sphere, morale is to all other factors as three is to one, but contradicted assertions of necessity by the military do not on the scales of justice bear a similarly disproportionate weight to sincere religious beliefs of the individual.

I respectfully dissent.*

LYNG v. NORTHWEST INDIAN CEMETERY PROTECTIVE ASSOCIATION
485 U.S. 439 (1988)

JUSTICE O'CONNOR delivered the opinion of the Court.

This case requires us to consider whether the First Amendment's Free Exercise Clause forbids the Government from permitting timber harvesting in, or constructing a road through, a portion of a National Forest that has traditionally been used for religious purposes by members of three American Indian tribes in northwestern California. We conclude that it does not.

I

As part of a project to create a paved 75-mile road linking two California towns, Gasquet and Orleans, the United States Forest Service has upgraded 49 miles of previously unpaved roads on federal land. In order to complete this project, the Forest Service must build a 6-mile paved segment through the Chimney Rock section of the Six Rivers National Forest. That section of the forest is situated between two other portions of the road that are already complete.

In 1977, the Forest Service issued a draft environmental impact statement that discussed proposals for upgrading an existing unpaved road that runs through the Chimney Rock area. In response to comments on the draft statement, the Forest Service commissioned a study of American Indian cultural and religious sites in the area. The Hoopa Valley Indian Reservation adjoins the Six Rivers National Forest, and the Chimney Rock area has historically been used for religious purposes by Yurok, Karok, and Tolowa Indians. The study concluded that constructing a road along any of the available routes "would cause serious and irreparable damage to the sacred areas which are an integral and necessary part of the belief systems and lifeway of Northwest California Indian peoples." Accordingly, the report recommended that the G-O road not be completed.

In 1982, the Forest Service decided not to adopt this recommendation, and it prepared a final environmental impact statement for construction of the road. The Regional Forester selected a route that avoided archaeological sites and was removed as far as possible from the sites used by contemporary Indians for specific spiritual activities. Alternative routes that would have avoided the Chimney Rock area altogether were rejected because they would have required the acquisition of private

---

*. **[Ed. Note.** In the wake of the *Goldman* decision, Congress enacted a statute providing that "a member of the armed forces may wear an item of religious apparel while wearing the uniform of the member's armed force." Pursuant to the new statute, items of religious apparel may be prohibited *only* if they would"interfere with the performance of the member's military duties" or if they are "not neat and conservative." See 10 U.S.C. § 774 (1988).]

land, had serious soil stability problems, and would in any event have traversed areas having ritualistic value to American Indians. At about the same time, the Forest Service adopted a management plan allowing for the harvesting of significant amounts of timber in this area of the forest. The management plan provided for one-half mile protective zones around all the religious sites identified in the report that had been commissioned in connection with the G-O road.

After a trial, the District Court issued a permanent injunction forbidding the Government from constructing the Chimney Rock section of the G-O road or putting the timber-harvesting management plan into effect. The court found that both actions would violate the Free Exercise Clause because they "would seriously damage the salient visual, aural, and environmental qualities of the high country." By a divided decision, the District Court's constitutional ruling was affirmed.

II

***

It is undisputed that the Indian respondents' beliefs are sincere and that the Government's proposed actions will have severe adverse effects on the practice of their religion. Respondents contend that the burden on their religious practices is heavy enough to violate the Free Exercise Clause unless the Government can demonstrate a compelling need to complete the G-O road or to engage in timber harvesting in the Chimney Rock area. We disagree.***

Whatever may be the exact line between unconstitutional prohibitions on the free exercise of religion and the legitimate conduct by government of its own affairs, the location of the line cannot depend on measuring the effects of a governmental action on a religious objector's spiritual development. ***

Even if we assume that we should accept the Ninth Circuit's prediction, according to which the G-O road will "virtually destroy the Indians' ability to practice their religion," the Constitution simply does not provide a principle that could justify upholding respondents' legal claims. However much we might wish that it were otherwise, government simply could not operate if it were required to satisfy every citizen's religious needs and desires. ***

Respondents attempt to stress the limits of the religious servitude that they are now seeking to impose on the Chimney Rock area of the Six Rivers National Forest. While defending an injunction against logging operations and the construction of a road, they apparently do not *at present* object to the area's being used by recreational visitors, other Indians, or forest rangers. Nothing in the principle for which they contend, however, would distinguish this case from another lawsuit in which they (or similarly situated religious objectors) might seek to exclude all human activity but their own from sacred areas of the public lands. The Indian respondents insist that "*[p]rivacy* during the power quests is required for the practitioners to maintain the purity needed for a successful journey." Similarly: "The practices conducted in the high country entail intense meditation and require the practitioner to achieve a profound awareness of the natural environment. Prayer seats are oriented so there is an unobstructed view, and the practitioner must be surrounded by *undisturbed* naturalness." No disrespect for these practices is implied when one notes that such beliefs could easily require *de facto* beneficial ownership of some rather spacious tracts of public property. Even without anticipating future cases, the diminution of the Government's property rights, and the concomitant subsidy of the Indian religion, would in this case be far from trivial: the District Court's order permanently forbade commercial timber harvesting, or the construction of a two-lane road, anywhere within an area covering a full 27 sections (i.e. more than 17,000 acres) of public land.

The Constitution does not permit government to discriminate against religions that treat particular physical sites as sacred, and a law forbidding the Indian respondents from visiting the Chimney Rock area would raise a different set of constitutional questions. Whatever rights the Indians may have to the use of the area, however, those rights do not divest the Government of its right to use what is, after all, *its* land. ***

Nothing in our opinion should be read to encourage governmental insensitivity to the religious needs of any citizen. The Government's rights to the use of its own land, for example, need not and should not discourage it from accommodating religious practices like those engaged in by the Indian respondents. Cf. *Sherbert*, 374 U.S., at 422-423 (Harlan, J., dissenting). ***

It is true that this Court has repeatedly held that indirect coercion or penalties on the free exercise of religion, not just outright prohibitions, are subject to scrutiny under the First Amendment. Thus, for example, ineligibility for unemployment benefits, based solely on a refusal to violate the Sabbath, has been analogized to a fine imposed on Sabbath worship.

This does not and cannot imply that incidental effects of government programs, which may make it more difficult to practice certain religions but which have no tendency to coerce individuals into acting contrary to their religious beliefs, require government to bring forward a compelling justification for its otherwise lawful actions. The crucial word in the constitutional text is "prohibit": [T]he Free Exercise Clause is written in terms of what the government cannot do to the individual, not in terms of what the individual can exact from the government."

Perceiving a "stress point in the longstanding conflict between two disparate cultures," the dissent attacks us for declining to "balanc[e] these competing and potentially irreconcilable interests, choosing instead to turn this difficult task over to the federal legislature." Seeing the Court as the arbiter, the dissent proposes a legal test under which it would decide which public lands are "central" or "indispensable" to which religions, and by implication which are "dispensable" or "peripheral," and would then decide which government programs are "compelling" enough to justify "infringement of those practices." We would accordingly be required to weigh the value of every religious belief and practice that is said to be threatened by any government program. Unless a "showing of 'centrality,'" is nothing but an assertion of centrality, the dissent thus offers us the prospect of this Court's holding that some sincerely held religious beliefs and practices are not "central" to certain religions, despite protestations to the contrary from the religious objectors who brought the lawsuit. In other words, the dissent's approach would require us to rule that some religious adherents misunderstand their own religious beliefs. We think such an approach cannot be squared with the Constitution or with our precedents, and that it would cast the judiciary in a role that we were never intended to play.

The decision of the court below, according to which the First Amendment precludes the Government from completing the G-O road or from permitting timber harvesting in the Chimney Rock area, is reversed. ***

JUSTICE KENNEDY took no part in the consideration or decision of this case.

JUSTICE BRENNAN, with whom JUSTICE MARSHALL and JUSTICE BLACKMUN join, dissenting.

* * *

I cannot accept the Court's premise that the form of the Government's restraint on religious practice, rather than its effect, controls our constitutional analysis. Respondents here have demonstrated that construction of the G-O road will completely frustrate the practice of their religion, for as the lower courts found, the proposed logging and construction activities will virtually destroy respondents' religion, and will therefore necessarily force them into abandoning those practices altogether. Indeed, the Government's proposed activities will restrain religious practice to a far greater degree here than in any of the cases cited by the Court today. None of the religious adherents in *Hobbie*, *Thomas*, and *Sherbert*, for example, claimed or could have claimed that the denial of unemployment benefits rendered the practice of their religions impossible; at most, the challenged laws made those practices more expensive. Here, in stark contrast, respondents have claimed—and proved—that the desecration of the high country will prevent religious leaders from attaining the religious power or medicine indispensable to the success of virtually all their rituals and ceremonies. [S]uch a showing, no less than those made out in *Hobbie, Thomas, Sherbert*, and *Yoder*, entitles them to the protections of the Free Exercise Clause.

In the final analysis, the Court's refusal to recognize the constitutional dimension of respondents' injuries stems from its concern that acceptance of respondents' claim could potentially strip the Government of its ability to manage and use vast tracts of federal property. In addition, the nature of respondents' site-specific religious practices raises the specter of future suits in which Native Americans seek to exclude all human activity from such areas. These concededly legitimate concerns lie at the very heart of this case, which represents yet another stress point in the longstanding conflict between two disparate cultures—the dominant western culture, which views land in terms of ownership and use, and that of Native Americans, in which concepts of private property are not only alien, but contrary to a belief system that holds land sacred. Rather than address this conflict in any meaningful fashion, however, the Court disclaims all responsibility for balancing these competing and potentially irreconcilable interests, choosing instead to turn this difficult task over to the Federal Legislature. Such an abdication is more than merely indefensible as an institutional matter: by defining respondents' injury as "nonconstitutional," the Court has effectively bestowed on one party to this conflict the unilateral authority to resolve all future disputes in its favor, subject only to the Court's toothless exhortation to be "sensitive" to affected religions. In my view, however, Native Americans deserve—and the Constitution demands—more than this. ***

JIMMY SWAGGART MINISTRIES v. BOARD OF EQUALIZATION OF CALIFORNIA

493 U. S. 378 (1990)

JUSTICE O'CONNOR delivered the opinion of the Court.

This case presents the question whether the Religion Clauses of the First Amendment prohibit a State from imposing a generally applicable sales and use tax on the distribution of religious materials by a religious organization.

I

California's Sales and Use Tax Law requires retailers to pay a sales tax "[f]or the privilege of selling tangible personal property at retail." *** The use tax, as a complement to the sales tax, reaches out-of-state purchases by residents of the State. It is "imposed on the storage, use, or other consumption in this state of tangible personal property purchased from any retailer," at the same rate as the sales tax (6 percent). Although the use tax is imposed on the purchaser, it is generally collected by the retailer at the time the sale is made. Neither the State Constitution nor the State Sales and Use Tax Law exempts religious organizations from the sales and use tax, apart from a limited exemption for the serving of meals by religious organizations.

From 1974 to 1981, appellant conducted numerous "evangelistic crusades" in auditoriums and arenas across the country in cooperation with local churches. During this period, appellant held 23 crusades in California—each lasting one to three days, with one crusade lasting six days—for a total of 52 days. At the crusades, appellant conducted religious services that included preaching and singing. Some of these services were recorded for later sale or broadcast. Appellant also sold religious books, tapes, records, and other religious and nonreligious merchandise at the crusades.

Appellant also published a monthly magazine, "The Evangelist," which was sold nationwide by subscription. The magazine contained articles of a religious nature as well as advertisements for appellant's religious books, tapes, and records. The magazine included an order form listing the various items for sale in the particular issue and their unit price, with spaces for purchasers to fill in the quantity desired and the total price.

Based on the sales figures for appellant's religious materials, the Board notified appellant that it owed sales and use taxes of $118,294.54, plus interest of $36,021.11, and a penalty of $11,829.45, for a total amount due of $ 166,145.10. Appellant did not contest the Board's assessment of tax liability for the sale and use of certain nonreligious merchandise, including such items as "T-shirts with JSM logo, mugs, bowls, plates, replicas of crown of thorns, ark of the covenant, Roman coin, candlesticks, Bible stand, pen and pencil sets, prints of religious scenes, bud vase, and communion cups." *** The trial court entered judgment for the Board, ruling that appellant was not entitled to a refund of any tax. The California Court of Appeal affirmed, and the California Supreme Court denied discretionary review. We noted probable jurisdiction and now affirm.

II

Appellant challenges the sales and use tax law under both the Free Exercise and Establishment Clauses.**

A

*** Our cases have established that "[t]he free exercise inquiry asks whether government has placed a substantial burden on the observation of a central religious belief or practice and, if so, whether a compelling governmental interest justifies the burden."

Appellant relies almost exclusively on our decisions in Murdock v. Pennsylvania, 319 U.S. 105 (1943), and Follett v. McCormick, 321 U.S. 573, 576 (1944).***

We reject appellant's expansive reading of *Murdock* and *Follett* as contrary to the decisions themselves. In *Murdock*, we considered the constitutionality of a city ordinance requiring all persons canvassing or soliciting within the city to procure a license by paying a flat fee.

*** Our decisions in these cases, resulted from the particular nature of the challenged taxes—flat license taxes that operated as a prior restraint on the exercise of religious liberty. In *Murdock*, for instance, we emphasized that the tax at issue was "a license tax—a flat tax imposed on the exercise of a privilege granted by the Bill of Rights," and cautioned that "[w]e do not mean to say that religious groups and the press are free from all financial burdens of government. We have here something quite different, for example, from a tax on the income of one who engages in religious activities or a tax on property used or employed in connection with those activities." In *Follett*, we reiterated that a preacher is not "free from all financial

---

. **[Ed. Note. The Court rejected an establishment clause claim in a separate part of its opinion, applying the *Lemon* test. (It found that neither the purpose nor the primary effect of the uniform 6% sales tax was to aid or to hinder religion; and neither did compliance with the reporting requirements of the law "excessively entangle" the state in the operations of the Swaggart Ministries.)]

burdens of government, including taxes on income or property" and, "like other citizens, may be subject to general taxation."

Significantly, we noted in both cases that a primary vice of the ordinances at issue was that they operated as prior restraints of constitutionally protected conduct. Our concern in *Murdock* and *Follett*—that a flat license tax would act as a precondition to the free exercise of religious beliefs—is simply not present where a tax applies to all sales and uses of tangible personal property in the State.

California's generally applicable sales and use tax is not a flat tax, represents only a small fraction of any retail sale, and applies neutrally to all retail sales of tangible personal property made in California. California imposes its sales and use tax even if the seller or the purchaser is charitable, religious, nonprofit, or state or local governmental in nature. Thus, the sales and use tax is not a tax on the right to disseminate religious information, ideas, or beliefs *per se*; rather, it is a tax on the privilege of making retail sales of tangible personal property and on the storage, use, or other consumption of tangible personal property in California. For example, California treats the sale of a bible by a religious organization just as it would treat the sale of a bible by a bookstore; as long as both are in-state retail sales of tangible personal property, they are both subject to the tax regardless of the motivation for the sale or the purchase. There is no danger that appellant's religious activity is being singled out for special and burdensome treatment. ***

Finally, because appellant's religious beliefs do not forbid payment of the sales and use tax, appellant's reliance on Sherbert v. Verner, 374 U.S. 398 (1963), and its progeny is misplaced, because in no sense has the State "'condition[ed] receipt of an important benefit upon conduct proscribed by a religious faith, or denie[d] such a benefit because of conduct mandated by religious belief, thereby putting substantial pressure on an adherent to modify his behavior and to violate his beliefs.'" Appellant has never alleged that the mere act of paying the tax, by itself, violates its sincere religious beliefs.

Although it is of course possible to imagine that a more onerous tax rate, even if generally applicable, might effectively choke off an adherent's religious practices, cf. *Murdock*, [319 U.S.], at 115 (the burden of a flat tax could render itinerant evangelism "crushed and closed out by the sheer weight of the toll or tribute which is exacted town by town"), we face no such situation in this case. Accordingly, we intimate no views as to whether such a generally applicable tax might violate the Free Exercise Clause. The judgment of the California Court of Appeal is affirmed.

EMPLOYMENT DIVISION, DEPARTMENT OF HUMAN RESOURCES OF OREGON v. SMITH

494 U.S. 872 (1990)

MR. JUSTICE SCALIA delivered the opinion of the Court in which REHNQUIST, C.J., and WHITE, STEVENS, and KENNEDY, JJ., joined.

This case requires us to decide whether the Free Exercise Clause of the First Amendment permits the State of Oregon to include religiously inspired peyote use within the reach of its general criminal prohibition on use of that drug, and thus permits the State to deny unemployment benefits to persons dismissed from their jobs because of such religiously inspired use. ***

The free exercise of religion means, first and foremost, the right to believe and profess whatever religious doctrine one desires. Thus, the First Amendment obviously excludes all "governmental regulation of religious beliefs as such." Sherbert v. Verner. *** But the "exercise of religion" often involves not only belief and profession but the performance of (or abstention from) physical acts: assembling with others for a worship service, participating in sacramental use of bread and wine, proselytizing, abstaining from certain foods or certain modes of transportation. It would be true, we think (though no case of ours has involved the point), that a State would be "prohibiting the free exercise [of religion]" if it sought to ban such acts or abstentions only when they are engaged in for religious reasons, or only because of the religious belief that they display. It would doubtless be unconstitutional, for example, to ban the casting of "statues that are to be used for worship purposes," or to prohibit bowing down before a golden calf.

Respondents in the present case, however, seek to carry the meaning of "prohibiting the free exercise [of religion]" one large step further. They contend that their religious motivation for using peyote places them beyond the reach of a criminal law that is not specifically directed at their religious practice, and that is concededly constitutional as applied to those who use the drug for other reasons. They assert, in other words, that "prohibiting the free exercise [of religion]" includes requiring any individual to observe a generally applicable law that requires (or forbids) the performance of an act that his religious belief forbids (or requires). As a textual matter, we do not think the words must be given that meaning. It is no more necessary to regard the collection of a general tax, for example, as "prohibiting the free exercise [of religion]" by those citizens who believe support of organized government to be sinful, than it is to regard the same tax as "abridging the freedom of the press" of those publishing companies that must pay the tax as a condition of staying in business. It is a permissible reading of the text, in the one case as in the other, to say that if prohibiting the exercise of religion (or burdening the activity of printing) is not the object of the tax but merely the incidental effect of a generally applicable and otherwise valid provision, the First Amendment has not been offended.

Our decisions reveal that the latter reading is the correct one. We have never held that an individual's religious beliefs excuse him from compliance with an otherwise valid law prohibiting conduct that the State is free to regulate. On the contrary, the record of more than a century of our free exercise jurisprudence contradicts that proposition. *** We first had occasion to assert that principle in Reynolds v. United States, 98 U.S. 145 (1879), where we rejected the claim that criminal laws against polygamy could not be constitutionally applied to those whose religion commanded the practice. "Laws," we said, "are made for the government of actions, and while they cannot interfere with mere religious belief and opinions, they may with practices. Can a man excuse his practices to the contrary because of his religious belief? To permit this would be to make the professed doctrines of religious belief superior to the law of the land, and in effect to permit every citizen to become a law unto himself."

*** The only decisions in which we have held that the First Amendment bars application of a neutral, generally applicable law to religiously motivated action have involved not the Free Exercise Clause alone, but the Free Exercise Clause in conjunction with other constitutional protections, such as freedom of speech and of the press, see Cantwell v. Connecticut, 310 U.S. at 304-307, or the right of parents, acknowledged in Pierce v. Society of Sisters, 268 U.S. 510 (1925), to direct the education of their children, see Wisconsin v. Yoder, 406 U.S. 205 (1972) (invalidating compulsory school-attendance laws as applied to Amish parents who refused on religious grounds to send their children to school).[2]

The present case does not present such a hybrid situation, but a free exercise claim unconnected with any communicative activity or parental right. Respondents urge us to hold, quite simply, that when otherwise prohibitable conduct is accompanied by religious convictions, not only the convictions but the conduct itself must be free from governmental regulation. We have never held that, and decline to do so now. There being no contention that Oregon's drug law represents an attempt to regulate religious beliefs, the communication of religious beliefs, or the raising of one's children in those beliefs, the rule to which we have adhered ever since *Reynolds* plainly controls. ***

Respondents argue that even though exemption from generally applicable criminal laws need not automatically be extended to religiously motivated actors, at least the claim for a religious exemption must be evaluated under the balancing test set forth in Sherbert v. Verner, 374 U.S. 398 (1963). *** In recent years we have abstained from applying the *Sherbert* test (outside the unemployment compensation field) at all. ***

Even if we were inclined to breathe into *Sherbert* some life beyond the unemployment compensation field, we would not apply it to require exemptions from a generally applicable criminal law. The *Sherbert* test, it must be recalled, was developed in a context that lent itself to individualized governmental assessment of the reasons for the relevant conduct. As a plurality of the Court noted in [Bowen v. Roy, 476 U.S. 693 (1986)], a distinctive feature of unemployment compensation programs

---

2. *** *Yoder* said that "the Court's holding in *Pierce* stands as a charter of the rights of parents to direct the religious upbringing of their children. And, when the interests of parenthood are combined with a free exercise claim of the nature revealed by this record, more than merely a 'reasonable relation to some purpose within the competency of the State' is required to sustain the validity of the State's requirement under the First Amendment."

is that their eligibility criteria invite consideration of the particular circumstances behind an applicant's unemployment: "The statutory conditions [in *Sherbert* and *Thomas*] provided that a person was not eligible for unemployment compensation benefits if, 'without good cause,' he had quit work or refused available work. The 'good cause' standard created a mechanism for individualized exemptions."

Whether or not the decisions are that limited, they at least have nothing to do with an across-the-board criminal prohibition on a particular form of conduct. We conclude today that the sounder approach, and the approach in accord with the vast majority of our precedents, is to hold the test inapplicable to such challenges. The government's ability to enforce generally applicable prohibitions of socially harmful conduct, like its ability to carry out other aspects of public policy, "cannot depend on measuring the effects of a governmental action on a religious objector's spiritual development." *Lyng*, [485 U.S.,] at 451. To make an individual's obligation to obey such a law contingent upon the law's coincidence with his religious beliefs, except where the State's interest is "compelling"—permitting him, by virtue of his beliefs, "to become a law unto himself," Reynolds v. United States, 98 U.S., at 167—contradicts both constitutional tradition and common sense.

The "compelling government interest" requirement seems benign, because it is familiar from other fields. But using it as the standard that must be met before the government may accord different treatment on the basis of race, see, *e.g.*, Palmore v. Sidoti, 466 U.S. 429, 432 (1984), or before the government may regulate the content of speech, see, *e.g.*, Sable Communications of California v. FCC, 492 U.S. 115, 126 (1989), is not remotely comparable to using it for the purpose asserted here. What it produces in those other fields—equality of treatment, and an unrestricted flow of contending speech—are constitutional norms; what it would produce here—a private right to ignore generally applicable laws—is a constitutional anomaly.[3]

Nor is it possible to limit the impact of respondents' proposal by requiring a "compelling state interest" only when the conduct prohibited is "central" to the individual's religion. Cf. *Lyng v. Northwest Indian Cemetery Protective Assn.* (BRENNAN, J., dissenting). It is no more appropriate for judges to determine the

---

3. [JUSTICE O'CONNOR] suggests that "[t]here is nothing talismanic about neutral laws of general applicability," and that all laws burdening religious practices should be subject to compelling-interest scrutiny because "the First Amendment unequivocally makes freedom of religion, like freedom from race discrimination and freedom of speech, a 'constitutional norm,' not an 'anomaly.'" But this comparison with other fields supports, rather than undermines, the conclusion we draw today. Just as we subject to the most exacting scrutiny laws that make classifications based on race, see *Palmore v. Sidoti*, 466 U.S. 429 (1984), or on the content of speech, see *Sable Communications*, 492 U.S. 115 (1989), so too we strictly scrutinize governmental classifications based on religion, see McDaniel v. Paty, 435 U.S. 618 (1978); see also Torcaso v. Watkins, 367 U.S. 488 (1961). But we have held that race-neutral laws that have the *effect* of disproportionately disadvantaging a particular racial group do not thereby become subject to compelling-interest analysis under the Equal Protection Clause, see Washington v. Davis, 426 U.S. 229 (1976) (police employment examination); and we have held that generally applicable laws unconcerned with regulating speech that have the *effect* of interfering with speech do not thereby become subject to compelling-interest analysis under the First Amendment. ***

"centrality" of religious beliefs before applying a "compelling interest" test in the free exercise field, than it would be for them to determine the "importance" of ideas before applying the "compelling interest" test in the free speech field. What principle of law or logic can be brought to bear to contradict a believer's assertion that a particular act is "central" to his personal faith? Judging the centrality of different religious practices is akin to the unacceptable "business of evaluating the relative merits of differing religious claims." United States v. Lee, 455 U.S., at 263 n.2 (STEVENS, J., concurring). ***[4]

If the "compelling interest" test is to be applied at all, then, it must be applied across the board, to all actions thought to be religiously commanded. Moreover, if "compelling interest" really means what it says (and watering it down here would subvert its rigor in the other fields where it is applied), many laws will not meet the test. Any society adopting such a system would be courting anarchy, but that danger increases in direct proportion to the society's diversity of religious beliefs, and its determination to coerce or suppress none of them. Precisely because "we are a cosmopolitan nation made up of people of almost every conceivable religious preference," Braunfield v. Brown, 366 U.S., at 606, and precisely because we value and protect that religious divergence, we cannot afford the luxury of deeming *presumptively invalid*, as applied to the religious objector, every regulation of conduct that does not protect an interest of the highest order. The rule respondents favor would open the prospect of constitutionally required religious exemptions from civic obligations of almost every conceivable kind—ranging from compulsory military service, see, *e.g.*, Gillette v. United States, 401 U.S. 437 (1971), to the payment of taxes, see, *e.g.*, *United States v. Lee,*; to health and safety regulation such as manslaughter and child neglect laws, and laws providing for equality of opportunity for the races, see, *e.g.*, Bob Jones University v. United States, 461 U.S. 574, 603-604 (1983). The First Amendment's protection of religious liberty does not require this.[5]

---

4. Nor is this difficulty avoided by JUSTICE BLACKMUN's assertion that "although *** courts should refrain from delving into questions of whether, as a matter of religious doctrine, a particular practice is 'central' to the religion, *** I do not think this means that the courts must turn a blind eye to the severe impact of a State's restrictions on the adherents of a minority religion." As JUSTICE BLACKMUN's opinion proceeds to make clear, inquiry into "severe impact" is no different from inquiry into centrality. He has merely substituted for the question "How important is X to the religious adherent?" the question "How great will be the harm to the religious adherent if X is taken away?" There is no material difference.

5. JUSTICE O'CONNOR contends that the "parade of horribles" in the text only "demonstrates *** that courts have been quite capable of strik[ing] sensible balances between religious liberty and competing state interests." *** But the cases we cite have struck "sensible balances" only because they have all applied the general laws, despite the claims for religious exemption. In any event, JUSTICE O'CONNOR mistakes the purpose of our parade: it is not to suggest that courts would necessarily permit harmful exemptions from these laws (though they might), but to suggest that courts would constantly be in the business of determining whether the "severe impact" of various laws on religious practice (to use JUSTICE BLACKMUN's terminology) or the "constitutiona[l] significan[ce]" of the "burden on the specific plaintiffs" (to use JUSTICE O'CONNOR's terminology) suffices to permit us to confer an

Values that are protected against government interference through enshrinement in the Bill of Rights are not thereby banished from the political process. Just as a society that believes in the negative protection accorded to the press by the First Amendment is likely to enact laws that affirmatively foster the dissemination of the printed word, so also a society that believes in the negative protection accorded to religious belief can be expected to be solicitous of that value in its legislation as well. It is therefore not surprising that a number of States have made an exception to their drug laws for sacramental peyote use. But to say that a nondiscriminatory religious-practice exemption is permitted, or even that it is desirable, is not to say that it is constitutionally required, and that the appropriate occasions for its creation can be discerned by the courts. It may fairly be said that leaving accommodation to the political process will place at a relative disadvantage those religious practices that are not widely engaged in; but that unavoidable consequence of democratic government must be preferred to a system in which each conscience is a law unto itself or in which judges weight the social importance of all laws against the centrality of all religious beliefs. ***

Because respondents' ingestion of peyote was prohibited under Oregon law, and because that prohibition is constitutional, Oregon may, consistent with the Free Exercise Clause, deny respondents unemployment compensation when their dismissal results from use of the drug. The decision of the Oregon Supreme Court is accordingly reversed.

JUSTICE O'CONNOR, with whom JUSTICE BRENNAN, JUSTICE MARSHALL, and JUSTICE BLACKMUN join as to Parts I and II, concurring in the judgment.

***

II

The Court today extracts from our long history of free exercise precedents the single categorical rule that "if prohibiting the exercise of religion is merely the incidental effect of a generally applicable and otherwise valid provision, the First Amendment has not been offended." Indeed, the Court holds that where the law is a generally applicable criminal prohibition, our usual free exercise jurisprudence does not even apply. To reach this sweeping result, however, the Court must not only give a strained reading of the First Amendment but must also disregard our consistent application of free exercise doctrine to cases involving generally applicable regulations that burden religious conduct.

A

The Free Exercise Clause of the First Amendment commands that "Congress shall make no law *** prohibiting the free exercise [of religion]." As the Court recognizes, however, the "free *exercise*" of religion often, if not invariably, requires

---

exemption. It is a parade of horribles because it is horrible to contemplate that federal judges will regularly balance against the importance of general laws the significance of religious practice.

the performance of (or abstention from) certain acts. Because the First Amendment does not distinguish between religious belief and religious conduct, conduct motivated by sincere religious belief, like the belief itself, must therefore be at least presumptively protected by the Free Exercise Clause.

The Court today, however, interprets the Clause to permit the government to prohibit, without justification, conduct mandated by an individual's religious beliefs, so long as that prohibition is generally applicable. But a law that prohibits certain conduct—conduct that happens to be an act of worship for someone—manifestly does prohibit that person's free exercise of his religion. A person who is barred from engaging in religiously motivated conduct is barred from freely exercising his religion. Moreover, that person is barred from freely exercising his religion regardless of whether the law prohibits the conduct only when engaged in for religious reasons, only by members of that religion, or by all persons. It is difficult to deny that a law that prohibits religiously motivated conduct, even if the law is generally applicable, does not at least implicate First Amendment concerns.

The Court responds that generally applicable laws are "one large step" removed from laws aimed at specific religious practices. The First Amendment, however, does not distinguish between laws that are generally applicable and laws that target particular religious practices. *** Our free exercise cases have all concerned generally applicable laws that had the effect of significantly burdening a religious practice. If the First Amendment is to have any vitality, it ought not be construed to cover only the extreme and hypothetical situation in which a State directly targets a religious practice. ***

To say that a person's right to free exercise has been burdened, of course, does not mean that he has an absolute right to engage in the conduct. Under our established First Amendment jurisprudence, we have recognized that the freedom to act, unlike the freedom to believe, cannot be absolute. Instead, we have respected both the First Amendment's express textual mandate and the governmental interest in regulation of conduct by requiring the Government to justify any substantial burden on religiously motivated conduct by a compelling state interest and by means narrowly tailored to achieve that interest. The compelling interest test effectuates the First Amendment's command that religious liberty is an independent liberty, that it occupies a preferred position, and that the Court will not permit encroachments upon this liberty, whether direct or indirect, unless required by clear and compelling governmental interests "of the highest order," *Yoder*, at 215. ***

B

In my view, the essence of a free exercise claim is relief from a burden imposed by government on religious practices or beliefs, whether the burden is imposed directly through laws that prohibit or compel specific religious practices, or indirectly through laws that, in effect, make abandonment of one's own religious or conformity to the religious beliefs of others the price of an equal place in the civil community.

Indeed, we have never distinguished between cases in which a State conditions receipt of a benefit on conduct prohibited by religious beliefs and cases in which a State affirmatively prohibits such conduct. The *Sherbert* compelling interest test applies in both kinds of cases. I would reaffirm that principle today: A neutral criminal law prohibiting conduct that a State may legitimately regulate is, if anything, *more* burdensome than a neutral civil statute placing legitimate conditions on the award of a state benefit.

*** Once it has been shown that a government regulation or criminal prohibition burdens the free exercise of religion, we have consistently asked the Government to demonstrate that unbending application of its regulation to the religious objector "is essential to accomplish an overriding governmental interest," or represents "the least restrictive means of achieving some compelling state interest." To me, the sounder approach—the approach more consistent with our role as judges to decide each case on its individual merits—is to apply this test in each case to determine whether the burden on the specific plaintiffs before us is constitutionally significant and whether the particular criminal interest asserted by the State before us is compelling. Even if, as an empirical matter, a government's criminal laws might usually serve a compelling interest in health, safety, or public order, the First Amendment at least requires a case- by-case determination of the question, sensitive to the facts of each particular claim. ***

Finally, the Court today suggests that the disfavoring of minority religions is an "unavoidable consequence" under our system of government and that accommodation of such religions must be left to the political process. In my view, however, the First Amendment was enacted precisely to protect the rights of those whose religious practices are not shared by the majority and may be viewed with hostility. The history of our free exercise doctrine amply demonstrates the harsh impact majoritarian rule has had on unpopular or emerging religious groups such as the Jehovah's Witnesses and the Amish. Indeed, the words of Justice Jackson in *West Virginia Board of Education v. Barnette* (overruling *Minersville School District v. Gobitis*) are apt:

> The very purpose of a Bill of Rights was to withdraw certain subjects from the vicissitudes of political controversy, to place them beyond the reach of majorities and officials and to establish them as legal principles to be applied by the courts. One's right to life, liberty, and property, to free speech, a free press, freedom of worship and assembly, and other fundamental rights may not be submitted to vote; they depend on the outcome of no elections.

III

The Court's holding today not only misreads settled First Amendment precedent; it appears to be unnecessary to this case. I would reach the same result applying our established free exercise jurisprudence.

A

There is no dispute that Oregon's criminal prohibition of peyote places a severe burden on the ability of respondents to freely exercise their religion. Peyote is a sacrament of the Native American Church and is regarded as vital to respondents' ability to practice their religion. See O. Stewart, Peyote Religion: A History 327-336 (1987); see also People v. Woody, 61 Cal. 2d 716, 721-722, 394 P. 2d 813, 817-818 (1964). ***. Under Oregon law, as construed by that State's highest court, members of the Native American Church must choose between carrying out the ritual embodying their religious beliefs and avoidance of criminal prosecution. That choice is, in my view, more than sufficient to trigger First Amendment scrutiny.

There is also no dispute that Oregon has a significant interest in enforcing laws that control the possession and use of controlled substances by its citizens. In light of our recent decisions holding that the governmental interests in the collection of income tax, *Hernandez*, 490 U.S., at 699-700, a comprehensive Social Security system, see *Lee*, 455 U.S., at 258-259, and military conscription, see *Gillette*, 401 U.S., at 460, are compelling, respondents do not seriously dispute that Oregon has a compelling interest in prohibiting the possession of peyote by its citizens.

B

Thus, the critical question in this case is whether exempting respondents from the State's general criminal prohibition "will unduly interfere with fulfillment of the governmental interest." Although the question is close, I would conclude that uniform application of Oregon's criminal prohibition is "essential to accomplish" its overriding interest in preventing the physical harm caused by the use of a Schedule I controlled substance. Oregon's criminal prohibition represents that State's judgment that the possession and use of controlled substances, even by only one person, is inherently harmful and dangerous. Because the health effects caused by the use of controlled substances exist regardless of the motivation of the user, the use of such substances, even for religious purposes, violates the very purpose of the laws that prohibit them. Moreover, in view of the societal interest in preventing trafficking in controlled substances, uniform application of the criminal prohibition at issue is essential to the effectiveness of Oregon's stated interest in preventing any possession of peyote. *** For these reasons, I believe that granting a selective exemption in this case would seriously impair Oregon's compelling interest in prohibiting possession of peyote by its citizens. Under such circumstances, the Free Exercise Clause does not require the State to accommodate respondents' religiously motivated conduct.

Respondents contend that any incompatibility is belied by the fact that the Federal Government and several States provide exemptions for the religious use of peyote. But other governments may surely choose to grant an exemption without Oregon, with its specific asserted interest in uniform application of its drug laws, being *required* to do so by the First Amendment. Respondents also note that the sacramental use of peyote is central to the tenets of the Native American Church, but I agree with the Court, that because "[i]t is not within the judicial ken to question the centrality of particular beliefs or practices to a faith," our determination of the constitutionality of Oregon's general criminal prohibition cannot, and should not, turn on the centrality of the particular religious practice at issue. ***

I would therefore adhere to our established free exercise jurisprudence and hold that the State in this case has a compelling interest in regulating peyote use by its citizens and that accommodating respondents' religiously motivated conduct "will unduly interfere with fulfillment of the governmental interest." Accordingly, I concur in the judgment of the Court.

JUSTICE BLACKMUN, with whom JUSTICE BRENNAN and JUSTICE MARSHALL join, dissenting.

*** I agree with JUSTICE O'CONNOR's analysis of the applicable free exercise doctrine, and I join [part II] of her opinion. As she points out, "the critical question in this case is whether exempting respondents from the State's general criminal prohibition 'will unduly interfere with fulfillment of the governmental interest.'" I do disagree, however, with her specific answer to that question.

I

In weighing the clear interest of respondents Smith and Black (hereinafter respondents) in the free exercise of their religion against Oregon's asserted interest in enforcing its drug laws, it is important to articulate in precise terms the state interest involved. It is not the State's broad interest in fighting the critical "war on drugs" that must be weighed against respondents' claim, but the State's narrow interest in refusing to make an exception for the religious, ceremonial use of peyote. Failure to reduce the competing interests to the same plane of generality tends to distort the weighing process in the State's favor. See Clark, Guidelines for the Free Exercise Clause, 83 Harv. L. Rev. 327, 330-331 (1969) ("The purpose of almost any law can be traced back to one or another of the fundamental concerns of government: public health and safety, public peace and order, defense, revenue. To measure an individual interest directly against one of these rarified values inevitably makes the individual interest appear the less significant").

The State's interest in enforcing its prohibition, in order to be sufficiently compelling to outweigh a free exercise claim, cannot be merely abstract or symbolic. The State cannot plausibly assert that unbending application of a criminal prohibition is essential to fulfill any compelling interest, if it does not, in fact, attempt to enforce that prohibition. In this case, the State actually has not evinced any concrete interest in enforcing its drug laws against religious users of peyote. Oregon has never sought to prosecute respondents, and does not claim that it has made significant enforcement efforts against other religious users of peyote. ***

The State proclaims an interest in protecting the health and safety of its citizens from the dangers of unlawful drugs. It offers, however, no evidence that the religious use of peyote has ever harmed anyone. *** The fact that peyote is classified as a Schedule I controlled substance does not, by itself, show that any and all uses of peyote, in any circumstance, are inherently harmful and dangerous. The Federal Government, which created the classifications of unlawful drugs from which Oregon's drug laws are derived, apparently does not find peyote so dangerous as to preclude an exemption for religious use.[5] *** The carefully circumscribed ritual context in which respondents used peyote is far removed from the irresponsible and unrestricted recreational use of unlawful drugs.[6]

Moreover, just as in *Yoder*, the values and interests of those seeking a religious exemption in this case are congruent, to a great degree, with those the State seeks to promote through its drug laws. Not only does the Church's doctrine forbid non-religious use of peyote; it also generally advocates self-reliance, familial responsibility, and abstinence from alcohol. Far from promoting the lawless and irresponsible use of drugs, Native American Church members' spiritual code exemplifies values that Oregon's drug laws are presumably intended to foster.

The State also seeks to support its refusal to make an exception for religious use of peyote by invoking its interest in abolishing drug trafficking. There is, however, practically no illegal traffic in peyote. See *Olsen*, 878 F. 2d, at 1463, 1467 (quoting DEA Final Order to the effect that total amount of peyote seized and analyzed by federal authorities between 1980 and 1987 was 19.4 pounds; in contrast, total amount of marijuana seized during that period was over 15 million pounds).

Finally, the State argues that granting an exception for religious peyote use would erode its interest in the uniform, fair, and certain enforcement of its drug laws. The State fears that, if it grants an exemption for religious peyote use, a flood of other claims to religious exemptions will follow. It would then be placed in a dilemma, it says, between allowing a patchwork of exemptions that would hinder its law enforcement efforts, and risking a violation of the Establishment Clause by arbitrarily limiting its religious exemptions. This argument, however, could be made in almost any free exercise case. See Lupu, Where Rights Begin: The Problem of Burdens on the Free Exercise of Religion, 102 Harv. L. Rev. 933, 947 (1989) ("Behind every free exercise claim is a spectral march; grant this one, a voice whispers to each judge, and you will be confronted with an endless chain of exemption demands from religious deviants of every stripe"). This Court, however, consistently has rejected similar arguments in past free exercise cases, and it should do so here as well. See Frazee v. Illinois Dept. of Employment Security, 489 U.S.

---

5. Moreover, 23 States, including many that have significant Native American populations, have statutory or judicially crafted exemptions in their drug laws for religious use of peyote. Although this does not prove that Oregon must have such an exception too, it is significant that these States, and the Federal Government, all find their (presumably compelling) interests in controlling the use of dangerous drugs compatible with an exemption for religious use of peyote.

6. In this respect, respondents' use of peyote seems closely analogous to the sacramental use of wine by the Roman Catholic Church. During Prohibition, the Federal Government exempted such use of wine from its general ban on possession and use of alcohol. However compelling the Government's then general interest in prohibiting the use of alcohol may have been, it could not plausibly have asserted an interest sufficiently compelling to outweigh Catholics' right to take communion.

829, 835 (1989) (rejecting State's speculation concerning cumulative effect of many similar claims); *Thomas*, 450 U.S., at 719 (same); *Sherbert*, 374 U.S., at 407.

The State's apprehension of a flood of other religious claims is purely speculative. Almost half the States, and the Federal Government, have maintained an exemption for religious peyote use for many years, and apparently have not found themselves overwhelmed by claims to other religious exemptions.[8]

II-III

Finally, although I agree with JUSTICE O'CONNOR that courts should refrain from delving into questions of whether, as a matter of religious doctrine, a particular practice is "central" to the religion, I do not think this means that the courts must turn a blind eye to the severe impact of a State's restrictions on the adherents of a minority religion. Cf. *Yoder*, 406 U.S., at 219 (since "education is inseparable from and a part of the basic tenets of their religion *** [, just as] baptism, the confessional, or a sabbath may be for others," enforcement of State's compulsory education law would "gravely endanger if not destroy the free exercise of respondents' religious beliefs").

Respondents believe, and their sincerity has never been at issue, that the peyote plant embodies their deity, and eating it is an act of worship and communion. Without peyote, they could not enact the essential ritual of their religion. If Oregon can constitutionally prosecute them for this act of worship, they, like the Amish, may be "forced to migrate to some other and more tolerant region." ***

For these reasons, I conclude that Oregon's interest in enforcing its drug laws against religious use of peyote is not sufficiently compelling to outweigh respondents' right to the free exercise of their religion. Since the State could not constitutionally enforce its criminal prohibition against respondents, the interests underlying the State's drug laws cannot justify its denial of unemployment benefits. Absent such justification, the State's regulatory interest in denying benefits for religiously motivated "misconduct," is indistinguishable from the state interests this Court has rejected in *Frazee, Hobbie, Thomas*, and *Sherbert*. The State of Oregon cannot, consistently with the Free Exercise Clause, deny respondents unemployment benefits.

I dissent.

---

8. Over the years, various sects have raised free exercise claims regarding drug use. In no reported case, except those involving claims of religious peyote use, has the claimant prevailed. See, e.g., Olsen v. Iowa, 808 F. 2d 652 (CA8 1986) (marijuana use by Ethiopian Zion Coptic Church); United States v. Rush, 738 F. 2d 497 (CA1 1984) (same), *cert. denied*, 470 U.S. 1004 (1985).

NOTE

1. The new doctrinal position taken by the five member majority in *Smith* produced a flurry of criticism.[1] Congress, too, responded to *Smith* and enacted The Religious Freedom Restoration Act of 1993.[2] There can be little doubt that it is meant to "overrule" the *Smith* standard and reinstate the *Sherbert-Yoder* standard as the general free exercise test adverted to in the *Smith* dissenting opinions and in the concurring opinion by Justice O'Connor.[3] Here are its principal provisions:

THE RELIGIOUS FREEDOM RESTORATION ACT OF 1993

* * *

SEC. 2. CONGRESSIONAL FINDINGS AND DECLARATION OF PURPOSES.

(a) Findings. — The Congress finds that —

(1) the framers of the Constitution, recognizing free exercise of religion as an unalienable right, secured its protection in the First Amendment to the Constitution;

(2) laws "neutral" toward religion may burden religious exercise as surely as laws intended to interfere with religious exercise;

(3) governments should not substantially burden religious exercise without compelling justification;

(4) in Employment Division v. Smith, 494 U.S. 872 (1990) the Supreme Court virtually eliminated the requirement that the government justify burdens on religious exercise imposed by laws neutral toward religion; and

(5) the compelling interest test as set forth in prior Federal court rulings is a workable test for striking sensible balances between religious liberty and competing prior governmental interests.

---

1. See, e.g., Michael W. McConnell, Free Exercise and the *Smith* Decision, 57 U.Chi.L.Rev. 1109 (1990); Douglas Laycock, The Remnants of Free Exercise, 1990 Sup.Ct.Rev. 1; Jesse H. Choper, The Rise and Decline of the Constitutional Protection of Religious Liberty, 70 Neb.L.Rev. 651 (1991). And the Oregon legislature, itself, soon wrote a religious use exception into the statute prohibiting peyote use. See Or. Rev. Stat. § 475.992 (1993). See also Carol M. Kaplan, *The Devil Is In the Details: Neutral, Generally Applicable Laws and Exceptions from Smith,* 75 N.Y.U. L.Rev. 1045 (2001). Not all commentators were hostile, however. Some were of the view that the majority position was, at least in part, an appropriate acceptance of Establishment Clause principles dating from the *Everson* case, as suggested in the Kurland synthesis (noted earlier): "[T]he religion clause of the first amendment *** should be read as a single precept that government cannot utilize religion as a standard for action or inaction because these clauses prohibit classification in terms of religion either to confer a benefit or to impose a burden." See, e.g., Mark Tushnet, "Of Church and State and the Supreme Court": Kurland Revisited, 1989 Sup.Ct.Rev. 373; Ira C. Lupu, Reconstructing the Establishment Clause: The Case Against the Discretionary Accommodation of Religion, 140 U.Pa.L.Rev. 555 (1991); William P. Marshall, In Defense of *Smith* and Free Exercise Revisionism, 58 U.Chi.L.Rev. 308 (1991).) For by far the most comprehensive review of Smith itself, see GARRETT EPPS, TO AN UNKNOWN GOD (2001).

2. 42 U.S.C. 2000bb (1993).

3. See Douglas Laycock, Free Exercise and the Religious Freedom Restoration Act, 62 Fordham L.Rev. 883, 895 (1994) ("The Religious Freedom Restoration Act is a response [to *Smith*].").

(b) Purposes. — The purposes of this Act are —

(1) to restore the compelling interest test as set forth in Sherbert v. Verner, 374 U.S. 398 (1963) and Wisconsin v. Yoder, 406 U.S. 205 (1972) and to guarantee its application in all cases where free exercise of religion is substantially burdened; and

(2) to provide a claim or defense to persons whose religious exercise is substantially burdened by government.

SEC. 3. FREE EXERCISE OF RELIGION PROTECTED.

(a) In General. — Government shall not substantially burden a person's exercise of religion even if the burden results from a rule of general applicability, except as provided in subsection (b).

(b) Exception. — Government may substantially burden a person's exercise of religion only if it demonstrates that application of the burden to the person—

(1) is in furtherance of a compelling governmental interest; and

(2) is the least restrictive means of furthering that compelling governmental interest.

(c) Judicial Relief. — A person whose religious exercise has been burdened in violation of this section may assert that violation as a claim or defense in a judicial proceeding and obtain appropriate relief against a government. Standing to assert a claim or defense under this section shall be governed by the general rules of standing under article III of the Constitution.

* * *

SEC. 5. DEFINITIONS.

As used in this Act —

(1) the term "government" includes a branch, department, agency, instrumentality, and official (or other person acting under color of law) of the United States, a State, or a subdivision of a State;

(2) the term "State" includes the District of Columbia, the Commonwealth of Puerto Rico, and each territory and possession of the United States;

(3) the term "demonstrates" means meets the burdens of going forward with the evidence and of persuasion; and

(4) the term "exercise of religion" means the exercise of religion under the First Amendment to the Constitution.

SEC. 6. APPLICABILITY.

(a) In General. — This Act applies to all Federal and State law, and the implementation of that law, whether statutory or otherwise, and whether adopted before or after the enactment of this Act.

(b) Rule of Construction. — Federal statutory law adopted after the date of the enactment of this Act is subject to this Act unless such law explicitly excludes such application by reference to this Act.

***

2. In which of the preceding cases, if any, would this act of Congress compel a different outcome?[4] In *Lyng*? In *Swaggart*? In *Goldman*? At least in *Smith* itself? Assuming the final case in this chapter (*Hialeah*) were to involve an ordinary anti-cruelty to animals general statute applied unexceptionally to "religious animal sacrifices" (i.e. not in any way specially targeting, but merely as not exempting such acts), would the new act apply to require the exemption of "*religious* animal sacrifices" from such laws? Or from some, but not all (if some, but not all, which ones, and why)?[5]

3. Assuming the Act may compel a different outcome in *Smith*, or at least a different outcome than the Court would otherwise reach under *Smith* in a significant number of other cases (even if not in *Smith* itself), what then? Does this raise any fundamental questions challenging Marbury v. Madison, 5 U.S. (1 Cranch) 157 (1803)?

What is the constitutional basis for the Religious Freedom Restoration Act? Is it section 5 of the fourteenth amendment (that "Congress shall have power to enforce, by appropriate legislation, the provisions of this article")? If so, what provision (of the fourteenth amendment) does the act "enforce" against the states?[6]

---

4. The Act itself refers to the "compelling interest test as set forth in *Sherbert v. Verner*." But as noted above the *Sherbert* "test" may subsequently have proven to be rather limited in its application. See Kenneth Karst, Religious Freedom and Equal Citizenship: Reflections on *Lukumi*, 69 Tulane L.Rev. 335, 357 (1994) ("A major doctrinal ambiguity in the RFRA left for the courts to resolve, is whether Congress has commanded the honest-to-goodness strict scrutiny of *Sherbert* itself and *Wisconsin v. Yoder*, or has adopted the not-so-strict scrutiny used by the Supreme Court in most free exercise cases during the pre-*Smith* era.").

5. As a further example, suppose a male prison inmate sues to enjoin the use of women guards (rather than only men guards) in cell shakedowns involving strip searches, the objection being a "privacy" objection of humiliation (the mirror image of a female inmate's equivalent objection to such searches being conducted by male guards); and the inmate objecting additionally on religious grounds (namely, that having to expose his naked body to female guards violates a "strong nudity taboo" of his Islamic faith). See Canedy v. Boardman, 16 F.3d 183, 186 n.2 (7th Cir. 1994). See also Werner v. McCotter, 49 F.3d 1476 (10th Cir. 1995) (remanding for consideration under the "compelling interest" standard a Native American Prisoner's claimed right to use a "sweat lodge"). Prior to the RFRA, the prisoner's claim would almost certainly have failed under the "reasonable relation" test of O'Lone v. Estate of Shabazz, 482 U.S. 342 (1987).

6. See Katzenbach v. Morgan, 384 U.S. 641 (1966); Robert Burt, *Miranda* and Title II: A Morganatic Marriage, 1969 Sup.Ct.Rev. 81, 83-84 ("In effect the Court is saying [in *Morgan*] that—at least in some circumstances—where Congress and the Court disagree about the meaning of the 14th Amendment, the Court will defer to Congress' version."). See also Daniel O. Conkle, The Religious Freedom Restoration Act: The Constitutional Significance of an Unconstitutional Statute, 56 Mont.L.Rev. 39 91995); Christopher L. Eisgruber & Lawrence C. Sager, Why the Religious Freedom Restoration Act Is Unconstitutional, 69 N.Y.U.L.Rev. 437 (1994); Ira C. Lupu, Of Time and the RFRA:

If the basis is some enumerated power vested in Congress to secure due judicial recognition of personal constitutional rights insufficiently accommodated by state law, but the Court itself has said that there is no "free exercise" right of personal exemption from otherwise valid, neutral state laws of general application, how can it be said that this act of Congress is merely appropriate legislation to "enforce" the fourteenth amendment? Is the act itself subject to constitutional objection: (a) on grounds that there is no authority to enact it; (b) on grounds that it violates separation of powers?

4. As was to be expected, the Religious Freedom Restoration Act (RFRA) was at once invoked as an alternative to the free exercise clause or the fourteenth amendment. Indeed, as a practical matter, the RFRA quietly became virtually a congressionally-supplied "replacement" for the free exercise clause (i.e. a replacement for the clause as interpreted and as applied in *Employment Division v. Smith*).[7] The effect of the RFRA was thus to make it of little consequence that a state law might, on its face and as applied, survive a fourteenth amendment free exercise clause challenge under the decision in *Smith.* For though that might be so, the law was still also examined under the more stringent "balancing" *Sherbert-Yoder* test, imposed by Congress under color of the RFRA.

As new cases continued to be filed, increasingly litigants no longer bothered to raise a free exercise claim as such, instead relying simply on the RFRA,[8] and requesting

---

A Lawyer's Guide to the Religious Freedom Restoration Act, 56 Mont.L.Rev. 171, 212-225 (1995).

7. *See Douglas Laycock & Oliver Thomas, The Religious Freedom Restoration Act*, 73 Tex. L.Rev. 209, 219 (1994) (describing the RFRA as meant to be "a *replacement* for the Free Exercise Clause," and "as universal [in the scope of its coverage] as the Free Exercise Clause") (emphasis added). Some courts even became confused by the RFRA, suggesting that whether a state shall be held to have "violate[d] the free exercise clause of the First Amendment *** must be analyzed under the standard set forth in the recently enacted Religious Freedom Restoration Act." See, e.g., *Lucero v. Hensley*, 920 F. Supp. 1067, 1072 (C.D. Cal. 1996). Clearly this was incorrect, however, for whether a state shall be held to have violated the free exercise clause, as distinct from having violated the RFRA, is not a determination to be made by the RFRA, but by the precedents of the Supreme Court in respect to the free exercise clause itself. (Still, the court's error was instructive, in indicating how dominant the RFRA had already become even to the point of suggesting that the Act itself determined the standard of judgment in every first amendment free exercise case.)

8. *See Douglas Laycock & Oliver Thomas, The Religious Freedom Restoration Act*, 73 Tex. L.Rev. 209, 219 (1994) (describing the RFRA as meant to be "a *replacement* for the Free Exercise Clause," and "as universal [in the scope of its coverage] as the Free Exercise Clause") (emphasis added). Some courts even became confused by the RFRA, suggesting that whether a state shall be held to have "violate[d] the free exercise clause of the First Amendment *** must be analyzed under the standard set forth in the recently enacted Religious Freedom Restoration Act." See, e.g., *Lucero v. Hensley*, 920 F. Supp. 1067, 1072 (C.D. Cal. 1996). Clearly this was incorrect, however, for whether a state shall be held to have violated the free exercise clause, as distinct from having violated the RFRA, is not a determination to be made by the RFRA, but by the precedents of the Supreme Court in respect to the free exercise clause itself. (Still, the court's error was instructive, in indicating how dominant the RFRA had already become even to the point of suggesting that the Act itself determined the standard of judgment in every first amendment free exercise case.)

that it be applied by the court as part of "the supreme Law of the Land," pursuant to Article VI of the Constitution. In this sense, therefore, it appeared to be irrelevant to try to understand what the Supreme Court may or may not regard as forbidden by the free exercise clause. Rather, it seemed important only to determine what was forbidden or not forbidden by the RFRA.[9] Determining when and how the RFRA applied, however, did not prove to be an easy task. There were substantial disagreements among the courts on what the RFRA requires.[10]

Additionally, however, with ever greater use being made of the RFRA, its constitutionality was increasingly called into question as well. The Supreme Court finally addressed that question in 1997.

CITY OF BOERNE v. FLORES
521 U.S. 507 (1997)

JUSTICE KENNEDY delivered the opinion of the Court.

---

9. Of course, litigants might still invoke both the first amendment and the RFRA. And it was still more common than not that they did. In such cases, however, the lesson was pretty much the same: the treatment of the first amendment issue became of relatively little importance, since virtually anything it would reach was also reached by the RFRA, but not vice-versa. See, e.g., *Smith v. Fair Employment & Housing Comm'n.*, 51 Cal.Rptr.2d 700 (Cal. 1996) (religiously-anguished landlord sought relief on first amendment and separately, on RFRA, grounds from state anti-discrimination statute exposing her to damages for refusing to rent to unmarried cohabiting couples), *cert. denied*, 521 U.S. 1129 (1997). *Hamilton v. Schriro*, 74 F.3d 1545 (8th Cir. 1995) (rejecting both first amendment and RFRA challenges by state prisoner to a prison regulation that restricted hair length and to the prison's lack of a suitable "sweat lodge," one judge dissenting partly on the ground that the hair length regulation violated the RFRA — i.e. that although the hair length regulation would pass muster under the first amendment, it could not survive an RFRA challenge), *cert. denied*, 519 U.S. 874 (1996).

10. The courts have not taken a uniform position with respect to the meaning of the requirement that persons invoking the RFRA must first show how compliance with the law would "*substantially*" burden them in respect to their religion. I.e. must it affect something "central" to their religion — and if so, just "how central"? Suppose the practice is not "mandated" by one's religion, but is part of an observant practice even close to the center of one's sense of a religiously-centered life? See *Lucero*, 920 F. Supp. at 1073 (noting that the Ninth and Tenth Circuits treat the matter differently, the Ninth Circuit having suggested that "the burdened practice [must] be [a practice] 'mandated' by one's religion" to meet the RFRA threshold, the Tenth Circuit having held it sufficient (to trigger the Act) that the regulation "significantly inhibit[s] or constrain[s] conduct or expression that manifest some central tenet" of an individual's religion, though it need not be conduct or expression actually mandated by his religion). The *Lucero* court observed that "[d]istrict courts in other circuits are split on whether to follow the religiously 'mandated' test or the religiously 'motivated' test."

Similarly, there is little agreement in respect to what suffices for a "compelling interest," and whether failure to force compliance with the law in a particular case would substantially (rather than only insubstantially) frustrate that compelling interest (such as it is). See, e.g., *Smith*, 51 Cal.Rptr.2d 700(court divided on the question whether, if only those landlords sincerely unable to reconcile their religious duty not to facilitate immoral acts by others (by renting them rooms) were exempt, such exemption would so undermine the state's anti-discrimination law (forbidding refusals to rent to unmarried cohabitants) as to work a serious frustration to the law).

A decision by local zoning authorities to deny a church a building permit was challenged under the Religious Freedom Restoration Act of 1993 (RFRA). The case calls into question the authority of Congress to enact RFRA. We conclude the statute exceeds Congress' power.

[I-II]

Situated on a hill in the city of Boerne, Texas, some 28 miles northwest of San Antonio, is St. Peter Catholic Church. Built in 1923, the church's structure replicates the mission style of the region's earlier history. In order to meet the needs of the congregation the Archbishop of San Antonio gave permission to the parish to plan alterations to enlarge the building.

A few months later, the Boerne City Council passed an ordinance authorizing the city's Historic Landmark Commission to prepare a preservation plan with proposed historic landmarks and districts. Under the ordinance, the Commission must preapprove construction affecting historic landmarks or buildings in a historic district.

Soon afterwards, the Archbishop applied for a building permit so construction to enlarge the church could proceed. City authorities, relying on the ordinance and the designation of a historic district (which, they argued, included the church), denied the application. The Archbishop brought this suit challenging the permit denial in the United States District Court for the Western District of Texas.

The Archbishop relied upon RFRA as one basis for relief from the refusal to issue the permit. The District Court concluded that by enacting RFRA Congress exceeded the scope of its enforcement power under § 5 of the Fourteenth Amendment. The court certified its order for interlocutory appeal and the Fifth Circuit reversed, finding RFRA to be constitutional. We granted certiorari, and now reverse.

Congress enacted RFRA in direct response to the Court's decision in *Employment Div., Dept. of Human Resources of Ore. v. Smith.* In [*Smith*], we declined to apply the balancing test set forth in *Sherbert v. Verner*, under which we would have asked whether Oregon's prohibition substantially burdened a religious practice and, if it did, whether the burden was justified by a compelling government interest. The application of the *Sherbert* test, the *Smith* decision explained, would have produced an anomaly in the law, a constitutional right to ignore neutral laws of general applicability. The anomaly would have been accentuated, the Court reasoned, by the difficulty of determining whether a particular practice was central to an individual's religion. We explained, moreover, that it "is not within the judicial ken to question the centrality of particular beliefs or practices to a faith, or the validity of particular litigants' interpretations of those creeds."

These points of constitutional interpretation were debated by Members of Congress in hearings and floor debates. Many criticized the Court's reasoning, and this disagreement resulted in the passage of RFRA. The Act's stated purpose [is]:

> (1) to restore the compelling interest test as set forth in *Sherbert v. Verner* and *Wisconsin v. Yoder* and to guarantee its application in all cases where free exercise of religion is substantially burdened; and
>
> (2) to provide a claim or defense to persons whose religious exercise is substantially burdened by government. § 2000bb(b).

The Act's universal coverage is confirmed in § 2000bb-3(a), under which RFRA "applies to all Federal and State law, and the implementation of that law, whether statutory or otherwise, and whether adopted before or after [RFRA's enactment]." ***

III

A

Congress relied on its Fourteenth Amendment enforcement power in enacting the most far reaching and substantial of RFRA's provisions, those which impose its requirements on the States. [R]espondent contends, with support from the United States as amicus, that RFRA is permissible enforcement legislation. Congress, it is said, is only protecting by legislation one of the liberties guaranteed by the Fourteenth Amendment's Due Process Clause, the free exercise of religion, beyond what is necessary under *Smith.* It is said the congressional decision to dispense with proof of deliberate or overt discrimination and instead concentrate on a law's effects accords with the settled understanding that § 5 includes the power to enact legislation designed to prevent as well as remedy constitutional violations. It is further contended that Congress' § 5 power is not limited to remedial or preventive legislation.

Congress' power under § 5, however, extends only to "enforc[ing]" the provisions of the Fourteenth Amendment. The design of the Amendment and the text of § 5 are inconsistent with the suggestion that Congress has the power to decree the substance of the Fourteenth Amendment's restrictions on the States.

While the line between measures that remedy or prevent unconstitutional actions and measures that make a substantive change in the governing law is not easy to discern, and Congress must have wide latitude in determining where it lies, the distinction exists and must be observed. There must be a congruence and proportionality between the injury to be prevented or remedied and the means adopted to that end. Lacking such a connection, legislation may become substantive in operation and effect. History and our case law support drawing the distinction, one apparent from the text of the Amendment.

1-2

The Fourteenth Amendment's history confirms the remedial, rather than substantive, nature of the Enforcement Clause. The Joint Committee on Reconstruction of the 39th Congress began drafting what would become the Fourteenth Amendment in January 1866. *** In February, Republican Representative John Bingham of Ohio reported the following draft amendment to the House of Representatives on behalf of the Joint Committee:

The Congress shall have power to make all laws which shall be necessary and proper to secure to the citizens of each State all privileges and immunities of citizens in the several States, and to all persons in the several States equal protection in the rights of life, liberty, and property.

The proposal encountered immediate opposition, which continued through three days of debate. Members of Congress from across the political spectrum criticized the Amendment, and the criticisms had a common theme: The proposed Amendment gave Congress too much legislative power at the expense of the existing constitutional structure. *** As a result of these objections having been expressed from so many different quarters, the House voted to table the proposal until April. The Amendment in its early form was not again considered. Instead, the Joint Committee began drafting a new article of Amendment, which it reported to Congress on April 30, 1866.

Section 1 of the new draft Amendment imposed self-executing limits on the States. Section 5 prescribed that "[t]he Congress shall have power to enforce, by appropriate legislation, the provisions of this article." Under the revised Amendment, Congress' power was no longer plenary but remedial. The design of the Fourteenth Amendment has proved significant also in maintaining the traditional separation of powers between Congress and the Judiciary. As enacted, the Fourteenth Amendment confers substantive rights against the States which, like the provisions of the Bill of Rights, are self-executing. The power to interpret the Constitution in a case or controversy remains in the Judiciary.

The remedial and preventive nature of Congress' enforcement power, and the limitation inherent in the power, were confirmed in our earliest cases on the Fourteenth Amendment. Recent cases have continued to revolve around the question of whether § 5 legislation can be considered remedial. ***

3

Any suggestion that Congress has a substantive, non-remedial power under the Fourteenth Amendment is not supported by our case law. In *Oregon v. Mitchell*, a majority of the Court concluded Congress had exceeded its enforcement powers by enacting legislation lowering the minimum age of voters from 21 to 18 in state and local elections. The five Members of the Court who reached this conclusion explained that the legislation intruded into an area reserved by the Constitution to the States. Four of these five were explicit in rejecting the position that § 5 endowed Congress with the power to establish the meaning of constitutional provisions.

There is language in our opinion in *Katzenbach v. Morgan*, 384 U.S. 641 (1966), which could be interpreted as acknowledging a power in Congress to enact legislation that expands the rights contained in § 1 of the Fourteenth Amendment. This is not a necessary interpretation, however, or even the best one. If Congress could define its own powers by altering the Fourteenth Amendment's meaning, no longer would the Constitution be "superior paramount law, unchangeable by ordinary means." It would be "on a level with ordinary legislative acts, and, like other acts, alterable when the legislature shall please to alter it." *Marbury v. Madison, 1 Cranch*, at 177. Under this approach, it is difficult to conceive of a principle that would limit congressional power. See Van Alstyne, The Failure of the Religious Freedom Restoration Act under Section 5 of the Fourteenth Amendment, 46 Duke L.J. 291, 292-303 (1996). ***

B

Respondent contends that RFRA is a proper exercise of Congress' remedial or preventive power. The Act, it is said, is a reasonable means of protecting the free exercise of religion as defined by *Smith.* It prevents and remedies laws which are enacted with the unconstitutional object of targeting religious beliefs and practices. ***

A comparison between RFRA and the Voting Rights Act is instructive. In contrast to the record which confronted Congress and the judiciary in the voting rights cases, RFRA's legislative record lacks examples of modern instances of generally applicable laws passed because of religious bigotry. Rather, the emphasis of the hearings was on laws of general applicability which place incidental burdens on religion. Much of the discussion centered upon anecdotal evidence of autopsies performed on Jewish individuals and Hmong immigrants in violation of their religious beliefs, and on zoning regulations and historic preservation laws (like the one at issue here), which as an incident of their normal operation, have adverse effects on churches and synagogues. It is difficult to maintain that they are examples of legislation enacted or enforced due to animus or hostility to the burdened religious practices or that they indicate some widespread pattern of religious discrimination in this country. Congress' concern was with the incidental burdens imposed, not the object or purpose of the legislation.

Regardless of the state of the legislative record, RFRA cannot be considered remedial, preventive legislation, if those terms are to have any meaning. RFRA is so out of proportion to a supposed remedial or preventive object that it cannot be understood as responsive to, or designed to prevent, unconstitutional behavior. It appears, instead, to attempt a substantive change in constitutional protections. Preventive measures prohibiting certain types of laws may be appropriate when there is reason to believe that many of the laws affected by the congressional enactment have a significant likelihood of being unconstitutional.

RFRA is not so confined. Sweeping coverage ensures its intrusion at every level of government, displacing laws and prohibiting official actions of almost every description and regardless of subject matter. RFRA's restrictions apply to every agency and official of the Federal, State, and local Governments. RFRA applies to all federal and state law, statutory or otherwise, whether adopted before or after its enactment. RFRA has no termination date or termination mechanism. Any law is subject to challenge at any time by any individual who alleges a substantial burden on his or her free exercise of religion. *** Simply put, RFRA is not designed to identify and counteract state laws likely to be unconstitutional because of their treatment of religion. In most cases, the state laws to which RFRA applies are not ones which will have been motivated by religious bigotry. *** In addition, the Act imposes in every case a least restrictive means requirement— a requirement that was not used in the pre-*Smith* jurisprudence RFRA purported to codify — which also indicates that the legislation is broader than is appropriate if the goal is to prevent and remedy constitutional violations.

*** When the Court has interpreted the Constitution, it has acted within the province of the Judicial Branch, which embraces the duty to say what the law is. *Marbury v. Madison*. When the political branches of the Government act against the background of a judicial interpretation of the Constitution already issued, it must be understood that in later cases and controversies the Court will treat its precedents with the respect due them under settled principles, including *stare decisis*, and contrary expectations must be disappointed. RFRA was designed to control cases and controversies, such as the one before us; but as the provisions of the federal statute here invoked are beyond congressional authority, it is this Court's precedent, not RFRA, which must control.

It is for Congress in the first instance to "determin[e] whether and what legislation is needed to secure the guarantees of the Fourteenth Amendment," and its conclusions are entitled to much deference. *Katzenbach v. Morgan*. Congress' discretion is not unlimited, however, and the courts retain the power, as they have since *Marbury v. Madison*, to determine if Congress has exceeded its authority under the Constitution. Broad as the power of Congress is under the Enforcement Clause of the Fourteenth Amendment, RFRA contradicts vital principles necessary to maintain separation of powers and the federal balance. The judgment of the Court of Appeals sustaining the Act's constitutionality is reversed.

JUSTICE STEVENS, concurring.

In my opinion, the Religious Freedom Restoration Act of 1993 (RFRA) is a "law respecting an establishment of religion" that violates the First Amendment to the Constitution.

If the historic landmark on the hill in Boerne happened to be a museum or an art gallery owned by an atheist, it would not be eligible for an exemption from the city ordinances that forbid an enlargement of the structure. Because the landmark is owned by the Catholic Church, it is claimed that RFRA gives its owner a federal statutory entitlement to an exemption from a generally applicable, neutral civil law. Whether the Church would actually prevail under the statute or not, the statute has provided the Church with a legal weapon that no atheist or agnostic can obtain. This governmental preference for religion, as opposed to irreligion, is forbidden by the First Amendment. ***

JUSTICE SCALIA, with whom JUSTICE STEVENS joins, concurring in part. [Omitted.]

JUSTICE O'CONNOR, with whom JUSTICE BREYER joins except as to a portion of Part I, dissenting.

[I]f I agreed with the Court's standard in *Smith,* I would join the opinion. As the Court's careful and thorough historical analysis shows, Congress lacks the "power to decree the substance of the Fourteenth Amendment's restrictions on the States." Rather, its power under § 5 of the Fourteenth Amendment extends only to enforcing the Amendment's provisions. In short, Congress lacks the ability independently to define or expand the scope of constitutional rights by statute. Accordingly, whether Congress has exceeded its § 5 powers turns on whether there is a "congruence and proportionality between the injury to be prevented or remedied and the means adopted to that end." This recognition does not, of course, in any way diminish Congress' obligation to draw its own conclusions regarding the Constitution's meaning. Congress, no less than this Court, is called upon to consider the requirements of the Constitution and to act in accordance with its dictates. But when it enacts legislation in furtherance of its delegated powers, Congress must make its judgments consistent with this Court's exposition of the Constitution and with the limits placed on its legislative authority by provisions such as the Fourteenth Amendment.

[But] *stare decisis* concerns should not prevent us from revisiting our holding in *Smith.* I believe that, in light of both our precedent and our Nation's tradition of religious liberty, *Smith* is demonstrably wrong. Moreover, it is a recent decision. As such, it has not engendered the kind of reliance on its continued application that would militate against overruling it. Accordingly, I believe that it is essential for the Court to reconsider its holding in *Smith* — and to do so in this very case. I would therefore direct the parties to brief this issue and set the case for reargument.

JUSTICE SOUTER, dissenting.

*** I have serious doubts about the precedential value of the *Smith* rule and its entitlement to adherence. I am not now prepared to join JUSTICE O'CONNOR in rejecting it or the majority in assuming it to be correct. In order to provide full adversarial consideration, this case should be set down for reargument permitting plenary reexamination of the issue.

JUSTICE BREYER, dissenting. [Omitted.]

NOTES

1. Five Justices (Rehnquist, C.J., Stevens, Thomas, Scalia, and Ginsburg, JJ.) expressly joined "the opinion of the Court" by Justice Kennedy, in holding that the RFRA exceeded Congress's power under § 5 of the fourteenth amendment (and may have overstepped the separation of powers). A seventh Justice, O'Connor, while dissenting on the disposition of the case (see her Opinion *supra* in text), declared that she, too, would "join the opinion," holding RFRA unconstitutional but for her disagreement with *Smith* (which she, Souter, and Breyer, JJ., merely declared should

be reconsidered in this very case or in an appropriate case newly challenging the Court's decision in *Smith* itself).

It thus appears to be very clear that the RFRA is "unconstitutional," in exceeding Congress's authority, a minimum of seven Justices of the Supreme Court having so concluded in this case. Accordingly, it appears to be equally clear that the RFRA therefore cannot now be successfully pleaded in lieu of, or additional to, a free exercise claim.

2. *Query,* however, whether this is necessarily true. **Note** that the RFRA applies to all "*Federal*" as well as to all "State" (and local) laws — and applies also to the "implementation" of all Federal laws "whether adopted before or after the enactment of this Act." **Note**, further, that the very next subsection of the Act (headed "Rule of Construction"), provides that "*Federal statutory law adopted after the date of the enactment of this Act is subject to this Act unless such law explicitly excludes such application by reference to this Act.*" (Emphasis added.) What is the status of these provisions today? Consider the following simple case.

Suppose a federal prisoner requests exemption from a federal prison rule of general application on one's length of hair (e.g., a Sikh claiming a religious requirement of longer hair or a Rastafarian with a similar claim). There is no suggestion the rule was instituted from religious animus or partiality. May the prisoner invoke the RFRA to assert a claim against the Warden of the federal prison (though clearly his counterpart, one held in a state prison, could not do so)? Is the power of Congress to provide the RFRA "accommodation" in respect to federal statutes derived from § 5 of the fourteenth amendment, or may it be derived from some other enumerated source of power, e.g, the "necessary and proper"clause in Article I? Is the RFRA a severable statute, such that its provisions in respect to federal statutes, past and future, are still applicable?"[25]

3. Within two years of the Court's decision in Boerne, Congress enacted a modified form of the same statute, Public Law 106-274 (Sept. 22, 2000), codified in 42 U.S. §2000cc. Titled "THE RELIGIOUS LAND USE AND INSTITUTIONALIZED PERSONS ACT OF 2000," this act re-enacts the RFRA standards still again. It directs that those standards now be applied in respect to "[any] land use regulation [that] imposes a substantial burden" on a person's or institution's "religious exercise," if the burden (a) affects, or removal of that burden would itself affect, interstate commerce; or if the burden (b) is imposed in a program or activity receiving any

25. *See Kikumura v. Hurley, 242 F. 3d. 950 (10th Cir. 2001); Setton v. Providence se. Joseph Med. (Tr., 192 f. 3d 826 (9th cir. 1999); Young v. Crystal Evangelical Free Church,*141 F.3d 854 (8th Cir. 1998); for a discussion of the application of RFRA to federal laws after *Boerne*, see Edward J.W. Blatkik, Note, *No RFRAF Allowed: The Status of the Religious Freedom Restoration Act's Federal Application in the Wake of City of Boerne v. Flores*, 98 Colum. L. Rev. 1410.

federal financial aid; or if the burden (c) is imposed in implementation of any regulation that permits individualized assessments of the proposed property use.[1]

CHURCH OF LUKUMI BABALU AYE, INC. v. CITY OF HIALEAH
113 S.Ct. 217 (1993)

JUSTICE KENNEDY delivered the opinion of the Court, except as to Part II-A-2.[*]

I

This case involves practices of the Santeria religion, which originated in the nineteenth century. When hundreds of thousands of members of the Yoruba people were brought as slaves from eastern Africa to Cuba, their traditional African religion absorbed significant elements of Roman Catholicism. The resulting syncretion, or fusion, is Santeria, "the way of the saints." The Cuban Yoruba express their devotion to spirits, called *orishas*, through the iconography of Catholic saints, Catholic symbols are often present at Santeria rites, and Santeria devotees attend the Catholic sacraments.

***

According to Santeria teaching, the *orishas* are powerful but not immortal. They depend for survival on the sacrifice. Sacrifices are performed at birth, marriage, and death rites, for the cure of the sick, for the initiation of new members and priests, and during an annual celebration. Animals sacrificed in Santeria rituals include chickens, pigeons, doves, ducks, guinea pigs, goats, sheep, and turtles. The animals are killed by the cutting of the carotid arteries in the neck. The sacrificed animal is cooked and eaten, except after healing and death rituals. The religion was brought to this Nation most often by exiles from the Cuban revolution. The District Court estimated that there are at least 50,000 practitioners in South Florida today.

Petitioner Church of the Lukumi Babalu Aye, Inc. (Church), is a not-for-profit corporation organized under Florida law in 1973. The Church and its congregants practice the Santeria religion. In April 1987, the Church leased land in the city of Hialeah, Florida, and announced plans to establish a house of worship as well as a school, cultural center, and museum. The prospect of a Santeria church in their midst was distressing to many members of the Hialeah community, and the announcement of the plans to open a Santeria church in Hialeah prompted the city council to hold an emergency public session on June 9, 1987. [T]he city council adopted Resolution 87-66, which noted the "concern" expressed by residents of the city "that certain religions may propose to engage in practices which are inconsistent

---

1. (A separate section re-enacts the RFRA standards, to make them govern any case involving a "substantial burden of the religious exercise of a person residing in or confined to an institution, as defined in §2 of the Civil Rights of Institutionalized Persons Act (42 U.S.C. § 1997)".)

*. THE CHIEF JUSTICE, JUSTICE SCALIA, and JUSTICE THOMAS join all but Part II-A-2 of this opinion. JUSTICE WHITE joins all but Part II-A of this opinion. JUSTICE SOUTER joins only Parts I, III, and IV of this opinion.

with public morals, peace or safety," and declared that "[t]he City reiterates its commitment to a prohibition against any and all acts of any and all religious groups which are inconsistent with public morals, peace or safety."

In September 1987, the city council adopted three substantive ordinances addressing the issue of religious animal sacrifice. Ordinance 87-52 defined "sacrifice" as "to unnecessarily kill, torment, torture, or mutilate an animal in a public or private ritual or ceremony not for the primary purpose of food consumption," and prohibited owning or possessing an animal "intending to use such animal for food purposes." Ordinance 87-71 defined sacrifice as had Ordinance 87- 52, and then provided that "[i]t shall be unlawful for any person, persons, corporations or associations to sacrifice any animal within the corporate limits of the City of Hialeah, Florida." The final Ordinance, 87-72, defined "slaughter" as "the killing of animals for food" and prohibited slaughter outside of areas zoned for slaughterhouse use. The ordinance provided an exemption, however, for the slaughter or processing for sale of "small numbers of hogs and/or cattle per week in accordance with an exemption provided by state law." All ordinances and resolutions passed the city council by unanimous vote.

Following enactment of these ordinances, the Church and Pichardo filed this action pursuant to 42 U.S.C. § 1983 in the United States District Court for the Southern District of Florida. Alleging violations of petitioners' rights under, *inter alia*, the Free Exercise Clause, the complaint sought a declaratory judgment and injunctive and monetary relief. [T]he District Court ruled for the city, finding no violation of petitioners' rights under the Free Exercise Clause. ***

II

* * *

In addressing the constitutional protection for free exercise of religion, our cases establish the general proposition that a law that is neutral and of general applicability need not be justified by a compelling governmental interest even if the law has the incidental effect of burdening a particular religious practice. *Employment Div., Dept. of Human Resources of Oregon v. Smith* [494 U.S. 872]. Neutrality and general applicability are interrelated, and, as becomes apparent in this case, failure to satisfy one requirement is a likely indication that the other has not been satisfied. A law failing to satisfy these requirements must be justified by a compelling governmental interest and must be narrowly tailored to advance that interest. These ordinances fail to satisfy the Smith requirements. We begin by discussing neutrality.

*** To determine the object of a law, we must begin with its text, for the minimum requirement of neutrality is that a law not discriminate on its face. A law lacks facial neutrality if it refers to a religious practice without a secular meaning discernable from the language or context. Petitioners contend that three of the ordinances fail this test of facial neutrality because they use the words "sacrifice" and "ritual," words with strong religious connotations. We agree that these words are consistent with the claim of facial discrimination, but the argument is not conclusive. The words "sacrifice" and "ritual" have a religious origin, but current use admits also of secular meanings. ***

There are further respects in which the text of the city council's enactments discloses the improper attempt to target Santeria. Resolution 87-66, adopted June 9, 1987, recited that "residents and citizens of the City of Hialeah have expressed their concern that certain religions may propose to engage in practices which are inconsistent with public morals, peace or safety," and "reiterate[d]" the city's commitment to prohibit "any and all [such] acts of any and all religious groups." No one suggests, and on this record it cannot be maintained, that city officials had in mind a religion other than Santeria.

It is a necessary conclusion that almost the only conduct subject to Ordinances 87-40, 87-52, and 87-71 is the religious exercise of Santeria church members. The texts show that they were drafted in tandem to achieve this result. We begin with Ordinance 87-71. It prohibits the sacrifice of animals but defines sacrifice as "to unnecessarily kill *** an animal in a public or private ritual or ceremony not for the primary purpose of food consumption." The definition excludes almost all killings of animals except for religious sacrifice, and the primary purpose requirement narrows the proscribed category even further, in particular by exempting Kosher slaughter. We need not discuss whether this differential treatment of two religions is itself an independent constitutional violation. It suffices to recite this feature of the law as support for our conclusion that Santeria alone was the exclusive legislative concern. The net result of the gerrymander is that few if any killings of animals are prohibited other than Santeria sacrifice, which is proscribed because it occurs during a ritual or ceremony and its primary purpose is to make an offering to the *orishas*, not food consumption. ***

We also find significant evidence of the ordinances' improper targeting of Santeria sacrifice in the fact that they proscribe more religious conduct than is necessary to achieve their stated ends. The legitimate governmental interests in protecting the public health and preventing cruelty to animals could be addressed by restrictions stopping far short of a flat prohibition of all Santeria sacrificial practice. If improper disposal, not the sacrifice itself, is the harm to be prevented, the city could have imposed a general regulation on the disposal of organic garbage. It did not do so. Under similar analysis, narrower regulation would achieve the city's interest in preventing cruelty to animals. With regard to the city's interest in ensuring the adequate care of animals, regulation of conditions and treatment, regardless of why an animal is kept, is the logical response to the city's concern, not a prohibition on possession for the purpose of sacrifice. The same is true for the city's interest in prohibiting cruel methods of killing.

Ordinance 87-72-unlike the three other ordinances does appear to apply to substantial nonreligious conduct and not to be overbroad. For our purposes here, however, the four substantive ordinances may be treated as a group for neutrality purposes. Ordinance 87-72 was passed the same day as Ordinance 87- 71 and was enacted, as were the three others, in direct response to the opening of the Church.

It would be implausible to suggest that the three other ordinances, but not Ordinance 87-72, had as their object the suppression of religion. We need not decide whether the Ordinance 87-72 could survive constitutional scrutiny if it existed separately; it must be invalidated because it functions, with the rest of the enactments in question, to suppress Santeria religious worship.

That the ordinances were enacted "'because of,' not merely 'in spite of,'" their suppression of Santeria religious practice is revealed by the events preceding enactment of the ordinances. The minutes and taped excerpts of the June 9 session, both of which are in the record, evidence significant hostility exhibited by residents, members of the city council, and other city officials toward the Santeria religion and its practice of animal sacrifice. The public crowd that attended the June 9 meetings interrupted statements by council members critical of Santeria with cheers and the brief comments of Pichardo with taunts. When Councilman Martinez, a supporter of the ordinances, stated that in prerevolution Cuba "people were put in jail for practicing this religion," the audience applauded.

Councilman Mejides indicated that he was "totally against the sacrificing of animals" and distinguished Kosher slaughter because it had a "real purpose." The "Bible says we are allowed to sacrifice an animal for consumption," he continued, "but for any other purposes, I don't believe that the Bible allows that." The president of the city council, Councilman Echevarria, asked, "What can we do to prevent the Church from opening?"

In sum, the neutrality inquiry leads to one conclusion: The ordinances had as their object the suppression of religion. The pattern we have recited discloses animosity to Santeria adherents and their religious practices; the ordinances by their own terms target this religious exercise; the texts of the ordinances were gerrymandered with care to proscribe religious killings of animals but to exclude almost all secular killings; and the ordinances suppress much more religious conduct than is necessary in order to achieve the legitimate ends asserted in their defense. These ordinances are not neutral, and the court below committed clear error in failing to reach this conclusion. ***

III

A law burdening religious practice that is not neutral or not of general application must undergo the most rigorous of scrutiny. *** It follows from what we have already said that these ordinances cannot withstand this scrutiny.

First, even were the governmental interests compelling, the ordinances are not drawn in narrow terms to accomplish those interests. As we have discussed, all four ordinances are overbroad or underinclusive in substantial respects. The proffered objectives are not pursued with respect to analogous non-religious conduct, and those interests could be achieved by narrower ordinances that burdened religion to a far lesser degree. The absence of narrow tailoring suffices to establish the invalidity of the ordinances.

Respondent has not demonstrated, moreover, that, in the context of these ordinances, its governmental interests are compelling. Where government restricts only conduct protected by the First Amendment and fails to enact feasible measures to restrict other conduct producing substantial harm or alleged harm of the same sort, the interest given in justification of the restriction is not compelling. It is established in our strict scrutiny jurisprudence that "a law cannot be regarded as protecting an interest 'of the highest order' when it leaves appreciable damage to that supposedly vital interest unprohibited." As we show above, the ordinances are underinclusive to a substantial extent with respect to each of the interests that respondent has asserted, and it is only conduct motivated by religious conviction that bears the weight of the governmental restrictions. There can be no serious claim that those interests justify the ordinances.

IV

The Free Exercise Clause commits government itself to religious tolerance, and upon even slight suspicion that proposals for state intervention stem from animosity to religion or distrust of its practices, all officials must pause to remember their own high duty to the Constitution and to the rights it secures. Those in office must be resolute in resisting importunate demands and must ensure that the sole reasons for imposing the burdens of law and regulation are secular. Legislators may not devise mechanisms, overt or disguised, designed to persecute or oppress a religion or its practices. The laws here in question were enacted contrary to these constitutional principles, and they are void.

Reversed.

JUSTICE SCALIA, with whom THE CHIEF JUSTICE joins, concurring in part and concurring in the judgment. [Omitted.]

JUSTICE SOUTER, concurring in part and concurring in the judgment.

This case turns on a principle about which there is no disagreement, that the Free Exercise Clause bars government action aimed at suppressing religious belief or practice. The Court holds that Hialeah's animal-sacrifice laws violate that principle, and I concur in that holding without reservation. *** [I]n a case presenting the issue, the Court should reexamine the rule *Smith* declared. ***

JUSTICE BLACKMUN, with whom JUSTICE O'CONNOR joins, concurring in the judgment.

*** I continue to believe that *Smith* was wrongly decided, because it ignored the value of religious freedom as an affirmative individual liberty and treated the Free Exercise Clause as no more than an antidiscrimination principle. Thus, while I agree with the result the Court reaches in this case, I arrive at that result by a different route.

When the State enacts legislation that intentionally or unintentionally places a burden upon religiously motivated practice, it must justify that burden by "showing that it is the least restrictive means of achieving some compelling state interest." A State may no more create an underinclusive statute, one that fails truly to promote its purported compelling interest, than it may create an overinclusive statute, one that encompasses more protected conduct than necessary to achieve its goal. In the latter circumstance, the broad scope of the statute is unnecessary to serve the interest, and the statute fails for that reason. In the former situation, the fact that allegedly harmful conduct falls outside the statute's scope belies a governmental assertion that it has genuinely pursued an interest "of the highest order." If the State's goal is important enough to prohibit religiously motivated activity, it will not and must not stop at religiously motivated activity. *** This case does not present, and I therefore decline to reach, the question whether the Free Exercise Clause would require a religious exemption from a law that sincerely pursued the goal of protecting animals from cruel treatment. The number of organizations that have filed amicus briefs on behalf of this interest, however, demonstrates that it is not a concern to be treated lightly.

———

Chapter 11

DEFINING "RELIGION"

INTRODUCTORY NOTE

How is "religion" to be understood within the first amendment? Exactly how generously or how stringently shall the differentiating key noun be taken in the clause that provides:

> Congress shall make no law respecting an establishment of *religion*, or prohibiting the free exercise thereof.

Consider the following assortment of dictionary definitions. Does the religion clause embrace them all? If not, at what point does it stop?

> *religion*:[1] 1. the personal commitment to and serving of God or a god with worshipful devotion; conduct in accord with divine commands especially as found in accepted sacred writings or declared by authoritative teachers; a way of life recognized as incumbent on true believers; and typically the relating of oneself to an organized body of beliefs; 2. one of the systems of faith and worship; 3. a personal awareness of or conviction of the existence of a supreme being or of supernatural powers or influences controlling one's own, humanity's, or all nature's destiny accompanied by or arousing reverence and a sense of duty to obey; 4. the body of institutionalized expressions of sacred beliefs, observances, and social practices found within a given cultural context; 5. a value held to be of supreme importance, a cause, principle, system of tenets held with ardor, devotion, conscientiousness, and faith; 6. any objective attended to or pursued with zeal or conscientious devotion.

A. The usual presumption in constitutional interpretation is the presumption of generous construction. (Assuredly this presumption was applied to the free speech and press clauses, was it not?) Applied here, that presumption might readily embrace *all* of these dictionary meanings, even if some of these were not necessarily generally recognized in common usage in 1787 or 1789. Is this what the first amendment does?

---

1. The noun "religion" is from Latin, derived from the verb *ligare*, meaning "to tie" or "to bind." We recognize it more familiarly in the noun "ligature"—something that ties (like a cord, a fastening, a binding). With the prefix *re* (also Latin), it is *religare*, to "tie back." One will find the same etymology in dictionaries under "rely." That is, both "rely" and "religion" are traced to *religare*, to tie back, *to bind to something preceding itself.* (Compare also the noun "religion" with the adjective "religious." The adjective springs even freer (in usage) than the noun, i.e. it ascribes a quality of attitude that struggles to close the distance between the actual (the *is*) and the ideal (the *ought*)—of holding with something that ties and that binds one, that identifies oneself with some value one holds even in the face of futility, even when one is alone...)

Note that some of these meanings are quite "earth bound," i.e. they are secular and even anti-spiritual. Marxism may be a religion within definition 5. or at least within definition 6., and this despite its own denunciation of immanence or of anything "up there" or "out there." Definition 4. is easily sufficient to include cults.[2] Are these also within the "religion" of the first amendment's purview?

Definition 3. itself does not rigorously require any sense of divinity or of God, whether personal or impersonal; it is enough that one hold some belief in "supernatural *** influences controlling one's *** destiny." Such a definition is quite consistent with one common view of astrology—without God, church, or any particularized articles of faith. Does the free exercise of astrology, and equally of Marxism on the other hand, bring the "religion" clauses of the first amendment into play?

B. Because the establishment clause may be thought to be principally concerned with disallowing government acts tending toward "*establishment* of religion," i.e. establishment of religion under government auspices, as distinct from the more general protection of "freedom of conscience"[3]—the preserve more particularly (though not exclusively) of the free exercise clause—there has been some inclination to view the word "religion" somewhat differently depending upon *which* clause is invoked, i.e. the establishment clause or the free exercise clause.[4]

---

2. Cf. Africa v. Pennsylvania, 662 F.2d 1025 (3d Cir. 1981), *cert. denied*, 450 U.S. 908 (1982) (discussing and delimiting "religion").

3. For works generally arguing for *this* construction of "religion" as protected by the first amendment, see Ronald Dworkin, Taking Rights Seriously 200-01 (1977); Milton Ridvas Konvitz, Religious Liberty and Conscience (1967); David A. J. Richards, Toleration and the Constitution 136-46, 238 (1986). Historically oriented scholarship tends to reject these claims, requiring at a minimum a belief in *some* transcendental extrapersonal or otherworldly source of personal duty, even if not identified to a concrete notion of God. See, e.g., Stanley Ingber, Religion and Ideology: A Needed Clarification of the Religion Clauses, 41 Stan.L.Rev. 233 (1989); Michael W. McConnell, The Origins and Historical Understanding of Free Exercise of Religion, 103 Harv.L.Rev. 1409, 1488-1500 (1990).

Professor Jesse Choper, a principal commentator on the religion clauses, suggests an additional requirement to qualify a free exercise claim—that the law would require an act or forbid an act the performance of which, or the forbearance from which, would at once imperil one in some extratemporal manner, i.e that it would carry post-death consequences which the state cannot control. Jesse H. Choper, Defining "Religion" in the First Amendment, 1981 U.Ill.L.Rev. 579. Similar though not the same is M. Sandel, Freedom of Conscience or Freedom of Choice, in Articles of Faith, Articles of Peace 74 (James Davison Hunter & Os Guiness eds. 1990) (the religiously impelled person does not choose, i.e he or she feels no freedom to do so; rather the religious person is an "encumbered" self). Sandel does not use the phrase, but his essay is insightful even in the literal definition of "religion" and *religare*, noted *supra*, in the sense of being literally tied, and not possessing choice. The reasoning person, idealized by the Enlightenment, may choose the good and wager all—including death itself—on its account. The dividing line is with the person who feels no power of election, i.e the matter (for him) is literally out of his hands.

4. E.g., Members or representatives of a group may sometimes designate the group as non-religious (e.g., as "Science") to avoid the strictures of the establishment clause, for example, to qualify for inclusion in public school curricula, or to qualify for federal grants. See, e.g., Edwards v. Aguillard,

The notion here is fairly obvious: the first clause seems to be principally concerned with ecclesiastical organizations, with churches, with official articles of faith, practice, and worship; the second clause may seem more spacious, i.e. more concerned with liberty—"religious" liberty— freedom of belief and of *personal conscience* needing breathing room from callous disregard by the secular state. So, for instance, it has been suggested that:

> [All] that is "*arguably religious*" should be considered religious in a free exercise analysis [and] anything "*arguably non-religious*" should not be considered religious in applying the establishment clause.[5]

Thus unless the state seems to seek to advance an organized church or a preferred religion or set of religions or their doctrines, the establishment clause should seldom be deemed to be drawn into play. But insofar as the thick layers of ordinary law may far more routinely create severe headwinds for conscience, often unnecessarily (or so it may be argued), the appropriate protection of the latter is conducive to a more generous view of "religion," more freely enabling one to state a free exercise claim.[6]

On the other hand, Justice Rutledge, in *Everson*, seemed to rule out this very bifurcation:

> "Religion" appears only once in the [First] Amendment. But the word governs two prohibition and governs them alike. It does not have two meanings, one narrow to forbid "an establishment" and another, much broader, for securing "the free exercise thereof." "Thereof" brings down "religion" with its entire and exact content, no more and no less, from the first into the second

482 U.S. 578 (1987) (holding invalid pursuant to the establishment clause a state statute mandating equal time for classroom instruction in "Creation Science" as for evolution); Malnak v. Yogi, 592 F.2d 197 (3d Cir. 1979) ("Science" of Creative Intelligence-Transcendental Meditation held to be essentially religious in character and thus ineligible for federal funding in public schools). Quite oppositely, Scientology (founded by L. Ron Hubbard) became the "Church of Scientology," gaining thereby the protections and exemptions of religions under statutes and under the free exercise clause. See, e.g:, Founding Church of Scientology v. United States, 409 F.2d 1146 (D.C. Cir. 1969).

5. Laurence H. Tribe, American Constitutional Law 848 (1977). Cf. Laurence H. Tribe, American Constitutional Law 1186 (2d ed. 1988) (abandoning former position). See also Note, Toward a Constitutional Definition of Religion, 91 Harv.L.Rev. 1056 (1978) (likewise proposing a "bifurcated" definition, with "religion" defined as embracing matters deemed of "ultimate concern" to the individual, under the free exercise clause, a narrower definition being applied in reviewing establishment clause objections or claims). (The "ultimate concern" suggestion is taken from Paul Tillich, The Shakings of Foundations 63-64 (1972); it is synonymous with whatever one "take[s] seriously without any reservation," whether or not related to any notion of God or of immanence as such.)

6. See also William W. Van Alstyne, Constitutional Separation of Church and State: The Quest for a Coherent Position, 57 Amer.Pol.Sci.Rev. 865, 873-75 (1963) (de facto the Court has been more receptive toward a broad view of "religion" in qualifying free exercise claims than in validating establishment clause objections).

> guaranty, so that Congress and now the states are as broadly restricted concerning the one as they are regarding the other.[7]

Perhaps it is just as well to see what has become of this issue in the Supreme Court.[8]

TORCASO v. WATKINS
367 U.S. 488 (1961)

MR. JUSTICE BLACK delivered the opinion of the Court.

Article 37 of the Declaration of Rights of the Maryland Constitution provides:

> [N]o religious test ought ever to be required as a qualification for any office of profit or trust in this State, other than a declaration of belief in the existence of God ***.

The appellant Torcaso was appointed to the office of Notary Public by the Governor of Maryland but was refused a commission to serve because he would not declare his belief in God. He then brought this action in a Maryland Circuit Court to compel issuance of his commission, charging that the State's requirement that he declare this belief violated "the First and Fourteenth Amendments to the Constitution of the United States."[1] The Circuit Court rejected these federal constitutional contentions, and the highest court of the State, the Court of Appeals, affirmed. ***

There is, and can be, no dispute about the purpose or effect of the Maryland Declaration of Rights requirement before us—it sets up a religious test which was designed to and, if valid, does bar every person who refuses to declare a belief in God from holding a public "office of profit or trust" in Maryland. The power and authority of the State of Maryland thus is put on the side of one particular sort of believers— those who are willing to say they believe in "the existence of God." It is true that there is much historical precedent for such laws. Indeed, it was largely

---

7. 330 U.S. 1, 32 (Rutledge, J., dissenting).

8. For additional suggestions and approaches, see George C. Freeman, III, The Misguided Search for the Constitutional Definition of "Religion," 71 Geo.L.J. 1519 (1983); Kent Greenawalt, Religion as a Concept of Constitutional Law, 72 Calif.L.Rev. 753 (1984); Timothy L. Hall, Note, The Sacred and the Profane: A First Amendment Definition of Religion, 61 Tex.L.Rev. 139 (1982); Gail Merel, The Protection of Individual Choice: A Consistent Understanding of Religion Under the First Amendment, 45 U.Chi.L.Rev. 805 (1978). More generally, see John Dewey, Intelligence in the Modern World 1036 (Joseph Ratner ed., 1939); Julian Huxley, Religion Without Revelation 20, 194 (1957); William James, Essays in Pragmatism 122-124 (A. Castell ed., 1952).

1. Appellant also claimed that the State's test oath requirement violates the provision of Art. VI of the Federal Constitution that "no religious Test shall ever be required as a Qualification to any Office or public Trust under the United States." Because we are reversing the judgment on other grounds, we find it unnecessary to consider appellant's contention that this provision applies to state as well as federal offices.

to escape religious test oaths and declarations that a great many of the early colonists left Europe and came here hoping to worship in their own way. It soon developed, however, that many of those who had fled to escape religious test oaths turned out to be perfectly willing, when they had the power to do so, to force dissenters from their faith to take test oaths in conformity with that faith. This brought on a host of laws in the new Colonies imposing burdens and disabilities of various kinds upon varied beliefs depending largely upon what group happened to be politically strong enough to legislate in favor of its own beliefs. The effect of all this was the formal or practical "establishment" of particular religious faiths in most of the Colonies, with consequent burdens imposed on the free exercise of the faiths of nonfavored believers.

There were, however, wise and far-seeing men in the Colonies—too many to mention—who spoke out against test oaths and all the philosophy of intolerance behind them. One of these, it so happens, was George Calvert (the first Lord Baltimore), who took a most important part in the original establishment of the Colony of Maryland. He was a Catholic and had, for this reason, felt compelled by his conscience to refuse to take the Oath of Supremacy in England at the cost of resigning from high governmental office. He again refused to take that oath when it was demanded by the Council of the Colony of Virginia, and as a result he was denied settlement in that Colony. A recent historian of the early period of Maryland's life has said that it was Calvert's hope and purpose to establish in Maryland a colonial government free from the religious persecutions he had known—one "securely beyond the reach of oaths ***."

Since prior cases in this Court have thoroughly explored and documented the history behind the First Amendment, the reasons for it, and the scope of the religious freedom it protects, we need not cover that ground again. ***

We repeat and again reaffirm that neither a State nor the Federal Government can constitutionally force a person "to profess a belief or disbelief in any religion." Neither can constitutionally pass laws or impose requirements which aid all religions as against non-believers and neither can aid those religions based on a belief in the existence of God as against those religions founded on different beliefs.[11] *** This Maryland religious test for public office unconstitutionally invades the appellant's freedom of belief and religion and therefore cannot be enforced against him. ***

Reversed and remanded.

---

11. Among religions in this country which do not teach what would generally be considered a belief in the existence of God are Buddhism, Taoism, Ethical Culture, Secular Humanism and others. See Washington Ethical Society v. District of Columbia, 249 F.2d 127; Fellowship of Humanity v. County of Alameda, 315 P.2d 394; II Encyclopaedia of the Social Sciences 293; 4 Encyclopaedia Britannica (1957 ed.) 325-327; 21 *id.*, at 797; Archer, Faiths Men Live by (2d ed. revised by Purinton), 120-138, 254-313; 1961 World Almanac 695, 712; Year Book of American Churches for 1961, at 29, 47. [**Ed. Note.** This footnote is itself part of Justice Black's "opinion of the Court." (i.e., it is Footnote 11. in *Torcaso v. Watkins*).]

MR. JUSTICE FRANKFURTER and MR. JUSTICE HARLAN concur in the result.

UNITED STATES v. SEEGER
380 U.S. 163 (1965)

MR. JUSTICE CLARK delivered the opinion of the Court.

These cases involve claims of conscientious objectors under § 6(j) of the Universal Military Training and Service Act, 50 U.S.C.App. § 456(j) (1958 ed.), which exempts from combatant training and service in the armed forces of the United States those persons who by reason of their religious training and belief are conscientiously opposed to participation in war in any form. The parties raise the basic question of the constitutionality of the section which defines the term "religious training and belief," as used in the Act, as "an individual's belief in a relation to a Supreme Being involving duties superior to those arising from any human relation, but (not including) essentially political, sociological, or philosophical views or a merely personal moral code." The constitutional attack is launched under the First Amendment's Establishment and Free Exercise Clauses and is twofold: (1) The section does not exempt nonreligious conscientious objectors; and (2) it discriminates between different forms of religious expression in violation of the Due Process Clause of the Fifth Amendment. ***

Seeger was convicted of having refused to submit to induction in the armed forces. He was originally classified 1-A in 1953 by his local board, but this classification was changed in 1955 to 2-S (student) and he remained in this status until 1958 when he was reclassified 1-A. He first claimed exemption as a conscientious objector in 1957 after successive annual renewals of his student classification. Although he did not adopt verbatim the printed Selective Service System form, he declared that he was conscientiously opposed to participation in war in any form by reason of his "religious" belief; that he preferred to leave the question as to his belief in a Supreme Being open, "rather than answer 'yes' or 'no';" that his "skepticism or disbelief in the existence of God" did "not necessarily mean lack of faith in anything whatsoever;" that his was a "belief in and devotion to goodness and virtue for their own sakes, and a religious faith in a purely ethical creed." He cited such personages as Plato, Aristotle and Spinoza for support of his ethical belief in intellectual and moral integrity "without belief in God, except in the remotest sense." His belief was found to be sincere, honest, and made in good faith; and his conscientious objection to be based upon individual training and belief, both of which included research in religious and cultural fields. Seeger's claim, however, was denied solely because it was not based upon a "belief in a relation to a Supreme Being" as required by § 6(j) of the Act.

At trial Seeger's counsel admitted that Seeger's belief was not in relation to a Supreme Being as commonly understood, but contended that he was entitled to the exemption because "under the present law Mr. Seeger's position would also include definitions of religion which have been stated more recently," and could be "accommodated" under the definition of religious training and belief in the Act. *** [T]he Court of Appeals [held] that the Supreme Being requirement of the section distinguished "between internally derived and externally compelled beliefs" and was, therefore, an "impermissible classification" under the Due Process Clause of the Fifth Amendment. ***

BACKGROUND OF § 6 (j)

The Draft Act of 1917 afforded exemptions to conscientious objectors who were affiliated with a "well-recognized religious sect or organization [then] organized and existing and whose existing creed or principles [forbade] its members to participate in war in any form." In adopting the 1940 Selective Training and Service Act Congress broadened the exemption afforded in the 1917 Act by making it unnecessary to belong to a pacifist religious sect if the claimant's own opposition to war was based on "religious training and belief." Those found to be within the exemption were not inducted into the armed services but were assigned to noncombatant service under the supervision of the Selective Service System. The Congress recognized that one might be religious without belonging to an organized church just as surely as minority members of a faith not opposed to war might through religious reading reach a conviction against participation in war. ***

[I]n 1948 the Congress amended the language of the statute and declared that "religious training and belief" was to be defined as "an individual's belief in a relation to a Supreme Being involving duties superior to those arising from any human relation, but (not including) essentially political, sociological, or philosophical views or a merely personal moral code." ***

INTERPRETATION OF § 6 (j)

Few would quarrel, we think, with the proposition that in no field of human endeavor has the tool of language proved so inadequate in the communication of ideas as it has in dealing with the fundamental questions of man's predicament in life, in death or in final judgment and retribution. This fact makes the task of discerning the intent of Congress in using the phrase "Supreme Being" a complex one. Nor is it made the easier by the richness and variety of spiritual life in our country. Over 250 sects inhabit our land. Some believe in a purely personal God, some in a supernatural deity; others think of religion as a way of life envisioning as its ultimate goal the day when all men can live together in perfect understanding and peace. There are those who think of God as the depth of our being; others, such as the Buddhists, strive for a state of lasting rest through self-denial and inner purification; in Hindu philosophy, the Supreme Being is the transcendental reality which is truth, knowledge and bliss. ***

Under the 1940 Act it was necessary only to have a conviction based upon religious training and belief; we believe that is all that is required here. Within that phrase would come all sincere religious beliefs which are based upon a power or being, or upon a faith, to which all else is subordinate or upon which all else is ultimately dependent. The test might be stated in these words: A sincere and meaningful belief which occupies in the life of its possessor a place parallel to that filled by the God of those admittedly qualifying for the exemption comes within the statutory definition. This construction avoids imputing to Congress an intent to classify different religious beliefs, exempting some and excluding others, and is in accord with the well- established congressional policy of equal treatment for those whose opposition to service is grounded in their religious tenets.

*** While the applicant's words may differ, the test is simple of application. It is essentially an objective one, namely, does the claimed belief occupy the same place in the life of the objector as an orthodox belief in God holds in the life of one clearly qualified for exemption? Moreover, it must be remembered that in resolving these exemption problems one deals with the beliefs of different individuals who will articulate them in a multitude of ways. In such an intensely personal area, of course, the claim of the registrant that his belief is an essential part of a religious faith must be given great weight. ***

APPLICATION OF § 6 (j) TO THE INSTANT CASE

As we noted earlier, the statutory definition excepts those registrants whose beliefs are based on a "merely personal moral code." The records in this case, however, show that at no time did [Seeger] suggest that his objection was based on a "merely personal moral code." Indeed at the outset [he] claimed in his application that his objection was based on a religious belief. We have construed the statutory definition broadly and it follows that any exception to it must be interpreted narrowly. The use by Congress of the words "merely personal" seems to us to restrict the exception to a moral code which is not only personal but which is the sole basis for the registrant's belief and is in no way related to a Supreme Being. It follows, therefore, that if the claimed religious beliefs meet the test that we lay down then their objections cannot be based on a "merely personal" moral code.

In *Seeger*, the Court of Appeals failed to find sufficient "externally compelled beliefs." However, it did find that "it would seem impossible to say with assurance that [Seeger] is not bowing to 'external commands' in virtually the same sense as is the objector who defers to the will of a supernatural power." *** The Court of Appeals also found that there was no question of the applicant's sincerity. He was a product of a devout Roman Catholic home; he was a close student of Quaker beliefs from which he said "much of [his] thought is derived"; he approved of their opposition to war in any form; he devoted his spare hours to the American Friends Service Committee and was assigned to hospital duty.

In summary, Seeger professed "religious belief" and "religious faith." He did not disavow any belief "in a relation to a Supreme Being"; indeed he stated that "the cosmic order does, perhaps, suggest a creative intelligence." He decried the tremendous "spiritual" price man must pay for his willingness to destroy human life. In light of his beliefs and the unquestioned sincerity with which he held them, we think the Board, had it applied the test we propose today, would have granted him the exemption. We think it clear that the beliefs which prompted his objection occupy the same place in his life as the belief in a traditional deity holds in the lives of his friends, the Quakers. We are reminded once more of Dr. Tillich's thoughts:

> "And if that word [God] has not much meaning for you, translate it, and speak of the depths of your life, of the source of your being, or your ultimate concern, *of what you take seriously without any reservation.* Perhaps, in order to do so, you must forget everything traditional that you have learned about God ***." Tillich, The Shaking of the Foundations 57 (1948). (Emphasis supplied.)

It may be that Seeger did not clearly demonstrate what his beliefs were with regard to the usual understanding of the term "Supreme Being." But as we have said Congress did not intend that to be the test. We therefore affirm the judgment. ***

MR. JUSTICE DOUGLAS, concurring.

If I read the statute differently from the Court, I would have difficulties. For then those who embraced one religious faith rather than another would be subject to penalties; and that kind of discrimination, as we held in Sherbert v. Verner, 374 U.S. 398, would violate the Free Exercise Clause of the First Amendment. It would also result in a denial of equal protection by preferring some religions over others—an invidious discrimination that would run afoul of the Due Process Clause of the Fifth Amendment. See Bolling v. Sharpe, 347 U.S. 497.

The legislative history of this Act leaves much in the dark. But it is, in my opinion, not a *tour de force* if we construe the words "Supreme Being" to include the cosmos, as well as an anthropomorphic entity. If it is a *tour de force* so to hold, it is no more so than other instances where we have gone to extremes to construe an Act of Congress to save it from demise on constitutional grounds. In a more extreme case than the present one we said that the words of a statute may be strained "in the candid service of avoiding a serious constitutional doubt." United States v. Rumely, 345 U.S. 41, 47. ***

WELSH v. UNITED STATES

398 U.S. 333 1970

MR. JUSTICE BLACK announced the judgment of the Court and delivered an opinion in which MR. JUSTICE DOUGLAS, MR. JUSTICE BRENNAN, and MR. JUSTICE MARSHALL join.

The petitioner, Elliott Ashton Welsh II, was convicted by a United States District Judge of refusing to submit to induction into the Armed Forces in violation of 50 U.S.C.App. § 462 (a), and was on June 1, 1966, sentenced to imprisonment for three years. One of petitioner's defenses to the prosecution was that § 6 (j) of the Universal Military Training and Service Act exempted him from combat and noncombat service because he was "by reason of religious training and belief *** conscientiously opposed to participation in war in any form." *** For the reasons to be stated, and without passing upon the constitutional arguments that have been raised, we vote to reverse this conviction because of its fundamental inconsistency with *United States v. Seeger*.

The controlling facts in this case are strikingly similar to those in *Seeger*. Both Seeger and Welsh were brought up in religious homes and attended church in their childhood, but in neither case was this church one which taught its members not to engage in war at any time for any reason. Neither Seeger nor Welsh continued his childhood religious ties into his young manhood, and neither belonged to any religious group or adhered to the teachings of any organized religion during the period of his involvement with the Selective Service System. At the time of registration for the draft, neither had yet come to accept pacifist principles. Their views on war developed only in subsequent years, but when their ideas did fully mature both made application to their local draft boards for conscientious objector exemptions from military service under § 6 (j) of the Universal Military Training and Service Act. That section then provided, in part:

> Nothing contained in this title shall be construed to require any person to be subject to combatant training and service in the armed forces of the United States who, by reason of religious training and belief, is conscientiously opposed to participation in war in any form. Religious training and belief in this connection means an individual's belief in a relation to a Supreme Being involving duties superior to those arising from any human relation, but does not include essentially political, sociological, or philosophical views or a merely personal moral code.

In filling out their exemption applications both Seeger and Welsh were unable to sign the statement that, as printed in the Selective Service form, stated "I am, by reason of my religious training and belief, conscientiously opposed to participation in war in any form." Seeger could sign only after striking the words "training and" and putting quotation marks around the word "religious." Welsh could sign only after striking the words "my religious training and." On those same applications, neither could definitely affirm or deny that he believed in a "Supreme Being," both stating that they preferred to leave the question open.[3] But both Seeger and Welsh affirmed on those applications that they held deep conscientious scruples against taking part in wars where people were killed. Both strongly believed that killing in war was wrong, unethical, and immoral, and their consciences forbade them to take part in such an evil practice. Their objection to participating in war in any form could not be said to come from a "still, small voice of conscience;" rather, for them that voice was so loud and insistent that both men preferred to go to jail rather than

---

3. In his original application in April 1964, Welsh stated that he did not believe in a Supreme Being, but in a letter to his local board in June 1965, he requested that his original answer be stricken and the question left open.

serve in the Armed Forces. There was never any question about the sincerity and depth of Seeger's convictions as a conscientious objector, and the same is true of Welsh. Seeger's conscientious objector claim was denied "solely because it was not based upon a 'belief in a relation to a Supreme Being' as required by § 6 (j) of the Act," while Welsh was denied the exemption because his Appeal Board and the Department of Justice hearing officer "could find no religious basis for the registrant's beliefs, opinions and convictions." Both Seeger and Welsh subsequently refused to submit to induction into the military and both were convicted of that offense.

*** In resolving the question whether Seeger and the other registrants in that case qualified for the exemption, the Court stated that "[the] task is to decide whether the beliefs professed by a registrant are sincerely held and whether they are, *in his own scheme of things*, religious." The reference to the registrant's "own scheme of things" was intended to indicate that the central consideration in determining whether the registrant's beliefs are religious is whether these beliefs play the role of a religion and function as a religion in the registrant's life. The Court's principal statement of its test for determining whether a conscientious objector's beliefs are religious within the meaning of § 6(j) was as follows:

> The test might be stated in these words: A sincere and meaningful belief which occupies in the life of its possessor a place parallel to that filled by the God of those admittedly qualifying for the exemption comes within the statutory definition.

What is necessary under *Seeger* for a registrant's conscientious objection to all war to be "religious" within the meaning of § 6 (j) is that this opposition to war stem from the registrant's moral, ethical, or religious beliefs about what is right and wrong and that these beliefs be held with the strength of traditional religious convictions. Most of the great religions of today and of the past have embodied the idea of a Supreme Being or a Supreme Reality—a God—who communicates to man in some way a consciousness of what is right and should be done, of what is wrong and therefore should be shunned. If an individual deeply and sincerely holds beliefs that are purely ethical or moral in source and content but that nevertheless impose upon him a duty of conscience to refrain from participating in any war at any time, those beliefs certainly occupy in the life of that individual "a place parallel to that filled by *** God" in traditionally religious persons. ***

In the case before us the Government seeks to distinguish our holding in *Seeger* on basically two grounds, both of which were relied upon by the Court of Appeals in affirming Welsh's conviction. First, it is stressed that Welsh was far more insistent and explicit than Seeger in denying that his views were religious. For example, in filling out their conscientious objector applications, Seeger put quotation marks around the word "religious," but Welsh struck the word "religious" entirely and later characterized his beliefs as having been formed "by reading in the fields of history and sociology." The Court of Appeals found that Welsh had "denied that his objection to war was premised on religious belief" and concluded that "[t]he Appeal Board was entitled to take him at his word." We think this attempt to distinguish *Seeger* fails for the reason that it places undue emphasis on the registrant's interpretation of his own beliefs. *** When a registrant states that his objections to war are "religious," that information is highly relevant to the question of the function his beliefs have in his life. But very few registrants are fully aware of the broad scope of the word "religious" as used in § 6 (j), and accordingly a registrant's statement that his beliefs are nonreligious is a highly unreliable guide for those charged with administering the exemption. Welsh himself presents a case in point. Although he originally characterized his beliefs as nonreligious, he later upon reflection wrote a long and thoughtful letter to his Appeal Board in which he declared that his beliefs were "certainly religious in the ethical sense of the word." He explained:

> I believe I mentioned taking of life as not being, for me, a religious wrong. Again, I assumed Mr. [Brady (the Department of Justice hearing officer)] was using the word 'religious' in the conventional sense, and, in order to be perfectly honest did not characterize my belief as 'religious.' ***

The Government also seeks to distinguish *Seeger* on the ground that Welsh's views, unlike Seeger's, were "essentially political, sociological, or philosophical views or a merely personal moral code." As previously noted, the Government made the same argument about Seeger, and not without reason, for Seeger's views had a substantial political dimension. In this case, Welsh's conscientious objection to war was undeniably based in part on his perception of world politics. In a letter to his local board, he wrote:

> I can only act according to what I am and what I see. And I see that the military complex wastes both human and material resources, that it fosters disregard for (what I consider a paramount concern) human needs and ends; I see that the means we employ to 'defend' our 'way of life' profoundly change that way of life. I see that in our failure to recognize the political, social, and economic realities of the world, we, *as a nation*, fail our responsibility *as a nation*.

We certainly do not think that § 6 (j)'s exclusion of those persons with "essentially political, sociological, or philosophical views or a merely personal moral code" should be read to exclude those who hold strong beliefs about our domestic and foreign affairs or even those whose conscientious objection to participation in all wars is founded to a substantial extent upon considerations of public policy. The two groups of registrants that obviously do fall within these exclusions from the exemption are those whose beliefs are not deeply held and those whose objection to war does not rest at all upon moral, ethical, or religious principle but instead rests solely upon considerations of policy, pragmatism, or expediency. ***

*** Welsh elaborated his beliefs in later communications with Selective Service officials. On the basis of these beliefs and the conclusion of the Court of Appeals that he held them "with the strength of more traditional religious convictions," we think Welsh was clearly entitled to a conscientious objector exemption. Section 6 (j) requires no more. That section exempts from military service all those whose consciences, spurred by deeply held moral, ethical, or religious beliefs, would give them no rest or peace if they allowed themselves to become a part of an instrument of war.

The judgment is [r]eversed.

MR. JUSTICE HARLAN, concurring in the result.

* * *

In my opinion, the liberties taken with the statute both in *Seeger* and today's decision cannot be justified in the name of the familiar doctrine of construing federal statutes in a manner that will avoid possible constitutional infirmities in them. *** I therefore find myself unable to escape facing the constitutional issue that this case squarely presents: whether §6 (j) in limiting this draft exemption to those opposed to war in general because of theistic beliefs runs afoul of the religious clauses of the First Amendment. For reasons later appearing I believe it does, and on that basis I concur in the judgment reversing this conviction, and adopt the test announced by Mr. Justice Black, not as a matter of statutory construction, but as the touchstone for salvaging a congressional policy of long standing that would otherwise have to be nullified. ***

The natural reading of § 6 (j), which quite evidently draws a distinction between theistic and nontheistic religions, is the only one that is consistent with the legislative history. In United States v. Kauten, 133 F.2d 703 (C.A.2d Cir. 1943), the Second Circuit, speaking through Judge Augustus Hand, broadly construed "religious training and belief" to include a "belief finding expression in a conscience which categorically requires the believer to disregard elementary self-interest and to accept martyrdom in preference to transgressing its tenets." This expansive interpretation of § 5(g) was rejected by a divided Ninth Circuit in Berman v. United States, 156 F.2d 377, 380-381 (1946). In the wake of this intercircuit dialogue, crystallized by the dissent in *Berman* which espoused the Second Circuit interpretation in *Kauten*, Congress enacted § 6 (j) in 1948. That Congress intended to anoint the Ninth Circuit's interpretation of § 5 (g) would seem beyond question in view of the similarity of the statutory language to that used by Chief Justice Hughes in his dissenting opinion in *Macintosh* and quoted in *Berman* and the Senate report. The report stated:

> This section reenacts substantially the same provisions as were found in subsection 5 (g) of the 1940 act. Exemption extends to anyone who, because of religious training and belief in his relationship to a Supreme Being, is conscientiously opposed to combatant military service or to both combatant and noncombatant military service. (See United States v. Berman [*sic*], 156 F.(2d) 377, certiorari denied, 329 U.S. 795.)

Against this legislative history it is a remarkable feat of judicial surgery to remove as did *Seeger*, the theistic requirement of § 6(j). ***

I cannot subscribe to a wholly emasculated construction of a statute to avoid facing a latent constitutional question, in purported fidelity to the salutary doctrine of avoiding unnecessary resolution of constitutional issues, a principle to which I fully adhere. [I]t is not permissible, in my judgment, to take a lateral step that robs legislation of all meaning in order to avert the collision between its plainly intended purpose and the commands of the Constitution. I therefore turn to the constitutional question.

The constitutional question that must be faced in this case is whether a statute that defers to the individual's conscience only when his views emanate from adherence to theistic religious beliefs is within the power of Congress. Congress, of course, could, entirely consistently with the requirements of the Constitution, eliminate all exemptions for conscientious objectors. Such a course would be wholly "neutral" and, in my view, would not offend the Free Exercise Clause, for reasons set forth in my dissenting opinion in Sherbert v. Verner, 374 U.S. 398, 418 (1963). See Kurland, Of Church and State and the Supreme Court, 29 U.Chi.L.Rev. 1 (1961). However, having chosen to exempt, it cannot draw the line between theistic or nontheistic religious beliefs on the one hand and secular beliefs on the other. Any such distinctions are not, in my view, compatible with the Establishment Clause of the First Amendment. See my separate opinion in Walz v. Tax Comm'n, 397 U.S. 664, 694 (1970). The implementation of the neutrality principle of these cases requires, in my view, as I stated in *Walz v. Tax Comm'n*, "an equal protection mode of analysis. The Court must survey meticulously the circumstances of governmental categories to eliminate, as it were, religious gerrymanders. In any particular case the critical question is whether the scope of legislation encircles a class so broad that it can be fairly concluded that [all groups that] could be thought to fall within the natural perimeter [are included]." The "radius" of this legislation is the conscientiousness with which an individual opposes war in general, yet the statute, as I think it must be construed, excludes from its "scope" individuals motivated by teachings of nontheistic religions,[8] and individuals guided by an inner ethical voice that bespeaks secular and not "religious" reflection. It not only accords a preference to the "religious" but also disadvantages adherents of religions that do not worship a Supreme Being. The constitutional infirmity cannot be cured, moreover, even by an impermissible construction that eliminates the theistic requirement and simply draws the line between religious and nonreligious. This in my view offends the Establishment Clause and is that kind of classification that this Court has condemned. ***

8. This Court has taken notice of the fact that recognized "religions" exist that "do not teach what would generally be considered a belief in the existence of God," Torcaso v. Watkins, 367 U.S. 488, 495 n. 11, e.g., "Buddhism, Taoism, Ethical Culture, Secular Humanism and others."

If the exemption is to be given application, it must encompass the class of individuals it purports to exclude, those whose beliefs emanate from a purely moral, ethical, or philosophical source.[9] The common denominator must be the intensity of moral conviction with which a belief is held. Common experience teaches that among "religious" individuals some are weak and others strong adherents to tenets and this is no less true of individuals whose lives are guided by personal ethical considerations.

[A]uthorities assembled by the Government, far from advancing its case, demonstrate the unconstitutionality of the distinction drawn in § 6 (j) between religious and nonreligious beliefs. Everson v. Board of Education, 330 U. S. 1 (1947), the Sunday Closing Law Cases, 366 U.S. 420, 582-599, and 617 (1961), and Board of Education v. Allen, 392 U.S. 236 (1968), all sustained legislation on the premise that it was neutral in its application and thus did not constitute an establishment, notwithstanding the fact that it may have assisted religious groups by giving them the same benefits accorded to non-religious groups.[12] To the extent that Zorach v. Clauson, 343 U.S. 306 (1952), and *Sherbert v. Verner*, stand for the proposition that the Government may (*Zorach*), or must (*Sherbert*), shape its secular programs to accommodate the beliefs and tenets of religious groups, I think these cases unsound.[13] ***

---

9. In Sherbert v. Verner, 374 U.S. 398 (1963), the Court held unconstitutional over my dissent a state statute that conditioned eligibility for unemployment benefits on being "able to work and *** available for work" and further provided that a claimant was ineligible "[i]f *** he has failed, without good cause *** to accept available suitable work when offered him by the employment office or the employer ***." This, the Court held, was a violation of the Free Exercise Clause as applied to Seventh Day Adventists whose religious background forced them as a matter of conscience to decline Saturday employment. My own conclusion, to which I still adhere, is that the Free Exercise Clause does not require a State to conform a neutral secular program to the dictates of religious conscience of any group. I suggested, however, that a State could constitutionally create exceptions to its program to accommodate religious scruples. That suggestion must, however, be qualified by the observation that any such exception in order to satisfy the Establishment Clause of the First Amendment, would have to be sufficiently broad to be religiously neutral. See my separate opinion in *Walz v. Tax Comm'n.* This would require creating an exception for anyone who, as a matter of conscience, could not comply with the statute. ***

12. *** Section 6 (j) speaks directly to belief divorced entirely from conduct. It evinces a judgment that individuals who hold the beliefs set forth by the statute should not be required to bear arms and the statutory belief that qualifies is only a religious belief. *** Congress, whether in response to political considerations or simply out of sensitivity for men of religious conscience, can of course decline to exercise its power to conscript to the fullest extent, but it cannot do so without equal regard for men of nonreligious conscience. It goes without saying that the First Amendment is perforce a guarantee that the conscience of religion may not be preferred simply because organized religious groups in general are more visible than the individual who practices morals and ethics on his own. Any view of the Free Exercise Clause that does not insist on this neutrality would engulf the Establishment Clause and render it vestigial.

13. That the "released-time" program in *Zorach* did not utilize classroom facilities for religious instruction, unlike McCollum v. Board of Education, 333 U.S. 203 (1948), is a distinction for me without Establishment Clause substance. At the very least the Constitution requires that the State not

Where a statute is defective because of underinclusion there exist two remedial alternatives: a court may either declare it a nullity and order that its benefits not extend to the class that the legislature intended to benefit, or it may extend the coverage of the statute to include those who are aggrieved by exclusion.

The appropriate disposition of this case, which is a prosecution for refusing to submit to induction and not an action for a declaratory judgment on the constitutionality of § 6 (j), is determined by the fact that at the time of Welsh's induction, notice and prosecution the Selective Service was, as required by statute, exempting individuals whose beliefs were identical in all respects to those held by petitioner except that they derived from a religious source. Since this created a religious benefit not accorded to petitioner, it is clear to me that this conviction must be reversed under the Establishment Clause of the First Amendment unless Welsh is to go remediless. *** Thus I am prepared to accept the prevailing opinion's conscientious objector test, not as a reflection of congressional statutory intent but as patchwork of judicial making that cures the defect of underinclusion in § 6 (j) and can be administered by local boards in the usual course of business. Like the prevailing opinion, I also conclude that petitioner's beliefs are held with the required intensity and consequently vote to reverse the judgment of conviction.

MR. JUSTICE WHITE, with whom THE CHIEF JUSTICE and MR. JUSTICE STEWART join, dissenting.

Whether or not United States v. Seeger, 380 U.S. 163 (1965), accurately reflected the intent of Congress in providing draft exemptions for religious conscientious objectors to war, I cannot join today's construction of § 6 (j) extending draft exemption to those who disclaim religious objections to war and whose views about war represent a purely personal code arising not from religious training and belief as the statute requires but from readings in philosophy, history, and sociology. ***

For me that conclusion should end this case. Even if Welsh is quite right in asserting that exempting religious believers is an establishment of religion forbidden by the First Amendment, he nevertheless remains one of those persons whom Congress took pains not to relieve from military duty. Whether or not § 6 (j) is constitutional, Welsh had no First Amendment excuse for refusing to report for induction. If it is contrary to the express will of Congress to exempt Welsh, as I think it is, then

---

excuse students early for the purpose of receiving religious instruction when it does not offer to nonreligious students the opportunity to use school hours for spiritual or ethical instruction of a nonreligious nature. Moreover, whether a released-time program cast in terms of improving "conscience" to the exclusion of artistic or cultural pursuits, would be "neutral" and consistent with the requirement of "voluntarism," is by no means an easy question. Such a limited program is quite unlike the broad approach of the tax exemption statute, sustained in *Walz v. Tax Comm'n*, which included literary societies, playgrounds, and associations "for the moral or mental improvement of men."

there is no warrant for saving the religious exemption and the statute by redrafting it in this Court to include Welsh and all others like him. ***

If I am wrong in thinking that *Welsh* cannot benefit from invalidation of § 6(j) on Establishment Clause grounds, I would nevertheless affirm his conviction; for I cannot hold that Congress violated the Clause in exempting from the draft all those who oppose war by reason of religious training and belief. *** I would not frustrate congressional will by construing the Establishment Clause to condition the exemption for religionists upon extending the exemption also to those who object to war on nonreligious grounds.

We have said that neither support nor hostility, but neutrality, is the goal of the religion clauses of the First Amendment. "Neutrality," however, is not self-defining. If it is "favoritism" and not "neutrality" to exempt religious believers from the draft, is it "neutrality" and not "inhibition" of religion to compel religious believers to fight when they have special reasons for not doing so, reasons to which the Constitution gives particular recognition? ***

The Establishment Clause as construed by this Court unquestionably has independent significance; its function is not wholly auxiliary to the Free Exercise Clause. It bans some involvements of the State with religion that otherwise might be consistent with the Free Exercise Clause. But when in the rationally based judgment of Congress free exercise of religion calls for shielding religious objectors from compulsory combat duty, I am reluctant to frustrate the legislative will by striking down the statutory exemption because it does not also reach those to whom the Free Exercise Clause offers no protection whatsoever.

I would affirm the judgment below.

NOTES AND QUESTIONS

Seeger and *Welsh* construed the language of an Act of Congress referring to "*religious* training and belief" very inclusively—to extend to *any* deeply seated compunction regarding one's personal participation in combatant training and service, if founded on "[a] sincere and meaningful belief that occupies in the life of its possessor a place *parallel to* that filled by the God of those admittedly qualifying for the exemption" (emphasis added). No conventional theology need be involved. In so construing the statute, moreover, Justice Clark declared that the Court did so in order to "avoid imputing to Congress an intent to classify different religious beliefs, exempting some and excluding others *** ."

Moreover, the Court suggested that were it to have given a more qualified (i.e. narrower) interpretation to the Act, as so construed the Act would have been vulnerable to an establishment clause objection. That would be so—the Court implied— because Congress would thereby have established a preference for some religions (those anchored in some sort of theism) over other religions (such as "secular humanism"?[9]) which have no such belief—and government favoritism *among* religions is disallowed by the establishment clause.

Likewise, the Court suggested, had it given a more confined definition of the scope of the exemption provided by the statute, the Act could have been subject to a valid fifth amendment due process objection on the ground that as thus construed, the Act "discriminate[d] between different forms of religious expression.'"

The plain suggestion is, again, that government *may* distinguish between "religion" and "nonreligion," and may grant a dispensation from the laws to the former without thereby being bound to grant the same dispensation to the latter;[10] but what it may not do is grant dispensation only to *some* religions (those of a sort it may favor—theistic religions) while withholding dispensation from *others* (i.e. those it may not favor— "religions" such as secular humanism that have no theology at all).

The interplay of: (a) what the establishment clause forbids (on the one hand); (b) what the free exercise clause requires (on the other hand); and (c) what the free exercise clause permits (though does not require[11]), is potentially complicated by how "religion" has been defined in these cases. For example, "inculcating religion" in the public schools is clearly forbidden under the establishment clause. But "inculcating moral values" is not only not forbidden by the establishment clause, rather, it is deemed among the more important functions of the public schools (according to the Court[12]). But given the manner in which "religion" has been defined, just what *is* it that can be "inculcated" and yet does not: (a) violate the establishment clause, (b) violate the free exercise clause; or (c) violate both?[13]

---

9. See *Torcaso*, n.11, where the Court rather matter-of-factly declared: "Among religions in this country, which do not teach what would generally be considered a belief in the existence of God are Buddhism, Taoism, *Ethical Culture, [and] Secular Humanism* *** " (emphasis added).

10. But see the very different approach reflected in Justice Harlan's concurring opinion in *Welsh*—not that Seeger or Welsh met the statutory requirement (to the contrary, in Harlan's view, neither met it), rather, that an act of Congress *cannot* confer a special advantage based on religion, for to do so is disallowed by the establishment clause; and that the equal protection of the fifth amendment entitles the *non*religious (but equally conscientious) objector to the same treatment as the religious objector. (See also Harlan's identical position on tax exemptions, in *Walz*, *supra* p. 866.) In this view, Congress did not incorrectly define a "religious conscientious objector," rather, it improperly favored religion over nonreligion as between persons having equally firm scruples against combatant training and service.

11. See *Smith*, p. 1048 *supra* (the free exercise clause generally does not require exceptions, rather, it merely permits them).

12. See, e.g., Ambach v. Norwick, 441 U.S. 68, 76-77 (1979).

13. See Edwards v. Aguillard, 482 U.S. 578 (1987) (Lousiana statute requiring equal time for "creation science"—as for "evolution science"—in public schools; *held*, violation of the establishment clause because Louisiana officials "identified no clear secular purpose"—indeed the "preeminent purpose of [the scheme] was clearly to advance the religious viewpoint"); Peloza v. Capistrano Unified Sch. Dist., 37 F.3d 517 (9th Cir. 1994), cert. denied 515 U.S. 1173 (1995) (public high school teacher challenged school district's requirement that he teach "evolutionism," on the ground that evolution is a "religious belief system" and that its teaching consequently violates the establishment clause; *held*, "neither the Supreme Court, nor this circuit, has ever held that evolutionism or secular humanism are 'religions' for Establishment Clause purposes"); Mozert v. Hawkins County Bd. of Educ., 827 F.2d

---

PROBLEM

As a final reprise on this problem and these issues, consider the following revision of an earlier case:

> The Texas Unemployment Compensation Fund is funded from payroll taxes collected from private employers in the state. The object of the Fund is to cushion the financial hardship to persons laid off or let go due to circumstances beyond their control. To that end, the plan provides that persons laid off without cause are eligible for 26 weeks unemployment compensation at 70% of their last regular wage, assuming that, despite due diligence, no alternative work for which they qualify can be found. Benefits are not available to employees who simply quit or to employees who are dismissed or replaced for just cause (e.g., employees dismissed for stealing or for failure to perform their jobs competently, or employees who simply fail to show up for work and are replaced in order that the employer's business can proceed as usual).

Recently, the following six people applied for unemployment compensation benefits at the appropriate state office. All are immediate former employees of Acme Meatpackers, Inc.:

1. **John Doe**. Doe was laid off because a downturn in Acme's business affected employees in his department. The state unemployment office reviewed current job listings and agreed with Doe that there is currently no job opportunity listed for which he might qualify.
2. **Jane Roe**. Roe was replaced at Acme following eight consecutive work days of unexcused failure to appear at work. Roe failed to appear because it was deer hunting season; she went off with her brother Pete, who persuaded her that deer hunting was more important than putting in her usual eight-hour day at Acme. Following her replacement at Acme, like Doe, Roe could find no other job opening elsewhere.

1058 (6th Cir. 1987), cert. denied, 484 U.S. 1066 (1988) (self-described "born again Christian" parents argued that Holt-Rinehart basic reading series contained themes offensive to their religious beliefs—for example, "secular humanism," "pacifism," "magic" and "women who have been recognized for achievements outside the home"—which thereby burdened students' free exercise of religion; *held*, government requirement that a person merely be *exposed* to ideas he or she finds objectionable on religious grounds does not constitute a *burden* on free exercise; students were not required to affirm or deny any beliefs, nor were they required to engage in or refrain from engaging in any conduct required or forbidden by their religion); Smith v. Board of School Comm'rs of Mobile County, 827 F.2d 684 (11th Cir. 1987) (parent argued that use of certain home economics, history and social studies textbooks advanced the "religion" of "Humanism" in violation of the establishment clause; *held*, "even assuming that secular humanism is a religion for purposes of the establishment clause," the challenged textbooks did not "convey a message of governmental approval of secular humanism or governmental disapproval of theism"—rather the textbooks were an "entirely appropriate" effort to "instill in Alabama public school children such values as independent thought, tolerance of diverse views, self-respect, maturity, self-reliance, and logical decision-making").

3. **Randy Pursley**. Pursley was likewise replaced at Acme following eight consecutive work days of unexcused failure to appear at work. Pursley's daughter was ill during this time, and Pursley placed his deep and abiding sense of obligation to care for her ahead of his job. (He would have returned to work once she no longer needed him at home.) Pursley had, however, already used the several days of excused absences provided by company rules for family hardship.
4. **Sarah Pratt**. Pratt was likewise replaced at Acme following eight consecutive work days of unexcused failure to appear at work. Pratt failed to appear after she learned that Acme made sustaining corporate contributions for the maintenance of a local memorial in honor of Jefferson Davis, the President of the Confederate States during the Civil War. Pratt, an African American, felt humiliated by this action of the Acme Board of Directions, and felt conscientiously unable to continue working for a company that spent in this way the profits she had helped to earn. Like the others, she could not find another job.
5. **Richard Parker**. Parker was likewise replaced at Acme following eight consecutive work days of unexcused failure to appear at work. Parker failed to show up because he concluded that his work at Acme was inconsistent with his being a zealous vegetarian, and equally inconsistent with his leadership in a statewide vegetarian advocacy group.
6. **Charles Goodweather**. Goodweather was likewise replaced after eight consecutive unexcused absences. Goodweather had recently converted to the Pantheism Faith, a central tenet of which is that all animal life is equally valued in God's sight, and that those who offend this precept (those who work in *meatpacking plants* surely do) will be cast out from Heaven when they die.

Just as had been the case with John Doe, the state unemployment office reviewed current job listings and agreed that there was no currently available job opportunity for which any of the remaining five was qualified.

I. Suppose that under the statute, among these six applicants, only John Doe is regarded as eligible for benefits. What constitutional complaint, if any, can be advanced by any of the other five persons, insofar as each is denied unemployment compensation benefits from the common fund? Should (or will) any of them prevail?[14] Why or why not?

---

14. If one says that Goodweather is to prevail, why is that? Has the state acted in any way to "penalize" his religion or his religious beliefs? (If Pratt and Pursley are not to be treated as eligible, why should Goodweather be regarded as constitutionally *more* entitled to financial subsidy from the state fund?)

II. Suppose the legislature amended the Act to make such persons as Goodweather eligible in addition to Doe.[15] Goodweather promptly applies for benefits under the amended act. At once, however:

a) Acme files suit to enjoin such payments to be made from the fund under the establishment clause of the first and fourteenth amendments. What result and why?[16]

b) Roe, Pratt, Pursley, and Parker all also file suit, each suing: to enjoin any payments to Goodweather, or in the alternative to mandate an equal payments to himself or herself. What result and why?[17]

III. Suppose in the original case the statute were applied such that, in addition to Doe, Pursley was deemed eligible, but none of the others were. Is the ineligibility of Goodweather, Roe, Pratt, or Parker now vulnerable on constitutional grounds? Why or why not?

IV. Suppose in the original case the Religious Freedom Restoration Act of 1993[18] had been in effect. And suppose that Goodweather had invoked this Act of Congress to assert an entitlement to benefits. Would the Act apply to so require payments to Goodweather from the state fund? If it did would it be constitutional, (and what makes it so)?

---

15. The amended statute declares that "persons unable to continue in a job due solely to its incompatibility with their religious beliefs shall receive unemployment compensation on the same terms as an employee who has been laid off."

16. Is this a permitted (or required) use of tax funds to "accommodate" the free exercise of religion, or is it a targeted direct subsidy of religious practice disallowed by the "no establishment" clause?

17. May Pratt and/or Parker be acting on considerations of conscience and belief as entitled to recognition as those of Goodweather? And so, too, Pursley as well? Why not?

18. See *supra* pp. 1059-1061. This is the Act of Congress that forbids government to act in a manner "that substantially burdens a person's exercise of religion even if the burden results from a rule of general applicability," except insofar as the law serves "a compelling government interest" by means constituting "the least restrictive means of furthering that governmental interest" under the circumstances of its application in each particular case.

Chapter 12

GOVERNMENT NEUTRALITY IN RELIGIOUS DISPUTES

INTRODUCTORY NOTE

A

The cases and materials we have already covered confirm several propositions. Some of these have been the object of continuing disagreement, but certainly not all. Among the *least* disputed is the proposition that the truth of a religious belief is not for any civil authority in this country to decide. This follows not only from the free exercise clause,[1] but also from the establishment clause and its separation of civil from religious authority. There can be no state religion and insofar as that is true, there can likewise be no such thing as a "heresy trial" conducted by the state.[2]

When one seeks the protection of the free exercise clause in order to claim an exemption from some law, however, consistent with the first amendment the *genuineness* of one's claim *is* subject to some degree of examination by civil authority, despite the separation of the church and the state. This is so, simply because were it otherwise, the free exercise clause would protect not merely "freedom of religion," but also "freedom of fraud." Because the Supreme Court is unwilling to read the free exercise clause as declaring that "Congress shall make no law *** prohibiting the free exercise of religious fraud,"[3] while it is true that the truth of a religious claim is not justiciable, the *sincerity* of the belief one claims to hold may well be. Indeed, when claims are asserted under the free exercise clause (or under statutes providing exemption if—and only if—compliance would require infidelity to one's religion), it is most often the bona fides of the claim that *will* be

---

1. United States v. Ballard, 322 U.S. 78, 86-87 (1944) ("Men may believe what they cannot prove. They may not be put to the proof of their religious doctrines and beliefs. Religious experiences which are as real as life to some may be incomprehensible to others. *** The religious views espoused by respondents might seem incredible, if not preposterous, to most people. But if those doctrines are subject to trial before a jury charged with finding their truth or falsity, then the same can be done with the religious beliefs of any sect.")

2. While "treason" or "sedition" may be a matter of concern to the state, "heresy" is not. (Rather, heresy is for the church, and where, as here, pursuant to the first amendment, the state and the church are separated, the state neither determines what constitutes heresy nor enforces the heresy findings of any church.)

3. United States v. Ballard, 322 U.S. 78 (1944) (*supra* p. 1008). Recall that Justice Jackson, in dissent, was willing to interpret the first amendment in this way, for he said that the constitutional question was "whether *misrepresentation* of religious experience or belief is prosecutable." He concluded that the wiser course was to hold that it was *not*—that one who solicits money from others to enrich himself, inducing them to believe in his powers of healing by faith (and to give him money on that account) cannot be prosecuted even though, if asked whether he actually believed he possessed such powers, he would smile and concede that of course he didn't believe any such nonsense.

the principal subject of trial, exactly as in *United States v. Ballard*, and any number of cases involving the military draft.[4]

B

As it is for individuals, so, too, moreover, one might suppose, it is for groups. That is, that insofar as a *group* of some sort seeks to secure an exemption from some regulation on the ground that compliance would be at odds with some requirement of *its* religious integrity, one might expect that the state may as readily press some inquiry equally to determine how and in what way compliance would in fact be compromising, just as in *Yoder*,[5] *Seeger*,[6] or *Prince*.[7] "In what manner would compliance compromise the religion of the group?" would be an unexceptional form of that question.

Inauthentic claims may as readily be made by groups as by individuals, so the question seems equally reasonable and the burden of responding convincingly, the same. Insofar as such a conflict is alleged to exist, the state might press as vigorously (albeit *no more* vigorously) here for evidence that the group *does* have the religious commitment it claims to have.[8] Up to a point, nothing appears ostensibly to warrant a different treatment in the courts to distinguish free exercise *claims* advanced by groups from those advanced by individuals.

---

4. Those who claim an exemption from combatant training and service on religious grounds may be denied the exemption if unable to show that they subscribe to a set of beliefs forbidding their participation in the required training or service. That is, the exemption, broad as it has been construed to be by the Supreme Court, is provided by Congress for the "*conscientious*" objector, not to the poseur—not to the false claimant who would trade on the exemption (provided for those genuinely experiencing the anguish of faith) in order to evade the common military draft. (**Note**, incidentally, that despite the latitude of the Supreme Court's treatment of the "religious" claims in United States v. Seeger, 380 U.S. 163 (1965), and Welsh v. United States, 398 U.S. 333 (1970), the Court has upheld a restriction disallowing an exemption when the conscientious objection is "war selective," i.e. not an objection to combatant training or service for any war purpose, but only in respect to certain ("unjust") wars. (The effect of the statute is thus to discriminate among religions.) See Gillette v. United States, 401 U.S. 437 (1971); see also Clay v. United States, 403 U.S. 698, 700 (1971) ("In order to qualify for classification as a conscientious objector, a registrant must satisfy three basic tests. He must show that he is conscientiously opposed to war in any form [citing *Gillette*]. He must show that this opposition is based upon religious training and belief, as the term has been construed in our decisions [citing *Seeger* and *Welsh*]. And *he must show that this objection is sincere*.") (emphasis added).

5. Wisconsin v. Yoder, 406 U.S. 205 (1972) (the Amish family school attendance case) (*supra* p. 10135).

6. United States v. Seeger, 380 U.S. 163 (1965) (the conscientious draft exemption case) (*supra* p. 1083).

7. Prince v. Massachusetts, 321 U.S. 158 (1944) (the child labor exemption case) (*supra* p. 1002).

8. Evidence, for example, that such wine as may be served as an incident of regular assemblages—despite a state or local prohibition law—is authentically part of a religious practice as such (that it is *not* a mere social "loss leader" to attract more attendance, that it is *not* served simply to provide a relaxed social atmosphere of boozy bonhomie for members who happen to like to drink).

C

Religious practices "by groups," however, are felt to be different from religious practices by individuals in two distinct respects. First, "*who* speaks for 'the group,'" is a question one ordinarily does not have in the individual case.[9] In sorting out "who speaks for the group," however, a court may scarcely dare ask, for fear that it may plunge itself into a dispute ongoing *within* the group itself. The cases examined in this chapter reflect the diffidence of the courts in getting drawn into such matters that were once the reserve of ecclesiastical courts, matters the first amendment itself is thought to withdraw from secular agencies even now, moreover, lest they appear to act to breach the proverbial wall separating the church from the state.

Second, there is in any event a sense of first amendment hazard in the conduct of state proceedings putting a religious organization on trial, so to account for itself in a secular inquisition probing for an authentication of the group's claim. This question is linked to the first question,[10] but has additional entangling elements of its own. Making demand of a religious group to "explain" seems inevitable whenever the authenticity of an alleged religious requirement is itself the main issue in litigation.[11]

But the very process of adversarial inquiry, the appearance of secular inquisition into a church, the examination (such as it may become), all seem threatening to many, both on and off the judicial bench. The case law reflects this uneasiness.[12] One may at once turn to the profile of principal Supreme Court cases (*infra*) to see how some of these matters have played out in the Court's innovation of specialized

---

9. The individual speaks for himself or herself (as to what he or she believes). (The distinction between "groups" and "individuals" may, however, not be all this clear cut. For example, in *Yoder*, had the mother and father agreed that their children should be reared in the Amish way, but genuinely disagreed as what that religious commitment meant (it being the mother's view that it did not mean the children must be withdrawn from public schooling, and the father's that it did), the court must decide "who speaks for *this family* in respect to what its observance of 'the Amish way' requires?" In a manner of speaking, we have a "religious schism" within the family itself. When that occurs, whose "voice" shall a court say *is* authoritative?)

10. For if different members *within* a community of faith don't even agree, how is an outside secular inquirer to figure it out?

11. For example, the "group" (the church) may have a set of written sacraments, none of which, however, makes even the slightest reference to *any* use of wine though the use of many other items is specified in exacting detail. The evidence before a court may indicate that wine is in fact dispensed rather freely at the church. Even so, the "church leaders" insist that it is a regular "religiously-expected observance" (and not a mere evasion of the prohibition law for the lubrication of its meetings); but inasmuch as nothing in the written list of church sacraments furnishes support for the claim, may the church leaders be queried to "explain to the court why, if, as you say, these uses of wine are regarded as enjoined in sacramental ways as part of your religion, there is not the slightest suggestion in this apparently definitive table of sacraments?"

12. For example, as one means courts have used to minimize the occasions for secular inquisition into ecclesiastical administration, even statutes of general application have sometimes been construed not to apply to ecclesiastical organizations unless the legislature has left virtually no room at all for such a possible construction. See, e.g., National Labor Relations Bd. v. Catholic Bishop, 440 U.S. 490 (1979) (construing National Labor Relations Act to find religious schools exempted).

first amendment doctrine in this area. The following case problem, however, also provides a concrete illustration one may find useful to consider either before or after that review.

PROBLEM

Title VII of the Civil Rights Act of 1964[13] forbids certain kinds of discrimination by employers. It applies to any employer of fifteen or more employees,[14] and its best known provision forbids *any* such employer "to fail or refuse to hire *** any individual ***because of such individual's race, color, religion, sex, or national origin."[15] With this background, suppose we put the case of a local Baptist church, the "Hard Rock Baptist Church." It has five hundred members, with some turnover in membership from time to time; and the church as such employs sixteen individuals including the minister. Suppose no woman will be considered for the position of minister. Accordingly, a woman, Anne Mather, who applies to be considered as minister is courteously but firmly turned away.[16] After following EEOC procedures, she files suit in federal court to enjoin the board from refusing to consider her application on the same terms as any other application received for the same post, *and to do so without reference to gender*, as required by Title VII.

The threshold question, of course, would be whether the Act provides an exemption for certain employers, and, more specifically, an exemption for a religious association or an incorporated (or unincorporated) church. If we stipulate here that the Act does *not* provide such an exemption,[17] then the remaining question is whether

---

13. 42 U.S.C. § 2000e *et seq.*

14. Literally, the Act applies only to employers of fifteen or more employees if "engaged in an industry affecting commerce," but "industry affecting commerce" is defined elsewhere in the Act to indicate Congress means to reach every employer whom it can (moreover, the Act is unequivocal that religious institutional employers are included).

15. 42 U.S.C. § 2000e-2(a).

16. Consider, parenthetically, the same situation arising with respect to another position to be filled by one rendering service within the church, such as that of janitor, gardener, or secretary ("ordinary" positions). It will be worthwhile to revisit this possibility later (see cases and discussion in nn. 17, 21 *infra*).

17. In fact, such an exemption would not be available. Section 2000e-1 of Title VII, provides only that "[t]his subchapter shall not apply to *** a religious corporation, association, educational institution, or society *with respect to the employment of individuals of a particular religion* to perform work connected with the carrying on by such corporation, association, educational institution, or society of its activities" (emphasis added). Thus the provision "exempts religious organizations from Title VII's prohibition against discrimination in employment *on the basis of religion*" (emphasis added), but *not* on the basis of race, national origin, or sex. Corporation of Presiding Bishop of The Church of Jesus Christ of Latter-Day Saints v. Amos, 483 U.S. 327, 329 (1987); Rayburn v. General Conference of Seventh-Day Adventists, 772 F.2d 1164, 1166 (4th Cir. 1985) ("Title VII does not confer upon religious organizations a license to make [hiring decisions] on the basis of race, sex, or national origin"), cert. denied, 478 U.S. 1020 (1986).

In other words, while Title VII exempts a church or parochial school which hires only members

the Act, as applied to the Hard Rock Baptist Church and its selection of its own minister, violates the free exercise clause insofar as it requires the church to make no distinction based on sex in the selection of its minister.

In phrasing its "free exercise" defense to Anne Mather's Title VII suit, the Church may argue that it is not possible, consistent with its tenets, scripture, tradition and beliefs, for a woman to serve as a minister of the faith.[18] If so, we appear to have just two questions to answer:

(a) *Is it true*?[19]

(b) Assuming it *is* true, insofar as this is the basis for their refusal to consider her application, does the free exercise clause (or the "no law respecting an establishment of religion" clause[20]) entitle them to prevail on a motion to dismiss the plaintiff's complaint?[21]

---

of its own *faith* even as janitors, gardeners, and secretaries (indeed, in *any* position, even one with no religiously-related job functions), it permits no exemption for discrimination on any *other* ground, regardless of the nature of the particular job. In respect to a particular job (in this case, church minister), the church's refusal to consider a woman would therefore have to be defended on first amendment grounds, and not on the basis that Title VII does not apply. See discussion, cases, and examples in Charles Sullivan et al., I Employment Discrimination 396-403 (2d ed. 1988).

Insofar as it allows religious organizations to discriminate on religious grounds even with respect to "ordinary" jobs (i.e. jobs involving no religious functions at all), incidentally, Title VII has been challenged—unsuccessfully—as a violation of the establishment clause of the first amendment. See Corporation of Presiding Bishop of The Church of Jesus Christ of Latter-Day Saints v. Amos, *supra* (sustaining the Act's exemption even as applied to such employment). But see Thorton v. Caldor, Inc., 472 U.S. 703 (1985) (striking state statute which permitted employees of private employers to miss whatever day of the week their religion required them to miss and which imposed a duty on employers to absorb the cost even when substantial, and holding that the state may only require employers to make "reasonable accommodation" of employee religious needs).

18. Obviously, if the religion is *not* one with any such idea, the church-employer may lose.

19. I.e. is it true that the doctrines of the church forbid such an appointment (as it is true of the ineligibility of women as priests of the hierarchical Catholic church)?

20. Note that, as applied to a church, Title VII itself is in the most direct and literal sense "a law respecting *an establishment* of religion" (for what could be more paradigmatically "an establishment of religion" than a church?).

21. In other words, is the church entitled to prevail because although Title VII applies in such a case (as much to the job of minister as to the job of janitor, gardener, or secretary), *as applied*, Title VII is invalid under the first amendment? May Congress compel a church (as employer) to give equal consideration to a woman applicant for minister, when to do so would be contrary to God's will as understood by the members of the church, or contrary to the articles of faith to which the church subscribes, and according to the gospels of which, just as Christ's original apostles were men, it is now and forever the case that God ordains that only men may preside over a congregation of the faithful?

Assume for now a favorable answer to the second question.[22] This leaves seemingly only one question in the immediate case: the truth (i.e. authenticity) of the

claim made by this church, the truth of the claim that it is indeed bound by articles of faith in the way it maintains, that it *is* a tenet of the faith constituted in *this* church[23] that only men may serve as ministers (gardeners, janitors, etc.). Just such a declaration has been put forward. Still, though it has been made, isn't it also subject to rebuttal? Surely one would think so.[24] If not, why not? What happens if the plaintiff claims, produces affidavits to support, and wants an opportunity to prove that the church's free exercise defense is *invalid* because it is simply *not true* (as the defendant alleges) that employment of women as ministers would be inconsistent with its articles of faith, its requirements of worship, organization, administration, or trust? The plaintiff wants to put on evidence, moreover, not just to try to persuade the court that "'the Baptist religion' as such does not in fact hold that women may not serve as ministers,"[25] but evidence of the following, more focused, sort:

a) That "the consistency of women as ministers of the gospel with the true will of God has been an uncertainty within the Baptist faith generally, and of the Hard Rock Baptist Church specifically, for many decades;"

---

22. The proposition seems so obvious as to be scarcely worth noting. (Surely, one would say, the Catholic Church cannot be compelled to employ women as priests against its doctrinal strictures!) Yet, is it possible the Hard Rock Baptist Church will lose on this claim, under the rule of Employment Division v. Smith, 494 U.S. 812 (1990) (*supra* p. 1048)? Note that Title VII, as presented here, is an act of general application. It addresses a general problem (namely, employment discrimination), and it addresses that problem by a single rule, applicable to all and all alike—*all* employers of 15 or more employees. Might a plaintiff prevail under such a law, and override the religious demurrer at least as to church *gardeners* (if not as to church ministers) even if the religious prohibition on women *as gardeners* is *equally* mandated by the articles of faith embraced by this particular church and its members? For an instructive comparison, see Bob Jones University v. United States, 461 U.S. 574 (1983) (sustaining denial of federal tax-exempt status (§ 501(c)(3)) to church-affiliated university operating under parietal rules forbidding interracial dating according to tenets of religion, despite admitted sincerity of religious requirement and virtual certainty that revocation of tax exempt status would compromise financial viability of the institution).

23. We know it is *not* the tenet of some religions (indeed, many admit women as ministers). Of course, religions need not hold the same view on such questions; the whole point of religious pluralism is that there may be as many "religions" as there are mere nuances of religious belief and of practice. We have often been told, for example, that for first amendment purposes, one may assuredly even have a "religion of one," a religion to which no one other than oneself subscribes.

24. For example, what if by civil discovery we secure the minutes of the deacons' meeting (in which the deacons resolved to recommend the male applicant to the church members), and the minutes disclose the fact that the sole reason for failing to recommend the better-trained, much more-experienced woman applicant was merely that, one of the deacons expressed a sense of discomfort in listening to sermons from women?

25. I.e. she seeks to contest what "the Baptist faith" does or does not hold; and she wants the court to agree with her that the local Baptist church has simply "got it wrong." (In effect, the state would be telling the church what its doctrines do and do not require.)

b) That "until 1985, it *was* deemed to be inconsistent, at least within the Hard Rock Baptist Church, if not in all churches calling themselves Baptist;"
c) That "in 1985, the subject came under prayerful consideration;" and
d) That "after prayerful consideration, meditation, review of scripture, etc., whereas previously only a *minority* of enrolled Hard Rock Baptist Church members believed it to be consistent with God's will that women, equally with men, were welcome in the sight of God to minister, in 1985, a *majority* concluded that the exclusion of women as ministers was scriptural error." Accordingly, and specifically, in a called meeting, with 420 of 510 enrolled members present, on report of a committee previously elected of the enrolled members to review and report on this subject, by vote of 280 to 120 (20 members present not voting), the scriptural error of past understandings of God's will was recognized by the [Name] Baptist church.

Relying on *this* evidence, plaintiff would seek a ruling by the federal court that the church's first amendment defense be rejected as a mere falsified claim.[26] But does this evidence show the claim to be falsified?

Maybe, surely on first impression one might think so, but not necessarily. After all, a "falsified" claim in the usual sense is a claim made by one who does not believe it to be true. Those asserting the claim here, however, may well believe it to be true—that the tenets of faith of the Hard Rock Baptist Church *do* preclude the appointment of women as ministers of the gospel, and that any such appointment would blaspheme against God, fatally estranging Him from a congregation presuming to receive God's word through a female narrator of scripture.

It is *their* position, moreover, that this proposition is not subject to some sort of "vote," rather, it is a matter of "revealed truth within the faith." "Matters capable of being appropriately decided by mere membership vote go to such *secular* incidents of Hard Rock Baptist Church actions as building, spending, and the like—whether to add a wing to the church building, for instance, or whether to start up a day school or purchase a bus." The attorney retained by the Hard Rock Baptist Church has pleaded the free exercise defense in good faith pursuant to instructions from the current *minister and deacons*[27] (not the "majority" of enrolled members[28]). *And who are the civil courts, to say that the deacons and minister are incorrect?*

---

26. In short, the Hard Rock Baptist Church, the plaintiff now suggests, is just like an individual seeking exemption from combatant training and service by qualifying as a "conscientious objector" under the appropriate federal law, but who, on review in an appropriate hearing, is determined to be a mere poseur.

27. Suppose the deacons were split 3/2 on this issue—3 siding with the minister, two siding with the majority of the enrolled members.

28. It is possible, of course, that another attorney may appear on the scene—namely one retained by members of the Hard Rock Baptist Church who "voted" their conviction that women *were* as eligible in the sight of God to minister as men, retained so that these members might seek intervenor status with the plaintiff. We may suppose that this is not merely possible, but that it happens.

We have enmeshed the court in a widening gyre of uncertainty and deepening intervention. We have arrived at still another pivotal question: Who is right? And, more to the point, given the evident internal conflict *within* the Hard Rock Baptist Church,[29] *what shall the court do*? May its involvement in this religious dispute within the Hard Rock Baptist church be precluded by the free exercise clause, construed to forbid secular courts from becoming engaged to proceed at all on the alleged merits of plaintiff's case? May the question we have arrived at itself be nonjusticiable (i.e. *necessarily* nonjusticiable, because any other position would at once engage the machinery of the secular state in deciding a religious dispute *within* a church, entangling the state with the church and imposing the state's decision regarding a dispute ongoing within the church)? Granted that this may happen, what shall the federal court do?[30]

PRESBYTERIAN CHURCH IN THE UNITED STATES v. MARY ELIZABETH BLUE HULL MEMORIAL PRESBYTERIAN CHURCH

393 U.S. 440 (1969)

Mr. Justice BRENNAN delivered the opinion of the Court.

* * *

Petitioner, Presbyterian Church in the United States, is an association of local Presbyterian churches governed by a hierarchical structure of tribunals which consists of, in ascending order, (1) the Church Session, composed of the elders of the local church; (2) the Presbytery, composed of several churches in a geographical area; (3) the Synod, generally composed of all Presbyteries within a State; and (4) the General Assembly, the highest governing body.

A dispute arose between petitioner, the general church, and two local churches in Savannah, Georgia—the respondents, Hull Memorial Presbyterian Church and

---

29. That is, the minister and a majority of the deacons hold that the lay members cannot "vote" propositions that are either true or not true (so to suppose is itself to suffer the secular confusion merely reflected in the meeting that took place), and the requirements of faith are today as they were yesterday.

30. Is this the proper answer: "[C]laims against religious entities under Title VII involving employees engaged in the religious mission of the church and the propagation of its ecclesiastical pursuits *must be dismissed* [whether they involve allegations of sex or of race discrimination, or not]"? Young v. Northern Ill. Conf. of United Methodist Church, 818 F.Supp. 1206, 1212 (N.D. Ill. 1993) (emphasis added), aff'd, 21 F.3d 184 (7th Cir., 1994), cert. denied, 115 S.Ct. 320 (1994). See also Minker v. Baltimore Annual Conf. of United Methodist Church, 894 F.2d 1354 (1990) (Age discrimination suit for denial of promotion as minister, pursuant to federal Age Discrimination in Employment Act, 29 U.S.C. §§ 621, 623 (1983), which provides no exemption for churches discriminating against a person as a minister merely because of his age, held, "the first amendment forecloses any inquiry into the Church's assessment of Minker's suitability for a pastorship, *even for the purpose of showing it to be pretextual*") (emphasis added). See also Combs v. Central Texas Annual Conference of the United Methodist Church, 173 F.3d 343 (5th Cir. 1999).

Eastern Heights Presbyterian Church—over control of the properties used until then by the local churches. In 1966, the membership of the local churches, in the belief that certain actions and pronouncements of the general church were violations of that organization's constitution and departures from the doctrine and practice in force at the time of affiliation,[1] voted to withdraw from the general church and to reconstitute the local churches as an autonomous Presbyterian organization. The ministers of the two churches renounced the general church's jurisdiction and authority over them, as did all but two of the ruling elders. In response, the general church, through the Presbytery of Savannah, established an Administrative Commission to seek a conciliation. The dissident local churchmen remained steadfast; consequently, the Commission acknowledged the withdrawal of the local leadership and proceeded to take over the local churches' property on behalf of the general church until new local leadership could be appointed.

The local churchmen made no effort to appeal the Commission's action to higher church tribunals—the Synod of Georgia or the General Assembly. Instead, the churches filed separate suits in the Superior Court of Chatham County to enjoin the general church from trespassing on the disputed property, title to which was in the local churches. The cases were consolidated for trial. The general church moved to dismiss the actions and cross-claimed for injunctive relief in its own behalf on the ground that civil courts were without power to determine whether the general church had departed from its tenets of faith and practice. The motion to dismiss was denied, and the case was submitted to the jury on the theory that Georgia law implies a trust of local church property for the benefit of the general church on the sole condition that the general church adhere to its tenets of faith and practice existing at the time of affiliation by the local churches.[2] Thus, the jury was instructed to determine whether the actions of the general church "amount to a fundamental or substantial abandonment of the original tenets and doctrines of the (general church), so that the new tenets and doctrines are utterly variant from the purposes for which the (general church) was founded." The jury returned a verdict for the local churches, and the trial judge thereupon declared that the implied trust had terminated and enjoined the general church from interfering with the use of the property in question. The Supreme Court of Georgia affirmed. We granted certiorari to consider the First Amendment questions raised. We reverse.

It is of course true that the State has a legitimate interest in resolving property disputes, and that a civil court is a proper forum for that resolution. Special

---

1. The opinion of the Supreme Court of Georgia summarizes the claimed violations and departures from petitioner's original tenets of faith and practice as including the following: "ordaining of women as ministers and ruling elders, making pronouncements and recommendations concerning civil, economic, social and political matters, giving support to the removal of Bible reading and prayers by children in the public schools, adopting certain Sunday School literature and teaching neo-orthodoxy alien to the Confession of Faith and Catechisms, as originally adopted by the general church." ***

2. This theory derives from principles fashioned by English courts. ***

problems arise, however, when these disputes implicate controversies over church doctrine and practice. The approach of this Court in such cases was originally developed in Watson v. Jones, 13 Wall. 679, 20 L.Ed. 666 (1872). *** There, as here, the disputes arose out of a controversy over church doctrine. There, as here, the Court was asked to decree the termination of an implied trust because of departures from doctrine by the national organization. The Watson Court refused pointing out that it was wholly inconsistent with the American concept of the relationship between church and state to permit civil courts to determine ecclesiastical questions. In language which has a clear constitutional ring, the Court said

> "In this country the full and free right to entertain any religious belief, to practice any religious principle, and to teach any religious doctrine which does not violate the laws of morality and property, and which does not infringe personal rights, is conceded to all. The law knows no heresy, and is committed to the support of no dogma, the establishment of no sect. *** All who unite themselves to such a body (the general church) do so with an implied consent to (its) government, and are bound to submit to it. But it would be a vain consent and would lead to the total subversion of such religious bodies, if any one aggrieved by one of their decisions could appeal to the secular courts and have them [*sic*] reversed. It is of the essence of these religious unions, and of their right to establish tribunals for the decision of questions arising among themselves, that those decisions should be binding in all cases of ecclesiastical cognizance, subject only to such appeals as the organism itself provides for."

The logic of this language leaves the civil courts no role in determining ecclesiastical questions in the process of resolving property disputes.

Later cases, however, also decided on nonconstitutional grounds, recognized that there might be some circumstances in which marginal civil court review of ecclesiastical determinations would be appropriate. The scope of this review was delineated in Gonzalez v. Roman Catholic Archbishop of Manila, 280 U.S. 1 (1929). There, Gonzalez claimed the right to be appointed to a chaplaincy in the Roman Catholic Church under a will which provided that a member of his family receive that appointment. The Roman Catholic Archbishop of Manila, Philippine Islands, refused to appoint Gonzalez on the ground that he did not satisfy the qualifications established by Canon Law for that office. Gonzalez brought suit in the Court of First Instance of Manila for a judgment directing the Archbishop, among other things, to appoint him chaplain. The trial court entered such an order, but the Supreme Court of the Philippine Islands reversed and "absolved the Archbishop from the complaint." This Court affirmed. Mr. Justice Brandeis, speaking for the Court, defined the civil court role in the following words:

> In the absence of fraud, collusion, or arbitrariness, the decisions of the proper church tribunals on matters purely ecclesiastical, although affecting civil rights,

are accepted in litigation before the secular courts as conclusive, because the parties in interest made them so by contract or otherwise.

In Kedroff v. St. Nicholas Cathedral of Russian Orthodox Church in North America, 344 U.S. 94 (1952), the Court converted the principle of Watson as qualified by Gonzalez into a constitutional rule. ***

Thus, the First Amendment severely circumscribes the role that civil courts may play in resolving church property disputes. It is obvious, however, that not every civil court decision as to property claimed by a religious organization jeopardizes values protected by the First Amendment. Civil courts do not inhibit free exercise of religion merely by opening their doors to disputes involving church property. And there are neutral principles of law, developed for use in all property disputes, which can be applied without "establishing" churches to which property is awarded. But First Amendment values are plainly jeopardized when church property litigation is made to turn on the resolution by civil courts of controversies over religious doctrine and practice. *** Hence, States, religious organizations, and individuals must structure relationships involving church property so as not to require the civil courts to resolve ecclesiastical questions.

The Georgia courts have violated the command of the First Amendment. The departure-from-doctrine element of the implied trust theory which they applied requires the civil judiciary to determine whether actions of the general church constitute such a "substantial departure" from the tenets of faith and practice existing at the time of the local churches' affiliation that the trust in favor of the general church must be declared to have terminated. This determination has two parts. The civil court must first decide whether the challenged actions of the general church depart substantially from prior doctrine. In reaching such a decision, the court must of necessity make its own interpretation of the meaning of church doctrines. If the court should decide that a substantial departure has occurred, it must then go on to determine whether the issue on which the general church has departed holds a place of such importance in the traditional theology as to require that the trust be terminated. A civil court can make this determination only after assessing the relative significance to the religion of the tenets from which departure was found. *** Plainly, the First Amendment forbids civil courts from playing such a role.

Since the Georgia courts on remand may undertake to determine whether petitioner is entitled to relief on its cross-claims, we find it appropriate to remark that the departure-from-doctrine element of Georgia's implied trust theory can play no role in any future judicial proceedings. The departure-from-doctrine approach is not susceptible of the marginal judicial involvement contemplated in Gonzalez.[7] Gonzalez' rights under a will turned on a church decision, the Archbishop's, as to church law, the qualifications for the chaplaincy. It was the archbishopric, not the

---

7. We have no occasion in this case to define or discuss the precise limits of review for "fraud, collusion, or arbitrariness" within the meaning of Gonzalez.

civil courts, which had the task of analyzing and interpreting church law in order to determine the validity of Gonzalez' claim to a chaplaincy. Thus, the civil courts could adjudicate the rights under the will without interpreting or weighing church doctrine but simply by engaging in the narrowest kind of review of a specific church decision—i.e., whether that decision resulted from fraud, collusion, or arbitrariness. Such review does not inject the civil courts into substantive ecclesiastical matters. In contrast, under Georgia's departure-from-doctrine approach, it is not possible for the civil courts to play so limited a role. Under this approach, property rights do not turn on a church decision as to church doctrine. The standard of departure-from-doctrine, though it calls for resolution of ecclesiastical questions, is a creation of state, not church, law. Nothing in the record suggests that this state standard has been interpreted and applied in a decision of the general church. Any decisions which have been made by the general church about the local churches' withdrawal have at most a tangential relationship to the state- fashioned departure-from-doctrine standard. A determination whether such decisions are fraudulent, collusive, or arbitrary would therefore not answer the questions posed by the state standard. To reach those questions would require the civil courts to engage in the forbidden process of interpreting and weighing church doctrine. Even if the general church had attempted to apply the state standard, the civil courts could not review and enforce the church decision without violating the Constitution. The First Amendment prohibits a State from employing religious organizations as an arm of the civil judiciary to perform the function of interpreting and applying state standards. Thus, a civil court may no more review a church decision applying a state departure-from-doctrine standard than it may apply that standard itself.

The judgment of the Supreme Court of Georgia is reversed, and the case is remanded for further proceedings not inconsistent with this opinion.

Mr. Justice HARLAN, concurring.

I am in entire agreement with the Court's rejection of the "departure-from-doctrine" approach taken by the Georgia courts, as that approach necessarily requires the civilian courts to weigh the significance and the meaning of disputed religious doctrine. I do not, however, read the Court's opinion to go further to hold that the Fourteenth Amendment forbids civilian courts from enforcing a deed or will which expressly and clearly lays down conditions limiting a religious organization's use of the property which is granted. If, for example, the donor expressly gives his church some money on the condition that the church never ordain a woman as a minister or elder, or never amend certain specified articles of the Confession of Faith, he is entitled to his money back if the condition is not fulfilled. In such a case, the church should not be permitted to keep the property simply because church authorities have determined that the doctrinal innovation is justified by the faith's basic principles.

On this understanding, I join the Court's opinion.

SERBIAN EASTERN ORTHODOX DIOCESE FOR THE UNITED STATES OF AMERICA AND CANADA v. MILIVOJEVICH
426 U.S. 696 (1976)

Mr. Justice BRENNAN delivered the opinion of the Court.

In 1963, the Holy Assembly of Bishops and the Holy Synod of the Serbian Orthodox Church (Mother Church) *** removed respondent Dionisije Milivojevich (Dionisije) as Bishop of the American-Canadian Diocese of that Church and appointed petitioner Bishop Firmilian Ocokoljich (Firmilian) as Administrator of the Diocese, which the Mother Church then reorganized into three Dioceses. In 1964 the Holy Assembly and Holy Synod defrocked Dionisije as a Bishop and cleric of the Mother Church. In this civil action brought by Dionisije and the other respondents in Illinois Circuit Court, the Supreme Court of Illinois held that the proceedings of the Mother Church respecting Dionisije were procedurally and substantively defective under the internal regulations of the Mother Church and were therefore arbitrary and invalid. The State Supreme Court also invalidated the Diocesan reorganization into three Dioceses. We granted certiorari to determine whether the actions of the Illinois Supreme Court constituted improper judicial interference with decisions of the highest authorities of a hierarchical church in violation of the First and Fourteenth Amendments. We hold that the inquiries made by the Illinois Supreme Court into matters of ecclesiastical cognizance and polity and the court's actions pursuant thereto contravened the First and Fourteenth Amendments. We therefore reverse.

I

The basic dispute is over control of the Serbian Eastern Orthodox Diocese for the United States of America and Canada (American-Canadian Diocese), its property and assets. ***

The Serbian Orthodox Church, one of the 14 autocephalous, hierarchical churches which came into existence following the schism of the universal Christian church in 1054, is an episcopal church whose seat is the Patriarchate in Belgrade, Yugoslavia. Its highest legislative, judicial, ecclesiastical, and administrative authority resides in the Holy Assembly of Bishops, a body composed of all Diocesan Bishops presided over by a Bishop designated by the Assembly to be Patriarch. The Church's highest executive body, the Holy Synod of Bishops, is composed of the Patriarch and four Diocesan Bishops selected by the Holy Assembly. The Holy Synod and the Holy Assembly have the exclusive power to remove, suspend, defrock, or appoint Diocesan Bishops. The Mother Church is governed according to the Holy Scriptures, Holy Tradition, Rules of the Ecumenical Councils, the Holy Apostles, the Holy Faiths of the Church, the Mother Church Constitution adopted in 1931, and a "penal code" adopted in 1961. These sources of law are sometimes ambiguous and seemingly inconsistent. ***

In 1913 and 1916, Serbian priests and laymen organized a Serbian Orthodox Church in North America. The 32 Serbian Orthodox congregations were divided into

4 presbyteries, each presided over by a Bishop's Aide, and constitutions were adopted. *** In 1927, Father Mardary called a Church National Assembly embracing all of the known Serbian Orthodox congregations in the United States and Canada. The Assembly drafted and adopted the constitution of the Serbian Orthodox Diocese for the United States of America and Canada, and submitted the constitution to the Mother Church for approval. The Holy Assembly made changes to provide for appointment of the Diocesan Bishop by the Holy Assembly and to require Holy Assembly approval for any amendments to the constitution, and with these changes approved the constitution. ***

Article 1 of the constitution provides that the American-Canadian Diocese "is considered ecclesiastically-judicially as an organic part of the Serbian Patriarchate in the Kingdom of Yugoslavia," and Art. 2 provides that all "statutes and rules which regulate the ecclesiastical-canonical authority and position of the Serbian Orthodox Church in the Kingdom of Yugoslavia are also compulsory for" the American-Canadian Diocese. ***

Respondent Bishop Dionisije was elected Bishop of the American-Canadian Diocese by the Holy Assembly of Bishops in 1939. He became a controversial figure; during the years before 1963, the Holy Assembly received numerous complaints challenging his fitness to serve as Bishop and his administration of the Diocese. *** [O]n June 12, 1962, the Holy Synod appointed a delegation to visit the United States. ***

The delegation remained in the United States for three months, visiting parishes throughout the Diocese. After completion of its survey, the delegation suggested to the Holy Synod that a commission be appointed to conduct a thorough investigation into the complaints against Dionisije. However, the Holy Assembly on May 10, 1963, instead recommended that the Holy Synod institute disciplinary proceedings against Dionisije. The Holy Synod thereupon met immediately and suspended Dionisije pending investigation and disposition of the complaints. The Holy Synod appointed petitioner Firmilian, Dionisije's chief episcopal deputy since 1955 and one of Dionisije's candidates for assistant bishop, as Administrator of the Diocese pending completion of the proceedings.

Dionisije's immediate reaction to these decisions of the Mother Church was to refuse to accept his suspension on the ground that it was not effectuated in compliance with the constitution and laws of the Mother Church. On May 25, 1963, he prepared and mailed a circular to all American-Canadian parishes stating his refusal to recognize these actions, and on May 27 he issued a press release stating his refusal to recognize his suspension and his intent to litigate it in the civil courts. He also continued to officiate as Bishop, refusing to turn administration of the Diocese over to Firmilian; in a May 30 letter to Firmilian, Dionisije repeated this refusal, asserted that he no longer recognized the decisions of the Holy Assembly and Holy Synod, and charged those bodies with being "communistic." ***

On June 13, the Holy Synod appointed such a commission, composed of two Bishops and the Secretary of the Holy Synod. On July 5, the commission met with

Dionisije, who reiterated his refusal to recognize his suspension or the Diocesan reorganization, and who demanded all accusations in writing. The commission refused to give Dionisije the written accusations on the ground that defiance of decisions of higher church authorities itself established wrongful conduct, and advised him that the Holy Synod would appoint a Bishop as court prosecutor to prepare an indictment against him.

On the basis of the commission's report and recommendations, which recited Dionisije's refusal to accept the decisions of the Holy Synod and Holy Assembly and his refusal to recognize the court of the Holy Synod or its competence to try him, the Holy Assembly met on July 27, 1963, and voted to remove Dionisije as Bishop. The minutes of the Holy Assembly meeting and the Patriarch's letter to Dionisije informing him of the Holy Assembly's actions made clear that the removal was based solely on his acts of defiance subsequent to his May 10, 1963, suspension, and his violation of his oath and loss of certain qualifications for Bishop under Art. 104 of the constitution of the Mother Church. ***

[T]he Holy Synod in October 1963 forwarded to Dionisije a formal written indictment based on the charges of canonical misconduct. In November 1963, Dionisije responded with a demand for the verified reports and complaints referred to in the indictment and for a six-month extension to answer the indictment. The Holy Assembly granted a 30-day extension in which to answer, but declined to furnish verified charges on the grounds that they were described in the indictment, that additional details would be evidentiary in nature, and that there was no legal or canonical basis for forwarding such material to an accused Bishop.

Dionisije returned the indictment in January, refusing to answer without the verified charges, denouncing the Holy Assembly and Holy Synod as schismatic and pro-Communist, and asserting that the Mother Church was proceeding in violation of its penal code and constitution.

The Holy Synod, on February 25, 1964, declared that it could not proceed further without Dionisije and referred the matter to the Holy Assembly, which tried Dionisije as a default case on March 5, 1964, because of his refusal to participate. The indictment was also amended at that time to include charges based on Dionisije's acts of rebellion such as those committed at the November meeting of the National Assembly which had declared the Diocese separate from the Mother Church. Considering the original and amended indictments, the Holy Assembly unanimously found Dionisije guilty of all charges and divested him of his episcopal and monastic ranks.

Even before the Holy Assembly had removed Dionisije as Bishop, he had commenced what eventually became this protracted litigation, now carried on for almost 13 years. Acting upon the threat contained in his May 27, 1963, press release, Dionisije filed suit in the Circuit Court of Lake County, Ill., on July 26, 1963, seeking to enjoin petitioners from interfering with the assets of respondent corporations and to have himself declared the true Diocesan Bishop. Petitioners countered with a separate complaint, which was consolidated with the original action, seeking declaratory relief that Dionisije had been removed as Bishop of the Diocese and *** injunctive relief granting petitioner Bishops control of the reorganized Dioceses and their property. After the trial court granted summary judgment for respondents and dismissed petitioners' countercomplaint, the Illinois Appellate Court reversed and remanded for a hearing on the merits.[4]

Following a lengthy trial, the trial court filed an unreported memorandum opinion and entered a final decree which concluded that "no substantial evidence was produced that fraud, collusion or arbitrariness existed in any of the actions or decisions preliminary to or during the final proceedings of the decision to defrock Bishop Dionisije made by the highest Hierarchical bodies of the Mother Church," *** and that "Firmilian was validly appointed by the Holy Episcopal Synod as temporary Administrator of the whole American Diocese in place of the defrocked Bishop Dionisije."

On appeal, the Supreme Court of Illinois reversed in part, essentially holding that Dionisije's removal and defrockment had to be set aside as "arbitrary" because the proceedings resulting in those actions were not conducted according to the Illinois Supreme Court's interpretation of the Church's constitution and penal code. Although the court denied rehearing, it amended its original opinion to hold that, although Dionisije had been properly suspended, that suspension terminated by operation of church law when he was not validly tried within one year of his indictment. Thus, the court purported in effect to reinstate Dionisije as Diocesan Bishop.

II

The fallacy fatal to the judgment of the Illinois Supreme Court is that it rests upon an impermissible rejection of the decisions of the highest ecclesiastical tribunals of this hierarchical church upon the issues in dispute, and impermissibly substitutes its own inquiry into church polity and resolutions based thereon of those disputes. Consistently with the First and Fourteenth Amendments

> civil courts do not inquire whether the relevant [hierarchical] church governing body has power under religious law [to decide such disputes]. *** Such a determination *** frequently necessitates the interpretation of ambiguous religious law and usage. To permit civil courts to probe deeply enough into the allocation of power within a [hierarchical] church so as to decide *** religious law [governing church polity] *** would violate the First Amendment in much the same manner as civil determination of religious doctrine. Md. & Va. Churches v. Sharpsburg Church, 396 U.S. 367, 369 (1970) (Brennan, J., concurring).

---

4. The Appellate Court initially held that the suspension, removal, and defrockment of Dionisije were valid and binding upon the civil courts but on rehearing directed that Dionisije should be afforded the opportunity at trial to prove that these were the result of fraud, collusion, or arbitrariness.

For where resolution of the disputes cannot be made without extensive inquiry by civil courts into religious law and polity, the First and Fourteenth Amendments mandate that civil courts shall not disturb the decisions of the highest ecclesiastical tribunal within a church of hierarchical polity, but must accept such decisions as binding on them, in their application to the religious issues of doctrine or polity before them.

Resolution of the religious disputes at issue here affects the control of church property in addition to the structure and administration of the American-Canadian Diocese. This is because the Diocesan Bishop controls respondent Monastery of St. Sava and is the principal officer of respondent property-holding corporations. Resolution of the religious dispute over Dionisije's defrockment therefore determines control of the property. Thus, this case essentially involves not a church property dispute, but a religious dispute the resolution of which under our cases is for ecclesiastical and not civil tribunals. ***

The principles limiting the role of civil courts in the resolution of religious controversies that incidentally affect civil rights were initially fashioned in Watson v. Jones, 13 Wall. 679, 20 L.Ed. 666 (1872). *** With respect to hierarchical churches, Watson held:

> [T]he rule of action which should govern the civil courts *** is that whenever the questions of discipline, or of faith, or ecclesiastical rule, custom, or law have been decided by the highest of these church judicatories to which the matter has been carried, the legal tribunals must accept such decisions as final, and as binding on them, in their application to the case before them." ***

Gonzalez v. Archbishop, 280 U.S. 1 (1929), applied this principle in a case involving dispute over entitlement to certain income under a will that turned upon an ecclesiastical determination as to whether an individual would be appointed to a chaplaincy in the Roman Catholic Church. The Court, speaking through Mr. Justice Brandeis, observed:

> Because the appointment (to the chaplaincy) is a canonical act, it is the function of the church authorities to determine what the essential qualifications of a chaplain are and whether the candidate possesses them. In the absence of fraud, collusion, or arbitrariness, the decisions of the proper church tribunals on matters purely ecclesiastical, although affecting civil rights, are accepted in litigation before the secular courts as conclusive, because the parties in interest made them so by contract or otherwise.

Thus, although *Watson* had left civil courts no role to play in reviewing ecclesiastical decisions during the course of resolving church property disputes, *Gonzalez* first adverted to the possibility of "marginal civil court review," Presbyterian Church v. Hull Church, 393 U.S. at 447, in cases challenging decisions of ecclesiastical tribunals as products of "fraud, collusion, or arbitrariness." However, the suggested "fraud, collusion, or arbitrariness" exception to the *Watson* rule was dictum only.

And no decision of this Court has given concrete content to or applied the "exception." However, it was the predicate for the Illinois Supreme Court's decision in this case, and we therefore turn to the question whether reliance upon it in the circumstances of this case was consistent with the prohibition of the First and Fourteenth Amendments against rejection of the decisions of the Mother Church upon the religious disputes in issue.

The conclusion of the Illinois Supreme Court that the decisions of the Mother Church were "arbitrary" was grounded upon an inquiry that persuaded the Illinois Supreme Court that the Mother Church had not followed its own laws and procedures in arriving at those decisions. We have concluded that whether or not there is room for "marginal civil court review" under the narrow rubrics of "fraud" or "collusion" when church tribunals act in bad faith for secular purposes,[7] no "arbitrariness" exception in the sense of an inquiry whether the decisions of the highest ecclesiastical tribunal of a hierarchical church complied with church laws and regulations is consistent with the constitutional mandate that civil courts are bound to accept the decisions of the highest judicatories of a religious organization of hierarchical polity on matters of discipline, faith, internal organization or ecclesiastical rule, custom, or law. For civil courts to analyze whether the ecclesiastical actions of a church judicatory are in that sense "arbitrary" must inherently entail inquiry into the procedures that canon or ecclesiastical law supposedly requires the church judicatory to follow, or else in to the substantive criteria by which they are supposedly to decide the ecclesiastical question. But this is exactly the inquiry that the First Amendment prohibits; recognition of such an exception would undermine the general rule that religious controversies are not the proper subject of civil court inquiry, and that a civil court must accept the ecclesiastical decisions of church tribunals as it finds them. ***

The constitutional evils that attend upon any "arbitrariness" exception in the sense applied by the Illinois Supreme Court to justify civil court review of ecclesiastical decisions of final church tribunals are manifest in the instant case. The Supreme Court of Illinois recognized that all parties agree that the Serbian Orthodox Church is a hierarchical church, and that the sole power to appoint and remove Bishops of the Church resides in its highest ranking organs, the Holy Assembly and the Holy Synod. ***

Yet having recognized that the Serbian Orthodox Church is hierarchical and that the decisions to suspend and defrock respondent Dionisije were made by the religious bodies in whose sole discretion the authority to make those ecclesiastical decisions was vested, the Supreme Court of Illinois nevertheless invalidated the decision to defrock Dionisije on the ground that it was "arbitrary" because a "detailed review of the evidence discloses that the proceedings resulting in Bishop Dionisije's removal and defrockment were not in accordance with the prescribed

7. No issue of "fraud" or "collusion" is involved in this case.

procedure of the constitution and the penal code of the Serbian Orthodox Church." Not only was this "detailed review" impermissible under the First and Fourteenth Amendments, but in reaching this conclusion, the court evaluated conflicting testimony concerning internal church procedures and rejected the interpretations of relevant procedural provisions by the Mother Church's highest tribunals. In short, under the guise of "minimal" review under the umbrella of "arbitrariness," the Illinois Supreme Court has unconstitutionally undertaken the resolution of quintessentially religious controversies whose resolution the First Amendment commits exclusively to the highest ecclesiastical tribunals of this hierarchical church. And although the Diocesan Bishop controls respondent Monastery of St. Sava and is the principal officer of respondent property-holding corporations, the civil courts must accept that consequence as the incidental effect of an ecclesiastical determination that is not subject to judicial abrogation, having been reached by the final church judicatory in which authority to make the decision resides. ***

IV

In short, the First and Fourteenth Amendments permit hierarchical religious organizations to establish their own rules and regulations for internal discipline and government, and to create tribunals for adjudicating disputes over these matters. When this choice is exercised and ecclesiastical tribunals are created to decide disputes over the government and direction of subordinate bodies, the Constitution requires that civil courts accept their decisions as binding upon them.

Reversed.

THE CHIEF JUSTICE concurs in the judgment.

Mr. Justice WHITE, concurring. [Omitted.]

Mr. Justice REHNQUIST, with whom Mr. Justice STEVENS joins, dissenting.

The Court's opinion, while long on the ecclesiastical history of the Serbian Orthodox Church, is somewhat short on the procedural history of this case. A casual reader of some of the passages in the Court's opinion could easily gain the impression that the State of Illinois had commenced a proceeding designed to brand Bishop Dionisije as a heretic, with appropriate pains and penalties. But the state trial judge in the Circuit Court of Lake County was not the Bishop of Beauvais, trying Joan of Arc for heresy; the jurisdiction of his court was invoked by petitioners themselves, who sought an injunction establishing their control over property of the American-Canadian Diocese of the church located in Lake County.

The jurisdiction of that court having been invoked for such a purpose by both petitioners and respondents, contesting claimants to Diocesan authority, it was entitled to ask if the real Bishop of the American-Canadian Diocese would please stand up. The protracted proceedings in the Illinois courts were devoted to the ascertainment of who that individual was, a question which the Illinois courts sought to answer by application of the canon law of the church, just as they would have attempted to decide a similar dispute among the members of any other voluntary association. The Illinois courts did not in the remotest sense inject their doctrinal preference into the dispute. They were forced to decide between two competing sets of claimants to church office in order that they might resolve a dispute over real property located within the State. Each of the claimants had requested them to decide the issue. Unless the First Amendment requires control of disputed church property to be awarded solely on the basis of ecclesiastical paper title, I can find no constitutional infirmity in the judgment of the Supreme Court of Illinois.

Unless civil courts are to be wholly divested of authority to resolve conflicting claims to real property owned by a hierarchical church, and such claims are to be resolved by brute force, civil courts must of necessity make some factual inquiry even under the rules the Court purports to apply in this case. We are told that "a civil court must accept the ecclesiastical decisions of church tribunals as it finds them." But even this rule requires that proof be made as to what these decisions are, and if proofs on that issue conflict the civil court will inevitably have to choose one over the other. In so choosing, if the choice is to be a rational one, reasons must be adduced as to why one proffered decision is to prevail over another. Such reasons will obviously be based on the canon law by which the disputants have agreed to bind themselves, but they must also represent a preference for one view of that law over another.

If civil courts, consistently with the First Amendment, may do that much, the question arises why they may not do what the Illinois courts did here regarding the defrockment of Bishop Dionisije, and conclude, on the basis of testimony from experts on the canon law at issue, that the decision of the religious tribunal involved was rendered in violation of its own stated rules of procedure. Suppose the Holy Assembly in this case had a membership of 100; its rules provided that a bishop could be defrocked by a majority vote of any session at which a quorum was present, and also provided that a quorum was not to be less than 40. Would a decision of the Holy Assembly attended by 30 members, 16 of whom voted to defrock Bishop Dionisije, be binding on civil courts in a dispute such as this? The hypothetical example is a clearer case than the one involved here, but the principle is the same. If the civil courts are to be bound by any sheet of parchment bearing the ecclesiastical seal and purporting to be a decree of a church court, they can easily be converted into handmaidens of arbitrary lawlessness. ***

The rule fairly implicit in the history of our First Amendment, is that the government may not displace the free religious choices of its citizens by placing its weight behind a particular religious belief, tenet, or sect. In *Hull*, the State transgressed the line drawn by the First Amendment when it applied a state-created rule of law based upon "departure from doctrine" to prevent the national hierarchy of the Presbyterian Church in the United States from seeking to reclaim possession and use of two local churches. When the Georgia courts themselves required an examination into whether there had been a departure from the doctrine of the church in order to apply this state-created rule, they went beyond mere application of neutral principles of law to such a dispute.

There is nothing in this record to indicate that the Illinois courts have been instruments of any such impermissible intrusion by the State on one side or the other of a religious dispute. There is nothing in the Supreme Court of Illinois' opinion indicating that it placed its thumb on the scale in favor of the respondents. Instead that opinion appears to be precisely what it purports to be: an application of neutral principles of law consistent with the decisions of this Court. Indeed, petitioners make absolutely no claim to the contrary. They agree that the Illinois courts should have decided the issues which they presented; but they contend that in doing so those courts should have deferred entirely to the representations of the announced representatives of the Mother Church. Such blind deference, however, is counseled neither by logic nor by the First Amendment. To make available the coercive powers of civil courts to rubber-stamp ecclesiastical decisions of hierarchical religious associations, when such deference is not accorded similar acts of secular voluntary associations, would, in avoiding the free exercise problems petitioners envision, itself create far more serious problems under the Establishment Clause. ***

JONES v. WOLF

443 U.S. 595 (1979)

Mr. Justice BLACKMUN delivered the opinion of the Court.

This case involves a dispute over the ownership of church property following a schism in a local church affiliated with a hierarchical church organization. The question for decision is whether civil courts, consistent with the First and Fourteenth Amendments to the Constitution, may resolve the dispute on the basis of "neutral principles of law," or whether they must defer to the resolution of an authoritative tribunal of the hierarchical church.

I

The Vineville Presbyterian Church of Macon, Ga., was organized in 1904, and first incorporated in 1915.

The property at issue and on which the church is located was acquired in three transactions, and is evidenced by conveyances to the "Trustees of [or 'for'] Vineville Presbyterian Church and their successors in office," or simply to the "Vineville Presbyterian Church." The funds used to acquire the property were contributed entirely by local church members. Pursuant to resolutions adopted by the congregation, the church repeatedly has borrowed money on the property. This indebtedness is evidenced by security deeds variously issued in the name of the "Trustees of the Vineville Presbyterian Church," or, again, simply the "Vineville Presbyterian Church."

In the same year it was organized, the Vineville church was established as a member church of the Augusta-Macon Presbytery of the Presbyterian Church in the United States (PCUS). The PCUS has a generally hierarchical or connectional form of government, as contrasted with a congregational form. Under the polity of the PCUS, the government of the local church is committed to its Session in the first instance, but the actions of this assembly or "court" are subject to the review and control of the higher church courts, the Presbytery, Synod, and General Assembly, respectively. The powers and duties of each level of the hierarchy are set forth in the constitution of the PCUS, the Book of Church Order, which is part of the record in the present case.

On May 27, 1973, at a congregational meeting of the Vineville church attended by a quorum of its duly enrolled members, 164 of them, including the pastor, voted to separate from the PCUS. Ninety-four members opposed the resolution. The majority immediately informed the PCUS of the action, and then united with another denomination, the Presbyterian Church in America. Although the minority remained on the church rolls for three years, they ceased to participate in the affairs of the Vineville church and conducted their religious activities elsewhere.

In response to the schism within the Vineville congregation, the Augusta-Macon Presbytery appointed a commission to investigate the dispute and, if possible, to resolve it. The commission eventually issued a written ruling declaring that the minority faction constituted "the true congregation of Vineville Presbyterian Church," and withdrawing from the majority faction "all authority to exercise office derived from the [PCUS]." The majority took no part in the commission's inquiry, and did not appeal its ruling to a higher PCUS tribunal.

Representatives of the minority faction brought this class action in state court, seeking declaratory and injunctive orders establishing their right to exclusive possession and use of the Vineville church property as a member congregation of the PCUS. The trial court, purporting to apply Georgia's "neutral principles of law" approach to church property disputes, granted judgment for the majority. The Supreme Court of Georgia, holding that the trial court had correctly stated and applied Georgia law, and rejecting the minority's challenge based on the First and Fourteenth Amendments, affirmed. We granted certiorari. ***

III

The only question presented by this case is which faction of the formerly united Vineville congregation is entitled to possess and enjoy the property located at 2193 Vineville Avenue in Macon, Ga. There can be little doubt about the general authority of civil courts to resolve this question. The State has an obvious and legitimate interest in the peaceful resolution of property disputes, and in providing a civil forum where the ownership of church property can be determined conclusively.

It is also clear, however, that the First Amendment severely circumscribes the role that civil courts may play in resolving church property disputes. Most importantly, the First Amendment prohibits civil courts from resolving church property disputes on the basis of religious doctrine and practice. Serbian Orthodox Diocese v. Milivojevich, 426 U.S. 696, 710 (1976); Maryland & Va. Churches v. Sharpsburg Church, 396 U.S. 367, 368 (1970). As a corollary to this commandment, the Amendment requires that civil courts defer to the resolution of issues of religious doctrine or polity by the highest court of a hierarchical church organization. Serbian Orthodox Diocese, 426 U.S., at 724-725. Subject to these limitations, however, the First Amendment does not dictate that a State must follow a particular method of resolving church property disputes. Indeed, "a State may adopt any one of various approaches for settling church property disputes so long as it involves no consideration of doctrinal matters, whether the ritual and liturgy of worship or the tenets of faith." Maryland & Va. Churches, 396 U.S., at 368. (BRENNAN, J., concurring) (emphasis in original).

At least in general outline, we think the "neutral principles of law" approach is consistent with the foregoing constitutional principles. The neutral-principles approach was approved in *Maryland & Va. Churches*, an appeal from a judgment of the Court of Appeals of Maryland settling a local church property dispute on the basis of the language of the deeds, the terms of the local church charters, the state statutes governing the holding of church property, and the provisions in the constitution of the general church concerning the ownership and control of church property. Finding that this analysis entailed "no inquiry into religious doctrine," the Court dismissed the appeal for want of a substantial federal question. 396 U.S., at 368. ***

The primary advantages of the neutral-principles approach are that it is completely secular in operation, and yet flexible enough to accommodate all forms of religious organization and polity. The method relies exclusively on objective, well-established concepts of trust and property law familiar to lawyers and judges. It thereby promises to free civil courts completely from entanglement in questions of religious doctrine, polity, and practice. Furthermore, the neutral-principles analysis shares the peculiar genius of private-law systems in general—flexibility in ordering private rights and obligations to reflect the intentions of the parties. Through appropriate reversionary clauses and trust provisions, religious societies can specify what is to happen to church property in the event of a particular contingency, or what religious body will determine the ownership in the event of a schism or doctrinal controversy. In this manner, a religious organization can ensure that a dispute over the ownership of church property will be resolved in accord with the desires of the members.

This is not to say that the application of the neutral-principles approach is wholly free of difficulty. The neutral-principles method, at least as it has evolved in Georgia, requires a civil court to examine certain religious documents, such as a church constitution, for language of trust in favor of the general church. In undertaking such an examination, a civil court must take special care to scrutinize the document in purely secular terms, and not to rely on religious precepts in determining whether the document indicates that the parties have intended to create a trust. In addition, there may be cases where the deed, the corporate charter, or the constitution of the general church incorporates religious concepts in the provisions relating to the ownership of property. If in such a case the interpretation of the instruments of ownership would require the civil court to resolve a religious controversy, then the court must defer to the resolution of the doctrinal issue by the authoritative ecclesiastical body. Serbian Orthodox Diocese, 426 U.S., at 709.

On balance, however, the promise of nonentanglement and neutrality inherent in the neutral-principles approach more than compensates for what will be occasional problems in application. *** We therefore hold that a State is constitutionally entitled to adopt neutral principles of law as a means of adjudicating a church property dispute.

The dissent would require the States to abandon the neutral-principles method, and instead would insist as a matter of constitutional law that whenever a dispute arises over the ownership of church property, civil courts must defer to the "authoritative resolution of the dispute within the church itself." It would require, first, that civil courts review ecclesiastical doctrine and polity to determine where the church has "placed ultimate authority over the use of the church property." After answering this question, the courts would be required to "determine whether the dispute has been resolved within that structure of government and, if so, what decision has been made." They would then be required to enforce that decision. We cannot agree, however, that the First Amendment requires the States to adopt a rule of compulsory deference to religious authority in resolving church property disputes, even where no issue of doctrinal controversy is involved. ***

The dissent also argues that a rule of compulsory deference is necessary in order to protect the free exercise rights "of those who have formed the association and submitted themselves to its authority." This argument assumes that the neutral-principles method would somehow frustrate the free-exercise rights of the members of a religious association. Nothing could be further from the truth. The neutral-principles approach cannot be said to "inhibit" the free exercise of religion, any more than do other neutral provisions of state law governing the manner in which churches own property, hire employees, or purchase goods. Under the neutral-principles approach, the outcome of a church property dispute is not foreordained. At any time before the dispute erupts, the parties can ensure, if they so desire, that the faction loyal to the hierarchical church will retain the church property. They can modify the deeds or the corporate charter to include a right of reversion or trust in favor of the general church. Alternatively, the constitution of the general church can be made to recite an express trust in favor of the denominational church. The burden involved in taking such steps will be minimal. And the civil courts will be bound to give effect to the result indicated by the parties, provided it is embodied in some legally cognizable form.

IV

It remains to be determined whether the Georgia neutral-principles analysis was constitutionally applied on the facts of this case. Here, the local congregation was itself divided between a majority of 164 members who sought to withdraw from the PCUS, and a minority of 94 members who wished to maintain the affiliation. Neither of the state courts alluded to this problem, however; each concluded without discussion or analysis that the title to the property was in the local church and that the local church was represented by the majority rather than the minority.

Petitioners earnestly submit that the question of which faction is the true representative of the Vineville church is an ecclesiastical question that cannot be answered by a civil court. At least, it is said, it cannot be answered by a civil court in a case involving a hierarchical church, like the PCUS, where a duly appointed church commission has determined which of the two factions represents the "true congregation." Respondents, in opposition, argue in effect that the Georgia courts did no more than apply the ordinary presumption that, absent some indication to the contrary, a voluntary religious association is represented by a majority of its members.

If in fact Georgia has adopted a presumptive rule of majority representation, defeasible upon a showing that the identity of the local church is to be determined by some other means, we think this would be consistent with both the neutral-principles analysis and the First Amendment. Majority rule is generally employed in the governance of religious societies. Furthermore, the majority faction generally can be identified without resolving any question of religious doctrine or polity. Certainly, there was no dispute in the present case about the identity of the duly enrolled members of the Vineville church when the dispute arose, or about the fact that a quorum was present, or about the final vote. Most importantly, any rule of majority representation can always be overcome, under the neutral-principles approach, either by providing, in the corporate charter or the constitution of the general church, that the identity of the local church is to be established in some other way, or by providing that the church property is held in trust for the general church and those who remain loyal to it. Indeed, the State may adopt any method of overcoming the majoritarian presumption, so long as the use of that method does not impair free-exercise rights or entangle the civil courts in matters of religious controversy.

Neither the trial court nor the Supreme Court of Georgia, however, explicitly stated that it was adopting a presumptive rule of majority representation.[6] Moreover,

---

6. The Georgia Code contains the following provision dealing with the identity of a religious corporation: "The majority of those who adhere to its organization and doctrines represent the church. The withdrawal by one part of a congregation from the original body, or uniting with another church or denomination, is a relinquishment of all rights in the church abandoned." Ga. Code § 22-5504 (1978). The trial court noted that the defendants (respondents here) did not claim any right of possession of the Vineville church property under this section. The Georgia Supreme Court did not mention the

there are at least some indications that under Georgia law the process of identifying the faction that represents the Vineville church involves considerations of religious doctrine and polity. Georgia law requires that "church property be held according to the terms of the church government," and provides that a local church affiliated with a hierarchical religious association "is part of the whole body of the general church and is subject to the higher authority of the organization and its laws and regulations." Carnes v. Smith, 222 S.E.2d, at 325, 328; see Ga.Code §§ 22- 5507, 22-5508 (1978). All this may suggest that the identity of the "Vineville Presbyterian Church" named in the deeds must be determined according to terms of the Book of Church Order, which sets out the laws and regulations of churches affiliated with the PCUS. Such a determination, however, would appear to require a civil court to pass on questions of religious doctrine, and to usurp the function of the commission appointed by the Presbytery, which already has determined that petitioners represent the "true congregation" of the Vineville church. Therefore, if Georgia law provides that the identity of the Vineville church is to be determined according to the "laws and regulations" of the PCUS, then the First Amendment requires that the Georgia courts give deference to the presbyterial commission's determination of that church's identity.

This Court, of course, does not declare what the law of Georgia is. Since the grounds for the decision that respondents represent the Vineville church remain unarticulated, the judgment of the Supreme Court of Georgia is vacated, and the case is remanded for further proceedings not inconsistent with this opinion.

Mr. Justice POWELL with whom, THE CHIEF JUSTICE, Mr. Justice STEWART, and Mr. Justice WHITE join, dissenting.

* * *

I

The Court begins by stating that "[t]his case involves a dispute over the ownership of church property," suggesting that the concern is with legal or equitable ownership in the real property sense. But the ownership of the property of the Vineville church is not at issue. The deeds place title in the Vineville Presbyterian Church, or in trustees of that church, and none of the parties has questioned the validity of those deeds. The question actually presented is which of the factions within the local congregation has the right to control the actions of the titleholder, and thereby to control the use of the property, as the Court later acknowledges.

Since 1872 disputes over control of church property usually have been resolved under principles established by Watson v. Jones, 80 U.S. [13 Wall.] (1872). Under the new and complex, two-stage analysis approved today, a court instead first must apply newly defined "neutral principles of law" to determine whether property titled to the local church is held in trust for the general church organization with which the local church is affiliated. If it is, then the court will grant control of the property to

---

provision.

the councils of the general church. If not, then control by the local congregation will be recognized. In the latter situation, if there is a schism in the local congregation, as in this case, the second stage of the new analysis becomes applicable. Again, the Court fragments the analysis into two substeps for the purpose of determining which of the factions should control the property.

As this new approach inevitably will increase the involvement of civil courts in church controversies, and as it departs from long-established precedents, I dissent.

The first stage in the "neutral principles of law" approach operates as a restrictive rule of evidence. A court is required to examine the deeds to the church property, the charter of the local church (if there is one), the book of order or discipline of the general church organization, and the state statutes governing the holding of church property. The object of the inquiry, where the title to the property is in the local church, is "to determine whether there [is] any basis for a trust in favor of the general church." The court's investigation is to be "completely secular," "rel[ying] exclusively on objective, well-established concepts of trust and property law familiar to lawyers and judges." Thus, where religious documents such as church constitutions or books of order must be examined "for language of trust in favor of the general church," "a civil court must take special care to scrutinize the document in purely secular terms, and not to rely on religious precepts in determining whether the document indicates that the parties have intended to create a trust." It follows that the civil courts using this analysis may consider the form of religious government adopted by the church members for the resolution of intrachurch disputes only if that polity has been stated, in express relation to church property, in the language of trust and property law. ***

This limiting of the evidence relative to religious government cannot be justified on the ground that it "free[s] civil courts completely from entanglement in questions of religious doctrine, polity, and practice." For unless the body identified as authoritative under state law resolves the underlying dispute in accord with the decision of the church's own authority, the state court effectively will have reversed the decisions of doctrine and practice made in accordance with church law. The schism in the Vineville church, for example, resulted from disagreements among the church members over questions of doctrine and practice. Under the Book of Church Order, these questions were resolved authoritatively by the higher church courts, which then gave control of the local church to the faction loyal to that resolution. The Georgia courts, as a matter of state law, granted control to the schismatic faction, and thereby effectively reversed the doctrinal decision of the church courts. This indirect interference by the civil courts with the resolution of religious disputes within the church is no less proscribed by the First Amendment than is the direct decision of questions of doctrine and practice.[2]

---

2. The neutral-principles approach appears to assume that the requirements of the Constitution will be satisfied if civil courts are forbidden to consider certain types of evidence. The First Amendment's Religion Clauses, however, are meant to protect churches and their members from civil

When civil courts step in to resolve intrachurch disputes over control of church property, they will either support or overturn the authoritative resolution of the dispute within the church itself. The new analysis, under the attractive banner of "neutral principles," actually invites the civil courts to do the latter. The proper rule of decision, that I thought had been settled until today, requires a court to give effect in all cases to the decisions of the church government agreed upon by the members before the dispute arose.

The Court's basic neutral-principles approach, as a means of isolating decisions concerning church property from other decisions made within the church, relies on the concept of a trust of local church property in favor of the general church. Because of this central premise, the neutral-principles rule suffices to settle only disputes between the central councils of a church organization and a unanimous local congregation. Where, as here, the neutral-principles inquiry reveals no trust in favor of the general church, and the local congregation is split into factions, the basic question remains unresolved: which faction should have control of the local church? ***

II

Disputes among church members over the control of church property arise almost invariably out of disagreements regarding doctrine and practice. Because of the religious nature of these disputes, civil courts should decide them according to principles that do not interfere with the free exercise of religion in accordance with church polity and doctrine. Serbian Orthodox Diocese v. Milivojevich, 426 U.S. 696, 709, 720 (1976). The only course that achieves this constitutional requirement is acceptance by civil courts of the decisions reached within the polity chosen by the church members themselves. The classic statement of this view is found in Watson v. Jones, 13 Wall., at 728-729:

> The right to organize voluntary religious associations to assist in the expression and dissemination of any religious doctrine, and to create tribunals for the decision of controverted questions of faith within the association, and for the ecclesiastical government of all the individual members, congregations, and officers within the general association, is unquestioned. All who unite themselves to such a body do so with an implied consent to this government, and are bound to submit to it. But it would be a vain consent and would lead to the total subversion of such religious bodies, if any one aggrieved by one of their decisions could appeal to the secular courts and have them reversed. It is of the essence of these religious unions, and of their right to establish tribunals

---

law interference, not to protect the courts from having to decide difficult evidentiary questions. Thus, the evidentiary rules to be applied in cases involving intrachurch disputes over church property should be fashioned to avoid interference with the resolution of the dispute within the accepted church government. The neutral-principles approach consists instead of a rule of evidence that ensures that in some cases the courts will impose a form of church government and a doctrinal resolution at odds with that reached by the church's own authority. ***

for the decision of questions arising among themselves, that those decisions should be binding in all cases of ecclesiastical cognizance, subject only to such appeals as the organism itself provides for.

Accordingly, in each case involving an intrachurch dispute—including disputes over church property—the civil court must focus directly on ascertaining, and then following, the decision made within the structure of church governance. By doing so, the court avoids two equally unacceptable departures from the genuine neutrality mandated by the First Amendment. First, it refrains from direct review and revision of decisions of the church on matters of religious doctrine and practice that underlie the church's determination of intrachurch controversies, including those that relate to control of church property. Equally important, by recognizing the authoritative resolution reached within the religious association, the civil court avoids interfering indirectly with the religious governance of those who have formed the association and submitted themselves to its authority.

III

Until today, and under the foregoing authorities, the first question presented in a case involving an intrachurch dispute over church property was where within the religious association the rules of polity, accepted by its members before the schism, had placed ultimate authority over the use of the church property.[6] The courts, in answering this question have recognized two broad categories of church government. One is congregational, in which authority over questions of church doctrine, practice, and administration rests entirely in the local congregation or some body within it. In disputes over the control and use of the property of such a church, the civil courts enforce the authoritative resolution of the controversy within the local church itself. The second is hierarchical, in which the local church is but an integral and subordinate part of a larger church and is under the authority of the general church. Since the decisions of the local congregation are subject to review by the tribunals of the church hierarchy, this Court has held that the civil courts must give effect to the duly made decisions of the highest body within the hierarchy that has considered the dispute. ***

A careful examination of the constitutions of the general and local church, as well as other relevant documents, may be necessary to ascertain the form of governance adopted by the members of the religious association. But there is no reason to restrict the courts to statements of polity related directly to church property. For the constitutionally necessary limitations are imposed not on the evidence to be considered but instead on the object of the inquiry, which is both limited and clear: the civil court must determine whether the local church remains autonomous, so that its members have unreviewable authority to withdraw it (and its property) from the

---

6. After answering this question, of course, the civil court must determine whether the dispute has been resolved within that structure of government and, if so, what decision has been made.

general church, or whether the local church is inseparably integrated into and subordinate to the general church.

IV

The principles developed in prior decisions thus afford clear guidance in the case before us. The Vineville church is presbyterian, a part of the PCUS. The presbyterian form of church government, adopted by the PCUS, is "a hierarchical structure of tribunals which consists of, in ascending order, (1) the Church Session, composed of the elders of the local church; (2) the Presbytery, composed of several churches in a geographical area; (3) the Synod, generally composed of all Presbyteries within a State; and (4) the General Assembly, the highest governing body." The Book of Church Order subjects the Session to "review and control" by the Presbytery in all matters, even authorizing the Presbytery to replace the leadership of the local congregation, to winnow its membership, and to take control of it. No provision of the Book of Church Order gives the Session the authority to withdraw the local church from the PCUS; similarly, no section exempts such a decision by the local church from review by the Presbytery.

Thus, while many matters, including the management of the church property, are committed in the first instance to the Session and congregation of the local church, their actions are subject to review by the Presbytery. Here, the Presbytery exercised its authority over the local church, removing the dissidents from church office, asserting direct control over the government of the church, and recognizing the petitioners as the legitimate congregation and Session of the church. It is undisputed that under the established government of the Presbyterian Church—accepted by the members of the church before the schism—the use and control of the church property have been determined authoritatively to be in the petitioners. Accordingly, under the principles I have thought were settled, there is no occasion for the further examination of the law of Georgia that the Court directs. On remand, the Georgia courts should be directed to enter judgment for the petitioners.

INDEX

References are to Pages

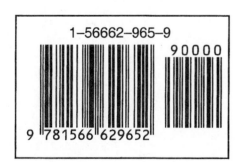
1–56662–965–9
90000
9 781566 629652